Y0-BXW-993

clinical cardiology

clinical cardiology

MAURICE SOKOLOW, MD
Professor of Medicine
Senior staff member, Cardiovascular Research Institute
formerly Chief of Cardiology and Program Director of
the USPHS Clinical Cardiology Training Program
University of California, San Francisco

MALCOLM B. McILROY, MD
Professor of Medicine
Senior staff member, Cardiovascular Research Institute
University of California, San Francisco

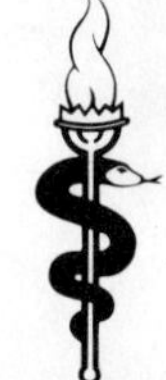

Los Altos, California 94022 LANGE Medical Publications

Lange Medical Publications

Drawer L Los Altos, California 94022

International Standard Book Number: *0-87041-230-2*
Library of Congress Catalogue Card Number: *77-88120*

A Concise Medical Library for Practitioner and Student

Clinical Cardiology $16.00

Current Medical Diagnosis & Treatment 1977 (annual revision). Edited by M.A. Krupp and M.J. Chatton. 1066 pp. 1977

Current Pediatric Diagnosis & Treatment, 4th ed. Edited by C.H. Kempe, H.K. Silver, and D. O'Brien. 1053 pp, *illus.* 1976

Current Surgical Diagnosis & Treatment, 3rd ed. Edited by J.E. Dunphy and L.W. Way. 1139 pp, *illus.* 1977

Current Obstetric & Gynecologic Diagnosis & Treatment. Edited by R.C. Benson. 911 pp, *illus.* 1976

Review of Physiological Chemistry, 16th ed. H.A. Harper, V.W. Rodwell, and P.A. Mayes. 681 pp, *illus.* 1977

Review of Medical Physiology, 8th ed. W.F. Ganong. 599 pp, *illus.* 1977

Review of Medical Microbiology, 12th ed. E. Jawetz, J.L. Melnick, and E.A. Adelberg. 542 pp, *illus.* 1976

Review of Medical Pharmacology, 5th ed. F.H. Meyers, E. Jawetz, and A. Goldfien. 740 pp, *illus.* 1976

Basic & Clinical Immunology. Edited by H.H. Fudenberg, D.P. Stites, J.L. Caldwell, and J.V. Wells. 653 pp, *illus.* 1976

Basic Histology, 2nd ed. L.C. Junqueira, J. Carneiro, and A.N. Contopoulos. 453 pp, *illus.* 1977

General Urology, 8th ed. D.R. Smith. 492 pp, *illus.* 1975

General Ophthalmology, 8th ed. D. Vaughan and T. Asbury. 379 pp, *illus.* 1977

Correlative Neuroanatomy & Functional Neurology, 16th ed. J.G. Chusid. 448 pp, *illus.* 1976

Principles of Clinical Electrocardiography, 9th ed. M.J. Goldman. 412 pp, *illus.* 1976

The Nervous System. W.F. Ganong. 226 pp, *illus.* 1977

Handbook of Psychiatry, 3rd ed. Edited by P. Solomon and V.D. Patch. 706 pp. 1974

Handbook of Obstetrics & Gynecology, 6th ed. R.C. Benson. 772 pp, *illus.* 1977

Physician's Handbook, 18th ed. M.A. Krupp, N.J. Sweet, E. Jawetz, E.G. Biglieri, and R.L. Roe. 754 pp, *illus.* 1976

Handbook of Pediatrics, 12th ed. H.K. Silver, C.H. Kempe, and H.B. Bruyn. 723 pp, *illus.* 1977

Handbook of Poisoning: Diagnosis & Treatment, 9th ed. R.H. Dreisbach. 559 pp. 1977

Lithographed in USA

This book is dedicated to
Margaret McIlroy and the memory of Ethel Sokolow

Table of Contents

Foreword

The sense of pleasure we always feel when we have the opportunity to place a new medical text in the medical school bookstores is a bit keener this time because of the special circumstances surrounding the development of *Clinical Cardiology,* by Dr Maurice Sokolow and Dr Malcolm McIlroy.

I have known these men personally for over twenty years. Fifteen years ago I first asked Dr Sokolow to consider writing such a book, and ever since then it has been taking form.

Dr Sokolow and Dr McIlroy have been colleagues for many years, making clinical cardiology rounds together frequently and discussing their findings with students, house staff, cardiology trainees, and other physicians. I am delighted to see their tremendous cumulative experience in the classroom, on the wards, and in the laboratory reflected in these pages.

The authors have spent the past three years developing this manuscript. In doing so they have stuck scrupulously to an agreement *not* to agree without first questioning and making sure; not to make hasty judgments on what is new, nor to cling without reason to what is old; but to work together in every patient's best interests and to make this book the best instructional material available.

The book has been reworked and refined right up to the printer's deadline with the most up-to-date and reliable information available, and we will publish a revised edition every two years.

Jack D. Lange, MD
President, Lange Medical Publications

Los Altos, California
October 1977

Preface

The purpose of *Clinical Cardiology* is to provide medical students, house staff, trainees in cardiology, internists, and other physicians in practice with a balanced, integrated, up-to-date account of the important aspects of adult cardiovascular diseases and the physiologic basis of their treatment. The clinical cardiologist's field of expertise has broadened in the past 25 years to add not only electrocardiography and radiology but also a host of noninvasive and invasive special investigations to the classic bedside skills of history-taking and physical examination. The modern physician must personally integrate the information derived from each of these technics into the specific clinical setting. It is no longer sufficient to leave the interpretation of specialized information to the specialist. Each physician's own interpretation, based on the whole clinical picture, must be compared and correlated with the narrower, more expert views of the electrocardiographer, radiologist, echocardiographer, and clinical physiologist.

It was not our intention to write a comprehensive or encyclopedic book. The allocation of space to different topics is intended to be roughly proportionate to our view of their importance. In general, we have attempted to put the main discussion of each subject in one place. When we have been forced to divide coverage of a subject between chapters, we have alerted the reader with cross-references. Research has expanded immensely in the past few years in some fields, and we have accordingly allotted more space and emphasized recent references where applicable. The reference lists are intended to provide a means of access to the literature rather than a comprehensive coverage of each subject. Books and monographs have been included in most instances.

Although each author initially took responsibility for writing individual chapters dealing with subjects within his own special field, each chapter was critically reviewed, discussed, and modified by the other author to provide a combined, considered opinion endorsed by both authors. We plan to keep the book current with biennial revisions, and we invite comments and criticisms from our readers.

We wish to thank our colleagues Dr Nelson B Schiller, Dr Norman Silverman, Dr Elias H Botvinick, Dr Oscar Rambo, Dr Erick Carlsson, Dr Gordon Gamsu, and Dr John Hutchinson for permission to reproduce echocardiograms, radioisotope studies, pathologic data, x-rays, and electrocardiograms from their files.

We are grateful to the University of California and to the United States Public Health Service for support of the academic teaching program in cardiology which has enabled us to continue to learn from our patients, students, and colleagues. Dr Julius H Comroe Jr, for many years Director of the Cardiovascular Research Institute at the University of California in San Francisco, has been an unselfish supporter of our careers, and we are happy to acknowledge our special debt to this great teacher. The senior author (Dr Sokolow) is particularly indebted to the physicians of the National Heart Hospital, London, and the staff of the Radcliffe Infirmary, Oxford, with whom he spent enlightening and pleasant sabbatical leaves.

We wish also to thank our publisher, Dr Jack Lange, and his editors, Dr James Ransom and Dr Milton Chatton, for invaluable advice and editing, and Mr William Bunker and Ms Mary Helen Stull for photographic and graphic help. Ms Laurel V. Schaubert contributed greatly to the teaching value of this book by providing anatomic drawings of high quality. Lastly, we want to express particular thanks to Mr Alan Venable and Ms Lorraine Matthews for skilled and loyal assistance in the manifold organizational tasks in preparation of the book. Mrs Lynda Crain, Ms Toby Garten, and Ms Karen Hogan also provided valuable secretarial assistance.

Maurice Sokolow
Malcolm B. McIlroy

San Francisco
December, 1977

1...
Physiology of the Circulatory System

ANATOMY OF THE HEART

The normal heart lies within its pericardial sac in the middle of the thorax slightly to the left of the midline. The low pressure right atrium and right ventricle occupy the anterior portion of the heart and the higher pressure left ventricle and atrium lie posteriorly. The long axis of the heart, from the apex of the left ventricle to the root of the aorta, runs upward and backward at an angle of about 30 degrees from the horizontal plane and 45 degrees from the sagittal plane of the body (Fig 1–1). The apex of the heart rests on the upper surface of the diaphragm, which lies close to the posterior and inferior surfaces of the heart. The lie of the heart varies with the build of the patient and with respiration. It assumes a more vertical position during inspiration and in tall, thin persons, and a more horizontal position during expiration and in persons of heavier build.

EXTERNAL APPEARANCE

Anterior Aspect

As viewed from the front (Fig 1–1), the largest area of the surface of the heart is formed by the tri-

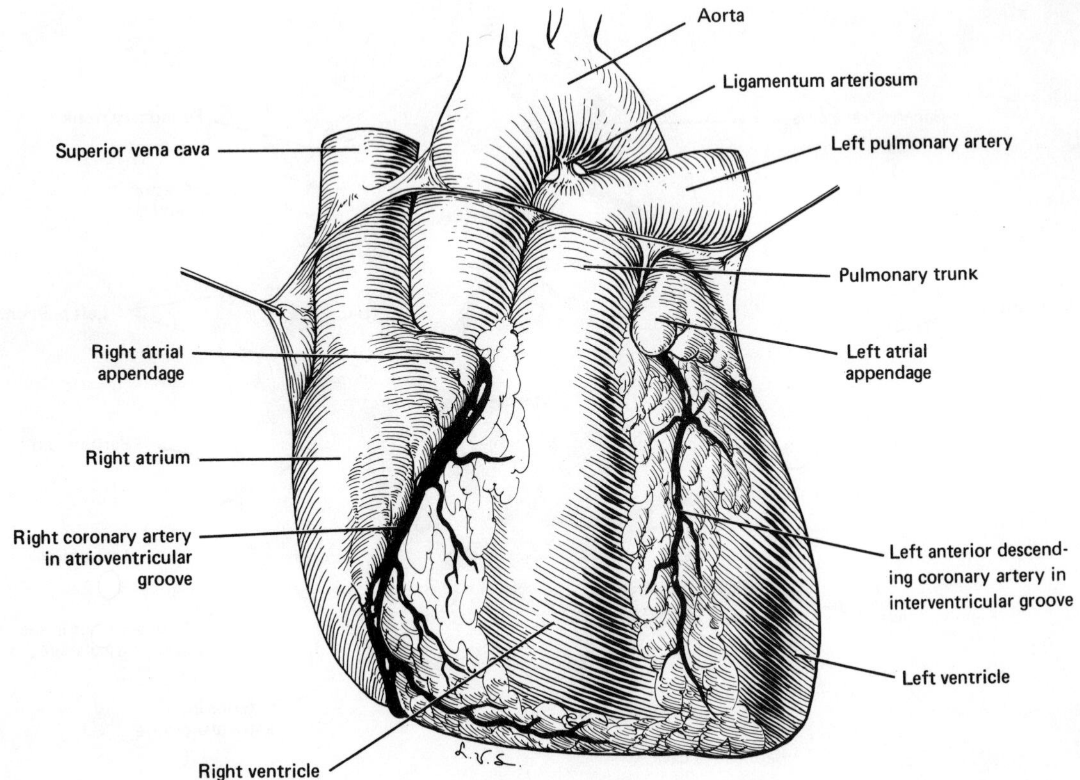

Figure 1–1. Anterior view of the heart.

angle-shaped right ventricle, with the pulmonary trunk arising from the apex of the triangle. Above and to the right of the right ventricle, one can see the right atrium—or, more specifically, the right atrial appendage—as an ear-shaped structure overlying the root of the aorta. The groove between the right atrium and ventricle (coronary sulcus) is often filled with fat and is occupied by the right coronary artery. Above the right atrium, the superior vena cava is seen entering the right atrium through the pericardium. The inferior vena cava lies on the diaphragmatic surface of the heart and enters the right atrium from the back. The anterior aspect of the heart reveals only a small part of the left ventricle, lying to the left of the right ventricle and forming the apex of the heart. The anterior interventricular sulcus often contains fat and is occupied by the anterior descending branch of the left coronary artery. The only portion of the left atrium visible from the front is the left atrial appendage, which lies above the ventricle and curves around the left side of the origin of the pulmonary trunk. The lungs normally cover most of the anterior surface of the heart, especially during inspiration, leaving only a small area apposed to the back of the sternum and left ribs.

Left-Sided Aspect

As viewed from the left side (Fig 1–2), the left ventricle and left atrium occupy most of the surface of the heart. The posterior interventricular groove separates the left ventricle above from the right ventricle below. The posterior descending branch of the right coronary artery lies in this groove. The atrioventricular groove runs almost vertically in this view, separating the left ventricle from the left atrium. The coronary sinus and the circumflex branch of the left coronary artery lie in this groove and complete the ring of blood vessels forming the base of the corona (crown) after which the blood vessels supplying the heart are named.

Posterior Aspect

The back of the heart mainly rests on the diaphragm and is largely occupied by the left atrium and ventricle plus portions of the right atrium and ventricle, as shown in Fig 1–3. The point at which all 4 chambers meet posteriorly is called the crux of the heart because of the cross-shaped pattern of blood vessels lying at the junction of the posterior interventricular groove and the atrioventricular groove. The vessels forming the cross are the coronary sinus and the posterior descending coronary artery. This latter vessel may be a branch of either the right or the circumflex branch of the left coronary artery depending on whether the right or left coronary artery is the larger (dominant) vessel. The pulmonary veins enter the back of the left atrium. The pattern may vary, but 2 right and 2 left pulmonary veins are normally present.

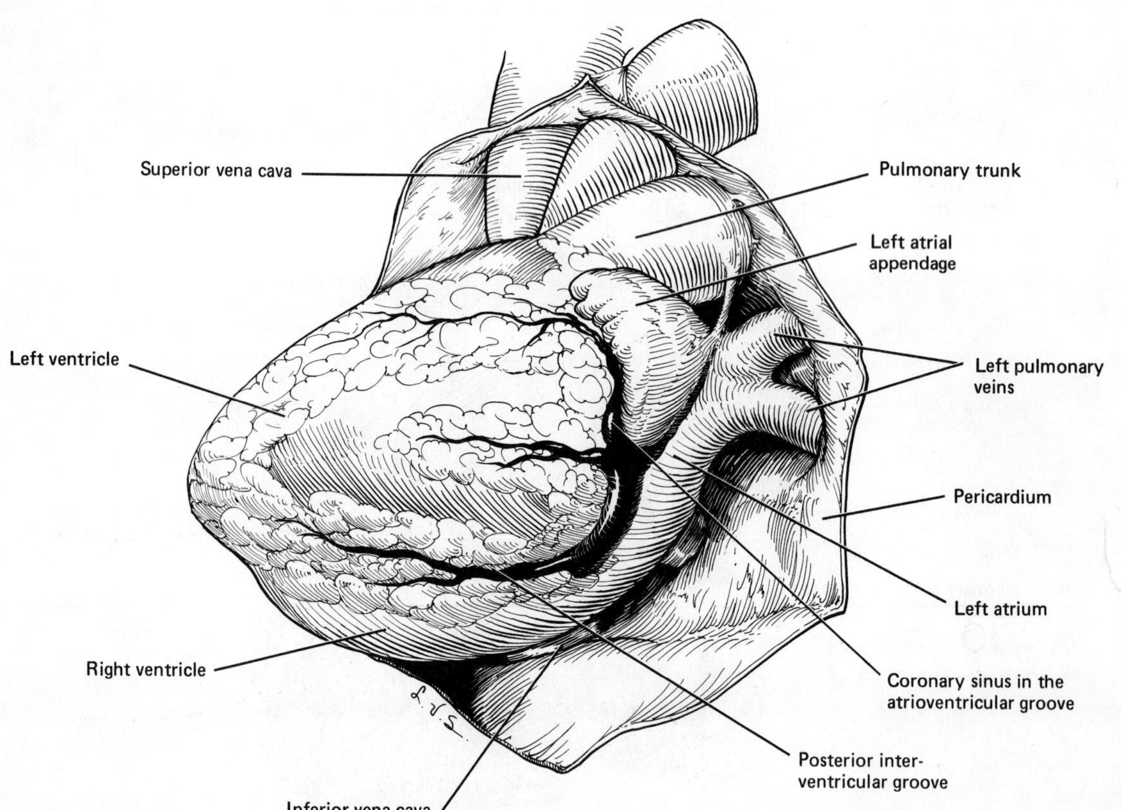

Figure 1–2. The heart viewed from the left side with the apex raised.

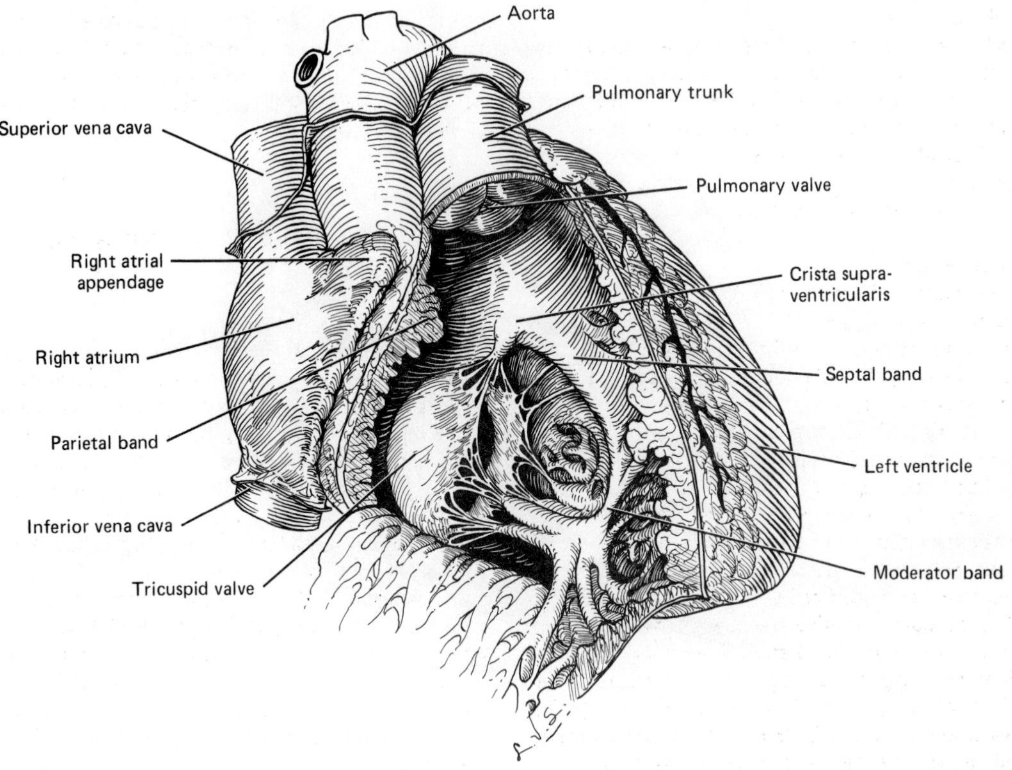

Figure 1–6. Anterior view of the heart with the anterior wall removed to show the right ventricular cavity.

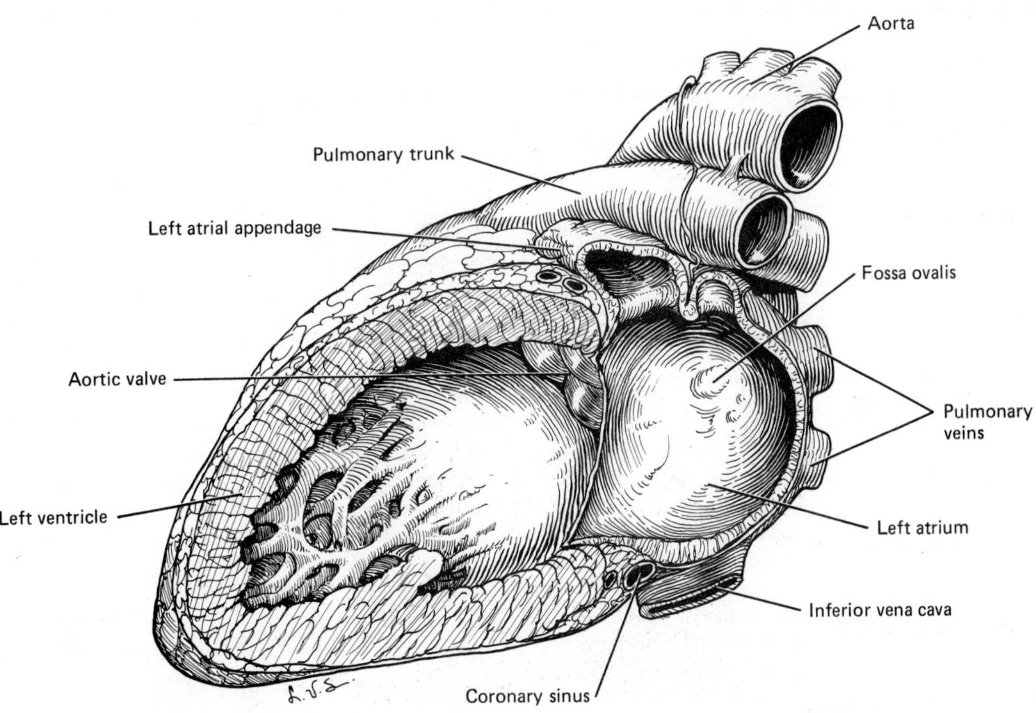

Figure 1–7. View of the left heart from the left side with the left ventricular free wall and mitral valve cut away.

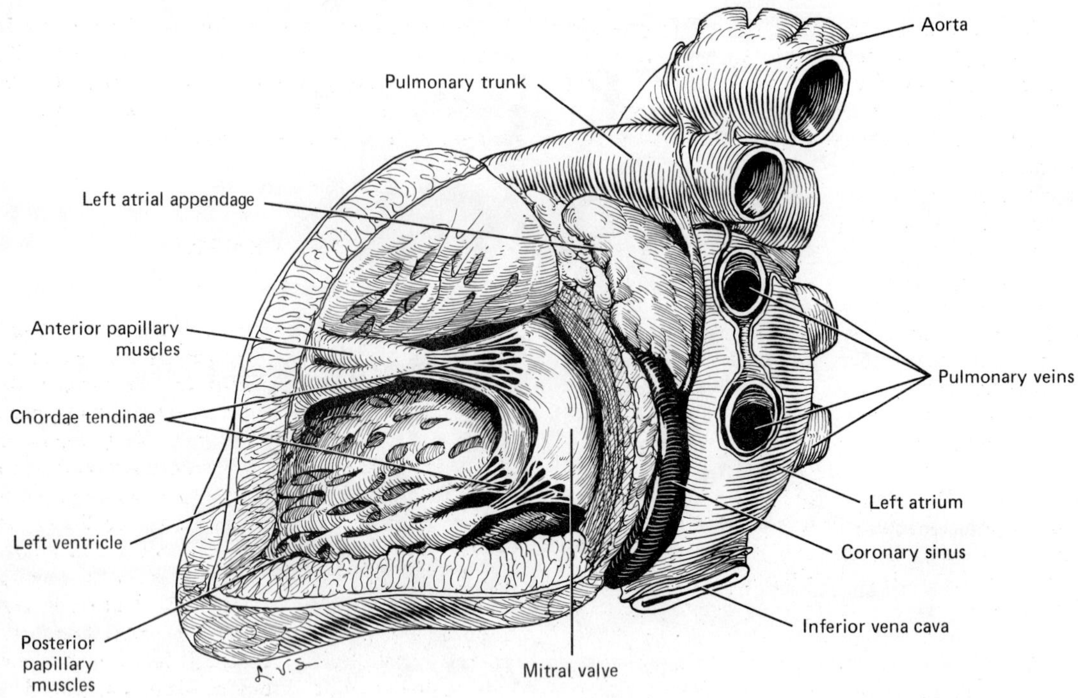

Figure 1–8. View of the left heart with the left ventricular wall turned back to show the mitral valve.

cuspid valve and its chordae, and an upper outflow tract from which the pulmonary trunk arises. The line of demarcation between the 2 portions consists of bands of muscle formed by the crista supraventricularis, the parietal band, the septal band, and the moderator band. The outflow tract of the right ventricle is derived from the embryologically distinct bulbus cordis–in contrast to the inflow portion, which arises from ventricular tissue.

The Left Atrium

The left atrium, like the right, is composed of a veinlike portion, into which the pulmonary veins drain, and a more muscular anterior portion, which includes the left atrial appendage. Its wall is slightly thicker than that of the right atrium, and the thinner area, corresponding to the fossa ovalis, can be seen on its right upper surface (Fig 1–7).

The Left Ventricle

The left ventricular cavity is shaped like an egg. The base of the egg is formed by the mitral valve ring. The wall of the left ventricle is 3–4 times as thick as that of the right ventricle and accounts for about 75% of the mass of the heart. The aortic and mitral valve rings lie close to one another, with the larger anterior mobile cusp of the mitral valve adjacent to the left and posterior cusps of the aortic valve. The posterior immobile cusp of the mitral valve is shorter and, together with the anterior cusp, is tethered to the anterior and posterior papillary muscles in a parachutelike fashion by chordae tendineae, some of which are shared by the 2 cusps as seen in Fig 1–8. The interventricular septum, which forms the anterior aspect of the left ventricle, bulges into the right ventricle, making the cross section of the mid portion of the left ventricle circular in shape.

CARDIAC VALVES

The *tricuspid valve* is a thin, filmy tripartite structure with anterior, posterior, and medial cusps. The membranous portion of the interventricular septum lies beside its medial cusp. The *mitral valve* is thicker than the tricuspid valve and is shaped like a bishop's hat (miter) in which the anterior surface (anterior cusp) is longer and wider than the posterior surface. The *pulmonary valve* is composed of pocketlike anterior right and left cusps. It is constructed of thinner tissue than the *aortic valve,* which lies farther down in the heart. It too has 3 cusps–the right (coronary), left (coronary), and posterior (noncoronary) cusps–associated with corresponding dilatations of the aorta called the aortic sinuses or sinuses of Valsalva.

THE CORONARY CIRCULATION

The coronary arteries are more variable in anatomic pattern than any other part of the cardiac anatomy. The 2 main coronary arteries—left and right—arise from the right and left aortic sinuses within the pockets of the aortic valve cusps. Either vessel may predominate and supply the posteroinferior portion of the heart. In 30% of persons the *left coronary artery* is the smaller of the 2. It runs behind the main pulmonary artery as a short main stem about 1 or 2 cm long before dividing into an *anterior* and a *circumflex branch.* The anterior branch usually has a *descending branch* which follows the interventricular groove. The circumflex branch follows the atrioventricular groove, curving around to the posterior surface of the heart. The area between these 2 vessels, each of which is defined by a course within a groove, is supplied by branches from one artery or the other. Thus, the left coronary artery usually consists of 3 branches, with the mid branch arising from one of the more readily definable arteries. The circumflex branch is larger in persons with a dominant left coronary pattern. In this case, the vessel may run as far as the crux of the heart and even give off the posterior descending branch, which runs in the posterior interventricular groove.

The right coronary artery runs in the atrioventricular groove, downward and to the right, before curving around to the back of the heart to reach the crux, giving off a posterior descending interventricular branch. An anterior right atrial branch usually arises near the origin of the right coronary artery. It usually supplies a branch to the sinoatrial node. The atrioventricular node is also commonly supplied by a branch of the right coronary artery that arises from the posterior descending branch.

Most of the coronary venous drainage is into the *coronary sinus.* The few veins that drain directly into the cardiac chambers are called thebesian veins. The main venous drainage of the left ventricle is via the great cardiac vein, which runs with the anterior descending branch of the left coronary artery before joining with the posterior cardiac vein to form the coronary sinus.

The anatomy of the coronary vessels is of great importance in the interpretation of coronary arteriograms and in coronary artery surgery. The subject is discussed in more detail in Chapter 8.

CONDUCTION SYSTEM

The *sinoatrial node,* which initiates the normal cardiac impulse, lies at the junction of the superior vena cava and the right atrium. The *atrioventricular node* is located in the right posterior portion of the interatrial septum near the base of the tricuspid valve. Poorly defined anterior, middle, and posterior atrial tracts connect the 2 nodes and conduct the cardiac impulse through the atrial tissue. The atrioventricular node is continuous with the *bundle of His,* which divides into a left and a right bundle branch at the top of the interventricular septum. The left branch divides again into anterior and posterior branches, and all 3 branches run subendocardially close to the septum before ramifying into the *Purkinje fibers,* which spread to all parts of the ventricular myocardium.

LYMPHATICS

The lymphatics of the heart are arranged in 3 plexuses: subendocardial, myocardial, and subepicardial. The drainage is outward to the subepicardial plexus where the vessels unite to form drainage trunks that follow the coronary arteries. They eventually form a single vessel which leaves the heart on the anterior surface of the pulmonary artery to reach a lymph node between the superior vena cava and the innominate artery. Few valves can be found in the cardiac lymphatics, and it appears that cardiac contraction provides the force which drives the lymphatic flow from the heart. No certain role for cardiac lymphatics has been established in disease. It has been suggested that endomyocardial fibrosis might be related to lymphatic obstruction. Cardiac transplantation, which inevitably severs the cardiac lymphatics, does not seem to produce any deleterious effect, but regeneration of lymphatic vessels is known to occur within 2 or 3 weeks after they have been divided.

CARDIAC NERVES

The heart is innervated both by cholinergic fibers from the vagus nerve and by adrenergic fibers arising from the thoracolumbar sympathetic system and passing through the superior, middle, and inferior cervical ganglions. The cholinergic supply is confined to the atria. Fibers from the right vagus nerve supply the sinoatrial node and serve to control the heart rate and the force of atrial contraction. Fibers from the left vagus nerve supply mainly the atrioventricular node, but there is usually some cross-innervation. The atria also receive sympathetic fibers, but most of the adrenergic nerves pass to the ventricles, where they serve to increase the force of cardiac contraction. The heart also has an autonomic sensory innervation via small, mainly nonmedullated sympathetic fibers. These are thought to respond to nociceptive stimuli and to constitute the pathway through which cardiac pain is mediated.

MICROSCOPIC ANATOMY OF THE HEART

The basic heart muscle cell forms part of a syncytium in which the individual cells are joined to-

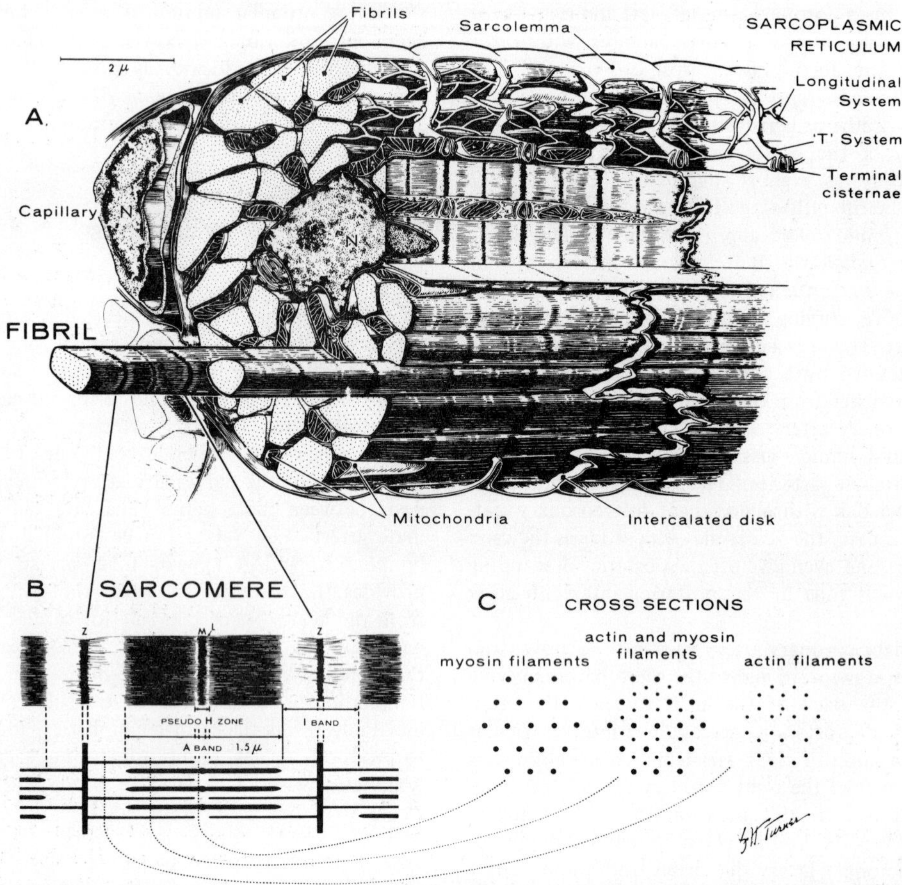

Figure 1–9. Diagram of cardiac muscle as seen under the electron microscope. *A:* A myocardial cell showing the arrangement of the multiple parallel fibrils. *B:* An individual sarcomere from a myofibril. A representation of the arrangement of myofilaments that make up the sarcomere is shown below. *C:* Cross sections of the sarcomere, showing the specific lattice arrangement of the myofilaments. N, nucleus. (Reproduced, with permission, from Braunwald E, Ross J Jr, Sonnenblick EH: Mechanisms of contraction of the normal and failing heart. N Engl J Med 277:794, 1967.)

gether in an irregular fashion in bands and spirals without the well-defined tendons and bony attachments characteristic of skeletal muscle. The heart muscle cell differs from the skeletal muscle cell also in that it possesses inherent rhythmicity. This property varies in different types of cardiac muscle; it is most marked in nodal tissue and least notable in peripheral muscle cells. The subcellular arrangement of cardiac muscle cells (Fig 1–9A) is similar to that of skeletal muscle. The cells are about 30 × 10 μm in size and contain about 20–50 fibrils. Each fibril is about 1 μm in diameter and is composed of a series of sarcomeres, the basic muscle units. The cell contains a nucleus and numerous mitochondria. The limiting membrane is the sarcolemma, from which a sarcoplasmic reticulum invaginates the cell to form a complex tubular (T) system surrounding each fibril. The electrical activity triggering the contraction of each sarcomere passes through this complex membranelike structure.

The Sarcomere

The structural unit of the sarcomere is shown in Fig 1–9B. Its banded appearance results from overlapping of the 2 major muscle proteins—actin and myosin—which accounts for the striated appearance. The wide dark A bands are formed by overlapping of the thicker myosin elements with the thinner, lighter actin filaments. The thinner dark Z lines indicate the end of one sarcomere and the beginning of the next. The lighter I bands are seen in areas in which only the actin filaments are present. The pattern of the sarcomere seen by electron microscopy varies with contraction and relaxation of the sarcomere. With contraction, as shown in Fig 1–10, the I band becomes shorter and the A band more dense. The Z lines come to lie closer together as the muscle contracts. When the muscle fibril is cut in cross section, a specific lattice pattern is seen (Fig 1–9C). In the zone in which the actin and myosin overlap (S zone), each thick myosin fiber is surrounded by 6 actin fibers. This hexagonal pattern is also seen in the lighter I band region. In the center of the sarcomere, where only myosin is present (M zone), the individual myosin filaments are connected in a lattice pattern. A similar pattern is seen at the Z lines.

? WHAT IS H ZONE!

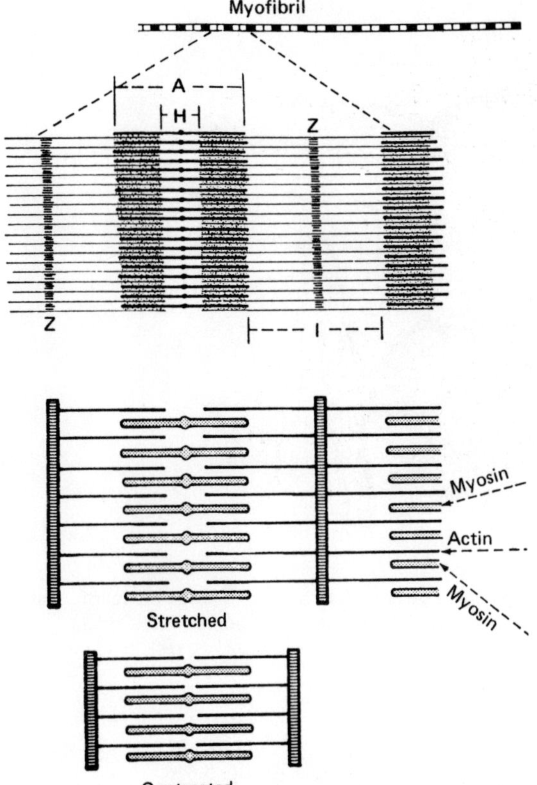

Figure 1–10. Muscular contraction. The myofibrils are composed of overlapping thick myosin filaments and thin actin filaments. The amount of overlap is diminished during stretching and increased during contraction. (Reproduced, with permission, from Rushmer RF: *Cardiovascular Dynamics,* 2nd ed. Saunders, 1970.)

EMBRYOLOGY OF THE HEART

The embryology of the heart is as complex as that of any organ in the body. The process of development of the heart takes place mainly during the period between the second and sixth weeks of gestation; thus, the factors responsible for the development of congenital heart lesions probably operate in most cases before the diagnosis of pregnancy is clinically certain.

Primitive Heart Tube

The heart is formed by the folding of the primitive vascular tube, which appears in the splanchnic mesodermal tissue near the pericardial cavity at about the start of the third week of gestation. At first the primitive heart tube is straight, but differential growth soon forms a cardiac loop, as shown in Fig 1–11. Three more or less distinct portions of the tube can be distinguished, and it is convenient to describe them separately even though their development proceeds in parallel. The 3 portions are (1) the sinus venosus, (2) the cardiac loop, and (3) the aortic and branchial arches.

The Sinus Venosus

The most caudad portion of the primitive heart tube gives rise to the sinus venosus. As shown in Fig 1–12, this is an independent chamber during the early stage of development of the heart. It originally consists of 2 horns, each receiving a duct of Cuvier. The umbilical veins are formed from this structure, which ultimately gives rise to the superior and inferior venae cavae, the pulmonary veins, the coronary sinus, and the posterior portions of the right and left atria.

The Cardiac Loop

The intermediate portion of the primitive heart tube bends to form the cardiac loop, which twists on itself to form 3 distinct portions: the primitive atrium, the ventricle, and, more distally, the bulbus cordis. In the process of twisting, the primitive heart comes to lie in close apposition to its surrounding pericardial sac, as shown in Fig 1–12. The cardiac chambers are at first single; septation to form separate right- and left-sided atria and ventricles occurs at a later stage.

Aortic Arches

The most distal portion of the primitive heart tube forms the aortic sac; distal to this sac, 6 paired aortic arches appear sequentially. Some disappear but others persist to give rise to the great vessels. The basic original pattern of arches is shown in Fig 1–13, with the persisting vessels outlined. The third arch persists as the internal carotid artery; the left fourth arch forms the arch of the aorta; and the sixth arch gives rise to the pulmonary arteries and the ductus arteriosus.

Septation

The most complex stage of cardiac embryology is septation of the various parts of the heart. Septation in

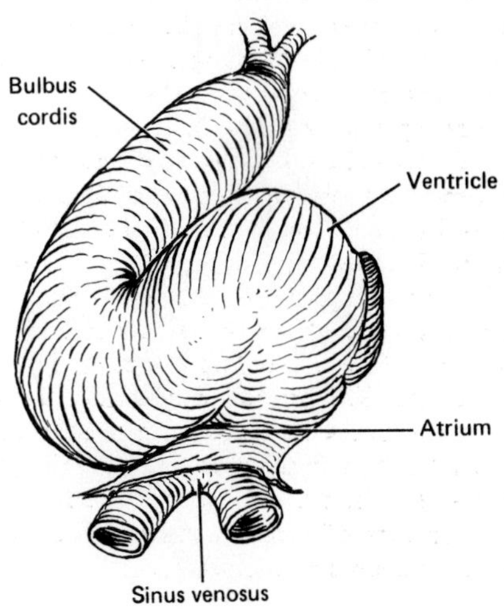

Figure 1–11. Formation of the cardiac loop.

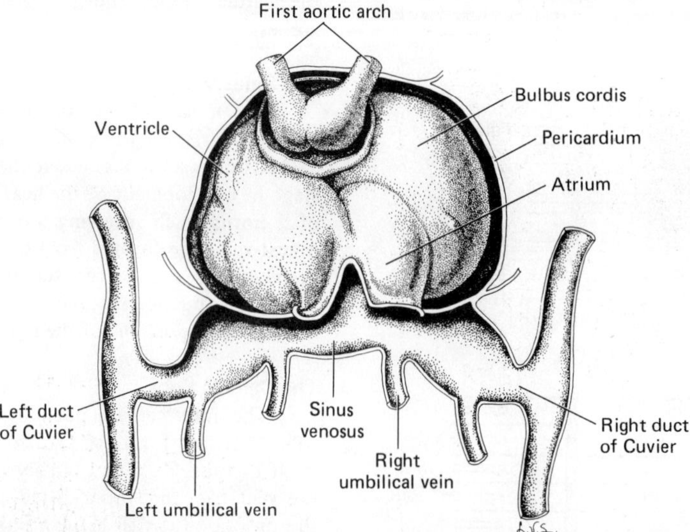

Figure 1–12. The sinus venosus, atrium, and ventricle as seen from the dorsal surface of an embryo at about the fourth week of gestation. (Modified and reproduced, with permission, from Davies J: *Human Developmental Anatomy.* Ronald Press, 1963.)

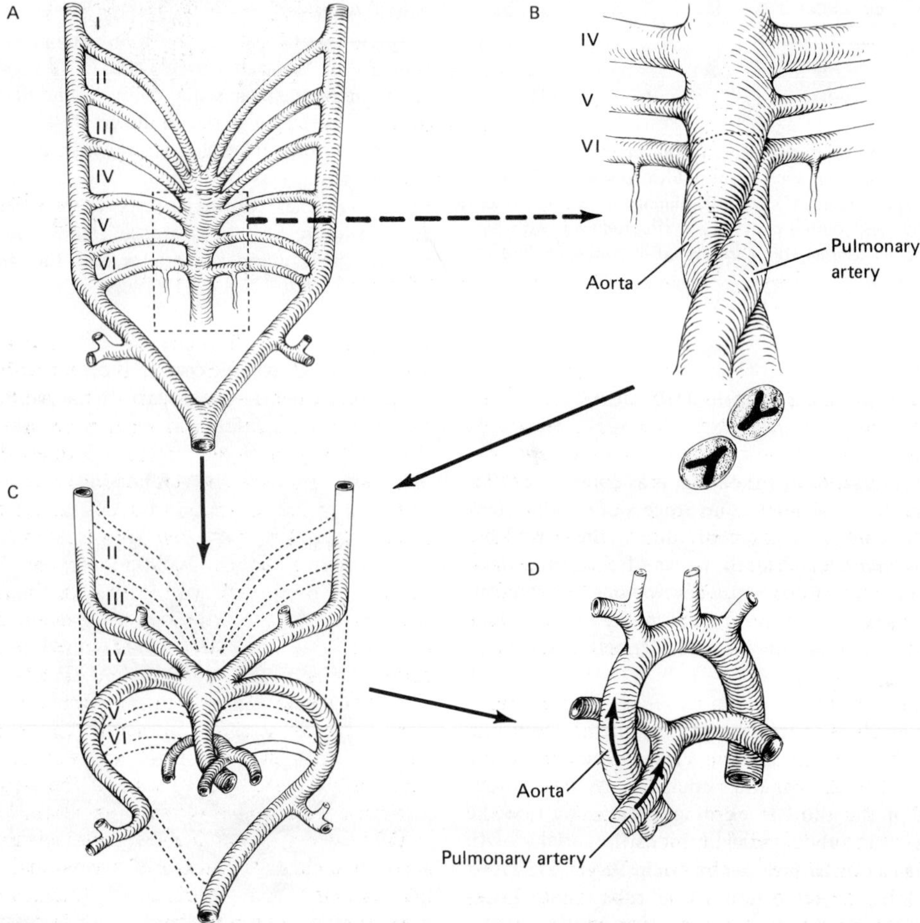

Figure 1–13. In *A*, the primitive arches are shown as paired structures. In *B*, the rotation and septation of the great vessels are seen. *C* shows the persistence of the third, fourth, and sixth arches to give the adult pattern shown in *D*.

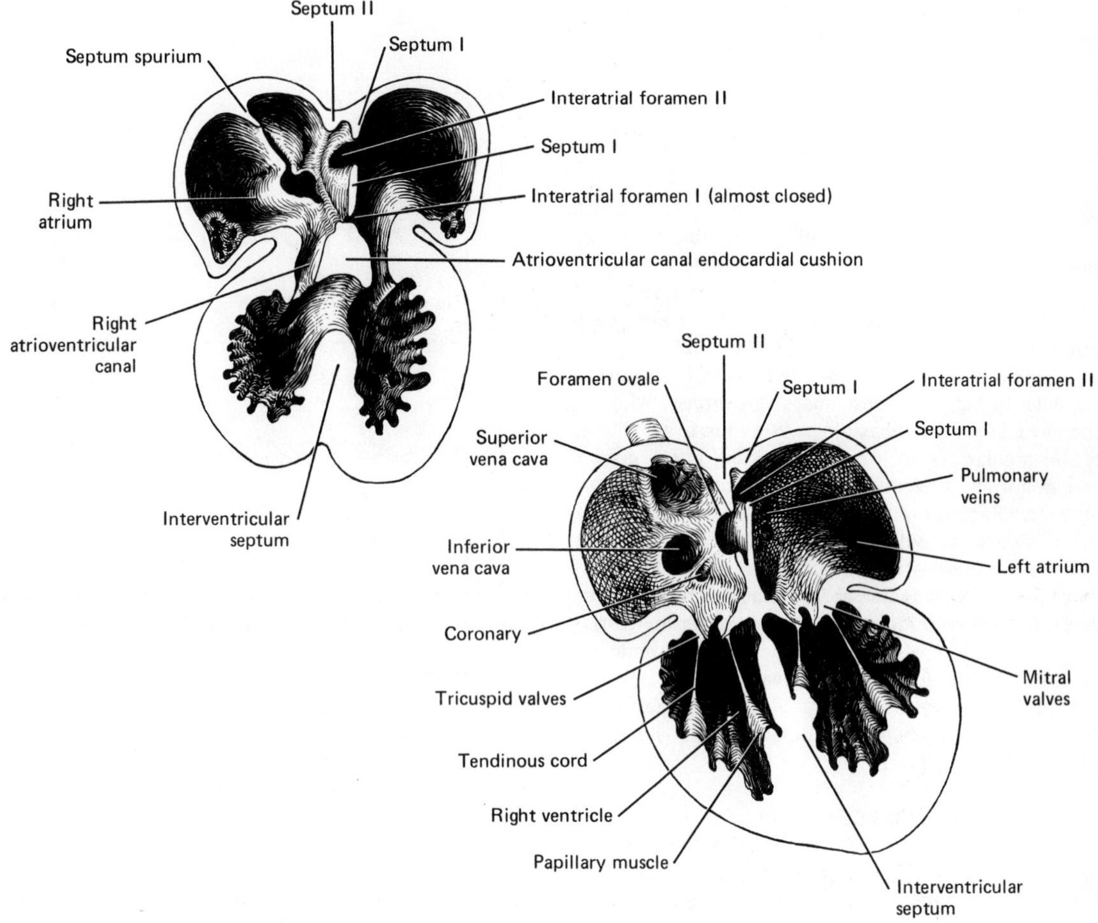

Figure 1–14. Early *(top)* and late *(bottom)* stages of atrial and ventricular septation.

the atrium is depicted in Fig 1–14. A septum extends downward and forward toward the center of the heart where the endocardial cushions are located and from which the atrioventricular valves subsequently develop. This is the septum primum. A second atrial septum—the septum secundum—grows on the right side of the septum primum. A hole develops in the septum primum in the middle of the atrium, and atrial septation is never complete. The septum secundum does not extend all the way forward and downward to the endocardial cushions, and a persistent interatrial communication between the 2 atrial septa persists as the foramen ovale until birth.

Separation of the primitive ventricle into right and left chambers is accomplished by the development of an interventricular septum, which grows from the anterior wall of the common ventricle. Its free margin is aligned slightly to the right of the midline, toward the region of the endocardial cushions.

The most distal part of the primitive ventricle, the bulbus cordis, dilates to form the truncus arteriosus, which develops between the ventricles and the aortic arches. A spiral septum forms within the bulbus cordis and grows downward toward the center of the heart, where the endocardial cushions are forming the atrioventricular valves and meeting the ventricular septum. The upper (membranous) part of the ventricular septum is formed in this area from endocardial cushion tissue. The spiral bulbar septum separates the truncus arteriosus into right and left portions forming the root of the aorta and the outflow tract of the right ventricle, respectively, along with their appropriate valves.

Abnormalities of septation account for a large number of congenital heart lesions. In the atrium, defects may occur in the septum primum or septum secundum, and associated abnormalities of the endocardial cushion (atrioventricular canal) area also occur. In the ventricle, the membranous portion of the septum is the site of almost all septal defects; and in the truncus arteriosus, abnormal septation accounts for transposition of the great vessels. The persistence of abnormal aortic arches gives rise to various lesions such as right-sided aortic arch and vascular anomalies of the aortic branches. Persistence of the normal fetal communications (ductus arteriosus and foramen ovale) also gives rise to congenital lesions, while developmental abnormalities of the sinus venosus account for anomalous pulmonary and systemic venous drainage patterns.

PHYSIOLOGIC FUNCTION OF THE CIRCULATION

Normal Metabolic Needs & Their Variations

The cardiovascular system consists of the heart, great vessels, arteries, capillaries, and veins, all of which function as an integrated circulatory system to supply amounts of blood adequate for the metabolic needs of the body during normal activity, at rest, and during periods of stress. The normal resting metabolic rate, measured as oxygen consumption, is about 250 ml/min. This figure can increase more than 10-fold in normal subjects during strenuous muscular exercise, which is the most important physiologic stimulus to which the cardiovascular system can be subjected. Other normal and abnormal stresses–excitement, emotion, changes in external temperature or gravitational force (posture), sexual activity, pregnancy, changes in body weight, salt deprivation or excess, anemia, and fever–all call for smaller increases in metabolic rate and cardiac output but seldom more than double the resting values. Transport of oxygen is the most conveniently measured overall index of cardiovascular function, but elimination of CO_2, transport of nutrient substances, and control of body temperature are also vital functions of the circulation.

Component Parts of the Circulation

The circulatory system counteracts the effects of gravity. A remarkably constant arterial pressure perfuses the aorta and its large branch arteries during all forms of activity, and these vessels act as almost pure transmission lines, carrying blood to the arteriolar bed of each specialized organ system (Fig 1–15). The ve-

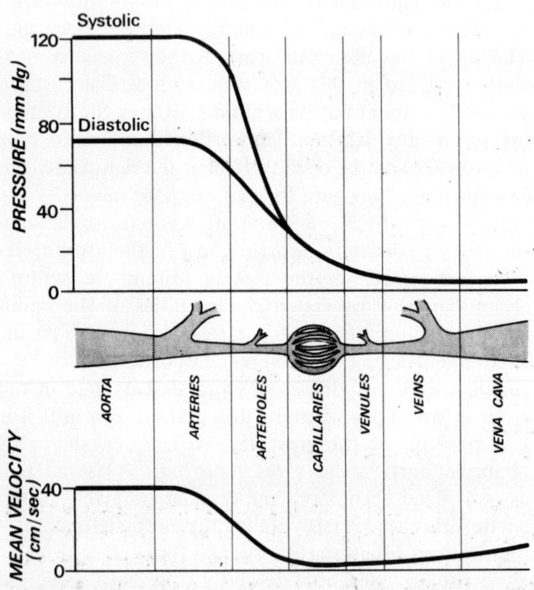

Figure 1–15. Changes in pressure and velocity as blood flows through the systemic circulation.

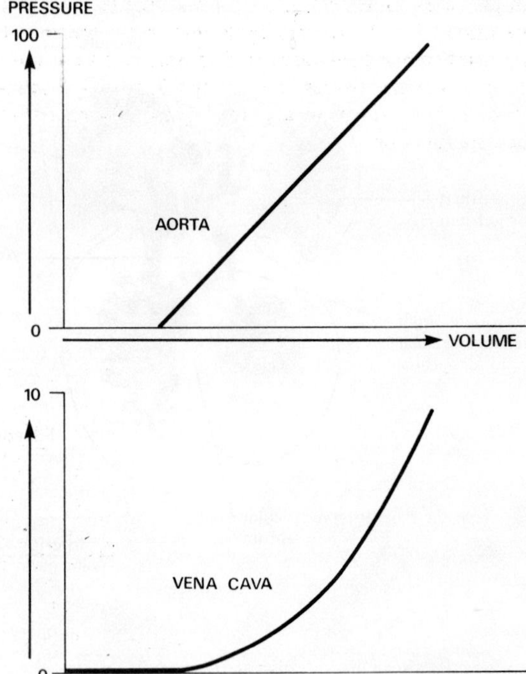

Figure 1–16. Pressure-volume curves for aorta and vena cava. The curves are plotted on the same arbitrary volume scale, but the pressure scale for the aorta is 10 times that for the vena cava.

locity of blood flow falls in the arterioles, which act as parallel resistance vessels controlling flow to each capillary bed, where gas exchange takes place. The veins act both as return vessels to the heart and as capacitance vessels whose high volume and marked distensibility play a major part in providing an adequate reservoir of blood for the heart (Fig 1–16). Since the resting output of the heart–about 5 liters/min–can increase with exercise 5- to 7-fold, the reserve capacity of the cardiovascular system is great; thus, in a person who leads a sedentary life, disease can make significant inroads into cardiac reserve without causing any symptoms.

Control Mechanisms

Adaptation of the circulation to the varying needs of the body is achieved by the interplay of many complex–often interrelated–regulatory control mechanisms which reinforce one another and have different response times. Neural control mechanisms act rapidly and over a short interval, whereas humoral adjustments come into play more slowly and remain active for longer periods. The various control systems support each other so effectively that reasonably satisfactory cardiovascular function can be maintained during exercise even after several important control mechanisms have been rendered inoperative. To the physician, the primary determinant of circulatory function is the heart itself. The physiologist views the circulatory system as a unit and thinks of the heart as a relatively simple pump that acts as a power source to maintain the circulation. Since this book deals with diseases of the heart rather than vascular disorders and their consequences in the tissues, it is reasonable to give emphasis to cardiac function and the control systems that regulate function.

THE CARDIAC CYCLE

The normal cardiac cycle, shown in Fig 1–17, involves a sequence of electrical, mechanical, hemodynamic, and molecular events which must be understood individually before the student can truly understand cardiac physiology.

The heart consists of a syncytium of striated muscle cells held together with fibrous tissue. Specialized muscle cells with a high degree of inherent rhythmicity

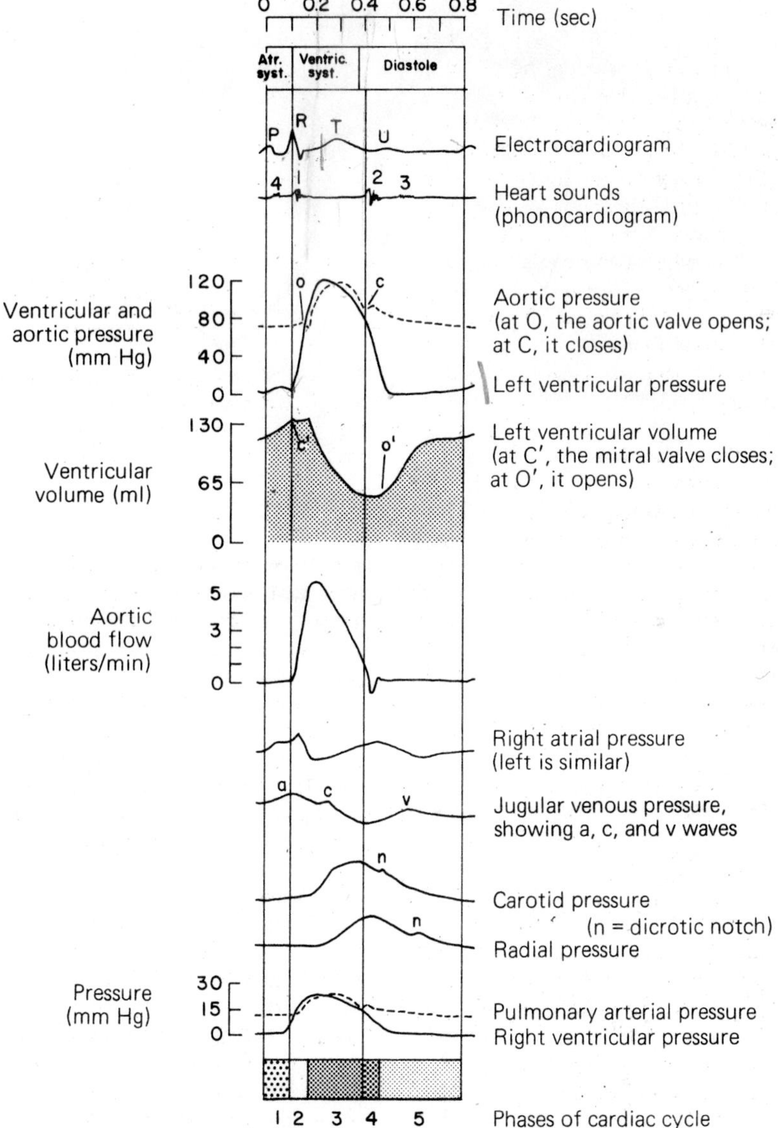

Figure 1–17. Events of the cardiac cycle at a heart rate of 75 beats/min. The phases of the cardiac cycle identified by the numbers at the bottom are: 1, atrial systole; 2, isometric ventricular contraction; 3, ventricular ejection; 4, isometric ventricular relaxation; 5, ventricular filling. Note that late in systole, aortic pressure actually exceeds left ventricular pressure. However, the momentum of the blood keeps it flowing out of the ventricle for a short time. The pressure relationships in the right ventricle and pulmonary artery are similar. Atr syst, atrial systole. Ventric syst, ventricular systole. (Reproduced, with permission, from Ganong WF: *Review of Medical Physiology,* 8th ed. Lange, 1977.)

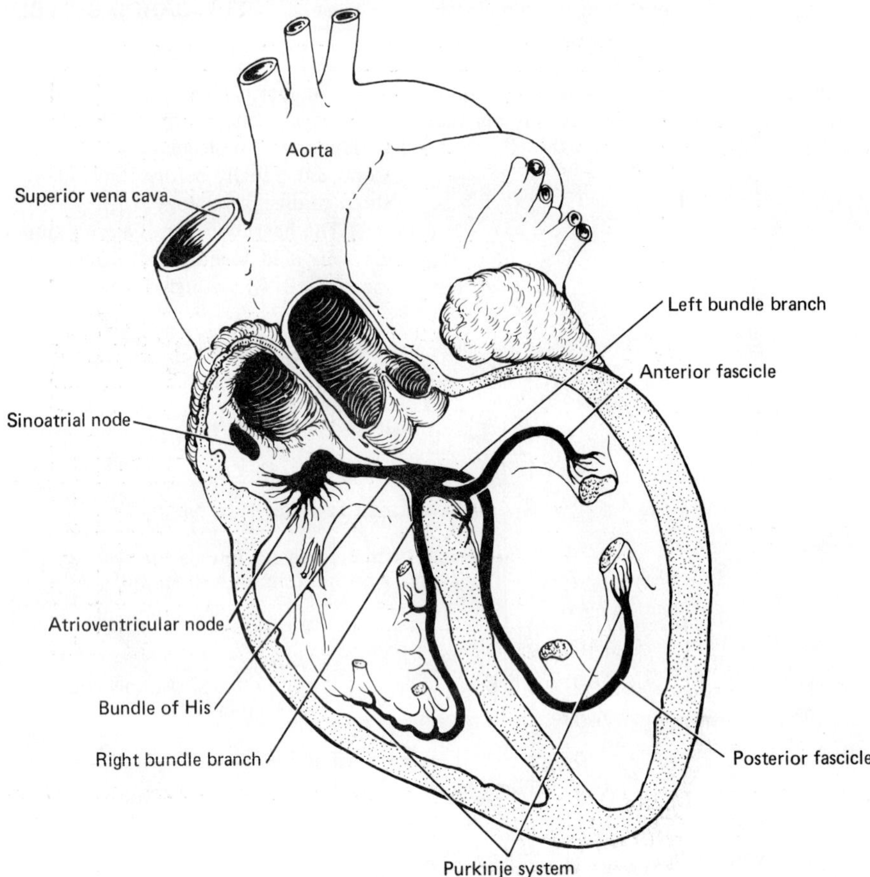

Figure 1–18. Diagram of the heart showing the impulse-generating and impulse-conducting systems. (Reproduced, with permission, from Junqueira LC, Carneiro J, Contopoulos AN: *Basic Histology,* 2nd ed. Lange, 1977.)

are present in conduction tissue (Fig 1–18) in the areas concerned with the generation and propagation of excitatory electrical activity.

Propagation of the Electrical Impulse

The cardiac cycle can be considered to start with sinoatrial firing, ie, the formation of an impulse in the sinoatrial node in the upper part of the right atrial muscle near the superior vena caval orifice. Electrical events precede mechanical events, and atrial contraction follows the P wave of the ECG and generates the atrial systolic activity (*a* wave). Activation proceeds in an orderly, repetitive fashion as the impulse spreads by several internodal pathways through both atria. When the impulse reaches the atrioventricular node, near the tricuspid valve, the cells of the bundle of His are activated and the impulse spreads via the Purkinje fibers to activate the ventricles, generating the Q, R, and S waves of the ECG. The impulse passes via the right and left bundle branches, the latter splitting into anterior and posterior divisions. Thus, there is a trifascicular ventricular conduction pathway through which the activating electrical impulse reaches each individual muscle cell at such a time that the result is an orderly sequence of ventricular contractions. The coordinated repetitive electrical consequences of atrial depolarization (P) and ventricular depolarization (QRS) and repolarization (T wave) of the heart can be displayed as an electrocardiographic signal (ECG), as shown in Fig 1–19, with P, QRS, and T waves of a shape and size virtually unrelated to the force of cardiac contraction. The ECG can be contrasted with the uncoordinated, asynchronous, variable, and disorderly electromyographic signals obtained from skeletal muscle during contraction. In skeletal muscle, the number of fibers taking part in a contraction depends on the force required to carry out that particular task, and recruitment of extra fibers, with a consequent increase in electrical activity, is seen when the force of muscular contraction is increased. In contrast, all cardiac muscle cells contract with each heartbeat, and any increase in the force of contraction is achieved by modulating mechanisms which involve each individual muscle cell.

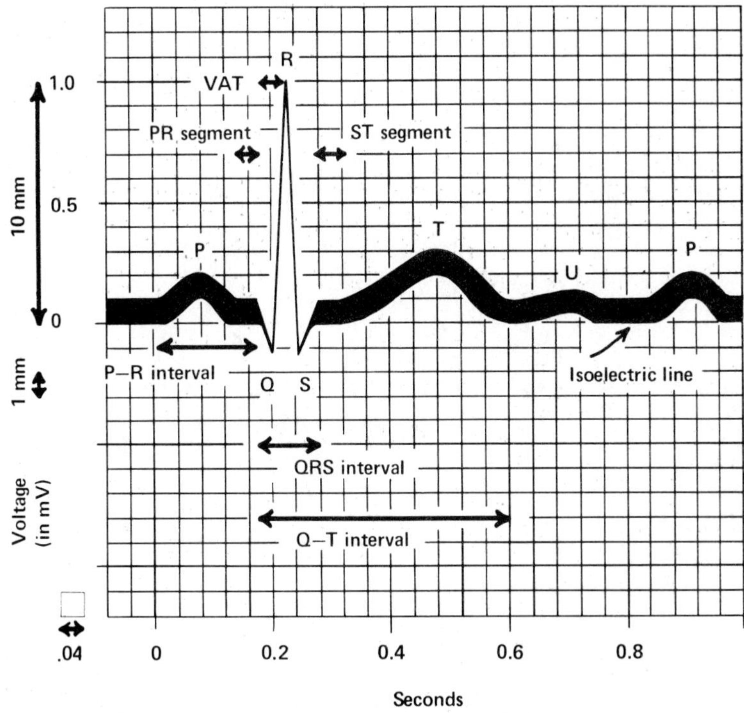

Figure 1–19. Diagram of electrocardiographic complexes, intervals, and segments. (Reproduced, with permission, from Goldman MJ: *Principles of Clinical Electrocardiography,* 9th ed. Lange, 1976.)

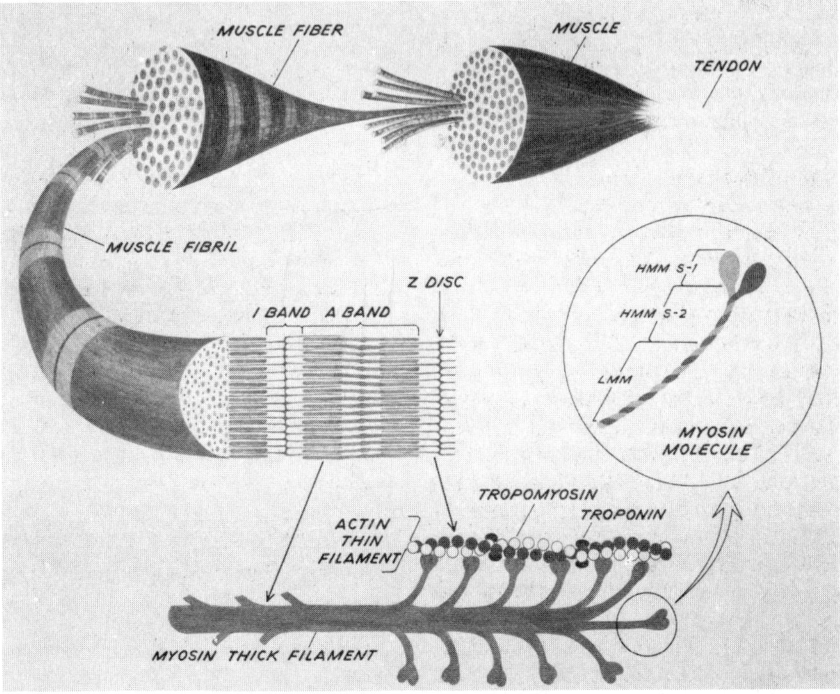

Figure 1–20. Structure of skeletal muscle. HMM, heavy meromyosin. LMM, light meromyosin.

CARDIAC CONTRACTION

Mechanism of Contraction

The electrophysiologic basis of the origin and spread of the impulse that excites cardiac contraction is described in Chapter 14. The molecular basis of contraction is similar to that in other types of muscle cell throughout the animal kingdom. The muscle cell, shown schematically in Fig 1–20, is composed of a number of muscle fibers that are in turn made up of muscle fibrils. The basic unit of the muscle fibril is the sarcomere, which lies between the Z lines. The sarcomere is the structural unit of which all striated muscle is composed. It consists of 2 main protein components–thick myosin filaments and thin actin filaments–which interdigitate with one another in parallel arrangement. A reaction between these 2 proteins at cross-bridges provides the mechanical force for contraction by mechanisms similar to those in skeletal muscle. The head of the myosin molecule is composed of heavy meromyosin, which can be split into 2 parts, whereas the tail consists of light meromyosin. Two separate proteins–tropomyosin and troponin–can be distinguished in the thin actin filament. The sliding filament hypothesis, which is shown diagrammatically in Fig 1–21, is now accepted as the most likely explanation of the phenomena associated with muscular contraction. The steps shown depict the influx of calcium as the action potential spreads via the transverse tubules. The actin filaments slide on the myosin filaments, and the Z lines move closer together. Calcium is then pumped back into the sarcoplasmic reticulum and the muscle relaxes.

Frank-Starling Law of the Heart

The sliding filament hypothesis can be used to explain the fundamental property of cardiac muscle referred to as the Frank-Starling law of the heart, which can be stated as follows: *The output of the heart increases in proportion to the degree of diastolic stretch of its muscle fibers.* This property of cardiac muscle, illustrated in Fig 1–22, is thought to depend on variations in the number of cross-bridges that can be formed between the actin and myosin filaments at any given muscle length. When a sarcomere is maximally shortened, the actin filaments overlap in the middle, covering up and eliminating from cross-linkage a number of active sites. As the sarcomere is stretched, more sites are uncovered and made available for cross-linkage, increasing the force that is developed. Further stretch beyond the normal range, which only occurs with injury or disease, reduces the amount of overlap and reduces the force of contraction by reducing the number of cross-bridges. The length-tension relationships of skeletal muscle have been studied experimentally for many years in preparations in which supramaximal tetanizing electrical stimuli are used to produce maximal muscular contraction. More recently, similar studies have been done using ventricular papillary muscle strips in an attempt to apply to cardiac muscle the principles developed from studying skeletal muscle. Because of the relatively long refractory period of cardiac muscle, it is not possible to produce a tetanizing contraction. While it can be clearly shown that the force of contraction of isolated papillary muscle does depend on the degree of stretch both before (preload) and during the contraction (afterload), the quantitative results of the studies, especially the extrapolated values for the maximal speed of contraction during minimal loading, are open to question.

The clearest expression of the law of the heart is

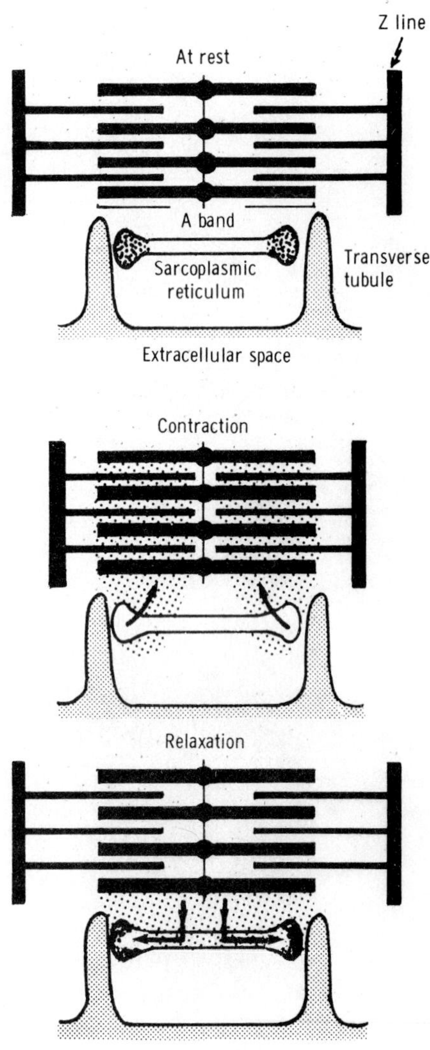

Figure 1–21. Muscle contraction. Calcium ions (represented by black dots) are normally stored in the cisterns of the sarcoplasmic reticulum. The action potential spreads via the transverse tubules and releases Ca^{2+}. The actin filaments (thin lines) slide on the myosin filaments, and the Z lines move closer together. Ca^{2+} is then pumped into the sarcoplasmic reticulum and the muscle relaxes. (Modified and reproduced, with permission, from Layzer RB, Rowland LP: Cramps. N Engl J Med 285:31, 1971.)

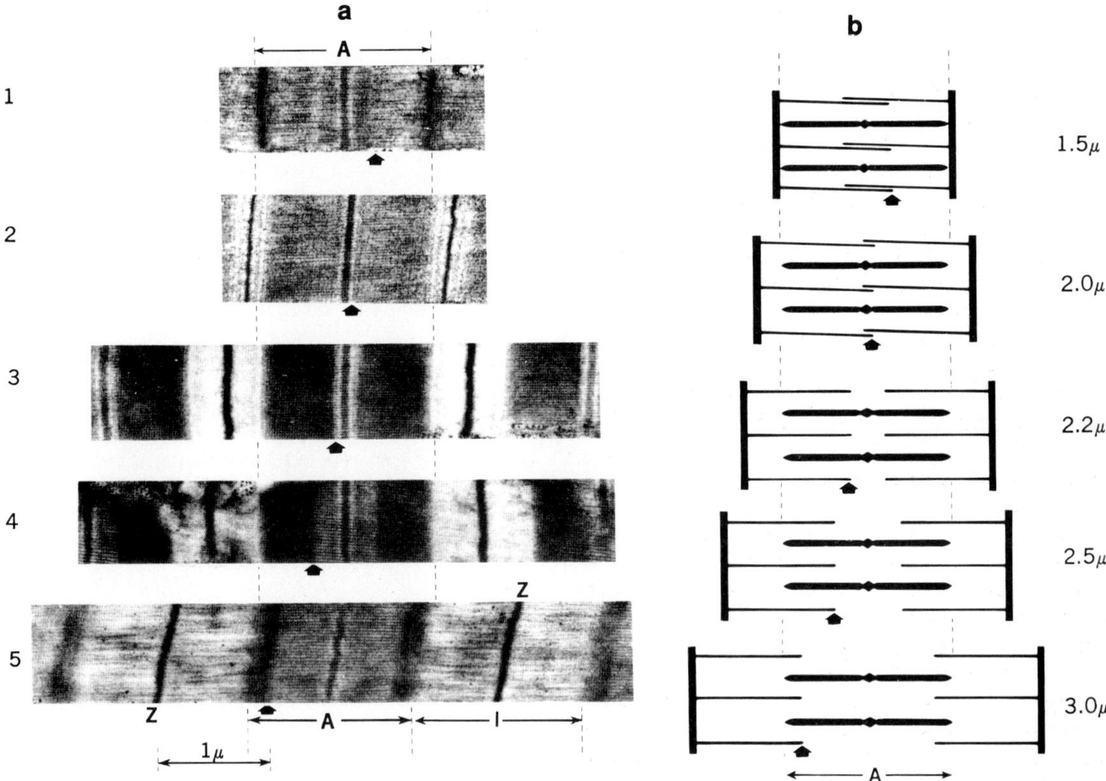

Figure 1–22. Panel *a* shows the band patterns resulting from an alteration of sarcomere length in skeletal muscle. Panel *b* shows the disposition of the thick and thin filaments that create these patterns. (Reproduced, with permission, from Sonnenblick EH: Myocardial ultrastructure in the normal and failing heart. Hosp Pract 5:35, April 1970.)

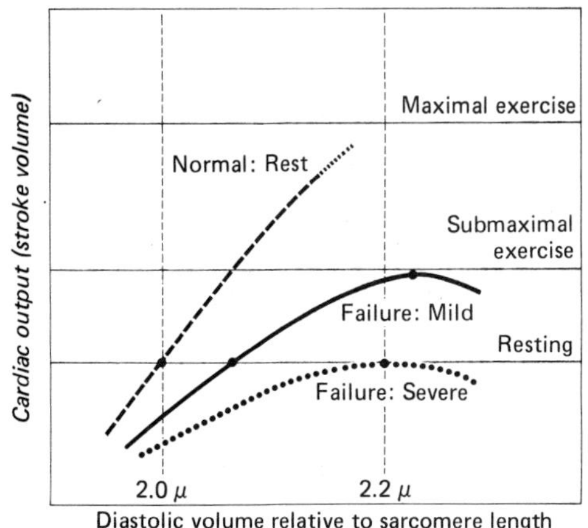

Figure 1–23. Curves representing the relationship between cardiac output and diastolic volume, which is related in turn to sarcomere length, in normal hearts and in hearts in mild and severe failure. A key point is that in the severe failure situation, exertion would produce increased diastolic volume but a fall in stroke volume. (Modified and reproduced, with permission, from Sonnenblick EH: Myocardial ultrastructure in the normal and failing heart. Hosp Pract 5:35, April 1970.)

given by plotting the ventricular diastolic volume relative to sarcomere length on the abscissa and the left ventricular stroke volume on the ordinate as shown in Fig 1–23. This graph takes no account of time and represents the result of a single beat. Time is secondarily involved because the ejection of a larger volume of blood in a single beat implies a more rapid ejection and a higher flow rate.

Length-Tension Relationships & Ventricular Pressure

The length-tension relationships of the individual sarcomeres must be viewed in light of the behavior of the whole heart. Two important considerations are involved. Tension must be converted into pressure and length into volume. The relationship between length, tension, and radius for a curved surface as stated by the law of Laplace is shown in Fig 1–24: For a sphere, *Pressure* = 2 × *Tension* ÷ *Radius.* In other words, thinking of the left ventricular cavity as a hollow sphere, the amount of tension that must be generated in the muscle of the wall to produce a given pressure in the cavity depends on the size of the ventricle. *Tension* = *Pressure* × *Radius* ÷ 2. If the ventricle increases in size, more tension must be generated to produce a given pressure. This physical principle indicates that there is more mechanical advantage in applying a force to contract a small than a large ventricular chamber. Thus, the larger and more dilated the ventri-

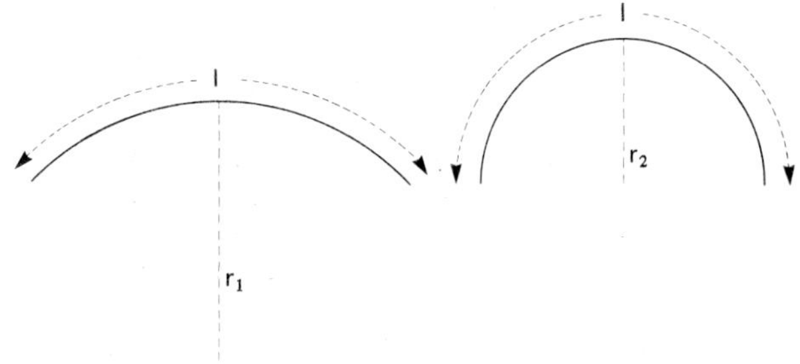

Figure 1–24. Relationship between length and tension underlying the law of Laplace. The tension in the rod of length *(l)* increases as the radius of curvature decreases from r_1 to r_2. For a sphere, pressure is inversely proportionate to the radius for a given tension.

cle, the larger its radius and the greater the tension which must be generated to achieve a given intracavitary pressure. The second conversion, from a change in length of the individual sarcomere to the change in volume of the whole ventricle, involves cubing the length change. This means that small changes in sarcomere length produce large changes in ventricular volume.

Excitation-Contraction Coupling

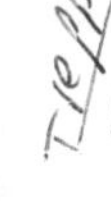

Changes in the speed of cardiac contraction are importantly involved in modulation of the force of cardiac contraction by an electrochemical interaction referred to as excitation-contraction coupling. In contrast to skeletal muscle, in which extra force is provided by recruitment of extra fibers, cardiac muscle relies on a modulating mechanism that involves an increase in the force generated by each individual fiber. It is best thought of as an increase in the rate of cross-bridge formation at any given sarcomere length. The 2 cardiac muscle proteins–tropomyosin and troponin–found in association with the thin actin filament play a regulatory role in actin-myosin interaction. The cross-bridges (heads of myosin molecules) attach to binding sites on actin and swivel when tropomyosin is displaced laterally by binding of calcium to troponin, as shown diagrammatically in Fig 1–25. Calcium enters and leaves the myocardial cell during the cardiac cycle, and its movement is associated with the slow inward current across the membrane as well as with both cardiac contraction and relaxation. The sarcoplasmic reticulum, which envelops the myofibrils within the cells, acts as a storage system for calcium and plays a part in the regulation of contraction. The increases in the force of cardiac contraction that occur with increase in heart rate, with sympathetic nervous stimulation, and with digitalis therapy are thought to be due to activation of the excitation-contraction coupling mechanisms. Changes in the force of cardiac contraction due to changes in the intensity of excitation-contraction coupling act independently of the basic Frank-Starling mechanisms, but the 2 are so closely linked that it is extremely difficult to carry out physiologic experiments in which the effects of either alone can be studied.

Increased Force of Cardiac Contraction

Any heartbeat in which the force of cardiac contraction is increased by enhanced excitation-contraction coupling tends to empty the heart more rapidly and to result in a smaller end-systolic volume. The result of more complete emptying depends on what happens during the subsequent diastole. If the volume of blood entering the ventricle during diastole is unchanged, the end-diastolic volume is less, and the force of contraction is decreased via the Frank-Starling mechanism, while still being enhanced by the excitation-contraction coupling mechanism.

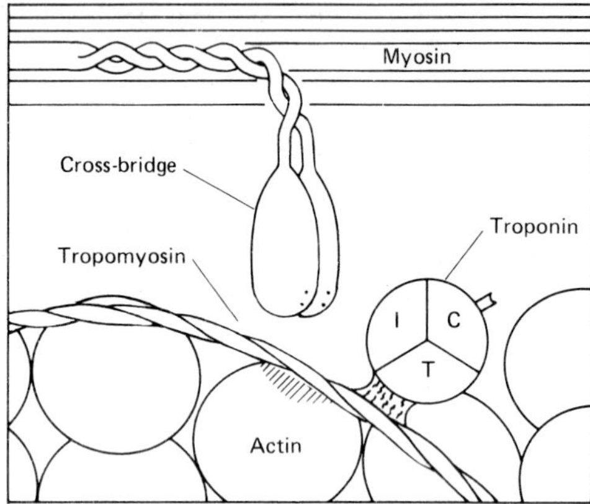

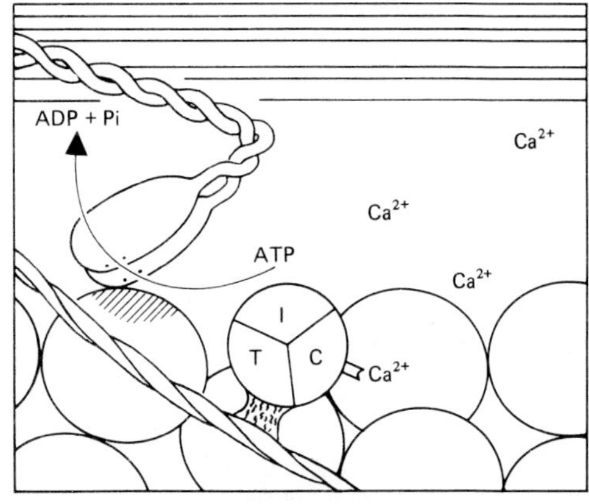

Figure 1–25. Initiation of muscle contraction by Ca^{2+}. The cross-bridges (heads of myosin molecules) attach to binding sites on actin (striped areas) and swivel when tropomyosin is displaced laterally by binding of Ca^{2+} to troponin C. (Modified from Katz AM: Congestive heart failure. N Engl J Med 293: 1184, 1975.)

Effect of Control Mechanisms

The circulatory control mechanisms respond to any change in cardiac output within a couple of beats and act to modify cardiac performance and change the hemodynamic state. It is thus difficult to determine the cause of changes in cardiac output on a beat-to-beat basis, and clear relationships between cardiac filling and stroke volume, which can be seen in isolated heart preparations in the laboratory, tend to be masked in patients. It is possible, however, to recognize the directions of change, and, if there is an increase in cardiac output with a decrease in filling pressure, this can clearly be seen to be beneficial whether it results from the Frank-Starling mechanism, from increased intensity of excitation-contraction coupling, or from both.

The Metabolic Cost of Cardiac Contraction

The metabolic cost of the 2 mechanisms for increasing the force of contraction is not the same in each case. There is evidence to indicate that increased excitation-contraction coupling costs more in terms of oxygen consumption of the myocardium than does increased output via the Frank-Starling mechanism. The metabolic measurements are difficult to make; even the beat-to-beat changes in cardiac output and cardiac volume cannot be measured with any great degree of accuracy in clinical circumstances. Thus, all that can be determined is the overall relationship between average cardiac output and filling pressure over several minutes, and it must generally be assumed that the circulatory control system has not changed its activity in the interim.

FUNCTIONAL CARDIAC ANATOMY

The basic molecular mechanisms of cardiac muscle contraction must be viewed against the background of the functional anatomy of the heart as it beats in the chest. The change in shape of the heart during each cycle is complex, and the approximation of the main bulk of the left ventricle by a sphere, or even an ellipse, is clearly an oversimplification, as is the description of its contraction as the change of one or 2 radii of curvature. Although an adequate description of the complex movements of the contracting left ventricle is not yet possible, a few important points can be made.

Change of Left Ventricular Axis With Contraction

The apex of the left ventricle remains relatively fixed during contraction, as does the ventricular septum. As shown in Fig 1–26, the left and posterior walls of the left ventricle move anteriorly and to the right during systole, and the main axis of the ventricular cavity, which lies in a direct line below the mitral valve during diastolic filling, shifts in an anterior direction during systole, bringing its long axis to a position during ejection in which the ventricular cavity now points directly into the ascending aorta.

Descent of the Base of the Heart

The base of the ventricle, formed by the mitral and aortic valve rings, moves downward toward the apex of the heart during systole, as shown in Fig 1–27. These changes, which occur with ventricular filling and emptying, are preceded by isometric relaxation and contraction phases in which changes in ventricular shape occur without any change in volume.

Right Ventricular Shape

The shape of the right ventricle is markedly different from that of the left. As shown in Fig 1–28, it has a narrow crescent-shaped cavity which lies on the anterior right-hand surface of the ventricular septum. The thin-walled right ventricle is more compliant and has a lower resting end-diastolic pressure than the left. Its volume is more susceptible to changes in intrapericardial and intrathoracic pressures than the left.

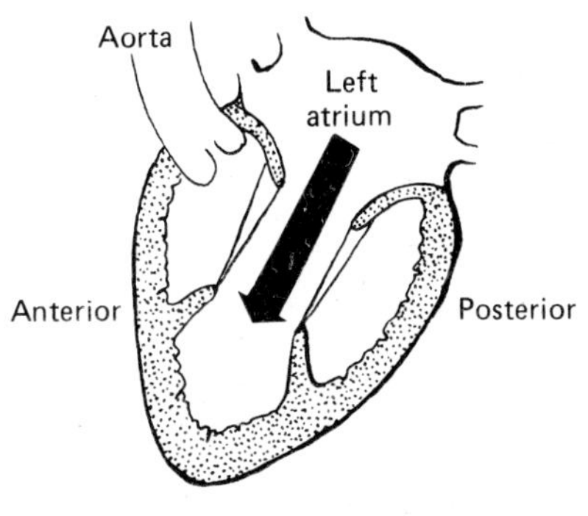

DIASTOLIC FILLING

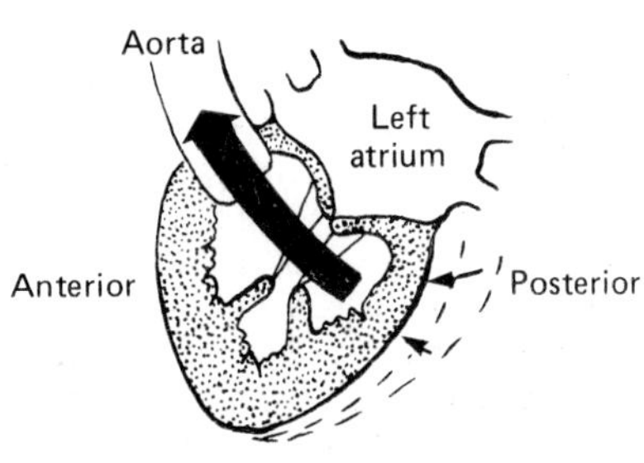

SYSTOLIC EMPTYING

Figure 1–26. Diagram of the heart in the left anterior oblique view showing change in axis of the left ventricle between diastolic filling and systolic emptying.

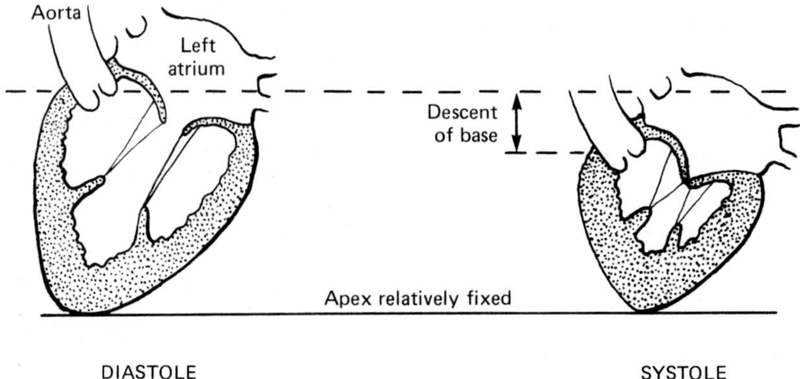

Figure 1–27. Diagram of the heart in the left anterior oblique view showing systolic descent of the base of the heart.

Atrial Anatomy

The atria are composed of even thinner muscle than the right ventricle and thus are even more compliant. The atrial musculature is thickest in the atrial appendages, which lie in the most anterior parts of the atria. The more posterior parts of the atria, around the sites of entry of the venae cavae, coronary sinus, and pulmonary veins, contain the least amounts of cardiac muscle and resemble veins in structure. Since there are no valves in the great veins on either side of the heart, the venae cavae on the right and the pulmonary veins on the left serve as reservoirs of blood for the ventricles. During ventricular diastole, as the base of the heart moves cephalad, the blood in the atria is transferred to the ventricles by the movement of the heart around it as well as by its own motion.

Ventricular Ejection

Both ventricles eject about the same proportion of their contents with each systole. Approximately two-thirds of the end-diastolic volume of about 100 ml/m^2 is delivered per beat, but this figure varies with cardiac filling and is influenced by postural changes in venous return.

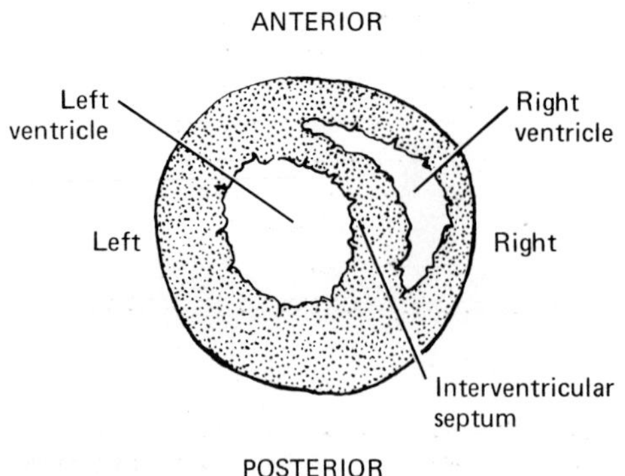

Figure 1–28. Cross section of the heart showing relative positions of the left and right ventricles.

A. Isometric Contraction: The rate of change of ventricular volume during ejection is a reflection of both cardiac filling and the force of cardiac contraction. It can be assessed by measuring the rate of change in left ventricular pressure during isometric ventricular contraction (dp/dt) as shown in Fig 1–29. The behavior of the heart during isometric contraction is influenced by the events of the previous diastole.

B. Preload and Afterload: The amount of filling (preload) influences the pressure developed during the next systole via the Frank-Starling mechanism. The output of the ventricle also depends on the resistance encountered by the contracting ventricle when the aortic valve opens during systole (afterload).

C. Aortic Velocity Pattern: The pattern of blood flow during the early part of ventricular ejection, shown in Fig 1–30, is normally one of a constantly increasing velocity (constant acceleration) which lasts

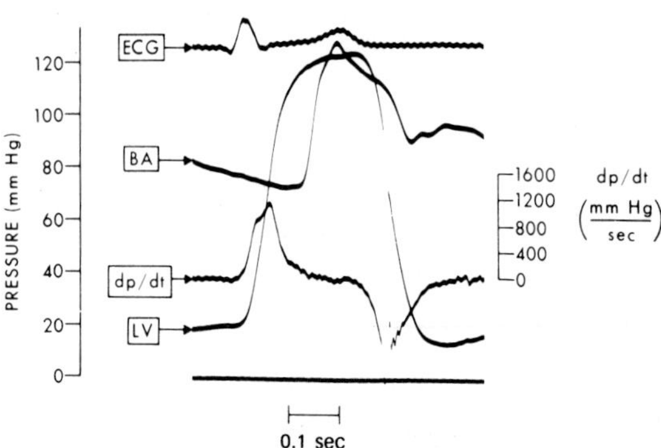

Figure 1–29. Pressure tracings and ECG showing the rate of change of left ventricular pressure. BA, brachial artery pressure; dp/dt, first derivative of left ventricular pressure; LV, high fidelity left ventricular pressure. (Reproduced, with permission of the American Heart Association, Inc., from: Kreulen TH & others: The evaluation of left ventricular function in man: A comparison of methods. Circulation 51:677, 1975.)

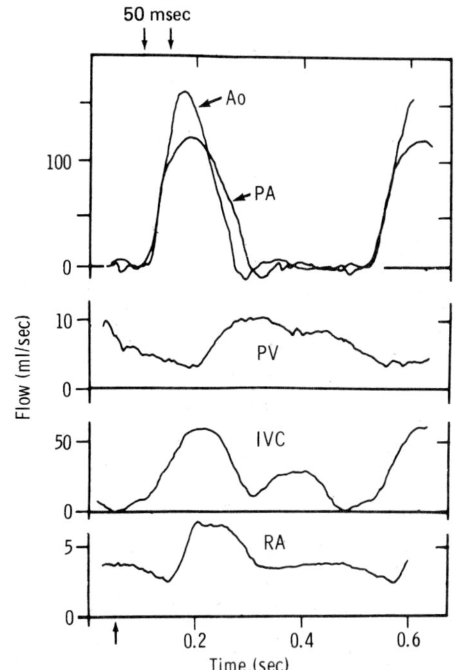

Figure 1–30. Changes in blood flow during the cardiac cycle in the dog. Systole at 0.2 and 0.6 sec. Flow patterns in man are similar. Ao, aorta; PA, pulmonary artery; PV, pulmonary vein; IVC, inferior vena cava; RA, renal artery. (Reproduced, with permission, from Milnor WR: Pulsatile blood flow. N Engl J Med 287:27, 1972.)

for approximately 50 msec. The pattern of flow at this time is "entry flow," and all the flowing elements of the stream of blood move with the same linear velocity, giving a blunt profile of flow across the vessel (Fig 1–31).

Laminar flow, with a parabolic velocity profile (Fig 1–32), does not develop for some distance down the aorta and until the later phase of ejection. It is thought that the pattern of flow late in systole is mainly dependent on conditions in the aorta.

D. Pattern of Ventricular Ejection: There is evidence that, as a first approximation, ventricular ejection can be thought of as occurring in 2 phases. In the first phase, radial shortening generates the force needed for the initial phase of ejection when aortic pressure builds up rapidly. In the second phase, the long axis of the ventricle shortens, and ejection continues for a length of time influenced by aortic impedance (afterload).

E. Pressure-Flow Relationships: Aortic pressure rises to a peak during ventricular ejection and comes to exceed left ventricular pressure relatively early during ejection. Thus, for about the latter half of systole, the pressure in the aorta actually exceeds that in the ventricle. It is the momentum of the blood flow that keeps up the flow in this phase of the cycle; when this falls off, the aortic valve closes.

F. Ventricular Relaxation: The period of ventricular relaxation that follows aortic valve closure lasts until the left ventricular pressure falls below left atrial pressure and is termed isometric ventricular relaxation. Its rate is linked to that of isometric contraction. Left ventricular filling starts when atrial pressure comes to exceed ventricular pressure and should be considered as an active process, whose rate depends on the rate of isometric relaxation. Filling is most rapid in the early part of diastole and ordinarily ceases before atrial contraction adds the extra tension that increases the force of the next ventricular contraction.

G. Myocardial Work and Oxygen Consumption: The heart is capable of putting out its largest amounts of work in conditions of normal aortic pressure, high flow, and small cardiac volume. High aortic pressure and increased ventricular volume are poorly tolerated. The most important indicator of cardiac work is the metabolic cost of cardiac activity, which is given by the oxygen consumption of the myocardium. This is extremely difficult to measure because it involves knowing both the total myocardial blood flow and the oxygen content difference between the blood in the

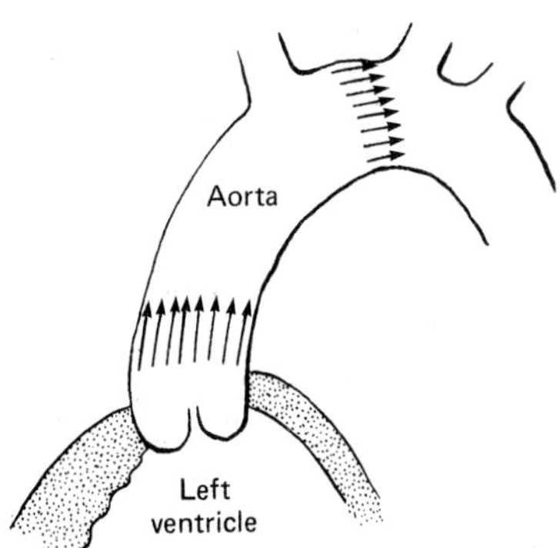

Figure 1–31. Diagram showing a blunt velocity profile in the aorta. All of the elements of the blood are traveling with the same velocity.

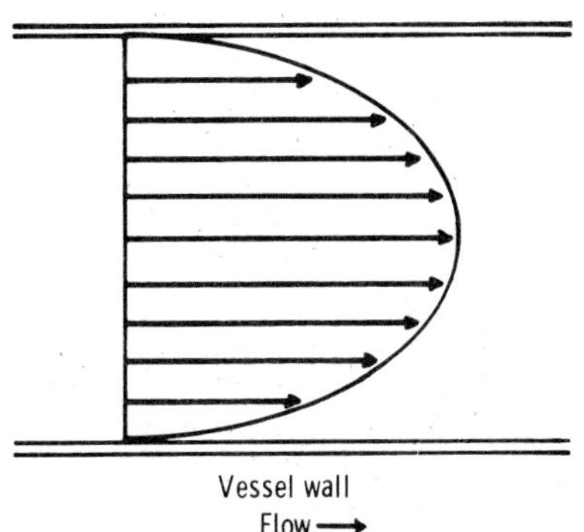

Figure 1–32. Diagram of the velocities of concentric laminas of a viscous fluid flowing in a tube, illustrating the parabolic distribution of velocities (laminar flow). (Reproduced, with permission, from Ganong WF: *Review of Medical Physiology,* 8th ed. Lange, 1977.)

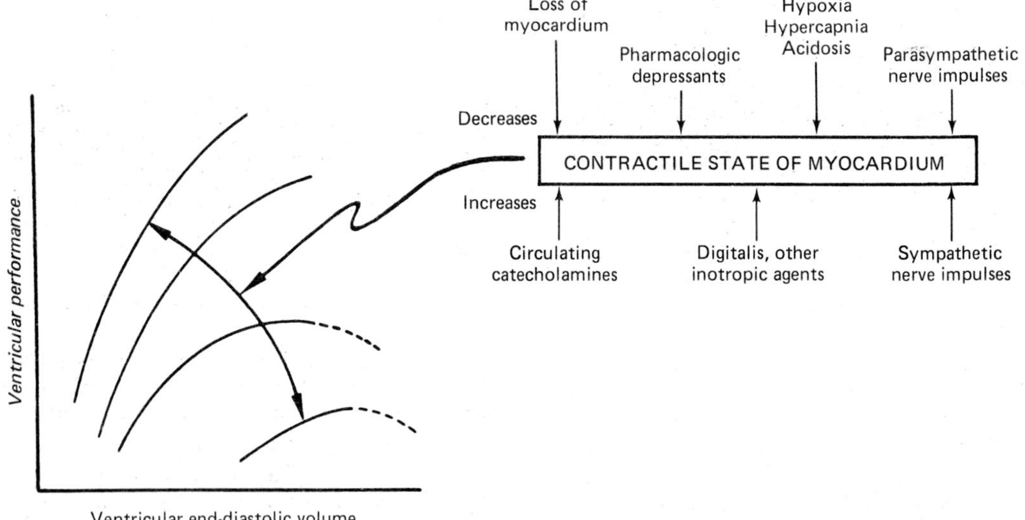

Figure 1–33. Effect of changes in myocardial contractility on the Frank-Starling curve. The major factors influencing contractility are summarized on the right. (Modified and reproduced, with permission, from Braunwald E, Ross J Jr, Sonnenblick EH: Mechanisms of contraction of the normal and failing heart. N Engl J Med 277:794, 1967.)

aorta and that in the coronary venous drainage. It has been shown in animals that the heart uses more oxygen in performing a given amount of external work against increased aortic pressure than in achieving an increase of aortic flow with a normal pressure. There is also evidence that increasing work via the Frank-Starling mechanism costs less oxygen than increasing work via the excitation-contraction coupling mechanism.

Myocardial oxygen consumption also depends on the mass of the heart muscle. Thus, when the heart hypertrophies in response to an increased mechanical load and the size of the individual muscle fibers increases, its oxygen consumption increases. This increases the need for coronary blood flow, and failure of coronary flow to keep up with the increased demands of a hypertrophied myocardium is a potential cause of myocardial ischemia.

H. Myocardial Contractility: It has become customary to think of myocardial performance in terms of "contractility." This is an ill-defined term which purports to describe the force of cardiac contraction in a way that is independent of preload and afterload and is illustrated in Fig 1–33. To date, none of the many proposed indices of cardiac contractility have proved adequate to describe the behavior of the heart in all circumstances, and it is probably best to reserve the term contractility for discussions of concepts of cardiac performance. The force of any given cardiac contraction is the result of so many factors that it is unrealistic to seek to describe it in terms of one specific measurement in the intact human heart, however specific it may be for an isolated heart muscle preparation.

CORONARY CIRCULATION

Coronary blood flow is an essential determinant of myocardial performance. Flow takes place during both systole and diastole (Fig 1–34) and is precisely adjusted to the needs of myocardial metabolism by the actions of multiple mechanisms. Left coronary artery flow is mainly diastolic; right coronary flow is more evenly spread between systole and diastole. The major coronary arteries lie on the surface of the heart, where they are exposed to the relatively low intrapericardial pressure. The branches that penetrate the walls of high-

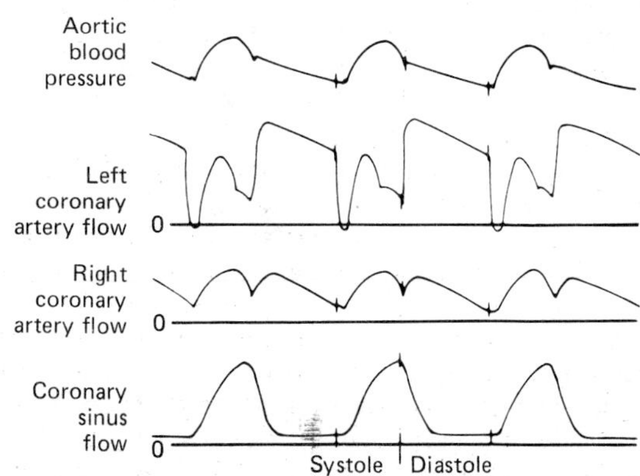

Figure 1–34. Schematic representation of blood flow in the left and right coronary arteries and the coronary sinus of the dog during phases of the cardiac cycle. (After Gregg DE. Reproduced, with permission, from: *Physiology and Biophysics,* 19th ed. Ruch TC, Patton HD [editors]. Saunders, 1965.)

pressure cavities, such as the left ventricle, are exposed to progressively greater systolic pressures as they pass deeper into the wall of the ventricle and come to lie closer to its lumen. It is difficult to see how the innermost subendocardial areas of the left ventricle can be perfused during ventricular systole, and it seems likely that there is a wide range of flows in different parts of the heart at different times during the cardiac cycle.

There is thus a gradient of vulnerability between the different layers of the myocardium. The subendocardial regions are more susceptible to ischemia than the superficial ones. Transmural myocardial infarction, manifested by deep Q waves in the ECG, is not usually seen when the coronary circulation is uniformly affected. Thus, in aortic valve disease, severe anemia, rapid arrhythmias, shock, and acute anoxia, evidence of diffuse subendocardial ischemia with widespread ST–T changes is likely to be found.

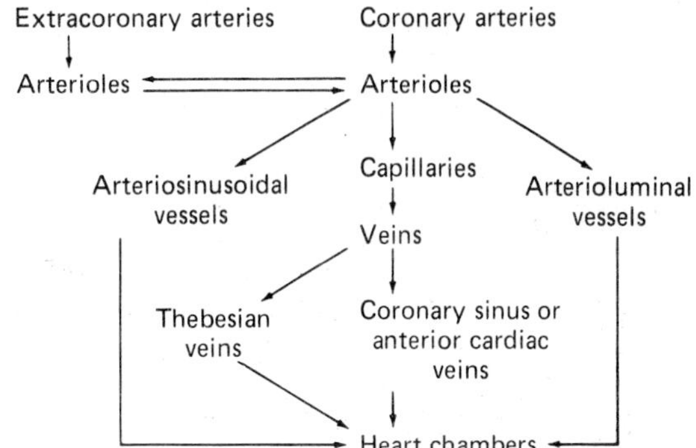

Figure 1–35. Diagram of the coronary circulation. (Based on Wearn JT & others: The nature of the vascular communications between the coronary arteries and the chambers of the heart. Am Heart J 9:143, 1933.)

Effect of Aortic Pressure

Aortic pressure is a major factor in coronary perfusion, and myocardial ischemia may occur in any situation in which blood pressure is acutely lowered, especially in older patients with coronary atherosclerosis.

Autoregulation

Autoregulation is important in maintaining coronary flow, which tends to be kept constant by inherent myocardial mechanisms thought to involve myogenic responses in arteriolar smooth muscle. Autonomic nervous system regulation of coronary blood flow is not thought to be a major factor, but it may induce coronary arterial spasm (also called Prinzmetal's syndrome).

Local Chemical Regulation

Local chemical regulation via vasodilator substances is important, and adenosine, formed by the breakdown of adenosine phosphate compounds, has recently been shown to play an important role. This substance is so rapidly built back into its parent compounds that it persists in the tissues for less than 1 sec.

Reactive Hyperemia

Adenosine is thought to play a part in the mediation of reactive hyperemia seen in actively metabolizing tissues such as cardiac muscle. Following any temporary interruption of blood flow, reactive hyperemia provides an increase in coronary blood flow, which can more than compensate for the deficiency resulting from the original ischemia. Reactive hyperemia provides a mechanism for maintaining coronary flow in response to local needs and is independent of autonomic nervous system control. It closely resembles the increase in coronary blood flow that occurs in response to vasodilator drugs such as amyl nitrite and nitroglycerin. These compounds paralyze smooth muscle in the walls of blood vessels by a direct action which cannot be blocked by any pharmacologic means.

Anastomotic Vessels

Coronary vessels drain both directly into the cardiac chambers and also via the coronary sinus (Fig 1–35). The arteries and arterioles anastomose freely with one another, and small collateral channels appear and grow in number and size when blood vessels are occluded by atherosclerotic changes. There is generally such a well-developed anastomotic network that it is impossible to be certain which major coronary vessel or vessels are involved when a given portion of the myocardium is the site of an infarct. It is also possible for more than one major coronary vessel to be occluded without resulting in an infarct. The rate of development of the lesions seems to be an important variable; if they develop slowly, major lesions may persist for years before symptoms occur.

CONTROL OF THE CIRCULATION

The circulatory system is made up of a systemic circuit (Fig 1–36) composed of multiple (parallel) pathways, each with its own local control mechanisms plus a pulmonary circulation which is essentially passive in the adult, and almost entirely concerned with gas exchange in the lungs. A hierarchy of systemic circuits exists and is based on how long life can be maintained in a given tissue when its circulation is cut off. In descending order of vital importance, these circuits are the cerebral, coronary, renal, visceral, muscular, skin, and reproductive organ circulations.

Dominance of the Cerebral Circulation

The cerebral circulation depends chiefly on the arterial blood pressure, and control of the circulation as a whole can be thought of as aimed primarily at providing the constant arterial pressure needed to maintain cerebral perfusion.

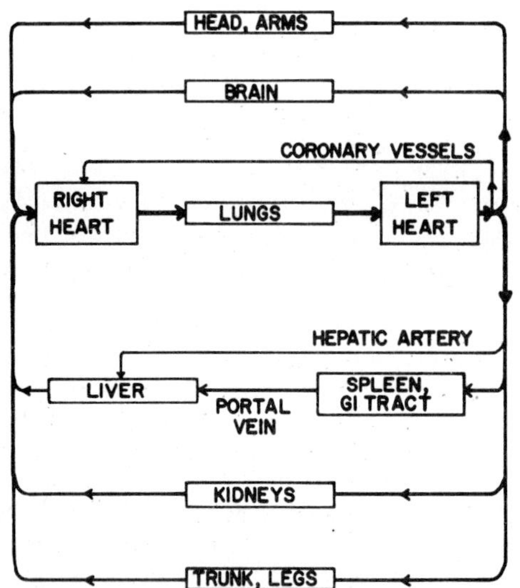

Figure 1–36. Diagram of the circulation in the adult. (Reproduced, with permission, from Ganong WF: *Review of Medical Physiology*, 8th ed. Lange, 1977.)

Controlled Variables: Aortic Pressure & Circulating Blood Volume

The 2 main controlled variables in the circulatory system are the central aortic pressure and the circulating blood volume. The servomechanisms that control aortic pressure are reasonably well understood, but the renal salt and water regulation mechanisms by which the blood volume is kept constant are not clear. They involve renin, angiotensin, aldosterone, vasopressin, and osmolality as well as purely physical factors.

Control of Arterial Pressure

A. Baroreceptor Mechanisms: Arterial pressure is kept constant by the baroreceptor servomechanism, which has multiple afferent sensory pathways and several efferent motor pathways. Arterial pressure is sensed via stretch receptors in the carotid sinuses near the bifurcations of the common carotid arteries in the neck (Fig 1–37) and by another set of stretch receptors in the arch of the aorta. Impulses from these receptors pass up the glossopharyngeal nerves to the medulla and provide a frequency-modulated input proportionate to the stretch of the vessel walls. Efferent impulses pass from the medullary centers via the vagus nerves to the sinoatrial (right vagus) and atrioventricular (left vagus) nodes. These impulses influence heart rate and modify the force of atrial contraction by inhibition of sympathetic activity. Other impulses pass via the sympathetic nerves to modify the level of arteriolar smooth muscle contraction in blood vessels in the limbs and in the visceral circulation via the thoracolumbar sympathetic outflow. The net effect of the system is to keep the mean arterial pressure almost constant. A rise in arterial pressure results in bradycardia, reduced force of atrial contraction, and release of peripheral arteriolar constriction. The active phase of the mechanism, which increases the frequency of impulses in the afferent nerves, is a rise in arterial pressure, and the response to a fall in pressure involves the inhibition of the reflex.

B. Speed of Response: The baroreceptor reflex represents a classic example of a short-term neural control mechanism. Heart rate changes take place within 1–2 sec, whereas changes in vasomotor control take 5 or 6 sec to act. Baroreceptor mechanisms are most readily brought into operation by changes in posture and also play a part in the increase in cardiac output that occurs in response to the start of exercise. They adapt to slow, prolonged changes in arterial pressure, and in systemic hypertension an abnormal level of blood pressure is kept constant on a short-term basis just as effectively as a normal level.

C. Effects of Disease: Normal baroreceptor function is impaired in disease affecting the autonomic nervous system; in conditions in which sensory input to the reflex is reduced, as in prolonged weightlessness; and after the administration of sympatholytic drugs.

D. Baroreceptor Brake-Sympathetic Nervous System Accelerator: The baroreceptor reflex is best thought of as a brake inhibiting the heart through the action of the vagus nerves and protecting the cerebral circulation from excessive increases in perfusion pressure. Conversely, the sympathetic nervous system is thought of as an accelerator which reciprocally comes into play when the baroreceptor brake is removed. The baroreceptor reflex has no direct action on the force of ventricular contraction, and ventricular function plays no direct part in the normal operation of the reflex. If arterial pressure falls because of impaired cardiac func-

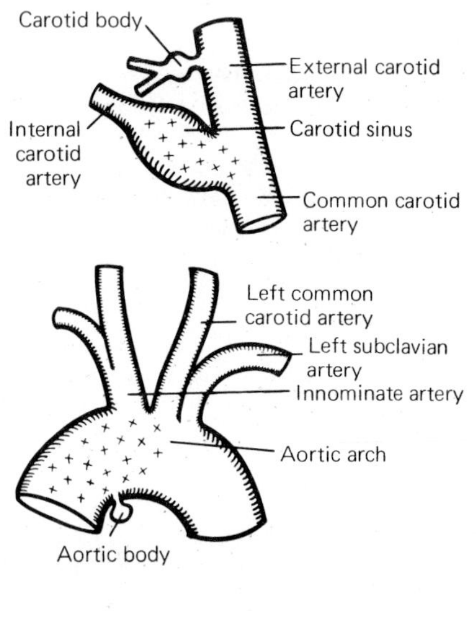

Figure 1–37. Baroreceptor areas in the carotid sinus and aortic arch. (Courtesy of Comroe JH Jr. Reproduced, with permission, from Ganong WF: *Review of Medical Physiology*, 8th ed. Lange, 1977.)

tion, the reflex will come into play to increase heart rate and constrict the arterial bed even at the expense of further decreasing cardiac function. This type of response is seen after myocardial infarction.

E. Effects of Sympathetic Nervous System on Cardiac Contraction: The force of cardiac contraction is influenced by the sympathetic nerves to the heart. Short-term stimulation of cardiac action occurs reflexly in response to arousal, alarm, excitement, anticipation of exercise, and pain. Any sudden stimulus—usually auditory, visual, or tactile—can cause a sudden increase in cardiac output within a second or less. The subsequent changes in cardiac output depend on whether a true or a false alarm has sounded and are influenced by baroreceptor responses. The circulatory response to isometric exercise is similar to that of arousal. Active muscular contraction causes an increase in heart rate and a disproportionate increase in arterial pressure. Thus, straining, as in lifting heavy objects, causes an increase in blood pressure; and, since the response is not directly related to the stimulus, even simple clenching of a fist can cause significant hypertension. The heart also responds to traumatic events such as interference with its blood supply, sudden and intolerable increases in arterial pressure, or obstruction to its output. Such stimuli are thought to affect nonmedullated afferent fibers from endings in the coronary vessels and to result in reflex bradycardia and hypotension mediated through the vagus nerves. They represent the Jarisch-von Bezold reflex which probably plays no part in the day-to-day physiologic regulation of the circulation.

Control of Blood Volume

One of the most remarkable features of the mammalian circulation (Table 1–1) is the small size of the circulating blood volume (5 liters) and the large proportion contained in the veins. Since the maximum cardiac output during exercise is normally 25 liters/min or more, a volume of blood equal to the total contents of the circulation must pass through the aortic valve on an average of once every 12 sec. Any change in blood volume is likely to have a marked effect on venous return and hence on cardiac output.

Table 1–1. Characteristics of various types of blood vessels in humans.*

	Lumen Diameter	Wall Thickness	All Vessels of Each Type: Approximate Total Cross-sectional Area (sq cm)	All Vessels of Each Type: Percentage of Blood Volume Contained†
Aorta	2.5 cm	2 mm	4.5	2
Artery	0.4 cm	1 mm	20	8
Arteriole	30 μm	20 μm	400	1
Capillary	6 μm	1 μm	4500	5
Venule	20 μm	2 μm	4000	
Vein	0.5 cm	0.5 mm	40	54
Vena cava	3 cm	1.5 mm	18	

*Data from Gregg, in: *The Physiological Basis of Medical Practice,* 8th ed. Best CH, Taylor NB (editors). Williams & Wilkins, 1966.

†In systemic vessels. There is an additional 12% in the heart and 18% in the pulmonary circulation.

A. Difficulty of Measurement: The measurement of blood volume, either as red cell or plasma volume, does not provide a clinically useful indication of the effective blood volume from a cardiovascular functional point of view. This is probably because mixing of the indicators used to measure blood volume with the contents of the circulation tends to be poor in the conditions in which disturbances of blood volume are important, ie, shock and heart failure.

B. Indirect Indications of Effective Blood Volume: Indirect evidence of the degree of filling of the circulation can be obtained by determining the effects of postural changes. When blood volume is large and the capacitance vessels are full, reducing venous return by standing up has little or no effect on the heart. The venous return does not decrease because there is no room for pooling of blood in the lower body and the level of blood in the venous reservoirs does not decrease sufficiently to lower the cardiac output. An adequate systemic arterial pressure can thus be maintained, and no baroreceptor adjustments are necessary. When the effective blood volume is reduced and the capacitance vessels are relatively empty, standing up leads to pooling of blood in the legs. This reduces venous return, which in turn reduces cardiac output, and the arterial pressure falls acutely. Fig 1–38 shows a tracing of arterial pressure in a normal subject in whom venous return is decreased by applying negative pressure to the lower part of the body. Systolic blood pressure falls while diastolic pressure is maintained, and heart rate increases via the baroreceptor system. When the negative pressure is discontinued, blood pressure rises and baroreceptor responses come into play within a couple of beats and restore the arterial pressure level by causing bradycardia and peripheral vasodilatation.

C. Effects of Posture: The simplest means of determining the adequacy of the circulating blood volume is to determine the effects of a simple change in posture on the patient's heart rate and blood pressure. The greater the increase in heart rate on standing, the smaller the effective blood volume. These changes have to be interpreted in light of the patient's build and the soundness of the autonomic control mechanisms. Tall persons are more subject to orthostatic changes, and any person in whom autonomic nervous paralysis is present will almost inevitably show a fall in blood pressure on standing.

D. Mechanisms of Control of Blood Volume: The mechanisms by which blood volume is kept constant are not completely understood. They involve the control of salt and water intake and excretion, transfer of fluid from extravascular to intravascular spaces, control of intracellular water, and hematopoiesis. The role of the kidneys is obviously of great importance, and additional contributions are made by the renin-angio-

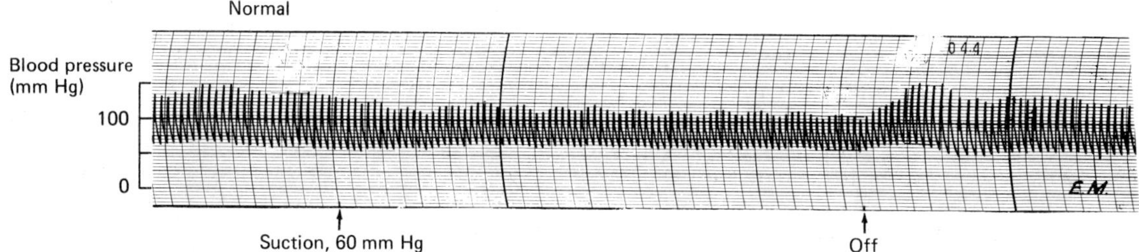

Figure 1–38. Brachial arterial blood pressure tracings in a normal subject. Venous return is reduced by applying suction to the lower half of the body. The baroreceptor reflexes maintain the mean level of arterial pressure, and there is overshoot of pressure when the venous return is restored.

tensin system, aldosterone secretion by the adrenal cortex, and atrial pressure receptors. It has recently been shown that there are important reflex mechanisms linking changes in atrial pressure to renal control mechanisms involving salt and water excretion. It had previously been thought that the atrial receptors only influenced urine flow by means of the effects of antidiuretic hormone from the posterior pituitary. The links between renal and adrenal control mechanisms in the regulation of blood volume and blood pressure will be discussed in Chapter 9.

DEVELOPMENT & AGING

The general physiologic principles set forth in the preceding pages are modified by growth and developmental influences from the fetal and neonatal period through adolescence and adult life up to the stage at which degenerative changes occur with aging. The special aspects of physiology of the fetus, infant, and growing child are outside the scope of this book, but aging is of increasing importance in cardiology in view of the increasing longevity of our population. Age appears to increase the differences between "normal" individuals, and the definition of normal and the establishment of ranges of normality become increasingly difficult in older subjects.

Degenerative Changes

Degenerative changes account for most cases of heart disease now seen in the Western world, and the inevitable aging processes seem to occur at widely differing rates in different people. Heart disease due to other causes does not protect patients from degenerative changes, and there is evidence that abnormally stressed tissues degenerate more rapidly than normally stressed ones. Patients with all forms of heart disease are coming to show more and more effects of the aging process as life expectancy increases and treatment to increase longevity becomes more effective.

SPECIAL CIRCULATIONS

Brain

The paramount importance of the cerebral circulation has already been mentioned. The blood supply to the brain, like that to the heart, is provided by an anastomosing system of arteries—the circle of Willis—and obstruction of a main vessel does not necessarily produce cerebral ischemia. As in the heart, it is not possible to be certain which cerebral or extracerebral vessel has been occluded in a patient in whom a particular part of the brain has been infarcted.

The principal factor influencing cerebral blood flow is the arterial CO_2 tension. Hyperventilation, by blowing off CO_2 in the lungs, decreases cerebral blood flow. Conversely, CO_2 administration increases cerebral blood flow. Autonomic reflex control of the cerebral circulation is not well developed, and cerebral perfusion is primarily dependent on the systemic arterial pressure, which is maintained by baroreceptor activity. The cerebral venous system contains no valves, and, since the cranial cavity is a closed space with rigid walls, cerebral circulation acts as a siphon to maintain blood flow by physical means.

Kidney

The renal circulation is under autonomic control, but mechanical and biochemical factors (probably bradykinin and prostaglandins) within the kidney play an important role in distributing flow preferentially to the cortex or medulla. The details of the intrinsic regulation of renal blood flow are not well understood. In normal circumstances, sodium excretion is regulated to maintain a balance between intake and output; however, in conditions of stress, when renal blood flow is compromised, sodium retention occurs. When the cause of inadequate renal perfusion is cardiac failure, the increased water retention that follows sodium retention increases blood volume and contributes to pulmonary and peripheral edema.

Other Viscera

Visceral blood flow is regulated by reflex hormonal and mechanical factors. The circulatory load imposed by visceral function is small and seldom compromises the general circulation.

Muscle

The circulation to the muscles is potentially the largest in the body, and its regulation to meet the metabolic demands of muscular exercise is complex. The degree of local autonomy is great, and each group of muscles can provide the necessary stimuli to bring about a perfusion adequate to meet its own metabolic needs. The overall cardiac output increases with muscular exercise as a result of sympathetic nervous activity. Any tendency for the blood pressure to fall as a result of the opening of muscle capillaries in response to muscular contraction causes release of the baroreceptor brake on the circulation and increases cardiac output. Increased muscular activity increases venous return to the heart, and this acts via the Frank-Starling mechanism to increase cardiac output. Local effects in the working muscles play an important role in the regulation of blood flow. Vasodilator substances—probably prostaglandins, bradykinin, potassium ions, inorganic phosphate ions, and breakdown products of ATP—are responsible for much of the marked local vasodilatation that occurs. The resistance to blood flow in the working muscles falls and local muscular blood flow increases. It is probable that local neural stimuli from muscle spindles, mediated via nonmedullated fibers, pass to the medulla and help to stimulate increases in cardiac output and ventilation. The hemodynamic changes during exercise vary with the subject's posture as shown in Fig 1–39. Cardiac output and stroke volume are higher in the recumbent position.

Skin

The principal role of the skin circulation is tem-

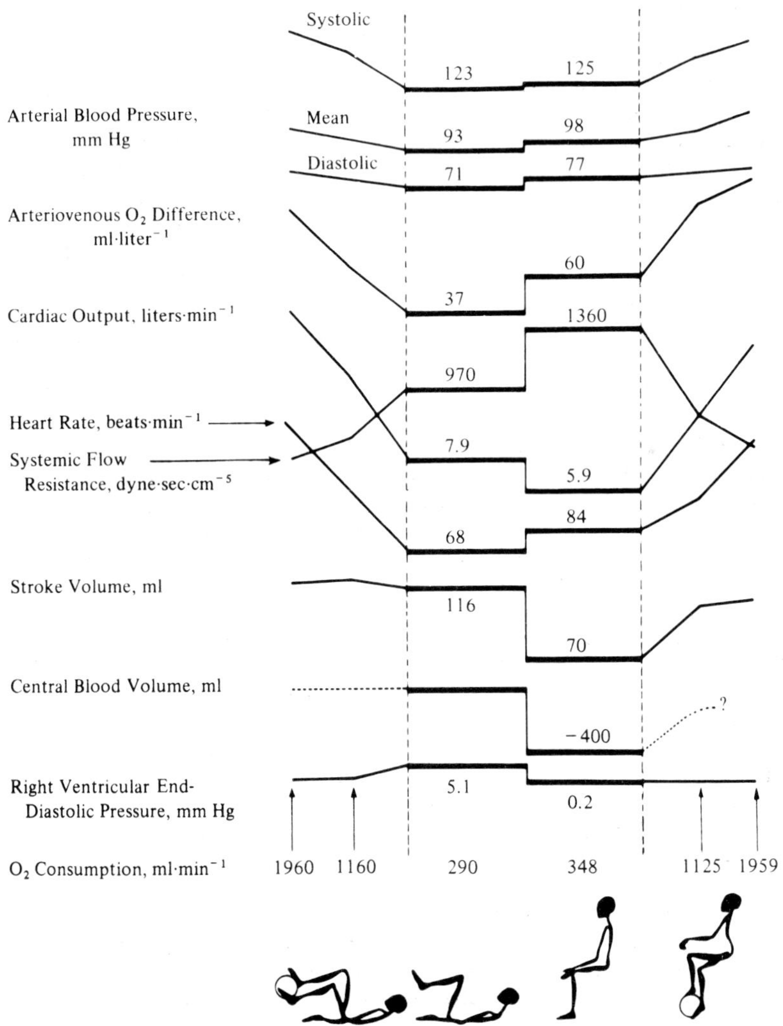

Figure 1–39. Hemodynamic changes during exercise in the recumbent and sitting positions in humans. Two work loads were used, corresponding to oxygen consumptions of approximately 1150–2000 ml/min^{-1}. The scales are linear, and changes during exercise may be estimated from the absolute figures given for the change from the recumbent to the erect position. (Reproduced, with permission, from Altman PL, Dittmer DS (editors): *Handbook of Respiration and Circulation.* Federation of American Societies for Experimental Biology, 1971.)

perature regulation. Since the mechanical efficiency of muscular work is only about 20–25%, large amounts of heat are generated during exercise. The skin acts as a radiator, and the evaporation of water from sweat acts as a means of cooling the blood perfusing the skin. This mechanism also comes into play in response to fever, with marked loss of heat occurring from the skin at times when the fever is subsiding. The converse occurs in response to low external temperatures and in periods when the body temperature is rising in febrile reactions. In this case, shivering and peripheral vasoconstriction act to generate and conserve heat. The demands of the skin circulation can become important in patients with severe heart disease when the cardiac reserves are seriously diminished.

Reproductive Organs

The circulation to reproductive organs is most important during pregnancy. The increased load of the placental circulation is sufficient to increase the resting cardiac output and blood volume. The peripheral resistance is lowered, and tachycardia and a wide pulse pressure can be noted as early as the middle of the second month of pregnancy.

DISTRIBUTION OF CARDIAC OUTPUT

All of these parallel systemic circulations compete for perfusion, and the total cardiac output reflects the sum of all their demands. Ordinarily, with normal cardiac function, enough blood flow is available for all circulations both at rest and during mild or moderate exercise. During severe exercise, however, the ability of other circulations to reduce their demands and thus free the maximal amount of blood for muscular perfusion is an important determinant of performance. The most important element in physical conditioning or exercise training is the development of mechanisms by which the greatest possible proportion of the available cardiac output is directed to the exercising muscles.

Pulmonary Circulation

Whereas appropriate distribution of cardiac output is the most important factor in systemic circulatory dynamics, maximal blood flow with minimal perfusion pressure is what is required in the pulmonary circulation. With increasing right ventricular output, eg, during exercise, there is an increase in the area of the pulmonary capillary bed and little or no increase in pulmonary arterial pressure. Reflex control of the pulmonary bed is minimal when compared to the systemic circulation. The principal factor influencing pulmonary arterial pressure is alveolar hypoxia. A lowered alveolar oxygen tension produces pulmonary arteriolar vasoconstriction. This probably serves as a local mechanism to divert pulmonary blood flow away from areas of the lung in which ventilation is inadequate. Increased CO_2 tension and hydrogen ion concentration are important in enhancing the response to hypoxia.

LIMITATION OF CARDIAC PERFORMANCE

Performance during sustained activity in normal subjects is always limited by the capacity of the heart to meet the demands of the circulation. Cardiac capacity increases after birth, during the period of growth and development, up to a peak in early adult life. With disease and the degenerative changes associated with aging, the capacity of the heart to perform work decreases and the maximum cardiac output, the maximum oxygen consumption, and the maximal heart rate decrease. Both the maximal values and the rates at which the maximal values are reached decrease with age. When the capacity of the heart to do work falls to a level at which renal or cerebral perfusion is compromised, a chain of events is initiated that leads to a vicious cycle resulting finally in a clinical syndrome known as heart failure. This condition is easy to recognize but difficult to define. It is best viewed as a derangement of the normal circulatory control mechanisms mediated through the autonomic nervous system and will be discussed in Chapter 10.

Failure of the heart to maintain its own circulation at an adequate level also leads to a vicious cycle which also results in what might just as well be called a form of heart failure but is in fact recognized as myocardial ischemia, discussed in Chapter 8.

The Heart as the Servant of the Circulation

The physiologic bases of these 2 forms of severe impairment of cardiac function—heart failure and myocardial ischemia—involve an understanding of the subservient role of the heart in relation to the overall circulation. The physiologic mechanisms involved in the maintenance of a normal blood pressure and blood volume so dominate the picture that when cardiac function is impaired, the autonomic nervous servomechanisms that ordinarily restore the status quo are activated even though the result is aggravation of the abnormal circulatory state.

Mechanisms of Heart Failure

"Inappropriate" physiologic mechanisms triggered by inadequate cardiac function are thus important in producing the vicious cycles that result in the clinical syndromes of heart failure and myocardial ischemia.

To cite specific examples, if the heart cannot maintain an adequate blood pressure, vasoconstriction mediated via the sympathetic nervous system occurs; this increases the work of the heart, causing a vicious cycle. If the heart cannot generate a blood pressure adequate to maintain renal perfusion, mechanisms physiologically appropriate for defense against loss of blood volume by dehydration, hemorrhage, or salt deprivation are set in motion. Retention of salt and water with blood volume expansion and restriction of urinary output then result in a vicious cycle by overloading the already damaged circulation, causing heart failure.

• • •

References

Bergel DH (editor): *Cardiovascular Fluid Dynamics.* 2 vols. Academic Press, 1972.

Berne RM, Levy MN: *Cardiovascular Physiology,* 3rd ed. Mosby, 1977.

Betz E: Cerebral blood flow: Its measurement and regulation. Physiol Rev 52:595, 1972.

Braunwald E: Determinants and assessment of cardiac function. N Engl J Med 296:86, 1977.

Braunwald E, Ross J Jr, Sonnenblick EH: *Mechanisms of Contraction of the Normal and Failing Heart,* 2nd ed. Little, Brown, 1976.

Brown E & others: Circulatory responses to simulated gravitational shifts of blood in man induced by exposure of the body below the iliac crests to subatmospheric pressure. J Physiol (Lond) 183:607, 1966.

Dawes GS: *Foetal and Neonatal Physiology.* Year Book, 1968.

Folkow B, Neil E: *Circulation.* Oxford Univ Press, 1971.

Ganong WF: *Review of Medical Physiology,* 8th ed. Lange, 1977.

Gauer OH & others: The effect of negative pressure breathing on urine flow. J Clin Invest 33:287, 1954.

Henry JP, Meehan JP: *The Circulation: An Integrative Physiologic Study.* Year Book, 1971.

Hertzman A: Vasomotor regulation of cutaneous circulation. Physiol Rev 39:280, 1959.

Heymans C, Neil E: *Reflexogenic Areas of the Cardiovascular System.* Churchill, 1958.

Hudson REB: *Cardiovascular Pathology.* 3 vols. Arnold, 1965–1970.

Huxley AF, Simmons RM: Proposed mechanisms for force generation in striated muscle. Nature 233:533, 1971.

Huxley HE: The mechanism of muscular contraction. Science 164:1356, 1969.

James TN: Anatomy of the coronary arteries in health and disease. Circulation 32:1020, 1965.

Johnson RA, Blake RM: Lymphatics of the heart. Circulation 33:137, 1966.

Jones RD, Berne RM: Intrinsic regulation of skeletal muscle blood flow. Circ Res 14:126, 1964.

Katz AM: *Physiology of the Heart.* Raven, 1977.

Keele CA, Neil E, Wright S: *Applied Physiology,* 11th ed. Oxford Univ Press, 1965.

Kirchheim HR: Systemic arterial baroreceptor reflexes. Physiol Rev 56:100, 1976.

Langer GA, Brady AJ: *The Mammalian Myocardium.* Wiley, 1974.

Langitt TW & others (editors): *Cerebral Circulation and Metabolism.* Springer-Verlag, 1975.

Linden RJ: Function of cardiac receptors. Circulation 48:463, 1973.

McDonald DA: *Blood Flow in Arteries,* 2nd ed. Williams & Wilkins, 1974.

Metcalfe J, Ueland K: Maternal cardiovascular adjustments to pregnancy. Prog Cardiovasc Dis 16:363, 1974.

Patterson SW, Piper H, Starling EH: The regulation of the heart beat. J Physiol 48:465, 1914.

Rowell LB: Human cardiovascular adjustments to exercise and thermal stress. Physiol Rev 54:75, 1974.

Sonnenblick EH, Skelton CC: Oxygen consumption of the heart: Physiological principles and clinical implications. Mod Concepts Cardiovasc Dis 40:9, 1971.

Yoffey JM, Cortice FC: Pages 272–277 in: *Lymphatics, Lymph, and the Lymphomyeloid Complex.* Academic Press, 1970.

Zelis R: *The Peripheral Circulation.* Grune & Stratton, 1975.

2...
History-Taking

A medical history carefully elicited by an understanding and competent clinician is essential to the evaluation of the patient with cardiovascular disease. Because of the great fear of heart disease by most patients, the physician's questioning should be unhurried and nonthreatening but nonetheless thorough. Skillful interrogation, appropriate to the urgency of the situation, must be matched by thoughtful listening. Questions should be as free as possible of the force of suggestion. The patient must be permitted to raise questions at appropriate times.

Artful history-taking brings the patient and physician close together. For this reason it is a critical factor not only in establishing the diagnosis but also in determining the outcome of subsequent therapy.

Subclinical Disease; Asymptomatic Patients

The modern tendency for patients with no symptoms to consult physicians for routine "checkup" examinations has increased the likelihood that doctors will cause unnecessary anxiety in their patients even though the intent of such examinations is to discover latent or developing illness. Since symptoms of disease are often exaggerations of normal findings (eg, dyspnea, fatigue), the borderline between normality and disease is often difficult to define. The problem becomes greater as the patient becomes older because the range of normality widens with advancing years. Some patients deny the existence of symptoms, fearing to be told that they are ill and may die; and some may exaggerate symptoms if being ill seems to have usefulness as a weapon or problem-solving device. Decreasing activity, failing memory, and wishful thinking may lead people to defer seeking advice until disease is far-advanced. Persons with no complaints are technically not "patients," and a distinction should be maintained between conditions discovered during routine examinations and the diseases of patients with true symptoms. Experience in dealing with clinical and laboratory information obtained from checkup examinations is relatively small, and physicians tend to forget that under such circumstances they are dealing with a presymptomatic phase of disease.

DYSPNEA

The difficulty of interpreting a symptom which may also be a normal physiologic response is perhaps most strikingly demonstrated in the case of the cardinal symptom of heart disease—dyspnea or shortness of breath. Shortness of breath on exertion is a normal phenomenon. In most cases, exercise performance is limited by shortness of breath rather than by fatigue, chest pain, leg pain, dizziness, or syncope. Dyspnea on progressively less severe exertion is also a normal accompaniment of the common modern combination of a sedentary life, increasing weight, and increasing age. The insidious onset of shortness of breath on exertion—a characteristic of heart disease—is thus more difficult to assess than some obviously abnormal symptom like hemoptysis or severe chest pain.

Mechanism of Dyspnea

The mechanism of dyspnea in normal and abnormal conditions is not always clear. "The unpleasant sensation of the need for increased ventilation" is the best description of dyspnea. Two main varieties have been distinguished. With the first variety, the patient feels that extra work on the part of the respiratory muscles is required to achieve adequate ventilation. With the second type, the patient is aware of a feeling of smothering and feels an urgent need to take another breath; the smothering sensation is akin to that associated with breath-holding. Dyspnea is a cortical sensation involving consciousness and must be distinguished from hyperpnea or increased ventilation, which may occur without any discomfort or distress and which may be seen in unconscious patients.

Dyspnea in Heart Disease

It is the dyspnea of patients with heart disease that most closely resembles the dyspnea of normal exertion. It is characteristically directly related to the degree of exertion. The patient complains that some effort that previously did not result in awareness of breathing now causes an unpleasant gasping sensation. The feeling of discomfort is in the chest but is not well localized to any single structure such as the diaphragm or the intercostal muscles.

In contradistinction to cardiac dyspnea, shortness

of breath at rest is more common in many lung diseases such as asthmatic attacks, bronchitis, pneumonia, or pneumothorax, but not in emphysema. Making the distinction between cardiac and pulmonary dyspnea can be extremely difficult. This is not surprising, since the mechanisms may be quite similar in certain circumstances.

A. Dyspnea Associated With Low Cardiac Output: When cardiac output is inadequate to meet the metabolic needs of the body, hyperventilation and subsequent dyspnea occur. Pulmonary congestion need not be present, although the dyspnea is similar to that occurring in pulmonary congestion and is quantitatively related to exertion. Nonmedullated sensory fibers arising from stretch receptors in muscle spindles monitor local metabolic conditions and cause reflex medullary ventilatory stimulation when flow to the exercising muscle is inadequate to meet metabolic needs. These nervous mechanisms involve primitive visceral sensory fibers that are highly resistant to blocking agents and therefore difficult to study.

B. Dyspnea Due to Pulmonary Congestion: Dyspnea on exertion is the cardinal symptom of pulmonary congestion. It results from a rise in left ventricular end-diastolic pressure or a raised left atrial pressure with a normal left ventricle in mitral valve disease. In both cases, increased pulmonary venous and pulmonary capillary pressures increase the stiffness of the lungs and the work of breathing by decreasing the compliance of the lungs, mainly by causing interstitial pulmonary edema. In addition to the mechanical changes, there is also a reflex autonomic visceral sensation, probably mediated through nonmedullated sensory fibers in the lungs and passing up the vagus nerves to the medulla, which contributes to dyspnea by direct autonomic sensory stimulation. In the early stages of heart disease, dyspnea only occurs with severe exertion, but as pulmonary congestion becomes more severe, permanent changes in the lungs occur: Resting lung compliance is reduced, and increased lymphatic drainage, thickening of interstitial tissues, and other compensatory changes occur. Such changes reduce the chances of acute pulmonary edema and enable the body to tolerate high pulmonary capillary pressures because of thickened barriers between the blood in the capillaries and the gas in the alveoli.

C. Dyspnea in Acute Pulmonary Edema: When pulmonary congestion is acute and severe, dyspnea occurs with minimal exertion, and pulmonary edema results as fluid is forced into the alveolar spaces by capillary congestion. This congestion may seriously interfere with gas exchange and cause hypoxia and respiratory acidosis with CO_2 retention.

D. Dyspnea Associated With Other Forms of Heart Disease: Dyspnea occurs in forms of heart disease other than those involving pulmonary congestion and low cardiac output. In cyanotic congenital heart disease, shunting of venous blood into the systemic circulation lowers arterial oxygen tension and contributes to dyspnea by stimulating the carotid bodies and increasing the ventilation needed for a given work load. In pulmonary embolism and pulmonary infarction, dyspnea may result from reflex stimulation of medullary centers by impulses from vagal nerve endings in the lungs and pulmonary arteries. Such dyspnea may be in addition to that due to inadequate cardiac output, which has already been described.

Dyspnea Resulting From Chemical Stimuli

Other mechanisms involved in dyspnea include chemical stimuli to ventilation mediated through hypoxia, increase in CO_2 (hypercapnia), and metabolic acidosis. The chemoreceptor cells of the carotid and aortic bodies respond primarily to hypoxia and secondarily to increased CO_2. The central chemosensitive areas in the medulla stimulate respiration primarily in response to acidosis resulting from CO_2 and only secondarily in response to hypoxia. Chemically mediated stimuli to ventilation provide slowly responding and long-lasting control mechanisms and are chiefly involved in controlling depth and rate of breathing rather than causing dyspnea. Hypoxia, as demonstrated by a lowered arterial oxygen tension breathing air at rest or during exercise ($P_{O_2} < 70$ mm Hg) is not generally found in dyspneic cardiac patients. Hyperventilation with low P_{CO_2}, low pH, and a normal or raised P_{O_2} is the usual finding. It is caused in cardiac patients by the release of acid metabolites from inadequately perfused tissues rather than by anxiety. Dyspnea also results from acute changes in the permeability of the pulmonary capillaries, as when pulmonary edema develops in heroin overdose, or on exposure to toxic fumes such as chlorine, phosgene, or other noxious gases.

Episodic Dyspnea

Episodic dyspnea and dyspnea at rest which is relieved by sitting up (orthopnea) are important indicators of severe disease. The mechanism of orthopnea involves an increase in pulmonary capillary pressure and a decrease in lung volume when lying flat. Lung compliance decreases and respiratory resistance increases to cause an acute increase in the work of breathing. Paroxysmal dyspnea classically occurs at night, often after a strenuous day or an evening out dancing, or after excessive salt or fluid intake. It characteristically wakes the patient up around 2:00 am and is so clearly relieved by sitting or standing and made worse by lying flat that a patient who has once experienced this symptom will often never sleep flat in bed again.

In acute pulmonary congestion in bedridden patients, the least exertion, such as eating, use of a bedpan or commode, washing, or the minor excitement of a visitor, may provoke an episode of dyspnea. The dyspnea of acute pulmonary congestion, if not relieved, will progress to acute pulmonary edema, which can cause circulatory collapse, with restlessness, anxiety, apprehension, sweating, tachycardia, tachypnea, and acute respiratory distress.

Dyspnea Associated With High Altitude Pulmonary Edema

Dyspnea due to pulmonary edema may occur in

persons acutely exposed to hypoxia at altitudes of 2000 m or more. The breathlessness usually comes on in the evening or during the night of the first day at high altitude. The patient often gives a history of unaccustomed exertion during the day. Even previously acclimatized persons returning to high altitude after a stay at sea level may be affected. Dyspnea, cough, frothy pink sputum, and circulatory collapse may develop if treatment is not forthcoming, and mountain climbers have died from the condition. Oxygen inhalation and returning to lower altitude are effective methods of treatment. The causative mechanism is almost certainly increased permeability of the alveolocapillary membrane of the lungs. The left atrial pressure has been shown to be normal in at least one person with the condition, and left heart failure is not the primary cause.

Diagnostic Value of Dyspnea

Certain features may occasionally help to show that dyspnea is due to specific forms of heart disease. In left ventricular failure, as opposed to pulmonary congestion, dyspnea is often associated with a heavy oppressive substernal discomfort, which tends to merge into angina of effort. Patients with mitral stenosis often complain of anginalike pain, but only when there is severe pulmonary hypertension. The distinction between dyspnea alone and angina plus dyspnea on the one hand, and between angina alone and dyspnea plus angina on the other, is difficult for both the patient and the physician to make. Acute left ventricular distention causes both severe discomfort in the chest and dyspnea resulting from acute pulmonary congestion. Similarly, acute imbalance between myocardial oxygen supply and demand often causes an acute rise in left ventricular end-diastolic pressure. In left ventricular failure, dyspnea appears first, and the discomfort never occurs without the dyspnea. The discomfort may radiate like anginal pain and is described as a sensation of heaviness, rather than pain, as in angina. Aortic valve disease, hypertension, and cardiomyopathy are the commonest causes of the discomfort. The basic mechanism is an increase in the work required from the left ventricle, and acute left ventricular distention may be involved.

Dyspnea in Normal Subjects

Dyspnea normally limits exercise performance in almost everyone. A person becomes conditioned to a certain level of discomfort arising from some particular task, such as walking up a familiar hill. The ease with which dyspnea is provoked varies with the amount of ventilation required for that task. This in turn depends on a person's physical condition, weight, age, and lifestyle. In sedentary persons, the ability of the circulation to distribute maximum blood flow to the exercising muscles while decreasing perfusion of relatively nonessential vascular beds (eg, adipose tissue, skin, and viscera) is impaired. A simple exercise program combined with weight reduction will often improve performance adequately within 4–6 weeks.

Dyspnea at Rest (Anxiety)

Dyspnea at rest commonly accompanies anxiety. The patient complains that normal breathing does not seem to satisfy his needs, and it is only by taking deep sighing breaths that relief is obtained. This form of dyspnea is not generally provoked by exertion and is associated with symptoms due to hyperventilation. The deep sighing breaths reduce alveolar and arterial P_{CO_2}, resulting in respiratory alkalosis. This provokes cerebral arterial vasoconstriction. Increased anxiety, headaches, dizziness, faintness, and even loss of consciousness can result. In addition, the ionized calcium level decreases with respiratory alkalosis, which can provoke numbness and tingling in fingers and lips, tetany, carpopedal spasm, and convulsions (hyperventilation syndrome). The cycle of anxiety resulting in hyperventilation and causing cerebral symptoms which in turn increase anxiety is extremely common and can be broken by the old-fashioned remedy of having the patient rebreathe expired air from a bag.

CHEST PAIN

Chest pain occurs in many varieties of heart disease and also in noncardiac diseases. Its correct interpretation is occasionally so difficult that it is almost impossible.

Ischemic Cardiac Pain (Angina Pectoris)

The classic ischemic pain of angina pectoris can be either so obvious that no one has the slightest difficulty in recognizing the symptom and arriving at a correct diagnosis, or so atypical that even after complete investigation, significant doubt about the nature of the pain still exists, although the latter is uncommon. The basic mechanism of ischemic pain is an increase in the demand for both coronary blood flow and oxygen delivery which exceeds the available supply.

A. Clinical Features: The original subjective description in the late eighteenth century by William Heberden of his own angina has not been surpassed. Angina of effort is described as a pain or tightness in the chest which is substernal, heavy, burning, and sharp (ie, severe but not stabbing). It may radiate (as shown in Fig 2–1) to the throat, anterior neck and lower jaw (never to the upper jaw), arms and upper back, but not to the lower spine or below the umbilicus, and rarely to the abdomen alone. It more often radiates to the left arm than to the right, and more commonly into both arms than to the right alone. It travels down the ulnar and volar surface of the arm to the wrist but only into the ulnar fingers, never down into the thumb or down the outer surface of the upper arm. Pain may occasionally start in the arms and move to the chest. It occurs more readily after a heavy meal, in cold, windy weather, and with excitement, anger, emotion, or tension. It sometimes comes on more readily with exercise

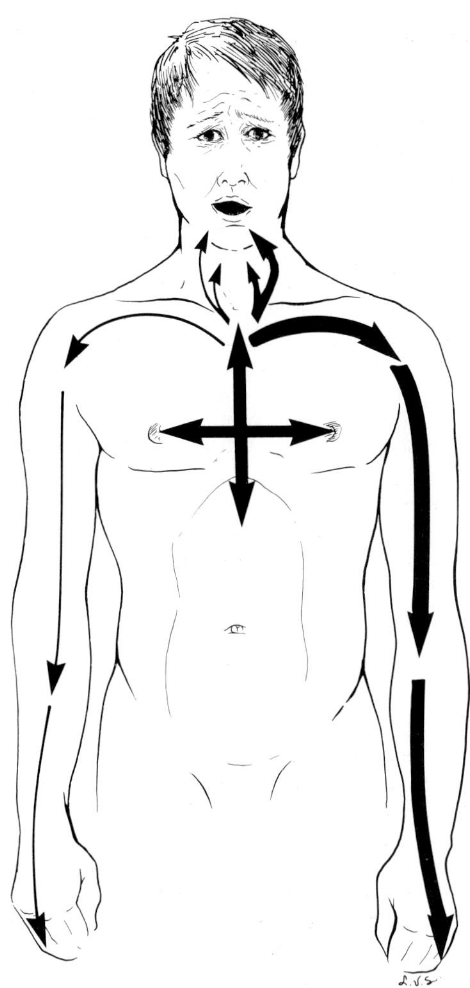

Figure 2–1. Principal areas of radiation of cardiac pain.

involving the arms. A patient attempting to describe the pain often subconsciously clenches the fists.

B. Effects of Temperature: In cold weather, walking against the wind with the face unprotected is likely to provoke anginal pain. Either hot or cold showers or baths may precipitate pain, and brisk toweling after a shower or bath may also provoke it. The sensory effects of temperature on the face are mediated through the fifth nerve and cause reflex autonomic changes in blood pressure and heart rate. Cold showers raise blood pressure and heart rate, and hot showers result in increased cardiac output in response to vasodilatation. Excitement, mental activity, and physical tension such as simple clenching of the fist raise arterial pressure and heart rate and increase the work of the heart. When the coronary circulation is severely diseased, even these minor circulatory changes are sufficient to provoke anginal pain. Anginal pain comes on more readily in the presence of fever, anemia, or arrhythmia, both bradycardia and tachycardia.

C. Mechanism of Cardiac Pain: The mechanism producing cardiac pain is not clearly understood. Nonmedullated, small sympathetic nerve fibers running with the coronary vessels are thought to provide the afferent pathway. The pain, like other forms of visceral sensation, is referred to the equivalent spinal segments C8 and T_{1-5}. Relief of angina following nonspecific surgical procedures such as thoracotomy, mammary artery ligation, and pericardial poudrage is well recognized but is not consistently found. Although it is thought to be a placebo effect, the severing of afferent autonomic nerves may play a role in relieving pain.

D. Ischemia Without Pain: Ischemia without pain is often demonstrable on ECG. In diabetic patients with autonomic nervous system disease, pain may be absent even though ischemia is severe. Chemical substances such as adenosine may provoke pain by stimulating sympathetic nerve endings. Certain compounds such as nicotine and lobeline provoke visceral sensations which resemble cardiac pain when they are injected into the circulation in normal subjects.

Pain of Myocardial Infarction

The pain of myocardial infarction is similar in type and distribution to that of angina of effort, but it is more severe, longer lasting, and associated at times with a feeling of impending death (angor animi) and also with circulatory collapse and shock. The patient may be short of breath, but pain ordinarily dominates the picture.

Pain in Acute Thoracic Disease

Pain similar to that of myocardial infarction also occurs with other acute intrathoracic disorders. *Aortic dissection* can cause severe chest pain. This frequently starts in the back or radiates to it. *Acute pulmonary embolism* also causes acute chest pain and shock which may be indistinguishable from that due to myocardial infarction. The cause is thought to be sudden acute right ventricular distention that stimulates ventricular receptors whose sensory representation resembles that of the left ventricle. Spontaneous pneumothorax and acute pleurisy, especially at the onset of lobar pneumonia, also cause chest pain and must be distinguished from pericardial disease, which causes a pain similar in distribution to other cardiac pains but more related to posture. Like pleural pain, pericardial pain is often worse with respiration, but relief obtained from sitting up and leaning forward or even from crouching on all fours face down is particularly suggestive of pericardial pain. Such maneuvers presumably alter tension on the pericardial sac. Like pleural pain, pericardial pain is often relieved when effusion develops.

Pain Associated With Anxiety States

The most troublesome pain to explain is the noncardiac pain of anxiety states and effort syndrome. The pain is stabbing, felt at the apex of the heart in the left inframammary region, and associated with a feeling of anxiety, breathlessness, and inability to take a satisfying deep breath (Da Costa's syndrome). It seems to be related to the sympathetic nervous system responses of fright. The more knowledge the patient has of heart disease, the more difficult it may be to interpret such pain because the description may be unconsciously molded to emphasize or minimize a possible cardiac illness.

Pain Associated With Herpes Zoster

The pain of herpes zoster classically precedes the rash, and the diagnosis should be borne in mind, especially in older persons. The pain is radicular in nature, gripping, tight, and constricting, and it may be severe. The diagnosis, which may be suspected when hyperesthesia is found in the affected area, becomes obvious when the eruption develops in a few days' time.

Musculoskeletal Pain

Musculoskeletal pain due to cervical or thoracic spinal bone or joint disease is readily confused with cardiac pain. Dorsal root pain (girdle pain) tends to be gripping and constricting and causes tightness. It is often associated with local tenderness, whereas angina is not. The presence of degenerative changes in spinal radiograms is no positive evidence of a musculoskeletal origin of the pain, any more than ST and T wave changes on the ECG indicate a cardiac origin. Provocation of the pain by movement, jarring, coughing, and sneezing, and relief of pain by means of massage, heat, and manipulation are useful in suggesting a musculoskeletal origin. Tenderness of the anterior rib cage suggests costochondritis (Tietze's syndrome).

Abdominal Pain

Abdominal pain sometimes occurs in patients with heart disease, especially in acute, severe right-sided failure. Hepatic distention is usually invoked as the causative mechanism. Abdominal pain also occurs in angina and in myocardial infarction, but the pain is never solely abdominal.

Esophageal spasm and pain associated with hiatal hernia can also be difficult to interpret. The esophagus and the stomach are innervated by the autonomic nervous system and are capable of causing visceral pain, having the same area of radiation as the heart. Any disease of the epigastric viscera can cause chest pain, which can be confused with cardiac pain. The pain of gallbladder disease is also difficult to distinguish from cardiac pain, and since gallbladder disease and coronary disease often coexist, accurate diagnosis of the cause of the pain may be extremely difficult.

PALPITATIONS

Awareness of the beating of the heart varies with the sensitivity of the patient and the severity of any disturbance of the force or rhythm of the heartbeat. The variation in these factors is great. Awareness of each ectopic beat or even of normal sinus rhythm may be extremely troublesome to some patients. Others may have an extremely forceful heartbeat owing to free aortic incompetence, or they may be subject to episodes of ventricular or supraventricular tachycardia with heart rates of over 180 beats/min without noticing anything. One must therefore differentiate between awareness of forceful heart action and an arrhythmia when the patient complains of palpitations. Most patients notice irregular rhythms more than they do regular tachycardia, but the more rapid the heartbeat, the more likely the patient is to notice an abnormality. In some cases, arrhythmia is only noticed during exercise when the heart rate is rapid.

Associated Symptoms

An important question is whether the palpitations are accompanied by any other symptoms such as dizziness, chest pain, or dyspnea. The functional effect of an arrhythmia may sometimes be a clue to its cause, as for example in mitral stenosis, in which dyspnea is almost always provoked when the arrhythmia occurs.

Examination & ECG Recording During an Attack

It is imperative to examine any patient with palpitations and record an ECG during an episode of palpitation. Until this has been done, it is essential to keep an open mind concerning the diagnosis. Palpitations often begin abruptly and cease gradually, and because the sinus tachycardia resulting from anxiety caused by the arrhythmia subsides only gradually, the patient may not be aware that the arrhythmia itself has stopped. The functional consequences of an episode of palpitations depend on the duration, the rapidity of the heart rate, and the state of the heart before the episode started. A paroxysm of tachycardia at a rate of about 140 beats/min may be well tolerated for a day or two, but any rapid arrhythmia with an acute onset and lasting for more than a week to 10 days is likely to provoke heart failure, even in healthy young persons. In older, sicker patients, especially those with anemia or hypoxia, a shorter time elapses before serious heart failure develops.

DIZZINESS & SYNCOPE

Dizziness and syncope are difficult symptoms to interpret if the patient's consciousness has been impaired and recollection of the events surrounding the attack is hazy. Dizziness and syncope both occur more commonly as benign manifestations than as symptoms of serious disease. They are most commonly due to noncardiac causes such as epileptic seizures, transient ischemic attacks due to cerebral or carotid vascular disease, and cerebrovascular accidents and vertigo due to vestibular disease rather than cardiac disease. A description of the episode from witnesses is of great value, but much can be learned from the circumstances surrounding the episode, as related by the patient. Dizziness is a frequent but not a necessary precursor of syncope, and one or both occur in 3 main types of conditions involving the cardiovascular system. The commonest form of cardiac syncope is simple vasovagal fainting resulting from certain autonomic nervous system effects. This is described in the chapter on hypotension (see Chapter 20). The next most common is cardiac syncope due to arrhythmia or cardiac standstill, in which the heartbeat does not maintain adequate blood flow to the brain. The least common is syncope on unaccustomed effort, in which the demand for systemic perfusion exceeds the supply during severe stress, and cerebral ischemia ensues. Cardiac syncope is described in the chapter dealing with arrhythmias, and effort syncope is described under the heading of aortic stenosis (see Chapter 13). Effort syncope can also occur in severe pulmonary stenosis and in primary pulmonary hypertension.

Fainting Attacks in Tetralogy of Fallot

A specific form of syncope occurs in patients with tetralogy of Fallot in whom infundibular obstruction is present. Spasm of the muscle of the outflow tract of the right ventricle results in an acute decrease in pulmonary blood flow. Right-to-left shunting of blood through the ventricular septal defect into the aorta increases as a result, and acute severe arterial hypoxemia occurs, leading to loss of consciousness. The factors precipitating the infundibular spasm are not known. Beta-blocking agents such as propranolol are the most effective remedies. The condition is most commonly seen in children but can occur in adults.

Carotid Sinus Syncope

Another rare cause of syncope is excessive sensitivity of the carotid sinus baroreceptor mechanism. Extreme bradycardia and peripheral vasodilatation may occur in response to minor mechanical stimulation of the neck, as in sharp turning of the head or pressure on the neck from too tight a collar. The condition is generally seen in older atherosclerotic men.

OTHER SYMPTOMS OF HEART DISEASE

Cough & Hemoptysis

Hemoptysis may occasionally be the first symptom of heart disease, and since there can be no hemoptysis without cough, cough is technically the presenting symptom. Mitral valve stenosis is the commonest condition in which hemoptysis is the presenting manifestation, and pulmonary congestion, frank pulmonary hemorrhage due to a ruptured vessel, and pulmonary infarction account for almost all cases. Cough without hemoptysis also occurs in any condition causing pulmonary congestion, and cough on exercise is sometimes seen in patients with mitral stenosis. Dry, unproductive cough is usually the earliest manifestation of impending pulmonary edema and precedes the profuse, watery, frothy pink sputum seen in the fully developed picture of acute pulmonary edema.

Cough may also occur as a manifestation of pressure on the bronchial tree in patients with cardiovascular disease. Left atrial enlargement may compress the left main bronchus in patients with mitral valve disease, and it may irritate the recurrent laryngeal nerve on the left side as it hooks under the aorta. Enlarging aortic aneurysms involving the aortic arch and tumors involving the heart may also cause cough when they compress mediastinal structures. Cough that occurs when the patient lies flat and is relieved when the patient sits up is particularly suggestive of pressure on the bronchial tree.

Fatigue

Fatigue is the most difficult cardiac symptom to evaluate. Whereas other symptoms of heart disease have associated outward manifestations, fatigue is entirely subjective. Although it is sometimes due to heart disease, fatigue is far more frequently due to noncardiac causes. Fatigue as a cardiac symptom is almost never of diagnostic value except as an indication of low cardiac output. It is rarely the first or the only symptom of significant organic heart disease, although it is a prominent symptom of neurocirculatory asthenia (Da Costa's syndrome). It commonly accompanies severe long-standing heart disease, especially chronic valvular disease with persistent right heart failure and low cardiac output. It is seen in patients with severe coronary artery disease after myocardial infarction, in mitral stenosis with marked increase in pulmonary vascular resistance, and in primary pulmonary hypertension. Dehydration due to excessive diuretic therapy and potassium depletion are 2 additional contributing factors.

Nocturia & Polyuria

Nocturia is occasionally the earliest symptom of raised left atrial pressure in left ventricular failure or mitral stenosis. The exact mechanism is not known, but transfer of fluid from the legs to the thorax when the patient lies down may play a part. Reflex connections have been demonstrated between left atrial receptors and the central nervous system, and the efferent pathway is known to involve the kidneys. Nocturia implies the passage of an abnormally large amount of urine at night, rather than an increased frequency of micturition at night, as occurs in prostatic disease. In the healthy state, the cardiac output is sufficient to provide adequate renal blood flow during the day, and urine flow at night is therefore conveniently reduced to a minimum. It may be that in early heart failure this mechanism breaks down because of inadequate cardiac output. There is also a connection between cardiac function and urinary output in patients with paroxysmal tachycardia due to any cause. Some patients note an increased urinary volume within 15–30 minutes of the start of an episode of tachycardia. The urine is of low specific gravity. The possibility of a reflex mechanism involving left atrial distention remains to be proved.

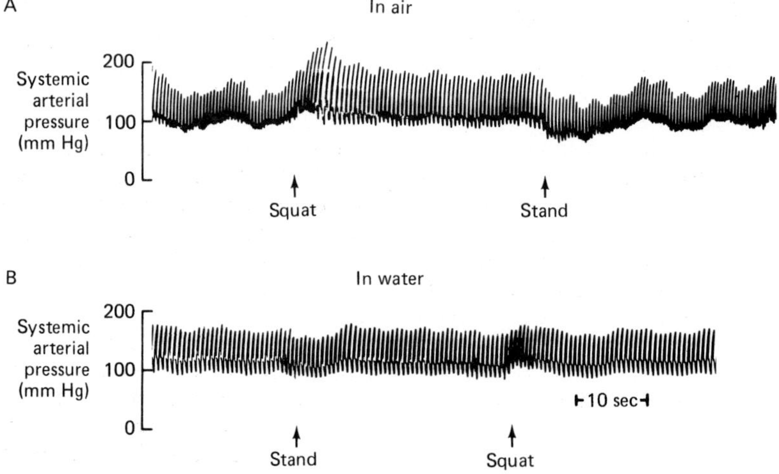

Figure 2–2. Systemic arterial pressure tracings from a normal subject, showing the effects of squatting *(A)* in air and *(B)* in water. The rise in arterial pressure on squatting and fall on standing do not occur in water.

Squatting

Exertional dyspnea that is relieved by squatting during recovery from exercise strongly suggests the diagnosis of tetralogy of Fallot. Squatting is seldom seen after puberty. It is a convenient means of increasing systemic venous return by lowering the patient's center of gravity and counteracting any tendency for blood to pool in the veins of the legs and pelvis. The central blood volume and pulmonary blood flow are both increased by squatting. It has been shown that it is the change in the amount of venous return and not the change in posture which is important, because squatting in water has no hemodynamic effect (as shown in Fig 2–2). Thus, in tetralogy of Fallot, squatting increases the arterial pressure and provides more blood flow to the lungs by decreasing the right-to-left shunt across the ventricular defect. It provides more pulmonary blood flow and a greater left ventricular inflow and also raises the arterial oxygen saturation by reducing the shunting effect. A similar result can be obtained by lying down, but children find it easier to squat after exertion. It is the pooling of blood in the legs in the upright position after stopping exercise that is the primary problem; if this does not occur, as in patients with a large pulmonary blood volume, the benefit from squatting is not seen. A tracing showing the time course of the changes in arterial pressure and arterial saturation on standing and squatting in a patient with tetralogy of Fallot is seen in Fig 2–3.

Hoarseness

Hoarseness as a manifestation of heart disease is seldom, if ever, a presenting symptom. It occurs in cardiac patients with gross left atrial enlargement in mitral valve disease, in giant left atrium, and in aortic aneurysms. All of these conditions cause pressure on the left recurrent laryngeal nerve and result in hoarseness. Hoarseness is also seen in patients with myxedema, in whom it may be the first clue to diagnosis.

Edema

Edema due to cardiac disease is seldom seen early because it is due to right heart failure, which is a late development in heart disease. A complaint of edema as a primary symptom implies a noncardiac cause such as venous stasis, thrombophlebitis, nephrotic syndrome, lymphedema, or idiopathic edema. Edema is seldom seen in patients with congestive heart failure under good medical control now that effective diuretic therapy is available. Right heart failure can be surprisingly severe, with hepatic enlargement, ascites, and a raised venous pressure, but no significant pitting edema of the ankles.

Cyanosis

Cyanosis is more a sign than a symptom, although patients do occasionally complain of blueness of the extremities, face, and lips. Cyanosis may be *peripheral* and associated with a low cardiac output, peripheral vasoconstriction, and a feeling of coldness. In this case, the blueness is due to a high concentration of reduced hemoglobin in the blood in the veins of the skin, and

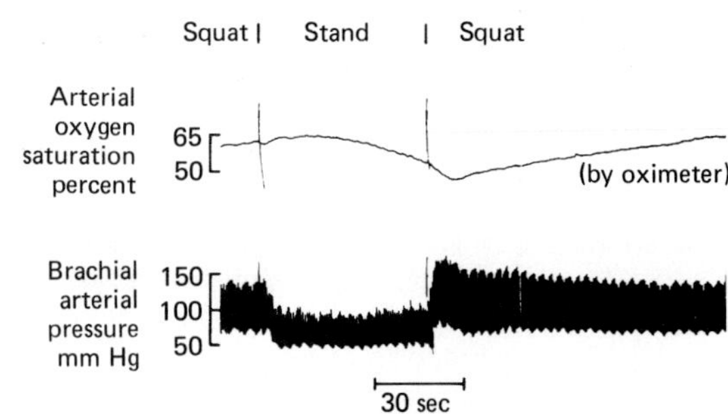

Figure 2–3. Changes in arterial oxygen saturation and blood pressure on standing and squatting in a patient with tetralogy of Fallot.

arterial saturation is normal. In true *central* cyanosis, the arterial oxygen saturation is reduced because of right-to-left shunting or lung disease. In this case, the patient's extremities are often warm, or, if they are made warm, the blue color does not disappear.

Loss of Weight (Cardiac Cachexia)

Loss of weight is not a presenting symptom of heart disease, but it does occur in chronically ill cardiac patients, especially when the cardiac output is low. It is probably related to secondary anorexia. The patient characteristically loses weight from the limbs and accumulates fluid in the abdomen. It is difficult to establish the true extent of the cachexia, because the accumulation of fluid tends to maintain total body weight.

FUNCTIONAL & THERAPEUTIC CLASSIFICATION OF HEART DISEASE

The patient's overall disability is conventionally expressed in terms of the New York Heart Association's criteria for functional capacity and therapeutic class.

Functional Capacity (Four classes.)

Class I: No limitation of physical activity. Ordinary physical activity does not cause undue fatigue, palpitation, dyspnea, or anginal pain.

Class II: Slight limitation of physical activity. Comfortable at rest, but ordinary physical activity results in fatigue, palpitation, dyspnea, or anginal pain.

Class III: Marked limitation of physical activity. Comfortable at rest, but less than ordinary activity causes fatigue, palpitation, dyspnea, or anginal pain.

Class IV: Unable to carry on any physical activity without discomfort. Symptoms of cardiac insufficiency, or of the anginal syndrome, may be present even at rest. If any physical activity is undertaken, discomfort is increased.

While this classification gives a good overall indication of the patient's status, many physicians prefer to subdivide class II into classes IIa and IIb. In class IIa, the patient can keep up with his peers walking on the flat but has limitation on more severe exercise such as climbing stairs. In class IIb, the patient has slight limitation on all forms of physical activity.

Therapeutic Classification (Five classes.)

Class A: Physical activity need not be restricted.

Class B: Ordinary physical activity need not be restricted, but unusually severe or competitive efforts should be avoided.

Class C: Ordinary physical activity should be moderately restricted, and more strenous efforts should be discontinued.

Class D: Ordinary physical activity should be markedly restricted.

Class E: Patient should be at complete rest, confined to bed or chair.

• • •

References

Barcroft H & others: Posthaemorrhagic fainting: Study by cardiac output and forearm flow. Lancet 1:489, 1944.

Heberden W: *Commentaries on the History and Cure of Diseases.* London, 1802.

Herrick JB: Clinical features of sudden obstruction of the coronary arteries. JAMA 59:2015, 1912.

Hultgren HN & others: Physiologic studies of pulmonary edema at high altitude. Circulation 29:393, 1964.

McIlroy MB: Breathlessness in cardiovascular disease. Pages 187–202 in: *Manchester Symposium on Breathlessness.* Blackwell, 1966.

O'Donnell TV, McIlroy MB: The circulatory effects of squatting. Am Heart J 64:347, 1962.

Parry CH: *An Inquiry Into the Symptoms and Causes of the Syncope Anginosa, Commonly Called Angina Pectoris: Illustrated by Dissections.* London, 1799.

Silverman ME: *Examination of the Heart.* Part 1: *The Clinical History.* American Heart Association, 1975.

Weiss S, Baker JP: The carotid sinus reflex in health and disease: Its role in the causation of fainting and convulsions. Medicine 12:297, 1933.

Wood P: Attacks of deeper cyanosis and loss of consciousness (syncope) in Fallot's tetralogy. Br Heart J 20:282, 1958.

Wood P: *Diseases of the Heart and Circulation,* 3rd ed. Lippincott, 1968.

Wood P: Polyuria in paroxysmal tachycardia and paroxysmal atrial flutter and fibrillation. Br Heart J 25:273, 1963.

3 . . .
Physical Examination

This chapter deals with only the more general or introductory aspects of the physical examination of the patient with heart disease. Details of the physical manifestations of cardiac disease appear under the description of each disease.

It is important to emphasize that examination of the cardiac patient is not confined to those parts of the body in which manifestations of cardiac disease are most commonly seen. Physicians should remember that cardiac disease can be associated with any disease from acromegaly to Zollinger-Ellison syndrome and that clues to the existence of noncardiac disorders which simulate, complicate, or merely coexist with heart disease may be apparent on methodic physical examination.

Approach to the Physical Examination

The general appearance and behavior of the patient are noted as the medical history is recorded. Similarly, the history-taking process may continue during the physical examination. The patient may be questioned about any findings and asked about awareness of signs and duration of such manifestations.

Examination of the patient usually starts from the head and proceeds downward. Inspection precedes palpation, percussion, and auscultation. The cardiologist traditionally feels the patient's pulse while carrying out the preliminary inspection, and many physicians start by recording the vital signs—pulse, temperature, and respiration—and blood pressure.

PULSES

The Radial Pulse

Palpation of the pulse wave that results from transmission of the pressure wave down the artery is classically performed on the patient's right wrist, with the examiner using the first 3 fingers of the right hand. The frequency, regularity, amplitude, rate of upstroke, and volume of the radial pulse require only one finger for their evaluation, but the rate of propagation of the wave (pulse wave velocity) and the thickness of the artery can only be properly examined with 3 fingers. The amplitude of the pulse (small or large) depends mainly on the pulse pressure and gives a rough indication of stroke volume. Thus the "small" pulse of severe mitral stenosis contrasts with the "large," jerky pulse seen in patients with mitral incompetence. In aortic stenosis, the rate of travel of the wave is slow; the "pulsus tardus" in this condition means that the pulse takes longer to pass under the examiner's fingers. The ease with which the pulse can be obliterated is felt by compressing the artery with the proximal finger and palpating with the other 2 in order to ascertain when the wave has disappeared. It is a rough indication of the systolic arterial pressure (Fig 3–1) and is less accurate than the measurement obtained by sphygmomanometry. The thickness of the undistended arterial wall can be felt using the middle finger to palpate while the proximal and distal fingers simultaneously occlude the vessel. It gives an indication of the degree of atherosclerosis.

Other Pulses

It is important to feel the pulse bilaterally to check for differences in timing and intensity. Brachial, radial, carotid, femoral, popliteal, and posterior tibial pulses are usually examined routinely. By this means, the physician may obtain clues about peripheral vascular disease, aortic dissection, and coarctation of the aorta. The closer the vessel lies to the heart, the more reliable the pulse is as an indicator of aortic pressure wave characteristics. Thus, the carotid arterial pulse is

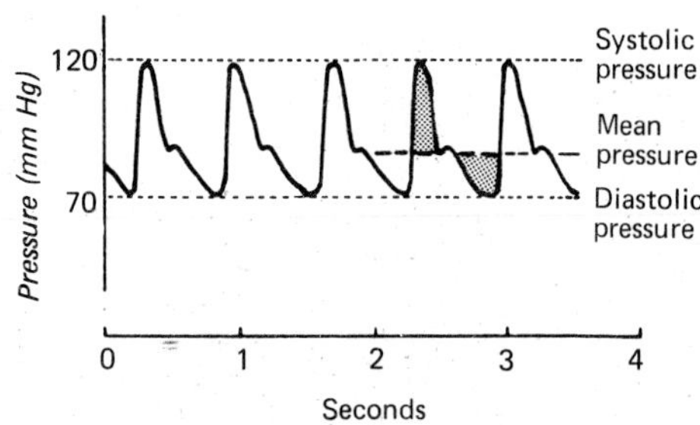

Figure 3–1. Brachial artery pressure curve of normal young person, showing the relation of systolic and diastolic pressure to mean pressure. The shaded area above the mean pressure line is equal to the shaded area below it. (Reproduced, with permission, from Ganong WF: *Review of Medical Physiology,* 8th ed. Lange, 1977.)

best for assessment of aortic valve disease. If there is a prominent pulse in the neck or if coarctation of the aorta is suspected for any other reason, it is important to feel the radial and femoral pulses simultaneously. In normal subjects, the 2 pulses are synchronous, whereas in coarctation of the aorta the femoral pulse is felt up to 0.15 sec after the radial.

BLOOD PRESSURE

Measurement Technic in the Arms

Indirect measurement of the systemic arterial pressure is conventionally performed using a sphygmomanometer on the right arm. A 12.5 cm cuff is wrapped around the upper arm and connected to a mercury or aneroid manometer. The arm is placed at heart level and the cuff is inflated to a level above the systolic pressure. The absence of a radial pulse is checked at the wrist. The cuff is slowly deflated (around 2 mm/beat) while the examiner feels the radial pulse. The pressure level at which the pulse is first felt is noted, and the cuff is reinflated. The cuff is then deflated a second time, with the examiner listening over the brachial artery with the stethoscope. The pressure level at which a sound is first heard over the artery is recorded as the systolic pressure. As deflation of the cuff continues, the sound arising from the vessel wall increases in intensity, decreases, becomes muffled, and finally disappears. Differences of opinion exist about the accuracy of considering the muffling or disappearance of sound as an indication of the diastolic pressure. Because the appropriate world cardiologic governing bodies are still undecided about whether it is the muffling of the sounds or their disappearance that is the "correct" level to use, both should be recorded. Correlation between direct arterial pressure measurement and sphygmomanometry has shown reasonable agreement between the 2 methods, especially in normal subjects, but the differences are sometimes marked in individual cases.

Blood pressure should be measured in both the standing and the supine positions in patients who might have hypotension or hypertension, and the pulse rate should always be measured and recorded along with the pressure. Blood pressure should be measured in both arms when the patient is first seen. On subsequent visits, it is taken in the right arm, except when the pulse in that arm is significantly reduced, as, for example, after a Blalock-Taussig operation for tetralogy of Fallot. The site of the measurement and position of the patient should be recorded.

Artifacts in Measurement

Artifacts in indirect measurement occur when the arm is large in relation to the cuff (Fig 3–2); when a patient has aortic incompetence, in which the indirectly measured diastolic pressure is usually falsely low; and when the patient is in shock. An erroneously low systolic pressure may be obtained in some hypertensive patients in whom the systolic pressure is not checked by palpation. An "auscultatory gap" may be present in such patients and in those with aortic stenosis and localized arteriosclerosis. The auscultatory gap is a range of pressures over which arterial sounds are absent even though arterial flow is present and the cuff pressure is not above the arterial pressure.

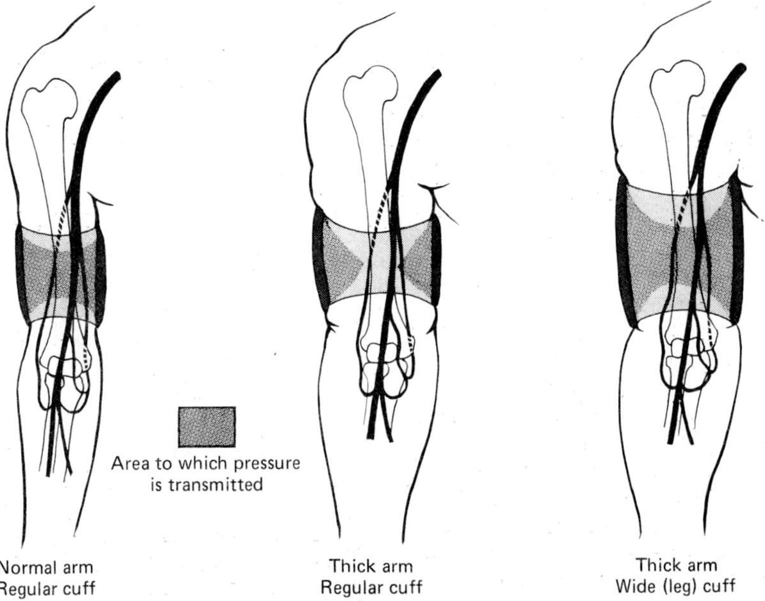

Figure 3–2. Diagram showing that pressure is not transmitted to the brachial artery when a regular cuff is used to measure blood pressure in a thick arm.

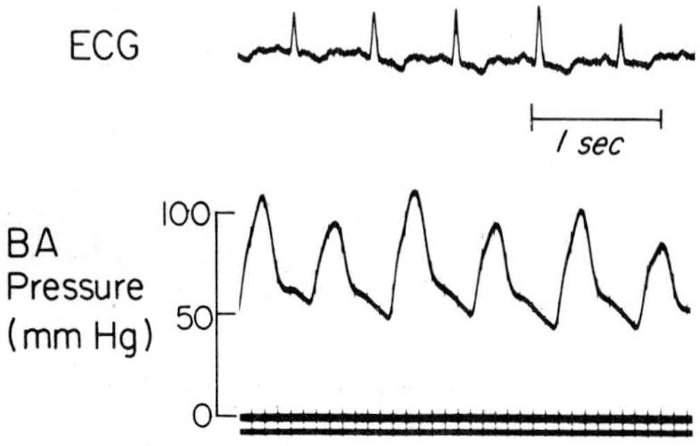

Figure 3–3. ECG and brachial arterial pulse pressure (BA) in a patient with pulsus alternans.

Blood Pressure in the Legs

The measurement of arterial pressure in both arms and both legs is advocated by some as a routine measure. If the leg pressure is to be measured, a special wide (20 cm) cuff is used; such a cuff is also needed for patients with thick or fat arms. The diagnosis of coarctation of the aorta is usually made on other grounds. In difficult cases, simultaneous brachial and femoral arterial tracings obtained during exercise may be needed.

Pulsus Alternans & Pulsus Paradoxus

Pulsus alternans and pulsus paradoxus should be sought when the blood pressure is measured. In pulsus alternans, every other heartbeat produces a higher systolic pressure. The mechanism is unknown although many theories have been proposed, and the finding, which is seen in left ventricular failure, carries a poor prognosis, especially if the heart rate is slow. Fig 3–3 shows an example of pulsus alternans in a brachial arterial pressure tracing in a patient with aortic stenosis.

Pulsus paradoxus is another incompletely understood phenomenon that is principally associated with pericardial disease in which cardiac filling is compromised. The abnormality shown in right and left ventricular pressure tracings in Fig 3–4 consists of an exaggeration of the normal respiratory fluctuation in systolic pressure. The arterial pressure (systolic, diastolic, and mean) normally falls by a few mm Hg when intrathoracic negative pressure increases during inspiration. If the systolic fall amounts to greater than 10 mm Hg (or more than 10% of the systolic pressure), pulsus paradoxus is present. The phenomenon can be due to an increase in the amplitude of intrathoracic pressure fluctuations resulting from changes in the mechanical properties of the lungs, as occurs in large pneumothorax, pleural effusion, or obstructive lung disease. It is more commonly due to decreased cardiac volume secondary to pericardial effusion, tamponade, or constriction. In this case, the reservoir of blood in the left heart is small, and when inspiration occurs, blood pools in the lungs, starving the left side of the heart of blood and causing a fall in cardiac output and arterial pressure.

EXAMINATION OF ORGANS & REGIONS OTHER THAN THE HEART

Examination of organs of the body other than the heart can provide important clues in the diagnosis of heart disease. Clinical findings and the symptoms and signs that may be noted on examination of various body structures are noted below.

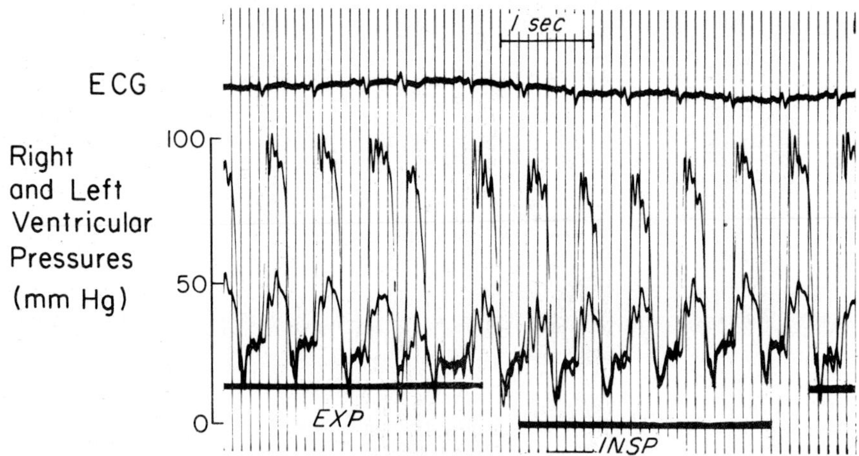

Figure 3–4. Pulsus paradoxus in right and left ventricular pressure tracings in a patient with constrictive pericarditis. EXP, expiration; INSP, inspiration.

EYES

Examination of the eyes may disclose petechial hemorrhages, which are evidence of embolism, or conjunctival pallor due to anemia. Examination of the ocular fundus is particularly important in patients with atherosclerotic vascular disease and especially in cases of hypertension. Direct visual examination of small arteries and arterioles in the fundus offers an important opportunity to assess the condition of the blood vessels, the retina, and the optic disk. The findings and their classification are discussed in Chapter 9. Hemorrhages and embolic phenomena (Roth spots) can also be seen in the retinas of patients with infective endocarditis.

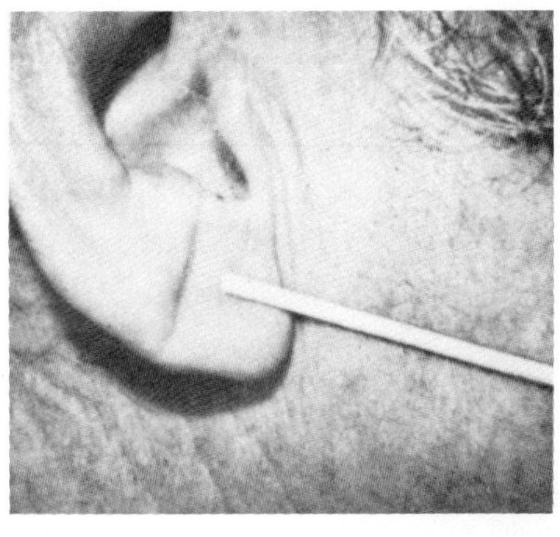

Figure 3–5. The earlobe sign—a deep crease in the lobular portion of the auricle. (Reproduced, with permission, from Frank ST: Aural sign of coronary-artery disease. N Engl J Med 289:327, 1973.)

MOUTH

The mucous membranes of the mouth and tongue can demonstrate reduced arterial oxygen saturation by their bluish color, but this physical sign is difficult to interpret and should always be checked by measuring arterial oxygen levels.

EARS

Inspection of the earlobe may reveal a deep crease in the lobe of the ear at the site shown in Fig 3–5. Ear

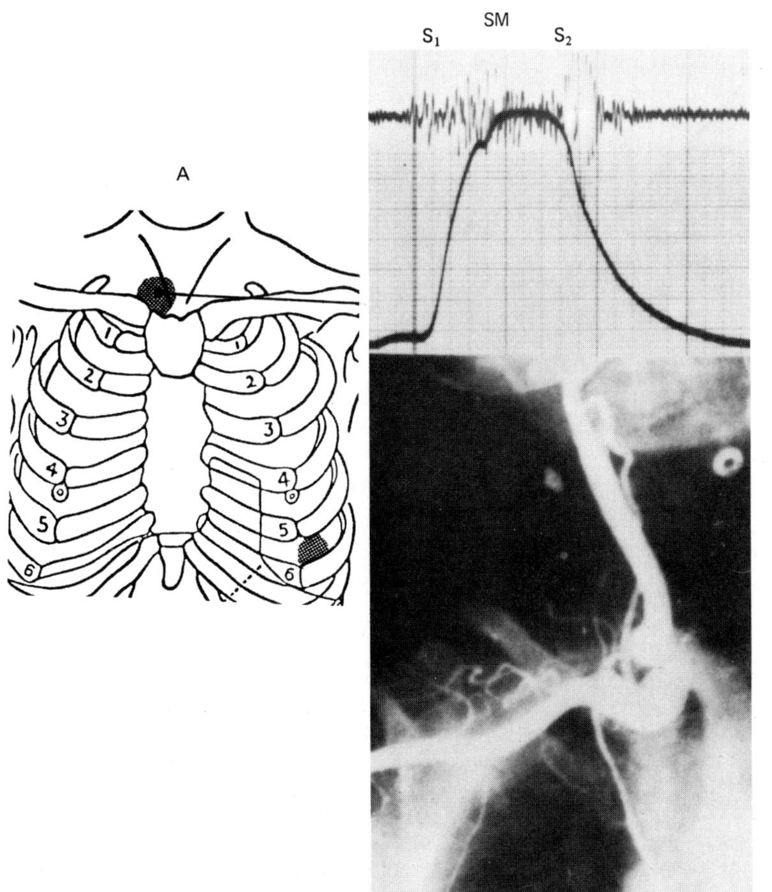

Figure 3–6. The chest wall diagram *(A)* shows 2 areas of heaving pulsation, marked by heavy shading. One, in the left fifth intercostal space, was caused by the apical thrust of a hypertrophic left ventricle. The other pulsating area is situated above the sternal end of the right clavicle. A graph of this pulsation is shown in *B.* It rises about 0.03 sec after the onset of S_1 and apparently represents an arterial pulse. Arteriography *(C)* reveals tortuosity and dilatation of the proximal portions of the right subclavian and common carotid arteries. A phonocardiogram taken from the pulsating swelling *(B)* shows a pansystolic murmur (SM). From a 50-year-old woman with hypertensive heart disease who had developed a pulsating swelling at the neck caused by kinked cervical arteries. (Reproduced, with permission, from Dressler W: *Clinical Aids in Cardiac Diagnosis.* Grune & Stratton, 1970.)

creases are associated with age and are present in most people over age 60. However, their occurrence in younger people is associated with a high incidence of premature atherosclerotic changes involving the cerebral, coronary, or aortoiliac vessels.

NECK

The venous pulse and pressure, the nature of the carotid pulse, and the presence of a goiter are sought in the examination of the neck. Accentuated pulsations of the carotid arteries are seen in coarctation of the aorta and aortic incompetence. In aortic stenosis, the carotid pulse is slow-rising and of small amplitude. Marked pulsation in the base of the neck on the right side is seen in elderly atherosclerotic people. It is due to kinking of the right carotid artery (Fig 3–6) resulting from dilatation of the aortic arch, which makes the aorta take a higher course in the mediastinum. This benign condition is more common in women.

Venous Pulse & Venous Pressure

The level of the venous pressure and the nature of the venous pulse are perhaps the most important observations to be made in the examination of the neck. The internal jugular vein should be examined because it lies deep to the sternocleidomastoid muscle and is in free communication with the right atrium. The external jugular vein is often easier to see, but it may be constricted as it passes through the fascial planes of the neck and may give an inaccurate assessment of venous events. The positioning of the patient is most important in examining the veins in the neck. The angle at which the patient is supported in the bed should be adjusted to bring the meniscus of blood in the vein to a level between the clavicles and the angle of the jaw (Fig 3–7). The higher the venous pressure, the more

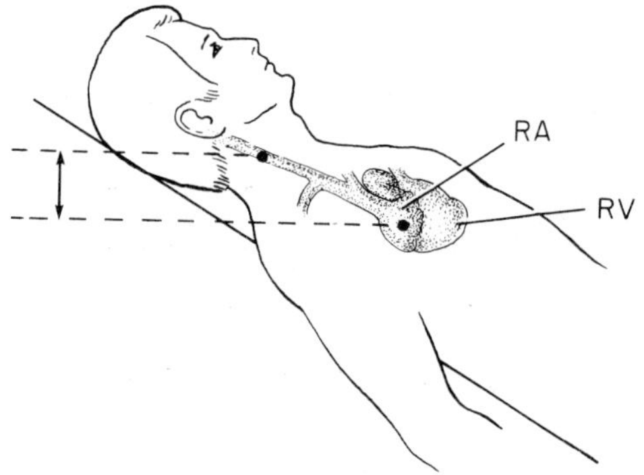

Figure 3–7. Examination of jugular venous pulse and estimation of venous pressure. RA, right atrium; RV, right ventricle.

erect the patient should be; patients with severe venous congestion may have to stand up and breathe in deeply in order to bring the level of the meniscus into view. The head should be comfortably supported in order to relax the neck muscles. Any movement of the earlobes should be noted, because this is always due to venous rather than arterial pulsation. Timing of the venous waves against the carotid pulse is carried out by feeling the artery on the opposite side of the neck or by listening to the heart, and not by feeling the radial pulse. Interpretation of the pulse wave pattern is sometimes facilitated by observing when the venous pressure falls. The first venous trough, the x descent, coincides with the carotid arterial pulse. Distinguishing arterial from venous pulses in the neck can be difficult. Venous pulses can be palpable; they are diffusely expansile and influenced by respiration.

Some authorities advocate exerting pressure over the abdomen to distend the neck veins—the results of which are shown in Fig 3–8. They maintain that the magnitude of the resulting venous distention (hepatojugular reflux) reflects the level of venous congestion.

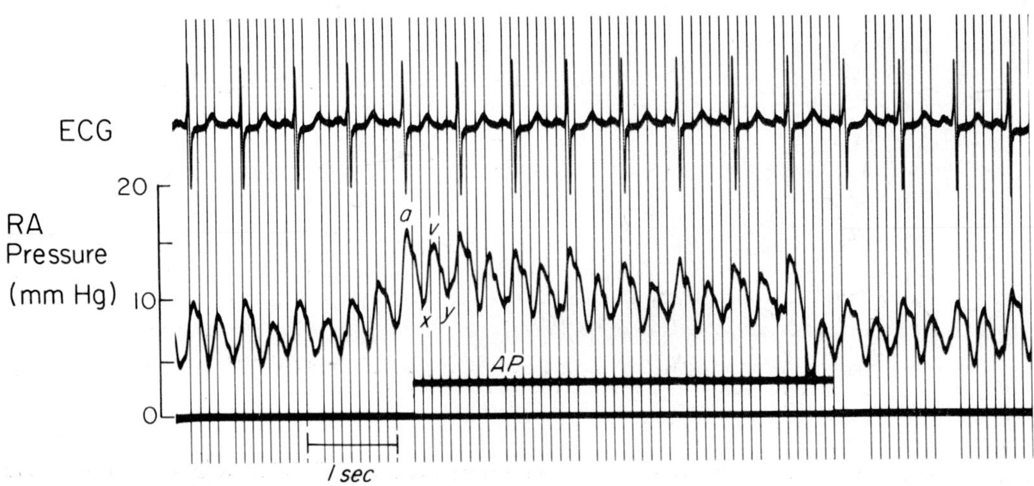

Figure 3–8. ECG and right atrial (RA) pressure in a normal subject showing the response to external abdominal compression (AP).

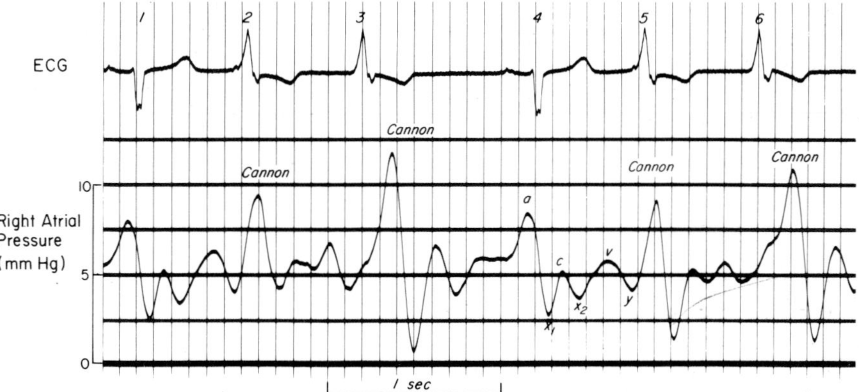

Figure 3–9. Right atrial pressure tracing in a patient with junctional ectopic beats. Beats 1 and 4 are sinus beats and produce normal venous pressure pulses. The other beats are junctional and give rise to cannon waves of varying sizes.

We believe that hepatojugular reflux can be seen in normal subjects and that proper positioning of the patient, relaxation with the mouth open, and quiet normal breathing are more important factors in evaluating venous pressure.

Direct bedside assessment of right atrial pressure requires skill and practice, but it can obviate the need for central venous pressure measurement, which requires use of a catheter. The level of the venous pressure is most important in distinguishing cardiac failure with edema and ascites from hepatic or renal disease with similar findings. Unfortunately, it is often in those patients with highest venous pressures that the examiner fails to note the raised pressure.

Normal Venous Pulse

The normal waves seen in the venous pulse in the neck are shown in the first and fourth beats in the tracing in Fig 3–9. The positive waves are *a, c,* and *v,* and the troughs are x_1, x_2, and *y*. The *a* wave is due to atrial contraction. It follows the P wave of the ECG and is absent in atrial fibrillation. The origin of the *c* wave is more controversial. It was originally noted in tracings of the venous pressure in the neck and attributed to the effects of carotid arterial pulsation. When it was also observed in right atrial pressure tracings, however, this explanation became untenable. It is now thought to be due to bulging of the tricuspid valve back into the atrium at the start of ventricular systole. The *v* wave is associated with atrial filling; pressure in the atrium rises to the *v* peak and falls as the tricuspid valve opens and the atrium empties into the ventricle. The x_1 and x_2 troughs are attributed to descent of the base of the heart during ventricular systole. The backward bulging of the valve interrupts this process to produce the *c* wave. The *c* wave is not always seen.

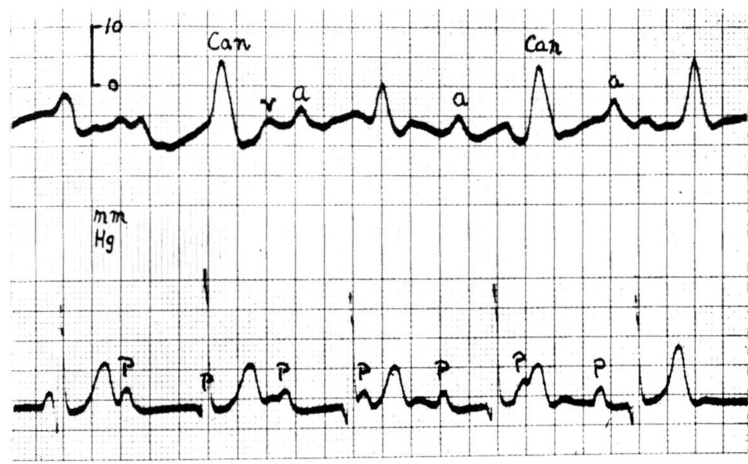

Figure 3–10. Irregular cannon waves in the central venous pulse in a case of complete heart block. Cannons (Can) are seen whenever P falls between Q and the peak of T on the ECG. (Reproduced, with permission, from Wood P: *Diseases of the Heart and Circulation,* 3rd ed. Lippincott, 1968.)

When it is absent, there is a single *x* descent. The *y* descent to the *y* trough is due to atrial emptying, and its rate is influenced by stenosis or insufficiency of the atrioventricular valve.

Abnormal or Exaggerated Waves

(1) Cannon waves: The magnitude of the *a* wave resulting from atrial contraction varies with the P–R interval. In the tracing shown in Fig 3–9, all but beats 1 and 4 are ectopic, with the P wave occurring at the start of the QRS complex. The *a* waves associated with these beats are larger and are referred to as *cannon waves* because of their explosive appearance when seen in the neck. The largest cannon waves are seen when atrial contraction occurs at a time when the tricuspid valve is closed, as in beats 3 and 6 in the tracing. Here the P wave is buried in the QRS complex, and large cannon waves can be seen. Irregular cannon waves of this type are also seen in complete heart block with atrioventricular dissociation (Fig 3–10). Regular cannon waves are seen in junctional tachycardia and in atrial tachycardia with rapid rates and a long P–R interval, as shown in Fig 3–11.

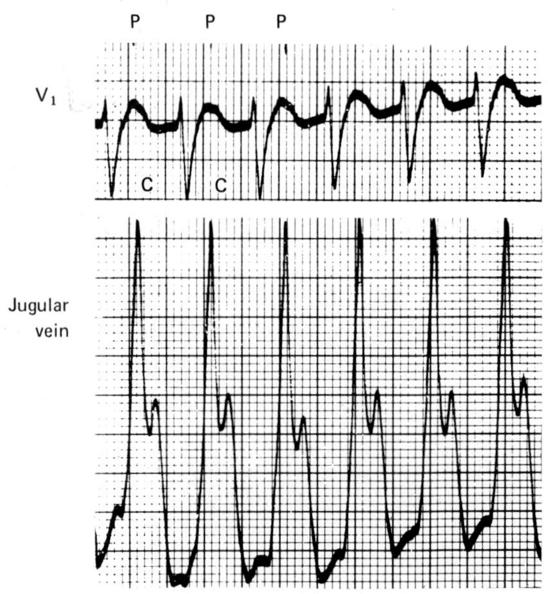

Figure 3–11. From a patient with rheumatic mitral stenosis who suffered attacks of paroxysmal atrial tachycardia. During such attacks, cannon waves were palpable over both the jugular veins and liver. The ECG (top) presents an atrial tachycardia at a rate of 154/min. The P waves fall on the preceding ventricular complexes and produce cannon waves (C). (Reproduced, with permission, from Dressler W: *Clinical Aids in Cardiac Diagnosis.* Grune & Stratton, 1970.)

(2) Giant *a* wave: The *a* wave is increased in force and amplitude in the presence of right ventricular hypertrophy. It is best seen as the "giant *a* wave" of pulmonary stenosis, shown in Fig 3–12, which is a short, sharp, flicking wave occurring just before ventricular systole. A large *a* wave is also seen in pulmonary hypertension and in tricuspid valve disease with stenosis.

(3) Giant *v* wave: A large *v* wave is seen in patients with tricuspid incompetence, especially when atrial fibrillation is present, as in the tracing in Fig 3–13. Tricuspid incompetence is seldom seen in patients with sinus rhythm, but when it occurs, *a, x, v,* and *y* peaks and troughs are present. The *x* descent is usually absent in patients with either tricuspid incompetence or constrictive pericarditis, and the *y* descent may be the principal event in the venous pulse.

(4) Effect of inspiration: Inspiration may stretch the tricuspid valve and increase the height of the *v* wave and the depth of the *y* trough, as shown in Fig 3–13. Inspiration also increases the height of the *a* wave and enhances the *x* descent, as shown in Fig 3–14 in a patient in sinus rhythm. The tracing superficially resembles that seen in Fig 3–13, but the timing of the peaks and troughs is different. The tracings

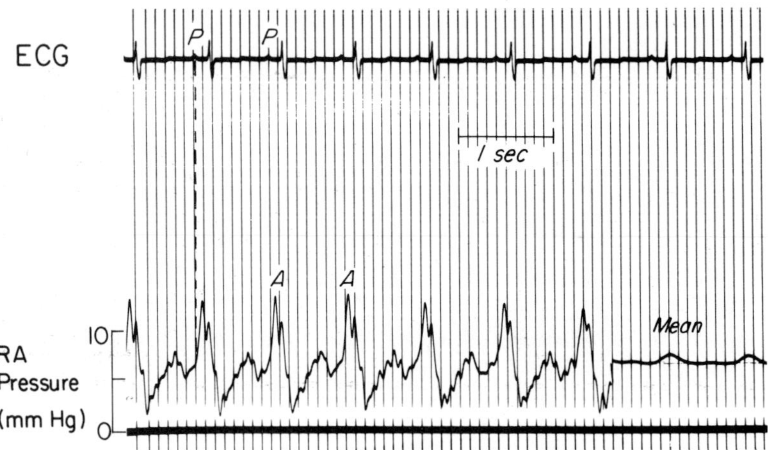

Figure 3–12. Right atrial (RA) pressure tracing showing giant *a* wave (A) in a patient with severe pulmonary stenosis. The *a* wave follows the P wave of the ECG.

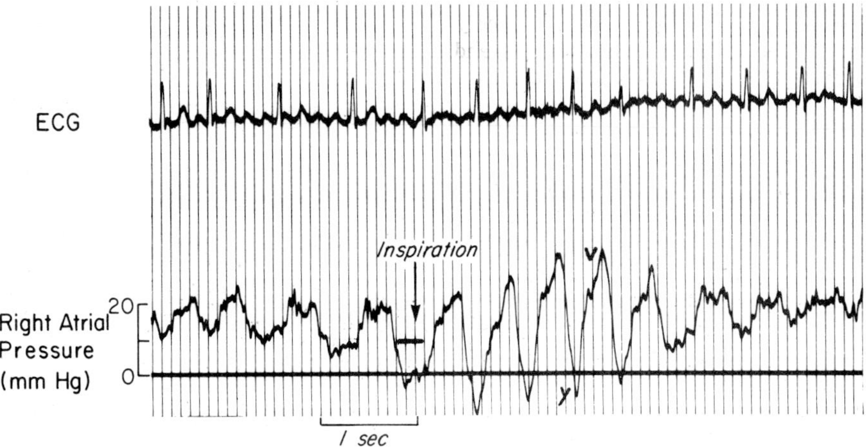

Figure 3–13. Right atrial (RA) pressure tracing in a patient with tricuspid incompetence and atrial fibrillation. The *v* peak and the *y* trough are exaggerated during inspiration.

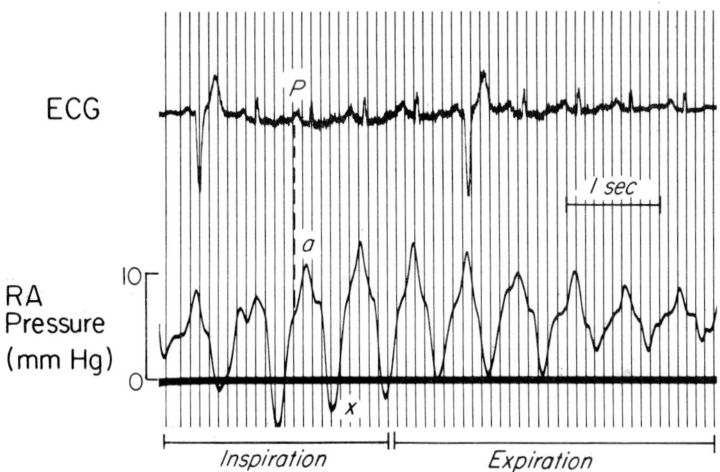

Figure 3–14. Right atrial (RA) pressure tracing showing increase in *a* wave and *x* descent with inspiration.

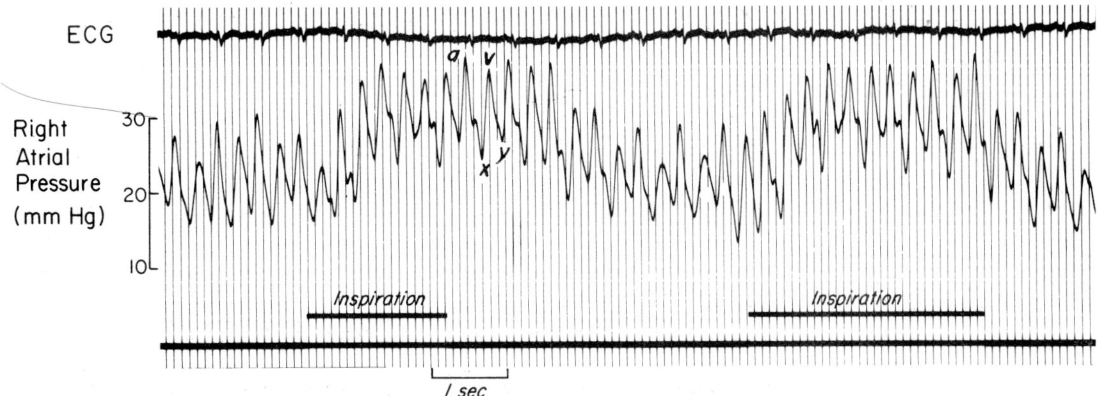

Figure 3–15. ECG and right atrial pressure (RA) tracings in a patient with constrictive pericarditis showing inspiratory increase in pressure (Kussmaul's sign).

point out the importance of accurate timing of events associated with cardiac contraction. When right heart filling is severely impaired, inspiration causes a rise in venous pressure, as shown in Fig 3–15. This is seen in constrictive pericarditis, cardiac tamponade, and severe right heart failure. In tricuspid incompetence, it is the amplitude of the pulsations that tends to increase (as in Fig 3–13), rather than the mean pressure, as in pericardial disease (Fig 3–15).

ARMS

Brachial and radial pulses should be compared between the 2 arms, and they should also be compared with the femoral pulses. The fingers, nails, and palms should be examined for evidence of embolism.

FINGERS

Clubbing of the fingers and nail beds (Fig 3–16) is seen in cyanotic congenital heart disease, in infective endocarditis, and in chronic lung disease, especially with cor pulmonale. Splinter hemorrhages in the nail beds should be sought as an indication of endocarditis, although it should be noted that similar findings may be seen in many normal people. Painful red, tender nodules in the pulp of the fingers or toes or on the palms or the soles are important evidence of embolism in infective endocarditis. They last for 4–5 days and gradually darken before fading and becoming painless. Such lesions seldom, if ever, suppurate. Other finger abnormalities associated with congenital heart disease include arachnodactyly, in which the fingers are long and spidery. This is seen in Marfan's syndrome and in some patients with atrial septal defect.

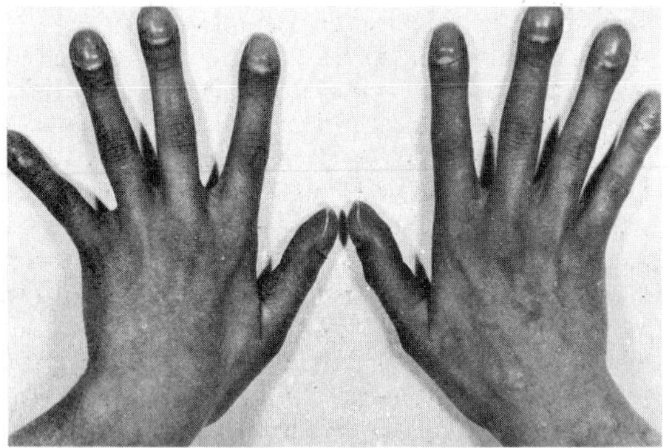

Figure 3–16. Clubbing of the fingers in a patient with congenital heart disease.

LUNGS

Examination of the lungs in patients with heart disease focuses on the detection of pleural fluid and a search for rales and crepitations, especially at the base of the lungs posteriorly. Such findings reflect raised pulmonary venous pressure. Added sounds are noted when there is fluid in the alveoli, but the signs are not specific, and they may be absent in some cases of obvious pulmonary edema. They are often due to other causes. Pleural effusion due to heart failure is usually bilateral; in unilateral cases, it is commoner on the side on which the subject habitually lies. Evidence of collapse of the left lower lobe should be sought in patients with marked left atrial enlargement.

BACK

Some cardiac murmurs are heard well in the back. The best examples are the murmurs of coarctation of the aorta, increased bronchial collateral flow, and peripheral pulmonary artery stenosis; the last is often heard well in the axilla as well. Evidence of systemic collateral vessels in coarctation of the aorta is also well seen and felt in the back. Large, pulsating vessels can be detected near the angles of the scapulas. Edema of the lumbar region and sacrum is also sought while the physician examines the patient's back.

ABDOMEN

In examining the abdomen, enlargement and tenderness of the liver and spleen should be sought as evidence of systemic venous congestion. The spleen may also be the site of a friction rub in infective endocarditis. Ascites and pitting edema of the ankles are also sought as evidence of congestive heart failure. Disproportionate ascites with minimal leg edema suggests constrictive pericarditis or prolonged diuretic therapy.

LOWER EXTREMITIES

In examining the lower extremities the physician palpates the femoral pulse; if its palpability is in question or if the patient is hypertensive, it is useful to look for delay between the radial and femoral pulse (see p 341). Absence of femoral pulsations and inequality between the 2 sides may suggest embolic disease or aortic dissection. Calf tenderness and pain on dorsiflexion of the foot (Homans' sign) are evidence of venous thrombosis. Clubbing of the toes is seen in cyanotic congenital heart disease, and differential cyanosis of the legs with clubbing, in the absence of similar findings in the arms, suggests patent ductus arteriosus with shunt reversal due to pulmonary hypertension. In addition to looking for edema of the sacrum, the examiner should check for edema in the flanks and medial aspects of the thighs in bedridden patients.

URINE

Examination of the urine is an important adjunct to the physical examination. Proteinuria should be sought in heart failure, in hypertensive patients, and in primary renal disease. Hematuria suggests renal infarction; if microscopic, infective endocarditis. Specific gravity should be recorded and the urinary sediment examined for casts and other abnormalities.

EXAMINATION OF THE HEART

INSPECTION

Examination of the chest starts with inspection of the shape and movements of the thorax and a search for visible pulsations. Chest deformities such as kyphosis and scoliosis may cause heart disease, but in general it is remarkable how a severe deformity can exist without causing cardiac embarrassment. Depressed sternum with pectus excavatum is obvious on inspection, and although it is often associated with benign heart murmurs, it is seldom of more than cosmetic importance. The left parasternal area sometimes bulges in patients who have had heart disease since early in life. Ventricular septal defect is the commonest lesion causing this sign.

Visible Pulsations

The cardiac impulse can sometimes be seen in normal subjects either in the area of the left nipple or in the epigastrium. Pulsation in the second or third left interspace over the right ventricular outflow tract can be seen in normal thin persons, but it can also suggest pulmonary hypertension or increased pulmonary blood flow. Pulsation to the right of the sternum is always abnormal, and, when seen in the second or third interspace, it indicates aneurysmal dilatation of the ascending aorta.

Periodic Breathing

Abnormalities of respiratory rhythm should be noted during inspection of the chest. The commonest abnormality is periodic breathing. This can occur in normal subjects at high altitude and may also be seen after head injuries. When it is due to heart disease, the cycle of hyperventilation followed by hypoventilation and apnea with subsequent gradual increase of ventilation lasts 40–120 seconds. The phenomenon results from oscillation of the feedback control mechanisms regulating respiration. In a patient with severe ventricular failure, there is an abnormal lag between the timing of the neurologic stimulus to breathe and the arrival back at the control center in the brain of the humoral signal resulting from respiratory changes in blood gases following the breath. This lag is thought to play an important part in the mechanism of periodic breathing. Periodic breathing is usually referred to as Cheyne-Stokes breathing. In the classic description, apnea was present, but this feature is not necessarily a component. The length of the lung-to-brain circulation time determines the length of the period of one cycle. By following this measurement, the examiner can note the progress of the patient's left ventricular failure. Periodic breathing is usually a manifestation of hyper- rather than hypoventilation and is generally abolished by giving oxygen, CO_2, or aminophylline. It tends to occur at night when sensory input is low and to disappear when a mouthpiece and nose clip are used to obtain spirometric tracings. In the example shown in Fig 3–17 from a patient with left ventricular failure, apnea was not present. The level of ventilation can be deduced from the CO_2 level in the expired air; it is lowest when end-tidal CO_2 is highest and vice versa. The respiratory rate varied during the cycle, which lasted about 45 sec. Arterial oxygen saturation is out of phase with ventilation; arterial pressure tends to fall when ventilation is low and tends to rise with hyperpnea.

PALPATION

Palpation of the chest is used to confirm the presence of pulsations that have been noted on inspection. The cardiac impulse is routinely sought and can be elicited by having the patient roll over to the left side. The examiner should note the nature of the impulse and distinguish between the feel of a large left ventricle and a right ventricle. The site where the impulse is felt is of primary importance in distinguishing the 2 impulses; in addition, the right ventricular impulse is more lifting than the left, is perceived as being farther from the hand, and less readily moves the examining fingers. The feel of a ventricle with a large stroke volume should be distinguished from the feel of a hypertrophied ventricle. Hypertrophy imparts a forceful thrust with relatively little movement of the examiner's hand, whereas increased stroke volume gives a more dynamic movement of greater amplitude. A "tapping" impulse is found in patients with mitral valve disease. This reflects the palpable vibrations of a loud first heart sound felt at the apex.

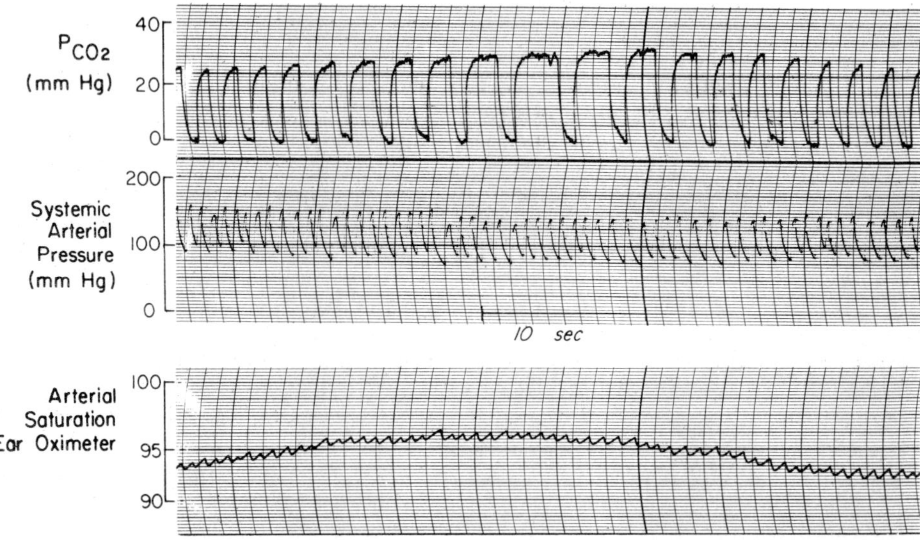

Figure 3–17. Periodic breathing in a patient with left ventricular failure.

Apex Beat

The position of the apex beat should always be located by palpation. It is the point farthest downward and outward at which the cardiac impulse can be clearly felt. Before the determination of cardiac size by chest radiography became routine, the position of the apex beat in the absence of lung disease was the most important measure of heart size. Its position should be described in relation to the intercostal space and to the distance from the midline, the nipple, or the mid-clavicular, anterior axillary, or midaxillary lines. These are imaginary lines drawn vertically through various planes, as shown in Fig 3–18. Palpation of the base of the heart may detect an impulse caused by closure of the aortic or pulmonary valves or arising from an aneurysm. The findings should be interpreted in light of the patient's build.

Thrills

The significance of palpable thrills is similar to that of cardiac murmurs and is discussed below (see Auscultation). Thrills are merely palpable, sustained high-frequency vibrations associated with the same disturbances of flow that cause heart murmurs. A murmur that is associated with a thrill is likely to have an organic cause.

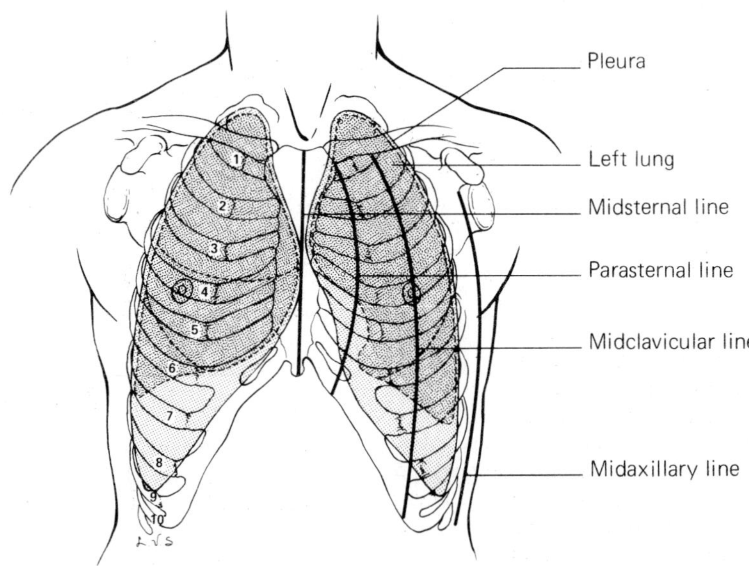

Figure 3–18. The thorax, showing rib cage, pleura, and lung fields. (Reproduced, with permission, from Dunphy JE, Way LW [editors]: *Current Surgical Diagnosis & Treatment,* 3rd ed. Lange, 1977.)

Palpable Impulses

Palpable impulses over the precordium must be interpreted in light of their associated findings; it is not always possible to be certain of their origin. In a patient with mitral incompetence, a substernal impulse may be due to systolic expansion of the left atrium rather than to right ventricular overactivity. It is also difficult to interpret epigastric pulsations. They may arise from the abdominal aorta or the right ventricle or be transmitted from the right atrium to an enlarged liver in tricuspid incompetence.

Paradoxic rocking impulses can sometimes be felt after myocardial infarction, especially when a left ventricular aneurysm is present. When the aneurysm involves the free ventricular wall, the outward motion of the aneurysmal sac can sometimes be felt in early systole.

Palpable Gallops

The vibrations produced by loud third and fourth heart sounds can often be felt. If the sounds are of very low pitch, the gallop may be easier to appreciate on palpation than on auscultation. In most cases in which a gallop is palpable, it is also audible.

PERCUSSION

Percussion of the heart has virtually no place in physical examination today because it is open to error and because the size of the heart is better determined by chest radiography. Before this method was routinely available, some confirmation of the estimate of heart size obtained by palpation was sought by percussion. Dullness to the right of the sternum was held to be evidence of pericardial effusion, and percussion of the left border was routinely advocated. Radiography has indicated that findings obtained by percussing the heart tend to be unreliable in all but the most skilled hands.

AUSCULTATION

Technic

Auscultation of the heart is performed with a properly fitting stethoscope that uses either an open bell or a closed diaphragm as the means of coupling the examiner's ear to the patient's chest. The diaphragm transmits more sound and is better for listening to high-pitched sounds (such as the second heart sound) and murmurs. The bell is better for low-pitched noises, and variation of the pressure of the bell on the skin can be used to alter the intensity of the sounds and murmurs heard. Auscultation focuses more on the timing of events within the cardiac cycle than on their intensity or the site at which they are heard best. Experienced physicians move the chest piece of the stethoscope to sites where they can best hear specific sounds. They do not restrict their examination to the classic "valvular" areas described in older textbooks. They also do not draw conclusions about the origin of events from the site at which they hear sounds and murmurs. The information obtained by auscultation must be integrated with that already obtained by inspection and palpation.

Heart Sounds

The timing of the different heart sounds is diagrammatically shown in Fig 3–19. First and second heart sounds are normally audible, and an early (diastolic gallop) third sound is often present in children and young adults. In addition, a fourth (atrial) sound can sometimes be recorded by phonocardiography.

A. First Heart Sound: The first heart sound (S_1) is attributed to closure of the mitral and tricuspid valves at the start of ventricular systole. The 2 components can sometimes be clearly distinguished, and although the right atrial and right ventricular contractions precede those of the left, the mitral valve closes before the tricuspid, and the first component of the first heart sound is mitral in origin. The position of the valve leaflets at the time of the start of systole influences the loudness of the first sound. In general, the first heart sound is louder, longer, and lower pitched than the second heart sound at the apex. In normal resting subjects, the atrioventricular valve leaflets have drifted into an almost closed position by the time

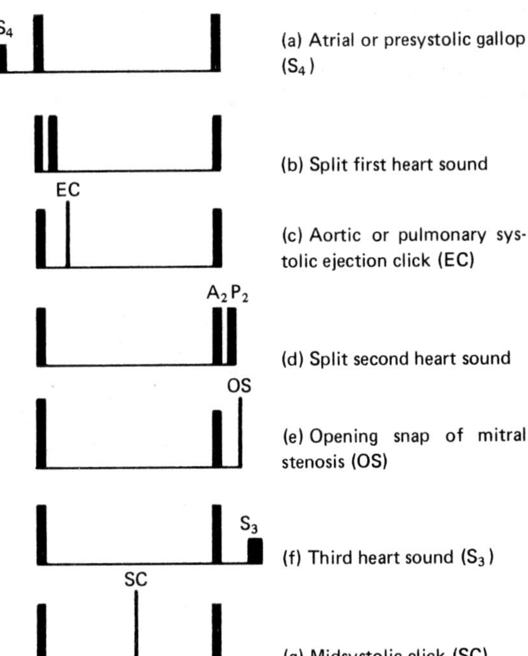

Figure 3–19. Timing of the different heart sounds and added sounds. (Reproduced in modified form, with permission, from Wood P: *Diseases of the Heart and Circulation,* 3rd ed. Lippincott, 1968.)

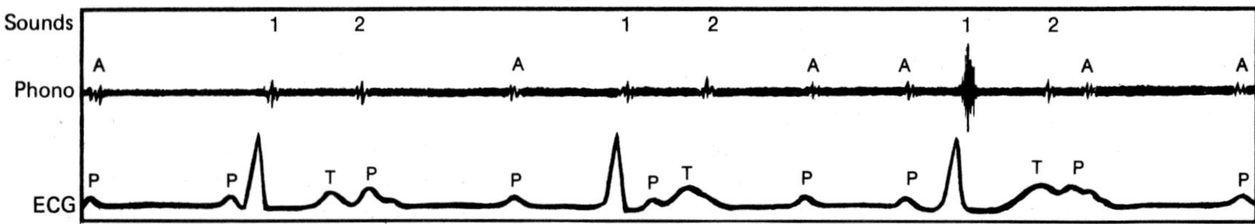

Figure 3–20. Phonocardiogram and ECG showing intensity of first sound varying with position of P wave on the ECG and atrial sound in complete heart block. (Courtesy of Roche Laboratories Division of Hoffman-La Roche, Inc.)

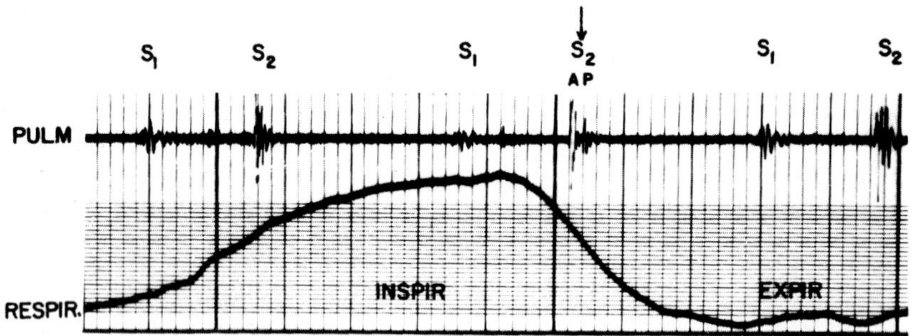

Figure 3–21. Phonocardiogram taken from the pulmonary area in a healthy 28-year-old man. It shows that splitting of the second sound becomes distinct after inspiration. The curve of respiration moves upward during inspiration. (Reproduced, with permission, from Dressler W: *Clinical Aids in Cardiac Diagnosis.* Grune & Stratton, 1970.)

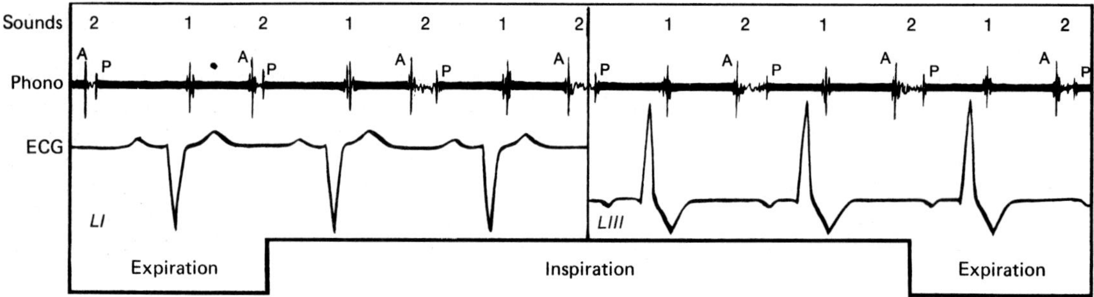

Figure 3–22. Phonocardiogram showing widely split second sound in right bundle branch block with P_2 even later on inspiration. (Courtesy of Roche Laboratories Division of Hoffman-La Roche, Inc.)

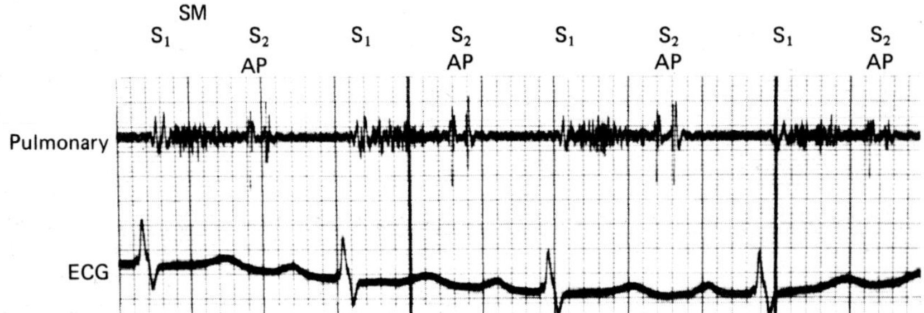

Figure 3–23. Phonocardiogram from the pulmonary area in a patient with ostium secundum atrial septal defect showing wide splitting of the second heart sound which remained constant although normal breathing was not interrupted while the phonocardiogram was obtained. (Reproduced, with permission, from Dressler W: *Clinical Aids in Cardiac Diagnosis.* Grune & Stratton, 1970.)

systole starts, because diastolic flow is more or less complete by late diastole. Atrial contraction tends to reopen the valves. Consequently, the length of the P–R interval affects the loudness of the first sound. When flow across an atrioventricular valve is increased for any reason or lasts longer than normally, the valve tends to shut from a more open position and produces more noise. The situation is similar to that encountered in closing an open door: the wider the door stands open before it is slammed shut, the louder the resulting noise. Thus, a loud first sound is heard in patients who are exercising, in patients with mitral stenosis in whom flow lasts throughout the whole of diastole, and in patients with left-to-right shunts and increased atrioventricular flow, eg, atrial septal defect. In complete heart block in which the P–R interval varies, the loudness of the first sound varies, being loudest when the P–R interval is slightly shortened to about 0.1 sec, as shown in Fig 3–20.

B. Second Heart Sound: The second heart sound (S_2) is due to closure of the semilunar valves and normally consists of 2 components (Fig 3–21). The earlier component is normally aortic in origin; the later one arises from the pulmonary valve (P_2). The location at which the second heart sound is best heard varies. It is normally heard well at the base and is almost always louder than the first sound in that area. It is sometimes necessary to listen at the apex or even in the epigastrium.

1. Splitting of the second heart sound—Right and left ventricular stroke volumes vary reciprocally with quiet respiration when there is adequate venous return. Inspiration favors right ventricular output, and expiration favors left ventricular output. Thus, in normal subjects resting quietly and breathing easily, the time of pulmonary valve closure with inspiration can be shown to move later in the cardiac cycle by 0.02–0.04 sec, as seen in Fig 3–22. Increased filling of the right heart is associated with a more negative pressure within the thorax during inspiration, which increases right ventricular output in accordance with the Frank-Starling mechanism. The extra output has a longer ejection time; consequently, the pulmonary valve closure sound is delayed. The opposite occurs with aortic valve closure during expiration, but the magnitude of the changes is less. Thus, although both the aortic and pulmonary components of the second heart sound move, the pulmonary component moves more. The net effect is that the interval between the 2 components of the second sound increases with inspiration and then decreases until the interval between the 2 sounds is not appreciable during expiration. The process is conventionally referred to as *physiologic splitting of the second heart sound.* When right ventricular systole is prolonged because of right bundle branch block, pulmonary valve closure is delayed. In this case, both the first and the second heart sounds tend to be split throughout the cardiac cycle, with the split widening further with inspiration (Fig 3–22). When right ventricular stroke volume is increased and venous return is high, as in atrial septal defect with large pulmonary blood flow, respiration has relatively little effect on right ventricular output. In this case, pulmonary valve closure is greatly delayed and the second sound is widely split; respiration has no effect, and the split is "fixed" even during expiration (Fig 3–23). Splitting of the second heart sound is almost always found in atrial septal defect with left-to-right shunt, but the finding of a *fixed* split is indicative of a significant left-to-right shunt. If the venous return is reduced when the patient stands up, the splitting of the second sound will become more normal, becoming either movable with respiration or less widely split.

2. Paradoxic splitting of the second sound—When left ventricular contraction is prolonged (eg, poor contractility, aortic stenosis), aortic valve closure is delayed and occurs after pulmonary closure. Aortic valve closure can be identified by timing it against the dicrotic notch of the carotid artery tracing (Fig 3–24). In paradoxic splitting, aortic and pulmonary valve clo-

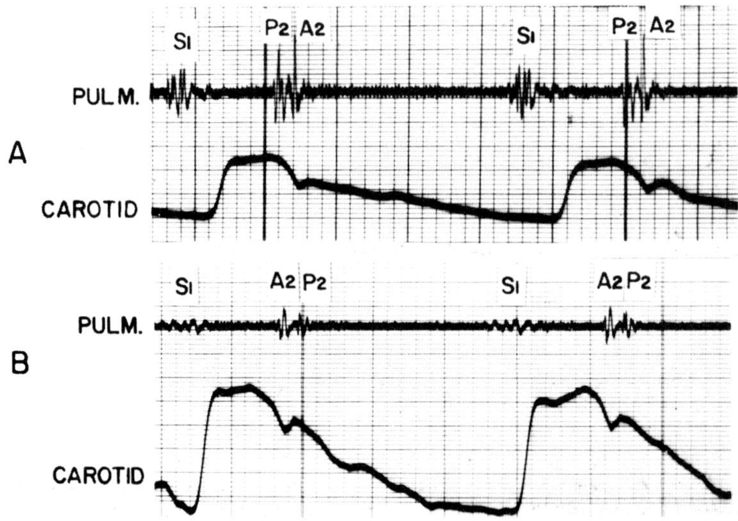

Figure 3–24. Paradoxic splitting of S_2 in a 55-year-old patient with Stokes-Adams syndrome with artificial pacing. *A:* The electrical pacemaker is in the right ventricle. The phonocardiogram shows splitting of the second sound. Comparison with the carotid pulse shows that the aortic element, which occurs 0.03 sec prior to the dicrotic notch, follows the pulmonary component. *B:* The electric pacemaker is in the left ventricle. The aortic element now precedes the pulmonary component of the second sound. (Reproduced, with permission, from Dressler W: *Clinical Aids in Cardiac Diagnosis.* Grune & Stratton, 1970.)

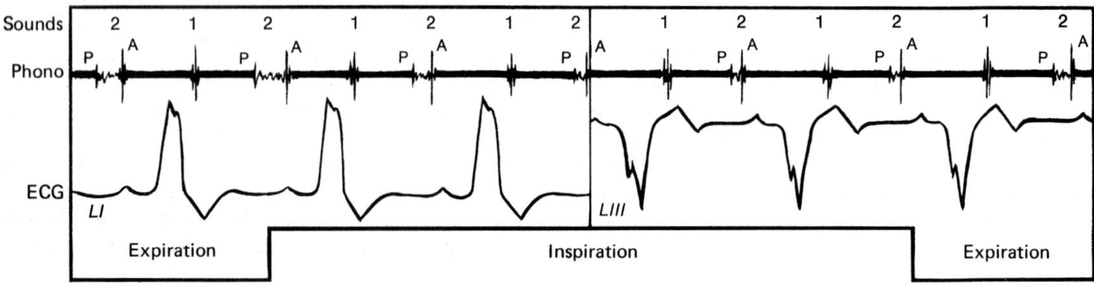

Figure 3–25. Phonocardiogram showing paradoxic splitting (split on expiration, closed on inspiration) in left bundle branch block. (Courtesy of Roche Laboratories Division of Hoffman-La Roche, Inc.)

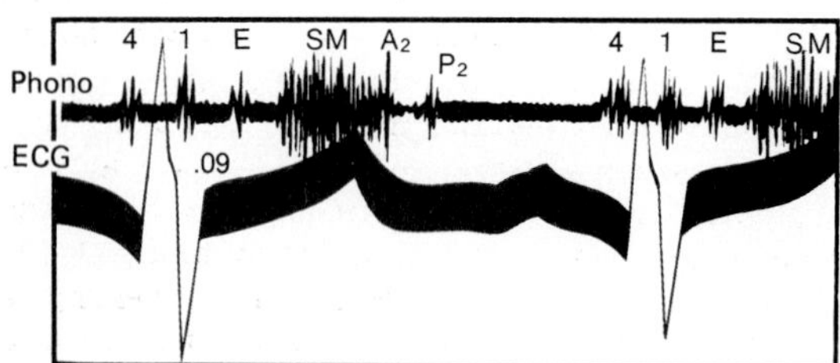

Figure 3–26. Phonocardiogram from a patient with pulmonary stenosis showing the typical presystolic gallop (4), ejection click (E), systolic murmur (SM), and delayed pulmonary valve closure sound (P_2). Recorded at left sternal border. (Courtesy of Roche Laboratories Division of Hoffman-La Roche, Inc.)

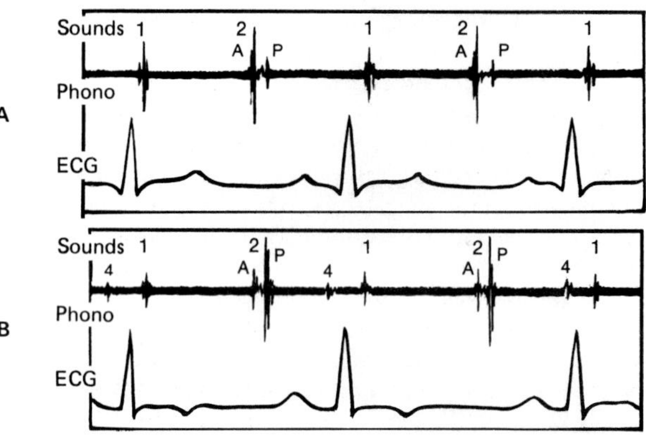

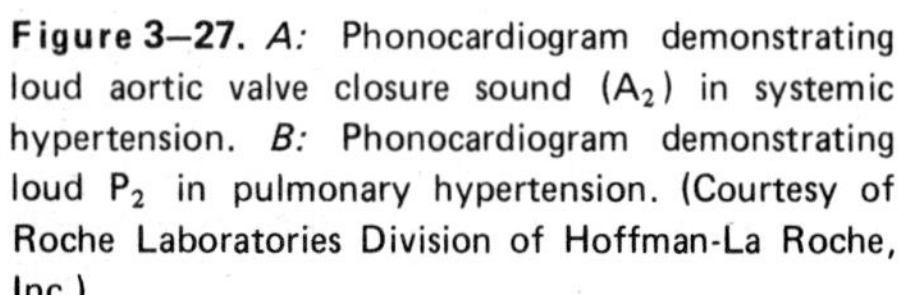

Figure 3–27. *A:* Phonocardiogram demonstrating loud aortic valve closure sound (A_2) in systemic hypertension. *B:* Phonocardiogram demonstrating loud P_2 in pulmonary hypertension. (Courtesy of Roche Laboratories Division of Hoffman-La Roche, Inc.)

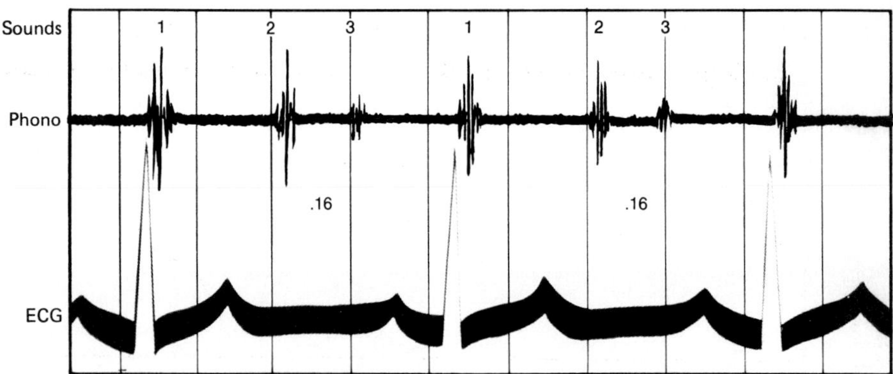

Figure 3–28. Phonocardiogram showing typical third heart sound (S_3). It follows the second sound (S_2) by 0.16 sec. (Courtesy of Roche Laboratories Division of Hoffman-La Roche, Inc.)

sure sounds coincide toward the end of inspiration, and splitting is greatest during expiration. This is also referred to as "reversed" splitting of the second sound and is found in patients with left bundle branch block, in aortic stenosis, and in any other condition that greatly overloads the left ventricle. The effect of respiration on the second heart sound in paradoxic splitting is shown in Fig 3–25. Aortic valve closure tends to be delayed and diminished in aortic stenosis and may be absent when the lesion is severe.

3. **Intensity**–The second heart sound is also important in patients with pulmonary stenosis. Here the timing and intensity of the sound vary with the severity of the stenosis. In mild cases, the second sound is normal. In cases with more severe stenosis, the second sound is delayed and diminished because pulmonary blood flow is less (Fig 3–26). Thus, in severe cases the sound of pulmonary valve closure is inaudible. However, it can usually be detected by phonocardiography and is shown to occur up to 0.12 sec after aortic valve closure. The loudness of each component of the second sound varies with the pressure in the corresponding vessel. Thus, a loud pulmonary valve closure sound is heard in pulmonary hypertension and a loud aortic second sound in systemic hypertension (Fig 3–27). Loudness of the components of the second sound is not an accurate indicator of pressure, which should be directly measured in doubtful cases. The character of the aortic valve closure sound is altered in patients with aortic disease. In patients with syphilitic aortitis and other diseases that dilate the root of the aorta, aortic valve closure has a high-pitched, drumlike, "tambour" quality. The reason for this is not known. In systemic hypertension, the aortic valve closure sound is not only loud but also clear and ringing.

C. **Third Heart Sound**: The third heart sound (S_3) shown in Fig 3–28 is associated with ventricular filling. It is not clear why it is normally present in young persons and disappears with age. An audible third heart sound is also found when there is an abnormally large diastolic flow into a normal ventricle, or a normal flow into an abnormal ventricle. The former occurs in patients with left-to-right shunt and also occurs in mitral or tricuspid incompetence. The latter is seen in patients with right or, more commonly, left ventricular disease. The third heart sound is a dull, low-pitched, localized sound occurring about 0.12–0.16 sec after the second sound. If the sound arises from the right heart, it increases in intensity during inspiration and is heard at the lower sternal edge. Conversely, a left-sided third sound increases on expiration.

D. **Fourth Heart Sound**: The fourth heart sound (S_4) results from atrial contraction and is thought to be a filling sound arising within the ventricle. Although it can often be recorded by phonocardiography, it is not normally audible. A fourth heart sound is heard shortly before the first heart sound in any condition in which the force of either the right or the left atrial contraction is increased. This means that atrial sounds are heard in conditions in which the ventricle is working against high pressure and the atria are contracting against increased resistance, as shown in Fig 3–29. Thus, pulmonary or aortic stenosis and pulmonary or systemic hypertension are the commonest causes of a fourth heart sound. A fourth heart sound is also often audible during an episode of angina pectoris. Here, too, the ventricular compliance is reduced, and the left atrium contracts against increased resistance. Right and left atrial sounds can often be distinguished on the basis of their response to respiration and the site where they are most clearly heard.

E. **Gallop Rhythm**: When a third or a fourth heart sound is present, the extra heart sounds give rise to a gallop or triple rhythm. When the extra sound is presystolic, it is difficult to distinguish the rhythm from that of a split first sound or even an ejection click following the first sound. The presystolic gallop is said to have the cadence of the word "Tennessee," whereas diastolic gallop has been likened to "Kentucky." In some cases, both third and fourth heart sounds can be heard. If the heart rate is rapid–about 120/min–the

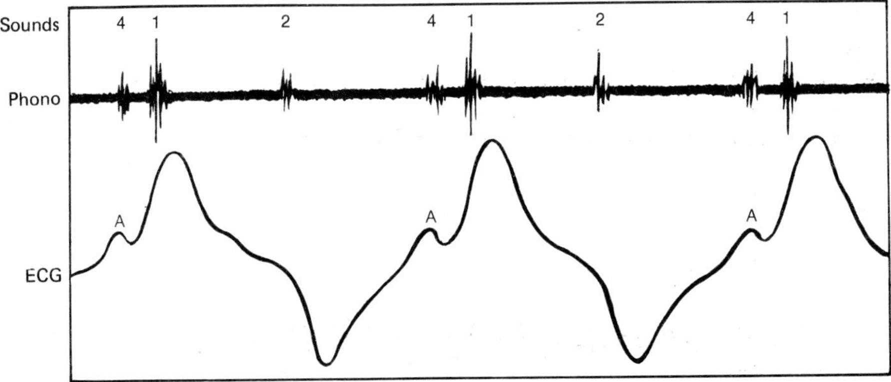

Figure 3–29. Phonocardiogram showing a fourth heart sound (4) and its relation to first sound (1). Below, an apexcardiogram shows the occurrence of the wave of atrial contraction together with the presystolic gallop sound. (Courtesy of Roche Laboratories Division of Hoffman-La Roche, Inc.)

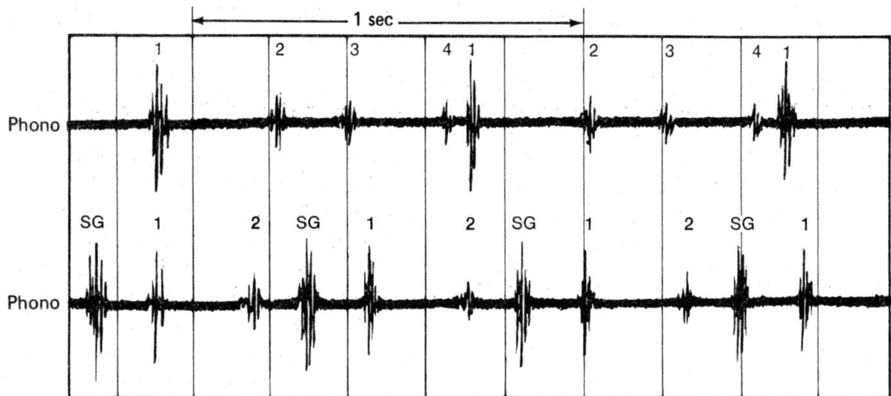

Figure 3–30. The phonocardiographic strip above shows separate presystolic and diastolic gallop; the strip below shows their fusion, which results in a summation gallop (SG). (Courtesy of Roche Laboratories Division of Hoffman-La Roche, Inc.)

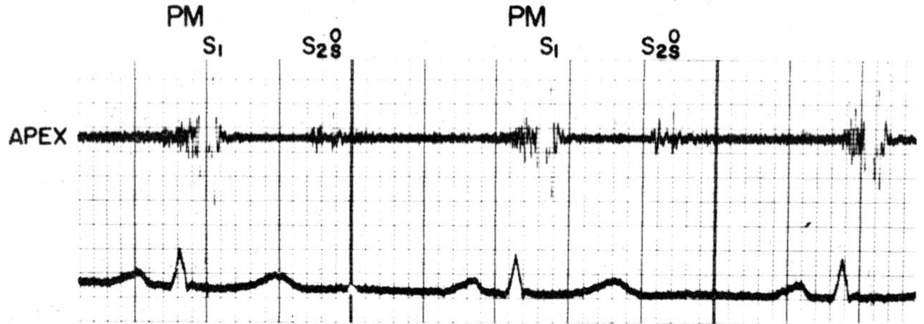

Figure 3–31. From a 24-year-old woman with mitral stenosis and sinus rhythm. The first sound (S_1) shows high amplitude vibrations that merge with a presystolic murmur (PM). There is also a mitral opening snap (OS). The opening snap occurs about 0.06 sec after the onset of S_2. (Reproduced, with permission, from Dressler W: *Clinical Aids in Cardiac Diagnosis.* Grune & Stratton, 1970.)

Figure 3–32. From a patient with rheumatic aortic regurgitation. The diastolic murmur is most distinct in the apical area. A phonocardiogram taken from that region shows a first sound of marked intensity. It is closely followed by a systolic murmur (SM) which starts with an ejection click (EC). The systolic murmur occupies the first half of systole. The second sound is immediately followed by a diastolic murmur which extends over the entire diastolic phase. (Reproduced, with permission, from Dressler W: *Clinical Aids in Cardiac Diagnosis.* Grune & Stratton, 1970.)

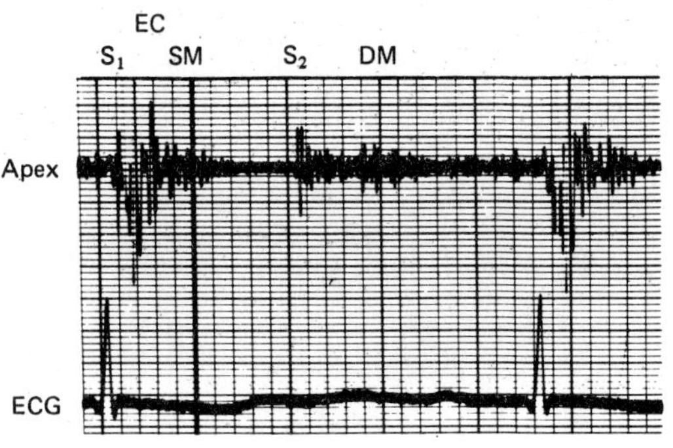

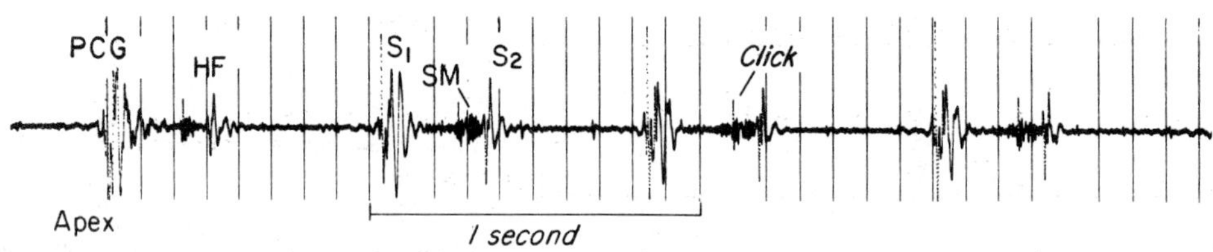

Figure 3–33. Apical high frequency (HF) phonocardiogram (PCG) showing late systolic click and murmur (SM) in a patient with hemodynamically insignificant mitral incompetence.

third and fourth sounds may be superimposed, giving rise to *"summation" gallop* (Fig 3–30). In this case, 2 inaudible sounds may combine to give an audible sound. It is possible to slow the heart rate by carotid sinus massage and listen to hear whether the gallop disappears or whether either the third or the fourth sound or both can be distinguished, which causes a quadruple rhythm. A prominent filling sound is also heard in patients with impaired ventricular filling in pericardial disease. This can be as loud a sound as the second heart sound and is sometimes called a "pericardial knock." It is thought to be caused by the sudden cessation of right ventricular filling.

F. Opening Snap: The opening snap of the atrioventricular valve heard in patients with rheumatic valvular disease is also considered as a heart sound. It is heard 0.06–0.12 sec after the second heart sound and is shown in Fig 3–31. (See further discussion under Mitral Stenosis, p 355.) It may be the loudest and most widely heard sound in the cardiac cycle and is heard best in the third or fourth left interspace in most cases.

G. Systolic Clicks: Extra intracardiac sounds are also heard during systole. These, like the opening snap, arise from valves. The commonest is the systolic ejection click, which can arise either from the aortic or the pulmonary valve. The click occurs early in systole, about 0.02 sec after the first sound. It usually ushers in a systolic ejection murmur, as shown in Fig 3–32. Ejection clicks commonly occur when dilatation of the great vessel (aorta or pulmonary artery) with which they are associated is combined with normal or increased flow through the vessel. They are louder during expiration, when the walls of the vessel are less taut, because the intrathoracic pressure is less negative. Ejection clicks are sometimes heard in normal subjects but are most common in patients with insignificant or mild stenosis of the associated valve. A different variety of systolic click is heard in patients with insignificant mitral incompetence, as shown in Fig 3–33. The clicks, which may be multiple, occur in mid or even

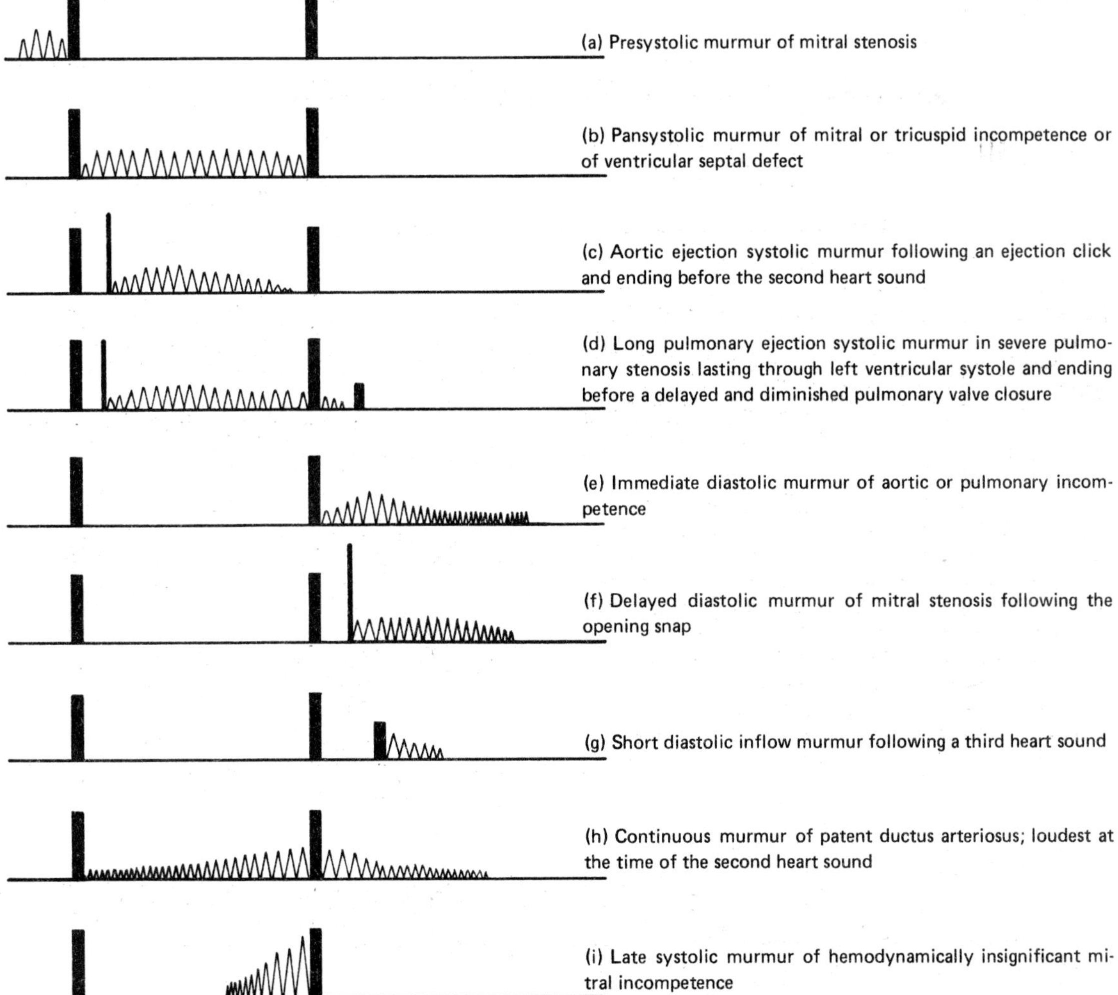

Figure 3–34. The timing of the principal cardiac murmurs. (Reproduced, in modified form, with permission, from Wood P: *Diseases of the Heart and Circulation,* 3rd ed. Lippincott, 1968.)

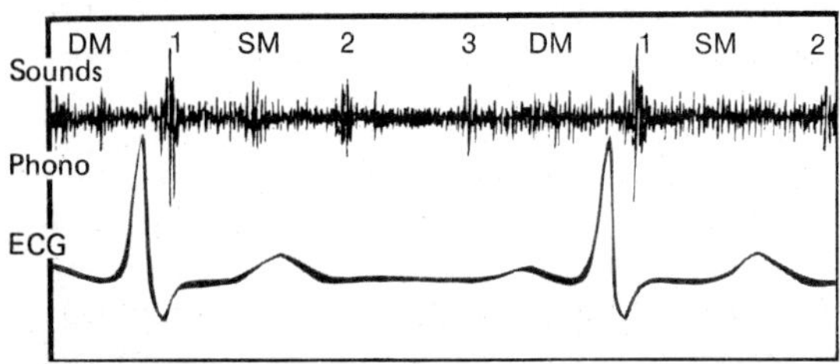

Figure 3–35. Phonocardiogram in atrial septal defect showing a systolic ejection murmur (SM), split second sound, and tricuspid diastolic murmur (DM). (Courtesy of Roche Laboratories Division of Hoffman-La Roche, Inc.)

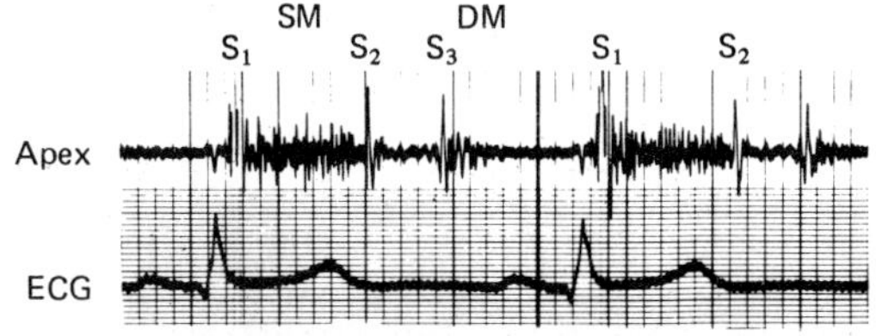

Figure 3–36. From a 25-year-old woman with a rheumatic lesion of the mitral valve. Mitral incompetence is dominant. The phonocardiogram shows a pansystolic murmur (SM) and a third heart sound (S_3) which is followed by a short diastolic murmur (DM). (Reproduced, with permission, from Dressler W: *Clinical Aids in Cardiac Diagnosis.* Grune & Stratton, 1970.)

late systole and may precede, follow, or accompany the late systolic murmur heard in this lesion. In some cases, the click occurs without any murmur. The basic lesion is prolapse of the mitral valve cusp, and although the sound is thought to originate in the valve, the exact mechanism of its production is not known.

Heart Murmurs

The timing of the principal heart murmurs is shown diagrammatically in Fig 3–34. Cardiac murmurs are thought to result from disturbances of normal blood flow patterns in the heart and great vessels. They are classified on the basis of their timing as systolic, diastolic, and continuous murmurs.

A. **Systolic Murmurs:** Systolic murmurs are generally less significant than diastolic murmurs and may occur in patients in whom no evidence of heart disease can be found.

1. **Ejection murmurs**–An abnormally large flow through a normal valve may cause a systolic murmur which is ejection in timing. An ejection murmur begins when flow starts in one of the great vessels and finishes before the time of valve closure. It thus starts after the first heart sound and ends before the second heart sound. Systolic ejection murmurs can be heard in high output states such as anemia, pregnancy, or thyrotoxicosis and also in patients with dilated aortic root due to atherosclerosis, hypertension, syphilis, or other forms of aortitis. They occur when there is a high stroke volume, as in complete heart block with bradycardia. Increased flow through the pulmonary valve occurs in patients with left-to-right shunts, especially in atrial septal defect, and a systolic ejection murmur is virtually always found in such conditions (Fig 3–35).

The most important causes of systolic ejection murmurs are aortic and pulmonary stenoses at a valvular level. The intensity and duration of such murmurs vary with the severity of the stenosis and with the stroke volume. When the stroke volume is low, the murmur may be of low intensity, and it does not last as long as it does when there is normal flow. Because a systolic ejection murmur can also occur when the stenosis is mild and the valve is merely thickened, it is unwise to base any assessment of the severity of the stenosis on the intensity of the murmur.

2. **Pansystolic murmurs**–Pansystolic (holosystolic) murmurs start with the first sound and continue up to the second sound, as shown in Fig 3–36. They are commonly due to incompetence of the mitral or tricuspid valve. The valve leaks throughout systole, and the relatively high pressure difference across the valve accounts for the murmur. The murmur is high-pitched and more musical (of purer tone) than an ejection murmur. A similar murmur is heard when there is flow across a ventricular septal defect with a large pressure difference between the 2 ventricles (Fig 3–37).

3. **Late systolic murmurs**–Mitral incompetence can also result in a late systolic murmur that increases in intensity up to the second sound, as shown in Fig 3–33. This murmur has a peculiar quality, and inexperienced observers may find it difficult to time. Once recognized, it is never forgotten. This late systolic murmur may become pansystolic when the degree of incompetence increases, eg, when peripheral resistance is increased during the overshoot that occurs following Valsalva's maneuver.

4. **Other systolic murmurs**–Although in theory it is easy to classify murmurs as ejection or pansystolic, it may be difficult to make this distinction in practice. In some cases, the murmur exhibits features of both varieties, and it varies in timing at different sites. In infundibular stenosis involving the outflow tract of the right ventricle or in hypertrophic obstructive cardiomyopathy, which produces a rather similar lesion in the left ventricle, there is usually a harsh murmur which lasts throughout systole but peaks in intensity in the middle of systole, when flow is greatest (Fig 3–38). Similarly, when pulmonary stenosis and ventricular septal defect

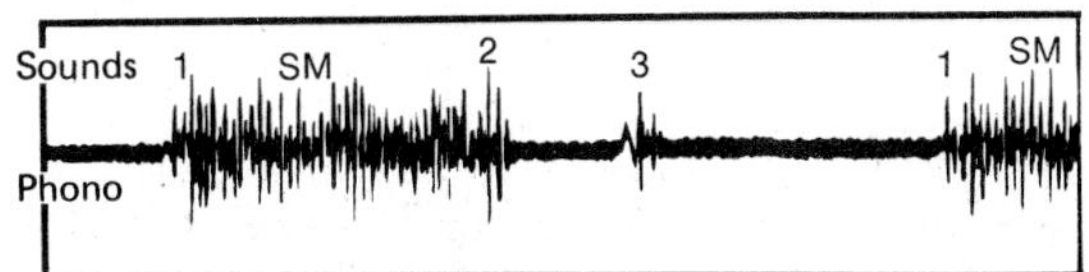

Figure 3–37. Pansystolic murmur (SM) and third heart sound (3) recorded at left sternal border in a patient with ventricular septal defect. (Courtesy of Roche Laboratories Division of Hoffman-La Roche, Inc.)

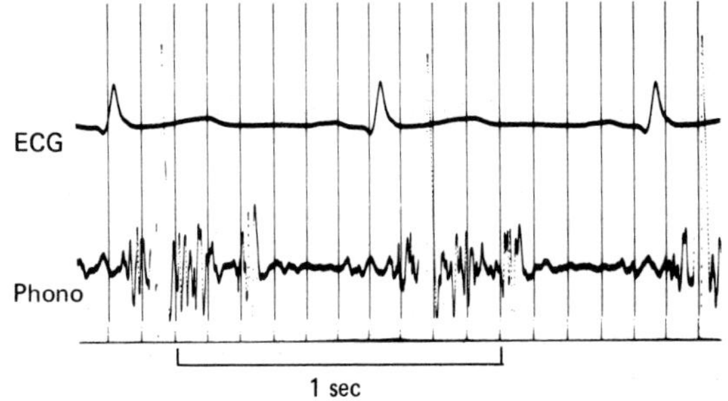

Figure 3–38. Long pansystolic ejection murmur in hypertrophic obstructive cardiomyopathy.

coexist, the murmur has characteristics of both pansystolic and ejection murmurs.

A special type of systolic murmur may occur in coarctation of the aorta or peripheral pulmonary arterial stenosis. In these conditions, there may be a murmur late in systole owing to the late peaking of flow across the narrowing in the vessel. In coarctation, there may also be a systolic murmur which lasts longer and is due to flow through collateral vessels in the chest wall which have developed in response to the lesion. This murmur is similar to that of bronchial collateral flow, which is heard in patients who have markedly reduced flow to the lungs via the pulmonary artery, as in pulmonary atresia. This systolic murmur also resembles the bruit heard over an arteriovenous fistula or over an extremely active toxic goiter. Systolic bruits are also heard over stenotic lesions in peripheral vessels. Carotid arterial and renal arterial stenotic lesions are the most important examples. These murmurs can be systolic or diastolic in timing and are ejection in character. They tend to occur late in the cardiac cycle.

B. Diastolic Murmurs: Diastolic murmurs are almost always due to significant lesions, although they can rarely occur in severe anemia. They are either *immediate,* caused by incompetence of the aortic or pulmonary valve, or *delayed,* caused by actual or relative mitral or tricuspid stenosis. A special form of diastolic murmur that is commonest in mitral stenosis is the *atrial systolic* or *presystolic murmur.*

1. Immediate (early diastolic) murmurs–Immediate or early diastolic murmurs start immediately after the time of closure of the appropriate valve, as shown in Fig 3–39. They decrease in intensity during diastole and are high-pitched and difficult to hear. They are heard best using the diaphragm of the stethoscope, with the subject sitting up and leaning forward and the breath held in expiration. These murmurs are heard on either side of the sternum in the third, fourth, and fifth interspaces. Their duration is roughly related to the severity of the valvular lesion. Similar murmurs are heard when there is diastolic flow from the aorta into any low pressure chamber, eg, the right ventricle or an atrium.

2. Delayed (middiastolic) murmurs–The delayed or middiastolic murmur does not start until the ventricular pressure has fallen below the level of the atrial pressure. There is thus a sound-free interval between the second heart sound and the start of the murmur, as shown in Fig 3–36. The murmur is low-pitched and rumbling, and its duration is related to the severity of the stenosis and the size of the stroke volume. Mitral stenosis is the commonest cause of such a murmur; patent ductus arteriosus and ventricular septal defect on the left side and atrial septal defect and tricuspid stenosis on the right side are other causes. An example of a tricuspid flow murmur in a patient with atrial defect is shown in Fig 3–35. Pure tricuspid stenosis is extremely rare, but mixed incompetence and stenosis does occasionally give rise to a delayed diastolic murmur. The right-sided murmurs increase with inspiration and are heard near the sternum. The left-sided murmurs are best heard with the patient lying in the left lateral position and the stethoscope applied directly over the point of maximal cardiac impulse.

3. Presystolic murmurs–Presystolic accentuation of a delayed diastolic murmur is characteristic of mitral stenosis. In some cases the presystolic murmur is all that can be heard at rest with the patient supine, as in Fig 3–31. The delayed diastolic murmur is often elicited by having the patient exercise and then lie on the left side. Presystolic accentuation of a murmur is also encountered in patients with severe aortic incompetence (Austin Flint murmur). The aortic cusp of the mitral valve tends to be caught between 2 streams of blood during diastole. One stream flowing from the aorta through the leaking valve encounters another from the left atrium during diastolic ventricular filling. The valve leaflet tends to vibrate in the 2 streams and cause what Austin Flint described as a blubbering murmur. This murmur may appear or become louder at the time of atrial systole and thus be confused with the murmur of mitral stenosis. In practice, the 2 lesions–mitral stenosis and aortic incompetence–are readily distinguished, and it is only when the lesions are thought to coexist that difficulties in diagnosis arise.

4. Continuous murmurs–Continuous murmurs arise when there is a pressure difference between 2 communicating vessels or chambers at all times in the cardiac cycle. The commonest example is that found in patent ductus arteriosus with left-to-right shunt (Fig 3–40). This lesion gives rise to a continuous "machin-

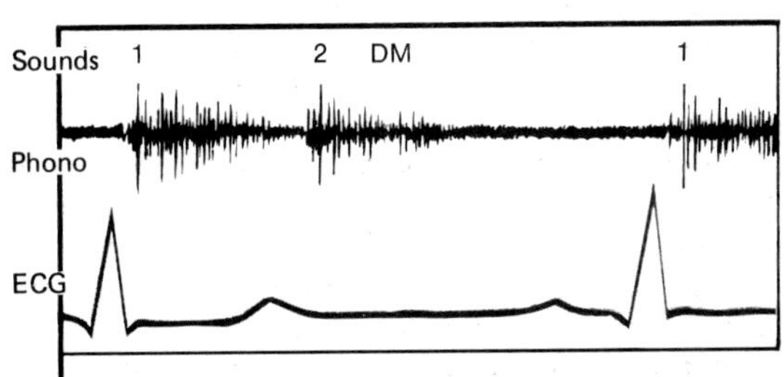

Figure 3–39. Phonocardiogram showing typical diastolic murmur in aortic incompetence and, in this instance, a systolic murmur although no aortic stenosis is present. (Courtesy of Roche Laboratories Division of Hoffman-La Roche, Inc.)

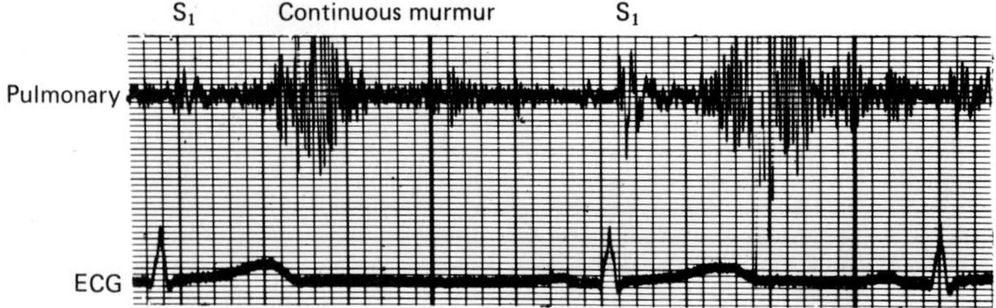

Figure 3–40. Patent ductus arteriosus characterized by a continuous murmur. The phonocardiogram, taken from the pulmonary area, shows a murmur which occupies the entire length of the cardiac cycle. It waxes at the end of systole and during early diastole, reaching at that point its highest frequency and intensity and enveloping the second sound. Only the first sound is distinctly visible. (Reproduced, with permission, from Dressler W: *Clinical Aids in Cardiac Diagnosis.* Grune & Stratton, 1970.)

ery" murmur. The characteristic feature of the murmur is that it is loudest at the time of the second heart sound. At this time, right ventricular ejection is coming to an end and pulmonary arterial pressure is falling, while aortic pressure is remaining high. Similar continuous murmurs are heard with aortopulmonary fistulas and after surgical creation of a shunt for the relief of tetralogy of Fallot (Blalock's operation).

C. Differential Diagnosis: Murmurs that come close to being continuous can be readily confused with the "machinery" murmur if their relationship to the second heart sound is not taken into account. In mixed aortic stenosis and incompetence, there is a to-and-fro systolic and diastolic murmur that can appear almost continuous. There is, however, a gap at the time of the second heart sound. Similarly, in patients with ventricular septal defect and aortic incompetence, the murmur may appear continuous. Coronary arteriovenous fistula and anomalous drainage of a coronary vessel into the pulmonary artery also give continuous murmurs, and in cases of rupture of a sinus of Valsalva aneurysm into a chamber with a lower pressure, the murmur is continuous or near continuous. The murmur of a patent ductus may only be heard high in the left chest below the left clavicle. In some patients, it may be confused with a venous hum. This is a sound that may be continuous and results from partial occlusion of a large vein. Such a bruit is abolished by pressure over the root of the neck or by a change in the patient's position. The hum is never loudest at the time of the second heart sound.

D. Factors Influencing Murmurs: The interpretation of the origin of murmurs can be assisted by determining the direction of transmission of the murmur. The stethoscope is moved over various areas of the precordium to determine where the murmur can still be heard. Murmurs arising from the mitral valve are transmitted toward the axilla. Aortic and pulmonary diastolic murmurs are transmitted down the sides of the sternum. Aortic stenotic murmurs are usually but not always transmitted into the neck. The information obtained from determining the direction of transmission of murmurs is only of secondary value, however. The tendency for right-sided murmurs to be accentuated with inspiration is of more significance than any tendency for a left-sided murmur to be louder during expiration. All intracardiac sounds tend to become less loud with inspiration simply because the stethoscope moves farther away from the origin of the sound and because lung tissue is likely to be interposed and decrease the sound transmission. Thus, exaggeration of a murmur by inspiration is of greater significance than an increase with expiration.

E. Effects of Drugs and Valsalva's Maneuver: Several simple devices and pharmacologic maneuvers have been advocated as aids in interpreting the origin of murmurs. Listening during the period of strain in Valsalva's maneuver or during the overshoot after release of the strain and determining the effect of amyl nitrite inhalation are perhaps the most popular methods. Right-sided murmurs disappear or diminish early during the strain and return early after release of pressure in Valsalva's maneuver. The increase in arterial pressure during the period of overshoot tends to accentuate the murmur of mitral incompetence and decrease the intensity of murmurs in aortic stenosis and hypertrophic obstructive disease. Similar results can be obtained with the use of phenylephrine infusion to raise the systemic arterial pressure. Amyl nitrite reduces systemic resistance and thus accentuates the murmurs of aortic stenosis and obstructive cardiomyopathy and decreases the murmur of mitral incompetence.

Pericardial Friction Rubs

Pericardial friction rubs are heard over the precordium as harsh, grating sounds related to the cardiac cycle and having a systolic component. When they have several components—most typically they have 3—it may be difficult to distinguish them from murmurs. They tend to vary with time, posture, and the phase of respiration. Their intensity tends to vary with the degree of pressure of the bell of the stethoscope on the chest, and they sound superficial, like the noise of hair rubbing against the diaphragm of the stethoscope.

. . .

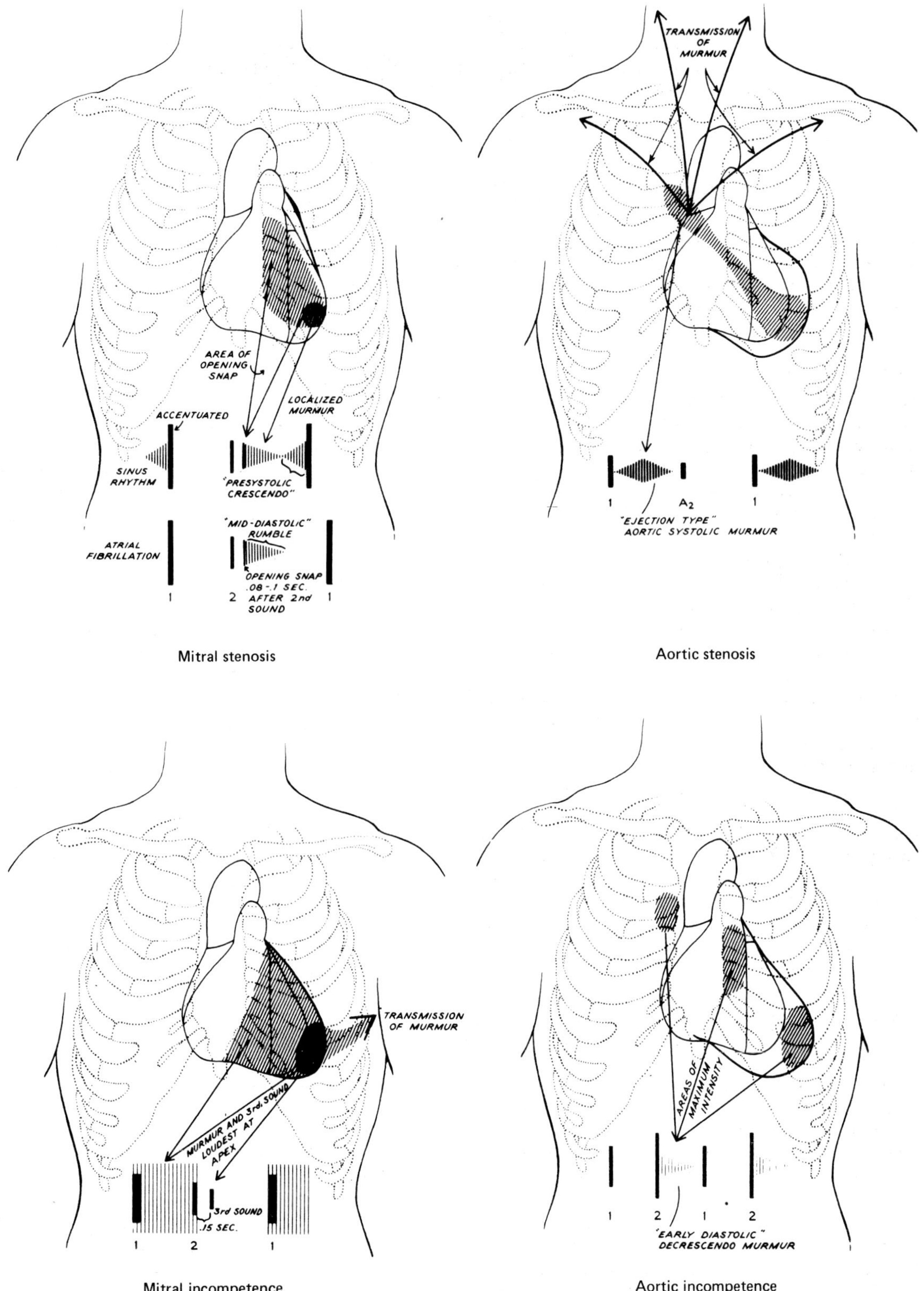

Figure 3–41. Murmurs and cardiac enlargement in common valve lesions. (Reproduced, with permission, from Krupp MA, Chatton MJ [editors] : *Current Medical Diagnosis & Treatment 1977.* Lange, 1977.)

INTEGRATION OF CARDIAC PHYSICAL FINDINGS

The findings on inspection, palpation, and auscultation must all be integrated to form an overall opinion of the likely clinical diagnosis. The heart sounds, clicks, snaps, and murmurs described in this chapter form the basis of the classic physical findings seen in the 4 commonest valvular lesions, illustrated in Fig 3–41.

• • •

References

Bruns DL: A general theory of the causes of murmurs in the cardiovascular system. Am J Med 27:360, 1959.

Dressler W: *Clinical Aids in Cardiac Diagnosis.* Grune & Stratton, 1970.

Flint A: On cardiac murmurs. Am J Med Sci 91:27, 1862.

Fowler NO: *Examination of the Heart.* Part 2: *Inspection and Palpation of Venous and Arterial Pulses.* American Heart Association, 1972.

Frank ST: Aural sign of coronary artery disease. N Engl J Med 289:327, 1973.

Hurst JW, Schlant RC: *Examination of the Heart.* Part 3: *Inspection and Palpation of the Anterior Chest.* American Heart Association, 1972.

Kincaid-Smith P, Barlow J: The atrial sound in hypertension and ischemic heart disease. Br Heart J 21:479, 1959.

Kirkendall WM & others: *Recommendations for Human Blood Pressure Determination by Sphygmomanometers.* American Heart Association, 1967.

Kussmaul A: Uber schwielige Mediastino-Pericarditis und den paradoxen Puls. (3 parts.) Berl Klin Wochenschr 10:433, 445, 461, 1873.

Lange RL, Hecht HH: The mechanism of Cheyne-Stokes respiration. J Clin Invest 41:42, 1962.

Leatham A: *Auscultation of the Heart and Phonocardiography,* 2nd ed. Churchill-Livingstone, 1975.

Leatham A: Splitting of the first and second heart sounds. Lancet 2:607, 1954.

Leatham A, Vogelpoel L: The early systolic sound in dilatation of the pulmonary artery. Br Heart J 16:21, 1954.

Leatham A, Weitzman D: Auscultatory and phonocardiographic signs of pulmonary stenosis. Br Heart J 19:303, 1957.

Leonard JJ, Kroetz FW: *Examination of the Heart.* Part 4: *Auscultation.* American Heart Association, 1967.

Mackenzie J: *The Study of the Pulse, Arterial, Venous and Hepatic, and of the Movements of the Heart.* Young J Pentland, 1902.

McDonald DA: Murmurs in relation to turbulence and eddy formation in the circulation. Circulation 16:278, 1957.

Mendel D, McIlroy MB: The mechanical properties of the lungs in patients with periodic breathing. Br Heart J 19:399, 1957.

Mounsey P: The early diastolic sound of constrictive pericarditis. Br Heart J 17:143, 1955.

Ravin A: *Auscultation of the Heart,* 2nd ed. Year Book, 1967.

Reid JVO: Mid-systolic clicks. S Afr Med J 35:353, 1961.

Vogelpoel L & others: The use of amyl nitrite in the diagnosis of systolic murmurs. Lancet 2:810, 1959.

Weitzman D: The mechanism and significance of the auricular sound. Br Heart J 17:70, 1955.

4 . . .
Clinical Physiology

Knowledge of the physiologic changes that occur in heart disease is essential for understanding and interpreting the results of diagnostic investigations in clinical cardiology and for assessing the results of treatment. An introductory discussion of the function and control of the normal cardiovascular system has been given in Chapter 1.

Clinical physiology is additionally concerned with 2 different but interrelated sets of measurements. The first set of measurements relates to overall circulatory function, more particularly to the transport systems for oxygen and CO_2. The second set comprises purely cardiac measurements such as cardiac output, intracardiac pressures, cardiac volumes, assessment of valvular stenosis and incompetence, intracardiac shunts, coronary blood flow, and assessment of cardiac function. Both applied physiology and normal basic physiology must be understood before the physician can develop a rational approach toward the special investigations undertaken for some patients and toward the interpretation of data obtained at the bedside or in the clinical laboratory. Practical experience in applying the clinical technics to patients is invaluable.

OXYGEN & CO_2 TRANSPORT

The basic mechanisms involved in cardiopulmonary function are oxygen uptake in the lungs, oxygen-CO_2 exchange in the tissues, and transport of CO_2 to the lungs for elimination.

Gas Tension

A. Partial Pressure: It is the partial pressure or tension of each gas that provides the force which determines how the gas will pass across the various membranes involved in gas transfer. The partial pressure of any gas in a mixture of gases is equal to the total pressure (barometric pressure) multiplied by the fraction of that gas in the mixture. Thus, since there is 20.9% oxygen in the atmosphere, the partial pressure of oxygen (P_{O_2}) in the atmosphere at normal barometric pressure (760 mm Hg) is (20.9/100) × 760, or 159 mm Hg. If any liquid such as blood is allowed to equilibrate with a gas, the partial pressure of the gas in the liquid will come to equal that in the gas. The amount of gas entering the liquid will depend on the solubility of the gas in the liquid and on any chemical reaction occurring between the gas and the liquid. If the barometric pressure is reduced, as at high altitude, the same fraction of oxygen in the atmosphere (20.9%) exerts a lower partial pressure because the total pressure is lower. Thus, at 3000 m the barometric pressure is about 525 mm Hg, and the partial pressure of oxygen is reduced to 110 mm Hg. Similarly, a gas mixture of higher oxygen content (50%) exerts a higher P_{O_2} at sea level ([50/100] × 760, or 380 mm Hg).

B. Oxygen Tension, Saturation, and Content: Hemoglobin, the respiratory pigment of blood, has an affinity for oxygen and combines reversibly with it. Hemoglobin exists in 2 forms, a red (oxygenated) form and a blue (reduced) form, depending on the oxygen content of the blood. The proportion of oxygenated blood can vary from 0–100%; this is the oxygen saturation of blood. Arterial oxygen saturation is reduced in cyanotic congenital heart disease and hypoxic patients. The complex relationship between oxygen tension and oxygen saturation is illustrated by the dissociation curve of hemoglobin shown in Fig 4–1 and is

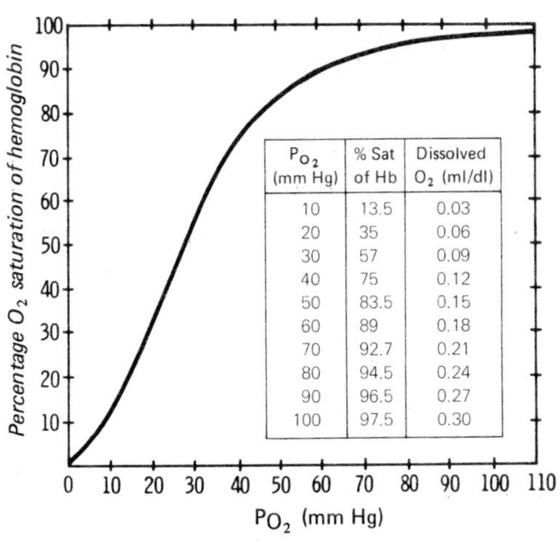

P_{O_2} (mm Hg)	% Sat of Hb	Dissolved O_2 (ml/dl)
10	13.5	0.03
20	35	0.06
30	57	0.09
40	75	0.12
50	83.5	0.15
60	89	0.18
70	92.7	0.21
80	94.5	0.24
90	96.5	0.27
100	97.5	0.30

Figure 4–1. Oxygen hemoglobin dissociation curve. pH 7.40, temperature 38 °C. (Redrawn and reproduced, with permission, from Comroe JH & others: *The Lung: Clinical Physiology and Pulmonary Function Tests,* 2nd ed. Year Book, 1962.)

influenced by the temperature and acidity of the blood. The hemoglobin concentration in blood varies with the degree of anemia or polycythemia, and the oxygen-carrying capacity is directly related to hemoglobin concentration. One gram of hemoglobin when fully saturated can carry 1.34 ml of oxygen. Thus, a normal person with 149 grams of hemoglobin per liter of blood has an oxygen capacity of 149 × 1.34, or 200 ml oxygen per liter of blood. Hemoglobin becomes fully saturated with oxygen at a P_{O_2} of 150–200 mm Hg. At this P_{O_2} there is a small amount (5–6 ml/l) of oxygen in solution in the plasma.

At a normal arterial P_{O_2} of 70–100 mm Hg, hemoglobin is about 97% saturated. Further increase in P_{O_2} to about 200 mm Hg will fully saturate hemoglobin and also result in an increase in the amount of oxygen in solution. Thus, on exposure to 100% oxygen, blood is fully saturated with oxygen and, in addition, contains about 21 ml/l of oxygen in solution, since solution of the gas in blood is directly proportionate to P_{O_2}.

It is important to distinguish between P_{O_2}, oxygen saturation, and oxygen content. P_{O_2} is the force driving oxygen across cellular membranes; oxygen saturation determines the color of the blood; and oxygen content is the volume of oxygen in the blood. The last measurement is most relevant to the cardiopulmonary transport of oxygen.

Oxygen content depends on hemoglobin level and is influenced by oxygen in solution, especially during oxygen breathing. Blood pH, temperature, and hemoglobin level must be known if oxygen content is to be accurately calculated from arterial P_{O_2}. The Severinghaus slide rule (shown in Fig 4–2) provides a convenient means of making this calculation.

CO_2 Transport

CO_2 production, which results from metabolism of substrates in the tissues, is the other aspect of gas exchange that equals oxygen consumption in importance. In addition, the regulation of the level of CO_2 in the blood plays a major role in determining the acid-base balance of the blood and of the body as a whole. It also sets the level of arterial pH (negative logarithm of the H^+ ion concentration). CO_2 is carried in the blood in 3 different ways. Like oxygen it dissolves in blood, but to a much greater degree (25 times greater, or about 27 ml/l) at a normal P_{CO_2} of 40 mm Hg in arterial blood. CO_2 is also carried as bicarbonate in the buffering system of the blood and in combination with hemoglobin as a carbamino compound. Arterial CO_2 tension is the most closely controlled variable in the respiratory system. The normal value of 40 mm Hg is equivalent to (40/760) × 100, or 5.25% CO_2 in the alveolar gas, and free equilibration takes place across the pulmonary membrane. Pulmonary ventilation is the most important determinant of arterial P_{CO_2}; hypoventilation raises the P_{CO_2} level. The level of ventilation is normally closely controlled by servomechanisms, and the arterial P_{CO_2} is maintained within a few mm of 40 mm Hg. The level of metabolism and the adequacy of tissue perfusion determine the pH and

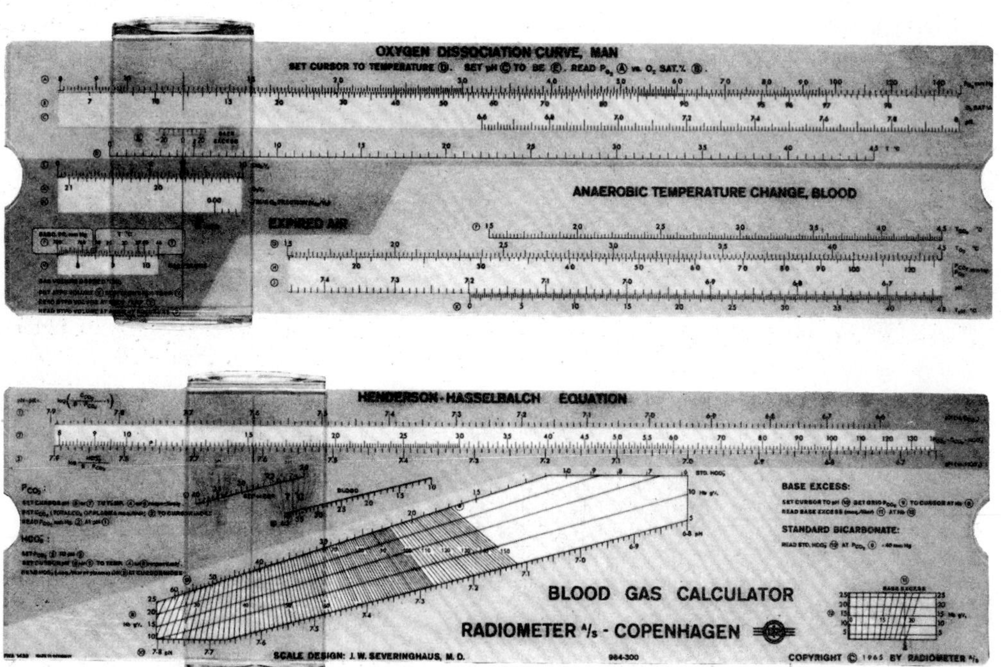

Figure 4–2. Blood gas calculator. On one side, the calculator has scales for acid-base balance. The other side includes the oxygen dissociation curve, anaerobic blood temperature change factors, and expired gas manipulations. (Reproduced, with permission, from the Radiometer Company, Copenhagen, and Severinghaus JW: J Appl Physiol 21:1109, 1966.)

P_{CO_2} of venous blood returning to the lungs, and the adequacy of ventilation determines the extent to which the products of metabolism are cleared from the blood by the lungs. Abnormalities of the arterial P_{CO_2} result both from abnormalities of ventilation and from disturbances of acid-base balance.

Relationship Between P_{CO_2} & pH

Alterations in the relationship between arterial P_{CO_2} and pH may be grouped into 4 categories, 2 of which are respiratory and 2 of which are metabolic.

Ventilation is the most important means of influencing P_{CO_2} and pH. (1) With hyperventilation, arterial pH rises and P_{CO_2} falls as CO_2 is washed out of the blood (respiratory alkalosis). (2) With hypoventilation, arterial pH falls and P_{CO_2} rises as CO_2 accumulates in the blood (respiratory acidosis).

Metabolism influences P_{CO_2} in the reverse direction. (1) In metabolic acidosis, although blood pH falls, the increased acidity of the blood stimulates ventilation so that arterial P_{CO_2} also falls. A low pH associated with a low P_{CO_2} is common in cardiac failure because inadequate tissue perfusion results in excessive anerobic metabolism and lactic acid accumulation. (2) In metabolic alkalosis, the arterial pH and P_{CO_2} are both elevated. This is by far the least common disturbance of the group and may occur as a result of alkali ingestion or following prolonged vomiting with loss of acid gastric contents.

	pH	P_{CO_2}
Respiratory acidosis	↓	↑
Respiratory alkalosis	↑	↓
Metabolic acidosis	↓	↓
Metabolic alkalosis	↑	↑

Assessment of Acid-Base Balance

Unless calculations are performed, it is not always easy to see the accommodation of pH level to changes in P_{CO_2}, both because renal compensatory forces may come into operation and because pH involves a logarithmic scale. The Severinghaus slide rule (Fig 4–2) is particularly helpful in calculating a value for base deficit or base excess from arterial P_{CO_2} and pH, and it takes into account the buffering properties of hemoglobin. Using it enables the clinician to accurately determine the acid-base balance of acutely ill patients and to plan appropriate therapy for acid-base disturbances. The various disturbances of blood gas tensions are commonly followed by measurements of the P_{O_2}, P_{CO_2}, and pH of arterial blood. These measurements are indicated in almost all acutely ill patients with cardiopulmonary disease and also in postoperative care of patients after major surgery, especially after cardiac surgery. These measurements are thus routinely available in most intensive care and coronary care units, where specially trained nurses and technicians can perform the analyses on the spot, without sending the specimen to a laboratory, and the information is available at any time.

MEASUREMENT OF CARDIAC OUTPUT

Cardiac output is one of the basic measurements in cardiac physiology. It is a required measurement in all cardiac catheterization studies and is also valuable in bedside catheterization of patients in coronary care units. Because the range of normal values is large, this measurement is most important in the interpretation of pressure measurements. The term cardiac output implies the measurement of systemic blood flow, which is essentially the same as pulmonary blood flow in normal subjects. In patients with intracardiac shunts, however, the pulmonary and systemic flows are not the same, and a clear distinction between the 2 must be made. At present, cardiac output is measured almost entirely by methods providing an average value over a 1- to 5-minute period. Instantaneous measurements of blood flow are only now coming into clinical use.

Fick Principle

Cardiac output is most commonly measured by the Fick principle, which states that the flow of blood through an organ (eg, the lungs) is equal to the amount of a substance (eg, oxygen) absorbed by the blood flowing through the organ, divided by the difference in oxygen concentration between the blood entering and blood leaving the organ. Thus, pulmonary blood flow is the oxygen consumption in ml/min divided by the arteriovenous difference across the lungs (pulmonary venous oxygen content minus pulmonary arterial oxygen content in ml/l). The same principle applies to systemic capillary beds of the entire systemic circulation. Thus, systemic blood flow is equal to the oxygen consumption of the body (equal in the steady state to the uptake in the lungs) divided by the difference in oxygen content between arterial blood going to the tissues and mixed venous blood (pulmonary arterial blood) returning to the lungs for oxygenation. In normal subjects, blood flow through the lungs is virtually equal to blood flow to the body, and no substantial right-to-left or left-to-right shunt is present.

In a normal subject the oxygen consumption is about 250 ml/min. The arterial oxygen content is about 200 ml/l, and the mixed venous (pulmonary arterial blood) content is about 150 ml/l. Thus, the cardiac output is 250/50 or 5 liters/min. This value in liters per minute is often adjusted to the size of the subject by dividing it by the body surface area derived from standard tables and expressed in m^2. The adjusted value is called the cardiac index; the normal value is about 4 liters/min/m^2.

Indicator Dilution Method

The Fick principle also forms the basis for the indicator dilution method of measuring cardiac output, which uses green dye (indocyanine green) or cold saline (thermodilution) injected into one place in the circulation and measured in another. A known amount of indicator is injected, usually into the right atrium, and the concentration of the indicator is subsequently measured at a downstream site after the indicator has thoroughly mixed with the blood. If cold saline is used, the temperature of blood in the pulmonary artery is usually measured continuously with a thermistor at the tip of a catheter (Swan-Ganz catheter). If green dye is used, the concentration is measured in systemic arterial blood by drawing a sample continuously through a photoelectric instrument (cuvette densitometer) that measures the optical density of blood at an appropriate wavelength. The cardiac output equals the amount of indicator injected, divided by its average concentration during its passage past the sampling site in the arterial blood (Fig 4–3). Of course, the indicator must not leave the circulation between the injection and the sampling sites, nor can it cause harmful effects or those that alter hemodynamic status.

In practice, when green dye is used, the logarithm of the concentration of dye is plotted against time as the concentration rises to a peak, falls, and then rises again as recirculation of dye occurs. With thermodilution, recirculation is negligible, and the disappearance follows an exponential pattern (straight line on a semilog plot). With dye, the exponential disappearance is interrupted by recirculation of dye, as shown in Fig 4–3, and the initial linear portion of the curve must be extrapolated to zero concentration to define the time-concentration curve during the first passage of the dye. Cardiac output is then calculated as shown in Fig 4–3. In practice, the indicator dilution method has recently been automated so that computers are used to extrapolate the curves and calculate cardiac output.

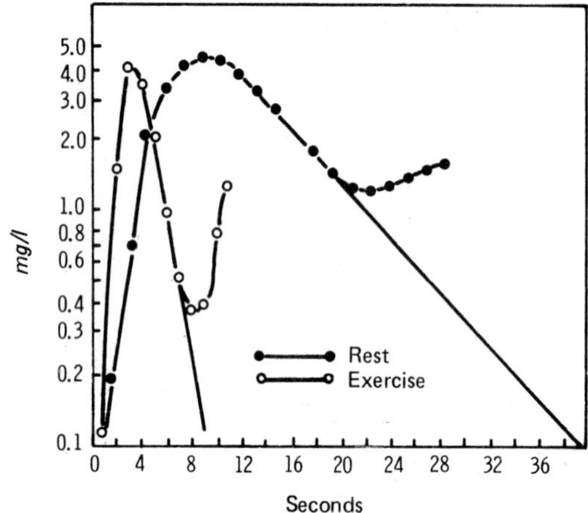

$$F = \frac{E}{\int_0^{\infty} C\,dt}$$

F = flow

E = amount of indicator injected

C = instantaneous concentration of indicator in arterial blood

In the *rest* example above,

$$\frac{\text{Flow in 39 sec}}{\text{(time of first passage)}} = \frac{\text{5 mg injection}}{\text{1.6 mg/l}}$$

(avg concentration)

Flow = 3.1 liters in 39 sec

$$\text{Flow (cardiac output)/min} = 3.1 \times \frac{60}{39} = 4.7 \text{ liters}$$

For the *exercise* example,

$$\text{Flow in 9 sec} = \frac{5 \text{ mg}}{1.51 \text{ mg/l}} = 3.3 \text{ liters}$$

$$\text{Flow/min} = 3.3 \times \frac{60}{9} = 22.0 \text{ liters}$$

Figure 4–3. Determination of cardiac output by indicator (dye) dilution. (Data and graph from Asmussen E, Nielsen M: The cardiac output in rest and work determined by the acetylene and the dye injection methods. Acta Physiol Scand 27:217, 1952.)

STROKE WORK

Stroke work is best defined as the external work done by the left ventricle. In its simplest sense, this represents the stroke volume × the mean systolic pressure with each contraction. In its strictest sense, however, it is defined as the area within the pressure-volume loop of the left ventricle. This is roughly calculated as the product of (systolic mean – mean left atrial pressure) × stroke volume × 0.0136. The conversion factor of 0.0136 represents the conversion from mm Hg pressure to the g-cm system. Stroke work is usually expressed on a per beat basis as gram-meters per square meter (g-m/m^2) of body surface area. The normalization of stroke work index per body surface area allows for comparison of one patient with another.

MEASUREMENT OF CARDIAC SHUNTS

Use of Fick Principle to Estimate Shunts

Methods based on the Fick principle can be used to estimate and investigate intracardiac and intrapulmonary shunts seen in congenital heart disease in which blood passes from one side of the circulation to another without traversing a capillary bed. Such shunts are either right-to-left, left-to-right, or bidirectional. In right-to-left shunts, venous blood bypasses the pulmonary capillary bed and enters the left side of the heart, reducing the arterial oxygen content and making the systemic blood flow greater than the pulmonary flow. In left-to-right shunts, oxygenated blood returning from the lungs passes through an abnormal communication to the right side of the heart and recirculates through the lungs without having passed through a systemic capillary bed. In this case, the pulmonary

Table 4–1. Derived hemodynamic indices used in this chapter.

Index	Normal Range of Values*
Mean systolic arterial pressure $(\overline{SAP}) = S - \frac{(S - D)}{3}$	80–107 mm Hg
Cardiac index (CI) $= \frac{CO}{BSA}$	2.8–4.2 liters/min/m^2
Stroke volume index (SVI) $= \frac{SV}{BSA}$	40–70 ml/m^2
Stroke work index (SWI)† $= SV \times (\overline{SAP} - \overline{PCW}) \times 0.0136$	40–80 g-m/m^2
Systemic vascular resistance (SVR) $= \frac{80\ (\overline{AP} - \overline{RA})}{CO}$	770–1500 dynes-sec-cm^{-5} ‡
Pulmonary vascular resistance (PVR) $= \frac{80\ (\overline{PA} - \overline{PCW})}{CO}$	20–120 dynes-sec-cm^{-5} ‡

Abbreviations in the equations

- S = peak systolic pressure (mm Hg)
- D = diastolic pressure (mm Hg)
- CO = cardiac output (l/min)
- BSA = body surface area (m^2)
- $\overline{AP}$ = mean arterial pressure (mm Hg)
- $\overline{RA}$ = mean right atrial pressure (mm Hg)
- $\overline{PA}$ = mean pulmonary artery pressure (mm Hg)
- $\overline{PCW}$ = mean pulmonary capillary wedge pressure (mm Hg)
- SV = stroke volume $\left(\frac{CO}{\text{heart rate}}\right)$ (ml)
- LV = left ventricular
- BP = blood pressure

*These normal values courtesy of Dr William W Parmley.

†More accurately, SWI $= \frac{(\text{mean LV systolic BP} - \text{mean LV diastolic BP}) \times SV \times 0.0136}{BSA}$

but left ventricular (LV) pressures are generally not readily available.

‡Divide by 80 to get mm Hg/l/min, used by many authorities.

flow is greater than the systemic. In bidirectional shunts, both processes coexist.

Right-to-Left Shunts

The characteristic feature of a right-to-left shunt is a reduction in systemic arterial saturation resulting from mixing of venous blood with oxygenated blood returning from the lungs. The right-to-left shunt can be calculated by applying the Fick equation to both the pulmonary and systemic circuits and subtracting the pulmonary flow from the systemic. As an example, in a patient with Fallot's tetralogy with mild polycythemia (hemoglobin 18.6 g/dl; oxygen capacity 250 ml/l; $\dot{V}_{O_2}$ 200 ml/min), pulmonary arterial (mixed venous) saturation might be 70% (oxygen content [70/100] × 250, or 175 ml/l); systemic arterial saturation 85% (oxygen content 212.5 ml/l); and end-pulmonary capillary saturation 97% (oxygen content 242.5 ml/l). The Fick principle can be used to calculate systemic flow ($\dot{Q}_S$):

$$\text{Systemic flow} = \frac{200}{(212.5 - 175)} = \frac{200}{37.5} = 5.3 \text{ liters/min}$$

The Fick principle can also be used to calculate pulmonary flow ($\dot{Q}_P$):

$$\text{Pulmonary flow} = \frac{200}{(242.5 - 175)} = \frac{200}{67.5} = 3.0 \text{ liters/min}$$

In this example, the right-to-left shunt is 5.3 – 3.0, or 2.3 liters/min.

Left-to-Right Shunts

The characteristic feature of left-to-right shunts is an increase in oxygen content and saturation in the chamber into which the shunt flows. In other words, the oxygen content is higher than in the immediately preceding cardiac chamber. The magnitude of left-to-right shunts can be calculated by applying the Fick equation to both the pulmonary and systemic circuits as illustrated above for right-to-left shunts.

For example, in a patient with an atrial septal defect, samples from the right heart chambers might show 85% saturation in the pulmonary arterial blood, 86% in the right ventricle, 83% in the right atrium, 67% in the superior vena cava, and 73% in the inferior vena cava. Arterial saturation and pulmonary venous saturation are 97% each. The oxygen capacity is 200 ml/l and the oxygen consumption 225 ml/min. The increase in this example occurs between the venae cavae and the right atrium; the venae cavae samples represent venous blood returning from the tissues, whereas the right atrial blood is of higher saturation because the blood shunted across the atrial defect is mixed with it. Assuming that the inferior vena cava drains two-thirds of the body and the superior vena cava one-third, the mixed venous saturation is

$$\frac{67 + (2 \times 73)\,\%}{3}$$

or 71% (oxygen content 144 ml/l). The Fick equation can be applied to calculate systemic flow ($\dot{Q}_S$):

$$\text{Systemic flow} = \frac{225}{(194 - 144)} = \frac{225}{50} = 4.5 \text{ liters/min}$$

The Fick principle can be similarly used to calculate pulmonary flow ($\dot{Q}_P$):

$$\text{Pulmonary flow} = \frac{225}{(194 - 166)} = \frac{225}{28} = 8 \text{ liters/min}$$

In this example, the left-to-right shunt is 8.0 – 4.5, or 3.5 liters/min.

Pulmonary to Systemic Flow Ratio

The size of left-to-right shunts is often expressed in terms of the ratio of pulmonary to systemic flows. In the example above, the ratio is (8.0/4.5) or 1.8:1. This is a small flow ratio, and values of 3 or 4:1 are not uncommon.

Accuracy of Shunt Estimations

The accuracy of shunt flow calculations based on intracardiac samples is not high. Bloodstreams tend not to mix fully in the right heart chambers, and, if there is valvular incompetence, blood from a more distal chamber can contaminate the next most proximal one. As the pulmonary arteriovenous oxygen difference becomes smaller in patients with large left-to-right shunts, the magnitude of the calculated pulmonary blood flow comes to vary widely in response to small differences in pulmonary arterial oxygen content. Blood oxygen content measurements are usually accurate to within ± 2 ml/l, and when the pulmonary arterial oxygen saturation is 90% or more, the pulmonary arteriovenous oxygen difference may be as low as 14 ml/l. Measurement errors then have a marked effect.

Bidirectional Shunts

The calculation of blood flow in bidirectional shunts in congenital heart disease is even more inaccurate than that in left-to-right shunts. The most satisfactory method of calculation is the measurement of "effective" blood flow. The concept of "effectiveness" of flow implies that any blood flow that fails to traverse a capillary bed is "ineffective." Thus, left-to-right shunt constitutes ineffective pulmonary flow and right-to-left shunt ineffective systemic flow. Effective flow ($\dot{Q}_{eff}$) is calculated from the Fick equation as

$$\text{Effective cardiac output} = \frac{\text{Oxygen consumption in ml/min}}{\text{Pulmonary venous} - \text{Mixed venous oxygen content in ml/l}}$$

In a patient with Eisenmenger's syndrome and a bidirectional shunt at ventricular level, samples from the right heart might show a pulmonary arterial saturation of 80%, right ventricle 78%, right atrium 65%, superior vena cava 63%, and inferior vena cava 67%. With oxygen consumption at 250 ml/min, oxygen capacity 210 ml/l, end-pulmonary capillary saturation 97%, and arterial saturation 92%, the systemic flow is calculated from the arterial and mixed venous (right atrial) samples as follows:

$$\text{Systemic flow} = \frac{250}{(193.2 - 136.5)} = \frac{250}{56.7} = 4.4 \text{ liters/min}$$

Pulmonary flow is calculated from end-pulmonary capillary and pulmonary arterial blood:

$$\text{Pulmonary flow} = \frac{250}{(203.7 - 168)} = \frac{250}{35.7} = 7.9 \text{ liters/min}$$

Effective flow is calculated from end-pulmonary capillary and mixed venous blood:

$$\text{Effective flow} = \frac{250}{(203.7 - 136.5)} = \frac{250}{67.2} = 3.7 \text{ liters/min}$$

The left-to-right shunt equals the difference between the pulmonary and effective flows (7.0 – 3.7) or 3.3 liters/min, and the right-to-left shunt equals the difference between the systemic and effective flows (4.4 – 3.7) or 0.7 liters/min. It is easy to see that these calculations may be subject to error when the arteriovenous difference becomes small and when mixing may be incomplete. It is important to realize that all shunt calculations must be regarded as semiquantitative measurements only.

End-Pulmonary Capillary Oxygen Saturation

The clinician must realize the importance of the value selected for end-pulmonary capillary saturation in all the calculations noted above. Pulmonary venous samples are seldom available, and arterial samples are not relevant if a right-to-left shunt is present. Therefore, the clinician must arbitrarily select a value for end-capillary saturation, and it is necessary to decide whether the conventional value of 97% is appropriate in any given case. The effect of oxygen breathing on arterial oxygen content provides some indirect evidence about the validity of assuming a normal end-pulmonary capillary saturation. If arterial oxygen is 97% or higher there is no problem, because end-capillary oxygen content must be normal and no significant right-to-left shunt can be present. When arterial saturation is low, however, it is not possible to tell whether arterial hypoxia is due to right-to-left shunt or to abnormal pulmonary function.

Effect of Oxygen Breathing

Breathing 100% oxygen eliminates oxygen exchange problems in the lungs and raises end-pulmonary capillary content to supernormal levels. If arterial hypoxia is due to lung disease, arterial oxygen content rises markedly with oxygen breathing. In patients with arterial hypoxia due to right-to-left shunt, end-pulmonary capillary saturation is normal and oxygen breathing has only a small and predictable effect on arterial oxygen content.

Breathing 100% oxygen raises end-pulmonary capillary oxygen content by increasing the amount of oxygen carried in solution in the blood. An increase of 18 ml/l in end-pulmonary capillary blood occurs if alveolar P_{O_2} changes from 100 mm Hg to 700 mm Hg. As long as the hemodynamic status of the patient remains unchanged, an equal increase of 18 ml/l in oxygen content will occur in all sites of the body. The rise of 18 ml/l corresponds to an increase in saturation of 9% if the oxygen capacity is 200 ml/l. If the oxygen capacity is higher than 200 ml/l, the percentage change in saturation is lower and vice versa.

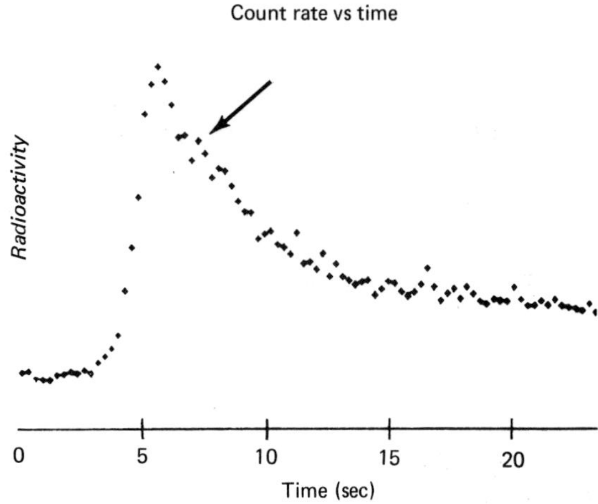

Figure 4–5. Indicator dilution curve in a patient with left-to-right shunt due to atrial septal defect (pulmonary/systemic flow ratio 2:1). Radioactivity is plotted on the ordinate and time on the abscissa. The hump on the disappearance curve results from early recirculation of shunted blood. (Courtesy of E Botvinick.)

Qualitative Estimation of Shunts by Indicator Dilution Methods

Indicator dilution curves provide qualitative information about shunts. In right-to-left shunts, a portion of the injected dose of indicator–which passes from an injection site in the right heart through the shunt–traverses a shorter path through the circulation than does the main bolus of dye, as shown in Fig 4–4. It thus appears earlier as a hump on the build-up phase of the dye curve recorded in the arterial tree. In left-to-right shunts, blood containing indicator recirculates abnormally early and produces a hump on the disappearance curve (Fig 4–5). The presence of shunts invalidates the normal method of analysis of cardiac output by indicator dilution. Although different patterns of indicator dilution curves can be observed in patients with different types of shunts, accurate measurement of flow cannot be obtained. For these reasons, and because of improvements in angiocardiographic technic, dye curves are now infrequently used in the investigation of patients with shunts.

Detection of Small Shunts

A number of methods are available for the detection of shunts that are too small to be detected from differences in the oxygen content of blood samples. These technics generally involve sampling blood from the right side of the heart after the patient has inhaled gaseous indicators such as hydrogen, nitrous oxide, or radioactive krypton that enter the pulmonary capillary blood. Hydrogen has the advantage that it can be detected with a platinum electrode at the tip of a catheter, thus eliminating the need for blood sampling. In practice, the detection of small shunts that are not discovered by means of right heart sampling of oxygen content or angiocardiography is of little clinical significance

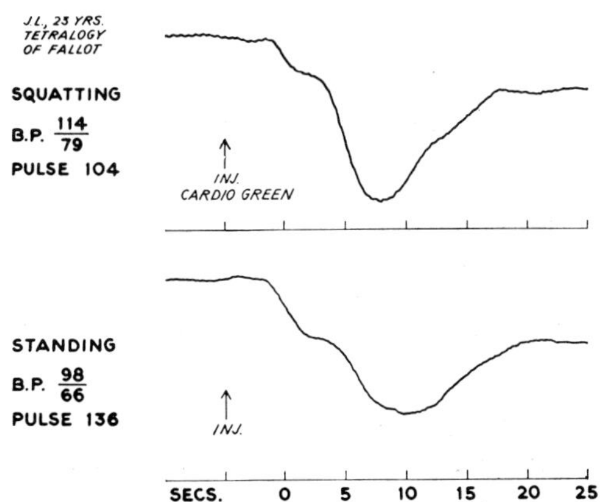

Figure 4–4. Indicator dilution curves showing early appearance of dye injected into the right atrium in a patient with Fallot's tetralogy. The size of the initial hump due to right-to-left shunt is greater in the standing position.

Other Methods for Measurement of Blood Flow

More direct methods for measuring instantaneous blood flow are available for research purposes and will probably become widely available within a few years. These methods generally measure the velocity of blood flow in the aorta or some other specific vessel, and their use depends on a knowledge of the cross-sectional area of the vessel for calculation of the actual volume of blood flowing past the instrument per unit of time. Electromagnetic and ultrasonic technics are most commonly used at present. Their most useful application is in the measurement of blood flow through aortocoronary grafts during surgical operations. Catheter tip blood velocity meters have been used in research studies, but their calibration remains a problem.

BLOOD VOLUME

The circulating blood volume can be determined either from measurements of red cell volume or from plasma volume plus hematocrit. The values, although statistically valid, are subject to considerable variation, and the range of normal values is wide. The principle in blood volume measurement is the injection of a tracer material which mixes with the total blood volume before it is excreted. The degree of dilution of the tracer is measured in a sample of blood drawn after mixing is complete. Commonly used tracers are radioactive chromium-labeled red cells, which measure red cell volume, or iodine-labeled albumin, which measures plasma volume. The total blood volume is calculated from the hematocrit:

$$\frac{\text{Red cell volume}}{\text{Red cell volume} + \text{Plasma volume}}$$

Thus, total blood volume equals

$$\text{Red cell volume} \times \frac{1}{\text{Hematocrit}}$$

or,

$$\text{Plasma volume} \times \frac{1}{1 - \text{Hematocrit}}$$

In practice, mixing of the indicator is not always complete before the indicator begins to be excreted, and incomplete mixing of indicator often gives falsely low values, especially in patients with heart disease in whom the cardiac output is low. The measurement of blood volume is consequently of less value than might be expected in cardiac patients.

Angiographic Measurements of Cardiac Chamber Volumes

Left ventricular volume is most commonly measured from cineangiograms recorded following the injection of iodine-containing contrast material into the ventricle during left heart catheterization. Ventricular volumes are calculated from the dimensions of opacified areas of individual films or cine frames exposed at the end of systole and the end of diastole.

The angiographic image of the left ventricle may be recorded in a single plane (usually the left anterior oblique) or in 2 planes: posteroanterior (shown in Fig 4–6) and lateral or 2 obliques. The examiner must make some assumption about the shape of the ventricle in the axis of revolution about the plane or planes in which measurements are made. The simplest assumption is to consider the left ventricle as a sphere, but the slightly more complex figure of a prolate ellipse is frequently used. Computer programs are commonly used to calculate left ventricular volume from a small number of specific angiographic measurements.

Errors of Method

The process of defining the edge of the ventricular shadow is often subjective. Blood trapped between the trabeculae carneae cordis, which form muscular projections into the body of the left ventricle, may not show up on end-systolic films as an opacity. The assumption made about a particular geometric shape for the ventricle introduces an unknown error. The end-diastolic volumes are more accurate than the end-systolic values, which are probably too small.

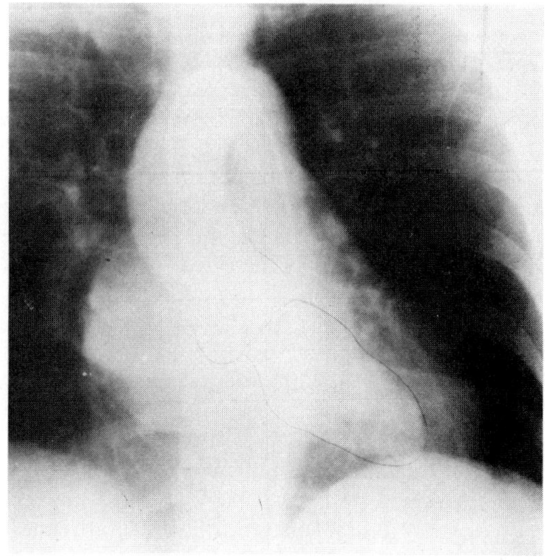

Figure 4–6. Posteroanterior view of the left ventricle following injection of contrast material. The outline of the ventricle from which volume was calculated is drawn on the radiogram.

Ejection Fraction

The ratio of stroke volume (end-diastolic minus end-systolic volume) to end-diastolic volume (the ejection fraction) has become the most widely accepted of all measurements assessing left ventricular function. It is a nondimensional number that expresses the percentage of blood in the ventricle that is ejected per beat. The normal value obtained from a measurement in 2 planes is 67 ± 9%. This value tends to be falsely high because the end-systolic volume from which it is calculated is falsely low. The injection of contrast material into the left ventricle is usually made with a catheter in the chamber, although less invasive methods using intravenous radioactive indicators or right-sided injections of contrast media are sometimes used. The injection of contrast media into the left ventricle often provokes ectopic beats, as shown in Fig 4–7. This can be significant in the evaluation of left ventricular function. A false idea of ejection fraction can also be obtained from the abnormally forceful left ventricular contraction that usually follows a run of ectopic beats.

Effects of Contrast Material

The contrast material itself also influences left ventricular function, mainly because of its hyperosmolarity. This factor is thought to be unimportant in the first few beats following injection, however, and it generally influences left ventricular end-diastolic pressure rather than ejection fraction. Left ventricular ejection fraction has proved to be a useful functional measure-

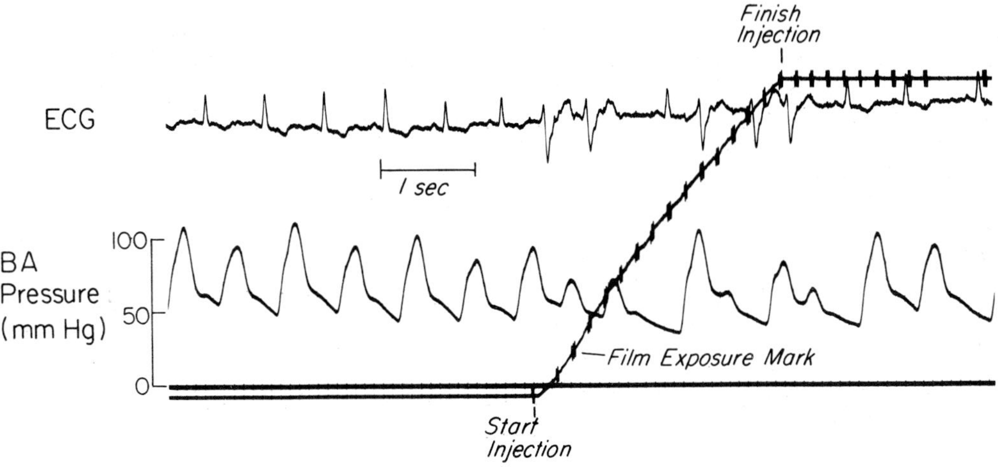

Figure 4–7. ECG and brachial arterial (BA) pressure tracing obtained during an injection of contrast material into the left ventricle in a patient with aortic stenosis. The timing of the angiographic film exposures is indicated. Pulsus alternans is present, and ectopic beats are seen during the injection.

ment that is greatly preferred to a visual impression of the force of contraction, which can be misleading. The right ventricle is of a completely different shape from the left and varies more in shape in disease. It is inappropriate to apply methods developed for computing left ventricular volume to the right side of the heart.

Measurement of Valvular Incompetence

Angiographic measurements of stroke volume include all the blood pumped by the ventricle, whereas methods based on the Fick principle measure only the blood that flows forward to the systemic arterial bed. It is thus possible by combining the 2 methods to measure the volume of blood returning to the ventricle or atrium through the incompetent aortic or mitral valve. The angiographic stroke volume minus the forward (Fick) stroke volume gives a measure of the amount of backflow, which is usually expressed as the "regurgitant fraction," the proportion of the angiographic stroke volume flowing back per beat. A value of 50% or more indicates severe valvular incompetence.

MEASUREMENT OF BLOOD PRESSURE

Direct measurements of the pressure in various cardiac chambers and great vessels are obviously of great importance in the diagnosis of various valvular and congenital heart lesions encountered in clinical cardiology. Direct measurements of systemic arterial and venous pressure are also often used in following the response to treatment in severely ill patients, eg, those with severe acute myocardial infarction.

Technic

Measurements of pressures in the heart and great vessels are almost always made through long small-bore catheters connected to electromanometers of the strain gauge type. Obtaining accurate pressure recordings presents significant problems, especially when the catheter is subject to motion because of the action of the heart. The only satisfactory solution is to use catheter tip manometers. Unfortunately, these are so expensive and the catheters to which they are attached are so unwieldy that their use outside research laboratories has not yet become practical. Experience and comparison of conventional and catheter-tip manometer tracings have made it possible to recognize high quality pressure tracings and know when serious artifacts are present. Excessive damping of pressure tracings resulting from leaky stopcocks, bubbles of air in the catheter or manometer, or blockage of the catheter should be easily recognized, as shown in Fig 4–8. Excessive overswing due to catheter fling in hyperdynamic hearts is more difficult to deal with. The problems in this case mainly relate to inertia and depend on the magnitude of the accelerative forces involved; they are thus greatest with rapidly changing pressure signals. Electrical and mechanical damping systems are of some help but are still not entirely satisfactory. Obtaining acceptable readings of intravascular pressure depends more on skill and experience in positioning the catheter than on any objective knowledge of the scientific principles. Part of the expertise of cardiac catheterization is recognizing an adequate tracing.

Configuration of Pressure Tracings

The pressures in each cardiac chamber are different. Examples are found in the sections on different diseases.

Systemic Arterial Pressure

Systemic arterial pressure is the most important pressure because it is the most closely controlled. Control is established mainly by the action of the baroreceptor system. The normal arterial wave form is shown

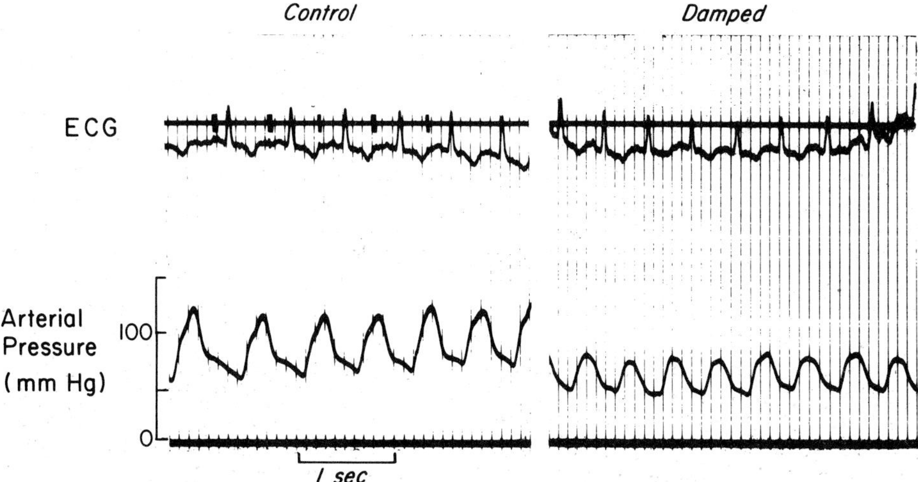

Figure 4–8. Control and damped brachial arterial pressure tracings obtained several minutes apart from a patient with aortic stenosis. Both the amplitude and the mean pressures decreased as the pressure was damped.

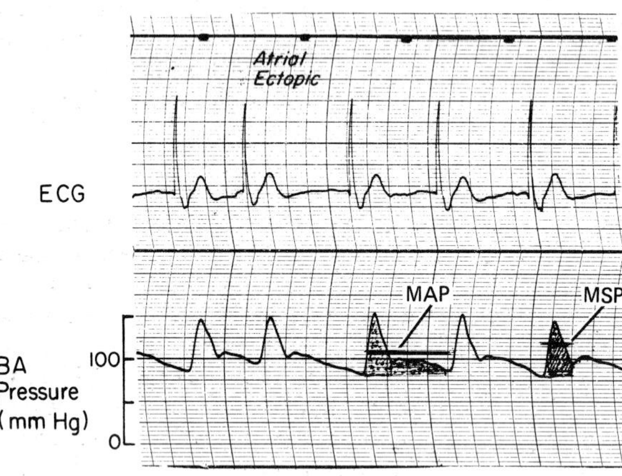

Figure 4–9. ECG and brachial arterial (BA) pressure in a normal subject. Mean arterial pressure (MAP) and mean systolic pressure (MSP) are indicated. One atrial ectopic beat is shown.

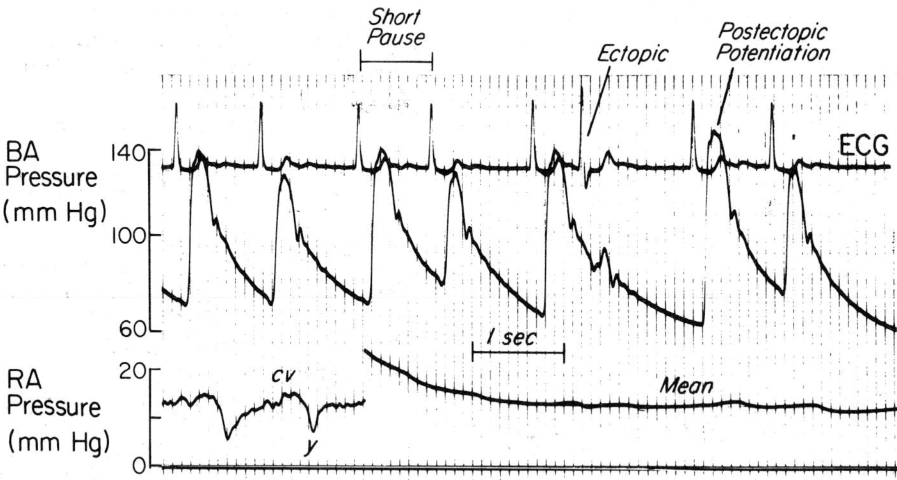

Figure 4–10. Brachial arterial (BA) and right atrial (RA) pressure tracings in a patient with mitral valve disease in atrial fibrillation. The effect of varying cycle lengths and an ectopic beat on arterial pressure are shown.

in Fig 4–9. Peak arterial pressure roughly coincides with the T wave of the ECG. There is often a prominent (dicrotic) notch on the downstroke associated with aortic valve closure. The normal values of 110–120 mm Hg peak systolic and 70–80 mm Hg minimal diastolic pressure change in response to physiologic stimuli such as exercise, excitement, mental stress, sleep, external temperature, posture, pregnancy, growth and development, and age. The range of normal values is wide and increases with age. Mean arterial pressure is usually recorded as the average pressure during the cardiac cycle and is obtained by electrically averaging the pressures recorded during the cycle. The pulse pressure (the difference between systolic and diastolic pressure) is usually about 40 mm Hg and mirrors stroke volume. It changes magnitude in the same direction as stroke volume in exercise, shock, or heart failure. The mean arterial pressure is roughly equal to the diastolic pressure plus one-third of the pulse pressure.

The mean systolic pressure (the average pressure during ventricular systole) can be measured by planimetry of an arterial pressure tracing, as shown in Fig 4–9. The mean systolic pressure gives an indication of the force against which the left ventricle must eject blood. This is not the same as the mean arterial pressure (also indicated in Fig 4–9), which is lower, because it is an average taken over the whole cardiac cycle. The systemic arterial bed senses the mean arterial pressure as the force pressing against the walls of the blood vessels and influencing the rate of wear and tear on vascular tissues. In atrial fibrillation, especially in association with mitral valve disease, the systolic arterial pressure varies with the R–R interval, being lower after a short pause and higher after a long pause, as shown in Fig 4–10. This reflects the effect of ventricular filling on the subsequent ventricular systole in accordance with the Starling mechanism. A similar effect is seen with an ectopic beat, even if it is atrial, as shown in Fig 4–9, in which the level of systolic arterial pressure in the beat after the pause following the ectopic beat is higher. When the ectopic beat is ventricular, the arterial pressure is increased by another mechanism. This is termed postectopic potentiation and involves the excitation-contraction coupling mechanism. It is seen in Fig 4–10, in which the beat following the ventricular ectopic beat shows the highest systolic arterial pressure in the strip. If regular ectopic beats are produced by pacing the heart after each normal beat (paired pacing), an increase in cardiac output results. This is not achieved without an increase in myocardial oxygen consumption.

Pressure Gradients

The pressure difference between different chambers or across valves constitutes a clinically important measurement. The difference between the peak systolic left ventricular pressure and the aortic systolic pressure is called the gradient across the aortic valve. Similarly, the difference between the diastolic left atrial or wedge pressure and the left ventricular diastolic pressure is the gradient across the mitral valve. The gradient is often used as an indication of the severity of stenosis of the affected valve.

The examiner must always take into account the blood flow at the time that pressure measurements are being made. The pressure difference across stenotic valves varies with the flow across the valve, and the relationship is nonlinear. Thus, doubling the blood flow does not merely double the pressure difference but produces closer to a 4-fold increase in pressure difference. These considerations are most important in patients with mitral and aortic stenosis, since they affect calculations concerning the severity of the stenosis. The situation in patients with stenosis is further complicated by changes in heart rate that alter the relative lengths of systole and diastole. Whenever possible, cardiac output and the differences in pressure between 2 chambers should be measured simultaneously. In some cases this is not practical and withdrawal tracings are obtained as the catheter is pulled from one chamber to another. Such tracings have the advantage that errors in calibrating 2 strain gauges are avoided since only one gauge is used. It is important to record the heart rate at the time that each pressure measurement is made as a rough indication that the hemodynamic status of the patient has not changed significantly.

Measurements of Valve Area

Hydraulic formulas have been adapted for use in estimating valve area based on pressure differences and flows across valves. The formulas are most commonly applied to stenotic lesions of the mitral and aortic valves. They are based on steady turbulent flow under stable conditions in smooth, cylindric pipes and should not be used when there is valvular incompetence unless the extra forward flow resulting from the incompetence can somehow be incorporated in the calculations. Although the assumptions underlying the formulas clearly do not apply to flow across cardiac valves, these valve area calculations represent the best available means of obtaining numerical estimates of valve orifice size and do take into account both pressure and flow.

The formula for mitral valve area (MVA) is

$$\text{MVA in cm}^2 = \frac{\text{Diastolic mitral flow in ml/sec}}{31 \times \sqrt{\Delta P} \text{ in mm Hg}}$$

where ΔP is the average pressure difference in mm Hg between the left atrium and the left ventricle during the period of diastolic flow. The value of 31 represents an arbitrary constant required to adjust the units appropriately.

The formula for aortic valve area (AVA) is

$$\text{AVA in cm}^2 = \frac{\text{Systolic flow in ml/sec}}{44.5 \times \sqrt{\Delta P} \text{ in mm Hg}}$$

where ΔP is the mean pressure difference across the valve during the time of systolic flow and 44.5 is the arbitrary constant.

CARDIAC MEASUREMENTS & ELECTRICAL ANALOGUES

Vascular Resistance

In describing the relationships between pressure and flow in the circulation, it is customary to measure vascular resistance as the ratio of pressure to flow. This is a simplistic application of Ohm's law, and it assumes that the circuits involved are linear and that there is a lack of phase difference between pressure and flow. In spite of these inaccuracies, pulmonary and systemic resistances are useful clinical measurements if their limitations are kept in mind.

Conductance (Calculations of Pulmonary & Systemic Vascular Resistance)

In some situations the reciprocal relationship—conductance—is used and the ratio of flow over pressure is calculated. Pulmonary vascular resistance (PVR) is a useful index of the degree of pulmonary vasoconstriction, especially in patients with pulmonary hypertension. It is calculated as follows:

$$\text{PVR in mm Hg/l/min} = \frac{\text{Mean pulmonary arterial pressure} - \text{Mean left atrial pressure}}{\text{Pulmonary blood flow}}$$

If pressure is expressed as dynes/cm^2 and flow in cm^3/sec, the units can be expressed as dynes-sec-cm^{-5}. However, these units do not show how the measurement is derived, and the equivalent units of mm Hg/l/min are preferable. One can convert mm Hg/l/min to dynes-sec-cm^{-5} by multiplying by 80. Systemic vascular resistance (SVR) is the analogous measurement in the systemic circulation. It is calculated as

$$\text{SVR in mm Hg/l/min} = \frac{\text{Mean arterial pressure} - \text{Mean right atrial pressure}}{\text{Systemic blood flow}}$$

Interpretation of Pulmonary Vascular Resistance

The pulmonary vascular resistance is raised in patients with mitral stenosis and in some patients in whom disproportionate pulmonary vasoconstriction occurs. The pulmonary artery pressure may be raised simply because of raised left atrial pressure, as in passive pulmonary hypertension. For example, if the left atrial mean pressure is 30 mm Hg, the mean pulmonary arterial pressure is 38 mm Hg, and the cardiac output is 5 liters/min, the pulmonary vascular resistance is 38 – 30 ÷ 5, or 1.6 mm Hg/l/min, which is in the normal range (< 2 mm Hg/l/min). If the pulmonary arterial pressure were 48 mm Hg, the left atrial pressure 18 mm Hg, and the cardiac output 2.5 liters/min, the pulmonary vascular resistance would be 48 – 18 ÷ 2.5, or 12 mm Hg/l/min, which is markedly raised. The pulmonary vascular resistance normally falls with exercise and is low in patients with uncomplicated left-to-right shunts. Thus, in a patient with an atrial septal defect, pulmonary arterial pressure might be 25 mm Hg, left atrial pressure 10 mm Hg, and pulmonary blood flow 15 liters/min. In this case, the pulmonary vascular resistance would be 25 – 10 ÷ 15, or 1 mm Hg/l/min, which is normal. If pulmonary hypertension develops, or if it has been present since an early age, as in Eisenmenger's syndrome, the pulmonary vascular resistance is increased. The systemic vascular resistance similarly serves to establish whether hypertension is wholly or partly the effect of increased output, or whether an abnormality of the vascular bed is present.

Vascular Compliance

Compliance is the term used in clinical physiology to describe the elastic behavior of elements involved in cardiovascular phenomena. It also refers to the storing of energy in a system, as in a spring. Like the term resistance, it is borrowed from the nomenclature of electrical theory, in which its analogue is capacitance. Compliance is the ratio of volume change to pressure change and is measured in terms of units of volume change per units of pressure change. Decreased compliance involves increased stiffness. Compliance when applied to the atria and ventricles refers to a change in pressure proportionate to a given amount of diastolic filling. If a chamber is compliant, it can accept a large volume with little rise in pressure. The word compliance first came into use in pulmonary physiology as a ratio expressing the volume of lung distention resulting from a given inflating transpulmonary pressure change. The term compliance is also used to describe the elastic behavior of the pulmonary and systemic arterial beds. A compliant bed can distend more with a given pressure change. The venous bed is referred to as a high compliance or high capacitance part of the circulation. The use of a single value to express the compliance of a structure implies a linear relationship between volume and pressure. This is seldom seen in the cardiovascular system. The left ventricle is more compliant at low volumes and becomes less compliant as it is distended. Thus, diastolic pressure tends to remain low until greater levels of distention occur, after which pressure rises more steeply. In general, acute heart failure causes higher diastolic ventricular pressures than do chronic lesions; thus, left ventricular compliance is said to increase with time as the ventricle distends in response to stretching. An indirect indication of ventricular compliance is given by the height of the *a* wave. If the ventricle is stiff and noncompliant, atrial contraction results in a larger pressure wave per given force of atrial contraction.

Time Constant

As a further extension of the electrical analogy it is possible to think in terms of the product of resistance and compliance. The units of this product are

$$\text{Time in min} = \frac{\text{mm Hg}}{\text{l/min}} \times \frac{1}{\text{mm Hg}}$$

The time constant is used in describing the change in left atrial pressure during diastole in a patient with mitral valve disease. In this case, the rate of left atrial pressure fall depends on both the resistance to flow across the mitral valve and the compliance (stiffness) of the left atrium. Either a high resistance to mitral valve flow (stenosis) or a large overdistended compliant atrium can increase the time constant of left atrial emptying. The time constant is the time taken for the pressure to fall to $1/e$ times (37%) the original value, where e is the base of natural logarithms (2.718). The time constants of the systemic and pulmonary circulations can also be determined from the diastolic fall of pressure in the system.

ASSESSMENT OF CARDIAC FUNCTION: "CONTRACTILITY"

One of the most important aspects of clinical cardiac physiology is the assessment of cardiac function. The reserve capacity of the heart is so large that disease must generally be far advanced before resting cardiac function is detectably impaired. Cardiac function normally deteriorates with age and is poor in sedentary people. Therefore, there is usually a mixed load on the heart in patients with cardiac symptoms. In addition to structural and mechanical problems there may be a functional myocardial factor and also an element of poor function owing to disuse. Assessment of cardiac function involves identifying each of these components in any individual patient, and it is most commonly required in patients in whom surgical correction of an anatomic defect is under consideration.

There are many measurements and indices available to assess cardiac dysfunction. None is entirely satisfactory. It is not possible to predict with certainty how a given patient's heart will function when a mechanical load such as valvular stenosis or incompetence is relieved. Thus, the severity of the cardiac lesion is of the greatest importance. There are a number of measurements which give an indication of ventricular function. They involve different levels of invasiveness. Although they are of value in prognosis, their results are almost never a complete contraindication to attempts to correct severe valvular lesions such as aortic stenosis.

Evidence of Impaired Ventricular Function

One of the most readily detectable indicators of poor ventricular function is pulsus alternans. In this condition, every other ventricular beat generates a lower pressure. The slower the heart rate and the bigger the pressure difference between alternate beats, the more significant the finding. The mechanism of mechanical pulsus alternans is unknown, and the finding is significant only if the heartbeat is regular.

An abnormally low cardiac output, usually reflected by an increased arteriovenous oxygen difference, is another finding that suggests myocardial disease, provided that an adequate venous return is present. These findings are not entirely reliable because healthy, well trained athletes often exhibit similar results, and resting values bear no necessary relationship to findings during exercise.

Valsalva's Maneuver

One of the most readily performed tests of cardiac function is to determine the patient's response to straining (Valsalva's maneuver), in which the subject blows against a mercury manometer to raise the intrapulmonary pressure to 40 mm Hg for 10 seconds. The height of the pressure and the duration of the period of strain can be varied, but 40 mm Hg and 10 seconds are conventionally used. The subject should not inhale deeply before straining; introducing a small leak into the system forces the subject to use the thoracic and abdominal muscles (rather than the cheeks) to generate the pressure. The sudden strain of the maneuver causes a complex sequence of mechanical and reflex changes in the circulation that depend on 2 factors, the level of cardiac function and effective central blood volume, and the speed and magnitude of the baroreceptor responses to a change in arterial pressure. The maneuver is best performed with a continuous recording of arterial pressure and is shown in Fig 4–11.

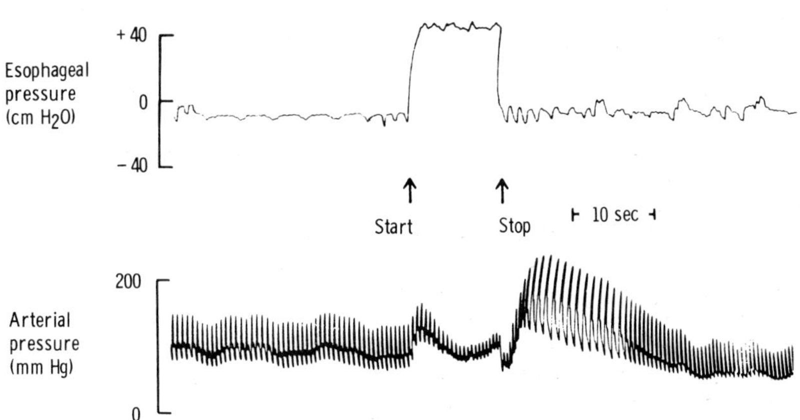

Figure 4–11. Tracing of the normal blood pressure and pulse response to straining (Valsalva's maneuver) in a normal man, recorded with a needle in the brachial artery.

A. Normal Response: The first effect is a rise in arterial pressure due to the transmission of applied pressure to the intrathoracic structures (heart and great vessels). The magnitude and speed of the rise depend on the suddenness and force of the strain. The arterial pressure then starts to fall, the pulse pressure narrows because the venous return is cut off, and the normal heart responds to a decrease in filling with a fall in output. The rate and magnitude of the fall during this period of strain reflect the size of the central blood volume.

B. Square Wave Response: In the extreme case of a large central blood volume, there is sufficient blood in the central circulation to maintain a constant pressure throughout the period of strain. This type of response is termed a square wave response and has in the past been incorrectly termed the heart failure response. It is seen in congestive heart failure but is also found in overhydrated normal subjects and in symptom-free patients with large left-to-right shunts, especially those with atrial septal defects. Fig 4–12 shows an example from a patient with atrial septal defect. The rate at which the heart empties during the period of straining depends on cardiac output. In congestive heart failure, the central circulation is overloaded and the cardiac output is low, so that the heart does not empty; thus, a square wave response is due to a combination of factors.

The reflex changes of Valsalva's maneuver depend on baroreceptor activity. In a normal response to Valsalva's maneuver, the fall in blood pressure and pulse pressure triggers reflex tachycardia within about 5–7 seconds and a rise in peripheral resistance a few seconds later. Thus, the arterial pressure stops falling and starts to rise toward the end of the period of strain. When the strain ends, the blood pressure falls and venous return is restored. The cardiac output increases and the blood pressure rises. The peripheral resistance is still raised in response to the previously low pressure, and the surge of blood into constricted vessels causes an overshoot of pressure. This overshoot in turn causes reflex bradycardia and vasodilatation which restore the pressure to normal.

The response to Valsalva's maneuver offers a convenient means of testing the reactivity of the baroreceptor reflex arc. It is primarily used in the investigation of patients with disease of the autonomic nervous system.

Left Ventricular Function

The size of the left ventricle, its ejection fraction, and the speed of ejection constitute the most reliable indices of ventricular function as determined by ventricular angiograms. Similar measurements can be obtained from echocardiograms, but these are much less reliable, although they do have the advantage of using noninvasive methods. It is important to remember that several crucial assumptions are made whenever these calculations are performed. For example, even the measurement of ventricular volume is likely to involve an assumption about the shape of the ventricle (spherical or ellipsoid), and if the measurement utilizes echocardiography, a single diameter is ordinarily measured and the radius cubed to give a volume measurement. Such measurements as the rate of circumferential shortening involve similar assumptions about ventricular shape which tend to be forgotten by those interpreting the studies.

Maximum dp/dt. The maximum rate of change of left ventricular pressure (dp/dt^{max}) during the phase of isometric contraction and relaxation is a popular and useful indicator of ventricular function. The measurement is valid only if a catheter tip manometer is used. Some authorities have advocated the measurement of $dp/dt^{max} \div p$, in which the maximal rate of change in pressure is divided by the actual pressure at that instant to give an index that has the units of sec^{-1}. The difficulty of defining "contractility" and the lack of any satisfactory means of measuring the force of cardiac contraction have already been mentioned in Chapter 1.

It seems clear that no assessment of ventricular function can predict how the heart will behave after a mechanical load is removed. Even retrospective analysis of preoperative studies cannot distinguish between those who will survive and those who will succumb to an operation. There is thus no alternative to accepting patients for surgical treatment even though operative risks may be high. Statistical analysis has shown that left ventricular function measurements are significant indicators of the prognosis, but they should not be used to make absolute predictions or to make the decision in individual cases. The most logical approach—although it is not easy to achieve—is to follow patients as closely as possible, recognize surgically treatable lesions at an early stage, and operate before severe myocardial damage occurs.

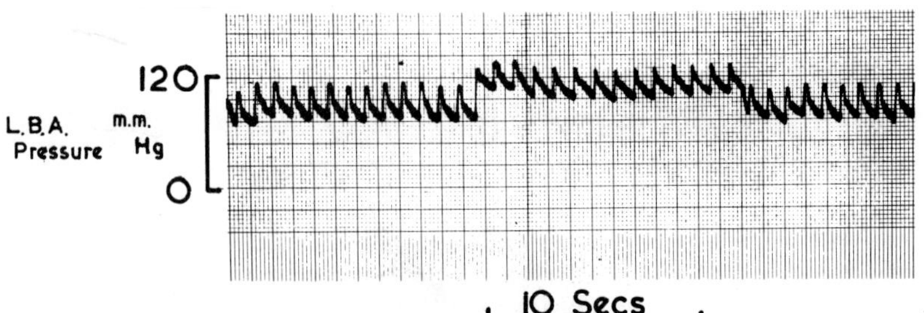

Figure 4–12. Arterial pressure tracing showing the response to Valsalva's maneuver in a patient with atrial septal defect and a large pulmonary blood flow. The pulse pressure is maintained during the period of strain, and there is no overshoot on release of the strain. LBA, left brachial artery.

Cardiac Work

The concept of measuring cardiac work is an appealing one and is now used more frequently as a means of expressing the response of the heart to different interventions (digitalization, afterload reduction, or cardioversion). The external mechanical work done by the heart can be expressed in rigorous physical terms as the integral of instantaneous intracardiac pressure with respect to volume. In practice, the less rigorous measurement of the mean arterial pressure multiplied by the average cardiac output in l/min (minute work in kg m/min) or stroke volume (stroke work in kg m/min) and work index or stroke volume index obtained by dividing these values by the calculated body surface area are commonly used. It is important to remember the short cuts that are necessarily made in deriving these values. As mentioned previously, work done against increased aortic pressure involves a greater expenditure of energy than work done to increase blood flow at normal pressure. The measurement of cardiac work lumps these 2 kinds of work together and fails to distinguish between them. Furthermore, any increase in cardiac work is likely to use more energy because of an increase in myocardial oxygen consumption. Any mechanism that increases cardiac work, as for example, therapeutic intervention following myocardial infarction, may not necessarily be beneficial.

Cardiac Function Curves

Measurements of stroke work or stroke work index can be plotted against end-diastolic pressure levels to give a clinically useful indication of changes in cardiac function. It is important to be aware of the assumptions made in the measurements and to take care not to overinterpret the data. Physicians who have not been directly concerned with the collection of basic information tend to be overly impressed by the "scientific" nature of clinical physiologic data, particularly when such information is presented in terms of work, power, and function curves. Clinical physiologic data must not be allowed to unduly influence the examiner when other forms of information point in another direction.

NORMAL VALUES

Rest

The normal resting cardiac output of about 6 liters/min (cardiac index about 4.05 liters/min/m^2) varies from about 3.5–7.5 liters/min. The values in the direct Fick equation which give this figure are blood oxygen capacity about 200 ml/l, arterial oxygen saturation 97%, arterial oxygen content 194 ml/l, mixed venous oxygen saturation 72%, mixed venous oxygen content 144 ml/l, arteriovenous oxygen content differences 50 ml/l, and oxygen consumption 300 ml/min.

The normal blood volume of about 5 liters is composed of about 2.75 liters of plasma and 2.25 liters of red cells to give a hematocrit of 2.25 ÷ 5, or 45%. The volume of blood in the heart and lungs (central blood volume) totals about 1.5 liters. About 0.9 liters are contained in the pulmonary arteries, capillaries, and veins, but only about 75 ml are in the pulmonary capillaries at any instant. The total volume of blood in the heart is about 0.6 liters. Left ventricular volume at the end of diastole is about 150 ml; with a stroke volume of 100 ml and an ejection fraction of 67%, the end-systolic volume is 50 ml. The conventional normal values for arterial pressure of 120 mm Hg systolic and 80 mm Hg diastolic should be thought of as normal for young adult subjects. Arterial pressure varies with age. The problem of deciding the upper limit of normal is dealt with in Chapter 9. Mean arterial pressure changes little with posture; systolic pressure may fall when the patient stands up after having been supine. Depending on the patient's effective blood volume, diastolic pressure rises, pulse pressure decreases, and heart rate increases.

The normal values for intracardiac pressures in mm Hg are shown in Table 4–2.

The normal mitral valve area is greater than 3 cm^2. Values of about 1.5 cm^2 indicate slight stenosis and 1.0 cm^2 or less, significant stenosis. Aortic valve area is greater than 2 cm^2. Values of about 1 cm^2 indicate mild stenosis and 0.7 cm^2 or less, significant stenosis. The normal pulmonary vascular resistance is

Table 4–2. Normal values for intracardiac pressures.

Site	Systolic Pressure (mm Hg)	Diastolic Pressure (mm Hg)	Mean Pressure (mm Hg)
Right atrium	*a* up to 7 *v* up to 5	*x* up to 3 *y* up to 3	Less than 5
Right ventricle	up to 25	End pressure before *a* up to 3 End pressure on *a* up to 7	Not applicable
Pulmonary artery	up to 25	Up to 15	Up to 18
Left atrium (direct or indirect wedge)	*a* up to 12 *v* up to 10	*x* up to 7 *y* up to 7	Up to 10
Left ventricle	120	End pressure up to 7 End pressure on *a* up to 12	Not applicable

less than 2 mm Hg/l/min, or less than 160 dynes-sec-cm^{-5}. The normal systemic resistance is less than 20 mm Hg/l/min, or less than 1600 dynes-sec-cm^{-5}.

The normal left ventricular work output at rest is about 1 watt or 6 kg-m/min. This value increases about 5-fold during exercise. The maximal rate of change of left ventricular pressure is about 1200 mm Hg/sec, and the corresponding figure for the right ventricle is about 250 mm Hg/sec.

The normal resting ventilation is about 5 liters/min. Normal arterial P_{O_2} is between 70 and 100 mm Hg, P_{CO_2} is 37–42 mm Hg; and pH is 7.36–7.43 units.

Exercise

During moderate exercise (sufficient to increase heart rate to about 120/min), oxygen consumption increases from about 250–300 ml/min to 1200–1500 ml/min. Arteriovenous oxygen difference increases from 50 ml/l to about 100 ml/l; and cardiac output to about 15 l/min. Blood gas tensions and pH do not change significantly. Ventilation increases to 30–40 l/min. Stroke volume increases to about 125 ml and arterial pulse pressure to about 60 mm Hg, with a systolic pressure of 130 mm Hg and a diastolic pressure of 70 mm Hg. With more severe exercise (oxygen consumption about 2500 ml/min) most untrained normal subjects show evidence of metabolic acidosis, with an increase in arterial lactate, a fall in pH, and a fall in arterial P_{CO_2} to about 35 mm Hg. The maximal heart rate in young adults of about 195/min falls to about 170 at the age of 60 years. Most patients with heart disease do not complain of dyspnea until their maximal oxygen consumption falls to less than 1200–1500 ml/min. By the time they are seriously disabled, their maximal cardiac output is about 10 liters/min.

• • •

References

Blink JR, Jewell BR: The meaning and measurement of myocardial contractility. Pages 225–285 in: *Cardiovascular Fluid Dynamics.* Vol 1. Bergel DH (editor). Academic Press, 1972.

Carlsson E: *Measurement of Cardiac Chamber Volumes and Dimensions by Radiographic Methods: A Methodological Study With Some Physiological Applications.* Univ of California Press, 1970.

Chaitman BR & others: Objective and subjective analysis of left ventricular angiograms. Circulation 52:420, 1975.

Cournand A & others: Measurement of the cardiac output in man using technique of catheterization of the right auricle or ventricle. J Clin Invest 24:106, 1945.

Dodge HT, Kennedy JW, Petersen JL: Quantitative angiocardiographic methods in the evaluation of valvular heart disease. Prog Cardiovasc Dis 16:1, 1973.

Dodge HT, Sandler H, Baxley WA: Usefulness and limitations of radiographic methods for determining left ventricular volume. Am J Cardiol 18:10, 1977.

Fick A: Ueber die Messung des Blutquantums in den Herzventrikeln: Sitzungsberichte der phys-med. Gesellschaft zu Würzburg 16, 1870.

Filley GF: *Acid-Base and Blood Gas Regulation.* Lea & Febiger, 1971.

Fry DL: Physiologic recording by modern instruments with particular reference to pressure recording. Physiol Rev 40:753, 1960.

Ganz W, Swan HJC: Measurement of blood flow by thermodilution. Am J Cardiol 29:241, 1972.

Goerke RJ, Carlsson E: Calculation of right and left cardiac ventricular volumes. Invest Radiol 2:360, 1967.

Gorlin R, Gorlin SG: Hydraulic formula for calculation of the area of the stenotic mitral valve, other cardiac valves, and central circulatory shunts. Am Heart J 41:1, 1951.

Greene DG & others: Estimation of left ventricular volume by one-plane cineangiography. Circulation 35:61, 1967.

Holmgren A: Circulatory changes during muscular work in man. Scand J Clin Lab Invest 8 (Suppl 24):1, 1956.

Hugenholz PG, Wagner HR, Sandler H: The in vivo determination of left ventricular volume. Circulation 37:489, 1968.

Jefferson K, Rees S: *Clinical Cardiac Radiology.* Butterworth, 1973.

Marshall RJ, Shepherd JT: *Cardiac Function in Health and Disease.* Saunders, 1968.

McIlroy MB: Pulmonary shunts. In: *Handbook of Physiology.* Vol 2. Fenn WO, Rahn H (editors). American Physiological Society, 1965.

Murray JF: *The Normal Lung: The Basis for Diagnosis and Treatment of Pulmonary Disease.* Saunders, 1976.

Ross J Jr: Afterload mismatch and preload reserve: A conceptual framework for the analysis of ventricular function. Prog Cardiovasc Dis 58:255, 1976.

Severinghaus JW: Blood gas calculator. J Appl Physiol 20:1108, 1966.

Severinghaus JW, Bradley AF: Electrodes for blood P_{O_2} and P_{CO_2} determination. J Appl Physiol 13:515, 1958.

Sharpey-Schafer EP: Effects of Valsalva's manoeuver on normal and failing circulation. Br Med J 1:693, 1955.

Starmer CF, McIntosh HD, Whalen RE: Electrical hazards and cardiovascular function. N Engl J Med 284:181, 1971.

Stewart GN: Researches on the circulation time and on the influences which affect it. J Physiol 22:159, 1897.

Swan HJC: Indicator-dilution methods in the diagnosis of congenital heart disease. Prog Cardiovasc Dis 2:143, 1959.

5...
Special Investigations: Noninvasive

INTRODUCTION

Special cardiologic investigations are dealt with under the headings of noninvasive and invasive studies. This chapter deals with noninvasive investigations, defined as procedures that do not involve cutting or puncturing the skin and implying an absolute absence of complications. The distinction is slightly blurred in the case of analyses of venous blood, such as enzyme determinations in myocardial infarction, and radioisotope studies, in which intravenous injections are made. These studies, together with standard laboratory tests involving venipuncture, are classified as noninvasive studies.

Routine Cardiologic Investigations

The clinical examination of all cardiac patients is incomplete without the recording of a 12-lead ECG and a chest x-ray, preferably a cardiac series consisting of posteroanterior, lateral, and right and left anterior oblique views. In some cases, fluoroscopy is substituted for chest x-rays, but this has the disadvantage of not providing a permanent record. The physician should interpret the ECG and chest x-rays independently before reading the opinions of the radiologist or electrocardiographer who may have provided a written interpretation of the findings. Both investigations form such an important aspect of the clinical evaluation of the patient's condition that a valid opinion about a case cannot be given until both have been seen by the physician.

Special Investigations

All investigations other than chest x-rays and the ECG are considered to be special studies indicated by some clinical finding. Standard laboratory tests of blood, urine, feces, sputum, bone marrow, and cerebrospinal fluid may be required in the diagnostic investigation of the patient with cardiovascular disease. The laboratory findings in each type of cardiac disease are covered in the chapters dealing with that disease.

Special Cardiovascular Studies

Two main types of information are sought by cardiologic studies: anatomic (structural) and physiologic (functional). While the relationship between structure and function is usually close, it is important to keep clearly in mind what specific information is being sought in any study. In many types of investigations, both structural and functional information is provided (eg, cardiac catheterization). In general, anatomic abnormalities relate to a specific diagnosis, whereas physiologic findings are more pertinent to degrees of functional impairment.

Most forms of cardiac investigation start as research procedures. Whether any new procedure will ultimately be accepted by the medical community is not usually decided for several years. The decisive factors include the clinical usefulness of the procedure, the prevalence of the conditions for which it is indicated, and economic factors such as cost of equipment that are outside the scope of this book. Not surprisingly, the current cardiologic literature is largely preoccupied with new forms of investigation which are still in the uncertain stage between research studies and standard procedures. It is virtually impossible to keep up with all of the available methods of cardiologic study, and an attempt will be made in this book to identify those procedures which the authors feel have reached the stage of being "standard" for each condition.

In all forms of investigation, it is important for the physician to bear in mind the cost to the patient in danger, discomfort, and expense and to make a clear distinction in his mind between clinically indicated studies and ancillary confirmatory procedures. In many cases an accurate diagnosis is required, and in cases in which cardiac surgery is contemplated an accurate diagnosis is in fact essential in every case. Because being right 85–90% of the time is not enough, studies must sometimes be done for confirmatory purposes even though the diagnosis is clinically almost certain.

The indications for the various special noninvasive investigations described in this chapter are discussed in the chapter dealing with specific types of heart disease. The present chapter is concerned with the principles involved in the investigations and with the procedures themselves, with only a brief account of their applications to patient care. The chapter starts with the 2 routine investigations required in all cardiac patients: ECG recording and interpretation of chest x-rays.

ECG RECORDING

Technic

The simplest diagnostic procedure with which every physician must be familiar is the taking of a standard 12-lead electrocardiogram (ECG). Modern electrocardiographs have become simple to use, and problems are most likely to be related to matching wall plugs, connecting the cables to the electrodes properly, and electrical interference. Nondisposable electrodes must be kept clean, and the use of an excessive amount of paste should be avoided because it interferes with specific precordial lead placement. With any type of electrode, providing adequate localized skin contact with the right amount of electrode paste is important. Correct and consistent precordial electrode placement is important, especially when serial records are needed. Interference from other electrical equipment, especially electric blankets in domiciliary practice, should be suspected when 60-cycle noise is encountered. Increased electronic filtering should not be used to eliminate this, as it will almost certainly decrease the frequency response of the equipment and give a damped and inaccurate ECG.

Each lead of the ECG should be properly calibrated.

Safety

The examiner should remain alert to the possibility of ground loops, which present a risk of electrocution when more than one electrical device is attached to the patient. Patients with temporary artificial pacemakers are particularly vulnerable, because currents as low as 10 microamperes applied directly to the endocardium via the pacemaker catheter can cause ventricular fibrillation.

Reporting Results; Display of Tracings

The tracing should be examined, mounted, reported, and the results returned to the patient's chart as soon as possible (within 24 hours). Care must be taken to correctly identify the ECG with the patient's name and hospital number. The role of the frontal plane axis in determining heart position is important. The interpretation should include the rhythm, rate, axis, duration of the P–R, QRS, and Q–T_c intervals, and description of P, QRS, and ST–T abnormalities in each lead, followed by an estimate of the significance of the findings. A statement of the clinical probabilities is desirable; pathognomonic findings are exceptional.

The degree of confidence the electrocardiographer has in the interpretation can be expressed by such phrases as "consistent with . . .," "suggestive of . . .," "probably due to . . .," etc. Serial records or comparisons with previous tracings are often necessary for proper interpretation. Records obtained over 1–5 minutes or 4- to 24-hour monitoring or those obtained during or after exercise or interventions such as carotid sinus massage may clarify the relationship between symptoms and ECG abnormalities. The role of medications and metabolic or electrolyte state must be considered in interpretation. For example, digitalis or quinidine therapy or hypokalemia or hyperkalemia can often be confused with primary myocardial disease (Figs 5–1 to 5–4).

One should be circumspect in interpretation. Every attempt should be made to recognize the diagnostic value of small abnormalities, but it is also necessary to avoid the dangers of "overreading" minor abnormalities.

Computer analysis of ECGs has not become widely accepted because of the variation in interpretations by different observers and the reliability of the computer program used.

Difficulties are encountered in the interpretation of arrhythmias and in comparison with previous records. Qualitative changes (eg, ST segment contours) are less well dealt with than quantitative ones.

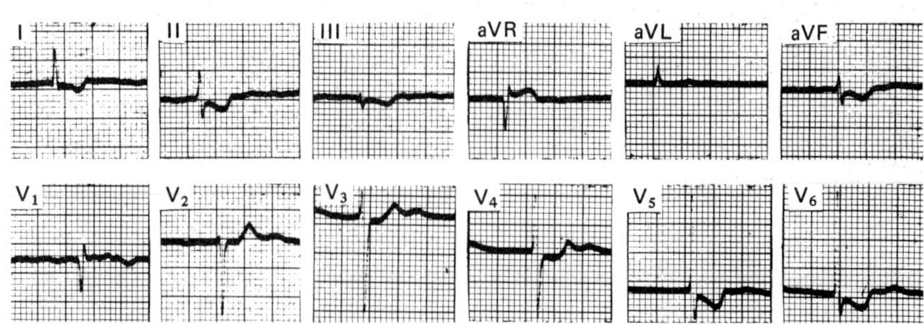

Figure 5–1. Digitalis effect. Note the ST segment depression. This produces an oblique downward configuration of the first portion of the ST in leads I, II, III, aVF, and V_{5-6}. There is a rounded ST segment depression in V_{3-4}. As a result, the T waves are "dragged" downward. There is reciprocal ST elevation in aVR. The above changes are indicative of digitalis effect but do not indicate digitalis toxicity. The rhythm is atrial fibrillation. (Reproduced, with permission, from Goldman MJ: *Principles of Clinical Electrocardiography,* 9th ed. Lange, 1976.)

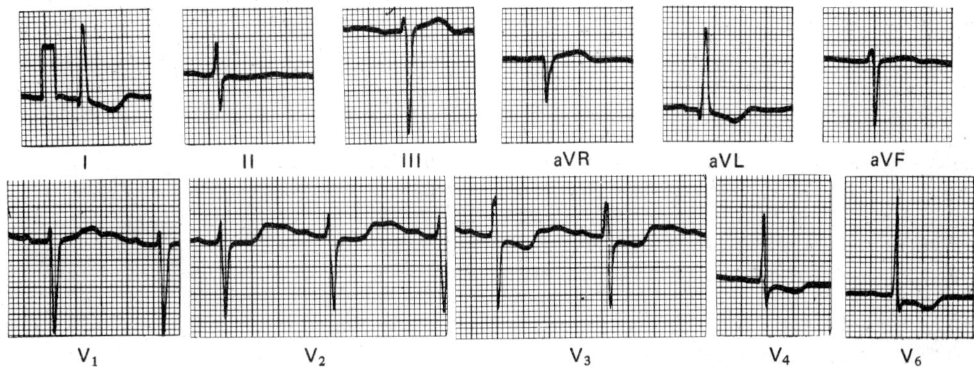

Figure 5–2. Effect of quinidine. The rhythm is regular sinus; P–R = 0.2 sec. The R in aVL = 14 mm. There is ST depression and T wave inversion in I, aVL, and V_{2-6}. The measured Q–T interval (see V_{2-3}) = 0.6 sec (Q–T_c = 0.65 sec). *Clinical diagnosis:* Aortic stenosis; quinidine therapy for previous ventricular arrhythmias. The R voltage in aVL and some of the ST–T changes are due to left ventricular hypertrophy. The long Q–T interval is due to quinidine. (Reproduced, with permission, from Goldman MJ: ***Principles of Clinical Electrocardiography,*** 9th ed. Lange, 1976.)

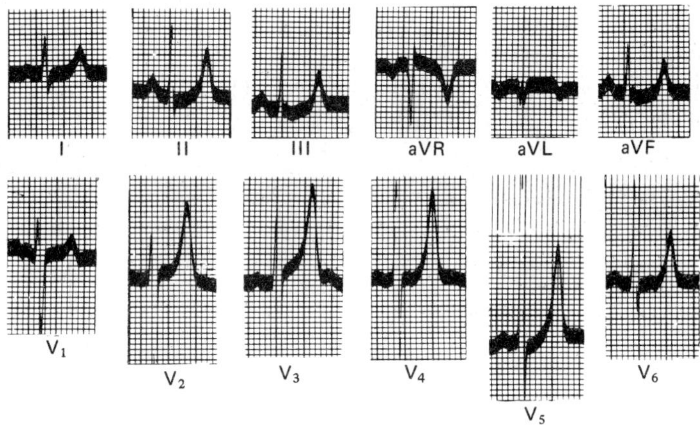

Figure 5–3. Hyperkalemia (chronic glomerulonephritis with uremia). Tall slender T waves are seen in I, II, III, aVF, and V_{2-6}. The rhythm is regular sinus; QRS interval = 0.09 sec. Serum potassium = 7.2 mEq/l. (Reproduced, with permission, from Goldman MJ: ***Principles of Clinical Electrocardiography,*** 9th ed. Lange, 1976.)

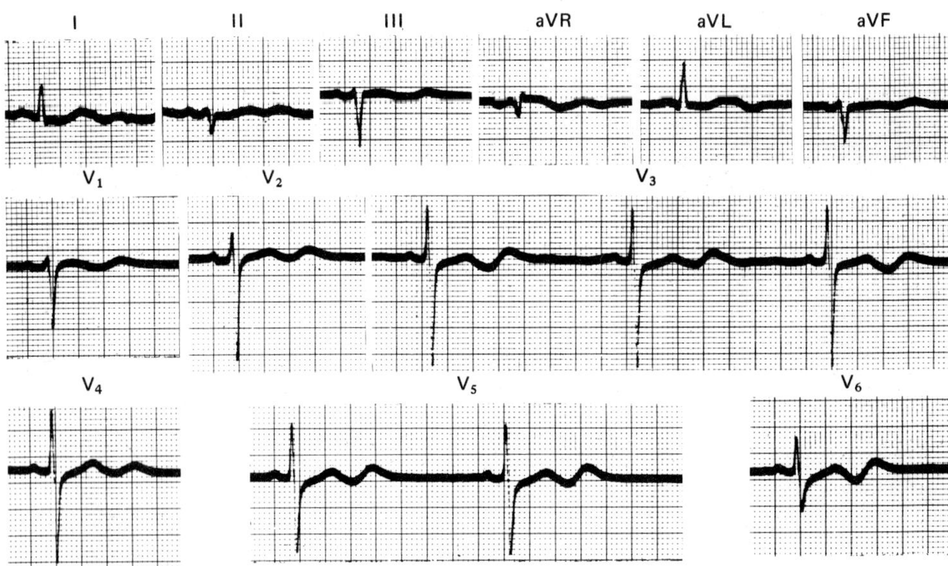

Figure 5–4. Hypokalemia (Cushing's syndrome). Regular sinus rhythm; P–R = 0.16 sec; QRS = 0.1 sec. The frontal plane QRS axis = –40 degrees. There is ST depression in leads I, aVL, and V_{3-6}. Prominent U waves are seen in all precordial leads. The measured Q–T interval = 0.51 sec, but when corrected for a heart rate of 37 the Q–T_C = 0.39 sec. Serum potassium = 2.5 mEq/l. (Reproduced, with permission, from Goldman MJ: *Principles of Clinical Electrocardiography,* 9th ed. Lange, 1976.)

CHEST X-RAYS

Size of Heart Shadow

A cardiac series of chest x-rays (posteroanterior, lateral, and left and right oblique views) should be obtained in all patients with suspected heart disease. In Fig 5–5 are shown the features visible in normal chest x-rays that indicate which cardiac structure forms the outline of the heart in each view. The posteroanterior chest x-ray should be taken with the x-ray tube 6 feet* from the x-ray so that distortion of heart size is avoided. This film is used for overall assessment of heart size. As a rough guide, the widest part of the heart should be less than half the diameter of the thorax. The Ungerleider tables, which relate the transverse diameter of the heart to the patient's height and weight, are probably more reliable than the simple measurement. Hearts larger than the correspondingly appropriate measures in the table are virtually always enlarged.

After looking at the heart size, one identifies the structures on the left border of the heart.

Shape of the Heart: Posteroanterior View (Fig 5–5A)

From above downward one sees the aortic knob or knuckle, the pulmonary artery, the left atrial appendage, and the rounded shadow of the left ventricle. The left atrial appendage is not normally visible as a bulge. The right border of the heart is formed by the superior vena cava or aorta above and by the right atrium below, and it is difficult to be sure whether the atrium is enlarged or displaced when the heart shadow is large. *Note: Differentiation between the left and right ventricle cannot always be made accurately on chest radiography; in doubtful cases, it is important to examine the ECG to obtain accurate evidence about ventricular dominance.* The ECG reflects hypertrophy, whereas the chest film reflects enlargement.

Shape of the Heart: Lateral View (Fig 5–5B)

The lateral chest x-ray is useful in assessing left ventricular and left atrial size. These 2 structures form the posterior wall of the heart, and marked posterior displacement of the cardiac shadow is usually seen best when the esophagus has been filled with barium. The downward sweep of the posterior part of the left ventricle passes below and behind the inferior vena cava when the left ventricle is enlarged. The right ventricle tends to lie close to the sternum when it enlarges. This sign is not specific, however, and displacement as well as enlargement may be responsible.

Shape of the Heart: Right Anterior Oblique View (Fig 5–5C)

The right anterior oblique view of the cardiac silhouette is most valuable in the assessment of enlargement of the right ventricular outflow tract and main pulmonary artery. These structures form the anterior border of the heart in this view, and absence or de-

*This distance varies in countries using the metric system.

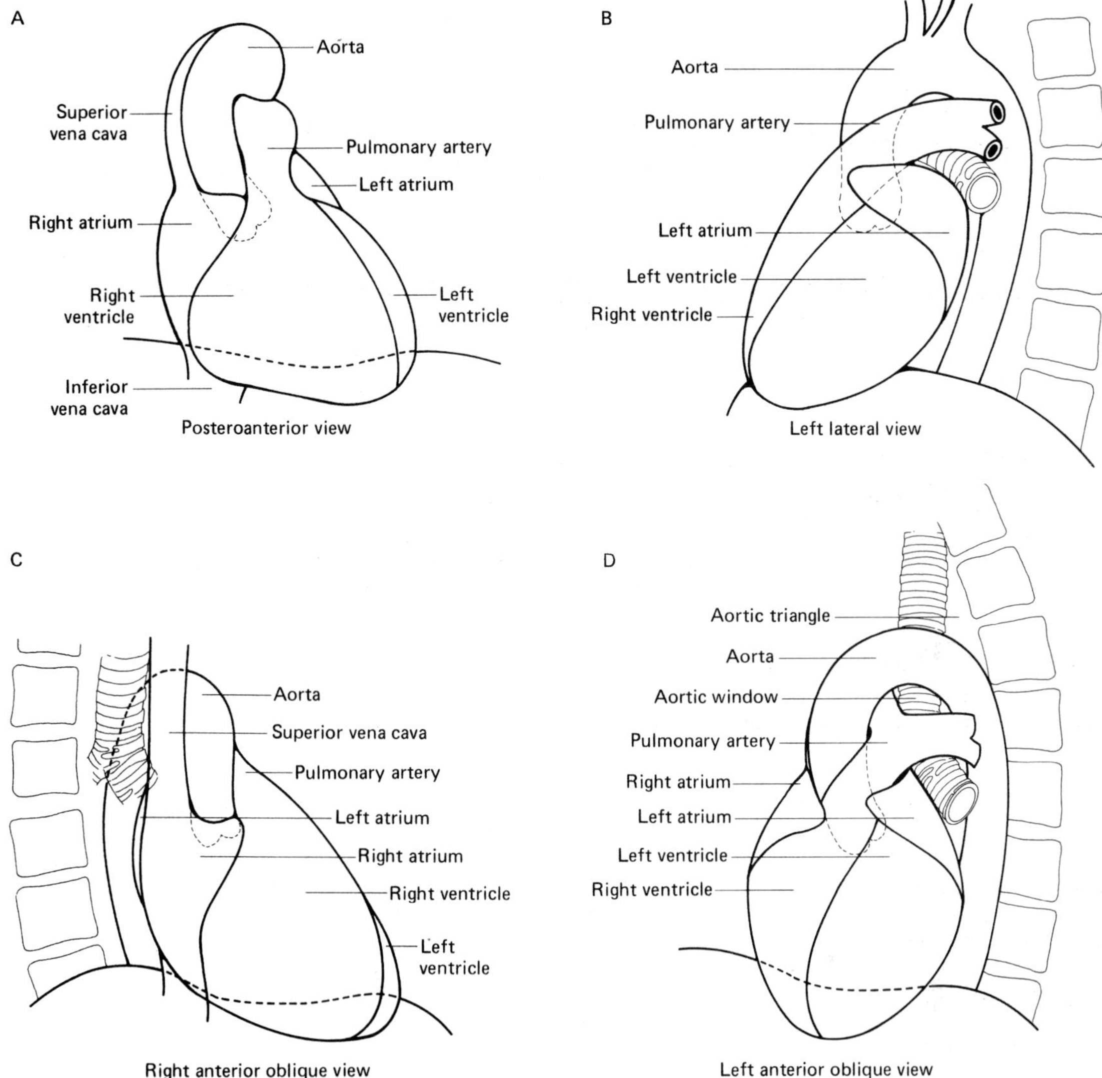

Figure 5–5. Diagrams showing radiologic features in a normal cardiac series. *A,* posteroanterior view; *B,* left lateral view; *C,* right anterior oblique view; *D,* left anterior oblique view.

crease in the size of the outflow tract, as in Fallot's tetralogy and pulmonary atresia, is also discernible.

Shape of the Heart: Left Anterior Oblique View (Fig 5–5D)

The left anterior oblique view is most valuable in left-sided lesions. The left atrium and left ventricle form the posterior edge of the cardiac shadow in this view, and the aortic arch is seen in its widest aspect, arching from front to back above the cardiac shadow. Two landmarks in this view are the aortic triangle above and the aortic window below the arch. Their boundaries are indicated in Fig 5–5D. Coarctation of the aorta and patent ducutus arteriosus are best seen in this view, which is also best for demonstrating dilatation of the ascending aorta. The degree of penetration which is optimal for cardiac x-rays is greater than that for pulmonary x-rays. Overpenetrating x-rays are sometimes useful, especially to demonstrate the size of the left atrium.

Lung Fields

Interpretation of the chest x-ray also involves examination of the lung fields for evidence of pulmonary congestion, redistribution of blood flow, pulmonary plethora in left-to-right shunts, and pulmonary oligemia with reduced pulmonary blood flow. Pulmonary edema tends to be central in origin and to spread out from the root of the lung. It is not infrequently asymmetric, perhaps because the patient lies on one side or the other. An example is shown in Fig 5–6.

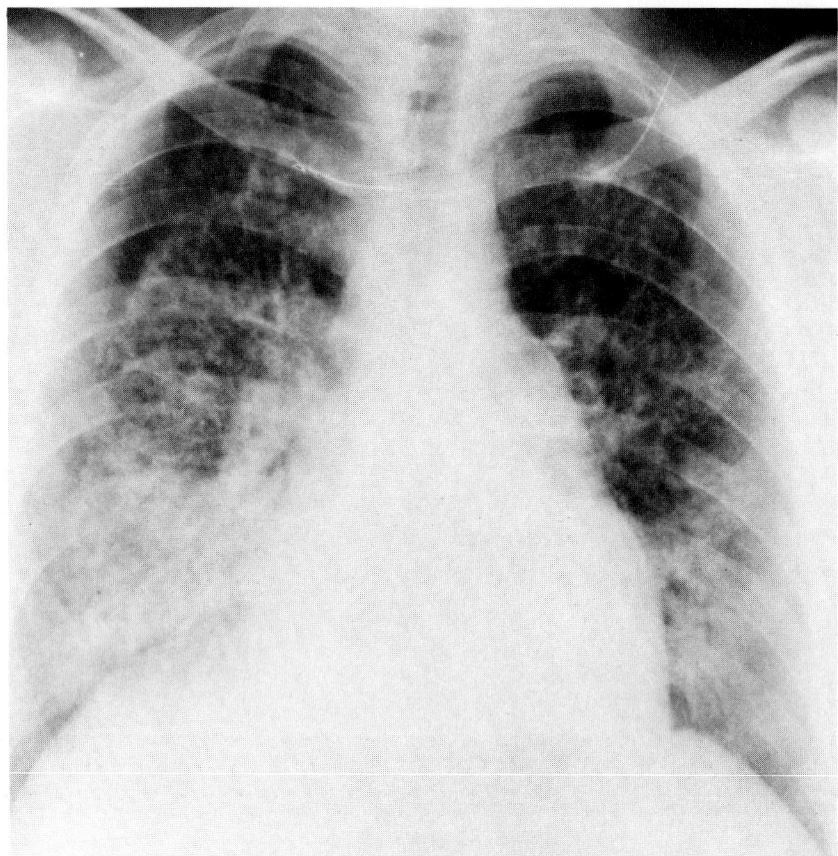

Figure 5–6. Chest x-ray of a patient with pulmonary edema showing perihilar ("bat's wing") distribution, especially on the right side. The lung periphery is relatively free of infiltrate.

ECHOCARDIOGRAPHY

Echocardiography has rapidly become a standard (though not routine) form of investigation of many kinds of heart disease. The apparatus required is moderately expensive, but the information gained is important enough to warrant having an instrument in every major hospital.

In all forms of ultrasonic examination, a piezoelectric crystal is intermittently excited electronically to transmit repeated bursts of sound waves. The standard cardiologic equipment uses 1000 bursts per second of ultrasound with a frequency of 2.25 megahertz (MHz) (2.25 million cycles per second). These waves penetrate tissues, and reflected waves of ultrasound travel back to the crystal. The time required for the reflected sound signals to return to the crystal varies with the distance traveled and provides a form of echo ranging. The transducer is switched to receive when it is not transmitting and puts out an electronic signal proportionate to the intensity of the echoes. Ultrasound is absorbed by bone and by air-containing lung tissue. Blood is a poor reflector in comparison with solid tissues such as muscle, vessel wall, and valvular tissue. Access to the heart for ultrasonic examination in adults is limited to areas where the heart abuts against the intercostal spaces, and it is the motion of the solid cardiac structures that is detected by echocardiography. The penetration of tissue by ultrasound depends on the basic frequency used. High-frequency ultrasound (10 MHz) penetrates poorly, but the standard cardiac echocardiographic frequency (2.25 MHz) provides adequate penetration to examine structures up to 20 cm (8 inches) from the surface. An aqueous gel is used to couple the transducer to the skin, and the transducers are focused usually at a depth of 5–10 cm. Several modes available for the display of the ultrasonic echoes received by the transducer are illustrated in Fig 5–7.

A Mode

In an A mode echo system, the intensity of the returning echo signal is displayed on the horizontal (X) axis of an oscilloscope, and the time required for the information to travel from the transmitter to the target and back to the receiver is displayed on the vertical (Y) axis. The highly reflective structures in the ultrasonic beam are thus shown, one above the other, with the nearest at the top and the farthest at the bottom of the

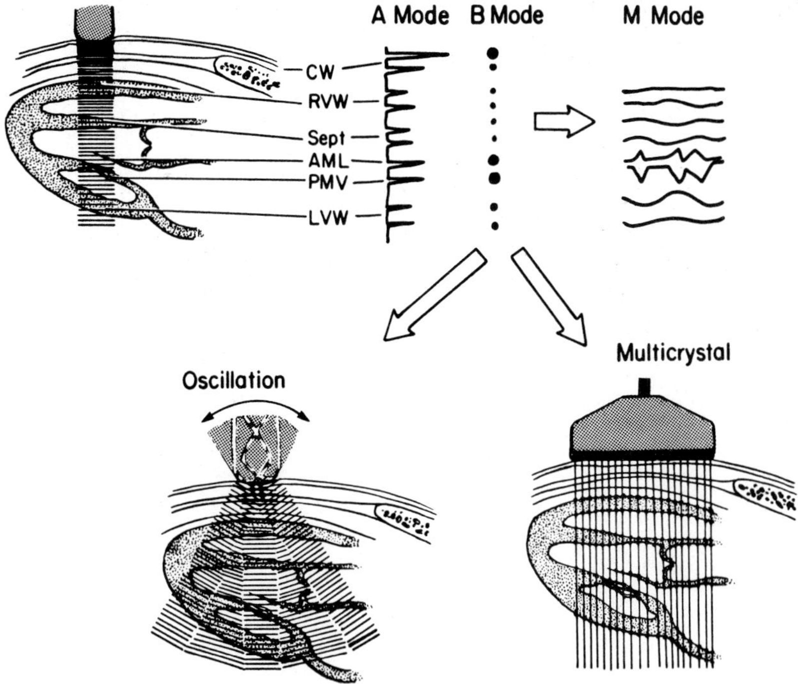

Figure 5–7. Diagram showing different modes of display of echocardiographic information. The structures depicted from front to back are the chest wall (CW), the right ventricular wall (RVW), the interventricular septum (Sept), the anterior mitral valve leaflet (AML), the posterior mitral valve leaflet (PMV), and the posterior wall of the left ventricle (LVW). (Courtesy of NH Silverman and NB Schiller.)

oscilloscope screen. Since the heart is moving, these echoes dance up and down during the cardiac cycle. The most rapidly moving structures are the valve leaflets, and in the view depicted in Fig 5–7 the anterior leaflet of the mitral valve is the most prominent structure. It abuts on the more fixed posterior mitral leaflet during systole and moves anteriorly during diastole. The basic A mode echo display system is seldom used in echocardiography today.

B Mode

In B mode echocardiography, the intensity of the echo signal is displayed on the Z (brightness) axis of the oscilloscope screen. A spot of brightness proportionate to the intensity of the echo signal is displayed on the screen, with distance from the transducer appearing on the Y axis. Pure B mode echoes are seldom used but form the basis of the standard M mode echocardiogram.

M Mode

In M mode (motion) echocardiography, a B mode echo signal is recorded on the Y axis and time on the X axis, either by sweeping the oscilloscope screen or by photographing the oscilloscope face on moving paper. Thus, the conventional M mode display, which is the most commonly used form of ultrasonic examination, shows time on the X axis, distance on the Y axis, and intensity of the echo on the Z axis. An ECG is recorded for timing, and the movement of the structures within the beam is displayed during the cardiac cycle. As shown in Fig 5–7, the movement of the mitral valve leaflets is readily seen, giving a pattern that is repeated with each heartbeat.

B Mode Scanners

A more advanced and much more expensive technic is now becoming available in which a B mode echographic tracing is rapidly and repeatedly scanned across a sector field at a rate sufficient to provide a continuous image to the unaided eye (frequency about 30/sec). The process depicted in Fig 5–7 can be either mechanical, with rapid oscillation of the transducer, or electronic, in which an array of crystals is sequentially and repeatedly excited to provide a similar form of scan. The B mode scanner provides a 2-dimensional pie-shaped image within which the reflective cardiac structures move in 2 dimensions which are at 90-degree angles to one another. By moving the transducer appropriately, transverse, sagittal, or coronal sections can be displayed and the scope of the ultrasonic examination greatly increased. The alternative (multicrystal) form of scanner illustrated in Fig 5–7 creates a 2-dimensional image by means of a linear array of crystals. This is valuable in examining stationary objects in a readily accessible field (eg, abdomen), but it is almost impossible to position a multicrystal scanner over the heart without having the field of a number of units

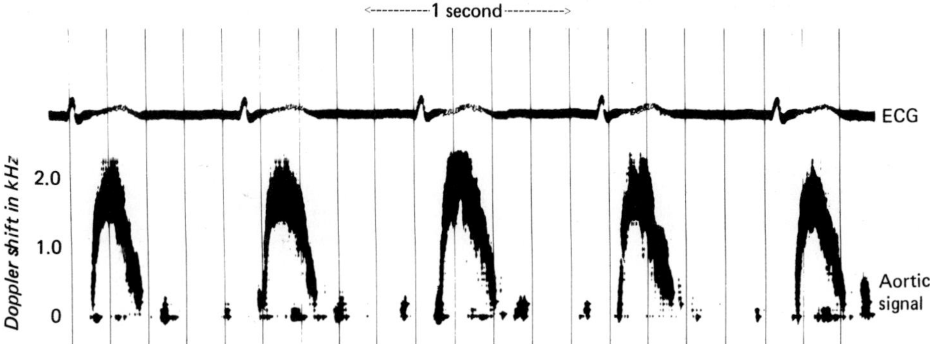

Figure 5–8. Doppler blood velocity signal and ECG recorded from the aorta in the suprasternal notch of a normal subject. The Doppler signal, which is proportionate to the velocity of blood flow, occurs during systole.

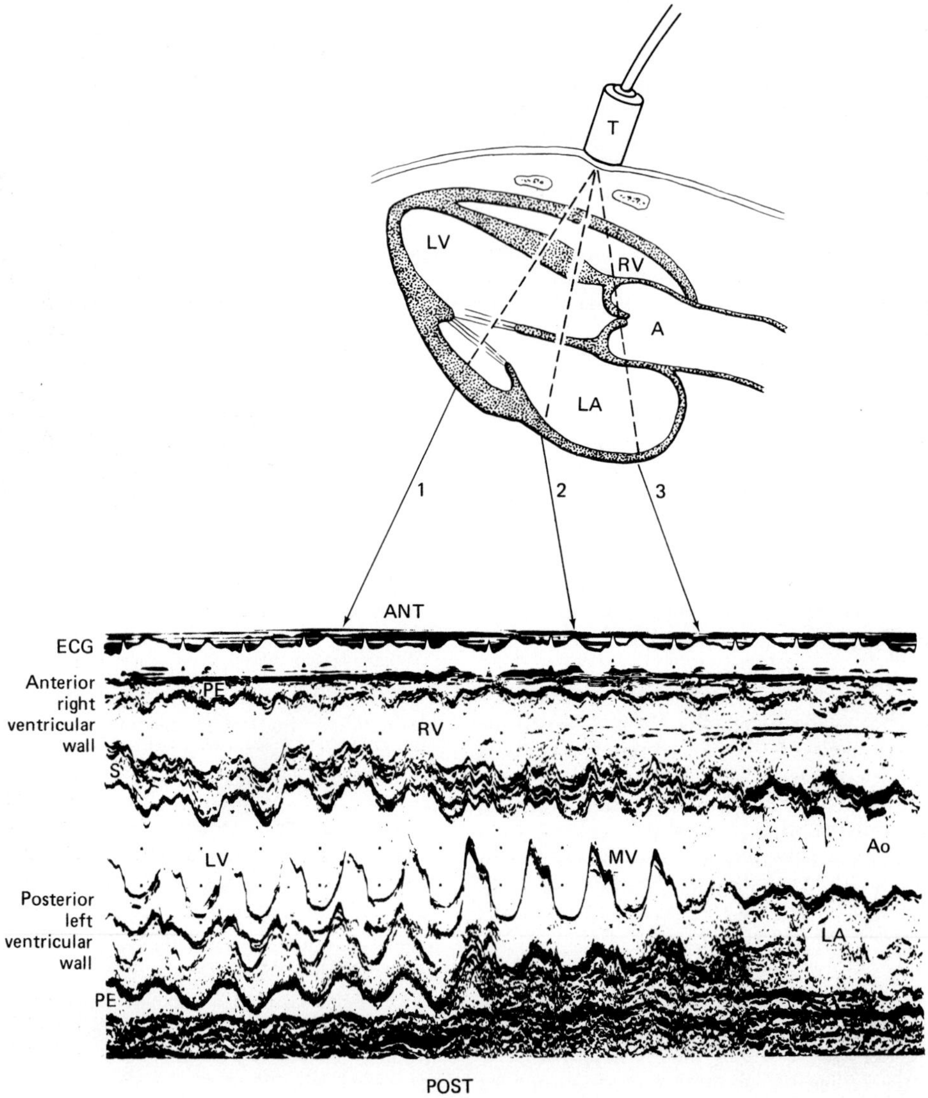

Figure 5–9. M Mode echocardiogram showing normal intracardiac structures in a patient with pericardial effusion. The transducer was moved from position 1 to position 3 during the recording. Ant, anterior; RV, right ventricular cavity; LV, left ventricular cavity; S, septum; MV, mitral valve; Ao, aorta; LA, left atrium; PE, pericardial effusion; POST posterior. (Courtesy of NB Schiller.)

blocked out by the ribs or sternum. Multicrystal scanners are thus of little value in cardiologic studies because of the limited access to the heart and the rapid motion of cardiac structures.

Limitations

The principal limitation of ultrasonic examination, as compared to radiography, is that sound has a slower velocity in tissue (about 1.5 km/sec) than x-rays (2.99×10^5 km/sec). The longer wavelength of the more slowly moving sound waves limits the resolution of ultrasonic examination. Ultrasound is, however, much less damaging to tissues than x-rays, and there is as yet no clinical evidence of ill effects despite extensive use of the technic over several years.

Doppler Blood Velocity Measurement

The velocity of blood flow can also be measured by ultrasonic methods. This technic (not yet standard) is a moderately expensive adjunct to M mode echocardiography. When ultrasound is reflected from a moving structure (eg, blood), there is a shift in the frequency of the reflected sound wave whose magnitude depends on—among other things—the speed at which the blood is traveling. Methods based on this principle have the potential for measuring aortic and pulmonary arterial blood velocity, and, if the cross-sectional area of the vessel involved can be measured, the method can be used to measure blood flow instantaneously by noninvasive means. There are still problems in calibrating the signals obtained, but they are not insurmountable. In combination with echocardiographic measurements, Doppler blood velocity measurements are helpful in the assessment of cardiac structure and function. A tracing of an aortic velocity signal obtained from the suprasternal notch in a normal subject is shown in Fig 5–8. The velocity of blood flow can be seen to increase in a linear manner (constant acceleration) during the rapid ejection phase of left ventricular systole.

Normal M Mode Findings

The structures that can be observed in what has come to be the basic echocardiographic scanning maneuver are shown in Fig 5–9.

A. Mitral Valve: With the transducer (T) in constant contact with the patient's skin through a layer of coupling jelly, the beam is aimed posteriorly through the fourth intercostal space to the left of the sternum. In position 1, indicated in Fig 5–9, the mitral valve leaflet echo is readily picked up. The beam intersects the right ventricular cavity, the interventricular septum, and the left ventricular cavity before passing through the mitral valve to reach the posterior wall of the left ventricle. In the example shown in Fig 5–9, there is an echo-free space anterior to the right ventricle and behind the left ventricle owing to pericardial effusion. Clearer pictures can usually be obtained when the heart is surrounded by fluid, which appears to act like aqueous coupling jelly to improve the quality of the signals. A more detailed picture of the mitral valve and its motions is shown in Fig 5–10. During systole, the anterior leaflet lies close to the posterior leaflet. Diastole starts from a point designated "d," and the anterior leaflet moves forward toward the septum, reaching the "e" point. As flow falls off in mid diastole, the anterior leaflet moves backward to a minimum point (f) before moving forward again as a result of atrial contraction to an "a" point. Throughout the whole of diastole, the posterior leaflet has remained close to the posterior wall of the left ventricle.

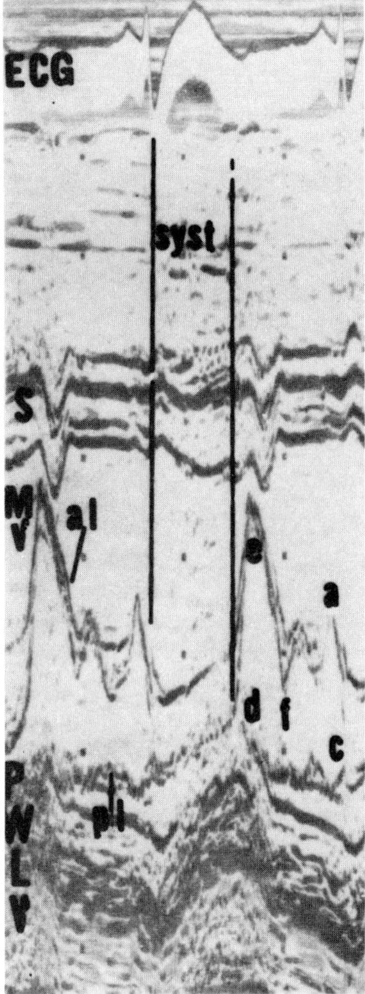

Figure 5–10. M mode echocardiogram showing details of the motion of a normal mitral valve. S, septum; syst, systole; MV, mitral valve; al, anterior leaflet; pl, posterior leaflet; PWLV, posterior wall of left ventricle. Points d, e, f, a, and c are peaks and troughs of mitral valve motion. (Courtesy of NB Schiller.)

B. Left Ventricle: By tilting the transducer in the direction of the feet, a picture of the left ventricular cavity is obtained. This is shown in detail in Fig 5–11. The posterior motion of the ventricular septum during systole, combined with the anterior motion of the posterior wall of the left ventricle, reduces the anteroposterior diameter of the ventricular cavity. The mitral valve is seen in this view, and in the patient in Fig

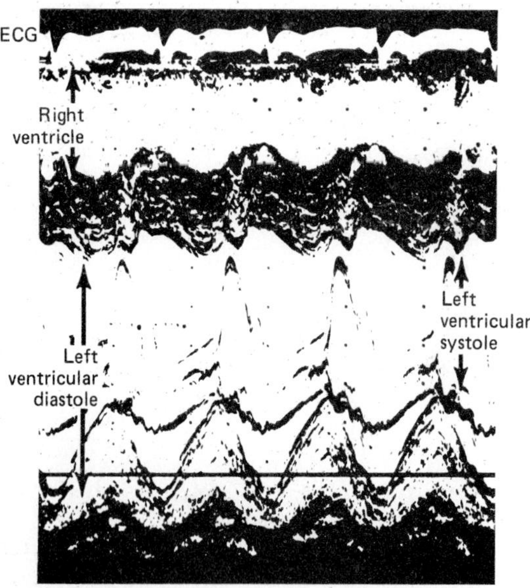

Figure 5–11. M mode echocardiogram showing the right and left ventricles in a patient with a high cardiac output. The arrows indicate the relative dimensions of the left ventricular systole and diastole. (Courtesy of NB Schiller.)

5–11 the range of motion of the heart wall and the valve is increased because of a high output state. The dominant left ventricle pulls the right ventricle posteriorly during systole, and the narrowing due to posterior systolic movement of the anterior wall of the right ventricle is not well shown.

C. **Aortic Valve**: Tilting the transducer upward and slightly medially through position 2 to position 3 in Fig 5–9 brings the aortic valve into view. The details seen in this view are illustrated in Fig 5–12. The right ventricular outflow tract comes to lie at the front of the display, and the left atrium, rather than the left ventricle, comes to lie behind the aorta as the mitral valve falls out of the picture. Its position in the center of the display is taken by the aorta, whose dense walls move forward during systole. The aortic valve leaflets can be seen during systole. They are less reflective than the mitral valve leaflets in normal subjects. The diastolic diameter of the aorta in Fig 5–12 is greater than normal because the patient had Marfan's syndrome. The left atrial diameter in this view is smaller than the aortic diameter. Normally, the left atrial dimension is greater than the aortic.

Clinical Uses of Echocardiography

The clinical value of echocardiography is now clearly established. Its main use is as a preliminary screening test, and it has not displaced cardiac cathe-

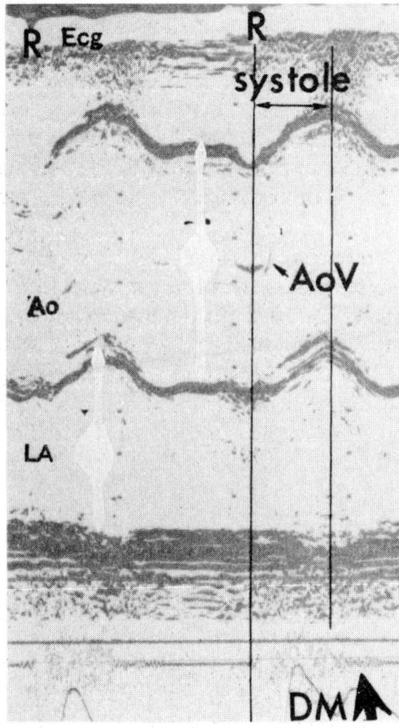

Figure 5–12. M mode echocardiogram showing the aortic valve (AoV) and the aorta (Ao) in a patient with Marfan's syndrome. The left atrium (LA) is seen to lie posteriorly. DM refers to an aortic diastolic murmur seen in the phonocardiogram.

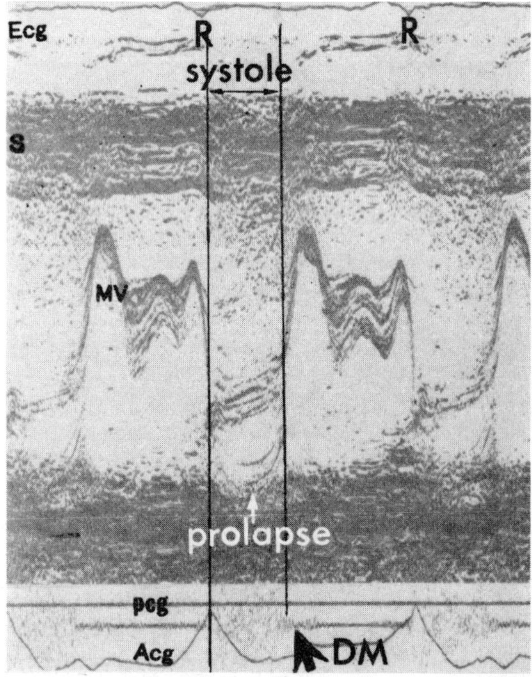

Figure 5–13. M mode echocardiogram of the mitral valve (MV) showing systolic prolapse in the same patient with Marfan's syndrome shown in Fig 5–12. A phonocardiogram (pcg) and apexcardiogram (Acg) are included, and the same diastolic murmur (DM) is shown. R, R wave of ECG; S, ventricular septum; ant, anterior leaflet; post, posterior leaflet. (Courtesy of NB Schiller.)

terization and angiography as a definitive preoperative diagnostic study. Echocardiography may be of value in evaluating nearly all the manifestations of heart disease (pericardial, valvular, congenital, hypertensive, coronary, and primary myocardial disease). It is of particular value in pericardial effusion (Fig 5–9) and in mitral valve disease—either incompetence or stenosis—especially in detecting prolapse of the valve leaflets during systole. An example is shown in Fig 5–13 from the same patient (with Marfan's syndrome) as in Fig 5–12. During systole, a gap appears between the anterior leaflet of the mitral valve and the posterior leaflet.

Another condition in which echocardiography is particularly valuable is hypertrophic obstructive cardiomyopathy. In this condition, as illustrated in Fig 5–14, there is systolic anterior motion of the mitral valve. The valve abuts against the hypertrophied interventricular septum during systole, and the motion coincides with the development of a systolic murmur.

The measurements made during echocardiographic examinations are valid in that they are calibrated in millimeters. There is, however, a certain element of skill and judgment in setting the controls which determine the intensity, and it is possible to blank out structures. The large step involved in calculating chamber volumes from single dimensions of cardiac chambers is likely to involve error. The technic, in spite of these minor disadvantages, has proved extremely useful in clinical cardiology, and the full potential of ultrasonic examination of the heart has yet to be realized.

Real Time B Mode Cardiac Scanning

The newer, more expensive, and more advanced technics which are available for scanning the heart give a 2-dimensional moving image. The display is a pie-shaped field 60–80 degrees wide and 15 cm or more deep. The 2 main views which are proving most useful are illustrated in Figs 5–15 and 5–16. In the apical view, the transducer is aimed upward and to the right from the cardiac apex. The 4 chambers of the heart can be seen in this view, with the atrioventricular valves separating the atria from the ventricles. The ECG serves to identify the phase in the cardiac cycle at which the single frame of the moving image was recorded. In the sagittal view, the transducer is placed on the front of the chest over the third or fourth intercostal space and scans a sector parallel to the long (apex to base) axis of the heart. The still pictures of the oscilloscope screen shown in Figs 5–15 and 5–16 do not do full justice to the technic because the motion of the heart cannot be shown. The full potential of this dynamic form of noninvasive examination, which uses very expensive equipment, has not yet been fully realized.

PHONOCARDIOGRAPHY

Phonocardiography is a standard (but not routine) study which is perhaps the most difficult and subjective of all noninvasive investigations. The apparatus is not expensive and is available in most large hospitals. Although modern bedside auscultation owes an enormous debt to phonocardiography, a recording of heart sounds is seldom of critical clinical importance. Phonocardiography is most valuable as a means of timing the events of the cardiac cycle and demonstrating their relationship to indirectly recorded pressure tracings such as the apexcardiogram (Fig 5–17), indirect carotid pulse tracings, external phlebograms, and stethographic recordings of respiration. It is of little value in analyzing the sound content of murmurs and heart sounds because the harmonic content of the recordings obtained is so dependent on the electrical filters used, the placing of the microphones, and the position of the patient. In consequence, phonocardiography is of most practical value in teaching auscultation and in settling differences of opinion. Its value in confirming the auscultatory findings is well established. Most people find it easier to appreciate sensory information when it is received simultaneously by 2 senses. Thus, listening to a patient's heart with a stethoscope and watching an oscilloscopic recording of the sounds at the same time is most valuable in teaching. After the student has become experienced in auscultation, the

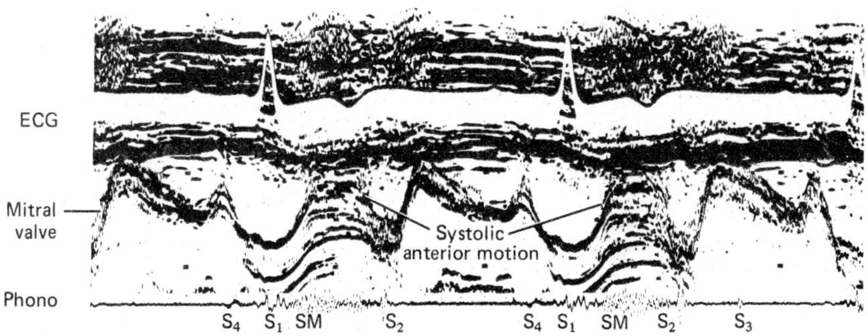

Figure 5–14. Echocardiogram, ECG, and phonocardiogram showing systolic anterior motion of mitral valve in a patient with hypertrophic obstructive cardiomyopathy. SM, systolic murmur. (Courtesy of NB Schiller.)

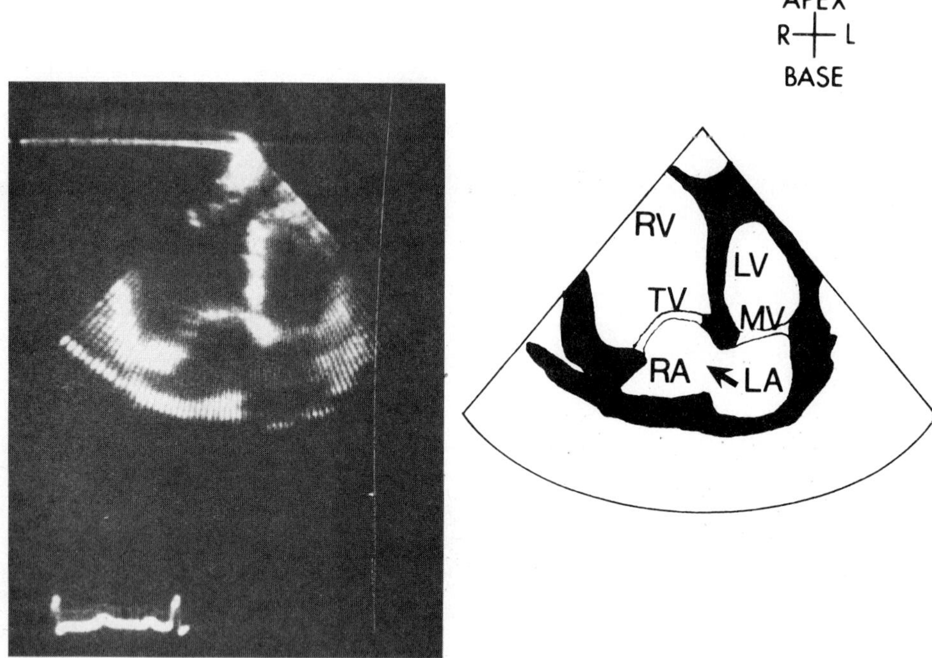

Figure 5–15. Sector scan of the heart in an apical view in a patient with atrial septal defect. An explanatory diagram is shown on the right. RV, right ventricle; TV, tricuspid valve; RA, right atrium; LV, left ventricle; MV, mitral valve; LA, left atrium with arrow pointing to the atrial defect. (Courtesy of NB Schiller.)

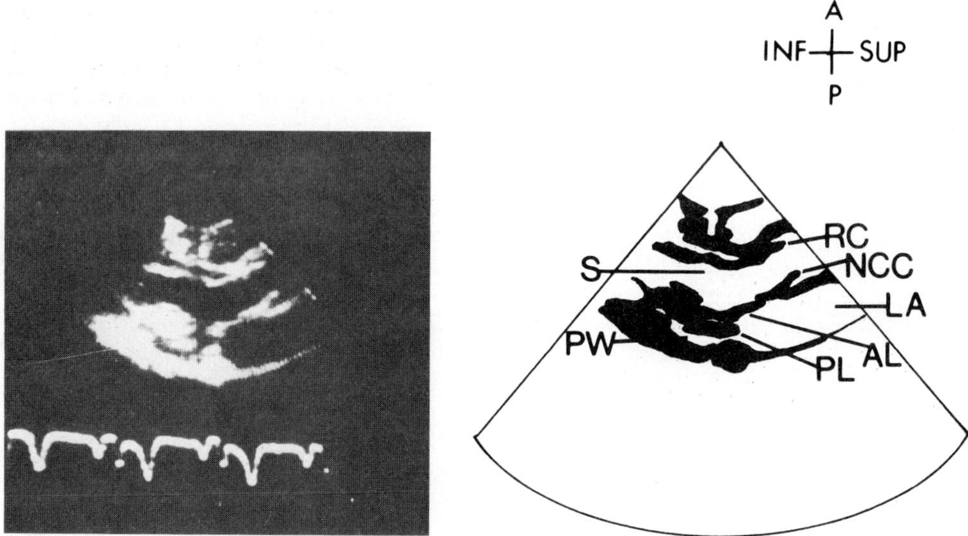

Figure 5–16. Sector scan of the heart in a sagittal view in a normal subject. An explanatory diagram is shown on the right. RC, right coronary aortic valve cusp; NCC, noncoronary cusp; S, ventricular septum; LA, left atrium; PW, posterior ventricular wall; AL, anterior mitral leaflet; PL, posterior leaflet. (Courtesy of NB Schiller.)

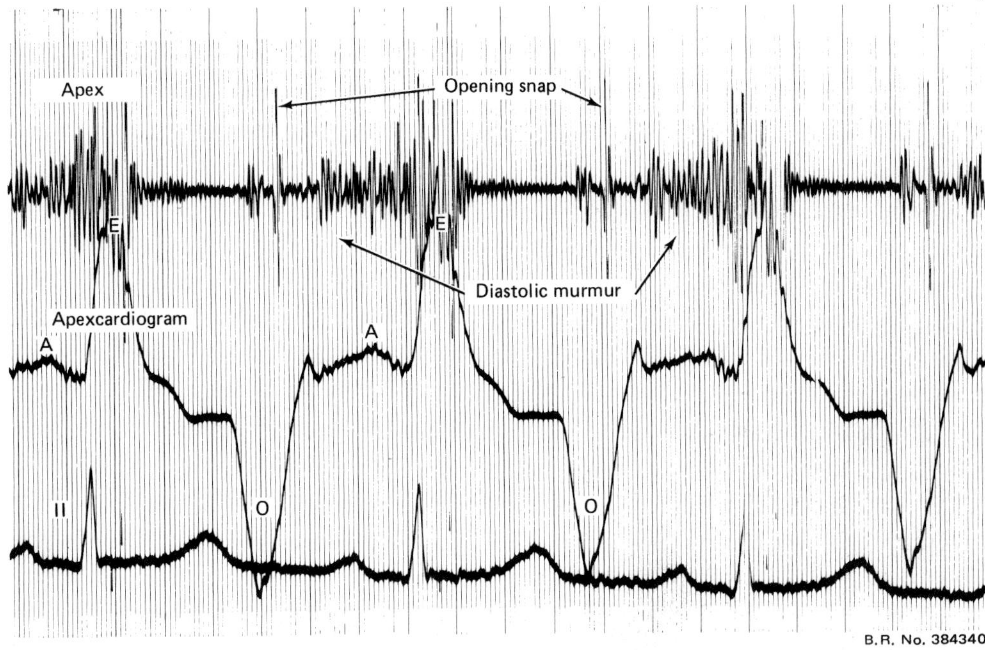

Figure 5–17. Phonocardiogram, apexcardiogram, and ECG of a patient with mitral stenosis. *A* represents the deflection due to atrial contraction, *E* the maximum systolic outward motion, and *O* the maximum diastolic inward motion. The phonocardiogram shows a clear opening snap followed by a diastolic murmur with presystolic accentuation.

phonocardiograph is less often needed. In practice, the principal reason for recording a phonocardiogram is to obtain a permanent tracing of the auscultatory findings. The tracing is thus an adjunct to and not a substitute for careful auscultation by a trained clinical observer. A possible exception to this generalization is in patients with artificial heart valves. Prosthetic valves give relatively clear sounds in which changes can indicate the development of thrombotic material on the valve, changes in ball size in a ball and cage device, or the early stages of valve dehiscence. Serial phonocardiography can be useful in following the postoperative course of patients with artificial valves on a long-term basis.

SPECIAL ELECTROCARDIOGRAPHIC INVESTIGATIONS

1. VECTORCARDIOGRAPHY

Vectorcardiography is a well-established electrocardiographic technic which has never achieved great popularity. The apparatus required is not expensive but differs from that needed for routine scalar electrocardiography. The electrical potentials generated by the heart during the cardiac cycle are displayed in a form which emphasizes their spatial orientation as vectors in the 3 conventional planes of the body: horizontal, sagittal, and frontal (Fig 5–18). Various lead systems are available, but the Frank lead system, using the X, Y, Z system, is most popular. The electrocardiographic signals are displayed on the X and Y axes of an oscilloscope, and the dimension of time is indicated by interrupting the ECG signal every 2 msec. The ECG signal traces out loops on the screen during the P, QRS, and T phases of the cardiac cycle. The standard 12-lead ECG was so well established by the time vectorcardiography became available that the dominant position of the ECG as an empirical pattern-recognition system has never been seriously challenged.

2. CONTINUOUS ECG MONITORING

Continuous electrocardiographic monitoring outside a laboratory has become a standard means of identifying arrhythmias, and this technic should be considered in any patient in whom an exact diagnosis of an arrhythmia or conduction defect has not yet been established. The apparatus required, which is moderately expensive, is available in most large hospitals. It is also routinely used in coronary care units to obtain the earliest possible indication of the onset of arrhythmia or to monitor the frequency of premature beats. Monitoring for up to 12 hours can readily be carried out in

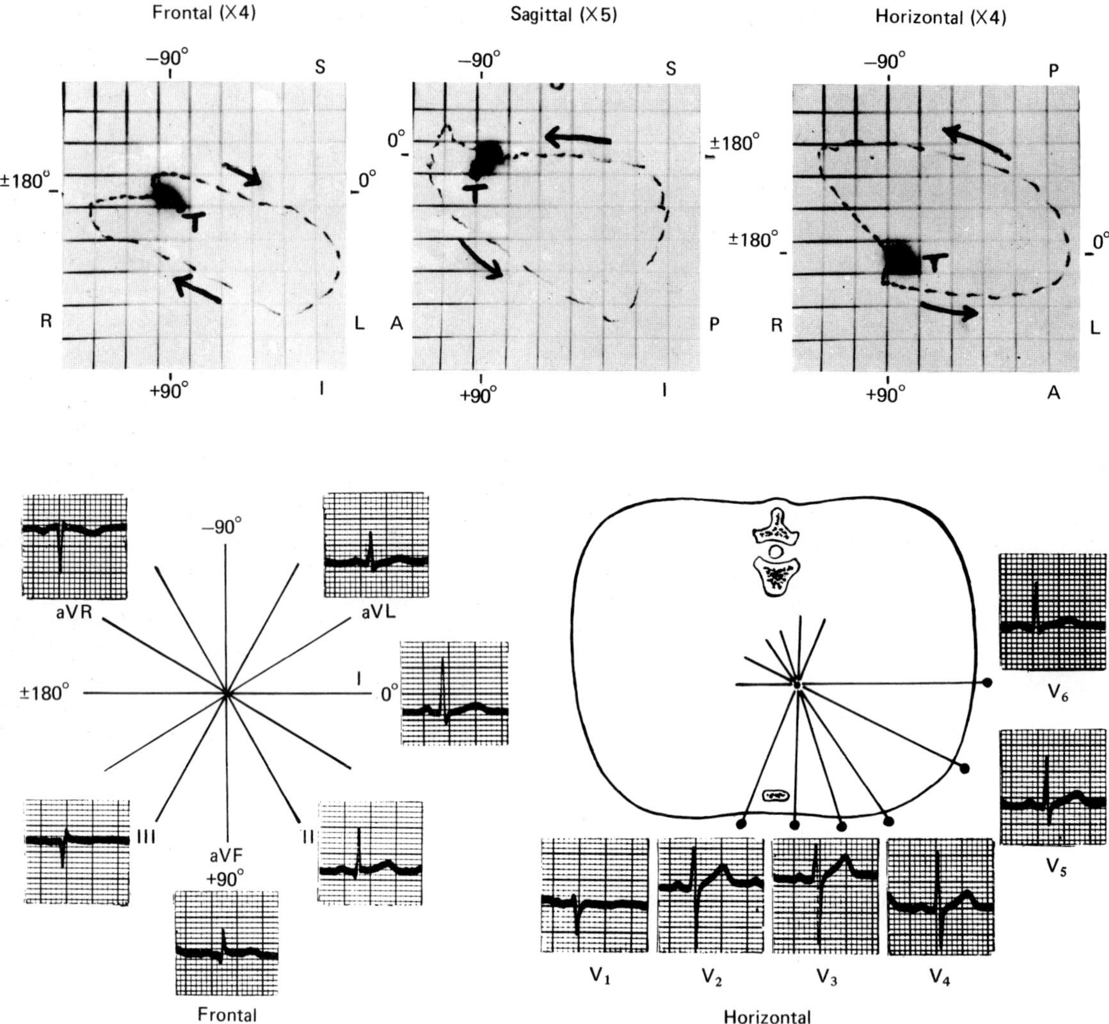

Figure 5–18. Normal adult vectorcardiogram. S, superior; I, inferior; R, right; L, left; A, anterior; P, posterior. The symbols (X4) and (X5) indicate the photographic magnification of the vector loop. (Reproduced, with permission, from Goldman MJ: ***Principles of Clinical Electrocardiography,*** 9th ed. Lange, 1976.)

patients going about their normal business. One lead of an ECG is usually recorded on a tape recorder which the patient carries strapped to his waist. The tape recording of the ECG is played back at speeds of 10–100 times the recording speed and scanned for abnormalities, either visually or using a special computer program. These areas of interest are then recorded at standard speed for analysis. Both arrhythmias and ST–T wave changes of ischemia can be detected in this way and the time of their occurrence correlated with events in the patient's life. In continuous monitoring in a coronary care unit, the ECG is usually continuously displayed on an oscilloscope and can be recorded on chart paper by simply pressing a button. Alarms are often arranged to provide a signal when the patient's heart rate falls outside a prescribed range. These are not always desirable, because displacement of ECG electrodes and disconnection of leads tend to trigger the alarm systems inappropriately. It is especially convenient to use a system that includes a memory loop. In this case, the immediate past portion (say the last 20 seconds) of the patient's ECG signal is continuously stored in a memory, which is continuously erased after 20 seconds. When some untoward event occurs, it is then possible to stop erasing the memory and examine the ECG during the period immediately preceding the untoward event.

3. EXERCISE ELECTROCARDIOGRAPHY

Exercise electrocardiography is a standard procedure for investigation of patients in whom a diagnosis of angina pectoris is being considered. It has come to replace the Master 2-step test, in which the ECG was recorded after rather than during exercise. The apparatus required is not expensive, and the test is available in many doctors' offices.

The technical aspects of ECG recording during exercise have largely been overcome, so that with improved electrodes it is now possible to obtain stable tracings even during severe exercise on a cycle ergometer or treadmill. Although various lead systems have been used, a single unipolar lead or a bipolar lead from the right subclavicular region to the apex beat, with an indifferent electrode on the head or left shoulder, will detect ischemic changes in the ECG during exercise almost as effectively as more complicated lead systems. Most exercise electrocardiography is carried out in patients with chest pain in whom a diagnosis of angina pectoris is being considered. The patient exercises at increasing loads, either on a treadmill or an ergometer, until his heart rate increases to 150–160 beats/min, until symptoms develop which force the patient to stop, or until ECG changes are noted which warrant stopping. The ECG is monitored continuously throughout the procedure, and a resting ECG is taken before and after the study. Exercise is conventionally performed in the upright position, and it is important to differentiate between ECG changes due to posture and those due to exercise by recording an ECG tracing with the patient standing before exercise. ***Caution:*** An exercise test of this type should never be carried out without a doctor present, and resuscitation equipment should always be available. The most recent ECG should always be compared with a preexercise tracing to make certain that a recent myocardial infarction has not occurred. The changes of myocardial ischemia shown in Fig 5–19 occur during exercise and are virtually always visible in the left ventricular leads (V_5 is probably the best). They consist of ST–T wave depression with T wave inversion. Junctional depression and upsloping ST segments, shown in Fig 5–20, are not significant, although ST depression of 2 mm and a duration of 0.08 sec are considered definite positive findings indicating ischemia. ST depression of 1–2 mm is deemed equivocal.

There is some relationship between the ease with which ECG changes can be provoked, their magnitude, and the severity and prognosis of the coronary lesions. Patients with significant left main coronary artery lesions often show marked ST depression with minimal

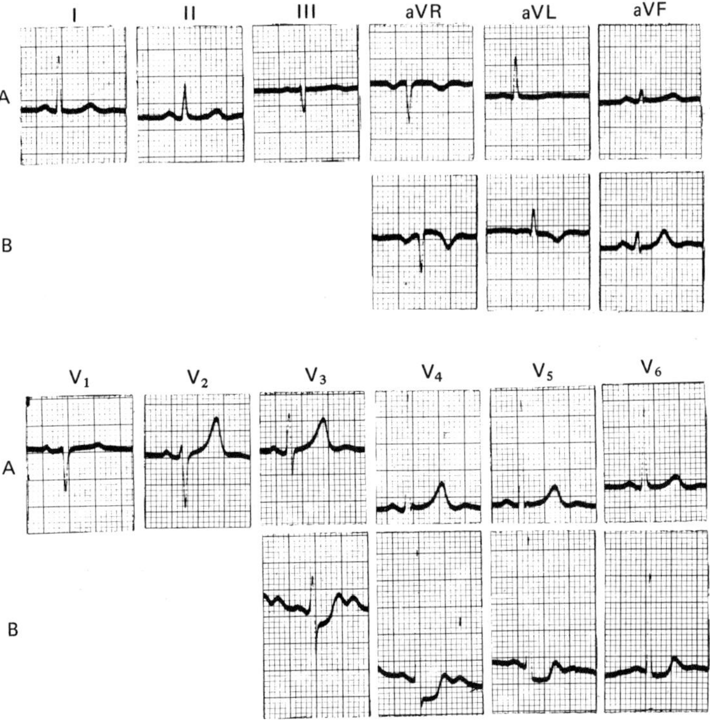

Figure 5–19. Effect of exercise (induced myocardial ischemia). *A:* Taken when patient was free of pain. The only suggestive abnormality is a flat T wave in aVL. *B:* Taken after exercise. There is minimal ST elevation in aVR and slight ST depression with T wave inversion in aVL. The most striking changes are seen in the precordial leads: There is 2 mm ST depression in V_3 and V_5; 3.5 mm in V_4; 1 mm in V_6. *Clinical diagnosis:* Arteriosclerotic heart disease; anginal syndrome. (Reproduced, with permission, from Goldman MJ: *Principles of Clinical Electrocardiography,* 9th ed. Lange, 1976.)

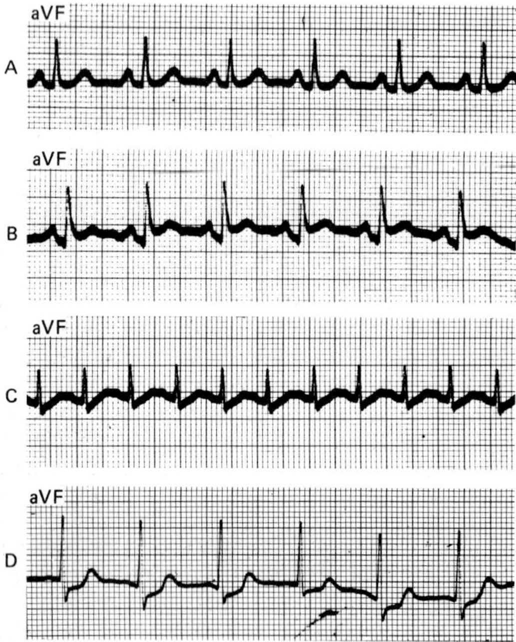

Figure 5–20. Pseudodepression versus coronary type of ST segment depression. *A:* Normal tracing; rate = 92; ST segment isoelectric. *B:* Prominent T_a waves; rate = 100; ST segment is isoelectric, being on the same level as the TP segment. *C:* Sinus tachycardia; rate = 168. ST segments appear depressed, but the ST segment displays a continuous ascent with upward concavity. This is typical of the pseudodepression associated with tachycardia and an exaggerated T_a wave. *D:* True ST segment depression associated with myocardial ischemia (postexercise record); the contour of the ST segment is that of horizontal depression. (Reproduced, with permission, from Goldman MJ: *Principles of Clinical Electrocardiography,* 9th ed. Lange, 1976.)

exercise. A positive exercise ECG showing myocardial ischemia undoubtedly occurs in patients with a normal coronary arteriogram. This finding, while it is uncommon, is most frequently seen in women with chest pain which is clinically compatible with angina pectoris. Conversely, a normal exercise ECG can be obtained in patients with obvious angina pectoris and severe coronary artery disease on angiography. In spite of these considerations, the specificity of an exercise test (correlation with angiographic findings of coronary disease) is about 70% while the sensitivity (ability to detect significant coronary artery disease) is of the same order. One must be cautious in interpreting exercise ECG tracings in patients taking digitalis and in patients with left ventricular hypertrophy; false-positive findings may occur, especially if one uses 1 mm of depression of the ST segment as the criterion for a positive response.

Exercise electrocardiography is of prognostic significance, especially if ischemic changes are associated with hypotension during exercise. This finding usually indicates multiple vessel coronary artery disease.

4. MYOCARDIAL ST SEGMENT MAPPING

This procedure, still in the research phase, is another form of investigation designed to follow the progress and assess the size of myocardial infarctions. It is moderately expensive and involves multiple ECG recordings from different sites of the precordium. In patients with anterior infarcts, the extent of the area over which ST elevation can be detected bears a relationship to the size of the infarcted area. By summing the total extent of ST elevation in 30 or so ECG leads placed in standard positions on the surface of the left chest, it is possible to obtain a numerical assessment which bears a relationship to infarct size. Unfortunately, changes in position of the heart and thickness of the chest wall vary greatly from patient to patient, and this detracts from the general usefulness of the technic.

MYOCARDIAL ENZYME DETERMINATIONS

A number of enzymes (eg, glutamic-oxaloacetic transaminase [GOT], lactate dehydrogenase [LDH], creatine phosphokinase [CPK]) are released into the blood following myocardial infarction. Necrosis of tissue with rupture of cell membranes and release of intracellular components must occur before the increased levels of enzyme are found. More specific enzymes and enzymatic fractions have now been identified, and the relatively specific myocardial MB ("myocardial band") fraction of creatine phosphokinase isoenzyme has become the standard test used to confirm that myocardial infarction has occurred. The level of this enzyme gives more specific information about myocardial necrosis than any other available at the moment. Attempts have been made to relate serial measurements of enzyme levels to the size of the infarction and the patient's clinical progress, with the examiner seeking evidence of healing on the one hand or extension with increasing enzyme levels on the other. Since the enzyme mixes with a large and potentially variable blood volume at an undetermined rate, such measurements tend to be relatively insensitive.

SPECIAL RADIOLOGIC INVESTIGATIONS

1. CINEFLUOROSCOPY

Cardiac fluoroscopy, which in the past was used almost routinely by clinical cardiologists, has now been replaced almost entirely by cinefluoroscopy in most medical centers. The latter has the advantage of obtaining a permanent record of the radiologic appearance of the heart and of its movement but is more expensive because of the costs of cinematography. Cinefluoroscopy is of greatest value in establishing the presence of calcification in the heart valves, the myocardium, the coronary arteries, or the pericardium or in recognizing paradoxic motion of a left ventricular aneurysm. It is also valuable in patients with prosthetic heart valves in whom the question of valve dehiscence is raised. A permanent postoperative record of artificial valve movement should therefore be obtained (if available) in all patients subjected to valve replacement for comparison with later studies if trouble arises.

2. OTHER TECHNICS

Special radiographic technics such as tomography and kymography are seldom used for examination of the heart today. Tomography may occasionally be useful in identifying the site of entry of pulmonary veins into the atria, in distinguishing between different sites of calcification in the heart, or in distinguishing a vascular shadow from a solid mass. Kymography as a means of measuring the magnitude of cardiac pulsations has long been superseded by cineradiography. The calculation of cardiac volumes by measurements derived from plain chest films is not routinely used outside the Scandinavian countries. Although the information obtained is statistically valid in distinguishing between groups of patients, it is not sufficiently accurate in individual cases to justify its use.

NUCLEAR MEDICAL INVESTIGATIONS

The various technics for investigating the heart by means of radionuclides fall into the general domain of radiology. They involve the injection of specially prepared radioactive materials which can be detected either in the bloodstream or the normal or abnormal myocardium. The apparatus required for recording the patterns of radioactivity is expensive, and the procedures have not yet become standardized.

Lung Scanning

Special gamma counting cameras can be used to scan the distribution of radioactivity in the lungs following intravenous injection of technetium-labeled albumin particles. This technic has proved valuable in localizing pulmonary arterial emboli and is most specific in patients with a normal chest x-ray. It is available in many large hospitals and is useful in pulmonary as well as cardiac disease.

Myocardial Imaging

Newer technics have been developed to scan the cardiac area by direct film images or computer-acquired views during the passage of intravenously injected radionuclides through the central circulation. The size and motion of the cardiac chambers can be determined, and information about localized areas of myocardium can be of value in shunt lesions. These methods provide a rather fuzzy substitute for angiocardiography at present and are not decisively diagnostic, but their potential for future usefulness is significant.

A. Perfused Areas: Scanning of the myocardium after the injection of potassium 45, rubidium 81, or thallium 201–isotopes which outline the perfused areas but not the unperfused ones–offers prospects of providing useful information about myocardial ischemia during exercise or myocardial scarring at rest. Thallium is coming to be most widely used. The indicators can be injected during exercise that is sufficient to provoke anginal pain, and the myocardial scanning can be carried out up to an hour later. An example showing ischemia during exercise is seen in Fig 5–21. Improvements in imaging technics will almost certainly enhance the quality of the pictures obtained with this method but may also increase the cost.

B. Infarcted Areas: Another form of myocardial imaging is used to delineate the extent of myocardial infarctions. Technetium-labeled pyrophosphate (^{99m}Tc), which is selectively taken up by infarcted cardiac tissue, can be detected by myocardial scanning within a few hours after injection. It provides an indication of the site and extent of the area of myocardial damage, as shown in Fig 5–22.

All these different forms of radiologic investigation appear likely to become significantly more useful as a result of the application of new technics of computer-assisted averaging and image enhancement. These should greatly improve the clarity and the definition of the images obtained and make possible the identification of structures whose presence can now only be inferred by the skilled specialist in the field.

CARDIOPULMONARY FUNCTION TESTING

Pulmonary function testing of varying degrees of complexity is available in most hospitals of moderate size. It is used mainly for the study of patients with lung disease, but, since pulmonary function is likely to be impaired in patients with heart disease, tests of pulmonary function are often needed in the assessment of cardiac patients. The 3 main elements of pulmonary function–ventilation, diffusion, and pulmonary blood flow–and the relationships between them need to be tested, both at rest and during exercise. The conventional measurements of vital capacity and maximum expiratory flow rate give an indication of the maximal ventilation the patient can achieve voluntarily. Maximal exercise ventilation may be a more relevant measurement, since it tests the response to natural stimuli rather than the ability to perform a respiratory maneuver. Diffusion of oxygen across the alveolar membrane

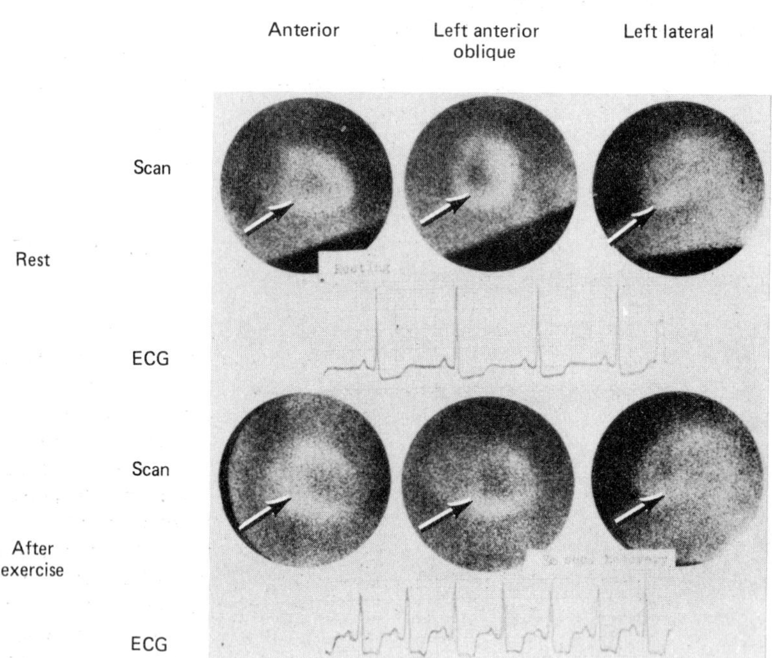

Figure 5–21. ECG tracings and anterior, left anterior oblique, and left lateral thallium 201 gamma camera scans of the heart in a patient with coronary artery disease studied at rest and after exercise which induced ST segment depression. An apical clear area (arrows) indicates the site of ischemia. (Courtesy of EH Botvinick.)

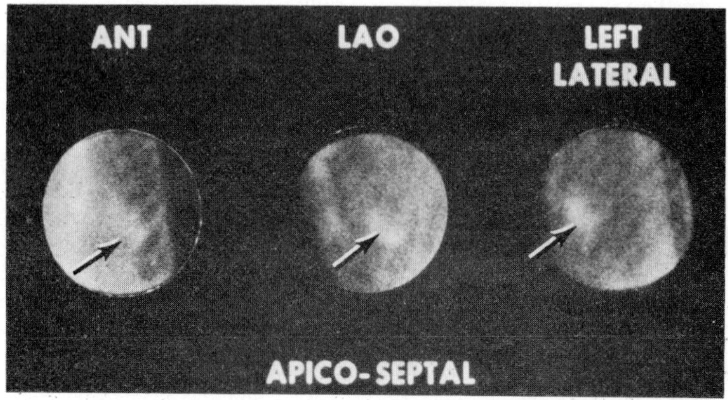

Figure 5–22. Anterior (ANT), left anterior oblique (LAO), and left lateral gamma camera scans of the heart after technetium-labeled pyrophosphate injection in a patient with a myocardial infarct. The apicoseptal infarct shows up as a light area (arrows). (Courtesy of EH Botvinick.)

is assessed by measuring the transfer of carbon monoxide into the blood. This process may be impaired in severe pulmonary congestion with edema. Measurement of the concentrations of physiologically relevant gases—oxygen and CO_2—or inert gases—usually helium—in the respired air at the mouth gives information about the adequacy of ventilation, its distribution, and its relationship to perfusion. Specific gas analyzers and flowmeters are now available with which to make appropriate measurements of cardiopulmonary function in patients at rest and during exercise. The mechanical properties of the lungs can be tested by measuring the force applied to the lungs (intrathoracic pressure) from esophageal pressure records using an air-filled balloon connected to a pressure transducer by a plastic tube. The compliance (stiffness) of the lungs and the resistance to air flow in the bronchial tree can be calculated. Arterial oxygen saturation can be measured noninvasively with an ear oximeter. The method is not in general use because of the difficulty in obtaining accurate measurements. The absorption of light transmitted through the illuminated ear is recorded at different wavelengths, and the concentration ratio of oxygenated and reduced hemoglobin is calculated. Arterial desaturation is more commonly found in lung disease but occurs in pulmonary edema and in patients with cyanotic congenital heart disease. Arterial oxygen tension can also be measured via the heated skin using an oxygen electrode. This technic is still in the developmental stage.

EXERCISE TESTING

Exercise testing, in which physiologic measurements are made, in addition to ECG recording, is not in routine use in the USA. The apparatus involved varies in complexity and in cost. The information obtained by exercise testing is almost entirely functional. Muscular exercise is the most significant, repeatable, and physiologically relevant stress to which a patient can be subjected. It can be conveniently performed either on a cycle ergometer or on a motor-driven treadmill. *An ECG must always be recorded, and resuscitation equipment must be available.* Standardized exercise tests are routinely done in cardiac patients in the Scandinavian countries. They provide objective evidence of the patient's work capacity and record work load, heart rate, ECG changes, and blood pressure. They are most helpful in following individual patients and assessing the effects of therapy and the progress of disease. Additional measurements such as ventilation, oxygen consumption, respiratory exchange ratio, cardiac output, and lung-to-ear circulation time by oximetry can be added to give additional physiologic information using noninvasive methods. Patients with heart disease show excessive exercise ventilation, a high respiratory exchange ratio due to disproportionate metabolic acidosis, a low maximal cardiac output, and a prolonged lung-to-ear circulation time.

OTHER GRAPHIC METHODS

Several other noninvasive graphic methods can be used to obtain information about cardiac function. None are standard, routine procedures, but all have their advocates.

1. BALLISTOCARDIOGRAPHY

Ballistocardiography, one of the oldest of these methods (Fig 5–23) purports to measure the accelerative forces imparted to the body by cardiac contraction. The procedure is not in common use, and it has been the difficulty encountered in standardization and calibration of the records obtained that has probably limited its usefulness. In principle, since the force of cardiac contraction is determined during the period of isovolumetric contraction, the accelerative forces during this period of constant ventricular volume are potentially of great functional significance. The technical problem involved in measuring the accelerative forces imparted to the body by the beating heart have not yet been mastered, and clinical ballistocardiography tends to be overly influenced by the effects of the damping properties of the body tissues. The method, therefore, is not always practical and is of little value in clinical cardiology.

2. APEXCARDIOGRAPHY

Apexcardiography attempts to record the same type of accelerative forces as ballistocardiography but

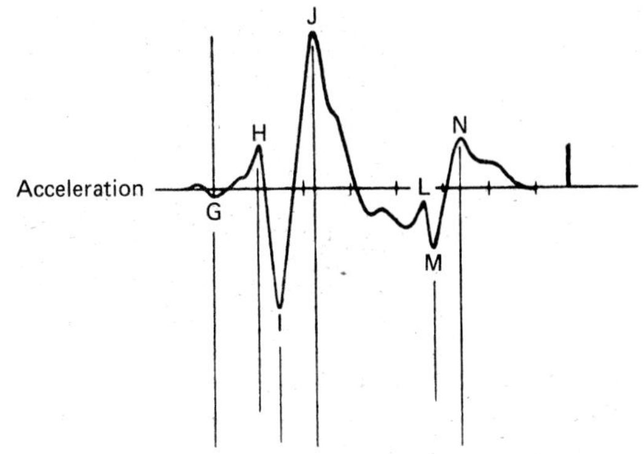

Figure 5–23. Ballistocardiographic tracing of a normal subject. The acceleration imparted by the heart gives rise to G, H, I, K, L, M, and N waves. (Reproduced, with permission, from Altman P, Dittmer DS [editors]: *Handbook of Respiration and Circulation.* Federation of American Societies for Experimental Biology, 1971.)

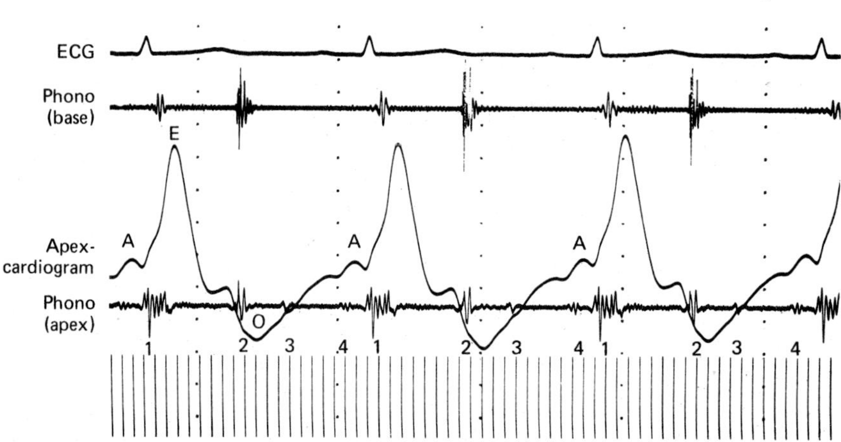

Figure 5–24. Apex- and phonocardiograms in a patient with 4 heart sounds (1, 2, 3, and 4). The atrial component in the apexcardiogram (A) is well seen.

concentrates on the displacement of the apex beat during the cardiac cycle. In the tracing shown in Fig 5–24 from a patient with prominent third and fourth heart sounds, outward movements of the left ventricle are recorded as positive deflections and occur during left atrial systole (A wave) and ventricular systole (E point). A negative deflection during early diastole (O point) is followed by a return of the tracing to the baseline during a rapid and then a slow filling phase. Apexcardiography is claimed by its advocates to help in understanding the hemodynamic events associated with cardiac filling and emptying, in distinguishing between an opening snap and a third heart sound, and in the investigation of patients with cardiomyopathy. The apparatus is not expensive, but the technic is not in routine use.

3. SYSTOLIC TIME INTERVALS

These noninvasive measurements do not require expensive apparatus but are not widely used. In systolic time interval measurements, the electrocardiogram, phonocardiogram, and an externally recorded carotid pulse tracing are used to provide a tracing from which specific time intervals are measured (Fig 5–25). The important intervals are the Q–A_2 interval, ie, the interval between the Q wave of the ECG and the aortic component of the second heart sound on the phonocardiogram, and the left ventricular ejection time (LVET), measured on the start of the upstroke of the carotid pulse tracing to the dicrotic notch on the downstroke. The difference between these 2 time intervals—the preejection period (PEP)—is the time from the Q wave to the start of the upstroke of the carotid arterial tracing. The PEP/LVET ratio is considered to reflect left ventricular function, the normal ratio of about 0.35 increasing to about 0.6 in patients with heart failure. The fidelity of the external recordings of carotid arterial pulsations is not high, and similar information can be obtained from echocardiographic recordings of aortic valve opening and closing. Systolic time intervals are most useful for following the progress of individual patients with left ventricular disease. As with other indirect methods, a definitive diagnosis or a serious decision, such as whether to submit a patient to cardiac surgery, would never be based solely on this measurement.

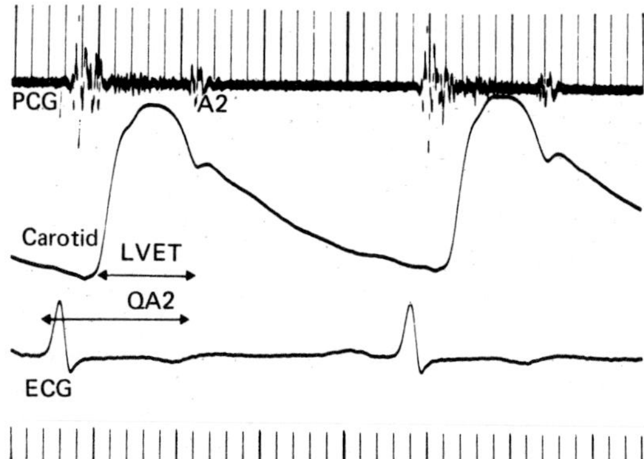

Figure 5–25. Phonocardiogram (PCG), indirect carotid tracing, and ECG from which systolic time intervals are measured. A_2, aortic valve closure. LVET, left ventricular ejection time; QA_2, time from Q wave to A_2. (Reproduced, with permission, from Oliver MF [editor]: *Modern Trends in Cardiology–3.* Butterworth, 1974.)

• • •

References

Ayotte B & others: Assessment of left heart function by noninvasive exercise test in normal subjects. J Appl Physiol 34:644, 1973.

Baily IK & others: Detection of coronary artery disease and myocardial ischemia by electrocardiography and myocardial perfusion scanning with thallium 201. Am J Cardiol 37:118, 1976.

Bates DV, Christie RV, Macklem PT: *Respiratory Function in Disease.* Saunders, 1971.

Botvinick EH & others: Myocardial stress perfusion scintography with rubidium-81 versus stress electrocardiography. Am J Cardiol 39:364, 1977.

Bruce RA: Exercise testing of patients with coronary heart disease: Principles and normal standards for evaluation. Ann Clin Res 3:323, 1971.

Chou T, Helm RA: *Clinical Vectorcardiography,* 2nd ed. Grune & Stratton, 1974.

Chung EK (editor): *Non-invasive Cardiac Diagnosis.* Lea & Febiger, 1976.

Comroe JH & others: *The Lung: Clinical Physiology and Pulmonary Function Tests,* 2nd ed. Year Book, 1962.

Feigenbaum H: *Echocardiography,* 2nd ed. Lea & Febiger, 1976.

Frank E: An accurate, clinically practical system for spatial vectorcardiography. Circulation 13:737, 1956.

Gibson TC & others: The A wave of the apexcardiogram and left ventricular diastolic stiffness. Circulation 49:441, 1974.

Goldman MJ: *Principles of Clinical Electrocardiography,* 9th ed. Lange, 1976.

Goldstein S, Killip T: Comparison of direct and indirect arterial pressures in aortic regurgitation. N Engl J Med 267:1121, 1962.

Henry WL & others: The differential diagnosis of anomalies of the great vessels by real-time, two-dimensional echocardiography. Circulation 51:283, 1975.

Hirschfeld DS, Schiller N: Localization of aortic valve vegetations by echocardiography. Circulation 53:280, 1976.

Holter NJ: New method for heart studies: Continuous electrocardiography of active subjects over long periods is now practical. Science 134:1214, 1961.

Jefferson K, Rees S: *Clinical Cardiac Radiology.* Butterworth, 1973.

Kleid JJ, Schiller NB: *Echocardiography Case Studies.* Med Exam Pub, 1974.

Leatham A: *Auscultation of the Heart and Phonocardiography,* 2nd ed. Livingstone, 1975.

Lebowitz E & others: 201-Tl for medical use. J Nucl Med 14:421, 1973.

Lipman BS, Massie E, Kleiger RE: *Clinical Scalar Electrocardiography,* 6th ed. Year Book, 1972.

Littmann D: *Examination of the Heart.* Part 5: *The Electrocardiogram.* American Heart Association, 1973.

Marriott HJL, Fogg E: Constant monitoring for cardiac dysrhythmias and blocks. Mod Concepts Cardiovasc Dis 39:103, 1970.

McDonald IG, Feigenbaum H, Chang S: Analysis of left ventricular wall motion by reflected ultrasound: Application to assessment of myocardial function. Circulation 46:14, 1972.

McIlroy MB: The clinical uses of oximetry. Br Heart J 21:293, 1959.

Mueller TM & others: Limitations of thallium-201 myocardial perfusion scintigrams. Circulation 54:640, 1976.

Muller JE, Maroko PR, Braunwald E: Evaluation of precordial electrocardiographic mapping as a means of assessing changes in myocardial ischemic injury. Circulation 52:16, 1975.

Mullins CB, Mason DT, Ashburn WL: Determination of ventricular volume by radioisotope angiography. Am J Cardiol 24:72, 1969.

Murray JF: *The Normal Lung: The Basis for Diagnosis and Treatment of Pulmonary Disease.* Saunders, 1976.

Oliver MF (editor): *Modern Trends in Cardiology–3.* Butterworth, 1974.

Patterson JA & others: Treadmill exercise in assessment of the functional capacity of patients with cardiac disease. Am J Cardiol 30:757, 1972.

Popp RL: Echocardiographic assessment of cardiac disease. Circulation 54:538, 1976.

Rapaport E: The fractional disappearance rate of the separate isoenzymes of creatine phosphokinase in the dog. Cardiovasc Res 9:473, 1975.

Reneman RS (editor): *Cardiovascular Applications of Ultrasound.* Elsevier, 1974.

Scherf D: The electrocardiographic exercise test. J Electrocardiol 1:141, 1968.

Sheffield LT, Reeves TJ: Graded exercise in the diagnosis of angina pectoris. Mod Concepts Cardiovasc Dis 34:1, 1965.

Sheffield LT & others: The exercise test in perspective. Circulation 55:681, 1977.

Sobel BE, Shell WE: Serum enzyme determinations in the diagnosis and assessment of myocardial infarction. Circulation 45:471, 1972.

Starr I, Noordegraaf A: *Ballistocardiography in Cardiovascular Research.* Lippincott, 1967.

Strauss HW & others: Thallium 201 for myocardial imaging: Relation of thallium 201 to regional myocardial perfusion. Circulation 51:641, 1975.

Ungerleider HE, Clark CP: A study of the transverse diameter of the heart silhouette with prediction table based on the teleroentgenogram. Am Heart J 17:92, 1939.

Wagner GS & others: The importance of identification of the myocardial specific isoenzyme of creatine phosphokinase (MB form) in the diagnosis of acute myocardial infarction. Circulation 47:263, 1973.

Wagner HN: Radioisotope scanning in pulmonary embolic disease. In: *Pulmonary Embolic Diseases.* Sasahara AA, Stein M (editors). Grune & Stratton, 1965.

Weissler AM: Current concepts in cardiology: Systolic-time intervals. N Engl J Med 196:321, 1977.

Weissler AM (editor): *Non-invasive Cardiology.* Grune & Stratton, 1974.

Whalen RE, Starmer CF: Electric shock hazards in clinical cardiology. Mod Concepts Cardiovasc Dis 36:7, 1967.

Willems JL, de Geest H, Kesteloot H: On the value of apex cardiography for timing intracardiac events. Am J Cardiol 28:59, 1971.

6 . . .

Special Investigations: Invasive

The descriptions of invasive investigations in this chapter are of a general nature, principally of the technics involved and not of the findings in different diseases. The latter are included in the chapters dealing with specific cardiac disorders. The varieties of investigation available, their indications and technics, precautions in their use, their complications, and some broad generalities about interpretation are offered in this chapter. An attempt has been made to show that a range of choices of approach is available, and it will be noted that the personal preference of the investigator, based upon a familiarity with a particular technic, plays a logical part in determining which procedure will be used.

It should be apparent from the term invasive that such investigations are carried out in hospitalized patients for valid indications and only after adequate preliminary appraisal. In many instances, however, invasive diagnostic methods provide important information which cannot be obtained by simpler methods of cardiac diagnosis. The patient should be advised about the nature, risks, and benefits of such procedures. It is necessary to obtain the patient's written informed consent before all studies.

BEDSIDE VERSUS LABORATORY PROCEDURES

Invasive investigations fall into 2 main categories: those carried out at the bedside in severely ill patients and those performed in a cardiac catheterization laboratory. There is some overlap between the two, but, in general, arterial and venous pressure monitoring and pulmonary arterial and wedge pressure recording with a Swan-Ganz catheter are done at the bedside. Formal diagnostic catheterization studies and angiography are performed in specially equipped laboratories.

BEDSIDE CATHETERIZATION

Whereas arterial blood sampling has become a routine procedure in most hospitals, arterial catheterization, together with central venous or pulmonary arterial pressure monitoring, is mainly confined to intensive care areas where specially trained personnel are constantly available to keep the catheters patent and make certain that they are appropriately positioned. This form of monitoring of the patient's hemodynamic status is only indicated in severe, life-threatening illnesses such as myocardial infarction with shock or heart failure and in acute pulmonary edema or in the postoperative period after cardiac surgery. The disturbance, loss of sleep, and psychologic effect on the patient must be weighed against the therapeutic benefit, ie, early recognition of complications and assessment of the effects of therapy.

The technics described under the heading of bedside catheterization are arranged in order of increasing complexity. Many are also used in the cardiac catheterization laboratory, where the principal difference is that sterility is more easily maintained and the catheter is not in place for as long as it is at the bedside.

ARTERIAL CATHETERIZATION

Arterial puncture is a standard and routine procedure used to obtain samples for blood gas analysis and for direct recording of arterial pressure. Arterial blood can be obtained from a number of different sites, and the principles involved are generally similar. Arterial puncture is more painful than venipuncture, and local anesthesia is advocated in all cases. The risks of hemorrhage and hematoma formation are much greater than with venipuncture, especially in patients receiving anticoagulant therapy, but infection of the puncture site and the development of blood-borne infections are much less apt to occur. Local thrombosis with consequent interruption of blood supply to the distal tissues is perhaps the greatest danger.

Single Samples

Single arterial blood samples can be taken with a fine (24 gauge) needle and a sterile syringe from the radial, femoral, or brachial arteries. The dead space of the syringe should be filled with heparin. The larger the vessel, the easier the procedure. Fixation of the artery is important, and the technic for achieving this varies with the puncture site. At the radial artery, the wrist is hyperextended; at the elbow, the forearm is extended and pronated, with a folded towel under the elbow. At the groin, the leg is extended and externally rotated. The needle is plunged firmly through the area where the artery is most easily felt, and suction is maintained on the barrel of the syringe during withdrawal. Firm pressure is applied to the puncture site for long enough to determine that hemorrhage will not occur. The time varies with the size of the needle and the efficiency of the patient's clotting mechanisms.

Percutaneous Arterial Catheterization

While single arterial samples can be satisfactorily obtained in the manner described above, the collection of repeated samples in acutely ill patients is greatly facilitated by an indwelling arterial catheter. This is usually a short (25 cm) polyethylene or Teflon tube whose proximal end holds a female adapter plus stopcock and whose distal end is tapered to fit snugly over a fine guide wire made of plastic fishing line about twice as long as the catheter. Commercially prepared sterile disposable kits have greatly simplified the procedure, which uses 3 basic components: a Cournand needle, the catheter, and a guide wire (fishing line).

The first step in insertion of the catheter is to cannulate the artery. This is generally performed with a Cournand needle, which has a sharp inner stylet which can be exchanged for a longer, blunt obturator. If an indwelling arterial catheter is to be left in situ for more than a day, the brachial artery is the site of choice because it is less painful or restricting than radial or femoral sites. In cannulating the brachial artery, the skin is cleaned and sterilized and draped with sterile towels. The arm is appropriately positioned, and local anesthetic is introduced into the skin to form a wheal at the puncture site. Anesthetic (1% lidocaine) is injected more deeply subcutaneously on either side of the vessel, taking care not to puncture the artery. The Cournand needle with the sharp stylet is firmly advanced, with the thumb over the end of the stylet, through the area where the artery is most clearly felt. The stylet is then withdrawn, and the needle is slowly withdrawn only until arterial blood spurts out. If no arterial blood has appeared by the time the needle has been fully withdrawn, the sharp stylet is reinserted and the procedure is repeated with the needle at a slightly different angle or position. The proper angle between the needle and the skin surface depends on the depth of the vessel being punctured. In superficial vessels such as the radial artery, the needle should be almost parallel to the skin; in cannulating the brachial artery, the appropriate angle is about 30 degrees; and for the femoral artery, 60 degrees in most persons but even more than that in obese or muscular people.

The second part of the procedure begins when arterial blood spurts out of the punctured vessel. The lumen of the needle is covered with the thumb, and the needle is threaded up the vessel if possible, with the operator taking care to maintain a full flow of blood. If this is not possible, the blunt obturator is inserted and the same procedure of threading is tried again. If this fails, the fishing line is threaded into the needle and an attempt is made to advance it up the needle and into the artery. If the patient experiences pain during this maneuver, it should be assumed that the fishing line is dissecting a path in the wall of the vessel. This is dangerous and must be avoided.

The third step begins when the fishing line has freely entered the vessel and passed well beyond the end of the needle. At this point, the needle is totally withdrawn while firm pressure is maintained over the puncture site to avoid hematoma formation. The tip of the intra-arterial catheter is then threaded over the fishing line until the end of the line, which should be about twice as long as the catheter, emerges from the connector at the hub. The line and catheter are then advanced together into the vessel, the line is withdrawn, and the catheter is left in the vessel. A stopcock is attached to the end of the catheter and the system flushed with sterile heparinized saline solution. The hub of the catheter is strapped to the patient's arm, and the puncture site is covered with a sterile dressing. A point along the catheter should be left uncovered in order to make certain that blood is not leaking back into the catheter. Regular flushing of the catheter or a continuous, high-pressure, slow (0.1 ml/min) infusion of heparinized saline (1000 units in 500 ml of saline) is required to ensure patency.

A similar technic is used for the percutaneous insertion of cardiac catheters. A longer plastic-coated metal guide wire—at least 1½ times as long as the catheter—is needed. Short plastic dilators are also available to enlarge the hole in the vessel, and plastic sheaths can be used to make it possible to insert catheters without end holes. A number of different approaches are available, and the operator's familiarity with one particular method usually determines what specific technic is used.

PERCUTANEOUS VENOUS & RIGHT HEART CATHETERIZATION

Venous puncture and venous catheterization present few problems in patients with large veins which have not previously been the site of multiple punctures. More peripheral, smaller veins should be used for infusions and for taking single blood samples. The larger veins in the antecubital fossa should be preserved for the introduction of catheters into the central circulation. Most difficulty is encountered in dealing with the veins of persons who habitually use intravenous drugs, especially heroin; in such patients it is sometimes necessary to make a cutdown to expose the venae comitantes of the brachial artery. Superficial veins can be made to relax by flicking the skin with a finger, by warming the arm, and, if necessary, by exercising the limb. The vein should be palpated rather than inspected to find a good puncture site, and the skin and the vein should be punctured sequentially. If a catheter is to be inserted, either a plastic fishing line or a catheter can be introduced through the needle. Successively larger catheters can be used to dilate the puncture site until a catheter with a large enough bore is introduced. For central venous pressure measurements, a plastic catheter equivalent to No. 5 French is sufficient, and a percutaneous approach is often successful.

Swan-Ganz Catheter

If a balloon-tipped catheter is to be placed in the pulmonary artery (Swan-Ganz catheter), a percutaneous technic is only feasible if the patient has large veins, and a cutdown over the vein is usually needed. Plastic venous catheters are easily severed, and the cut distal end can enter the circulation. Special care is needed in handling such catheters, and the importance of sterility and the prevention of venous thrombosis should be stressed. The standard balloon-tipped catheter used to monitor pulmonary and indirect left atrial (wedge) pressure can be introduced without fluoroscopic control in most cases. The length of catheter which has been introduced should be carefully measured. When it is felt that the tip is in the right atrium, the balloon is partially inflated and the catheter allowed to float forward through the right ventricle with the bloodstream. *ECG monitoring is mandatory*, and if fluoroscopic control is not available, a record of pressure at the tip is essential in order to check the position of the catheter.

Pressure Recording

Arterial and venous pressures are usually recorded at the bedside with a strain gauge pressure transducer. The operator should be familiar with the steps required to balance the gauge and set the operating pressure range appropriately. Provision must be made for calibrating the manometer against a column of water or mercury, setting the zero level at the middle of the thorax, and providing a drip of heparinized normal saline to flush the catheter. The physician should be familiar with the characteristics of the pressure tracings in each of the right heart chambers. The recording of indirect left atrial (wedge) pressure is checked by observing the appropriate change in the tracing when the balloon is inflated. If there is any doubt, a blood sample can be obtained. It should show high P_{O_2} (about 100 mm Hg) and a low P_{CO_2} ($<$ 30 mm Hg) in normal subjects.

Thermodilution Catheters

Special catheters are available for the recording of cardiac output by thermodilution. Cold saline is injected through a proximal lumen which lies in the right atrium. The resulting temperature change is recorded at the tip of the catheter in the pulmonary artery with a thermistor bead embedded in the wall of the catheter.

Complications of Bedside Catheterization

The complications of bedside arterial and venous catheterization increase with the length of time the catheter is left in place. It is difficult to maintain sterility, especially when an incision is made in the skin. Infection is much more readily introduced through a venous than an arterial catheter, and infection of arterial puncture sites virtually never occurs. Thrombophlebitis, pulmonary embolism, and endocarditis can all occur following venous catheterization, and, if phlebitis occurs, removal of the catheter and reinsertion in another site should be undertaken without delay. The catheter itself may be accidentally severed and may enter the right heart if care is not taken to secure it properly. Air embolism is a possible hazard, especially when the jugular vein is the site used and when the slow drip of heparinized saline used to maintain patency is exhausted and the bottle empty.

The main dangers of arterial catheterization are hemorrhage and thrombosis of the artery. Hematoma formation due to leakage of blood from the puncture site must always be looked for. It can occur from the posterior wall of the vessel and track insidiously via fascial planes, eg, retroperitoneally following femoral puncture. Small platelet thrombi often form at the tip of the catheter and break off to cause peripheral emboli in the extremities. Splinter hemorrhages and Osler's nodes, similar to those seen in infective endocarditis, commonly occur and are harmless. The greatest danger of vascular occlusion occurs when an arterial catheter is being removed. It is a mistake to press heavily over the puncture site while removing the catheter. This can readily scrape off a film of incompletely formed thrombotic material, mainly platelets. This material may be sufficient to form an embolus which can block the vessel and seriously interfere with the blood supply to the region.

ELECTIVE DIAGNOSTIC CARDIAC CATHETERIZATION

Cardiac catheterization has become a standard procedure for the diagnosis and assessment of severity of cardiovascular disease. It is now almost always combined with some sort of angiographic procedure. The range of possible investigations is wide, and the morbidity and mortality rates of the different procedures vary widely with the age of the patient, the severity of the disease, and the skill and experience of the operator. *Cardiac catheterization should only be undertaken by a physician who has personally seen and evaluated the patient's problem clinically before the study.* The technics require constant practice, and the procedure should not be done occasionally in laboratories that are only used once or twice a week. The study combines anatomic diagnosis with functional assessment, and, especially in congenital heart disease, it cannot be known what information should be obtained until the procedure is actually under way. Thus, it is not always a routine procedure in which a previously decided list of data must be obtained but rather an investigation in which the operator should be continuously aware of what has been established and what remains to be done. The study optimally requires the cooperation of a cardiologist, a radiologist, a nurse, and a technician.

Indications for Diagnostic Cardiac Catheterization

Cardiac catheterization is indicated in preparation for all cardiac surgical procedures in order to make the diagnosis as certain as possible and thereby to provide maximum help to the surgeon. What procedure is chosen depends to some extent on the facilities available as well as on the preference of the investigator. In general, combined right and left heart catheterization with angiography has gradually come to be the most widely used approach. In some centers, thoroughness of the investigation, using all types of studies that could possibly throw light on the problem, is the preferred approach, but in the authors' opinion excessively prolonged procedures expose the patient to unnecessary risks. For example, we do not believe that coronary arteriography is routinely indicated in all patients on the chance that surgically important lesions will be identified. Cardiac catheterization should rather be looked on as an investigation with about the same importance as the history, physical examination, ECG, and chest x-ray.

It is possible to obtain misleading information from cardiac catheterization, and the possibility that an error has been made in a laboratory investigation should not be discounted when collateral facts support that inference.

Selection of Studies

It is often more difficult to decide what studies should be undertaken in a given patient than to decide which patient should be studied. The operator must consider how much the patient can tolerate, especially the time involved in any given procedure. High-risk patients—eg, those with severe mitral stenosis, pulmonary hypertension, recent myocardial infarction, or severe aortic stenosis—are much more likely to suffer complications from prolonged procedures. It is often better to postpone part of the study to a later date than to add a procedure such as coronary arteriography to the end of a 3-hour session. The operator must always bear in mind the primary aim of the study, which may be to establish a diagnosis in a patient with congenital heart disease, measure the pressure difference and flow across an aortic valve, or measure the pulmonary vascular resistance in a patient with pulmonary hypertension.

RIGHT HEART CATHETERIZATION

Technic

The conventional approach is via the right medial basilic vein at the bend of the elbow, but almost any vein in the arm or leg can be used. The cephalic vein often takes an awkward bend at the shoulder, and it is impossible to enter the thorax by this route in about one-third of patients. The vein is usually isolated by means of a small skin incision using 1% lidocaine anesthesia, and the catheter is inserted via a small incision in the vein.

Entering the Thorax

The catheter is advanced to the shoulder or neck as soon as possible; if it catches on valves, it can be freed by slight twisting. Deep inspiration sometimes helps the catheter enter the chest.

Entering the Pulmonary Artery

The catheter is advanced into the pulmonary artery under fluoroscopic vision. A loop is conventionally made in the right atrium by pointing the catheter tip to the right and advancing it until its tip catches on the right atrial wall. When pushed farther, the catheter tip will point cephalad. This loop is then rotated through 180 degrees until it points to the left, and, as it passes through the tricuspid valve, the catheter is advanced rapidly through the right ventricle. If the catheter is pointing caudad, it will enter the apex of the right ventricle and probably provoke ectopic beats. As the catheter is rotated, it may enter the coronary sinus and point in a straight line toward the left shoulder. The coronary sinus position can be confirmed by finding a low oxygen saturation (30–40%). It should always be possible to enter the pulmonary artery except in patients with tricuspid atresia. Difficulty is most commonly encountered in patients with a large right atrium or corrected transposition of the great vessels.

Wedging the Catheter in a Branch of the Pulmonary Artery

When the catheter enters the pulmonary artery, a wedge pressure is obtained by advancing the catheter firmly until its tip becomes wedged in the tapering vessel. A tracing is obtained, and *a* and *v* waves are sought if the patient is in sinus rhythm or a *v* wave if the patient is in atrial fibrillation. The right lower lobe of the lung is the usual site for wedging the catheter. The tracing obtained is called a pulmonary capillary (PC) or wedge pressure tracing.

Validity of Wedge (PC) Pressure

In the 25 years since wedge pressure was first introduced, it has been repeatedly shown to give an accurate measure of left atrial pressure, delayed by about 0.1 sec. An example of simultaneous left atrial and pulmonary capillary tracings is shown in Fig 6–1. Experience and judgment are needed to determine whether a satisfactory measurement of wedge pressure has been obtained, especially in patients with pulmonary hypertension, mitral stenosis, or acute mitral incompetence. The best way to determine that the catheter is wedged is by recording the pressure change as it is withdrawn. It "pops out" of the wedge position and

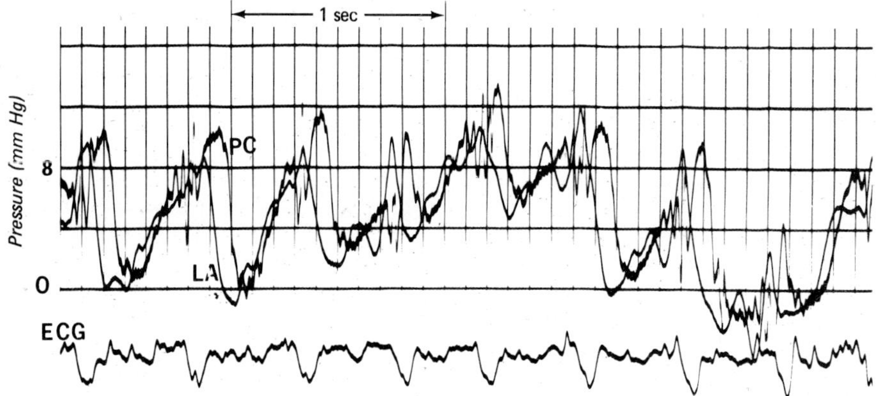

Figure 6–1. Simultaneous left atrial (LA) and wedge (PC) pressure tracings in a patient with aortic stenosis obtained during simultaneous transseptal and right heart catheterization. The patient is in atrial fibrillation, and the PC pressure can be seen to lag about 0.1 sec behind the LA pressure. The wave forms are similar.

pressure rises at that instant, changing from a wedge to a pulmonary arterial configuration as shown in Fig 6–2. A catheter in the wedge position can be flushed easily, but withdrawal of blood samples may be difficult. In any case, the sample obtained is physiologically irrelevant, since the blood obtained equilibrates with an overventilated and underperfused area of lung on the way to the sampling catheter. However, the characteristic high P_{O_2}, low P_{CO_2}, and high pH found in wedge samples are a good means of confirming that the catheter has been properly placed to obtain a satisfactory wedge pressure tracing. It is also possible in a patient with an atrial septal defect to pass a catheter through the defect and to wedge the catheter in the reverse direction by pushing the catheter far out from the left atrium into a pulmonary vein. The pressure obtained resembles that seen in the pulmonary artery, but the measurement is liable to be incorrect in the presence of pulmonary hypertension.

PRESSURE RECORDINGS

Pulmonary Artery

Phasic and mean pulmonary arterial tracings should always be recorded in the main pulmonary artery. The right pulmonary artery is more readily entered than the left, and the lower lobes of the lungs are more easily catheterized than the upper lobes.

Right Ventricle

Right ventricular pressure tracings are convention-

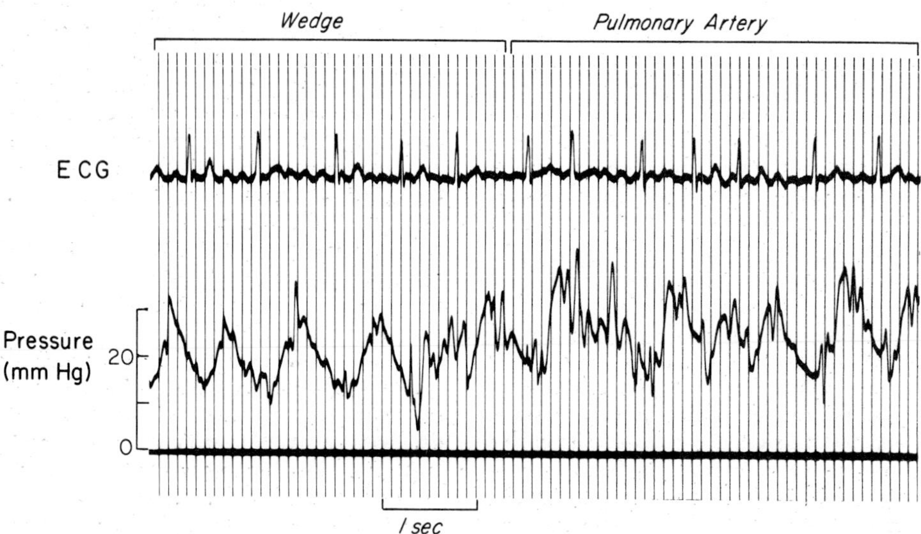

Figure 6–2. Pressure tracing and ECG showing withdrawal of a catheter from the wedge to the pulmonary artery in a patient with mitral valve disease in atrial fibrillation.

ally recorded on withdrawal of the catheter from the pulmonary artery. Mean ventricular pressures are not obtained. Right ventricular tracings are particularly liable to be interrupted by ectopic beats, and it is difficult to place a catheter in the right ventricle in a stable position.

Blood Sampling

At the time that withdrawal tracings from the pulmonary artery are obtained, blood samples are taken from each chamber, especially if there is any question of a left-to-right shunt. A sample from the superior vena cava should be followed by a high caval or innominate vein sample if an atrial defect is suspected, because anomalous venous return into the superior vena cava must be excluded. Opinions differ about the importance of obtaining a sample from the inferior vena cava. We believe that a sample should be taken after positioning the catheter approximately 2.5 cm below the diaphragm and pointing to the left, away from the hepatic vein. This may be difficult, and streams of blood from the renal vein tend to give falsely high saturations if the catheter is placed too low.

Measurement of Cardiac Output

Cardiac output is ordinarily measured during right heart catheterization when the right heart catheter is in the main pulmonary artery (mixed venous blood) and an arterial sample is available from a systemic artery. A 3-minute expired gas collection is made, and simultaneous pulmonary arterial and systemic arterial samples are drawn during the gas collection and analyzed for oxygen content and capacity. Van Slyke analysis, rather than oximetry, is recommended for maximum accuracy, and an ECG tracing is obtained during the gas collection to record the heart rate and to make sure that the patient is in a steady state.

LEFT HEART CATHETERIZATION

Left heart catheterization is usually carried out in combination with right heart studies. The right heart data are generally obtained first.

Indications for Left Heart Catheterization

Left heart catheterization has come to be widely used in all forms of heart disease affecting the left heart, eg, mitral and aortic valve disease, coronary artery disease, and cardiomyopathy. It is not necessarily indicated in most forms of congenital heart disease, especially when the catheter can be passed from the right heart through a defect into the left heart. In some centers an attempt is routinely made to enter all cardiac chambers in all patients. We feel that the operator should exercise judgment in choosing procedures and should tailor the study to the particular needs of each patient.

Different Approaches to Left Heart Catheterization

There is no general agreement about the correct way to approach the left side of the heart. Four methods are in common use in adults: (1) retrograde percutaneous femoral artery catheterization, (2) retrograde brachial arterial catheterization via arterial cutdown, (3) transseptal left heart catheterization via the femoral vein, and (4) direct percutaneous left ventricular puncture.

Almost all laboratories use more than one approach to the left heart since no one approach is always appropriate, feasible, or successful. The choice depends partly on personal preference and partly on the method used for coronary angiography in that particular laboratory which in turn depends on the equipment used.

Selection of Method

The nature of the patient's disease plays an important part in the choice of method. Most problems are encountered in patients with aortic stenosis in whom it is difficult to pass a catheter in a retrograde fashion across the aortic valve. If at all possible, the entire left heart study is performed by a single route in an attempt to minimize complications. Thus, the fact that a brachial arteriotomy will be needed to perform coronary arteriography by the Sones technic leads to the selection of the retrograde brachial arterial approach, while the need for a study by the Judkins technic for coronary angiography would lead to the selection of a retrograde femoral approach. Transseptal catheterization requires more skill and constant practice than any other form of left heart catheterization and is consequently becoming less popular. It is probably the approach of choice in aortic stenosis, but in order to maintain one's skill in the technic it must be used in other conditions as well.

Retrograde Percutaneous Femoral Artery Catheterization Technic

The method used to introduce the catheter is similar to that used in coronary arteriography by the Judkins technic. The femoral artery is punctured with a Cournand needle about 2.5 cm below the inguinal ligament in the groin. A guide wire is threaded via the needle to the abdominal aorta, and the needle is removed. A short (25 cm) dilator is advanced over the wire into the artery and pushed in and pulled out of the artery 2 or 3 times. The dilator is removed and replaced by an end-hole catheter. The catheter and the wire are advanced under fluoroscopic control to the ascending aorta in the position shown in Fig 6–3. Several varieties of catheter are available for entering the left ventricle. If the aortic valve is normal, a pigtail catheter can usually be advanced into the left ventricle without a guide wire. Any straight end-hole, nontapered catheter should always be used with a soft guide wire projecting 3–10 cm from its tip because the unoccluded tip may damage the aortic valve when pushed firmly against it. The guide wire rather than the

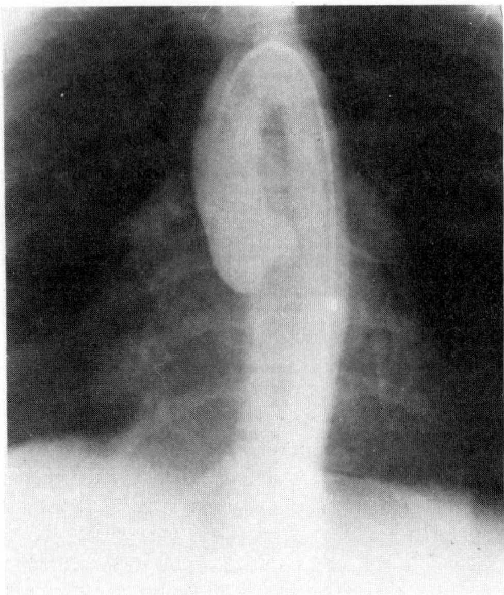

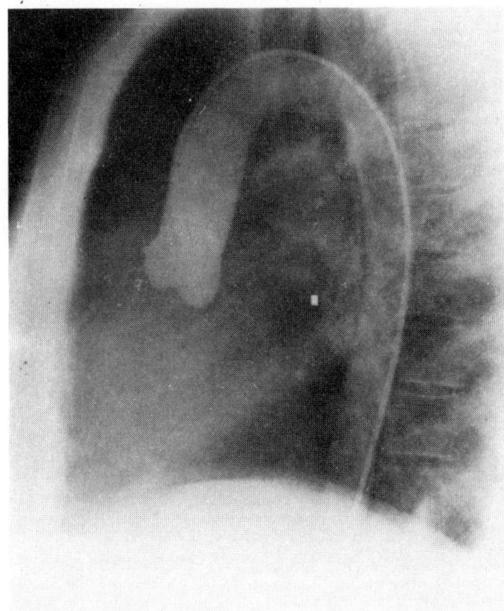

Figure 6–3. Posteroanterior *(left)* and lateral *(right)* views of an aortic angiogram following supravalvular injection of contrast material in a patient with mitral stenosis. The aorta is normal.

catheter is manipulated to enter the ventricle, the catheter is then advanced over the wire, and the wire is withdrawn. Because it has a curve near the tip, a right coronary artery Judkins catheter is a useful alternative to the standard Gensini Teflon catheter for entering the left ventricle.

Contraindications

This approach is not advocated when the patient has iliofemoral atherosclerosis or has had peripheral vascular surgery, with or without prosthetic replacement. When aortic stenosis is present, retrograde femoral catheterization is unsuccessful in a significant number of patients (15–20%), and in many laboratories another approach is used from the start of the procedure.

Retrograde Arterial Catheterization Via a Brachial Arterial Cutdown Technic

Cutting down on the brachial artery and exposing it for 1.5–2.5 cm is the method of choice from the arm since the vessel is usually too small for percutaneous catheterization. Generous use of local anesthesia, complete familiarity with the anatomy, and an ability to distinguish between the brachial artery and the median nerve are important factors in the success of this approach, which is also used for coronary arteriography by the Sones technic. Adequate exposure through a 5 cm incision, checking for position of the vessel by palpating its pulse, and identification of the tendinous expansion of the brachialis muscle and its retraction laterally are helpful in the dissection, which usually takes 15–20 minutes. Two plastic tapes are placed around the vessel for control of hemorrhage, and the catheter is inserted either through an arteriotomy or via a puncture site which has been dilated with a tapering plastic cannula. It is helpful to put a loose pursestring suture around the site of entry into the vessel before opening it, using 5-0 silk. The hole in the vessel can then be quickly closed by tightening this suture at the end of the procedure.

A straight, closed-tip catheter with multiple side holes—either a Lehman catheter with a tapered tip, a Sones catheter, or an NIH catheter—is usually used from the arm. Negotiating the bend in the subclavicular area is sometimes a problem in elderly atherosclerotic patients, but the degree of control of the catheter is much greater than with the femoral approach. Crossing the aortic valve is more readily accomplished using the brachial artery than the femoral route. Patients with aortic stenosis present the main problem.

Transseptal Catheterization

Transseptal left heart catheterization provides an alternative approach which is preferred in many centers. A long (> 35 cm) needle with a curved tip is introduced into a catheter in the right femoral vein and passed into the right atrium. The catheter, which also has a curved tip and is shaped to fit snugly over the needle, has been placed in the vein either through a cutdown over the saphenous vein or percutaneously. The catheter is advanced until it impinges on the fossa ovalis in the middle of the atrial septum, and the needle is then advanced to puncture the atrial septum. The procedure is carried out under fluoroscopic vision and with a continuously visible pressure record. Once the tip has entered the left atrium, the catheter is advanced over the needle to lie in the left atrium. The catheter itself, or a smaller one passed through it, is then advanced into the left ventricle in the position

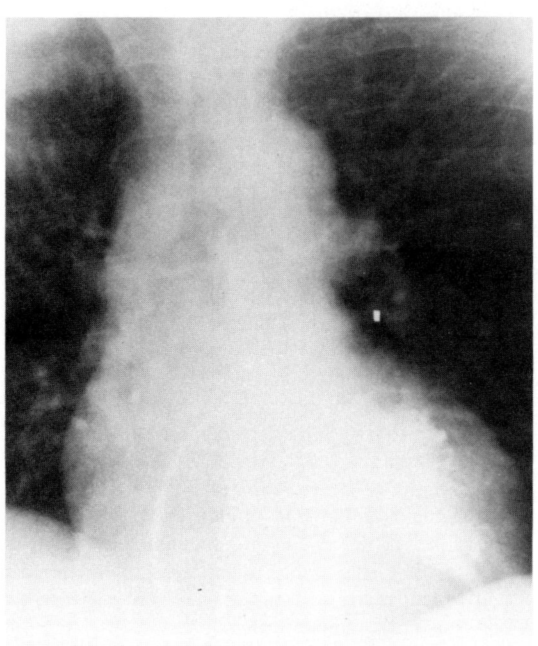

Figure 6–4. Single frame from left ventricular angiography carried out via a catheter passed transseptally into the left atrium and left ventricle.

shown in Fig 6–4. The principal indication for the use of transseptal catheterization is in patients with aortic stenosis in whom a retrograde aortic catheter fails to enter the left ventricle.

Contraindications

The procedure is likely to cause problems in patients with kyphoscoliosis, left atrial thrombus, left atrial myxoma, or giant left atrium. The success rate in entering the left ventricle from the atrium is not 100%, and the fact that aortography and coronary arteriography are now so commonly performed has tended to reduce the number of transseptal studies being done.

Left Ventricular Puncture

Percutaneous transthoracic left ventricular puncture is indicated only when a catheter cannot be passed across the aortic valve in a retrograde manner, as in a patient with calcific aortic stenosis. This procedure is easier to perform and less dangerous than might be expected and is described in Chapter 13.

Measurements During Left Heart Catheterization

Left ventricular and aortic pressures constitute the principal measurements to be obtained during left heart catheterization. In investigating patients with mitral disease, the left ventricular pressure is measured together with the wedge pressure (via right heart catheterization) in order to assess the pressure difference across the mitral valve. The wedge pressure is inevitably delayed by about 0.1 sec and so lags behind the left ventricular pressure. This fact, illustrated in Fig 6–5, must be taken into account in analyzing the tracings and calculating valve area. During transseptal catheterization, the gradient across the mitral valve is recorded on pulling the catheter back across the valve.

Simultaneous arterial or aortic and left ventricular pressures are recorded during transseptal catheterization to assess aortic valve hemodynamics. In retrograde catheterization, the pressures are recorded on pullback. Pressure differences within the ventricle are best sought in retrograde studies on withdrawal of the catheter from the body of the ventricle to the outflow tract. In transseptal catheterization, the operator should be careful to avoid confusing valvular and subvalvular obstructions, which tend to give superficially similar tracings.

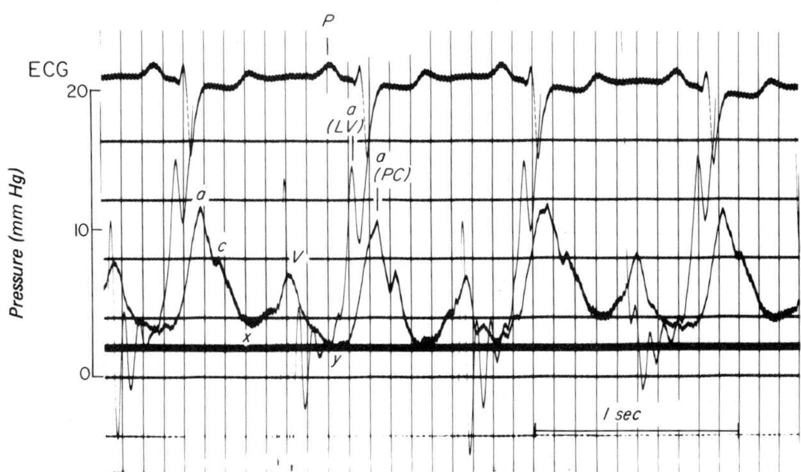

Figure 6–5. Simultaneous wedge (PC) pressure measured by the right heart route and left ventricular (LV) pressure measured by retrograde left heart catheterization. The delay in the PC tracing can be seen at the time of the *a* wave. The systolic LV pressure is "off scale," and the tracings show the diastolic events only.

ANGIOCARDIOGRAPHY

Angiocardiography has come to play a major role in the clinical assessment of cardiac lesions in the last 20 years. The advent of image intensifiers and cineangiography has greatly improved the quality of the pictures obtained. Left ventricular angiography has come to be an important means of assessing left ventricular function. The performance of the left ventricle can be assessed either by observing the speed and extent of contraction or by measuring the ventricular ejection fraction (see p 68).

Technic

Pressurized injectors are conventionally used, and the dosage of contrast material and the rate of injection vary with the size of the catheter used and the size of the patient. Angiography (other than coronary angiography) requires the use of a multiple-hole catheter, preferably with a closed tip (Lehman or NIH). A small preliminary injection is always given to ensure that the catheter is appropriately positioned. This prevents the injection of large amounts of contrast material into the myocardial tissue. This complication can be serious if it occurs either in the right or the left ventricle when the catheter tip is embedded in trabeculae.

Effects of Contrast Material

A major reason for the more widespread use of angiocardiography has been the refinement in the contrast material used. Multiple injections of up to 2 ml/kg can now be given without fear of complications. The contrast material always affects ventricular function, so that an increase in ventricular diastolic pressure is often seen after an injection. This finding is particularly likely to occur in patients in whom ventricular function is impaired. It may last for half an hour or more and occasionally interferes with assessment of the severity of a lesion.

Quality of Angiograms

Angiocardiography provides the best pictures when the dose of contrast material is large and the dye remains highly concentrated in the heart. Thus, sequential pictures of the chambers of the right and left heart are best taken when cardiac function is good. Conversely, if the contrast material is injected directly into a chamber whose function is poor (eg, the left ventricle in cardiomyopathy), the chamber tends to be well outlined because the dye stays so long in the ventricle. In general, the most satisfactory pictures are obtained in small patients with small hearts in whom the catheter is positioned close to the area of interest. In patients with large left-to-right shunts with large hearts and deep chests, the results are less satisfactory.

Coronary Angiography

Coronary angiography has come to be an extremely important investigation which is indicated in all patients with coronary artery disease in whom surgical treatment is contemplated. It is also indicated in older patients with other lesions in whom the presence of associated coronary disease is suspected. *Coronary arteriography is not useful in the diagnosis of angina pectoris, which is based principally on the history and the ECG changes that occur with the onset of the pain.* Abnormalities in the coronary arteriogram can be present without symptoms, and the presence of lesions in an arteriogram cannot be used to show that a given patient's pain is due to ischemia.

Two methods are in common use for coronary angiography. The older Sones method involves a brachial arterial cutdown using a catheter with a tapered tip. This catheter is manipulated into the aortic root by technics that require considerable skill in order to enter the right and left coronary arteries. Small (5–10 ml) injections of contrast material are made by hand, and cineangiographic films are taken of the coronary circulation. Multiple views are obtained, and the procedure is made easier if the patient lies strapped in a cradle in which he can be turned at different angles to the x-ray apparatus. Biplane angiograms are seldom obtained by this method because access to the arm is needed to manipulate the catheter.

The more modern technic introduced by Judkins uses a percutaneous femoral arterial approach. Specially shaped catheters are used for the right and left coronary arteries. The left coronary catheter enters the left coronary ostium quite readily, and little skill is needed for its placement. The right coronary catheter is slightly more difficult to place, but less skill is needed than for the Sones method. Injections of contrast material are again made by hand, and, since the arms are free to be placed above the head, biplane angiography can be readily performed. The number of injections of contrast medium, the duration of the procedure, and the severity of the coronary disease determine the morbidity and mortality rates of the Judkins technic.

Left ventricular angiography should always be performed as an adjunct to coronary arteriography. Left ventricular volume and ejection fraction are measured, and localized areas of abnormal ventricular motion are sought.

Videotape Recorders

It is important to make certain that adequate coronary arteriographic films have been obtained and that it will not be necessary to repeat the studies. Videotape recorders are used in many laboratories to view the results immediately and decide whether the pictures are adequate. The underlying anatomy and the distribution of atherosclerotic disease are so variable that it is difficult to be sure all aspects of the lesion have been demonstrated if only a single pass of the study on a television screen is seen. With experience, the adequacy of the films can be assessed while the cineangiogram is being filmed, and the extra time taken to view the films during the procedure, with the catheters still in place—which increases the morbidity rate of the study—can be avoided.

OTHER STUDIES

Exercise During Cardiac Catheterization

Exercise is sometimes used during cardiac catheterization to evaluate the effect of stress on the hemodynamic state. However, it is difficult to do physiologic studies in supine patients lying under a fluoroscopic screen with catheters in several vessels. The use of a femoral approach generally restricts the studies to a single leg raising, which does not provide much stress. If the brachial approach is used, the patient can pedal a cycle ergometer attached to the foot of the table, but even this form of exercise is less satisfactory than upright exercise on a cycle ergometer or treadmill. Exercise is most commonly used in patients with mitral valve disease and usually consists of a short, nonsteady state period of leg raising.

Coronary Sinus Catheterization & Atrial Pacing

Functional information about the adequacy of coronary perfusion can be obtained by coronary sinus catheterization and by right atrial pacing. It is difficult to use exercise to induce angina in the cardiac catheterization laboratory, and the less "physiologic" stress of progressive levels of tachycardia produced by atrial pacing is more frequently employed. Unfortunately, the electrocardiographic tracing and the level of left ventricular pressure provide unreliable indications of the effects of myocardial ischemia during pacing. The onset of pain and the level of lactate in the coronary sinus blood are the most valuable indicators of ischemia. Selective catheterization of different cardiac venous segments via the coronary sinus and its branches provides some degree of localization of the area of ischemia.

His Bundle Recordings

Intracardiac electrocardiography is occasionally used in the elucidation of difficult cardiac arrhythmias, eg, in distinguishing supraventricular and ventricular arrhythmias. His bundle recording is mainly used for research purposes and seldom provides information that affects management of the patient. Intracardiac electrograms are obtained from the conduction system as it runs in the interventricular septum near the tricuspid valve. A special catheter with 4 separate electrodes at different distances from the tip is positioned in the right heart after introduction through a right femoral vein approach. A second catheter is often inserted from the arm to pace the heart by right atrial stimulation. The timing of the electrical signals from the different electrodes against a conventional ECG is used to identify the recording site, and recordings can be obtained from the bundle of His and the right bundle. (See Chapters 14 and 15.)

COMPLICATIONS OF CARDIAC CATHETERIZATION

The complications of these invasive studies vary with the complexities of the investigations, the length of time the studies last, and the basic disease from which the patient is suffering. Some of the complications are common to all types of study; others are confined to particular types of procedures and particular diseases.

COMPLICATIONS COMMON TO ALL FORMS OF CATHETERIZATION

Vessel Spasm

Spasm of the vessel into which a catheter is inserted—either an artery or a vein—almost invariably results from excessive trauma, often due to the use of too large a catheter for the size of the vessel. It is more common in young, nervous persons, and prior sedation, which is not needed routinely, may help to minimize it.

Vasovagal Attacks

Vasovagal attacks with bradycardia, hypotension, and ultimately loss of consciousness can occur in any study but are sufficiently common in coronary arteriography (especially when the catheter is near the orifice of the right coronary artery) so that atropine, 0.4–0.8 mg intravenously, is recommended as a routine form of premedication. In other studies, it is sufficient to watch for the early signs—bradycardia, often associated with yawning—and raise the patient's legs and give atropine via the catheter.

Pulmonary Edema

Cardiac catheterization involves keeping the patient lying flat for several hours. If the patient has pulmonary congestion, this may provoke pulmonary edema. The first hint of its development is often restlessness, with a dry cough.

Arrhythmia

Atrial or ventricular arrhythmias are commonly provoked during cardiac catheterization. Fortunately, they usually subside upon removal of the catheter, which is thought to be responsible for their provocation by direct mechanical stimulation. Atrial arrhythmias are common when the catheter is in the right atrium in patients with atrial septal defect or mitral valve disease. Runs of ventricular ectopic beats are particularly frequent when the catheter is in the right ventricle. If the patient has left bundle branch block and electrical activation of the heart depends solely on the right bundle branch, cardiac standstill often takes the place of the run of ectopic beats. A pacemaker should always be available in the laboratory but is seldom needed. Ventricular tachycardia and ventricular fibrillation are rarely seen in right heart catheterization. They are most likely to occur during coronary arteriography (incidence about 1%). A sharp blow on the chest—or, if that is not successful, direct current countershock—should restore sinus rhythm. A defibrillator should be available in the room where cardiac catheterization is being done for use in an emergency. In some centers, a pacemaker catheter is kept in the right ventricle during coronary angiography for use in an emergency, but we do not feel that this is necessary. The pacemaker catheter may itself cause arrhythmia.

Prevention of Complications

In general, the sooner the onset of a complication is recognized, the easier it is to restore the patient's status to normal and complete the study. Most complications are due to the study, and stopping the procedure is usually an effective but unsatisfactory method of treatment.

SPECIAL COMPLICATIONS OF PARTICULAR PROCEDURES

Right Heart Catheterization

Right heart catheterization should result in minimal morbidity and a zero mortality rate in adults. Adequate data should be obtainable in 99% of cases. Venous spasm is probably the most common problem, and anatomic variations in venous anatomy may interfere with the passage of the catheter to the right atrium.

Left Heart Catheterization

Percutaneous femoral catheterization is the procedure most likely to lead to arterial occlusion. Thrombus forms on the outside of the catheter, and as the catheter is withdrawn from the vessel a sheath of thrombus is pulled off which coils up and blocks the artery. This complication, which is described on p 100, is likely to occur when the catheter is left for a long time in the arterial tree. A low cardiac output and a small femoral artery, as seen in thin female patients with mitral stenosis and raised pulmonary vascular resistance, favor the occurrence of the complication.

Following brachial arterial arteriotomy, control of hemorrhage is sometimes a problem. It usually responds to prolonged pressure over the vessel. On removal of the catheter at the end of the study, a jet of blood should spurt from both the proximal and distal ends of the artery. When this does not happen, the presence of a blood clot should be suspected. Gently probing the vessel with a soft plastic catheter often dislodges soft thrombus. Passage of a Fogarty balloon catheter is the next step, and a vascular surgeon should be summoned when these measures do not meet with success. Since the brachial artery can usually be tied off without compromising the circulation to the hand and arm, the complications of the brachial approach are seldom serious, but the median nerve may be damaged.

In transseptal catheterization, it is possible to puncture the free wall of the right atrium, the aortic wall, or the tricuspid valve inadvertently, and complications can be serious. Hemorrhage and tamponade are the most common causes of death from the procedure.

In direct left ventricular puncture, the principal complication is pneumothorax. If the procedure is done only in patients with severe left ventricular hypertrophy due to aortic stenosis, the danger of intrapericardial hemorrhage and tamponade is minimized.

The dangers associated with all forms of left heart catheterization are about 10 times greater than those of right heart studies. Systemic embolism from thrombus forming on catheters in the left heart is much more dangerous than in the lesser circulation. It is important to flush catheters in the left side of the circulation frequently and forcefully. The catheters used almost always have multiple openings, and a slow drip of heparinized saline, which is used to keep single-hole catheters patent, should not be used with multiple-hole catheters. It is possible for the drip to pass through one of the holes, leaving the others to become clogged with thrombus. The correct procedure is to flush multiple-hole catheters forcefully every 2 minutes or so.

Coronary Angiography

Ventricular fibrillation or ventricular tachycardia occurs during coronary angiography in about 1% of patients with coronary disease. A sharp blow on the chest or direct current countershock should restore sinus rhythm, and in many laboratories coronary angiography is continued after this treatment has been successful. Coronary angiography is now the commonest precipitating cause of death in the cardiac catheterization laboratory in adults. The procedure is most dangerous in patients with severe 3-vessel or left main coronary disease, those with previous myocardial infarction and heart failure, and those with a low systolic and high diastolic left ventricular pressure. Progressive hypotension during and after the procedure—rather than arrhythmia—is the usual problem. Precipitation of myocardial infarction is another complication of the procedure. This may be due to embolism, trauma to the coronary ostium, or impaction of the catheter, which occludes the ostium completely.

It is important to monitor the pressure at the catheter tip at all times when the catheter is in a coronary vessel. This obviously is not possible during injection, but arrangements should be made to switch off the pressure tracings for the minimal time. Progressive damping of the pressure tracing is an important indication of the need to reposition the catheter. Spasm of the proximal part of a coronary artery can occur during coronary angiography and is usually attributed to mechanical effects of the catheter. Sublingual nitroglycerin is used for prevention and treatment. In some laboratories, it is routinely given before the study; in others, it is withheld until some indication of spasm is recognized.

The contrast material used in angiography tends to act as an osmotic load and increase the blood volume. This can lead to complications, especially in patients on the verge of pulmonary edema. It is unwise to inject large amounts of contrast material into the pulmonary arteries of patients with mitral stenosis, especially if the pulmonary vascular resistance is raised. The patient is likely to develop pulmonary edema, and the quality of the pictures obtained from the left atrium and ventricle is likely to be poor.

Hypersensitivity responses to the iodine in the contrast material are rare. It seems that injections into the left side of the heart, bypassing the lungs, cause less trouble than intravenous injections, as in intravenous urography.

RISKS OF CARDIAC CATHETERIZATION

Most of the risks of cardiac catheterization have already been mentioned. In our experience, death on the catheterization table has been due to uncontrollable hypotension in patients with severe ischemic heart disease in heart failure; to hemorrhage following perforation of the aorta during transseptal catheterization; or to ventricular fibrillation which did not respond to resuscitation. Later complications leading to death have included severe febrile reactions in severely ill patients. These are generally attributed to the pyrogenic effects of traces of blood left in catheters after cleaning. Ultrasonic cleaners and more widespread use of disposable catheters have reduced the incidence of this complication.

Peripheral embolism resulting from the dislodgement of intracardiac thrombus or calcific material from the aortic valve has occasionally contributed to severe disability and even death. Air embolism is a potential hazard but has never been recognized as an important factor in our experience. Paradoxic embolism can occur in patients with right-to-left shunts; and cerebral embolism, which is a spontaneous complication in Fallot's tetralogy, can occur following catheterization.

Any form of arrhythmia or conduction defect can occur during cardiac catheterization. Fortunately, removal of the catheter usually restores normal rhythm. If it does not, direct current countershock is almost always effective for correcting a tachyarrhythmia if resuscitation is efficiently carried out. Vasovagal episodes should never cause serious problems provided the complication is recognized in its early stages and atropine is available.

The development of pulmonary edema should not cause serious problems if its early manifestations are quickly recognized and steps taken to treat them by sitting the patient up and giving oxygen. Local complications such as arterial occlusion, hemorrhage, venospasm, and phlebitis are relatively common but should not cause serious problems.

It is of interest that infective endocarditis is virtually unknown following cardiac catheterization, and its presence is no bar to study.

Morbidity & Mortality Rates

Patients in whom trouble is to be expected include those with severe mitral stenosis with or without pulmonary hypertension, patients with pulmonary hypertension due to any cause, pulmonary or aortic stenosis of severe degree, Ebstein's malformation, left bundle branch block, and severe ischemic heart disease with heart failure. The mortality and morbidity statistics are highly dependent on the types of patients studied and the experience of the operator. A rate of serious complications (eg, embolism, arrhythmia, and hemorrhage) of more than 3% and a mortality rate of more than 0.3% call for review of the operations and standard procedures in selecting and studying patients by means of these technics.

• • •

References

Abrams HL: *Angiography*, 2nd ed. 2 vols. Little, Brown, 1971.

Bahler RC, MacLeod CA: Atrial pacing and exercise in the evaluation of patients with angina pectoris. Circulation 43:407, 1971.

Bernéus B & others: Percutaneous catheterization of peripheral arteries as method for blood sampling. Scand J Clin Lab Invest 6:217, 1954.

Braunwald E, Swan HJC (editors): Cooperative study on cardiac catheterization. Circulation 37 (Suppl 3), 1968.

Brewster H, McIlroy MB: Blood gas tensions and pH of pulmonary "wedge" samples in patients with heart disease. J Appl Physiol 34:413, 1973.

Brock RC & others: Percutaneous left ventricular puncture in the assessment of aortic stenosis. Thorax 11:163, 1956.

Brown R & others: The effect of angiocardiographic contrast medium on circulatory dynamics in man. Circulation 31:234, 1965.

Damato AN, Gallagher JJ, Lau SH: Application of His bundle recordings in diagnosing conduction disorders. Prog Cardiovasc Dis 14:601, 1972.

Damato AN & others: Study of atrioventricular conduction in man using electrode catheter recordings of His bundle activity. Circulation 39:287, 1969.

DeSanctis RW: Diagnostic and therapeutic uses of atrial pacing. Circulation 43:748, 1971.

Fogarty TJ & others: A method for extraction of arterial emboli and thrombi. Surg Gynecol Obstet 116:241, 1963.

Forssmann W: Die sondierung des rechten Herzens. Klin Wochenschr 8:2085, 1929.

Friesinger GG & others: Hemodynamic consequences of the injection of radiopaque material. Circulation 31:730, 1965.

Gensini GG: *Coronary Arteriography*. Futura, 1975.

Grossman W (editor): *Cardiac Catheterization and Angiography*. Lee & Febiger, 1974.

Hellems HK & others: Pulmonary capillary pressure in man. J Clin Invest 27:540, 1948.

Judkins MP: Selective coronary arteriography. 1. A percutaneous transfemoral technic. Radiology 89:815, 1967.

Kory RC, Tsagiris TJ, Bustamente R: *Catheterization*. Thomas, 1965.

Mendel D: *A Practice of Cardiac Catheterization*, 2nd ed. Blackwell, 1974.

Rackley CE, Russell RO Jr: *Coronary Care–Invasive Techniques for Hemodynamic Measurements*. Am Heart Association, 1973.

Rapaport E, Scheinman M: Rationale and limitations of hemodynamic measurements in patients with acute myocardial infarction. Mod Concepts Cardiovasc Dis 38:55, 1969.

Ross J & others: Transseptal left heart catheterization: A new diagnostic method. Prog Cardiovasc Dis 2:315, 1959.

Selzer A: *Principles of Clinical Cardiology*. Saunders, 1975.

Sones FM, Shirey EK: Cine coronary arteriography. Mod Concepts Cardiovasc Dis 31:735, 1962.

Swan HJC & others: Catheterization of the heart in man with use of a flow-directed balloon-tipped catheter. N Engl J Med 283:447, 1970.

Zimmerman HA: *Intravascular Catheterization*. Thomas, 1966.

7...
Therapeutic Procedures

This chapter deals with the technics of some of the special therapeutic procedures commonly used in the management of cardiac disorders. The procedures may be applied to many different clinical situations, and, since they are therapeutic, they must often be done at the bedside. Whenever possible, the patient's status should be monitored by the methods described in Chapters 5 and 6 to observe the response to therapy. However, since therapeutic procedures are often needed in emergency situations, the technics described must on occasion be used in circumstances that are less than ideal.

CARDIOPULMONARY RESUSCITATION

All physicians should be familiar with the emergency procedures involved in cardiopulmonary resuscitation. These vary with the nature of the emergency and the circumstances surrounding the episode. Resuscitation in a highly equipped area such as an intensive care or coronary care unit differs significantly from that carried out in the street or in some other public place.

The principles involved are similar in all circumstances, and speed in applying the appropriate treatment is of paramount importance. Establishment of the nature and, if possible, the cause of the emergency is essential.

The situations encountered in practice in public are (1) sudden collapse without warning, (2) choking on food in the airway (in restaurants), and (3) epileptic seizures.

Resuscitation in a Public Place

When a patient falls to the ground or is found incapacitated, the presence of a pulse should be sought at the carotid artery in the neck and the presence of a heartbeat determined by direct palpation or auscultation. At the same time, the state of consciousness should be established by determining whether the patient can respond to simple commands. The cortical state of consciousness and cerebration should be checked by observing the size of the pupils and testing their response to light. The circumstances surrounding the collapse should be determined, if possible, by questioning witnesses, but nothing should delay the start of resuscitative measures if breathing has stopped and cardiac function is ineffective. It is important in this preliminary assessment to establish whether the patient is breathing and whether the airway is patent, for this determines the priorities of treatment, especially when no help is available.

A. Pulseless, Breathing Patient: If the patient is pulseless and breathing, closed chest cardiac resuscitation should be started. A sharp blow on the lower sternum sometimes stops ventricular arrhythmia or restarts the heart after sudden cardiac arrest (it is equivalent to an electric shock of about 1 joule). The patient must be placed on a firm support, usually on the floor, and rhythmic pressure applied to the lower sternum sufficient to move the rib cage one-fifth of the anteroposterior diameter of the chest with every stroke (Fig 7–1). The rate of massage should be about 80–100/min. The patient's head should be as low as possible to encourage cerebral perfusion, and a carotid or femoral pulse should be sought during the procedure if possible. The patient's breathing should be observed to make certain it is being maintained.

B. Pulseless Patient Not Breathing: If neither pulse nor respiration is present, the mouth and pharynx must be cleared of obstructions such as blood, vomitus, mucus, or a bolus of food to open the airway so that mouth-to-mouth resuscitation can be started. The nostrils are pinched closed, the airway kept clear by backward and upward pressure on the chin, and the lungs inflated by forced expiration, as shown in Fig 7–2. After a few inflations, closed chest cardiac massage is begun. Combined cardiac and pulmonary resuscitation is given in alternating fashion, 15 strokes of cardiac massage to every 2 or 3 lung inflations. When help arrives, someone else should take over one of the resuscitative tasks. When qualified and specially equipped persons come on the scene, a plastic airway (Fig 7–3) and a bag with a one-way valve of the type shown in Fig 7–4 may be substituted for mouth-to-mouth resuscitation and arrangements can be made to move the patient to an appropriate place for further care as needed.

C. Patient With Pulse But Not Breathing: If the patient is not breathing but has a pulse, the procedures described above to open the airway should be followed

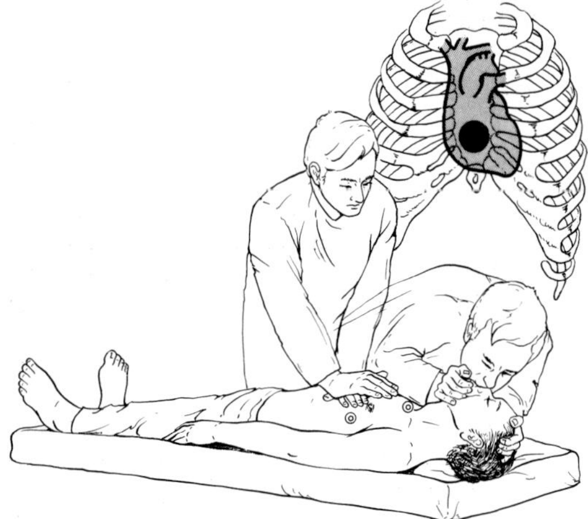

Figure 7–1. Technic of closed chest cardiac massage. Heavy circle in heart drawing shows area of application of force. Circles on supine figure show points of application of electrodes for defibrillation. (Reproduced, with permission, from Krupp MA & others: *Physician's Handbook,* 18th ed. Lange, 1976.)

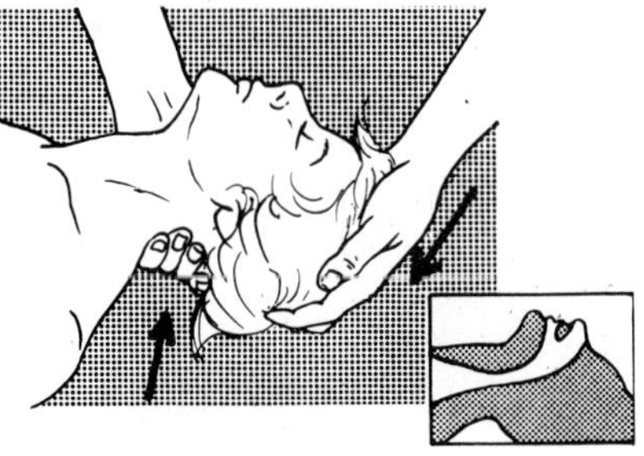

(1) The operator takes his position at the patient's head.

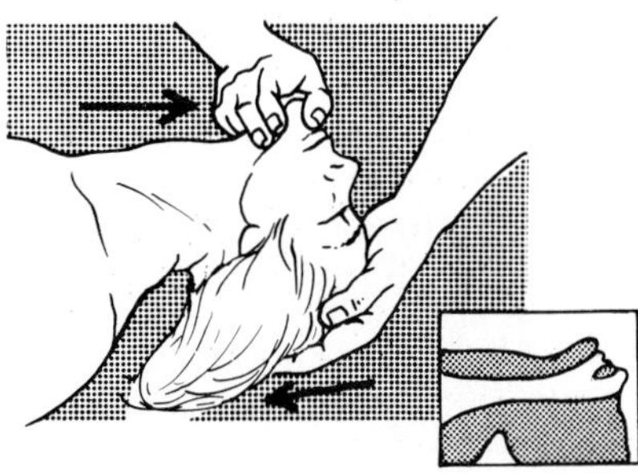

(2) With the right thumb and index finger he displaces the mandible forward by pressing at its central portion, at the same time lifting the neck and tilting the head as far back as possible.

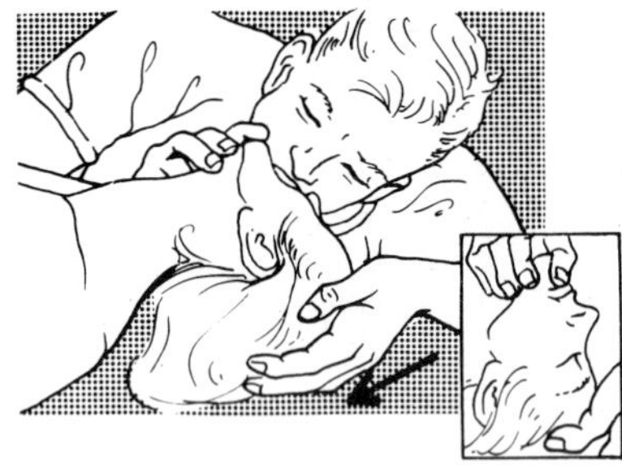

(3) After taking a deep breath, the operator immediately seals his mouth around the mouth (or nose) of the victim and exhales until the chest of the victim rises.

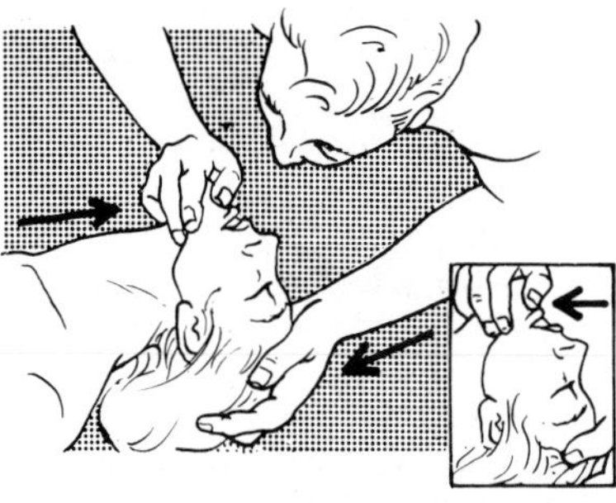

(4) The victim's mouth is opened by downward and forward traction on the lower jaw or by pulling down the lower lip.

Figure 7–2. Technic of mouth-to-mouth insufflation. (Reproduced, with permission, from Benson RC: *Handbook of Obstetrics & Gynecology,* 6th ed. Lange, 1977.)

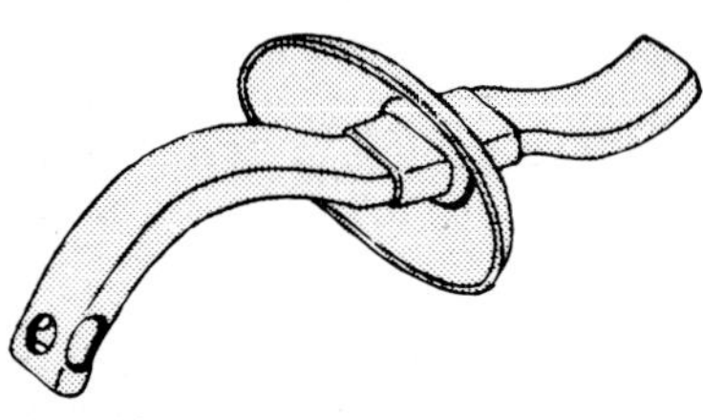

Figure 7–3. Airway for use in mouth-to-mouth insufflation. The larger airway is for adults. The guard is flexible and may be inverted from the position shown for use with infants and children. (Reproduced, with permission, from Krupp MA & others: *Physician's Handbook,* 18th ed. Lange, 1976.)

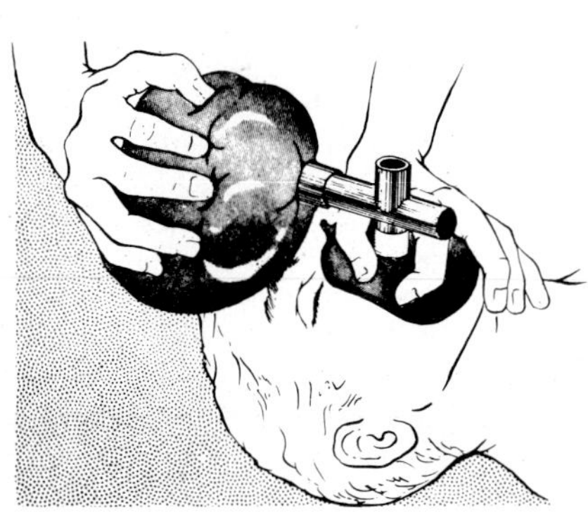

Figure 7–4. Portable manual resuscitator. (Reproduced, with permission, from Krupp MA & others: *Physician's Handbook,* 18th ed. Lange, 1976.)

and mouth-to-mouth resuscitation performed. The state of the circulation must be checked at intervals in order to determine that adequate cardiac function is being maintained.

Choking on Food

Choking on food is commonly seen in restaurants in persons who have overindulged in alcohol. It is also a risk in nursing homes among elderly, debilitated, edentulous patients who may be oversedated. Acute respiratory distress associated with airway obstruction due to blockage by food is often apparent because the patient stands up, coughs and sputters, and shows clear signs of respiratory distress. The rescuer first takes up a position behind the victim, who stands still in the upright position. The rescuer's arms are then placed around the victim's waist, with the hands formed into fists against the victim's epigastrium, and pulled in forcibly on the victim's abdomen several times. The forced expiratory airflow will usually dislodge the obstruction, at least partially, and it may then be possible to grasp it with the fingers down the throat and remove it if the patient cannot spit it out. If the victim is lying on the floor, the rescuer should kneel astride the victom's body and attempt to expel the obstruction with a forceful blow with the fist to the epigastrium. If these simple maneuvers fail, emergency tracheostomy may have to be performed using the sharpest knife available.

Epileptic Seizure

Make certain that the pulse and respiration are present and that the airway is patent. Lay the patient on a flat surface and support the chin to maintain a free airway. Place the best available padded object between the teeth to prevent tongue biting. Try to establish a diagnosis and summon assistance.

Resuscitation in a Hospital Setting

All hospitals should have an emergency resuscitation team available at all times capable of responding to a telephone call for assistance anywhere in the hospital. The emergency is usually announced over a public address system, and the appropriate persons—usually a cardiologist, an anesthetist, and a surgeon—should go as quickly as possible to the scene. The emergency procedures are instituted by persons already at the scene as described above for resuscitation in a public place. In a hospital setting, it is usually easier to make a rapid diagnosis because the reasons for the patient's hospitalization will be known. The same principles apply in deciding whether closed chest cardiac massage or mouth-to-mouth resuscitation (or both) is required, and, since more than one person is usually present, one must take charge and direct operations, maintaining resuscitative measures until further assistance arrives. Note should be made of the time the resuscitation team arrives on the scene since this will be important in deciding when to abandon resuscitation efforts if they are unsuccessful.

Three basic questions must be considered when the full team is assembled: (1) What is the nature of the problem? (Arrhythmia? Asystole? Respiratory failure?) (2) What is the underlying cause of the problem and is it correctable? (Myocardial infarction? Pulmonary embolism? Hemorrhage? Trauma?) (3) What further measures are needed?

During this period, someone should be attaching electrocardiograph leads, starting an intravenous drip if one is not already set up, preparing the DC defibrillator, preparing drug doses in appropriate syringes for immediate use, and taking an arterial blood sample for analysis of P_{O_2}, P_{CO_2}, and pH.

Emergency Defibrillation

If ventricular fibrillation or tachycardia is the cause of the emergency, direct current defibrillation should be carried out with a minimum of delay. AC defibrillators are no longer used. In emergency situations, a DC shock of 400 joules is routinely given and repeated as necessary. The paddles, which should already have been liberally smeared with ECG electrode paste, are applied, one over the cardiac apex and the other over the base of the heart, in the positions shown in Fig 7–1. Everyone except the holder of the paddles breaks physical contact with the patient, and the shock is administered by pressing the button to complete the circuit and discharge the electric impulse through the patient. Since the patient is already unconscious, no anesthetic is required. The instant of the shock is clearly visible as the patient's body jerks because of electrical stimulation of the thoracic muscles. When the response to the shock has been determined, a decision is made whether to restart cardiac massage and ventilation, whether to try to improve the state of perfusion and oxygenation by some other means, or whether to try another shock.

Further Measures

If defibrillation is unsuccessful, one should consider the possibility of giving lidocaine, 50 mg, as an intravenous bolus, and repeating the DC shock. The drug can be repeated up to a total dose of 500 mg. If asystole is present and a pacemaker is not immediately available, intravenous or intracardiac epinephrine (0.5 mg, or 5 ml of a 1:10,000 aqueous solution) should be tried. The drug may start cardiac contractions and produce ventricular fibrillation which can then be treated by DC countershock. Acidosis develops rapidly with cardiac arrest and inhibits cardiac contractility. Since closed chest cardiac massage provides only 15-20% of a normal output, acidosis must be treated in all cases which do not respond within 3–5 minutes. Sodium bicarbonate solution, 3.75 g (44.6 mEq), should be given intravenously and the dose repeated every 5 minutes until the circulation is restored. A slow infusion of 5% sodium bicarbonate at 100-150 drops/min is often more convenient. The effect of the infusion should be monitored by arterial blood gas measurements whenever possible.

If asystole is present, calcium chloride, 10 ml of a 10% solution, should be tried as a cardiac stimulant. If this fails, the question of cardiac pacing arises. External cardiac pacemakers require high voltage (up to 100 volts) to stimulate cardiac contraction using electrodes at the cardiac apex and right second interspace. External pacing is sometimes effective in primary asystole, but it is traumatic and not tolerable in a conscious patient. It is sometimes possible to stimulate the heart to contract by tapping the precordium rhythmically about 60 times per minute with the ulnar edge of the hand, using a modified "karate chop"; if this is successful, it is much preferred to external pacing. External pacing is only used as an emergency procedure to bridge the gap until a temporary transvenous pacemaker can be inserted. If bradycardia is present after DC countershock, atropine (0.4–0.8 mg intravenously) should be tried.

Isoproterenol is often used as a general supportive measure when the heart rate is slow. It is given as an intravenous drip with 1 mg of the drug in 500 ml of 5% dextrose in water at a rate of 0.03 mg per 5 minutes. If the patient recovers, he should be carefully examined, transferred to an intensive care area, and observed for the development of shock and for complications arising from the precipitating cause of the original circulatory collapse.

Follow-Up Measures

After the patient has responded to resuscitative measures, evaluation of central nervous system function deserves careful consideration. Each case must be treated on its merits, and it must be decided whether the physician is prolonging life or simply prolonging dying in patients with serious brain damage. Apparently complete central nervous system recovery has been reported in a few patients who have remained unconscious for up to a week after resuscitation.

Hypothermia at 30 °C for 2–3 days may lessen the degree of brain damage. It is also important to look for complications of resuscitation, such as broken ribs, ruptured abdominal viscera, or pneumothorax.

OXYGEN THERAPY

Oxygen therapy should be considered in all patients in whom hypoxia is present and in those who are dyspneic at rest. The objective is to maintain an arterial P_{O_2} > 60 mm Hg. Oxygen is ordinarily available as the pure 100% gas either from a cylinder or via a wall outlet in intensive care areas. The technics used for administration of the gas at ambient pressure are shown in Table 7–1. The ease with which the patient tolerates oxygen therapy depends on the benefit derived from its use. When dyspnea and hypoxia are severe at rest, as in acute pulmonary edema or in lung disease, and the oxygen both raises the arterial P_{O_2} and relieves the dyspnea, the patient tolerates the therapy well. If the dyspnea is not relieved by oxygen, as in right-to-left shunts, severe low cardiac output states, and shock, the patient often tolerates the mask or catheter poorly.

Table 7–1. Oxygen therapy equipment at ambient pressure.*

Equipment	Flow (l/min)	Approximate O_2 Concentration Delivered (Percent)	Remarks
Nasal cannula (prongs)	2–6	30–40	Nasal obstruction interferes.
Nasal catheter	2–6	30–40	Misplaced catheter may cause gastric dilatation.
Mask (with exhalation valve)	6–8 8–12	35–45 45–65	May be difficult to fit and uncomfortable for prolonged use.
Mask (with bag)	6–8 8–12	40–60 60–90	
Venturi mask (Venti-Mask)	4–8	24,28,35†	Reasonably accurate concentrations delivered by Venturi principle. Light plastic mask.

*Reproduced, with permission, from Krupp MA & others: *Physician's Handbook,* 18th ed. Lange, 1976.
†Disposable mask for each concentration.

It is difficult to achieve an alveolar oxygen level of more than 40% by the use of masks or nasal catheters, especially in dyspneic patients, and thus it is mainly in those patients in whom a small increase in alveolar P_{O_2} produces a large increase in arterial P_{O_2} that oxygen therapy is effective.

It is possible to achieve higher alveolar oxygen levels by careful administration of oxygen with a qualified person in constant attendance and constant monitoring available; 100% oxygen increases the oxygen content of blood leaving the lungs in patients with normal lung function by increasing the amount of oxygen carried in solution in the blood. This effect is small in patients with normal levels of hemoglobin, amounting to 17 ml/l (hemoglobin level 14.9 g/dl) or equivalent to about an 8.5% increase in saturation in a person with an oxygen capacity of 200 ml/l. This extra oxygen does not generally produce a significant clinical effect in patients in heart failure with a low cardiac output and normal lungs. In anemic patients, however, the effects are greater, amounting to the equivalent of a 34% increase in oxygen saturation in a patient with an oxygen capacity of 50 ml/l (hemoglobin level 3.7 g/dl).

Effective oxygen therapy is not without its dangers, since alveolar collapse (atelectasis) is likely to occur if nitrogen is eliminated from the lungs. Since it is so difficult to achieve alveolar oxygen levels of 90% or more in clinical practice, atelectasis is seldom a problem except when increased barometric pressures are used. It is the danger of lung damage that contraindicates the use of hyperbaric chambers for the delivery of increased amounts of oxygen in the treatment of heart disease.

Oxygen Therapy in Specific Conditions

Oxygen therapy is indicated in the treatment of high-altitude pulmonary edema, especially when the patient cannot return to a lower altitude. It should be tried in all patients with myocardial infarction in whom severe myocardial damage has occurred. Ventilation-perfusion mismatching may be present, and hypoxia is not infrequently seen.

If oxygen therapy is well tolerated, it can increase the oxygenation of marginally perfused tissues. If the patient is disturbed by the mask or catheter used for its administration, the resulting increase in cardiac output may offset the benefits obtained. Oxygen is indicated in any patient with pulmonary edema irrespective of the underlying cause. Oxygenation of the blood leaving the lungs is incomplete in pulmonary edema, and oxygen is usually effective and well tolerated in all but the most restless patients.

It is in patients with lung disease, especially those with cor pulmonale, that oxygen is most clearly indicated. Oxygen often reduces the pulmonary artery pressure by reversing hypoxic pulmonary arterial vasoconstriction. This may break the vicious cycle responsible for right heart failure and thus play a major part in the patient's recovery.

Respiratory depression due to oxygen therapy can occur in patients who have lost their respiratory sensitivity to CO_2 (eg, in emphysema and chronic bronchitis). In such patients, oxygen therapy can result in respiratory depression and CO_2 retention, with loss of consciousness due to "CO_2 narcosis." The cerebral blood flow increases, the blood pressure rises, and the cerebrospinal fluid pressure may also increase, leading to papilledema and convulsions. However, the chance of this sequence of events occurring has been exaggerated, and it rarely occurs even in patients with chronic pulmonary disease. Artificial or assisted ventilation can be used if any tendency to hypoventilation develops in such patients.

Positive Airway Pressure

Maintenance of a continuous positive airway pressure and the use of positive pressure to inflate the lungs have a place in the treatment of pulmonary edema. Positive end-expiratory pressure (PEEP) can be achieved by having the patient breathe from a mask fitted with a demand valve, breathing out into a tube the end of which is submerged in water to a level of several centimeters. The extra end-expiratory pressure serves to increase the lung volume and, by increasing the intra-alveolar pressure, prevents the transudation of fluid into the alveoli. A similar effect can be obtained by the use of patient-cycled respirators. The aim of their use in pulmonary edema is not to assist in lung inflation but to provide a constant positive pressure airway throughout the respiratory cycle and maintain a normal alveolar volume. They can be used with either air or oxygen, and a considerable amount of cooperation is required from the patient. This form of therapy is preferable to continuous positive pressure breathing, in which active lung inflation is produced by an artificial respirator. The patient is much more likely to struggle and fight the respirator when it is used to inflate the lungs.

VENESECTION

Venesection is a traditional means of treating cardiac failure which is seldom used today. Venous blood is ordinarily removed from an antecubital vein with the patient semirecumbent. Blood should not be removed rapidly, and a total of 500 ml is removed in about 15 minutes through a large (16 gauge) needle. If the patient shows any evidence of distress, the foot of the bed can be raised and venous return improved. The great increase in the effectiveness of diuretic drugs has markedly reduced the need for this procedure. It is now almost confined to the treatment of hemochromatosis and of polycythemia in adult patients with cyanotic congenital heart lesions in whom cardiac surgery is not indicated (eg, Eisenmenger's complex).

Bloodless Venesection

The use of tourniquets applied to the limbs in rotation to reduce venous return has been advocated in the treatment of acute pulmonary edema. Blood pressure cuffs are inflated on 3 limbs to a level of about 40 mm Hg (between venous and arterial pressure) in order to trap blood in the periphery. The cuff is removed and reapplied on another limb in rotation every 15 minutes. Up to 700 ml of blood can be trapped in the limbs by this means.

BLOOD TRANSFUSION IN CARDIAC PATIENTS

Blood transfusion is seldom indicated in the treatment of heart disease but is not infrequently needed when anemia occurs for other reasons. The patient should always receive the transfusion in the supine position so that the earliest manifestations of pulmonary congestion can be readily recognized. The patient can then sit up to relieve pulmonary congestion while the transfusion is slowed or stopped. Packed cells should be routinely used, and transfusion should be given as slowly as possible after taking into account the underlying reason for the transfusion. The use of sodium citrate as the anticoagulant imposes a severe load on the circulation, and the use of heparinized blood is preferable.

AFTERLOAD REDUCTION

The use of vasodilator drugs to combat the peripheral vasoconstriction seen in acute forms of heart failure provides a useful emergency means of relieving the load on the left ventricle. This technic is particularly helpful in patients with acute aortic or mitral incompetence, which often cause acute pulmonary edema. The treatment also has a place in some cases of acute myocardial infarction with heart failure. The dose of the vasodilator drug must be carefully titrated against its effects on the systemic arterial pressure, heart rate, and cardiac output, and direct monitoring of arterial and wedge pressure is mandatory. The benefits of reducing the load against which the left ventricle must eject blood must be weighed against any increase in cardiac output that may result from increase in heart rate. When valvular incompetence is present, the additional benefit resulting from the decrease in backflow across the incompetent valves provides an important indication for the use of afterload reduction as an emergency measure to tide the patient over until surgery can be performed. The use of the treatment in chronic left heart failure is advocated by some, but the results are less dramatic.

There is no entirely satisfactory drug with which to produce systemic vasodilatation. Phentolamine, which acts as an alpha-adrenergic blocking agent, can be used either intravenously or orally. Sodium nitroprusside is relatively short-acting and is given intravenously, and hydralazine can be given by mouth. The optimal dosage of all of these drugs must be determined by trial and error in each individual patient. The most satisfactory regimen is to start with a small dose (5 mg of phentolamine, 15 μg/min of nitroprusside, or 25 mg of hydralazine) while monitoring the hemodynamic status closely and to gradually increase the medication until a full hemodynamic response is obtained. The dose is then reduced by 15–20% to a maintenance level.

Several other drugs have been tried in an attempt to obtain longer-lasting effects. Sublingual or topical nitroglycerin and sublingual or oral isosorbide dinitrate have been shown to be effective, but their effects on capacitative vessels (veins) are greater, and a fall in output may occur. Their absorption and consequently their therapeutic effects are less predictable than those of intravenous drugs.

PERICARDIOCENTESIS

This procedure is more commonly required in chronic than in acute pericardial effusion. It is best carried out in a cardiac catheterization laboratory under fluoroscopic control. In traumatic cases and after thoracic surgical procedures when tamponade is suspected, it is best combined with surgical exploration, which is needed to check for bleeding points. The puncture site of choice is in the subxiphoid region, with the subject semirecumbent, but any precordial site can be used. The needle used should not be too small (18 gauge or larger), especially if purulent effusion is suspected, and should have a short bevel. The procedure is much more safely carried out if the exploring (chest) electrode of an ECG is connected to the needle by means of a sterile wire with alligator clips at each end. By this means, any contact between the needle tip and the myocardium can be detected as a sudden elevation of the ST segment, and inadvertent cardiac puncture can be avoided. The procedure is done under local anesthesia similar to that used in thoracocentesis, and precautions should be taken to avoid the intercostal blood vessels that run behind the lower edges of the ribs. It is advantageous to have a central venous pressure recording available at the time of removal of pericardial fluid. A significant fall in central venous pressure indicates that relief of tamponade has occurred, and the final pressure gives an indication of the state of right ventricular function and the level of blood volume. All pericardial taps should be regarded as diagnostic as well as therapeutic procedures, and fluid should always be sent for appropriate laboratory examination, including culture. If a large volume of fluid is to be removed, it is helpful to insert a soft plastic catheter through the needle to avoid myocardial and coronary artery injury. In some cases, fluid may be replaced by air in an attempt to prevent adhesion with possible later constriction.

ELECTIVE CARDIOVERSION

Restoration of sinus rhythm by direct current countershock applied to the chest, when carried out electively, is always performed with the patient under anesthesia. The procedure is sufficiently painful that analgesia with morphine or meperidine is not sufficient. The indications for the use of this treatment are similar to those for restoration of sinus rhythm by means of drugs and are dealt with elsewhere (see p 481). An antiarrhythmia agent, either quinidine by mouth (0.2 g 4 times daily) for 2 days before, or intravenous procainamide (0.2 g) immediately, is given before the procedure. This premedication is intended to reduce the tendency for the rhythm to revert to the precardioversion state. The premedication may on occasion restore sinus rhythm and make countershock unnecessary. An adequate 12-lead ECG should be taken at the start of the procedure. The rhythm should be identified and a lead chosen in which the characteristics of the arrhythmia are clearly seen. Lead V_1 or V_2 is usually best for patients with atrial fibrillation. The patient's recent medication must be accurately known, especially the level of digitalis dosage and, if possible, the digitalis blood level. If there is any possibility of an element of digitalis toxicity, elective cardioversion should be postponed until digitalis toxicity is resolved, or the first shock after the patient has been anesthetized should be small (about 5 joules). At least 3 persons should be in attendance: a nurse, an anesthesiologist, and a cardiologist. The anesthesiologist chooses the method of anesthesia; the nurse runs the ECG recording, which should also be displayed on a monitor oscilloscope if possible; and the cardiologist applies the paddles to the chest and administers the shock. The large current passing through the body must not be allowed to feed back through the ECG leads and damage the ECG machine. Everyone except the holder of the paddles breaks physical contact with the patient in order to avoid an electric shock. The paddles are insulated. The minimum shock necessary to restore sinus rhythm varies. In most cases an initial dose of 80 joules is used in atrial fibrillation except when digitalis has been given. In that case, a trial dose of 5 joules is given and the shock is gradually increased. Atrial flutter usually responds to lower doses. Electrical countershock almost always restores sinus rhythm for at least a few beats, but in many instances the abnormal rhythm recurs. If the first shock is ineffective, a second shock with a larger dose should be given. If multiple shocks (6 or more) are not effective, the physician should consider leaving the patient in the abnormal rhythm, especially if it is atrial fibrillation. The dosage of antiarrhythmia drug, usually quinidine, is continued after the procedure if sinus rhythm is restored.

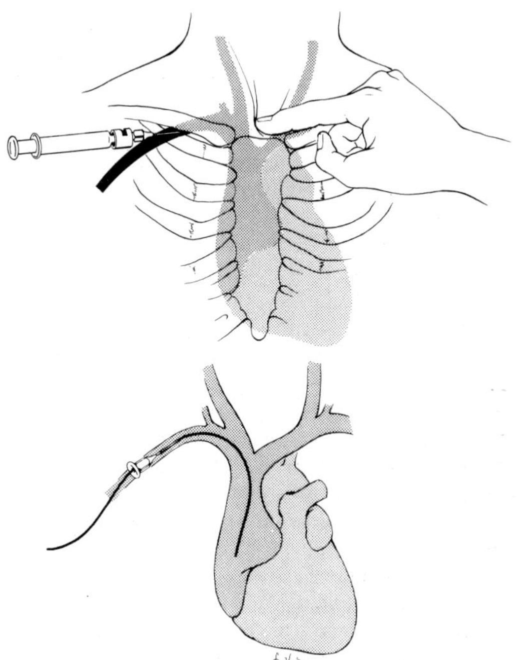

Figure 7–5. Percutaneous subclavian catheterization. (Reproduced, with permission, from Dunphy JE, Way LW [editors]: *Current Surgical Diagnosis & Treatment,* 3rd ed. Lange, 1977.)

PACEMAKERS

Insertion of a Temporary Pacemaker

This procedure should be done under strict sterile conditions, preferably in a well-equipped cardiac catheterization laboratory. In dire emergencies it may be done without fluoroscopic control in the patient's bed in a ward or a coronary care unit. The right subclavian vein in the supraclavicular fossa is the best place in which to insert the pacemaker catheter, and the procedure is performed percutaneously at this site, as shown in Fig 7–5. If the operator is not familiar with this approach, a cutdown over the medial basilic vein in the right antecubital fossa should be used. The pacemaker catheter must be advanced until its tip catches in the trabeculae at the apex of the right ventricle. The control box used to supply the pacing impulse is usually encased in a sterile rubber glove, so that it can be handled by the operator and connected to the catheter under the most sterile conditions. An electrocardiograph must always be available, and, when the catheter is thought to be embedded in the apex of the right ventricle on fluoroscopic examination, an attempt is made to pace the heart. The control box is set to provide a rate of about 70/min–faster than the patient's rate–and the output gradually increased. Electrical signals on the ECG will indicate the timing and magnitude of the pacemaker signal as a spike on the tracing. If the pacemaker catheter is appropriately positioned, the threshold at which the pacemaker will take over will be at an output of 1–2 mA. The pacemaker output is generally left at a level 2–3 times the threshold, using a "demand" mode. The catheter is secured to the skin at the entry site by sutures and the area kept as sterile as possible. Use of the subclavian route of entry leaves the patient's arms free and is less likely to result in dislodgement of the catheter than the antecubital route. A temporary pacemaker should be either removed or replaced by a permanently implanted pacemaker within a week at most for fear of phlebitis. Insertion of a temporary pacemaker for life-threatening bradycardia is recommended as a safety measure in all patients in whom a permanent pacemaker is to be used. The extra control available from the temporary instrument during the operation for placing the permanent pacemaker is most valuable.

Permanent Pacemaker Implantation

Permanent pacemakers are almost always placed via the transvenous route except when epicardial pacing leads are left in position at the time of surgery. The pulse generator (control box) is placed in the right infraclavicular fossa. This avoids a thoracotomy. The pacemaker catheter may be bipolar, with the anode and the cathode within the heart, or unipolar, with the cathode in the heart and the anode at the pulse generator. Competitive fixed rate pacemakers are no longer in general use, having been replaced by noncompetitive demand pacemakers. Fixed rate pacemakers had the disadvantage of interacting with the patient's own rhythm, so that the paced impulse could fall in the vulnerable phase of the cardiac cycle (on the T wave) and set off fatal ventricular arrhythmias. Demand (R

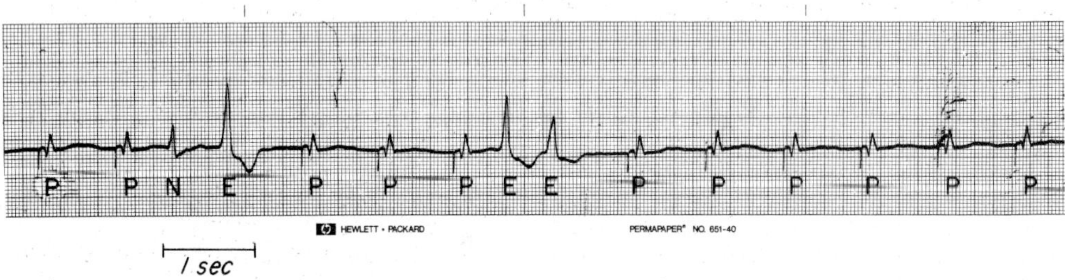

Figure 7–6. ECG from a patient with a demand (R-inhibited) pacemaker. P, paced beat; N, normal beat; E, ectopic beat. The pacemaker fires about 0.8 sec after a naturally occurring R wave, giving a heart rate of 75 beats/min.

wave-inhibited) pacemakers avoid this complication by generating a pacing impulse only when no intrinsic cardiac impulse has occurred within a preset period. Ventricular demand pacemakers are most commonly used, and the interval that elapses before an impulse occurs is usually about 1 sec, as shown in Fig 7–6.

Complications of Pacemaker Therapy

The pacemaker may fail because of fracture of its leads or displacement of the intracardiac electrodes. Displacement is more likely to occur soon after implantation because fibrosis provoked by the foreign material tends to anchor the electrode with time. The electrode may erode through the right ventricular wall and come to rest in the pericardium. This is usually associated with an increase in the threshold required for stimulation. This can in some instruments be increased transcutaneously by means of a special tool. It is also possible to change the mode of operation of a demand pacemaker to a fixed rate mode with an external magnet in order to test its function and decide whether battery replacement is needed.

Battery failure is the commonest and the inevitable ultimate cause of pacemaker failure. Most units with mercury batteries require replacement after about 4 or 5 years. Impending battery failure can be inferred from a decrease in the rate of the pacemaker. The impulse recorded from a standard ECG is ordinarily adequate for this form of analysis, which can be carried out over a telephone line with the appropriate equipment. Newer lithium batteries are expected to last up to 10 years, and improvements in the technic of powering the pacemaker will probably make battery replacement during the patient's lifetime unnecessary in the future. Externally rechargeable batteries are now available in which a charging period of 1 hour a month is all that is needed.

INTRA-AORTIC BALLOON PUMPING

This specialized circulatory support technic is used only in intensive care areas. The principle is to reduce the load on the heart and increase coronary perfusion by lowering the systolic and raising the diastolic pressure. A plastic balloon connected to a catheter is placed in the thoracic aorta and alternately inflated and deflated in time with the heartbeat. Inflation takes place in diastole and deflation during systole. The technic involves exposure and arteriotomy of the aortoiliac arterial area.

This procedure is effective as a short-term measure but is not widely used except in specialized centers. It may have a place in the postoperative management of cardiac surgical patients. Its medical use has been almost entirely confined to patients with cardiogenic shock following myocardial infarction.

• • •

References

Chardack WM: Heart block treated with implantable pacemaker. Prog Cardiovasc Dis 6:507, 1964.

Chatterjee K, Parmley WW: The role of vasodilator therapy in heart failure. Prog Cardiovasc Dis 19:301, 1977.

Goldberg AH: Cardiopulmonary arrest. N Engl J Med 290:381, 1974.

Gordon AS (chairman): Standards for cardiopulmonary resuscitation (CPR) and emergency cardiac care (ECC). JAMA 227 (Suppl):837, 1974.

Heimlich HJ: A life-saving maneuver to prevent food-choking. JAMA 234:398, 1975.

Jude JR, Nagel EL: Cardiopulmonary resuscitation, 1970. Mod Concepts Cardiovas Dis 39:133, 1970.

Kaltman AJ: Indications for temporary pacemaker insertion in acute myocardial infarction. Am Heart J 81:837, 1971.

Kleiger R, Lown B: Cardioversion and digitalis: Circulation 33:878, 1966.

Lamberti JJ & others: Intra-aortic balloon counterpulsation: Indications and long-term results in postoperative left ventricular power failure. Arch Surg 109:766, 1974.

Lown B: Electrical reversion of cardiac arrhythmias. Br Heart J 29:469, 1967.

Lown B & others: New method for terminating cardiac arrhythmias. JAMA 182:548, 1962.

Scherf D, Bornemann C: Thumping of the precordium in ventricular standstill. Am J Cardiol 5:30, 1960.

Sowton E: Hemodynamic studies in patients with artificial pacemakers. Br Heart J 26:737, 1964.

Wright KE Jr, McIntosh HD: Artificial pacemakers: Indications and management. Circulation 47:1108, 1973.

8...

Coronary Disease

Coronary heart disease is perhaps the most important fatal disease in the industrialized countries. In the USA, it is the cause of one-third to one-half of all deaths and 50–75% of all cardiac deaths; approximately 500,000 people a year die from the disease. The disease affects men in the prime of life; the average age at the time of the first myocardial infarction is in the mid fifties. Women are spared for about 10 years relative to men.

Coronary heart disease has apparently increased in frequency since the early 1930s, especially in younger people. The data are hard to evaluate because death in a younger person is more apt to be followed by autopsy diagnosis, whereas the cause of death in an older person, especially one with known coronary disease, is often not specifically confirmed at autopsy. Data from death certificates are notoriously unreliable, in part as a result of changing fashions in diagnostic nomenclature (Morgan-Jones, 1970).

The importance of coronary heart disease extends beyond the high morbidity and mortality rates associated with the disorder because clinical manifestations are unpredictable or absent and apparently random in occurrence; because the course is variable; and because in one-third to one-half of patients death is sudden and unexpected ("sword of Damocles"). The recognition of coronary heart disease in any of its clinical forms raises the possibility of sudden death, and even minimal symptoms may portend more serious disease.

In about 99% of cases, coronary artery disease is due to atherosclerotic changes. Other vascular diseases such as syphilis and connective tissue disorders (eg, systemic lupus erythematosus) are rare causes. The discussion here will be limited to atherosclerotic coronary heart disease.

ATHEROSCLEROSIS

Robbins and Angell (1976) define atherosclerosis as follows: "Basically, the disorder comprises the development of focal fibrofatty elevated plaques or thickenings, called atheromas, within the intima and inner portion of the media. As the disorder advances, the atheromas undergo a variety of complications—calcification, internal hemorrhages, ulceration, and sometimes superimposed thrombosis."

The clinical manifestations of atherosclerosis have become more common and occur at an earlier age in recent years, but the pathologic process of atherosclerosis itself has not changed. Atherosclerosis is an age-related degenerative process, increasing progressively in frequency with advancing age. Yet it is not inevitable, because some octogenarians have minimal or no evidence of coronary atherosclerosis on postmortem examination.

Atherosclerosis may begin early in life. During the Korean War, evidence of atherosclerosis was found in about three-fourths of young soldiers killed in battle, and about one-fourth had stenosis of at least 50% of one coronary artery. In various studies, the extent of coronary atherosclerosis is greater in those who have more severe clinical manifestations of coronary heart disease, but the correlation is far from perfect. With the exception of the left main coronary artery, isolated stenosis of one coronary artery is rarely the cause of sudden death in coronary heart disease. Extensive disease of 2 or 3 arteries is usually found at autopsy.

There has been a tremendous outpouring of atherosclerosis research during the past 10 years, with emphasis on pathogenesis and epidemiology, prevention by recognition of predisposing factors, physiologic and hemodynamic studies, and new methods of diagnosis, prognosis, and treatment.

The clinical disease coronary heart disease (ischemic heart disease) must be differentiated from its underlying pathologic process, coronary atherosclerosis. Other causes of coronary disease include various forms of arteritis, coronary embolism, and lupus erythematosus and similar connective tissue disorders. In some instances, coronary spasm alone may be the cause of myocardial ischemia, although more frequently coronary spasm complicates coronary atherosclerosis.

NEW CLINICAL INVESTIGATIONS

New methods of clinical investigation have greatly extended the range of studies available. The basis of clinical diagnosis, however, today as heretofore, is the history of angina pectoris, myocardial infarction, cardiac failure, or arrhythmias. A family history of coronary disease may be present, and atherogenic factors such as lipid disorders or hypertension should be sought. Coronary arteriography can be used if needed to study the anatomy of the coronary arteries. Left ventricular cineangiograms permit estimation of left ventricular size and function, ejection fraction, and wall motion. Quantitative graded exercise ECG studies have largely replaced the 2-step Master test (Master, 1968) as a means of inducing myocardial ischemia for diagnostic purposes. Echocardiography is a noninvasive technic for estimating the size and configuration of ventricular dimensions, identifying contraction abnormalities, determining the systolic ejection fraction, and diagnosing or ruling out mitral or aortic disease, pericarditis, and left atrial myxoma. Exercise can be performed during cardiac catheterization or after myocardial imaging with radioactive isotopes combined with electrocardiographic recordings to diagnose ischemia or infarction. During exercise, one can determine changes in left ventricular end-diastolic pressure and myocardial lactate production by sampling blood from the coronary sinus. One can simulate the effects of exercise by atrial pacing or infusions of isoproterenol; as the heart rate and myocardial oxygen consumption increase, angina pectoris and evidences of left ventricular ischemia may appear.

These procedures document the abnormality of the coronary circulation by demonstrating ischemic changes in the ECG or changes in compliance or pressure in the left ventricle. But coronary angiograms are required to define the anatomy of the coronary arteries, their branches, and collateral circulation; and left ventricular angiography is most reliable for determining left ventricular ejection fraction and the presence of abnormalities such as aneurysm or impaired contractility in localized areas.

Evaluation of the patient with coronary disease is a complex, sophisticated procedure and ideally involves teams of specially trained physicians and technicians, including physiologists, cardiologists, radiologists, anesthesiologists, and surgeons.

GENERAL CLASSIFICATION OF CORONARY HEART DISEASE

The classification of coronary heart disease by type and degree is arbitrary and unsatisfactory because the clinical manifestations merge into each other and represent a diverse spectrum of progressive ischemia, necrosis, fibrosis, and left ventricular dysfunction. Any of the manifestations may be the first one to appear, and the patient may present with one, develop another, and then stabilize at either level. Fig 8–1 illustrates the presenting clinical manifestations in the Framingham Study. Furthermore, the disease can have acute and chronic phases, and the patient may be critically ill during one phase and capable of full activity a few months later with or without another manifestation. The correlation between symptoms, clinical manifestations, and pathologic findings is so imprecise that one cannot be predicted on the basis of the other. On discussing the clinical expression of the various phases of coronary heart disease, it is wise to recall

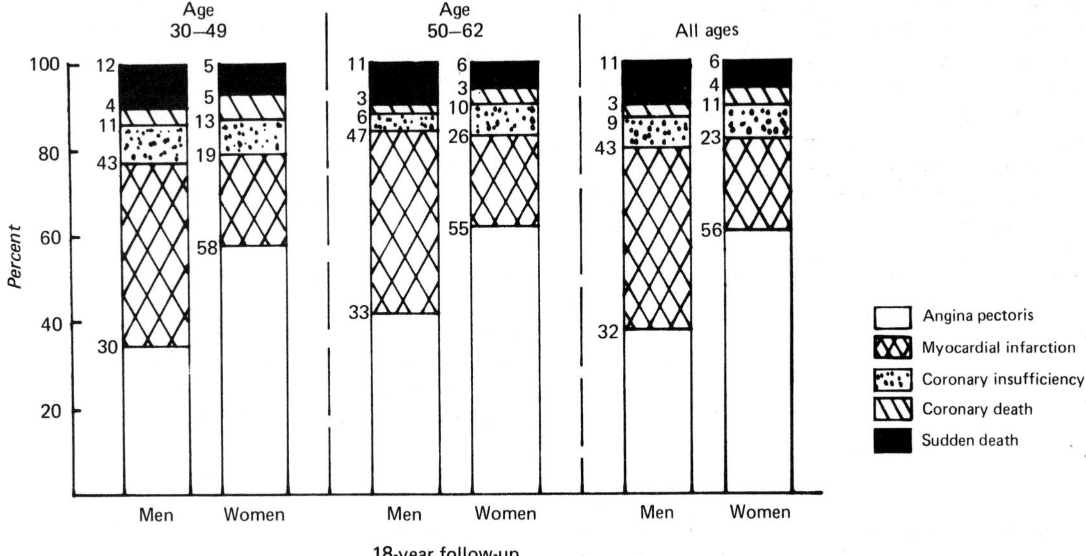

Figure 8–1. Presenting clinical manifestations of coronary heart disease: Framingham Study, men and women age 30–62 years at entry. (Reproduced, with permission, from Kannel WB: Some lessons in cardiovascular epidemiology from Framingham. Am J Cardiol 37:269, 1976.)

that they are not self-limited or specific. In coronary heart disease, therefore, the patient may present with—or may develop—any of the following:

(1) Asymptomatic or presymptomatic coronary disease.

(2) Sudden death.

(3) Acute myocardial infarction.

(4) Angina pectoris of effort.

(5) Unstable angina pectoris (coronary insufficiency, intermediate coronary syndrome).

(6) Cardiac failure.

(7) Cardiac arrhythmias or atrioventricular conduction defects.

Each of these clinical features will be discussed along with the pathophysiologic mechanism that distinguishes one from another and the special investigations useful in their evaluation that have been developed during the past 5–10 years. An attempt will be made to indicate where each one fits into the clinical approach to the problem. Treatment of coronary heart disease will be discussed as a whole rather than under each individual subheading.

We shall attempt also to relate the prognosis of coronary heart disease to different clinical manifestations, describing special methods of investigation that have clarified our concepts of prognosis in recent years.

PATHOGENESIS OF CORONARY HEART DISEASE

Certain factors have been identified in recent years that have clarified the pathologic process responsible for coronary heart disease. Epidemiologic studies of large population groups, especially the Framingham Study, were designed by Dawber, Kannel, and their associates (Dawber, 1958) to determine the factors influencing the development of coronary heart disease in the adult population of Framingham, Massachusetts. It was begun around 1949 with a representative sample of 2282 men and 2845 women age 30–62 who were found to be clinically free of coronary heart disease at that time. Through clinical examinations at 2-year intervals and other methods of follow-up over more than 20 years, the study has traced the natural history of the various manifestations of coronary disease, as well as stroke and peripheral artery disease, and has meticulously related their development to host and environmental factors. The study has provided an elaborate epidemiologic survey of coronary disease and has explored risk factors which increase the likelihood of developing coronary disease. The established risk factors are hypertension, hyperlipidemia, diabetes, a family history of early atherosclerosis, age, male sex, and perhaps obesity. Factors deemed less important are behavior pattern, sociocultural factors, decreased physical activity, cigarette smoking, and emotional "stress of modern life."

Risk Factors in Atherosclerosis

Any attempt to explain the pathogenesis of coronary heart disease must take into account those conditions leading to atherosclerosis as well as factors that convert underlying atherosclerosis into clinical disease. There are 2 major schools of thought about the pathogenesis of atherosclerosis: (1) the hypothesis of Rokitansky, revived by Duguid (1946), which postulates that coronary artery thrombosis is the initiating event and that the atheroma is the result of the healing process combined with infiltration of lipids; and (2) the hypothesis that intimal injury caused by elevated pressure, deposition of lipid, and infiltration of hypertrophied smooth muscle cells from the media leads to obstruction of the coronary artery, fibrosis, lipid deposition, and atheroma formation (Ross, 1976).

Hypertension, hyperlipidemia (especially decrease in high density lipoproteins and increase in low density lipoproteins, serum cholesterol, and triglycerides), a positive family history of atherosclerosis, diabetes, and cigarette smoking increase the prevalence and incidence of atherosclerosis. Combinations of risk factors greatly enhance the probability of a cardiovascular event; in the Framingham Study, the probability of a cardiovascular event occurring within 8 years increased from 2% in patients with no risk factors to 49% when 5 risk factors were present. The probability was an intermediate one when fewer risk factors were present (Kannel, Am J Cardiol 38:46, 1976). In individuals age 70 with no other risk factor, the combination of age and systolic blood pressure increases 3-fold the probability of cardiovascular disease within 8 years as the systolic pressure rises from 105 mm Hg to 195 mm Hg; in people 35–45 years of age, the probability increases only 25–30% at the higher pressure ranges.

The mechanisms by which these risk factors operate to enhance the likelihood of atherosclerosis are not precisely known, nor is the pathogenesis of the disease itself.

A. Hyperlipidemia: Hyperlipidemia is thought to foster atherogenesis by increasing the deposition of lipid in the intima because of its increased concentration in plasma. The importance of lipid disorders is strikingly emphasized by the course of coronary disease in hypercholesterolemia. Myocardial infarction has been shown to occur in 85% of subjects by age 60—in contrast to 20% of the population at large. Most subjects with homozygous hypercholesterolemia develop myocardial infarction by age 30. Forty percent of women who survived acute myocardial infarction had type II hyperlipoproteinemia (Fredrickson, 1972), as compared to no type IIs among age-matched control subjects (Mann, 1975). (See below for comments on classification.)

The classification of hyperlipidemias has been the subject of "confusion and controversy" (Havel, 1977). It is likely that the Fredrickson classification, valuable when introduced, is no longer adequate because of the emergence of new information regarding the genetic and metabolic aspects of hyperlipidemic states. As we have learned more about the familial hyperlipidemic

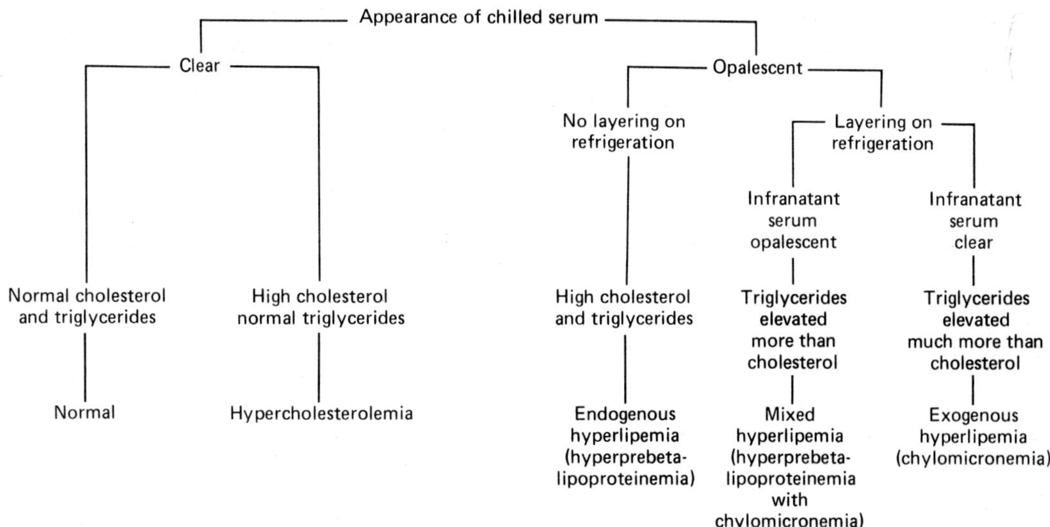

Figure 8–2. Evaluation of hyperlipoproteinemias with simple technics. (Modified and reproduced, with permission, from Havel RJ: Pathogenesis, differentiation and management of hypertriglyceridemia. In Stollerman GH [editor]: Adv Intern Med 15:117, 1969. Copyright © 1969, Year Book Med Pub Inc., Chicago.)

syndromes, for example, it has become possible to better define the specific patterns of individual patients (Havel, 1977). A pattern does not mean merely a specific disease but can also be influenced by diet and alcohol consumption, even in essentially normal lipidemic subjects. Furthermore, treatment cannot be determined on the basis of phenotyping but depends on the cause of the hyperlipidemia.

Fig 8–2 describes a *beginning* simplified approach to the evaluation of the hyperlipidemias.

Serum lipids are not constant quantities and can be altered by various means such as substituting unsaturated vegetable fats for animal fats or adding beta-sitosterol to interfere with the absorption of cholesterol (Farquhar, 1958). The estimated sex- and age-adjusted plasma cholesterol and triglyceride levels in control subjects were found by Goldstein (J Clin Invest, 1973) to be, respectively, 270 and 147 mg/dl at the 90th percentile; 285 and 165 mg/dl at the 95th percentile; and 134 and 200 mg/dl at the 99th percentile. Approximately one-third of the cholesterol and triglyceride values in survivors of myocardial infarction were above the 80th percentile of the levels found in control subjects. Increases in mean total cholesterol plasma levels and mean triglyceride levels are both positively correlated with increasingly severe and multiple coronary artery stenosis (Murray, 1975).

Newer studies (Miller, 1975; Gordon, 1977) suggest that a decrease in high density lipoproteins (HDL) is more important than an increase in low density lipoproteins (LDL) or total cholesterol in the pathogenesis of atherosclerosis (Fig 8–3). HDL increase the absorption of cholesterol from peripheral tissues, including the arterial wall ("scavenger" effect), and transport it to the liver, where metabolic breakdown and excretion occur. The cholesterol in atheroma is derived from that

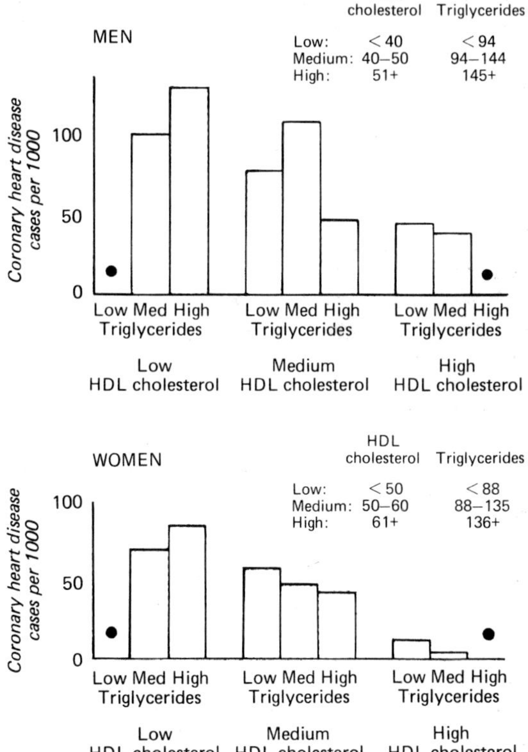

Figure 8–3. Incidence of coronary heart disease by level of HDL (high density lipoprotein) cholesterol and triglycerides, Framingham Study. (Reproduced, with permission, from Gordon T & others: High density lipoprotein as a protective factor against coronary heart disease: The Framingham Study. Am J Med 62:707, 1977.)

in the plasma, whereas that in the arterial wall is normally synthesized in situ. Decreased HDL may impair the clearance of cholesterol from the arterial wall, leading to an imbalance between filtration of cholesterol from plasma and its clearance, thereby causing increased deposition of cholesterol.

B. Hypertension: Hypertension increases the filtration of lipid from plasma to the intimal cells by virtue of increased arterial pressure, especially in the presence of elevated plasma lipids. Hypertension as well as hyperlipidemia may injure the intima, leading to proliferation of smooth muscle cells in the media as a "protective" mechanism. Increased susceptibility to injury from shear forces, torsion, and lateral wall pressure changes may also be important. Hypertension is now the most common and most important risk factor in the pathogenesis of atherosclerosis; atherosclerotic complications constitute the most common causes of death in hypertensive patients.

The average degree of coronary artery sclerosis in a large group of routine autopsies was grade 9 (on a scale of 1–10) in hypertensives in the 40- to 49-year age group, whereas this degree of coronary sclerosis was not reached in nonhypertensives until age 60–70 years (Lober, 1953). Purely hypertensive complications (cardiac failure, accelerated or malignant hypertension, hemorrhagic stroke, and renal failure) have been sharply reduced by present-day antihypertensive treatment, but this is not true of atherosclerotic complications (myocardial and cerebral infarction), possibly because reduction of elevated pressures is begun too late in life.

C. Diabetes: The asymptomatic hyperglycemia of adult patients with diabetes mellitus has been reported to be a risk factor independent of and additive to the effect of blood pressure and serum lipids. Diabetes affects the capillary basement membrane (microangiopathy) of all tissues. It produces abnormalities in small coronary vessels as well as in the major arteries. Pathologically, atherosclerosis occurs more frequently and at an earlier age in diabetic patients. Patients with diabetes have been shown to have a 2- to 3-fold greater incidence of coronary disease than nondiabetics (Lober, 1953), but, for unknown reasons, small vessel rather than large vessel disease is often the cause. It is not rare to see angina and myocardial infarction in young people with juvenile onset diabetes. Control of hyperglycemia in maturity onset diabetes has not been shown to influence subsequent coronary disease. Rigid control of juvenile onset diabetes has been claimed by some to be preventive, although this opinion has been challenged.

D. Family History: A positive family history may reflect (1) genetic predisposition to the development of hypertension, hyperlipidemia, or diabetes or (2) environmental influences such as diet, stress, and lifestyle.

For men under age 55, a coronary death in a first-degree male relative under age 55 increases the risk of coronary death to 3 times that of the general population. For women under age 65, a coronary death in a first-degree male relative under age 55 increases the risk of coronary death to 5 times that of the general population (Slack, 1968). The risk of coronary death in these cases is greater than it is in middle-aged men with elevated serum cholesterol or blood pressure. Men with risk of dominantly inherited familial hypercholesterolemia have a 15-fold increase in risk, and 50% die of coronary heart disease before age 60 (Slack, 1969). Slack suggests that family history as a risk factor for early coronary death has been underappreciated and that it might be used in selecting individuals for screening as a high-risk subset in lieu of screening the total population (Slack, 1977).

E. Cigarette Smoking: The principal importance of cigarette smoking is that it precipitates arrhythmias and that it is a factor in sudden death in patients with coronary artery disease. In addition, smoking is a definite risk factor in promoting atherosclerosis. The mechanism of atherogenesis due to cigarette smoking is not clear, but the clinical reality is apparently firmly established by epidemiologic studies.

The frequency of cigarette smoking is high in patients with atherosclerosis; at the outset of the Framingham Study, in 1949, 60% of the men and 40% of the women were smokers. Cigar and pipe smoking are considerably less important as risk factors.

The major components of cigarette smoke that have been considered as factors in atherogenesis are carbon monoxide and nicotine. Nicotine elevates plasma norepinephrine and epinephrine within a few minutes after inhaling, which also increases the free fatty acids. Smoking also increases blood pressure and pulse rate, which increase myocardial oxygen consumption. The electrophysiologic effect of sympathetic stimulation includes lowering of the ventricular fibrillation threshold. Coronary vasoconstriction may also occur.

The sudden death mortality rate in heavy smokers (more than 20 cigarettes a day) is 5 times that of nonsmokers, as illustrated in Fig 8–4.

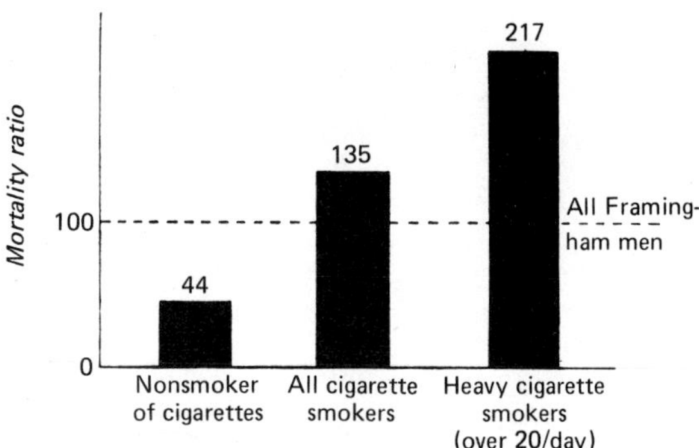

Figure 8–4. Framingham Study 12-year follow-up mortality ratios for sudden death in nonsmokers, all smokers, and heavy smokers among men originally aged 30–62. (Modified and reproduced, with permission, from Kannel WB: *Habits and Coronary Heart Disease: The Framingham Heart Study.* Public Health Service Publication No. 1515, National Heart Institute, 1966.)

F. Physical Inactivity: A sedentary habit of life may produce its effects through associated obesity, which may predispose to diabetes and possibly hypertension. Preliminary data suggest that because inactive people have fewer collateral coronary vessels, physical inactivity may merely decrease the chance for survival when myocardial infarction occurs; it does not influence the atherosclerotic process itself. The high incidence of myocardial infarction in vigorous northeastern Finns who consume a diet high in saturated fats and cholesterol suggests that exercise affords only minimal protection against coronary disease. (A comprehensive study is under way in Finland to evaluate the role of exercise, diet, and other risk factors.)

G. Personality Factors: Rosenman and Friedman (1976) have postulated that personality and behavior characteristics such as pressure of time and work, competitiveness, and aggressiveness (type A) are variables independent of other risk factors. They found that the incidence of coronary disease was lower in type B (more relaxed) individuals. Their work has not been fully accepted by other investigators, although, interestingly, large segments of the public believe that these behavioral characteristics are significant causes of coronary disease. The interaction of personality and sociocultural factors may be more significant (Biörck, 1975).

H. Other Factors: Softness or hardness of natural water, once considered to be important, has recently been shown by epidemiologic studies to have little or no importance as a risk factor. Gout, hyperuricemia, and hypothyroidism have been mentioned in the past but at most are minor factors.

Each risk factor discussed above is not only significant in itself but is also additive and perhaps synergistic when combined with one or more other risk factors. Hypertension and atherosclerosis, for example, are independent disease processes, yet hypertension accelerates atherosclerosis.

PATHOLOGY OF ATHEROSCLEROSIS

The pathology of atherosclerosis and acute myocardial infarction is a complex subject, and the reader should study the many excellent monographs and textbooks devoted to the subject for further details. See especially Robbins (1976) and Anderson (1971). In this section, a summary of the pathologic features will be presented, with a brief discussion of controversial aspects. Photographs illustrating the pathologic features of coronary atherosclerosis are presented in Figs 8–5 and 8–6.

The term atherosclerosis refers to arteriosclerosis in the muscular arteries, including, among others, the large and middle-sized vessels: the aorta and the coronary, femoral, iliac, internal carotid, and cerebral arteries. The term nodular arteriosclerosis is preferred by Pickering, but atherosclerosis is the term in common use in the USA.

The typical lesion of atherosclerosis is the fibrous plaque, which grossly is dull white and slightly elevated and impinges on the arterial lumen but, when uncomplicated, rarely occludes it. Histologically, it is characterized by a protrusion of smooth muscle cells containing lipids surrounded by a matrix of connective tissue cells, collagen, elastic fibers, and mucopolysaccharides. As the fibrous plaque enlarges, it may become calcified, may undergo necrosis, may bleed internally, and may develop a superimposed mural thrombus–and in these ways may ultimately partially or completely occlude the artery. Hemorrhage into old atherosclerotic plaques in the coronary arteries was found by Roberts (1971) to have occurred in about one-fourth of patients with fatal acute myocardial infarction or "sudden death," although in many of his specimens there was no associated superimposed thrombus. The lesions are focal, tend to occur at points where the arteries branch, and do not impair flow through the artery until stenosis exceeds 70% of the lumen of the artery.

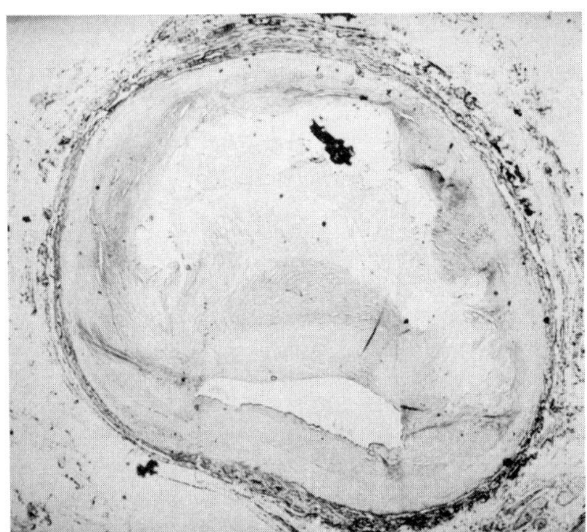

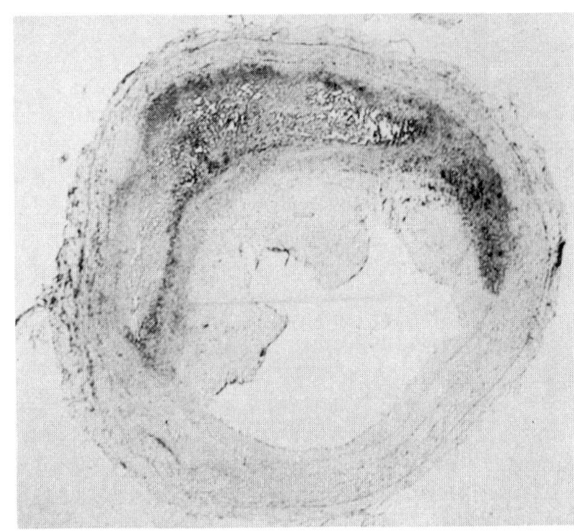

Figure 8–5. Two examples of coronary atherosclerosis in adults. (Courtesy of O Rambo.)

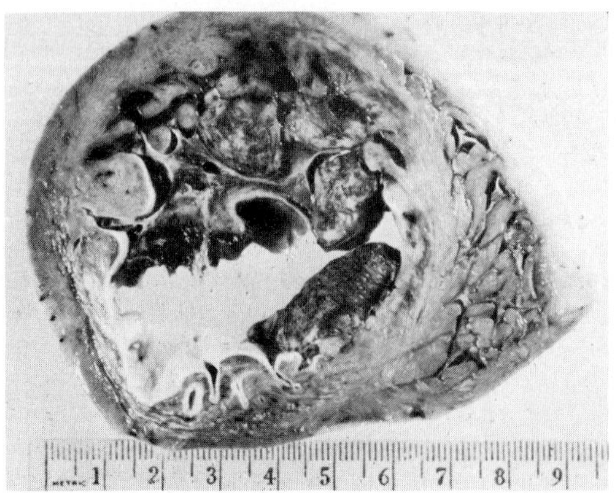

Figure 8–6. Mural thrombosis of the heart superimposed on underlying atherosclerosis. (Courtesy of O Rambo.)

Relationship Between Coronary Thrombosis & Myocardial Infarction

The relationship between mural thrombosis of the coronary arteries and myocardial infarction has been the subject of considerable debate. For many years it was thought that the 2 were synonymous, but, as will be discussed later, either one may occur without the other. The first descriptions of nonfatal acute myocardial infarction by Herrick (1912) and by Levine (1929) were based on the assumption that coronary thrombosis and acute myocardial infarction were identical, but Roberts (1971) has shown that coronary thrombosis is present in only about half of patients with acute myocardial infarction who come to necropsy. The extent of thrombosis is a function of the time between onset of symptoms and death. A study of cases examined by the coroner showed 3 times as many coronary thromboses in patients surviving 24 hours as in those who died within 1 hour after onset of symptoms (Spain, 1960). The question to be resolved is whether coronary thrombosis is the usual cause of acute myocardial infarction or whether it is the result of the infarction and complicates a hemorrhage or ulceration within an atherosclerotic plaque or other mechanism. Ridolfi and Hutchins (1977) believe that coronary thromboses are precipitated by focal atherosclerotic ulcerations and that the thrombosis precedes and causes myocardial infarction.

Structure of a Normal Artery & One With a Fibrous Plaque

The structure of a normal muscular artery is illustrated in Fig 8–7A. The effect of endothelial injury and the subsequent deposition of platelet aggregates (microthrombi) and infiltration of smooth muscle cells into the damaged intima from the media are illustrated in Fig 8–7B and C. The lipid particles that accumulate in the fibrous plaque arise from the plasma lipid flowing through the artery, as shown by the similarity of the lipid composition of the plasma and of the atherosclerotic plaque.

Endothelial Damage Theory

The pathogenesis of atherosclerosis has been the subject of conflicting theories which need not be discussed in detail here. Ross and Glomset (1976) offer evidence that atherosclerosis is a response of the intima to endothelial injury, resulting in platelet aggregation on the damaged endothelial surface and proliferation and extension of smooth muscle cells from the media

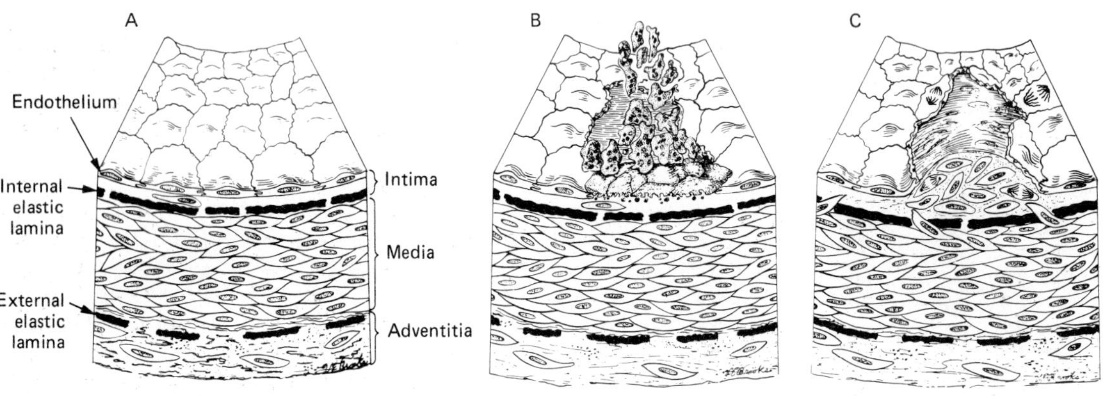

Figure 8–7. Mechanisms of production of atheroma. *A:* Structure of normal muscular artery. The adventitia, or outermost layer of the artery, consists principally of recognizable fibroblasts intermixed with smooth muscle cells loosely arranged between bundles of collagen and surrounded by proteoglycans. It is usually separated from the media by a discontinuous sheet of elastic tissue, the external elastic lamina. *B:* Platelet aggregates, or microthrombi, which may form as a result of adherence of the platelets to the exposed subendothelial connective tissue. Platelets that adhere to the connective tissue release granules whose constituents may gain entry into the artery wall. Platelet factors thus interact with plasma constituents in the artery wall and may stimulate events shown in the next illustration. *C:* Smooth muscle cells migrating from the media into the intima through fenestrae in the internal elastic lamina and actively multiplying within the intima. Endothelial cells regenerate in an attempt to recover the exposed intima, which thickens rapidly owing to smooth muscle proliferation and formation of new connective tissue. (Reproduced, with permission, from Ross R, Glomset JA: The pathogenesis of atherosclerosis. [Part 1.] N Engl J Med 295:369, 1976.)

into the intima. This produces the fibrous plaque, which may then undergo calcification, hemorrhage, and thrombosis. Endothelial injury may result from a number of physical and biochemical factors. One such physical factor is the shearing stress of hypertension. Damage by substances such as excess low density lipoproteins (LDL) or homocystine may, if not corrected by measures aimed at reduction of the plasma lipid concentration, lead to infiltration of lipid particles through the damaged endothelium and in this way set in motion the series of reactions leading to the development of the complicated fibrous plaque of atherosclerosis (Harker, 1976).

Culture of Endothelium in Vitro

Arterial endothelial cells have recently been cultured in the laboratory, allowing direct study of their behavior and the possible factors that damage them and allow platelet adherence. Further study is required to determine whether the "response to injury" hypothesis explains how the so-called risk factors enhance the likelihood of development of atherosclerosis in susceptible subjects. Recent work by Brown and Goldstein (1976) has provided further explanation of how biochemical substances may injure the cell by demonstrating in human fibroblasts that a receptor for low density plasma lipoproteins is absent in patients with familial hypercholesterolemia; in this way, serum cholesterol may rise, and the absence of the receptor permits penetration of the cell by cholesterol, with resulting endothelial damage.

Pathologic Lesions & Serum Lipoprotein Studies

Pathologic examination following death due to symptomatic coronary heart disease in patients in whom serum lipoprotein typing had been performed during life has confirmed the observations of Blumgart (1960) that in practically all patients with fatal coronary heart disease, at least one major coronary artery is more than 75% stenotic and that as a rule 3 major coronary arteries are stenotic. A lesser extent of narrowing of the lumen of the coronary arteries is also found in patients who during life had normal serum lipoproteins. Abnormalities of lipoprotein are therefore not essential to the development of atherosclerosis, but persons with normal serum lipoproteins have fewer and less severe atherosclerotic lesions. Severe atherosclerosis is found not only in fatal cases of acute myocardial infarction and in those who died suddenly but also in patients studied within the first year following onset of ischemic symptoms. Coronary arteriograms revealed stenotic lesions in 1–3 coronary arteries in patients with recent onset of symptoms, indicating that extensive coronary atherosclerosis is usually present when symptoms appear. This pathologic fact complicates clinical studies of coronary heart disease because the stenotic pathologic lesion may be well developed before symptoms occur; therefore, the absence of symptoms cannot be equated with the absence of stenosis, and it does not rule out even complete occlusion of a coronary artery.

Cardiac Hypertrophy

Cardiac hypertrophy is uncommon in uncomplicated coronary heart disease but develops if myocardial infarction with cardiac failure ensues or if hypertension has been present. The average heart weight in fatal cases of acute myocardial infarction is just over 400 g, slightly higher than normal.

Rupture of the Heart

Rupture of the heart (usually involving the free wall of the left ventricle) occurs in about 5% of patients with acute fatal myocardial infarction but may be due to rupture of a false aneurysm in an area of dyskinesia. True aneurysm of the left ventricle may cause cardiac failure or arrhythmias (see section on clinical aspects of acute myocardial infarction), but rupture of a true aneurysm is uncommon. Rupture of the heart usually occurs within the first few days after an acute myocardial infarction, but often the early symptoms of the infarction are missed. About one-third of patients with rupture of the heart have a perforated ventricular septum or papillary muscle, the latter causing acute mitral regurgitation with the abrupt development of cardiac failure.

The prognosis is poor because of the extensive hemopericardium, the hemodynamic effects of the cardiac tamponade, and the sudden catastrophic nature of most such ruptures.

In some patients, rupture of the heart is not abrupt, as is a "blowout," but may be gradual, owing to slitlike perforation of the ventricular wall with increasing hemopericardium. Pericardial tamponade can be diagnosed antemortem, and surgical treatment may be successful if the diagnosis of a gradual perforation is made promptly.

Coronary Arteriography & Pathology of the Coronary Arteries

Pathologic examination has shown that coronary arteriography, which is used clinically to delineate the anatomy of the coronary arteries, usually underestimates the extent and degree of coronary stenosis. There is usually good agreement between the radiologic interpretation of the coronary arteriogram and the findings of the pathologist if the stenosis exceeds 85%; if the stenosis is less than this, or if the lesions are peripheral, there is great variation in opinion about the degree of stenosis. Furthermore, the lesions may be obscured in one radiologic plane, and multiple views with different projections are required to avoid missing or underestimating the lesions. Irregular narrowing of the arteries seen on coronary arteriograms is often found by pathologic study to be due to multiple stenoses of moderate degree. Proximal lesions are more prevalent than distal ones—a fact of considerable operative significance. Not only do proximal lesions more adversely affect blood flow to the myocardium, but the beneficial effect of bypassing a proximal stenosis is correspondingly greater. Collateral vessels between a relatively normal coronary artery and a companion coronary artery distal to a stenosis are found in practically all cases of severe stenoses—compensating, in part, for the decreased flow through the stenotic channel.

PATHOLOGIC PHYSIOLOGY

The relationship of the pathologic process of atherosclerosis to clinical coronary heart disease is poorly understood, although recent work on the roles of degree of obstruction, integrity of left ventricular function, and the presence and adequacy of collateral vessels has offered valuable prognostic insights. The exact reasons for the apparently haphazard onset of angina, myocardial infarction, ventricular arrhythmias, or sudden death are often unknown.

Onset of Myocardial Infarction

Two mechanisms have been postulated to explain the onset of myocardial infarction: coronary thrombosis and subintimal hemorrhage. The latter has been found to be uncommon, and the former has been rejected vigorously by Roberts (1971), who asserts that thrombosis is secondary and not primary in the usual case of myocardial infarction. Even if thrombosis is primary, the reason for its development is unclear; possible explanations include ulceration of an atherosclerotic plaque, deficiency in fibrinolytic mechanisms, abnormalities in platelet adhesiveness, slowed coronary flow from progressive narrowing of the arteries, and abnormalities in the balance of various locally produced prostaglandins.

Ventricular Arrhythmias

Fibrosis and chronic ischemia of subendocardial fibers ("blighted zone") containing Purkinje cells induce variable excitability, automaticity, velocity of conduction, refractory periods, and repolarization in neighboring fibers, leading to electrical instability with ventricular fibrillation and sudden death. Ventricular fibrillation has been found to be the chief mechanism of cardiac arrest in apparently healthy individuals and in those with known coronary disease who have been resuscitated after apparent death in cardiac arrest. Sudden death is rarely due to conduction defects or Stokes-Adams attacks in the absence of acute anterior myocardial infarction. Emotional factors, with intense sympathetic discharge from the central nervous system, have been incriminated in some patients who have developed ventricular tachycardia or fibrillation or acute myocardial infarction. Vagal stimulation may decrease the heart rate and lead to an increased incidence of arrhythmia, aggravated by sympathetic stimulation.

The threshold for ventricular fibrillation has been lowered in animals following hypothalamic and stellate ganglion stimulation, suggesting that autonomic impulses from the hypothalamus favor the development of ventricular fibrillation (Lown, 1977). The fact that ventricular premature beats are often absent during sleep suggests a similar mechanism in humans (Lown, 1973; Ryan, 1975).

Table 8–1. Prevalence of prodromal symptoms in patients with acute myocardial infarction.*

Symptoms	Incidence: In Hospital (112 Patients) Percent	Out of Hospital (88 Patients) Percent
Chest pain	67	35
	$P < 0.001$	
Dyspnea	36	39
Arm and other pain	14	10
Fatigue and weakness	38	42
Dizziness and syncope	10	8
Anorexia and nausea	14	17
Emotional changes	14	20
Ankle edema and ascites	1	7
General malaise	16	17
Miscellaneous	9	16

*Reproduced, with permission of the American Heart Association, Inc., from Alonzo AA, Simon AB, Feinleib M: Prodromata of myocardial infarction and sudden death. Circulation 52:1056, 1975.

Premonitory Symptoms

Reports of premonitory symptoms such as weakness, shortness of breath, and vague chest discomfort days or weeks before the event in 50–75% of patients with acute myocardial infarction suggest that progressive myocardial ischemia, with worsening balance between supply and demand of oxygen in the myocardium, is the most frequent mechanism of acute myocardial infarction and that the onset is not as "unexpected" as was once thought. Prodromal symptoms are listed in Table 8–1.

Unusual demands (unaccustomed severe exertion, rapid ventricular rates, intense emotion, acute hypoxemia, severe anemia or blood loss) on a myocardium already compromised by decreased flow from coronary artery stenoses may precipitate local chemical and pathophysiologic events in patients with coronary atherosclerosis and may explain unexpected myocardial infarction.

Variable Postinfarction Health

The long period of good health that often follows an initial episode of angina or myocardial infarction is largely unexplained. Some patients may have no symptoms whatever despite normal physical activity after well-documented myocardial infarction not apparently precipitated by an unusual episode. It is difficult to reconcile such a benign course with the downhill course of patients who, following acute myocardial infarction, have progressively worsening symptoms and recurrent myocardial infarctions. The coronary anatomy may differ in patients with such discrepant courses and thus explain the confusion.

ASYMPTOMATIC (LATENT) CORONARY HEART DISEASE

Coronary disease can sometimes be diagnosed early by subjecting the patient to stress to induce an imbalance between oxygen supply and demand in the myocardium, ie, by exercising the patient to a level not spontaneously achieved without urging.

Initial Symptoms in Latent Coronary Heart Disease

Sudden death may be the only clinical manifestation of coronary heart disease, which means that asymptomatic coronary heart disease must have existed in the time immediately preceding this event.

Middle-aged individuals may present not with angina but with ventricular arrhythmias or atrioventricular or bundle branch conduction defects that may be the first manifestation of coronary heart disease. Asymptomatic atrial fibrillation is rarely such a manifestation because it is uncommon even in patients with stable angina pectoris. Stokes-Adams attacks in patients with complete atrioventricular block usually occur during the initial phase of acute myocardial infarction or in the months following an acute anterior myocardial infarction, but Stokes-Adams attacks occur infrequently as an isolated manifestation of coronary disease in asymptomatic patients. Short bouts of ventricular premature beats or tachycardia are a more important manifestation and may be the precursors of ventricular fibrillation and sudden death. Ventricular premature beats, however, are so common and variable in the older population at large that it is difficult to classify them as manifestations of asymptomatic coronary disease. Furthermore, various studies have shown that premature beats in the absence of clinical coronary disease do not presage sudden death.

Myocardial ischemia is usually more easily induced by exercise in patients prone to develop coronary heart disease, such as those with type II hyperlipidemia or diabetes, than in normal control subjects. Some physicians believe that all such patients should be subjected to coronary angiography for prognostic purposes. Patients with normal coronary angiograms have a good prognosis for at least 5 years (Bruschke, 1973). In individuals who have vague symptoms or ECG changes that might be due to coronary heart disease, especially in those whose occupations involve hazards to others (eg, airline pilots), asymptomatic disease may be unmasked by appropriate stress tests and invasive coronary arteriographic studies. Radioisotope perfusion scans with thallium 201 and other radiopharmaceuticals and wall motion studies (see below), with and without exercise, may prove helpful in these situations.

Special Investigations

A. Electrocardiography (Routine and Stress): (See also Chapter 5.) The most common manifestation of asymptomatic coronary heart disease is an ECG abnormality found on routine examination. Since stenosis of the coronary arteries usually develops gradually, it is logical to assume that there is a preclinical phase in which one may recognize the presence of obstructive lesions which might prevent adequate increases in flow to meet increases in demand. Acute myocardial infarction may occur without symptoms, or the symptoms may be so atypical that the diagnosis of "old infarction" can only be made on the basis of ECG abnormalities noted later. In the Framingham Study, this atypical history of presentation accounted for 20% of all acute myocardial infarctions.

1. Routine ECG–Routine electrocardiography may reveal the characteristic features of infarction, with typical abnormal Q waves or unequivocal ST–T abnormalities, or may show ST–T changes that are so typical in the absence of Q waves that the diagnosis of previous infarction is strongly suspected. There may be borderline Q waves in the absence of ST–T changes, and vectorcardiography may be helpful.

2. Stress ECG–If the ECG is normal at rest, typical horizontally depressed and downward-sloping ST contours lasting at least 0.08 sec, characteristic of myocardial ischemia, may be induced with exercise (Table 8–2) and persist for at least 3 minutes. In studies of large numbers of apparently healthy middle-aged males, typical ischemic ST segment changes have been evoked by exercise, and the prevalence of the changes increases with the age of the population studied. J point depression must be differentiated from the horizontal downward-sloping ST depression because the former has no prognostic significance. In some cases, ischemic changes are associated with typical anginal pain induced by the exercise, but the ECG changes can appear in the absence of symptoms.

Ischemic ST changes induced in apparently healthy men who have normal resting ECGs have prognostic significance for the prediction of subsequent clinical coronary disease. Robb and Seltzer (1975) found a 3-fold increase in those with an ischemic response (ST segment depressed 1–1.9 mm) to the double Master test (twice the number of steps climbed in a given time). Multistage treadmill exercise testing by various authors has shown a 3- to 5-fold increase in the incidence of coronary disease, the greater increase occurring in men with more than 1.5 mm ST depression with exercise.

When the ischemic ST depression equals or exceeds 2 mm, not only is the prognosis correspondingly worse but the likelihood of a lesion of the main left coronary artery or double or triple vessel disease increases. Conclusions based on the magnitude of the ST

Table 8–2. Criteria for diagnosis of coronary disease with exercise stress test (assuming normal baseline ECG and no digitalis).

Criteria
Horizontal downsloping ST depression $\geq$ 2 mm.
Duration of ST depression > 3 min.
Angina pectoris during or immediately after the test.
Exercise associated with hypotension or blood pressure < 130 mm Hg.

depression call for caution because the reproducibility of the ischemic changes on different occasions of examination is far from perfect, especially if the amount of exercise demanded of the patient is not the same and the increase in pulse rate is not close to maximal.

Graded exercise can be performed using either a treadmill or a cycle ergometer in which the amount of work load can be measured; the work of the heart can also be increased by progressive atrial pacing from a catheter in the right atrium. A variety of other methods of stress have been utilized, such as maximum isometric hand grip, progressively increasing doses of isoproterenol, induced hypoxia, and rapid injection of contrast medium into the coronary arteries to note the characteristics of the resulting increase in coronary flow. Ischemia, hypoperfusion, or induction of anginal pain by stress is considered to represent asymptomatic subclinical coronary heart disease. Nonspecific ST–T changes before or after exercise have been shown pathologically to be due in many cases to subendocardial fibrosis from previous necroses, many of which were unrecognized, especially in diabetic patients; it is therefore possible to infer the existence of a presymptomatic phase of coronary heart disease, but this diagnosis is less certain. One must always distinguish between coronary atherosclerosis and coronary heart disease because, although the latter follows from the former, the former may occur in the absence of the latter.

The criteria for the recognition of myocardial ischemia using exercise tests have caused considerable controversy over the years and have often forced the examiner to choose between test sensitivity and test specificity. If specificity is wanted, a typical ST depression of 2 mm or more and lasting at least 3 minutes, especially if angina or hypotension is induced in a patient who has not received digitalis or diuretic agents, is a highly specific indication of myocardial ischemia. Conversely, if one wishes to increase the sensitivity of the test, the magnitude of the ST change may be reduced to 1 mm or more so long as the typical ST contour is present and persists for at least 3 minutes. False-positives are increased when strict criteria are relaxed, although sensitivity is increased. Specificity is greater in groups of patients with known coronary disease than in asymptomatic subjects.

Exercise testing is also useful in the assessment of left ventricular function, especially if the history is of doubtful accuracy or the symptoms seem out of proportion to other clinical findings. Comparison of the functional capacity of the ventricles during exercise and at rest may reveal the onset of angina, dyspnea, or hypotension on slight effort of short duration and is therefore an important index of cardiac function. Noting ECG changes and maximal oxygen uptake during exercise also gives useful information about cardiovascular function. For many years Bruce (1977) has performed submaximal and maximal exercise tests both in asymptomatic middle-aged men and in patients with coronary heart disease. He has related the findings on exercise to noninvasive observations of the size of the heart, the duration of exercise, and the maximum systolic pressure during exercise in over 1600 men with coronary heart disease (Fig 8–8). The mortality rate from coronary heart disease increased markedly when

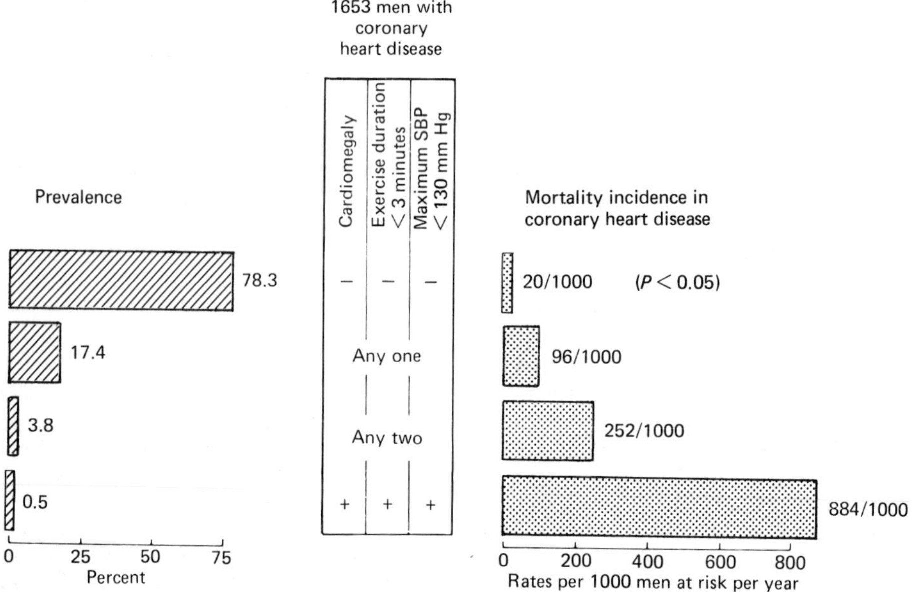

Figure 8–8. Mortality incidence in men with coronary heart disease (CHD), according to the presence or absence of 3 predictors: cardiomegaly, peak systolic pressure less than 130 mm Hg, and exercise duration not exceeding 3 min. *P* for the first row applies in combination with the second, third, and fourth rows and is based on Poisson confidence intervals. SBP, systolic blood pressure. (Reproduced, with permission, from Bruce RA: Exercise testing for evaluation of ventricular function. N Engl J Med 296:671, 1977.)

all 3 noninvasive observations during exercise were abnormal. The mortality rate increased from 20 per 1000 (2%) per year in patients in whom all 3 variables were normal to 884 per 1000 (88.4%) when all 3 were positive. The prognostic value of the determination of the 3 predictors allowed Bruce to separate low-risk from high-risk patients.

Submaximal or maximal exercise has more than prognostic value. Serial observations permit investigators to accumulate data on progressive abnormalities and their relationship to prognosis with medical treatment versus surgical treatment. The method also allows comparative observations on the benefit of various methods of treatment. Progressive increase in the magnitude of the ST depression, especially if associated with exertional hypotension, conduction defects, and complex ventricular arrhythmias, justifies the inference that the lesion is either in the left main coronary artery or in the left anterior descending artery proximal to its first septal branches.

B. Cineangiograms: (See also Chapter 6.) Cineangiograms performed as part of the diagnostic work-up of a patient with murmurs or valvular heart disease may demonstrate areas of hypokinesia or left ventricular contraction abnormalities or even a left ventricular aneurysm resulting from previous unsuspected myocardial infarction. Such invasive studies may also show enlargement of the left ventricle or evidences of left ventricular dysfunction with decreased ejection fraction, but these signs are conclusively related to coronary heart disease only if segmental wall motion abnormalities or associated severe stenosis of the coronary arteries during coronary arteriograms is present.

C. Coronary Angiograms: (See also Chapter 6.) Coronary angiograms, performed in some clinics in patients being evaluated for certain types of valvular heart disease such as aortic stenosis, may reveal areas of stenosis in the coronary arteries which represent coronary atherosclerosis, but the changes are not considered diagnostic of functionally significant coronary heart disease in the absence of induced myocardial ischemia or evidence of prior myocardial infarction. Approximately 20% of patients in the older age group with aortic valvular disease have significant coronary stenoses (> 75%).

D. Correlation of ECG and Coronary Angiography: Ischemia has been assumed to be the result of disproportion between coronary blood flow and the myocardial demand for oxygen. Recent evidence that classic positive exercise tests may be reported when no significant obstructive lesions can be demonstrated on coronary angiography has been very disturbing. Even if it is assumed that the informant was credible and the examiner experienced, such findings are not common either in asymptomatic patients or in patients with angina pectoris. Nevertheless, there are well-documented instances in which reliable patients with negative angiograms give classic positive histories of angina or so-called false-positive exercise stress tests. One may postulate that patients with false-positive tests have small vessel disease such as occurs in diabetes mellitus or in various forms of arteritis; that the coronary angiogram was technically unsatisfactory; that the disease is in vessels too small to be visible on the angiogram; that a coronary embolus has recanalized; or that coronary vasoconstriction was induced by the exercise. Coronary spasm has been documented angiographically, and coronary vascular resistance has been increased in humans following stimuli such as the cold pressor test, which produces systemic vasoconstriction. Alpha-adrenergic blocking agents such as phentolamine abolish the increased coronary vascular resistance during the cold pressor test—further evidence of the probable role of adrenergic mechanisms in episodic myocardial ischemia (Mudge, 1976). Pathologically, it has been shown that coronary angiograms give a conservative estimate of the degree and extent of coronary obstructive lesions. Furthermore, the resolution of the films is often inadequate.

False-negative exercise tests are more common and easier to explain. In many instances they occur because the exercise is not severe enough to induce myocardial ischemia; when the amount of exercise is increased, ischemia can be induced. False-negative exercise tests may also occur when the patient is in a phase of stabilized coronary disease with good collateral flow; the patient may have a negative exercise test during a stable phase and a positive test during an unstable phase of coronary disease. These observations apply more to exercise testing of patients with angina pectoris of effort or unstable angina than to testing of those with asymptomatic coronary heart disease.

The term myocardial ischemia has been used loosely to refer to residual ST–T abnormalities that follow myocardial infarction, ie, when the ECG changes reflect scarring or fibrosis and not current ischemia. The term induced myocardial ischemia is preferred to chronic ischemia except when the intention is to denote a collection of cells in the neighborhood of an old scar that may be viable but are permanently inadequately perfused. It is difficult to see how such a process could persist for weeks or months in a patient with stable angina.

SUDDEN DEATH

Sudden death is the initial and only clinical manifestation of coronary heart disease in about one-fourth of all patients. Most sudden deaths are not totally unexplained or unexpected; in many cases, the patient is known to have had coronary or hypertensive heart disease or has recently sought medical care or noticed the onset of symptoms, which were subsequently disregarded or misinterpreted. The recurrence rate of ventricular fibrillation—the mechanism of the "sudden death syndrome"—is high: about 30% in the first year and 50% by 3 years (Cobb, 1975). Survivors of out-of-hospital ventricular fibrillation who were subsequently studied by cardiac catheterization and coronary arte-

Table 8–3. Distribution of prodromal symptoms in the 2 weeks before death among 208 ASHD sudden deaths and data on whether the symptom was increasing in frequency.*

Symptom	Total		Increasing in Frequency	
	Number	Percent	Number	Percent
Chest pain	77	37	28	13
Shortness of breath	88	42	38	18
Coughing	64	31	25	12
Fainting	10	5	4	2
Dizziness	29	14	19	9
Palpitations	22	11	9	4
Undue fatigue	116	56	78	38
Difficulty sleeping	59	28	28	13

*Reproduced, with permission, from Kuller L, Cooper M, Perper J: Epidemiology of sudden death. Arch Intern Med 129:714, 1972.

Table 8–4. Selected clinical findings on admission among 92 deaths in hospital.*†

On Admission	Number	Percent
Clinical shock	32	35
Pulmonary edema	30	33
Coma	13	14
Ventricular fibrillation	6	7
Ventricular tachycardia	1	1
Complete heart block	4	4
Left bundle branch system block	6	7
At least one of the above	56	61

*Reproduced, with permission, from Kuller L, Cooper M, Perper J: Epidemiology of sudden death. Arch Intern Med 129:714, 1972.

†Excludes 2 incomplete cases.

riography demonstrated a high prevalence of advanced coronary atherosclerosis (almost all had severe stenosis in one or more of the major coronary arteries), and three-fourths had abnormalities of left ventricular wall motion. Over a 2-year period, those who experienced recurrences of ventricular fibrillation or died suddenly had a significantly higher prevalence of 3-vessel disease, a lower ejection fraction, and more severe abnormalities of left ventricular wall motion (Weaver, 1976). Vigorous antiarrhythmia drug therapy combined with management of adverse psychologic factors may reduce the recurrence rate of ventricular fibrillation and the likelihood of sudden death in this subset of patients. With a combination of monthly 24-hour ECG monitoring and daily telephone transmission ECGs, asymptomatic complex ventricular arrhythmias have been recorded in three-fourths of patients who have been resuscitated following unexpected cardiac arrest in the community (Myerburg, 1977). Carefully controlled high-dosage antiarrhythmia drug therapy, monitored by blood level measurements, decreased the 1-year mortality rate from 30%, previously recorded by Cobb, to 10% even though all ventricular arrhythmias were not abolished by the treatment.

Although the episode of ventricular fibrillation leading to sudden death was often unsuspected, about one-third of the patients had seen a physician within 2 weeks before death complaining of various prodromal symptoms, as shown in Table 8–3. Clinical findings in patients who were initially resuscitated but who subsequently died in the hospital are shown in Table 8–4.

One-fourth of all deaths of patients with coronary disease in the USA and UK are investigated by a coroner. Autopsy usually discloses severe atherosclerosis involving 2 or 3 coronary arteries even though the patient had had no prior symptoms. Rarely, isolated stenosis of only one artery is found. Table 8–5 shows the causes of death in patients who died within an hour of onset of the acute episode. The principal causes (other than coronary disease) of sudden death in adults are shown in Table 8–6.

Coronary atherosclerosis is the major finding, but fresh coronary thrombosis, intramural or subintimal hemorrhage, and recent myocardial infarction are also found, suggesting that sudden death is due to arrhythmia, probably ventricular fibrillation. This hypothesis is reinforced by the ECGs obtained by mobile coronary ambulance crews, who have been able to demonstrate ventricular fibrillation in most patients who have collapsed and were apparently "dead." If and when these patients are resuscitated and subsequently studied, myocardial infarction can be demonstrated in half of them at most, but a history of cardiovascular disease can be elicited in about three-fourths of patients even

Table 8–5. Causes of death in consecutively performed autopsies on white men who died unexpectedly and suddenly from natural causes within one hour of onset of acute fatal episode.*†

Cause of Death	Age in Years									Total	
	31–35	36–40	41–45	46–50	51–55	56–60	61–65	66–70	Over 70	Number	Percent
Coronary artery disease	6	54	64	69	72	67	41	26	23	422	91
Other	0	5	3	6	9	6	4	2	6	41	9
Total	6	59	67	75	81	73	45	28	29	463	100

*Reproduced, with permission of the American Medical Association, from Spain DM, Bradess VA, Mohr C: Coronary atherosclerosis as a cause of unexpected and unexplained death. JAMA 174:384, 1960.

†Acute episodes were witnessed. These include all cases in which autopsy was performed and which fell within the above described category and were reported to the medical examiner's office of Westchester County from March 9, 1949, to December 31, 1959.

Table 8–6. Principal conditions other than coronary artery disease associated with or causing sudden death in adults.*

Cardiovascular
Rheumatic heart disease
Bacterial endocarditis
Myocarditis
Cardiomyopathies (primary myocardial disease)
Ruptured aortic aneurysm
Aortic dissection
Coronary embolism
Coronary microembolism
Respiratory
Pulmonary thromboembolism
Pneumonias
Asthma
Bilateral midline fixation of cricoarytenoid joint
Central nervous system
Intracerebral hemorrhage
Subarachnoid hemorrhage
Meningitis
Encephalomyelitis
Gastrointestinal
Gastrointestinal hemorrhage
Peritonitis associated with perforated peptic ulcer
Alcoholism and nutritional fatty liver or cirrhosis
Other
Trauma
Poisoning and drug reactions
Fulminating infections, including meningococcemia
Amniotic embolism
Air embolism
Fat embolism
Myxedema
Amyloidosis
Hemochromatosis
Endocrine dysfunction
Leukemia

*Reproduced, with permission, from Schwartz CJ, Walsh WJ: The pathologic basis of sudden death. Prog Cardiovasc Dis 13:465, 1971.

though ventricular fibrillation was the first manifestation of coronary heart disease in one-fourth. The age-adjusted incidence of sudden death increases with increasing blood pressure, serum cholesterol, relative weight, and cigarettes smoked per day at the time of the initial examination in the Framingham Study (Kannel, 1975).

It must be assumed that some emotional or physical event induced the ventricular fibrillation and that acute myocardial infarction or coronary thrombosis did not occur as the primary event. Interviews with relatives of people who died indicate that the most significant relationship between sudden death and other identifiable factors was that with acute psychologic stress (Myers, 1975).

A differentiation has sometimes been made between instantaneous death and sudden death within an hour. Patients who are not accustomed to strenuous physical exertion should be warned of its risks, especially in a setting of emotional stress or on unusually cold or unusually hot, humid days. Shoveling snow after dinner and pushing stalled automobiles in cold weather are particularly dangerous activities. Hot, humid weather increases the blood flow to the skin and increases the work of the heart.

Differential Diagnosis

In deaths investigated by the coroner's office, sudden unexpected, unexplained deaths which occur within 1 hour after onset of symptoms are almost always due to coronary heart disease. When death is delayed more than 2 hours, coronary disease is less commonly the cause but is still the cause in at least half of cases. Other causes are overwhelming sepsis; other cardiac disorders such as myocarditis, cardiomyopathy, or aortic stenosis; cerebral hemorrhage; shock due to any cause; bowel obstruction; and aortic dissection. The so-called "café coronary," which is due to tracheal obstruction by food while eating, may be confused with sudden death from coronary disease.

Prevention of "Sudden Death"

Since most deaths from coronary heart disease occur suddenly, usually owing to ventricular fibrillation, successful resuscitation depends upon how quickly trained persons can institute appropriate measures to sustain the patient until defibrillation can be accomplished. Efforts to prevent sudden death have been concentrated in preventing the electrical instability in patients who in many cases have a known high risk of ventricular fibrillation. Two approaches have been used to prevent or combat "sudden death" outside the hospital: (1) vigorous use of antiarrhythmia agents in patients at high risk, especially those with known coronary heart disease with complex ventricular arrhythmias or previous episodes of ventricular fibrillation; and (2) community efforts to provide specially equipped and trained ambulance and fire department personnel who can reach the patient within 2–3 minutes, recognize arrhythmias, administer atropine or lidocaine, and accomplish defibrillation. There is no doubt that lives have been saved in communities where such services are available.

Examination of the data summarized in Tables 8–3 and 8–4 shows that about two-thirds of patients who are resuscitated subsequently testify to having had premonitory symptoms in the preceding 1–2 weeks, and one-fourth of them saw a physician in the preceding 1–2 days, not necessarily for a recognizable cardiac complaint. Because so many "sudden deaths" are unwitnessed or occur so soon after the development of acute symptoms that the mobile coronary care team cannot arrive in time, most patients with ventricular fibrillation do not survive. However, in one study, the mobile fire department coronary care approach allowed discharge from the hospital of about 20% of 1106 patients found to be in ventricular fibrillation by the mobile team, although over 40% were initially resuscitated (Cobb, 1975). Thus, resuscitation during the acute phase does not mean that the patient will survive. In some small communities where the mobile unit has been able to reach the scene in response to the patient's call within 5 minutes, patients with acute myocardial infarction who might develop a fatal arrhythmia within 30 minutes can be treated appropriately by trained ambulance or fire department personnel. This means that some deaths that occur in ambulances not equipped for resuscitation may be preventable.

The fatality rate in patients with acute myocardial infarction with ventricular fibrillation in the first hour is higher than in those who do not fibrillate.

Data from Sweden suggest that beta-adrenergic blocking agents may prevent the onset of sudden death in patients with coronary heart disease. Wilhelmsson (1974) showed that there were 4 times as many deaths in a placebo group as in a treated group given beta-blockers over a 2-year period. This promising approach to prevention of sudden death awaits confirmation.

The use of allied health personnel, including ambulance drivers and firemen trained in the use of lidocaine and atropine injections, is increasing, but data are not yet available regarding the benefit of this "mobile unit" approach to the use of drugs at the onset of acute myocardial infarction.

A. Cigarette Smoking: The relationship between cigarette smoking and sudden death has been extensively documented. In cases studied by the coroner's office, for example, sudden deaths from coronary heart disease are 2–3 times as common in smokers as in nonsmokers, which suggests that cigarette smoking may predispose to ventricular fibrillation in susceptible individuals. Although sudden death occurs at an older age in women than in men, it occurs in younger women who are heavy smokers. The electrophysiologic mechanism by which smoking causes ventricular fibrillation in patients with coronary artery disease is not fully understood. Coronary disease is progressive, and there may come a point at which obstruction is neatly balanced with respect to supply and demand, so that smoking may result in less successful perfusion of myocardial cells and in this way produce the electrical instability that results in ventricular fibrillation.

B. Physical Activity: As mentioned earlier, the very high incidence of both coronary disease and coronary deaths in the lumberjacks of northeastern Finland indicates that hard physical activity does not effectively protect against coronary heart disease. The increased physical activity may lead to increased food intake, and there is some evidence that serum cholesterol is slightly higher in eastern than in western Finland, where the coronary mortality rate in men is half as high as in eastern Finland.

Emergency Measures

A. Resuscitation: (See also Chapter 7.) The value of resuscitation efforts on behalf of patients with ventricular fibrillation has been demonstrated in a number of community studies in which the 1-year survival rate of those who were resuscitated was about 70%. Resuscitated patients with primary ventricular fibrillation are often able to return to work with adequate left ventricular function. There is an increased likelihood of recurrence of ventricular fibrillation within the next year, and the long-term prognosis is guarded unless antiarrhythmia agents and attention to social, psychologic, and environmental factors are employed to reduce adrenergic impulses operating "through the mind" that may produce coronary vasoconstriction.

B. Patient Education: The high mortality rate from ventricular fibrillation in acute myocardial infarction and the high incidence of sudden death within 1–3 hours after the acute ischemic episode have highlighted the need for shortening the interval between onset of symptoms and admission to a coronary care unit. There should be no delay in getting the patient to the hospital, and this means within 1 hour at most after onset of symptoms. The best advice is to get to the hospital and *then* call the personal physician unless it is known that the physician can be contacted without delay. Education of the patient's family in the technics of resuscitation—especially in patients with known coronary heart disease—may save lives, and encouraging results have followed the vigorous educational efforts of the National Committee for Emergency Coronary Care chaired by Dr Hilliard Katz (Shapter, 1974).

In spite of public education efforts, even patients with previous coronary heart disease and those who have been told to seek immediate care should new symptoms or a change of symptoms appear sometimes delay seeking medical care, perhaps because patients fail to realize the significance of the symptoms or try to combat the fear of death with the psychologic mechanism of denial.

As has been stated previously, sudden death may be the only manifestation of the disease; it may occur early or late in the course of acute myocardial infarction; it may complicate stable or unstable angina pectoris; and it may be the terminal event in a patient with ischemic cardiomyopathy and cardiac failure. The possibility of sudden death therefore tends to dominate the thinking of every patient with coronary disease and is a constant source of dread for both the patient and the family. Although excessive physical activity or intense emotion may be responsible in some instances, especially when death is instantaneous (within seconds), most sudden deaths occur during the patient's usual activities and not as a result of some determinable unusual event.

Delays in treatment in the emergency room must be minimized. Emergency rooms should be equipped for immediate monitoring and resuscitation. These remarks bear primarily on emergency management of patients who have developed acute myocardial infarction, in whom sudden death is common within the first hour, but they apply also to patients who have collapsed from primary ventricular fibrillation, ie, not preceded by shock or cardiac failure. (Although it is usually preceded by ventricular arrhythmias of less severe type, it may occur de novo.)

C. Reversibility of Sudden Death: There is no doubt that sudden death due to primary ventricular fibrillation is reversible in many cases. Many of these survivors have had no episodes of acute myocardial infarction after resuscitation, as shown by serial enzyme and electrocardiographic examination. Most have the same left ventricular function 1 year later as they had before the episode of fibrillation. Furthermore, when cardiac arrest occurs during ECG monitoring of these patients, the arrhythmia is ventricular fibrillation rather than ventricular standstill. Therefore, major public health effort should be directed toward identifying groups of people most likely to have primary ventricular fibrillation and devising methods of preventing the attacks. The most important of these preventive measures is treatment of ventricular arrhythmias in patients with known coronary heart disease. Unfortunately, ventricular premature beats that occur either singly, from multifocal sites, or even in short runs are so common in middle-aged people with or without known coronary heart disease that it is difficult to identify individuals likely to develop ventricular fibrillation. The frequency and characteristics (multifocal, paired, early in diastole, short runs) of complex ventricular premature beats occurring during 12 hours of continuous ECG recording, as well as those induced by exercise, correlate positively with the development of ventricular fibrillation, but the relationship has not been sufficiently close to warrant vigorous treatment with antiarrhythmia agents of all patients with ventricular premature beats. This is reinforced by the observation that the currently available antiarrhythmia agents (quinidine, procainamide, phenytoin, and propranolol) are of limited effectiveness and often produce side-effects that make continued therapy difficult (Jelinek, 1974). The value of beta-blockers must be confirmed. Lown (1977) has studied the relationship between ventricular premature beats and sudden death and has attempted to grade their severity on the basis of their frequency and whether they are multifocal, occur in runs, or occur early in diastole during the vulnerable or supernormal phase of excitability. He found treatment unsatisfactory because approximately 60% of patients receiving procainamide developed a lupuslike sensitivity reaction within the year, about one-third of patients receiving quinidine had side-effects, and phenytoin was ineffective. (See below under Acute Myocardial Infarction, p 153.)

D. Defibrillation: When ventricular fibrillation occurs in coronary care units, it often is preceded by ventricular tachycardia or multifocal ventricular premature beats. A small electric shock during this period may depolarize the reentry circuit, terminating the ventricular tachycardia. A sharp thump on the chest is not quite as effective but may do the same. Electrophysiologic studies have demonstrated that myocardium which has been damaged by fibrosis or by ischemic episodes has a variable recovery of excitability and duration of refractoriness in neighborhood cells; this can lead to multiple reentry circuits, which in turn may initiate ventricular fibrillation. Prompt treatment of ventricular tachycardia in susceptible patients may prevent ventricular fibrillation.

E. Café Coronary: See Differential Diagnosis.

ACUTE MYOCARDIAL INFARCTION

General Considerations

In myocardial infarction there is ischemic necrosis of a variable amount of myocardial tissue as a result of an abrupt acute decrease in coronary flow or an equivalent abrupt increase in myocardial demand for oxygen which cannot be supplied by an obstructed coronary artery. Coronary flow may be impaired by a thrombus in one of the coronary arteries or hemorrhage within or beneath an atherosclerotic plaque, or decreased flow may be due to shock, dehydration, or hemorrhage, leading to poor perfusion of all tissues, including the myocardium. Rapid ventricular rates due to ventricular tachycardia or uncontrolled atrial fibrillation may also contribute to myocardial ischemia because of the decreased diastolic filling time. Transient temporary ischemia is reversible, but persistent ischemia (approximately 1 hour) results in a central area of complete necrosis which is surrounded by an area of ischemia in cells that are viable but not necrotic. The histologic pattern is illustrated in Fig 8–9 (Bishop, 1976).

Abrupt occlusion of a coronary artery in the dog is followed by marked reduction and altered distribution of blood flow, with the subendocardium most severely affected. By 24 hours—and especially by 96 hours—there is a significant increase in collateral blood flow which decreases the size of the central core of necrosis (Bishop, 1976). Hamby and others (1976) have demonstrated that collateral vessels are protective and decrease the size of the infarct. Infrequently, de-

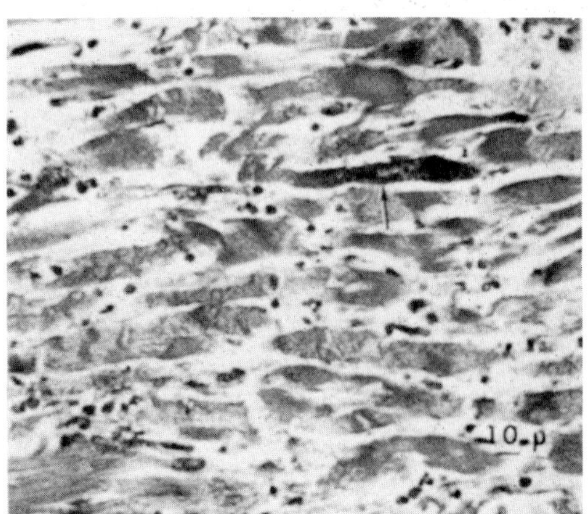

Figure 8–9. Photomicrograph of myocardium in peripheral region 96 hours after coronary artery occlusion. Note extensive myofibril degeneration and necrosis with many contraction bands, fragmented fibers, and loss of myofibrils, with edema and polymorphonuclear neutrophil infiltration. Occasional cells contain mineral deposits (arrow). Hematoxylin and eosin stain. (Reproduced, with permission of the American Heart Association, Inc., from Bishop SP, White FC, Bloor CM: Regional myocardial blood flow during acute myocardial infarction in the conscious dog. Circ Res 38:429, 1976.)

creased coronary flow may result from occlusion of a coronary artery by an embolus, coronary ostial stenosis from syphilis, or acute vasculitis in connective tissue disorders.

A. Location and Extent of Infarction: The site and extent of necrosis depend upon the degree of occlusion of the coronary artery, the disproportion between flow and demand resulting from the anatomic distribution of stenoses within the coronary vessels, the adequacy of the collateral circulation between neighborhood coronary arteries, and the presence and extent of previous infarctions. The infarct may involve the full thickness of the myocardium from endocardium to epicardium (transmural infarction) or may be confined to the subendocardium (nontransmural or subendocardial infarction). Coronary thrombosis, formerly thought to be the usual event precipitating acute myocardial infarction, is now regarded by some as an uncommon event, occurring in perhaps one-fifth of cases; the coronary thrombosis found in previous studies at autopsy is considered to be a consequence rather than the cause of the poor perfusion. *Coronary occlusion and acute myocardial infarction are therefore independent entities.* A thrombus may occlude a branch of the coronary artery without producing myocardial infarction, which may occur in the absence of coronary thrombosis. One must keep in mind the 3 distinct entities: (1) coronary atherosclerosis (a pathologic finding that may or may not be associated with coronary heart *disease*), (2) coronary thrombosis, and (3) myocardial infarction.

B. Arteries Occluded: The left anterior descending artery is most commonly occluded and results in infarction of the anteroseptal portion of the left ventricle. Less commonly, occlusion of the right coronary artery leads to infarction of the inferior and posterior left ventricle. Least common is occlusion of the left circumflex artery, producing anterolateral myocardial infarction. When occlusion of the left main coronary artery occurs (rarely without severe disease of its branches), massive infarction of the left ventricle usually results. Decrease in coronary flow in occlusive disease of the coronary artery usually implies occlusion of at least 80% of the artery (because it has been shown that coronary blood flow is not decreased until occlusion exceeds 75%).

C. Radioisotope Studies of Myocardial Perfusion: Analyses of coronary perfusion in patients with previous myocardial infarction utilizing a radioisotope such as thallium 201 have shown that even with significant stenosis the myocardium supplied by the artery may have normal coronary blood flow at rest but hypoperfusion or altered distribution of flow under the stress of exercise, with atrial pacing, or with the increased coronary blood flow that follows the injection of contrast medium into the coronary artery. The complex relationship between occlusion and infarction depends on the net effect of multiple forces and factors such as the number, degree, and location of stenoses, the adequacy of the blood flow distal to the stenosis, the runoff via collateral channels, the adequacy of the blood flow and the presence of stenoses in the associated coronary arteries, and left ventricular function, in addition to more general factors such as anemia, hypoxia, and tachycardia.

Thallium isotopic perfusion scans do not show small perfusion defects, and reproducibility is variable unless maximum exercise is performed. Resolution of isotopic scans is imperfect, but the reliability of scanning may be improved by the use of computer technics. Further study by more refined technics is necessary in order to develop methods of distinguishing (1) hypoperfusion resulting from scar; (2) ischemic but viable myocardium: the ischemic process is potentially reversible by drugs such as nitroglycerin or by coronary bypass surgery; and (3) viable resting cells that are made ischemic by stress.

In contrast to thallium 201, which reveals defects in perfusion ("cold spots"), technetium Tc 99m pyrophosphate has the advantage of being actively taken up by acutely infarcted myocardial cells, producing discrete, well-localized "hot spots" in transmural acute infarction. Technetium pyrophosphate has limitations in nontransmural incomplete subendocardial infarction because diffuse uptake can be seen. Such uptake may also occur in the absence of infarction, and it will cause false-positive interpretations. On the other hand, the positive localized uptake of pyrophosphate demonstrates recent myocardial infarction more effectively than the failure of uptake of thallium by scarred or ischemic cells following induced ischemia. Radioisotope myocardial scans are being performed with increasing frequency in many centers, with promising results of practical importance. Combinations of agents that reflect both defects in perfusion (thallium) and increased activity after myocardial necrosis (pyrophosphate) may give additional information and allow the physician to recognize ischemia as well as old and new infarctions and to demonstrate the effect of various therapeutic agents and interventions on viable but ischemic myocardial cells.

As imaging technics improve, especially with 3-dimensional computer processing, it is becoming possible to more accurately determine the size of an infarct, especially if it is anterior, and to correlate the quantitative estimate of the size of the infarct with serial serum enzyme determinations and hemodynamic measurements. This will allow noninvasive technics to supersede invasive ones. Thallium 201 myocardial perfusion studies after exercise either in asymptomatic individuals or in patients with suspected angina pectoris are often more reliable than treadmill or bicycle exercise testing; ischemic ST segment change may not occur with the exercise. The reverse is occasionally true, ie, the perfusion study is negative but the exercise ECG or 12- to 24-hour ECG monitoring shows characteristic ST segment abnormalities. The methods are complementary, and both should be used. In patients with old myocardial infarction or myocardial scars, image perfusion defects may be diagnostic of an old infarction or scar at a time when only nonspecific ST segment abnormalities without Q waves are present in the resting ECG. If image defects following exercise do not change, it confirms that the defect seen at rest is due to an old scar.

The usual method of administration of thallium is by intravenous injection. Recent studies have shown that when the radioisotope is injected directly into the coronary artery (rather than into the general circulation) during coronary arteriography, resolution is better and wall motion abnormalities can be more clearly seen, and this technic may prove to be an important addition to the diagnostic evaluation of coronary disease. In some cases pyrophosphate scans are the earliest diagnostic indicator in acute myocardial infarction, preceding diagnostic serum enzyme abnormalities. Newer radioimmunoassay technics for determining myocardial band isoenzymes of creatine phosphokinase may improve the diagnostic sensitivity of the serum enzymes and allow earlier diagnosis of myocardial infarction than do pyrophosphate scans.

One of the most promising of the newer radiopharmaceutical technics being tested is the use of radioiodinated fragments of antimyosin antibody, which allows discrete myocardial uptake in dogs who have had induced coronary occlusion (Beller, 1977). Infarcted myocardial cells have increased membrane permeability and permit the intracellular concentration of the specific antibody to myosin. Haber and his associates (Beller, 1977) showed excellent localization precisely in the area of absent blood flow, as determined by the distribution of radioactive microspheres which demonstrate an inverse relationship between blood flow and concentration of the radiolabeled myosin-specific antibody. When the radioiodinated fragments were injected intravenously, discrete uptake required approximately 72 hours, but when the isotope was injected into the coronary artery, clear images were demonstrated as early as 7 hours after occlusion. The area of uptake was verified by killing the animal and demonstrating that the region concentrating the antibody fragments corresponded to the infarcted area. Isotopes of hydrogen and of fatty acids such as palmitate are also being employed, the former for earlier recognition of acute myocardial infarction and the latter to take advantage of the metabolic requirement of the myocardium for fatty acids (Resnekov, 1977; Sobel, 1977). Examples of radioisotopic scans in coronary heart disease are given in Figs 8–10 and 8–11.

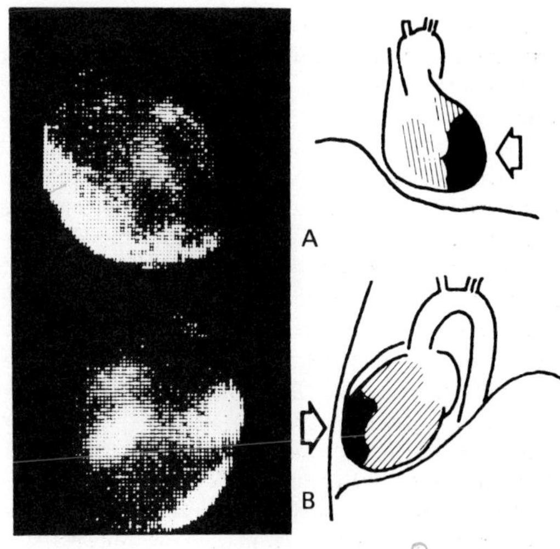

Figure 8–10. Anterolateral infarction. The frontal *(A)* and left lateral *(B)* scintiscans show an area of diminished activity (arrows) at the site of infarction. (Reproduced, with permission, from Wackers FJT & others: Noninvasive visualization of acute myocardial infarction in man with thallium-201. Br Heart J 37:741, 1975.)

D. Size of Myocardial Infarct: As a result of the factors mentioned earlier that influence myocardial ischemia, the artery occluded in an extensive myocardial infarction cannot always be predicted accurately; anterior infarction can follow occlusion of a right coronary artery if collaterals from the right, secondary to previous left coronary artery occlusion, supplied the anterior myocardium. Although we describe myocardial infarction as a disease entity, it is more useful to consider it as a continuum of increasing necrosis from a few cells to massive infarction. The former results in a mild illness typically characterized almost exclusively by the presence of cardiac pain (see below) without disturbance in left ventricular function and with minimal systemic manifestations or serum enzyme elevations, although the ECG pattern may be diagnostic. When necrosis involves many cells and a large area, especially if there has been previous infarction with segmental scars, the clinical picture is confounded and complicated by the presence of ventricular arrhythmias, cardiogenic shock, left ventricular dysfunction with cardiac failure, heart block, cardiac arrest, and death. The physician therefore must attempt to estimate the extent of the infarction in terms of its impact on the circulation as well as its site and size. The former is a function of the extent of the previous as well as the current myocardial infarction, which limits left ventricular function. If the amount of previous irreversible myocardial scarring and fibrosis is extensive, with borderline left ventricular function, even a small additional myocardial infarction may be sufficient to produce severe clinical manifestations of cardiogenic shock and failure.

Methods for measuring the size of the myocardial infarction include the following: (1) determination of the extent of ECG abnormalities and location of the Q, ST, and T wave changes, whether they occur in just a few leads over the lateral chest or extend across the entire anterior precordium and perhaps the inferior wall as well; (2) ST mapping, in which the magnitude and persistence of ST segment elevation using multiple precordial leads are added up and averaged over a period of days; (3) serial determinations of myocardial band (MB) isoenzymes of creatine phosphokinase (CPK) released into the serum by necrosing myocardial cells; (4) pyrophosphate and thallium radioisotope uptake studies; (5) hemodynamic studies; and (6) cineangiography.

The greater the isoenzyme rise or increased up-

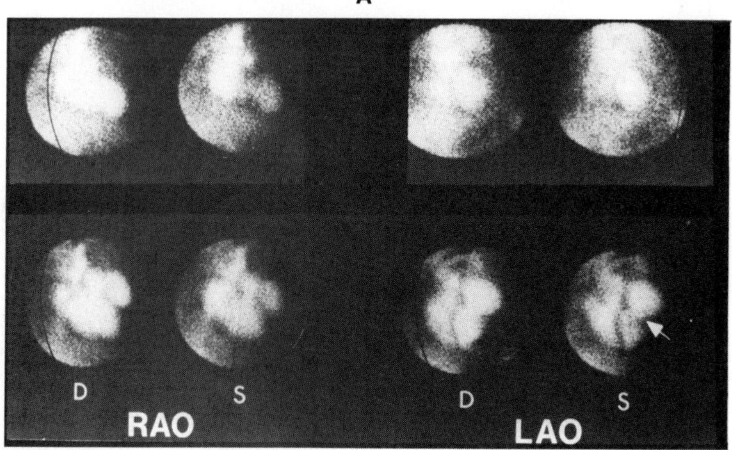

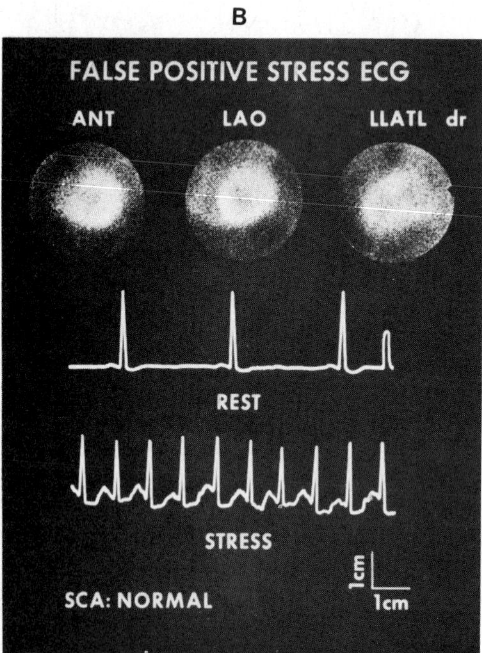

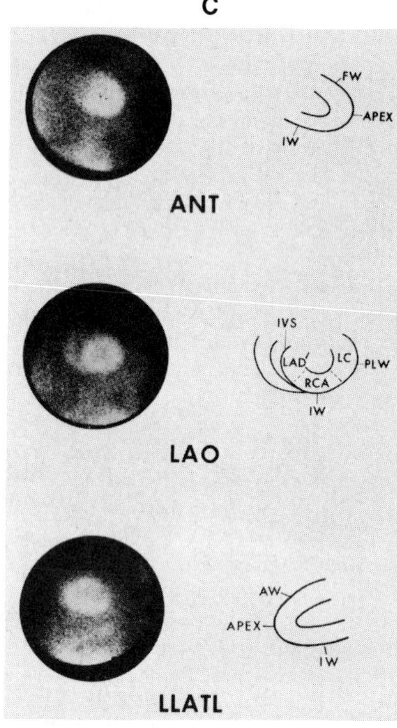

Figure 8–11. Isotopes in coronary heart disease. *A:* Top, true aneurysm; bottom, false aneurysm. *B:* Positive stress test (? false-positive) with normal image and normal coronary angiogram—not on digitalis. *C:* Normal thallium 201 perfusion image. *D:* Thallium study showing a positive exercise test. There is a defect in the septum at rest in the left anterior oblique position, and the left lateral anterior wall shows a defect. After exercise, the entire previously normal anterior apical wall and the posterior wall become abnormal. The septal abnormality is more obvious. Angiography shows triple-vessel disease chiefly affecting the left anterior descending and circumflex arteries, and the left anterior descending artery fills from the right. *E:* Man age 58 with a negative treadmill test but showing, at rest, a residual old infarct abnormality, worse with exercise after thallium. Selective angiogram shows left anterior oblique artery 80% stenotic and right carotid artery 90% stenotic. *F:* Discrete acute apical and anterior infarct (in image 3) 2 hours after injection of technetium stannous pyrophosphate. White area in image 3 in lateral view lights up with acute infarct. The anterior view in 1 is normal. The anterior view in 2 shows haziness in both anterior and lateral views (diffuse uptake), but in both anterior and lateral views the light area shows an acute infarct. (*A* is reproduced, with permission, from Botvinick EH & others: Noninvasive diagnosis of the false left ventricular aneurysm with radioisotope gated cardiac blood pool imaging: Differentiation from true aneurysm. Am J Cardiol 37:1089, 1976. *C* and *D* are reproduced, with permission, from Botvinick EH & others: Thallium 201 myocardial perfusion scintigraphy clarifying normal, abnormal, and equivocal stress tests. Am J Cardiol, Jan 1978. [In press.] *B* and *F* are courtesy of EH Botvinick. *E* is reproduced, with permission, from Botvinick EH & others: Myocardial stress perfusion scintigraphy with rubidium 81 versus stress electrocardiography. Am J Cardiol 39:364, 1977.)

D

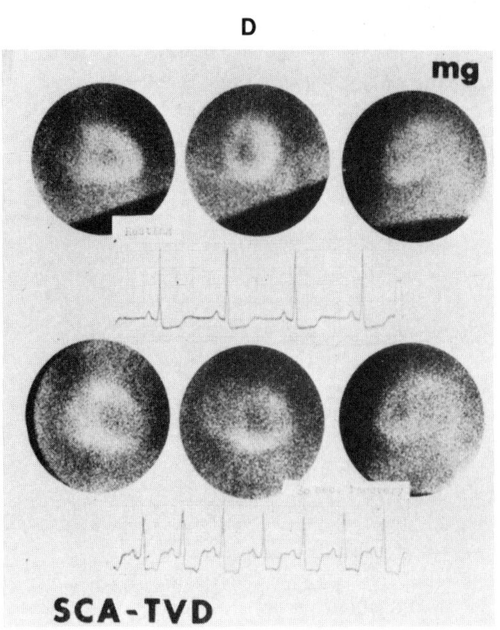

E

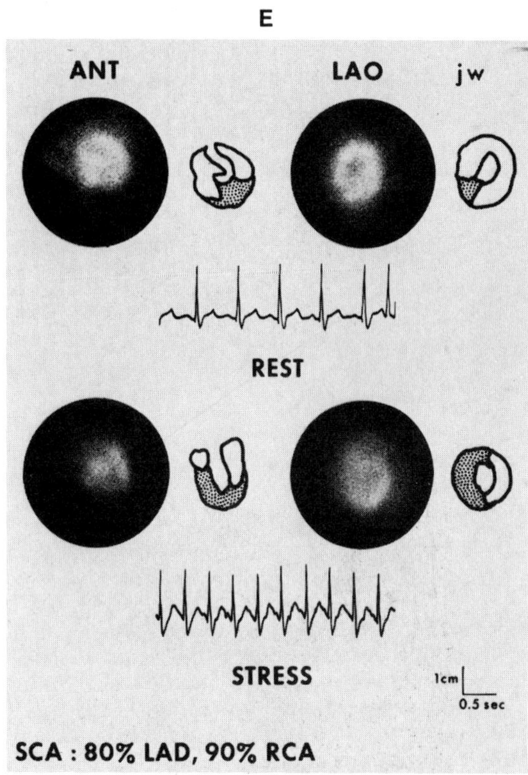

F

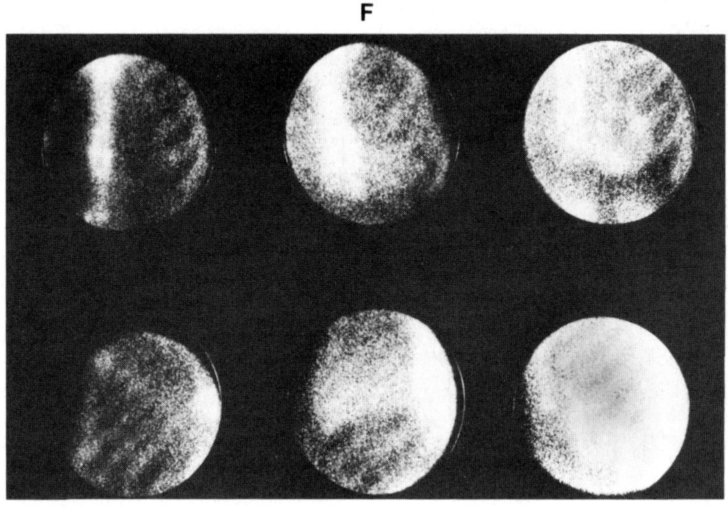

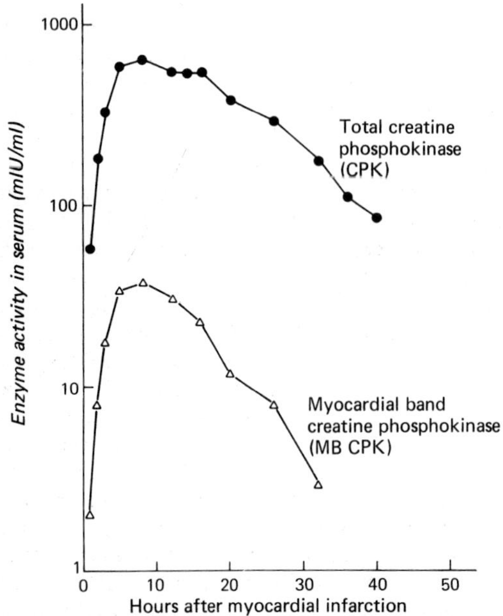

Figure 8–12. Serial changes in total serum CPK activity and serum MB CPK activity in a patient with hemodynamically uncomplicated acute myocardial infarction. The disappearance rate of MB CPK activity exceeded the corresponding rate for total CPK. MB denotes myocardial band of CPK. (Reproduced, with permission, from Sobel BE, Roberts R, Larson KB: Estimation of infarct size from serum MB creatine phosphokinase activity: Applications and limitations. Am J Cardiol 37:474, 1976.)

take of pyrophosphate (or factors of uptake of thallium), the greater the number of necrosed myocardial cells. It is important to measure specifically the MB isoenzymes because other CPK enzymes may also arise from skeletal muscle tissue and because intramuscular injections given for the relief of pain may produce a rise in muscle CPK isoenzymes. Evolution of a major infarct takes hours (Fig 8–12). More recently, recognition of the presence and extent of acute myocardial infarction has been estimated by radioisotope perfusion studies using ^{99m}Tc pyrophosphate, which is selectively and rapidly taken up by necrosing cells and can demonstrate as little as 4 g of infarcted muscle. The isotope is injected intravenously, and myocardial uptake imaging, obtained by an external counter, reflects acute necrosing cells but not old scar. Old fibrotic areas as well as new areas of infarction may be identified using different isotopes such as thallium 201, which is not taken up by scarred, necrosed, or fibrosed areas and can be demonstrated by so-called "cold" areas of decreased uptake following intravenous injection. A combination of isotopes can indicate the magnitude of old as well as recent myocardial infarction.

E. Determination of Wall Motion Abnormalities and Left Ventricular Function by Radioisotope Studies: The extent of myocardial damage can also be estimated by radioisotope gated blood pool scans (equilibrated in the total blood pool and "gated"—synchronized—to the ECG for both end-systole and end-diastole) that utilize intravenous injection of technetium Tc 99m-labeled human albumin to estimate left ventricular ejection fraction and wall motion abnormalities. The frequency of diminished left ventricular ejection fraction and abnormalities of left ventricular contraction such as hypokinesia can be demonstrated by serial scanning observations in patients with acute myocardial infarction or in patients who have recovered from a myocardial infarction but continue to have disability resulting from angina or dyspnea.

F. Minor Myocardial Infarction: As indicated later in the section on unstable angina, it is often difficult to recognize minor myocardial infarction, and patients thought to have unstable angina without infarction may in fact have had a small myocardial infarction which was not heralded by the appearance of new Q waves. It was once thought that the prognosis in myocardial infarction was better if patients had only ST–T abnormalities but not Q waves, but more recent data have shown that this is not always the case. These "nontransmural" myocardial infarctions often, when examined at autopsy, have transmural islands of infarcted tissue, although the major areas of necrosis are subendocardial (Scheinman, 1973).

The diagnosis of minor myocardial infarction is often obvious only in retrospect when one reviews the entire sequence of events of the illness. Slight increases in serum enzymes, relatively minor ST–T abnormalities, slight fever, the presence of transient gallop rhythm, and serial radioisotopic scans may permit the diagnosis of slight myocardial infarction. It is hazardous, however, to make this diagnosis when the patient is first seen because the myocardial infarction may extend and hemodynamic manifestations may worsen, and a patient who originally presented with what appeared to be minor myocardial infarction may develop a more severe variety. Furthermore, even a small area of myocardial necrosis may induce ventricular arrhythmias or conduction defects, with resultant worsening of the clinical picture. Hemodynamic abnormalities may appear slight when the patient is first seen, but they require caution in estimating prognosis and the ultimate size of the myocardial infarction. Table 8–7 describes the relative sensitivity and specificity of diagnostic tests in nontransmural infarction.

G. Hemodynamic Studies: Hemodynamic studies during the acute phase of acute myocardial infarction are being used with increasing confidence to estimate

Table 8–7. Rank order sensitivity and specificity of noninvasive tests in the diagnosis of acute nontransmural myocardial infarction.

Sensitivity	Specificity
1. Serial ECGs	1. Serum enzymes
2. Wall motion studies	2. Pyrophosphate focal uptake
3. Serum enzymes	3. Serial ECGs
4. Thallium 201 defect at rest	4. Thallium 201 defect at rest
5. Pyrophosphate focal uptake	5. Wall motion studies

the impact of the infarction on left ventricular function. Patients with slight infarction may show normal left ventricular filling pressures, cardiac output, pulmonary artery pressure, and stroke work index. These patients usually have an ejection fraction exceeding 60%, and their prognosis is good. They may present with an initial clinical picture of severe prolonged pain and typical ECG abnormalities but rarely are in cardiogenic shock or cardiac failure, and hemodynamic studies are normal. Elevated left ventricular filling pressure, especially in association with a falling stroke work index, indicates worsening of left ventricular function, and the whole train of adverse clinical features such as hypotension, severe ventricular arrhythmias, cardiac failure, and shock may develop. In many coronary care units, patients with moderate to severe myocardial infarction undergo special investigations such as invasive monitoring of arterial pressure, measurement of left ventricular filling pressure, and determination of cardiac output by the thermodilution method in order to correlate stroke work index and left ventricular filling pressure and so permit therapeutic interventions which may increase the chance of survival (see below).

Left ventricular dysfunction may reflect damage to the left ventricle with ischemic cardiomyopathy and does not necessarily indicate myocardial infarction per se unless there are abrupt left ventricular changes in the presence of an acute clinical episode of ischemia. With the increasing use of invasive technics such as left ventricular cineangiography and coronary arteriography in acute myocardial infarction, identification of abnormalities in left ventricular wall motion, cardiac volume, and ejection fraction to evaluate prognosis and to judge appropriate treatment permits a more reliable estimate of the extent of myocardial muscle damage than do ST mapping or enzyme changes. These invasive studies may ultimately be superseded by radioisotopic scans. Echocardiography can supplement isotopic studies and demonstrate left ventricular size and the magnitude of septal and posterior left ventricular dimensions and contraction; it also provides an estimate of ejection fraction that correlates reasonably well with that determined by left ventricular cineangiography, especially if 2-dimensional echoes are obtained.

H. Systemic Manifestations: An indirect measure of the amount of necrotic tissue is the magnitude of the systemic response to acute infarction as evidenced by fever, tachycardia, leukocytosis, and acceleration of the sedimentation rate. These systemic signs of tissue necrosis usually appear 24–48 hours after the onset of the initial pain and are related to the amount of tissue that has undergone necrosis. They therefore serve as an estimate of the extent of infarction. The delayed systemic response is also helpful in differentiating acute myocardial infarction from such conditions as pneumonia or acute pericarditis, in which systemic abnormalities are present at the onset of illness.

Clinical Findings

A. Symptoms:

1. Pain—Pain is the classic dominant feature of acute myocardial infarction that compels the patient to seek help. It is similar in quality to angina pectoris (p 164) and may be described as a heaviness or tightness or a great weight sitting on the chest. The pain is similar to ordinary angina in location and radiation, although it may radiate more widely than angina of effort, and the patient recognizes that the discomfort has changed in its distribution. Not only may it radiate more widely to the lower jaw and teeth, neck, left shoulder, upper back, or down the left arm to the 2 fingers innervated by the ulnar nerve (which of course it may do with angina of effort), but it may also involve the upper posterior thoracic area, and the patient may think he has an orthopedic problem. The pain is more severe than that of angina of effort, does not subside with rest, builds up rapidly but not instantaneously, may wax and wane, and may reach maximum severity in a few minutes. Nitroglycerin has little or no effect, which will be obvious to a patient with angina who has previously found nitroglycerin to be effective in less than 1 minute. The pain may last for hours if unrelieved by narcotics and may be unbearable. The severity of the chest pain is not related to the severity of the infarct or to its size, and the physician must not be misled into considering the event a minor one because the symptoms are not devastating.

2. Sweating, weakness, and apprehension—The patient often breaks out into a cold sweat, feels weak and apprehensive, and moves about, seeking a position of comfort—in contrast to the discomfort of angina of effort, in which the patient's instinct is to stand still or to sit or lie down.

3. Lightheadedness, dyspnea, and hypotension—In association with the pain and sweating, the patient may feel weak, faint, and lightheaded. Syncope may occur if there is a rapid onset of ventricular tachycardia or fibrillation or an atrioventricular conduction defect with a Stokes-Adams attack. Syncope and manifestations of cerebral infarction are presumably the effects of decreased cardiac output on a compromised carotid or cerebral arterial supply to the brain.

The presence or absence of pain is important in evaluating the significance of hypotension, especially at the onset of acute myocardial infarction. The vasomotor response to acute pain is hypertension in some individuals but abrupt decrease in cardiac output and vasodilatation in muscles and skin in others, resulting in hypotension with poor tissue perfusion manifested by cold, clammy skin, a gray appearance, sighing respirations, tachycardia, and low blood pressure. These signs must not be taken as evidence of cardiogenic shock until pain is relieved by appropriate medication (see below).

Ventricular arrhythmias in the first few hours after an acute infarction may cause hypotension because of the pain and fear engendered by the infarct. The myocardium often responds to acute ischemia with variable electrophysiologic changes of excitability and refractoriness, increased vulnerability to ventricular ectopia, and ventricular fibrillation.

4. Nausea, vomiting, and "indigestion"—Nausea

and vomiting are not rare and may be due to severe pain, vagal stimulation, or the abrupt fall in cardiac output, with resulting general cellular hypoperfusion. The discomfort may extend into the epigastrium and be associated with sensations of indigestion and bloating, and the patient may think he has acute indigestion and take antacids without benefit. In retrospect, he may often be aware that he had similar milder discomfort in the central chest hours, days, or sometimes a week or so prior to the acute severe event.

5. Pulmonary edema and left ventricular failure—In 10–20% of cases, the pain is minor and may be misinterpreted or overshadowed by the presence of acute pulmonary edema, rapidly developing left ventricular failure, profound weakness, shock, dyspnea, or cough or wheezing of acute left ventricular failure.

6. Retrospective diagnosis—In perhaps 10% of cases, the initial symptoms are mild enough so that the diagnosis is only recognized in retrospect, when an ECG is taken months later and evidence of previous acute infarction is discovered that was not previously present. This is particularly true in patients with autonomic nervous system dysfunction due to diabetes mellitus. The patient may fail to realize that myocardial infarction has occurred because the pain lasts only 30 minutes and is unrelated to effort, with onset at rest or even during sleep. A patient with previous angina of effort will recognize the unusual features, particularly the severity, radiation, and duration of the discomfort and its failure to respond to nitroglycerin; however, a patient who has not had angina of effort may interpret the discomfort as indigestion or musculoskeletal disease or may merely complain of feeling unwell.

B. Signs: The signs of acute myocardial infarction may be trivial, or the patient may be at the point of death when first seen. The clinical picture is related to the size and extent of the infarction, the presence of previous infarction with left ventricular dysfunction, and the adequacy of the collateral circulation.

1. Initial signs—The initial signs may be more severe than those found 1–2 hours later, especially if the patient has had a ventricular arrhythmia, marked bradycardia with poor output, or abrupt left ventricular failure which subsided as compensatory reflex mechanisms came into play.

2. Signs in mild cases—In mild cases the patient may appear well, the skin may be dry, and the pulse and blood pressure normal, and there may be no signs of failure, the patient complaining only of prolonged substernal discomfort.

3. Signs in more severe cases—In more severe cases the patient appears acutely ill, may have marked hypotension with low cardiac output, tachycardia, cold, clammy, sweaty skin, and a gray (ashen) appearance due to peripheral cyanosis. If cerebral perfusion is impaired, the patient may be mentally dull and confused and may have either tachycardia or bradycardia depending upon whether the baroreceptor response to low cardiac output predominates or impairment of perfusion to the sinus node or vagal reflexes produces sinus bradycardia. At the onset of acute myocardial infarction, the temperature is usually normal. Fever is delayed for 24–72 hours and is due to myocardial necrosis, which takes time to develop.

4. Combination of shock and cardiac failure—A patient with clinically apparent shock with a systolic pressure less than 80 mm Hg and a urine output less than 20 ml/hour may show signs of left ventricular failure with a diastolic gallop rhythm, pulsus alternans, and bilateral rales. The gallop and rales may rapidly progress to acute pulmonary edema or right-sided congestive heart failure or may remain the same. The chest x-ray confirms left ventricular failure by haziness in the central lung fields if there is transudation into the alveoli or redistribution of flow to the upper lobe if there is interstitial edema. Kerley's B lines may also occur after some days but may be out of phase with the clinical signs, and there may be hemodynamic evidence of raised pulmonary artery diastolic pressure. At any time there may be a discrepancy between the radiologic evidence of left ventricular failure and the pulmonary artery diastolic pressure. Although the radiologic signs lag behind the hemodynamic ones, x-ray offers valuable evidence of cardiac failure. When the pulmonary artery wedge pressure is normal, the great majority of patients have no radiographic evidence of left ventricular failure or pulmonary congestion. When patients have a high degree of raised wedge pressure (more than 25 mm Hg), radiologic changes of pulmonary congestion are almost always present (Kostuk, 1973).

The venous pressure may be raised but may be difficult to recognize because of the venous constriction resulting from the intense sympathetic discharge caused by the low cardiac output; yet when hemodynamic studies are done, the right atrial pressure is elevated. If the signs of shock are delayed, venous constriction out of proportion to arteriolar constriction may lead to transudation of fluid out of the capillaries, and the patient may be hypovolemic, in which instance the right atrial pressure is low and volume repletion is indicated.

C. Laboratory Findings:

1. White count and ESR—The white blood count and sedimentation rate are normal at onset and rise with the fever as myocardial necrosis occurs. As the necrotic area of myocardium extends toward the epicardium, pericarditis may be recognized by pericardial friction rub, but this is often delayed until at least the second day and is transient, usually lasting not more than 2–4 days, and may be intermittent. Depending upon the size of the infarct, the fever, white count, and sedimentation rate may be only slightly raised or may be quite profoundly affected, with fever of 40 °C lasting 3–7 days. High fever and leukocytosis indicate extensive infarction in the absence of pneumonia or other diseases. The sedimentation rate often remains elevated for 2–3 weeks after the white blood count and temperature have returned to normal.

2. Myocardial enzymes—With necrosis of cells, myocardial enzymes appear in the serum and may be noted within 4 hours in the case of the MB isoenzymes

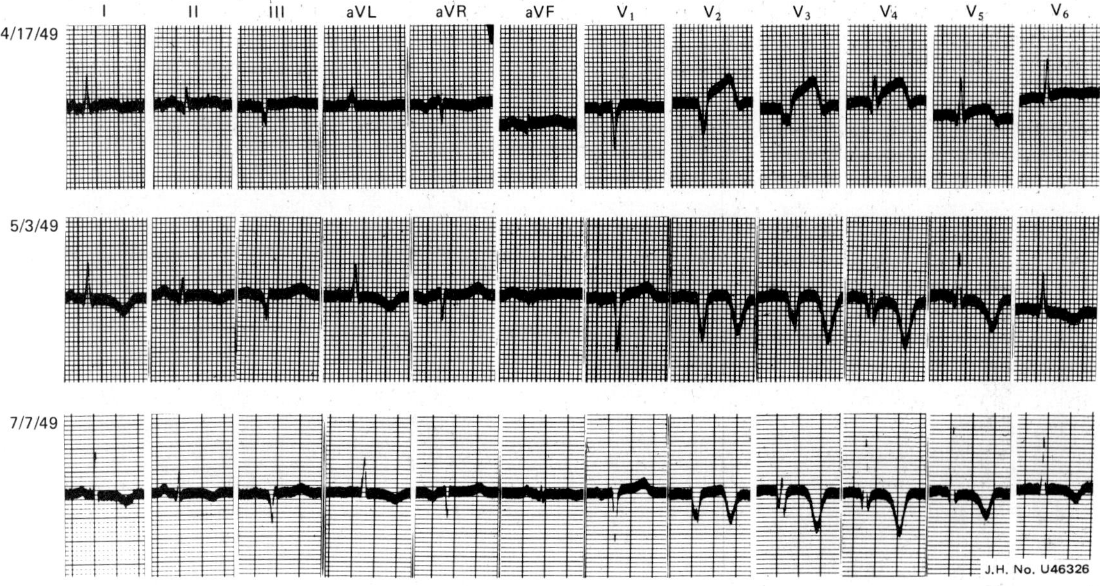

Figure 8–13. ECG of a 65-year-old man with myocardial infarction. Pain in the posterior aspect of the upper chest awakened him from sleep and required injection of analgesic. The pain recurred the next day and spread to the anterior chest. Recurrent pain at rest occurred for another month. Note appearance of R in V_3 and V_4 and serial ST–T changes, especially in V_{2-5}, indicating anteroseptal myocardial infarction extending laterally.

of CPK, derived exclusively from myocardial cells, as compared with other bands of CPK, which may enter the serum from muscle, brain, or liver. Serum glutamic-oxaloacetic transaminase may not rise for 6–12 hours and returns to normal in 5–7 days; CPK is usually normal in 4–6 days. Serum lactate dehydrogenase may remain elevated for 7–9 days. Serial determinations of enzymes every 2 hours make it possible to determine the area under the time curve of the increase and decrease in the enzyme and thus enable the physician to estimate the magnitude of the infarction and discern whether extension of infarction has occurred.

D. Electrocardiographic Findings: A myocardial infarction of significant size, especially if transmural and anterior, produces characteristic ECG changes in about 95% of patients. Five examples of the ECG changes in myocardial infarction are seen in Figs 8–13 to 8–17.

1. Early unchanged ECG–At the onset of infarction the ECG may be within normal limits, especially if there is no previous record for comparison; *it is essential that a normal ECG at this stage should not rule out the diagnosis.*

2. Early ECG changes–The characteristic pattern may be delayed for hours or days, and the initial slightly convex ST elevation seen over septal leads V_{2-4} in anteroseptal myocardial infarction, over lateral leads V_{5-6} in anterolateral infarction, and in inferior leads II, III, and aVF in inferior infarction may be subtle and difficult to distinguish from the normal variant of early repolarization. Over a period of hours or days, however, the characteristic evolution occurs with subsequent symmetric inversion of T waves in the leads that initially showed convex elevated ST segments.

3. Evolving ECG–If characteristic broad Q waves are present in leads with convex elevated ST segments

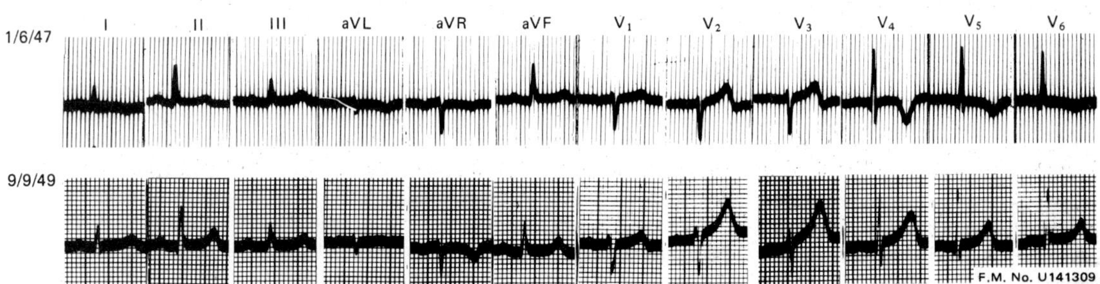

Figure 8–14. ECG of a 63-year-old man with myocardial infarction. The ECG abnormalities characteristic of myocardial infarction on the first tracing have completely disappeared in the second tracing obtained 2 years later.

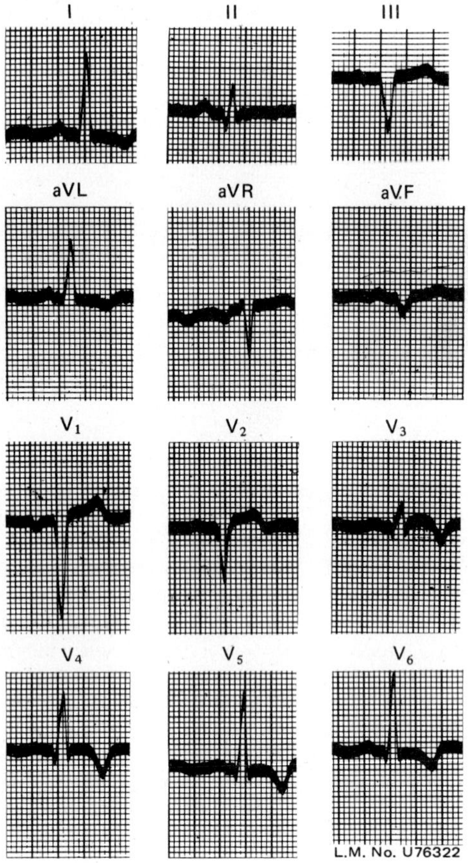

Figure 8–15. ECG of a 59-year-old man showing old inferior myocardial infarction and more recent anteroseptal myocardial infarction with associated left ventricular conduction defect.

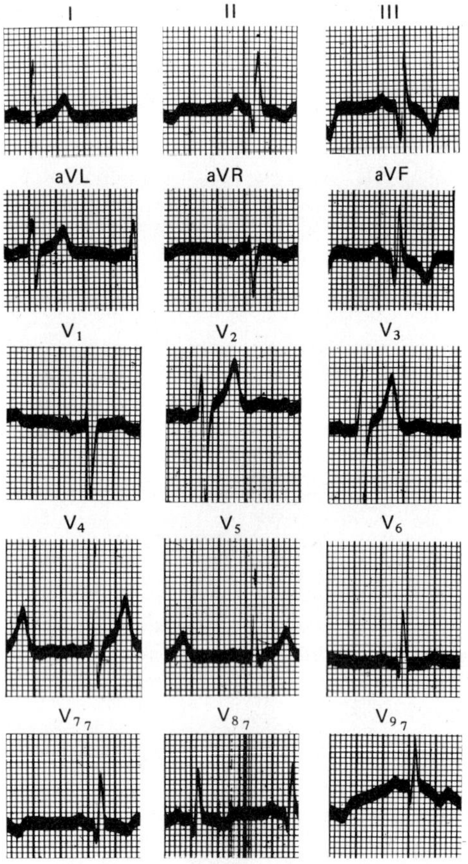

Figure 8–17. An example of inferior myocardial infarction with typical findings in leads II, III, and aVF and in the posterolateral leads (V_{7-9}) in the seventh interspace but no diagnostic findings in the routine lateral leads (V_{4-6}).

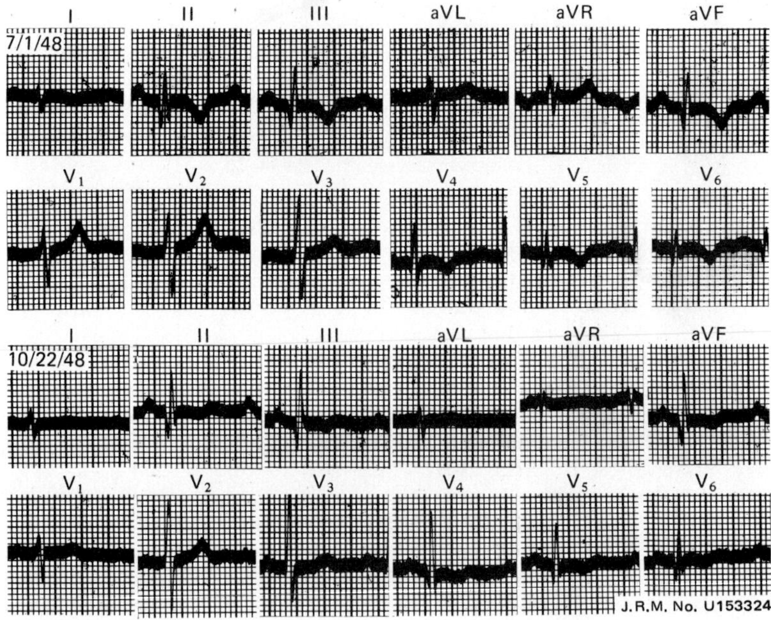

Figure 8–16. ECG of a 59-year-old man with inferolateral myocardial infarction who had dyspnea on exertion for 6 months as well as angina of effort and anginal pain on awakening that lasted about 2 weeks (up until 2 months before the time of the first tracing). Blood pressure was 140/90.

that subsequently evolve to symmetrically inverted T waves, an unequivocal diagnosis can be made. Q waves are more significant than QS complexes, particularly in the right precordial (V_{1-3}) or septal leads (V_{3-4}) or in the inferior leads (II, III, aVF) in horizontal heart position with left axis deviation. If there is a broad ($\geqslant$ .04 sec) slurred, wide Q wave with an amplitude exceeding 30% of that of the succeeding R wave, which is slightly slurred in its upstroke–and especially if a previous ECG did not show the Q waves–the diagnosis is strongly supported.

4. **Serial changes**–The diagnosis is less certain if there are no diagnostic Q waves, as is the case with nontransmural infarctions. In these instances, serial changes with waxing and then waning of the ST–T abnormalities are more reliable than static changes. If the patient is seen after the infarction has been present for some days and there is no previous ECG for comparison, the initial ST–T changes may appear nonspecific and further serial records over days to weeks may be necessary before one can interpret the ECG changes as diagnostic.

5. **ECG in presence of old infarct**–If the patient has had previous myocardial infarction, if there is left bundle branch block or significant conduction defects in the peripheral Purkinje system, or if there is underlying left ventricular hypertrophy or digitalis effect, the interpretation is more difficult and the presence of diagnostic Q waves or characteristic serial evolution of the ST–T abnormalities is required to establish the ECG diagnosis of myocardial infarction. Radioisotopic methods may be especially useful in these situations.

6. **Return to normal ECG**–The usual evolution of the ST–T changes takes several weeks, but in minor infarction this may occur within 10 days. When the acute infarction is characterized only by ST–T changes, the ECG may return completely to normal in about 20–30% of patients; a normal ECG therefore does not exclude a previous infarction.

7. **Abnormal Q waves**–Q waves, defined as initial negative deflections followed by positive deflections–in contrast to QS complexes, which are negative deflections not followed by positive ones–have greater diagnostic value, when abnormal, than ST–T abnormalities. A Q wave of 0.04 sec, especially if slightly slurred and followed by a slurred upstroke of the R wave, is considered diagnostic of anterior infarction when it occurs in the precordial leads and of inferior infarction when it occurs in lead aVF. One-half to two-thirds of patients with Q waves demonstrate localized segmental wall motion abnormalities by left ventricular angiography in the area of the Q wave representing infarction. It is now believed that the immediate subendocardial area does not contribute to the Q waves but that they are the result of necrosis of the mid- and subepicardial areas. The Q waves may be transient and due to functional impairment resulting from hypoxia or ischemia or the development of collateral blood flow and may disappear as the infarct heals. When myocardial infarction occurs in dogs as a result of coronary occlusion, one-third to one-half of the animals lose their Q waves over a period of 5–10 minutes. The presence of a Q wave, therefore, does not mean myocardial scar, death of cells, or permanent damage, because during left ventricular angiography the Q waves may disappear and segmental areas of hypokinesia or asynergy may contract more normally when the load on the myocardium is decreased following administration of nitroglycerin or hydralazine.

Conduction defects that alter pathways of activation may influence the appearance and course of Q waves. The Q waves may disappear when left bundle branch block develops, only to reappear when the conduction delay disappears in intermittent block, as sometimes occurs during the course of an acute infarction.

It was once thought that persistent Q waves, especially when associated with elevated ST segment abnormalities, were a reliable sign of ventricular aneurysm. However, recent correlative studies utilizing left ventricular angiograms have shown that some ventricular aneurysms are not associated with Q waves and that many patients with Q waves do not have aneurysms, although they may have segmental localized contraction abnormalities.

The interpretation of a significant Q wave in aVF as a sign of an inferior infarction is often difficult; most reliable is a Q wave 0.04 sec wide with a depth of at least 30% that of the succeeding R wave and an associated significant Q wave in lead II. In old inferior infarction, the Q waves often become smaller and nondescript, and diagnosis is doubtful. Small Q waves may appear in aVF in a vertically placed heart in normal individuals. A Q wave in aVF is more significant if the patient has a horizontally placed heart (left ventricular potentials transmitted to the left arm) than when it is present in a vertically placed heart (left ventricular potentials transmitted to the left leg). When typical evolutionary serial ECG changes occur in the presence of progressive increases in serum enzymes (particularly the MB isoenzymes of CPK) and a compatible clinical history, the diagnosis is considered to be firmly established.

E. **Radioisotope Studies**: Radioisotope perfusion studies with technetium Tc 99m pyrophosphate (which is taken up by acutely necrosed myocardial cells) allow recognition of the presence and size of acute myocardial infarction provided the study is performed within about the first 6 days. Thallium 201 can be used to demonstrate old infarcts with defects of perfusion because the isotope is not taken up by actively necrosing or necrotic cells or by ischemic areas with "cold" spots induced by exercise. The combination may demonstrate the necrotic area by increased uptake of pyrophosphates or failure of uptake of thallium.

After the patient has recovered from acute myocardial infarction, radioisotope studies utilizing thallium and gated blood pool scans, at rest and after exercise, are valuable for identifying perfusion defects, for determining left ventricular size and function, and for identifying wall motion abnormalities, including true and false aneurysm, and for aiding in prognosis and treatment (see p 136).

Computer analysis of the magnitude of the radioisotope uptake using myocardial imaging with an external counter has made this kind of study easier to quantify. However, despite this improvement, technical resolution of imaging is still relatively insensitive. Myocardial imaging is not yet established as a routine method of clinical study.

Course & Complications

Table 8–8 compares the complications in patients with acute myocardial infarction with those in patients with acute coronary insufficiency (unstable angina). Late mortality rate is 4–15% per year depending on the number of vessels involved and the degree of left ventricular dysfunction.

In mild cases, after chest pain is relieved by morphine or one of its analogues, the course is uneventful, with no evidences of arrhythmia, cardiac failure, or cardiogenic shock. In more severe infarction, and even in some milder cases, the most common finding is the development of arrhythmias, usually ventricular premature beats, ventricular tachycardia, or ventricular fibrillation (see below). Less commonly, atrial premature beats or atrial fibrillation may occur; paroxysmal atrial tachycardia is least common. There may be junctional tachycardia, especially if there is impairment of perfusion of the sinus node or increased vagal reflexes causing sinus bradycardia. Atrioventricular conduction defects with partial or complete atrioventricular block and Stokes-Adams attacks, pulmonary edema, or congestive heart failure may develop over hours or days, but the most lethal development is cardiogenic shock, which carries a high mortality rate. Extension of the infarcted area to the epicardium causes pericarditis in about 10% of cases, usually causing pericardial pain in the first few days combined with a pericardial friction rub. The rub is usually transient, lasting only a few days to a week.

A. Arrhythmias:

1. **Tachyarrhythmias**–(See also Chapter 15.) ECGs examined within hours after an episode of acute myocardial infarction show ventricular arrhythmias (usually ventricular premature beats) in 80–90% of cases, ventricular tachycardia in 10–15%, and ventricular fibrillation in 5–10% (Table 8–9). The ventricular premature beats may be single or may occur in salvos; may occur frequently or only occasionally; or may be repetitive and lead to ventricular tachycardia or fibrillation. The ischemic cells, which are inadequately perfused, are usually the sites of onset of abnormal activation leading to arrhythmia. These surviving Purkinje fibers have abnormal electrophysiologic changes which foster arrhythmias. Severe ventricular arrhythmias are 10–20 times more common in the first 4 hours than they are on the second day; for this reason, patients are ideally admitted as soon as possible to a coronary

Table 8–8. Comparison of complications and hospital course in patients with acute coronary insufficiency (unstable angina) and a group of 359 concurrently admitted patients with definite acute myocardial infarction.*

	Definite Myocardial Infarction (359 Patients)	Acute Coronary Insufficiency (Unstable Angina) (100 Patients)
Average age (years)	62	62
Men:women	2.5:1	1.8:1
Complications		
Hypotension (<90 mm Hg systolic)†	34%	4%
Bradycardia	16%	12%
Atrial premature beats	15%	15%
Ventricular premature beats†	61%	35%
Ventricular tachycardia†	25%	6%
Atrioventricular block		
First to second degree†	13%	5%
Third degree†	7%	1%
Bundle branch block	11%	7%
Congestive heart failure†		
Mild to moderate	39%	20%
Severe	16%	6%
Acute mortality		
Coronary care unit†	16%	0
Hospital outside coronary care unit†	5%	1%
Average length of stay		
Coronary care unit	6.6 days	4.6 days
Hospital	21 days	14 days

*Reproduced, with permission, from Krauss KR, Hutter AM, DeSanctis RW: Acute coronary insufficiency (unstable angina). Arch Intern Med 129:808, 1972.

†$P < .05$.

Table 8–9. Incidence of dysrhythmias among 284 patients seen within the first hour, 1966–69.*

Dysrhythmia	Number of Patients				Total Number of Patients
	Within 1 Hour	Within 2 Hours	Within 3–4 Hours	After 4 Hours	
Bradyarrhythmia	88 (31%)	10 (3.5%)	6 (2%)	21 (7%)	125 (44%)
Ventricular ectopic beats	70 (25%)	36 (13%)	16 (6%)	41 (14%)	163 (57%)
Ventricular fibrillation	28 (10%)	12 (4%)	2 (0.7%)	12 (4%)	54 (19%)
Ventricular tachycardia	10 (3.5%)	16 (6%)	6 (2%)	55 (19%)	87 (31%)
Atrial fibrillation/flutter	11 (4%)	0	0	15 (5%)	26 (9%)
Supraventricular tachycardia	1 (0.4%)	0	0	10 (3.5%)	11 (4%)

*Reproduced, with permission, from Adgey AA & others: Acute phase of myocardial infarction. Lancet 2:501, 1971.

unit with specially trained nurses and medical personnel and equipment permitting continuous ECG monitoring. The great frequency of early ventricular arrhythmias explains the high mortality rate before the patient receives treatment. The severity of early arrhythmias is related to the size of the infarct and the presence of ventricular asynergy or aneurysm. The abrupt development of ventricular tachycardia or ventricular fibrillation may result in cardiac arrest, which in patients in the coronary care unit is usually due to ventricular fibrillation.

a. **Ventricular fibrillation**–When ventricular fibrillation or cardiac arrest follows the development of shock or heart failure, it is considered secondary to the poor left ventricular function and not to primary electrical instability of the ischemic myocardium. Prompt recognition and treatment of ventricular arrhythmias in the coronary care unit (see Treatment, below) has been a major factor in reducing the mortality rate of acute infarction in the hospital and in mobile ambulance units. Continuous monitoring of the patient, with a monitor both at the bedside and at the nursing station, permits immediate recognition of the abnormal rhythm, which must be treated promptly (within 30 seconds) in order to prevent irreversible cardiac or cerebral damage. Sudden cardiac death in acute ischemia is usually due to ventricular fibrillation, and at autopsy most patients have severe coronary disease with 2- or 3-vessel involvement; occasionally, only a single vessel is diseased.

b. **Other tachyarrhythmias**–(See also Chapter 15.) Accelerated idioventricular rhythm occurs in about 15–25% of patients. It is usually due to enhanced automaticity but may be an "escape" rhythm. Idioventricular rhythms are "benign" because the heart rate is usually relatively slow (60–100/min) and because they infrequently lead to ventricular tachycardia with more rapid rates (150–180/min) or ventricular fibrillation. This is not always true, however; close observation is required, and the possibility of ventricular tachycardia must be considered when ventricular rates exceeding 100–110/min occur. As with the usual rapid ventricular tachycardias, the idioventricular rhythm is often heralded in the first few days by ventricular premature beats with varying coupling intervals combined with sinus bradycardia.

Table 8–10. Frequency of supraventricular arrhythmias (222 instances in 154 patients).*

Type of Arrhythmia	Alone	Combined	Total	Incidence	Mortality
	(Number)			(Percent)	
Supraventricular premature contractions	70	58	128	36	24
Supraventricular tachycardia	20	35	55	16	25
Atrial flutter or fibrillation	5	34	39	11	41

*Reproduced, with permission, from Cristal N, Szwarcberg J, Gueron M: Supraventricular arrhythmias in acute myocardial infarction: Prognostic importance of clinical setting; mechanism of production. Ann Intern Med 82:35, 1975.

Atrial arrhythmias, including paroxysmal atrial fibrillation or tachycardia, are less common, usually short-lived, and do not require rigorous treatment (such as cardioversion) unless symptoms appear or hemodynamic deterioration occurs. Their frequency is illustrated in Table 8–10.

When the ventricular rate is rapid–exceeding 140–150 beats/min in atrial fibrillation or atrial tachycardia–coronary perfusion may be decreased and cardiac output may fall. If the patient has incipient left ventricular failure it may worsen, and the adverse hemodynamic effects may increase the area of infarction, with the possible development of conduction defects, hypotension, cardiac failure, or cardiogenic shock. In these situations, cardioversion should be used promptly in order to reverse the clinical and hemodynamic abnormalities. If the ventricular rate is slower and the patient is tolerating it well, without symptoms or hemodynamic change, one may use conventional antiarrhythmia agents such as digitalis–or edrophonium or rapid atrial stimulation if digitalis toxicity is a possibility. Atrial stimulation must not be used in fibrillation.

2. **Bradyarrhythmias**–(See Table 8–11 and Chapter 15.) At the onset of acute infarction, sinus bradycardia or sinus standstill may occur in 10–20% of cases, causing junctional escape or idioventricular rhythms. Bradycardia is due to the Jarisch-von Bezold vagal reflex, a chemoreflex triggered by chemical

Table 8–11. Incidence of bradyarrhythmia among 284 patients related to time after onset of symptoms and site of infarction, 1966–69.*

Site of Infarction	Number of Patients				Total Number of Patients
	Within 1 Hour	Within 2 Hours	Within 3–4 Hours	After 4 Hours	
Sinus or nodal bradycardia	75 (26%)	9 (3%)	5 (2%)	19 (7%)	108 (38%)
Anterior infarct	24 (18%)	5 (4%)	1 (0.7%)	2 (1.5%)	32 (24%)
Posterior infarct	48 (36%)	4 (3%)	3 (2%)	16 (12%)	71 (53%)
Atrioventricular block, second degree or complete	17 (6%)	2 (0.7%)	1 (0.4%)	8 (3%)	28 (10%)
Anterior infarct	1 (0.7%)	0	1 (0.7%)	1 (0.7%)	3 (2%)
Posterior infarct	15 (11%)	2 (1.5%)	0	7 (5%)	24 (18%)

*Reproduced, with permission, from Adgey AA & others: Acute phase of myocardial infarction. Lancet 2:501, 1971.

stimuli (possibly histamine) from the left ventricular wall or coronary artery causing bradycardia or hypotension. Involvement of the sinoatrial nodal artery in right coronary artery occlusion with inferior or posterior myocardial infarction may also cause bradycardia. Slow heart rates allow for a greater degree of nonhomogeneity of excitability and refractoriness in neighborhood fibers, and arrhythmias are thus more common in patients with slow heart rates. When bradycardia is associated with ventricular premature beats and evidence of poor cardiac output and hypotension at the onset of acute myocardial infarction, increasing the sinus rate with atropine (0.3–0.6 mg intravenously) is often salutary but may produce sinus tachycardia and ventricular arrhythmias if high or repetitive doses of atropine are used. The appropriate dosage and, indeed, the usefulness of this treatment are being reevaluated.

B. Atrioventricular Conduction Defects: Atrioventricular conduction defects are common in acute myocardial infarction, occurring in about 10% of patients, and are associated with a mortality rate of about 50% in third degree or Mobitz type II block. (For further details, see Chapter 14.)

1. Conduction defects in anterior infarction–Atrioventricular and intraventricular conduction defects are more hazardous in the presence of anterior myocardial infarction because they represent widespread necrosis in the ventricular septum, often involving the bundle of His and its branches and frequently resulting in impaired left ventricular function and hypokinesia. The conduction defect may be recognized early during ECG monitoring in the coronary care unit. The patient may develop a left anterior hemiblock with left axis deviation of –45 to –60 degrees, indicating damage to the left anterior superior fascicle of the left bundle with or without right bundle branch block.

2. Stokes-Adams attacks–The patient may also develop partial atrioventricular block with prolongation of the P–R interval (> 0.21 sec) or may have second degree atrioventricular block with dropped beats (Mobitz type II). The change from a first degree atrioventricular block or a left anterior hemiblock to second degree atrioventricular block and then complete atrioventricular block with Stokes-Adams attacks may occur within hours, and immediate prophylactic placement of a temporary artificial pacemaker is essential. When complete atrioventricular block occurs in anterior infarction, the ventricular escape pacemaker is usually below the area of destruction in the septum, in one of the branches of the left or right bundle, or even in the ventricular myocardium; as a result, the QRS complex is usually wide (> 0.12 sec) and the rate of discharge of the ectopic pacemaker in one of the fascicles is usually slow and unreliable.

3. Conduction defects in inferior infarction–The situation is more favorable when atrioventricular conduction defect occurs in inferior myocardial infarction because the damage is usually to the atrioventricular node and is more ischemic than destructive, resulting from partial occlusion of the branch of the right coronary artery to the atrioventricular node. In such instances, although there are exceptions, the patient may have a partial atrioventricular block with a prolonged P–R interval or may have second degree atrioventricular block with partial progressive atrioventricular block–so-called Wenckebach phenomenon or Mobitz type I–rather than 2:1 atrioventricular block with dropped beats, Mobitz type II (see Chapter 14).

4. Infrequency of Stokes-Adams attacks in inferior infarcts–When complete atrioventricular block occurs in the presence of inferior myocardial infarction, the pacemaker is just below the atrioventricular node, the QRS is usually narrow (< 0.11 sec), and the heart rate is faster (about 60/min) because the cardiac pacemaker is high in the conduction system. The infrequency of Stokes-Adams attacks in the presence of complete atrioventricular block with inferior myocardial infarction and a narrow QRS complex has led to a conservative approach with continued monitoring rather than insertion of a temporary right ventricular pacemaker, although this decision must be individualized and must be considered tentative at present.

5. Complete infranodal block–Complete infranodal block is uncommon in patients with *preexisting* bundle branch block, but in about one-fourth of patients, right bundle branch block or left anterior hemiblock *develops* during acute myocardial infarction. Prophylactic pacing is advised in these latter instances because of the suddenness with which complete block may occur, especially if the H–V interval in the His bundle recording (see Chapter 14) exceeds 70 msec. The abrupt appearance of bundle branch block is an unfavorable sign and is associated with an increased frequency of both atrioventricular block and cardiac failure, with a higher mortality rate than in patients who do not develop bundle branch block.

6. Bilateral bundle branch block–Bilateral bundle branch block is diagnosed when block of either the right or the left bundle is associated with any degree of atrioventricular (bifascicular) block or when there are conduction defects in both branches. The mortality rate is high in these patients; but, as with other types of ventricular conduction defects in acute myocardial infarction, the prognosis is worse when the conduction defect develops following the acute myocardial infarction than when it preexisted. Because severe ventricular conduction defects in acute myocardial infarction reflect a large area of myocardial necrosis, ventricular arrhythmias and cardiac failure are the usual causes of death rather than complete atrioventricular block; for this reason, insertion of temporary prophylactic pacemakers may not contribute much to ultimate survival.

His bundle recordings may be helpful in making the decision whether or not to insert a pacemaker in bilateral bundle branch block because complete atrioventricular block is more common if the H–V interval exceeds 70 msec even if the P–R interval is normal. The mortality rate is greater in patients with bifascicular or bilateral bundle branch block with a prolonged H–V interval than when this interval is normal. The data are confusing because some patients with prolongation of the H–V interval in this situation do not develop atrioventricular block and hence are not at risk for Stokes-Adams attacks.

Because of the current conflicting reports on the significance of prolonged H–V intervals and of the likelihood of complete atrioventricular block with Stokes-Adams attacks in bilateral bundle branch block, especially the block preceding the acute myocardial infarction, prophylactic pacemaker insertion is not advised until further prospective studies substantiate its value or unless progressive atrioventricular block or symptoms of syncope develop.

The indications for *permanent* ventricular pacing in patients who have developed complete atrioventricular block during acute myocardial infarction are controversial. Some authors have asserted that patients with bifascicular block who develop complete atrioventricular block during the acute infarction are at high risk of recurrent complete atrioventricular block with sudden death if permanent pacing is not performed. In contrast, survival is improved if these patients are permanently paced despite the high mortality rate of about 50% over the next 1–2 years (Ritter, 1976). Further prospective studies are required to determine whether death can be prevented by insertion of a permanent demand pacemaker in this specific subset of patients.

C. Cardiac Failure:

1. Acute left ventricular failure—Acute left ventricular dysfunction resulting from acute myocardial infarction may lead to unremitting pump failure or may be transient and associated with acute pulmonary edema, subsiding with relief of pain and the development of compensatory mechanisms such as opening of collateral channels. Cardiac failure is the cause of death in two-thirds of hospital deaths except for those deaths occurring in the first 4 hours; arrhythmias, sudden death, and conduction defects account for the remainder.

2. Milder cases of left ventricular failure—In less severe cases, the existence of left ventricular failure can be inferred on the basis of dyspnea, pulmonary rales, gallop rhythm, pulsus alternans, raised venous pressure, radiologic evidence of pulmonary venous congestion or redistribution of fluid to the upper lobes, or, less often, the presence of Kerley's B lines. If there is alveolar edema, bat's wing infiltrates near the hilar areas of the lungs may be seen.

3. Bedside hemodynamic monitoring—Monitoring of right atrial and pulmonary artery wedge pressure during the course of acute infarction has been made possible by the development of a balloon-tipped catheter by Swan and Ganz (1970) that allows repeated measurements of pressure and oxygen saturation in the right side of the heart in the coronary care unit with little disturbance to the patient. Serial determinations of cardiac output utilizing thermodilution (see Chapters 4 and 6) and computerized technics also make it possible for patients with left ventricular dysfunction to be monitored intermittently for the purpose of determining right atrial pressure, pulmonary arterial pressure, pulmonary arterial wedge pressure, and cardiac output. Treatment can be individualized on the basis of abnormalities disclosed by these studies. Serial determinations of indices of left ventricular performance such as cardiac output, stroke output, or stroke work index can be compared with left ventricular filling pressure by inflating the balloon at the tip of the catheter wedged into the pulmonary artery. One can then determine whether left ventricular function is improving or deteriorating.

Hemodynamic studies have shown that with more severe manifestations on presentation—varying from an uncomplicated course to one with mild or severe left ventricular failure or cardiogenic shock—the mean pulmonary artery wedge or diastolic pressure (the left ventricular filling pressure) increases, the left ventricular end-diastolic volume increases, the ejection fraction falls, and the cardiac output decreases. Subsets of acute myocardial infarction in cardiac failure have been defined by relating the left ventricular filling pressure to stroke work or cardiac index, which describes left ventricular performance. When the end-diastolic pressure is high and the stroke work index is low, the prognosis is worse (Forrester, 1977). Only 25% of patients with an uncomplicated acute myocardial infarction have an abnormal (> 12 mm Hg) left ventricular filling pressure, but the percentage rises progressively to 70% when left ventricular failure is more definite (Ross, 1972).

4. Bedside echocardiography—Echocardiography at the bedside can complement hemodynamic studies and allow estimation of left ventricular dimensions and wall motion, septal and posterior myocardial wall contraction, size of the left atrium, and ejection fraction. Echocardiography can support the diagnosis of severe left ventricular failure in acute myocardial infarction by showing greatly increased left ventricular dimensions and a wide E-point separation between the maximum excursion of the anterior mitral valve leaflet and the ventricular septum (see Fig 10–7).

5. Factors precipitating cardiac failure—Although cardiac failure may develop progressively and insidiously, it may appear abruptly following an arrhythmia or pulmonary infarction or following complications such as perforation of the ventricular septum or dysfunction of the papillary muscle with the development of acute mitral regurgitation. When either of the latter 2 complications develops, a loud, harsh systolic murmur and thrill suddenly appear over the lower left parasternal area in the case of septal perforation or at the apex in the case of mitral regurgitation. In both instances, severe cardiac failure may develop rapidly. A perforated ventricular septum gives rise to the abrupt development of very large *v* waves on the wedge tracing and a high oxygen content in the right ventricle, which can be demonstrated by using the Swan-Ganz catheter. Minor degrees of papillary muscle dysfunction are commonly found (about 50% of cases) if careful auscultation is done daily to search for the pansystolic or late systolic murmur of slight mitral insufficiency that accompanies the lesion.

6. **Evaluating left ventricular function**–The ejection fraction, which can be estimated serially by radioisotope study or by echocardiography, can be used to estimate the size of the infarct and the effectiveness of left ventricular function and helps to determine prognosis.

D. Cardiogenic Shock: Cardiogenic shock with hypotension and poor tissue perfusion with oliguria and cerebral obtundation may be present at the onset of a massive infarction or may develop insidiously over the next few days. It is more apt to occur when there has been previous infarction or when the current infarction is so massive that at least 50% of the myocardium is destroyed. Three-vessel coronary artery disease, severe proximal left anterior descending artery stenosis, or left main coronary artery stenosis is frequently present in patients with cardiogenic shock. Cardiogenic shock is more common than congestive failure in patients dying from "pump failure" after acute myocardial infarction. It is the most frequent cause of death in the hospital following acute infarction. The large area of damaged myocardium frustrates successful medical treatment, although, as will be seen later, modern therapy with circulatory assist devices, eg, intra-aortic balloon counterpulsation, intravenous vasodilator drugs, and other types of treatment made safer by intracardiac pressure monitoring can decrease the acute mortality rate.

Hemodynamic studies in patients with cardiogenic shock demonstrate a high left ventricular filling pressure, low cardiac output, low stroke work index, severe hypotension, and no evidence of hypovolemia. Severe cardiogenic shock is a dread event, and patients usually die within a few days. The prognosis is poor even in somewhat milder cases, and aggressive therapy is warranted. In some centers, following stabilization by temporary circulatory assist mechanisms such as aortic balloon counterpulsation, vasodilator therapy, and inotropic agents, coronary arteriography and left ventricular cineangiography are performed with a view to possible emergency operation. Cineangiography may also demonstrate the presence of perforation of the ventricular septum or gross mitral regurgitation as well as evidence of hypokinesia or akinesia or left ventricular aneurysm which may require surgical treatment. At autopsy, most patients with cardiogenic shock have severe coronary disease and destruction of at least 50% of the myocardium. Even when salvage during the acute episode is possible by heroic effort, 1- or 2-year survivals are infrequent because of the severity of myocardial disease. The low survival rate is also due to the frequency of the late complications of dyskinesia and akinesia, with or without true aneurysm, which occur commonly in patients with severe acute myocardial damage. Left ventricular asynergy with dyskinesia is more common than true aneurysm and occurs in most patients after transmural infarction. In patients who have recovered from cardiogenic shock or cardiac failure after an acute infarction, search for akinetic segments or ventricular aneurysm should be performed by noninvasive technics with radioisotopes (Fig 8–24) or 2-dimensional echocardiography. If the patient has persistent or recurrent symptoms of cardiac failure or recurrent ventricular arrhythmias after successful initial management, left ventricular angiography is usually required. (See section on ventricular aneurysm, p 159.) It is often difficult to differentiate dyskinetic (abnormal type of motion) segments from true aneurysm; localized paradoxic motion of the dyskinetic segment is essential to confirm the diagnosis. At times, what appears to be an akinetic segment response to nitroglycerin with more adequate wall motion, indicating that the myocardial cells were viable and not scarred and dead. Mitral regurgitation from papillary and free wall muscle dysfunction and ventricular septal defect from perforation of the septum should always be considered with a view to possible surgical treatment in patients who have had cardiogenic shock or cardiac failure.

E. Arterial Embolism: An uncommon occurrence during the course of acute infarction, which may be delayed for days, weeks, or months, is systemic embolism to various arteries (cerebral, coronary, visceral, or peripheral) resulting from dislodgement of a portion of mural thrombus which has developed over the endocardium at the site of myocardial infarction. For reasons that are not clear, this complication is seen less frequently today. This is true even though anticoagulant therapy during acute myocardial infarction is less commonly used today than in the past. Perhaps earlier ambulation plus measures now taken to prevent venous thrombosis after acute infarction may be factors.

F. Phlebothrombosis and Pulmonary Embolism: These complications are also less common now than when prolonged bed rest was routinely recommended following acute infarction, even though anticoagulants given to prevent these "venous" complications are used less frequently than formerly.

Phlebothrombosis with or without pulmonary embolism occurs in approximately 10% of patients with acute myocardial infarction. Fatalities are rare, perhaps because of anticoagulant therapy.

G. Cerebral Infarction: The fall of arterial pressure associated with acute infarction in a patient with a compromised cerebral arterial blood supply may produce cerebral infarction. One should suspect acute myocardial infarction in all patients who develop cerebral infarction; it is surprising how frequently an ECG will reveal an unsuspected myocardial infarction in patients who present with cerebral infarction. Cerebral embolism secondary to a mural thrombus in the left ventricle may also cause cerebral infarction, but the event is usually later in the course of acute myocardial infarction and is of sudden onset.

H. Rupture of the Heart: This is an uncommon event (5%) and may cause sudden death due to acute hemopericardium and tamponade. Rupture may not be an immediate "blowout" but may be "subacute," with slight penetration of the epicardium to the pericardium, escape of blood, and worsening of the clinical picture, but with sufficient warning in some patients to allow surgical treatment. Fig 8–18 shows a myocardial

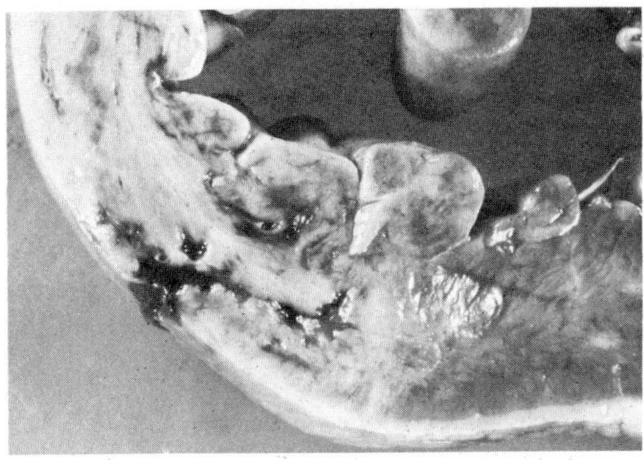

Figure 8–18. Myocardial infarction with early rupture of the left ventricular wall. (Courtesy of O Rambo.)

infarction with early rupture of the left ventricular wall.

Penetration of a weakened epicardial wall with pericardial effusion may be recognized by a change in symptoms and by echocardiography, and immediate surgery has been successful in some patients. Cardiac rupture is more common during the first week, but it can occur later. It is more common in first episodes than in recurrent myocardial infarction.

I. Acute Renal Failure: Following marked hypotension and prolonged shock, patients may develop acute tubular necrosis with oliguria, anuria, and acute renal failure. Renal failure is uncommon unless the shock is profound and lasts several hours. It may also occur if vasodilator therapy with sodium nitroprusside is unusually vigorous, producing prolonged hypotension.

J. Pericarditis: Extension of the transmural infarct to the epicardial surface may result in inflammatory changes in the pericardium, possibly with hemopericardium, especially if anticoagulants have been used. Pericarditis can be suspected when the patient develops a different type of pain following subsidence of the pain of acute infarction. The pain differs in that it is affected by movement in bed and by swallowing and is often relieved by leaning forward. Definitive diagnosis depends upon recognition of a pericardial friction rub (in about 15% of patients), which may be triphasic if the heart rate is slow but may appear to be uniphasic if the rate is more rapid. The rub is usually heard along the left sternal border, is harsh and grating in quality, may be intermittent, and may last only a few days.

Prevention

There are no known methods of prevention of myocardial infarction other than prevention of coronary artery atherosclerosis by avoiding as many risk factors as possible. Unusual physical or psychologic stress has been thought to precede acute myocardial infarction in some cases, but retrospective studies do not as a rule disclose any activities that might explain the cardiac event.

Treatment

Patients are ideally treated at the onset of myocardial infarction in a coronary care unit equipped for continuous monitoring of the ECG, with alarm signals, arterial and venous pressure recording, pacemaker insertion and resuscitation equipment, and specially trained nurses and physicians in attendance. Facilities for introduction of bedside Swan-Ganz balloon catheters for determination of intracardiac pressures and oxygen content in the right heart, pressure transducers for determination of direct intra-arterial pressure, and equipment to determine the cardiac output by the thermodilution method are valuable in the individualized management of severe manifestations occurring during the course of acute myocardial infarction. Equipment for taking bedside chest films, an echocardiograph, and perhaps equipment to determine the wall motion and perfusion status of the myocardium utilizing radioisotopes are also desirable, either in the unit or nearby. Details of the design and equipment of coronary care units are discussed in articles included with the references at the end of this chapter.*

In the following discussion it is assumed that coronary care unit facilities, equipment, and personnel are available. Of course the authors realize that there are hospitals where all of these resources may not be available. Physicians caring for patients under such circumstances should attempt to offer, to the extent possible, the kind of care available in better equipped centers, particularly by making every effort to recognize arrhythmias early. Reliance must be placed upon the clinical examination to recognize and treat complications of acute myocardial infarction that would otherwise be diagnosed by direct hemodynamic monitoring. In areas where trained coronary care unit nurses are not available, "sitters" can be taught to recognize changes in a patient's appearance or symptoms, or changes on an oscilloscopic monitor if one is available, and call for help immediately should an arrhythmia or other changes appear. All such medical facilities should have available at least one nurse and one physician who could then begin appropriate therapy or defibrillation. If no defibrillation equipment is available, one must rely on cardiac massage and intravenous drugs such as lidocaine in hope of reversing the ventricular fibrillation. The minimum requirements are constant surveillance and a trained person who can respond immediately if arrhythmias or other complications occur.

In smaller hospitals with coronary care units but with limited bed capacity and nursing support, criteria for admission to the coronary care unit must be established to select patients who will benefit most from the services available. The major benefit of the coronary care unit is that it makes possible early recognition of severe ventricular arrhythmias, which may be the prelude to ventricular fibrillation and sudden death. These ominous arrhythmias are frequent in patients with extensive myocardial infarction with hypotension, impaired perfusion of the cerebrum and kidney, and car-

*See Day (1968), Lown (1969), and Whalen (1971).

diac failure. Patients in these categories, therefore, have priority status. Patients with very mild initial episodes of myocardial infarction are at lesser risk, although a minor infarction may become more extensive and arrhythmia may then develop. Ventricular fibrillations can occur early in patients with minor myocardial infarction.

A patient with very severe myocardial infarction or one who has had multiple infarction in the past may present with cardiogenic shock. These patients have the highest mortality rates, but the treatment of "pump failure" associated with cardiogenic shock is difficult and the prognosis poor, not only within the next few days but also within the first year. Bedside hemodynamic monitoring and therapy directed toward the specific type of hemodynamic abnormality (as will be discussed later) increases survival during hospitalization, but the 1-year mortality rate is still very high. The introduction of intra-aortic balloon assist devices increases survival, but again the 1- or 2-year mortality rate is very high because such a large area of myocardium is destroyed. Utilizing the analogy of the battlefield, one might say that these patients' prospects for survival are so limited that they should be given a lower priority than patients with severe myocardial infarction not in cardiogenic shock, but both groups require intensive therapy. On the other hand, some writers maintain that the opportunity to at least improve some patients temporarily so that they can be discharged from the hospital and perhaps survive several years should give patients with cardiogenic shock a higher priority than those with mild myocardial infarction (Chatterjee, 1973).

Some writers believe that relatively mild myocardial infarction should be treated in the home as was routinely done years ago. They reason that the psychologic impact of admission to the coronary care unit may induce adrenergic stimuli that increase the likelihood of ventricular arrhythmias, particularly ventricular fibrillation. Where coronary care units are not available, home care for patients with initially mild acute myocardial infarction is acceptable if the minimum requirement for constant surveillance and ready availability of effective treatment of arrhythmias can be met.

A. Immediate Measures: (See Emergency Measures in section on sudden death, p 134.) The risk of ventricular fibrillation and sudden death is greatest in the first 4 hours. Patients with acute myocardial infarction should enter the coronary care unit as soon as possible so that defibrillation can be done if needed. The extension of coronary care capability to specially equipped ambulances and fire department vehicles manned by personnel trained in defibrillation and resuscitation (so-called pre-coronary care) may reduce the number of deaths in the first hour after the attack.

Arrival at emergency room. Upon arrival at the emergency room, the ECG should be monitored and the patient sent immediately to the coronary care unit unless the emergency room has equivalent facilities. Monitoring should be continued during transfer to the coronary care unit. Upon arrival in the unit, the adequacy of ECG recording should be verified and monitoring continued during the evaluation procedure. A slow intravenous drip of glucose and water is begun so that an open intravenous line will be in place if needed. As a rule, no other routine measures are indicated.

B. Relief of Pain: Relief of pain is the first requirement if cardiac rhythm is satisfactory. Pain may cause nausea and vomiting, hypertension, or hypotension. If the pain is severe and the systemic response is marked, sinus tachycardia, sweating, a feeling of impending doom, and restlessness due to acute anxiety may occur.

If the pain is severe or if the patient is in shock, give morphine sulfate, 5–10 mg slowly intravenously, repeated every 15 minutes until pain is relieved, or, less desirably, meperidine (pethidine; Demerol), 25–50 mg intravenously, repeated in 15 minutes if necessary. If the pain is not severe but bad enough to be disturbing, give morphine, 10–15 mg intramuscularly, repeated in 1 hour if necessary; or meperidine, 50–100 mg intramuscularly. Monitoring of respirations is necessary in determining when to repeat the dose of morphine or meperidine; the injection should not be repeated if respirations are less than 12/min. The patient should be kept supine following injection of morphine because venous pooling and decreased venous return, decrease of left ventricular filling pressure, and decreased cardiac output may cause severe hypotension and fainting.

If the pain is not relieved by opiates or oxygen (see below), aminophylline, 0.5 g slowly intravenously at a rate of 1–2 ml/min, may be helpful in relieving pain. Pentazocine is not recommended as an alternative analgesic for pain of myocardial infarction because it increases left ventricular filling pressure and cardiac work. Nitroglycerin sublingually or isosorbide dinitrate orally may relieve pain, but one must be careful to stop the drug if tachycardia or hypotension develops.

C. Rest:

1. Sedation–Patients with acute myocardial infarction are apprehensive and anxious and often have a feeling of impending doom. Opiates, in addition to relieving pain, produce physical and mental rest by allaying anxiety; if they are ineffective, drugs such as diazepam (Valium), 5–10 mg orally every 6 hours, may be helpful. If pain is not a problem and patients are restless and unable to sleep, sedatives should be used as necessary because adequate sleep is vital for physical and mental rest.

2. Bedside care–During the first days, patients with myocardial infarction should not be allowed to feed or care for themselves unless the attack is mild. Diet should be mild, low caloric, and low residue, with multiple small feedings. Most patients find that a bedside commode, with help getting on and off, requires less effort than use of a bedpan. After the first few days, patients can feed themselves and move about in bed, but even in mild cases bed rest is advisable for at least the first week. Chair privileges are then allowed, beginning with 30–60 minutes depending on individual responses (see Table 8–13, p 162).

3. **Early ambulation**—Studies are being done in some centers to determine the safety of allowing patients with mild infarctions and no complications to walk about after 5 days and go home after 7–9 days. Preliminary data indicate that delayed complications are not more frequent in patients *without complications* who are mobilized this early (Hutter, 1973).

D. **Oxygen**: The decreased cardiac output and pulmonary venous congestion associated with acute myocardial infarction often result in decreased arterial P_{O_2}; levels as low as 50 mm Hg breathing room air are not uncommon. Hypoxemia of this degree may contribute to the development of ventricular arrhythmias, hypotension and shock, unrelieved chest pain, and aggravation of any tendency to develop left ventricular failure. Oxygen by face mask at flow rates of 6–10 liters/min is preferable to an oxygen tent or intranasal oxygen. Positive pressure breathing is often resisted by the patient, decreases venous return and cardiac output, and may aggravate myocardial ischemia. Other procedures for the management of left ventricular failure with dyspnea are preferable (see below).

E. **Anticoagulant Therapy**: Anticoagulant therapy during the acute phase is controversial. Anticoagulants are not used routinely in patients with mild attacks in whom chest pain is rapidly relieved, signs of myocardial necrosis are minimal, and shock and cardiac failure are absent. In older patients with cardiac failure or cardiogenic shock in whom prolonged bed rest is anticipated, anticoagulation with heparin and coumarin drugs is often given to prevent venous thrombosis and possible pulmonary emboli unless there are contraindications such as a history of bleeding, peptic ulcer, or hepatic insufficiency. Anticoagulants can be stopped when patients are fully ambulatory. Miniheparin is not advised because it is less effective. Randomized studies favor continuous rather than intermittent heparin therapy because major bleeding episodes appear to be more common when boluses of heparin are given intravenously at 4-hour intervals than when heparin is given as a continuous intravenous drip. The drip should average about 1000 units/hour, although a loading dose of 5000 units is often given in order to keep the activated partial thromboplastin time between 40 and 60 sec. The 24-hour dose is prepared by mixing 20–25 thousand units of heparin in 500–1000 ml of 5% dextrose.

F. **General Clinical Observation**: After the patient has been relieved of pain, reassured, sedated, given oxygen, and made comfortable in bed with monitoring devices in place, further therapy depends on the presence or absence of complications.

Regardless of the severity of the myocardial infarction, the prognosis is always guarded. The patient is naturally frightened after this brush with death. A calm, reassuring manner may relieve anxiety and help the patient to accept the required therapy.

The physician must be prepared to deal with the patient's regression, denial, anger, and hostility as well as anxiety because emotional stress complicates medical management, adversely affects the course of the disease, and may be instrumental in producing ventricular arrhythmias. The physician's manner is most important in minimizing emotional responses to the illness. Neither excessive gravity nor excessive optimism is warranted; realistic optimism is always both justified and therapeutic.

Alert clinical observation by the physician at hourly intervals during the first day is required to make certain that pain does not return and that hypotension, cardiogenic shock, ventricular arrhythmias, and cardiac failure do not occur. The function of constant observation by special coronary care nurses is to alert the physician to any new symptoms such as dyspnea, embolism, palpitations, mental confusion, oliguria, syncope or near syncope from heart block, or arrhythmias.

Treatment of Sequelae

A. **Arrhythmias**:

1. **Ventricular arrhythmias**—(See also Chapter 15.) The most common adverse event (approximately 90% of cases) during the course of acute myocardial infarction is the development of an arrhythmia, usually ventricular. Ventricular premature beats are common and must be recognized and treated promptly; they indicate either increased irritability from enhanced spontaneous depolarization of the damaged myocardial cells or reentry phenomena from currents of injury set up by impaired conduction and delayed repolarization in neighborhood fibers. Ventricular premature beats or ventricular tachycardia may be associated with atrioventricular conduction defects; may rapidly change to ventricular fibrillation; may decrease cardiac output and coronary perfusion and aggravate myocardial ischemia; or may increase the size of the infarct and foster the development of cardiac failure or cardiogenic shock. Lidocaine, 50–100 mg intravenously, followed by an intravenous infusion at a rate of 1–2 mg/min, is the initial therapy of choice. In some centers, lidocaine is begun immediately upon admission to the coronary care unit as a prophylactic measure. If lidocaine produces central nervous system symptoms of confusion or excitement (which rarely follow the dose noted above but may occur when the drug is given at a higher rate of infusion), alternative drugs may be used. If lidocaine is ineffective, as occasionally happens, alternative drugs are procainamide, 50 mg/min intravenously up to a total dose of 1 g, or quinidine gluconate, 0.8 g diluted in 100–200 ml of glucose and water given at a rate of 1 ml/min. It can be repeated if necessary, controlled by blood levels. Do not exceed 6 μg/ml in the steady state infusion. If the patient has been receiving digitalis or has hypokalemia resulting from diuretic therapy, potassium salts may be given orally or intravenously depending upon the urgency of need. Prompt treatment of ventricular arrhythmias is indicated to prevent ventricular fibrillation and cardiac arrest, but one cannot depend on the warning manifestations of premature beats because ventricular fibrillation may occur without warning early in the course of the disease.

2. Ventricular tachycardia and fibrillation—Ventricular tachycardia is an emergency and, if not rapidly converted with intravenous lidocaine, should be terminated by electrical cardioversion. Ventricular fibrillation should be instantly recognized by the alarm system at the nursing station, and defibrillation should be accomplished within 30 sec. If a physician is not immediately available, defibrillation should be performed by specially trained nurses, because delay compromises not only cardiac function but also cerebral function. After defibrillation, lidocaine is given by constant intravenous infusion in a dosage of 1–2 mg/min in order to prevent recurrence. This may be discontinued in 24–48 hours if there is no recurrence.

3. Other ventricular or junctional arrhythmias—Nonparoxysmal ventricular tachycardia (accelerated idioventricular rhythm) or atrioventricular dissociation with junctional tachycardia and aberrant conduction may occur early in the course of acute myocardial infarction and may be confused with either ventricular tachycardia or complete atrioventricular block. Because the prognosis with these arrhythmias is better than that of ventricular tachycardia in general, supportive care is usually sufficient and defibrillation is rarely needed if the differential diagnosis can be made.

4. Atrial arrhythmias—Atrial arrhythmias occur less frequently (about 15% of cases) than ventricular ones. The most common atrial arrhythmia is fibrillation. It is usually transient, lasting hours or 1–2 days, and, unless the ventricular rate is rapid and hemodynamic deterioration occurs with resultant worsening of congestive failure or recurrence of anginal pain, treatment consists of digitalization or, if the situation is more urgent, cardioversion. Conservative therapy is usually more desirable because of the transient nature of the atrial fibrillation and because experience has shown that the prognosis is more closely related to the underlying problem than to the arrhythmia. If frequent atrial premature beats occur—especially if they produce hemodynamic deterioration with resultant symptoms—they should be treated with quinidine sulfate, 0.3 g orally every 4–6 hours. Frequent premature beats often presage atrial fibrillation and may result in a fall in arterial pressure which decreases coronary perfusion and may increase the size of the infarct.

5. Late ventricular fibrillation—The frequency of ventricular fibrillation (10% overall) decreases with time and with healing of the infarction. Persistence of an ischemic zone between necrotic and normal myocardium may account for late ventricular arrhythmias during the first 1–2 days as a result of reentry circuits or increased automaticity, and ECG monitoring should be continued for several days after the last episode of ventricular arrhythmia. This is particularly important in patients who are transferred to general medical wards without monitoring equipment after 3 or 4 days in the coronary care unit. Ideally, patients should be transferred to an intermediate unit where they can be monitored for another week or so until it is clear that ventricular arrhythmias are not recurring.

B. Cardiac Failure and Cardiogenic Shock: Left ventricular performance is impaired to some degree in all patients with acute myocardial infarction, and the extent and degree of functional loss depend on such factors as the status of the myocardium if there has been previous myocardial ischemia or infarction, the extent of the new infarction, and the presence of preexisting left ventricular disease as a result of hypertension or other cardiac disorders. A first myocardial infarction of minor extent in a patient with no underlying cardiac disease usually produces little or no impairment of left ventricular performance as judged by symptoms and signs and by hemodynamic monitoring of cardiac output, left ventricular filling pressure, and arterial pressure, but it may cause hypokinesia on radioisotope wall motion studies. Experiments in dogs have shown that the area of infarction "balloons" after occlusion of coronary artery, causing localized hypokinesia. If the infarction is large and occurs in an area of previous infarctions with large areas of scar and borderline compensation, the patient may rapidly go into severe cardiac failure. In the presence of hypotension and impaired perfusion of the vital organs, cardiogenic shock may occur. Possibilities thus range from no clinical evidence of impaired cardiac function to cardiogenic shock with a very high (80%) mortality rate. It is thus appropriate to discuss the subject as a continuum with treatment individualized according to the degree of severity (Table 8–12).

1. Mild and moderate cardiac failure—Some degree of cardiac failure, usually left ventricular failure, can be detected in 20–50% of patients with acute myocardial infarction unless the attack is mild. The findings are usually not overt. The patient may or may not have dyspnea; clinical examination may reveal pulmonary rales, diastolic gallop rhythm, and accentuated hilar congestion on chest x-ray. The typical central congestion with bat's wing densities does not occur

Table 8–12. Acute myocardial infarction: Suggested therapeutic measures in relation to hemodynamic indices.*

Left Ventricular Stroke Work Index	Left Ventricular Filling Pressure	Therapy
Normal	Normal	Observation
Normal	Raised	Diuretics
Decreased	Decreased or normal	Volume expansion
Moderately decreased	Raised	Afterload reducing agents with or without diuretics
Markedly decreased (cardiogenic shock)	Raised	Intra-aortic balloon counterpulsation and afterload reducing agents. Use of inotropic agents if other measures do not increase cardiac output, eg, dopamine or dobutamine.

*Modified and reproduced, with permission, from Chatterjee K, Swan HJC: Hemodynamic profile of acute myocardial infarction. Chapter 6 in: *Myocardial Infarction.* Corday E, Swan HJC (editors). Williams & Wilkins, 1973.

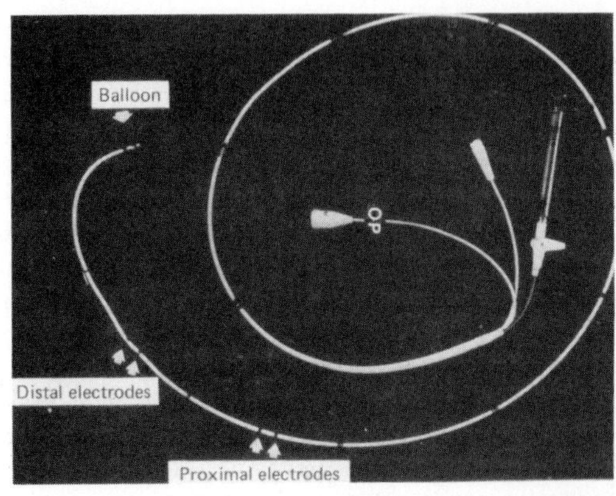

Figure 8–19. Balloon flotation electrode catheter for cardiac monitoring and emergency pacing. The distance from the tip is marked in 10 cm intervals. The position of the proximal (25 and 26 cm) and distal (17 and 18 cm) electrode pairs is indicated by arrows. The proximal end of the catheter consists of the lumen for inflation of the balloon, the distal lumen, and the special adapter for the electrode cables. (Reproduced, with permission, from Chatterjee K & others: Use of a balloon-tipped flotation electrode catheter for cardiac monitoring. Am J Cardiol 36:56, 1975.)

unless the patient develops acute pulmonary edema. The development of Kerley's B lines occurs later, with chronic failure, and may not be present even though the pulmonary wedge pressure is elevated. The increased pulmonary congestion in the upper lobes is usually part of generalized pulmonary venous congestion during this phase, but if the process continues there may be reversal of the normal flow pattern, ie, upper lobe congestion and lower lobe oligemia, as pulmonary arterial constriction occurs in the lower lobes. The radiologic findings may be out of phase with the clinical findings because they take longer to develop and to regress. It is valuable to obtain serial portable (not lying, but upright for 10 minutes) chest x-rays in order not to miss otherwise unsuspected pulmonary venous congestion. In patients who are being monitored by means of a bedside Swan-Ganz catheter, elevated pulmonary venous wedge pressure may be noted before the radiologic changes occur.

If left ventricular failure is minimal or subclinical, treatment can be conservative, with oral diuretics (eg, hydrochlorothiazide, 50–100 mg orally), oxygen, and avoidance of sodium-containing fluids and food. Hemodynamic intracardiac monitoring is *not necessary* because the left ventricular filling pressure is usually normal (< 12 mm Hg) and the cardiac index is also normal (> 2.5 liters/min/m^2). The prognosis is good (mortality rate ± 6%) (Chatterjee, 1973).

2. **More severe cardiac failure**–Left ventricular failure not promptly relieved by diuretic therapy requires more aggressive management, *beginning* with hemodynamic monitoring of the arterial pressure, pulmonary venous wedge pressure (left ventricular filling pressure), and cardiac output utilizing the floating balloon catheter (Fig 8–19). (See also p 100, Chapter 6, for discussion of the Swan-Ganz catheter.) Stroke work index can be computed from these measurements, and rational therapy can be given on the basis of the specific hemodynamic abnormality found. It is hazardous to continue to use potent therapeutic agents unless hemodynamic monitoring is available so that the results can be observed and drug dosages adjusted as needed.

Hypotension is often the first sign that cardiac failure may be more severe than is suggested by slight dyspnea and pulmonary rales, especially if it persists after pain is relieved.

a. **Volume replacement**–When monitoring reveals that left ventricular filling pressure is low (< 12 mm Hg) and cardiac output is normal despite the low arterial pressure, hypovolemia is the most probable cause. Treatment consists of volume replacement by the intravenous route in 100 ml increments beginning with dextrose, salt-poor albumin, plasma, or other similar fluids (eg, dextran). Further increments can be given every 5–10 minutes until the left ventricular filling pressure rises to 18 mm Hg. If cardiac output does not increase as the left ventricular filling pressure rises to 15–20 mm Hg, volume replacement should be stopped to prevent pulmonary edema, which may occur abruptly.

b. **Diuresis**–If the only hemodynamic abnormality is a raised left ventricular filling pressure but blood pressure and cardiac output are normal, more vigorous diuresis can be obtained with large doses (80–160–320 mg) of furosemide. Excessive diuresis must be avoided because the patient may become dehydrated, and, although the filling pressure may fall, the blood pressure may also fall, so that further volume repletion will be needed.

c. **Vasopressors**–Some patients with acute myocardial infarction have hypotension with impaired tissue perfusion primarily due to failure of compensatory peripheral vasoconstriction without a substantial change in filling pressure or cardiac output; these patients often respond with a rise in arterial pressure to the inotropic action of sympathetic amines (norepinephrine, dopamine, or dobutamine) that stimulate the beta-adrenergic receptors of the heart. These drugs should be considered a temporary measure to allow the use of vasodilators or intra-aortic balloon assist (see below). They should be infused at a slow rate to avoid tachycardia, marked increases in blood pressure, and ventricular arrhythmias. The physician's aim is not only to maintain the blood pressure but also to prevent arrhythmias.

d. **Vasodilator therapy**–When cardiac dysfunction is more severe, with reduced cardiac output, increased left ventricular filling pressure (above 20 mm Hg), and arterial blood pressure at or above 90 mm Hg, vasodilator therapy can be cautiously started while the hemodynamic result is monitored. Drugs such as sodium nitroprusside, trimethaphan, and phentolamine, given by intravenous drip, decrease the impedance to left ventricular ejection, reduce left ventricular volume and filling pressure, decrease myocardial oxygen consumption, improve perfusion to the brain (Fig 8–20), kidneys, and heart, and may improve left ventricular stroke work index. Striking changes have been observed by Chatterjee and Parmley (1977), and temporary improvement may tide the patient over a critical period. Vasodilator therapy should not be used if the fall in blood pressure is severe, but dopamine or dobutamine should be tried in low output states.

Nitroglycerin given sublingually in the acute phase of acute myocardial infarction may decrease the wedge pressure but may also produce arterial hypotension with or without bradycardia (Fig 8–21), as was first shown by Proger and Ayman (1932). The same effect may occur with intravenous sodium nitroprusside, but the dose can be carefully titrated to try to avoid hypotension. In less severe cases, nitroglycerin ointment (see p 174 on angina pectoris) can be used with appropriate safeguards in acute myocardial infarction. The ointment may reduce the left ventricular filling pressure with only a slight fall in arterial pressure. Its long duration of action (3–6 hours) makes this method of administration of nitroglycerin preferable when close minute-to-minute observation with intravenous medication is not possible or after it has been shown that intravenous medication is hemodynamically beneficial.

Efforts must be made to raise arterial pressure to about 100 mm Hg with vasopressors before vasodilator therapy.

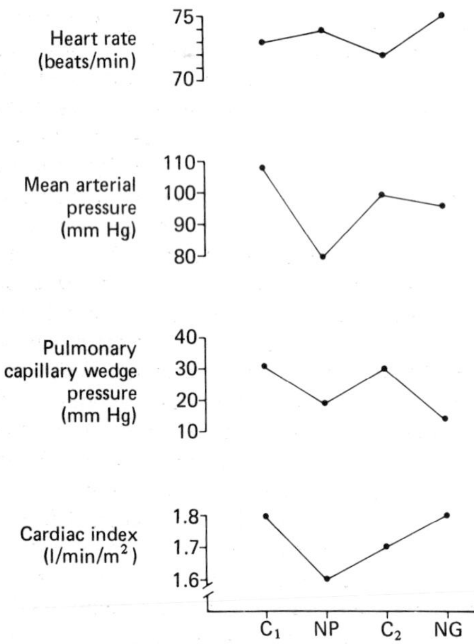

Figure 8–20. Hemodynamic changes following administration of nitroprusside (NP) and nitroglycerin (NG) in a patient with acute myocardial infarction. C_1 and C_2 refer to control periods. (Adapted and reproduced, with permission of the American Heart Association, Inc., from Armstrong PW & others: Vasodilator therapy in acute myocardial infarction: A comparison of sodium nitroprusside and nitroglycerin. Circulation 52:1118, 1975.)

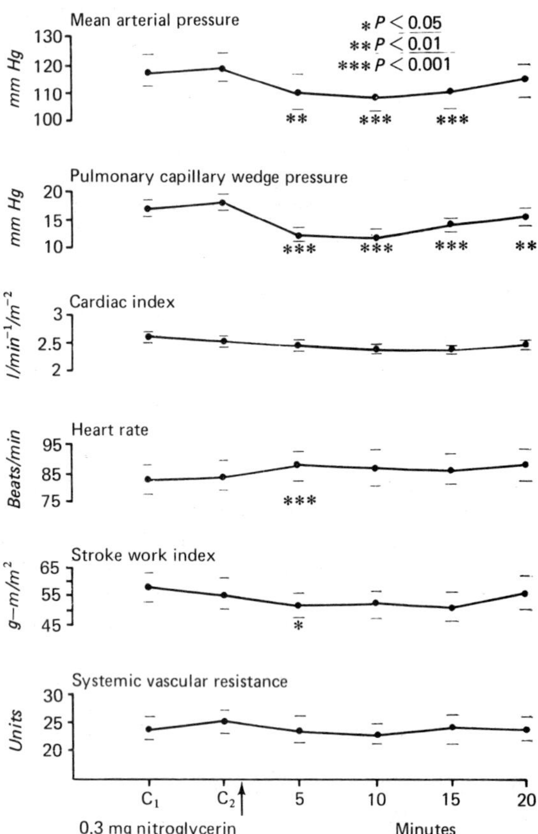

Figure 8–21. Hemodynamic effects of 0.3 mg sublingual nitroglycerin in 14 patients with acute myocardial infarction. The mean values and standard errors are shown during 2 control observations, C_1 and C_2, separated by 20 minutes, and after nitroglycerin. (Reproduced, with permission, from Delgado CE & others: Role of sublingual nitroglycerin in patients with acute myocardial infarction. Br Heart J 37:392, 1975.)

e. Aortic balloon counterpulsation—If it is not possible to raise blood pressure with vasopressors without worsening left ventricular filling pressure, decreasing cardiac output, and aggravating cardiac failure, aortic balloon counterpulsation is a dramatically effective temporary method of raising arterial pressure so that vasodilator therapy can be started. Counterpulsation removes blood from the aorta during systole and returns it in diastole. Expulsion of blood during systole with a deflated balloon decreases impedance to left ventricular ejection, reducing the afterload and the work of the left ventricle, and results in a fall in left ventricular filling pressure similar to that achieved by vasodilators. However, blood is returned during diastole, raising the diastolic blood pressure, increasing coronary perfusion, and improving left ventricular function by decreasing myocardial ischemia.

f. Combination of aortic balloon counterpulsation and vasodilator therapy—Parmley (1974) found that external counterpulsation followed by vasodilator therapy with sodium nitroprusside significantly improved left ventricular "pump" function in acute myocardial infarction with cardiogenic shock and thus reduced the mortality rate in his series. External counterpulsation is rarely effective unless nitroprusside is used concomitantly. It has been replaced in most centers by invasive intra-aortic balloon counterpulsation. The newer treatment with hydralazine, nitroprusside, and dopamine may make counterpulsation unnecessary in some patients. The long-term prognosis in patients who have been successfully treated by balloon assist for cardiogenic shock is still poor (approximately 10% survival after 1 year) because of the extensive underlying disease implied by the presence of cardiogenic shock.

g. **Counterpulsation as prelude to cardiac surgery**–Invasive balloon counterpulsation can be used as a temporary measure to tide the patient over acute "pump failure" and make it possible to perform coronary angiograms as well as to explore the feasibility of coronary bypass surgery if accessible sites of severe coronary artery stenosis are identified. The surgical mortality rate in patients recovering from cardiogenic shock is high, and further data are required for a definite conclusion about the feasibility and desirability of operative therapy.

h. **Hemodynamic parameters guiding treatment**–The poor response to medical as well as surgical therapy in patients with cardiogenic shock following myocardial infarction can be appreciated when one considers that at least half of the left ventricle has been shown to be damaged in autopsy studies of such patients. Left ventricular stroke work is usually less than 20 g-m/m^2 and often less than 15 g-m/m^2, and hypoxemia with P_{O_2} of less than 40–50 mm Hg is frequently found. The high wedge pressure (left ventricular filling pressure) induces dyspnea; impaired peripheral perfusion resulting from the decreased cardiac output is recognized clinically by cold, pale, clammy skin, cerebral obtundation, poor urine output, and evidence of venous constriction.

i. **Value of hemodynamic monitoring in prognosis**–Monitoring of the hemodynamic parameters mentioned previously is valuable in prognosis because patients with left ventricular filling pressures under 15 mm Hg and stroke work indices of more than 35–40 g-m/m^2 have a good prognosis (mortality rate, 6%), whereas if the filling pressure exceeds 20 mm Hg and the stroke work index is less than 15–20 g-m/m^2, the mortality rate is 80% (Chatterjee, 1973). In patients with intermediate values, with moderately decreased left ventricular function and a raised left ventricular filling pressure, the stroke work index is about 35 g-m/m^2 and the mortality rate about 25%. In patients with a poor prognosis, aggressive therapy is warranted before severe deterioration occurs. The various drugs and forms of therapy discussed should be considered as therapeutic trials. The physician should maintain close clinical and hemodynamic observation and should be prepared to adjust or stop therapy depending upon the clinical and hemodynamic responses. The response of the patient determines the drugs used and their dosages, and these are varied as treatment proceeds. If the blood pressure falls, the physician cannot continue administration of the sodium nitroprusside; he must stop the infusion and use pressor agents to raise the blood pressure, if possible, before resuming nitroprusside infusion. Alternatively, the drug can be stopped completely and other measures instituted.

j. **Digitalis**–Digitalis, the time-honored inotropic agent, is infrequently used today in the treatment of cardiac failure due to acute myocardial infarction, principally because of its tendency to cause ventricular arrhythmias and its relative low order of effectiveness against severe left ventricular pump failure. When cardiac failure is severe, requiring inotropic agents, digitalis should certainly be tried. However, in milder types of cardiac failure, the drug should probably be withheld, chiefly because if ventricular arrhythmias develop it is difficult to decide whether they are due to digitalis therapy or myocardial ischemia. Digitalis should be used if the patient has atrial fibrillation with a rapid ventricular rate or clinical or hemodynamic deterioration that is *not* due to Wolff-Parkinson-White syndrome.

C. **Conduction Defects:**

1. **Stokes-Adams attack with heart block**–(See Chapter 14.) *This is an emergency!* Complete heart block complicates acute myocardial infarction in 6–10% of cases; it has a high mortality rate (about 60% untreated), usually lasts less than a week, and often can be treated by artificial pacing through a transvenous catheter placed in the right ventricle. Pacing at a rate of 70–80/min may greatly improve cardiac output and tissue perfusion and prevent Stokes-Adams attacks. Death during a Stokes-Adams attack with syncope is rare in the presence of inferior myocardial infarction because the atrioventricular conduction damage is nodal and the result of transient ischemia due to occlusion of a branch of the right coronary artery. When atrioventricular conduction defects occur in anterior infarction, however, they usually represent widespread necrosis of the septum and the conduction system, involving the bundle of His or the bundle branches, usually with decreased left ventricular function and ventricular asynergy. Progression of the ECG changes of heart block may be rapid and lead to complete atrioventricular block and Stokes-Adams attacks. A temporary artificial demand pacemaker should therefore be introduced if atrioventricular conduction delay or bifascicular block develops acutely in anterior infarction. The atrioventricular conduction defects are usually transient and subside within a week. Temporary pacemakers are usually left in place for a week after the atrioventricular conduction becomes normal. A permanent pacemaker may be advisable in anterior infarction associated with Stokes-Adams attacks because the frequency of sudden death within a year after leaving the hospital is high in patients who have had complete atrioventricular block during the episode of acute infarction but have left the hospital without the protection of a pacemaker. The mortality rate has been said to be reduced by half if a permanent pacemaker is used in patients with acute anterior myocar-

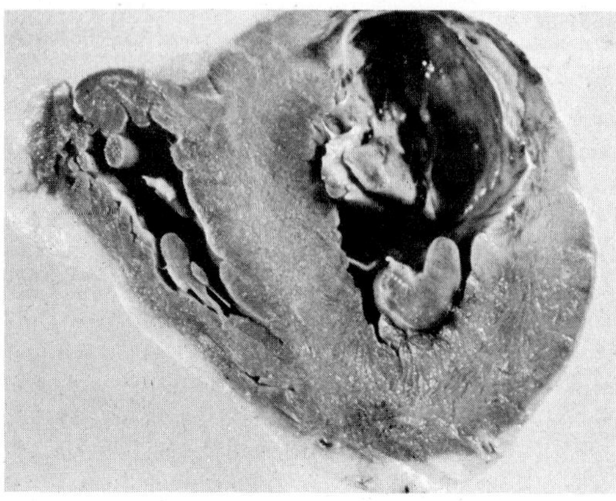

Figure 8–22. Cardiac aneurysm of the posterior wall of the left ventricle following acute myocardial infarction. (Courtesy of O Rambo.)

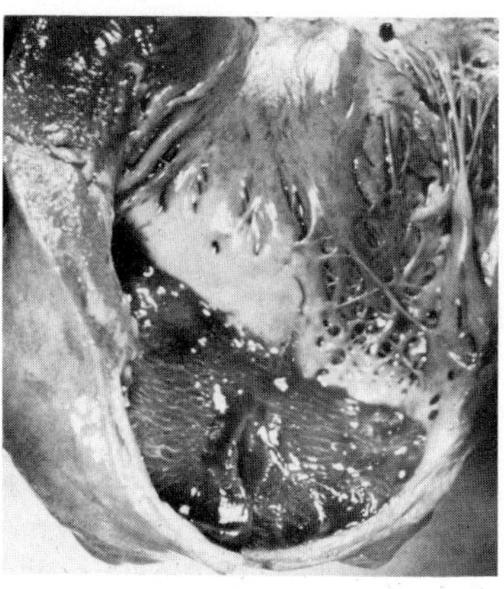

Figure 8–23. Old myocardial infarction with left ventricular aneurysm and associated mural thromboses at the apex of the left ventricle. (Courtesy of O Rambo.)

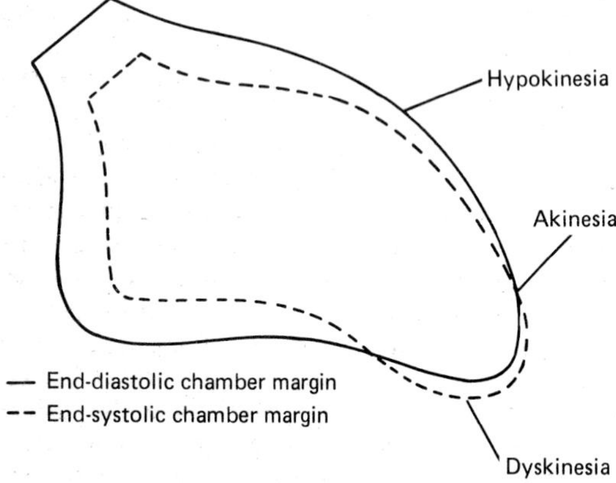

Figure 8–24. Segmental wall motion is analyzed by superimposing end-systolic chamber outline on end-diastolic chamber outline from left ventricular angiograms. Inward excursion is qualitatively estimated as mild, moderate, or severe hypokinesia, akinesia (no systolic motion), and dyskinesia (paradoxic outward systolic motion). (Reproduced, with permission, from Alderman EL: Angiographic indicators of left ventricular function. JAMA 236:1055, 1976. Copyright © 1976, American Medical Association.)

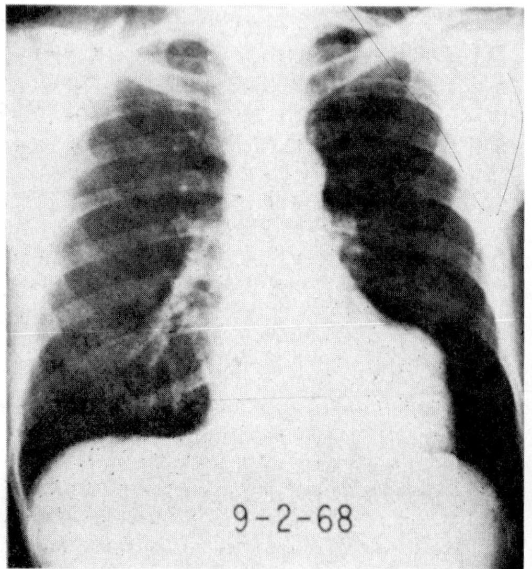

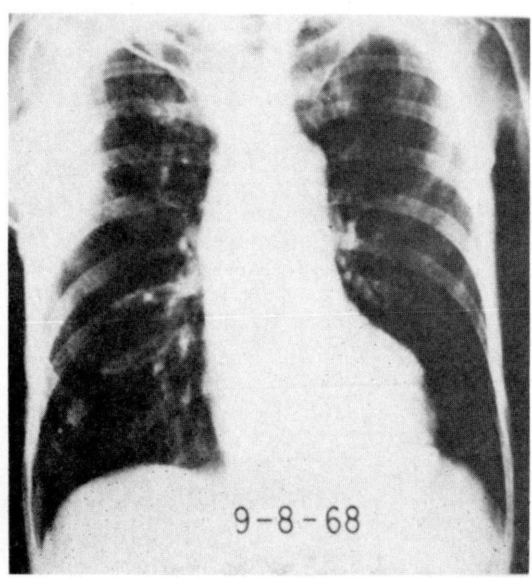

Figure 8–25. *Left:* Classic x-ray findings of a discrete left ventricular aneurysm. *Right:* Film from a patient who at autopsy was found to have diffuse thinning and aneurysmal dilatation of the entire apical region of the left ventricle. (Reproduced, with permission, from Davis RW, Ebert PA: Ventricular aneurysm: A clinical-pathologic correlation. Am J Cardiol 29:1, 1972.)

dial infarction who have developed complete atrioventricular block in association with bifascicular block during the acute attack. The data supporting these statements are still incomplete and contradictory, however, and further experience may modify this opinion.

2. Second degree heart block; Mobitz I and II—(See Chapter 14.) Second degree atrioventricular block with Wenckebach pauses (see below) (Mobitz I) and *narrow* QRS complexes is not routinely paced if the patient has inferior infarction. His bundle recordings have demonstrated that if the conduction defect is in the atrioventricular node, above the bundle of His (the usual finding in inferior infarctions), Stokes-Adams attacks are uncommon in inferior infarction with narrow QRS complexes even if complete block develops. They are common in anterior infarction with wide QRS complexes. This is in contrast to the atrioventricular conduction defect that occurs in anterior infarctions, in which His bundle recordings and pathologic data show that the block is usually distal to the atrioventricular node, within the bundle of His or in the bundle branches with *wide* QRS complexes (Mobitz II); Stokes-Adams attacks with fatalities occur if the patient is not protected by a pacemaker.

3. Prophylactic demand pacemakers in Mobitz II block—(See Chapter 14.) Because asystole may occur unpredictably, electrode catheters should be placed prophylactically in patients with anterior infarctions who have bifascicular block, complete atrioventricular block, or type II Mobitz atrioventricular block or in those who have inferior infarctions with complete atrioventricular block. Infusions of lidocaine should be given to prevent ventricular fibrillation if atrioventricular block subsides and competition occurs with the patient's own pacemaker.

4. Demand pacemaker versus fixed rate pacemaker—Ventricular fibrillation is the major hazard associated with pacing in acute myocardial infarction because of competition between the patient's own pacemaker and that of the artificial pacemaker and perhaps because of contact of the pacemaker with the ventricular wall. For this reason, patients with first degree atrioventricular block or with type I second degree atrioventricular block with Wenckebach pauses and narrow QRS complexes in inferior infarction are not routinely paced. Demand pacemakers are activated by a delay in the appearance of the QRS complex. When atrioventricular conduction is unstable, intermittent competition between the normal and artificial pacemaker will not occur.

5. Sinus bradycardia—Sinus bradycardia, especially in inferior infarction, may precede atrioventricular block and provide a setting in which ventricular arrhythmias can occur. Furthermore, when hypotension and decreased cardiac output occur with bradycardia in acute myocardial infarction, perfusion of the vital organs may be inadequate. Atropine, 0.25–0.6 mg intravenously, is desirable in such situations, with close observation to determine its effectiveness and side-effects since ventricular arrhythmias may result. If atropine is ineffective or if the bradycardia is marked or associated with sinoatrial or atrioventricular block, a temporary prophylactic transvenous demand pacemaker should be inserted into the right ventricle.

D. Treatment of Complications:

1. Thromboembolic phenomena—Thromboembolic phenomena are usually manifested by phlebothrombosis resulting from enforced bed rest. Pulmonary embolism and arterial emboli from mural thrombi in the left ventricle occur infrequently. Anticoagulants (heparin, coumarins) should be administered promptly (see Chapter 7).

2. Renal failure—During the early phases, the treatment of oliguria and anuria is that of the cardiogenic shock that induced it; late renal failure may be due to persistence of cardiogenic shock or to prolonged hypotension from vasodilator therapy. Early vigorous treatment of cardiogenic shock and caution in the use of vasodilator agents should decrease the incidence of renal failure. If renal failure with acute tubular necrosis develops after the patient has been stabilized with respect to cardiogenic shock and left ventricular failure, hemodialysis or peritoneal dialysis is indicated.

3. Perforation of the interventricular septum and mitral insufficiency due to papillary muscle and left ventricular wall dysfunction or rupture—These complications may occur together but are usually separate untoward events. Either may result in abrupt worsening of left ventricular failure. Hemodynamic studies are usually required to establish the nature of these lesions. Whenever possible, surgical repair of the ventricular septal defect or replacement of the mitral valve should be delayed for 4–10 weeks after the lesion has been stabilized by vigorous treatment of cardiac failure (see Chapter 10). Patients with acute mitral insufficiency with acute left ventricular failure requiring surgery have marked pulmonary venous congestion, a very high *v* wave, raised mean pulmonary capillary wedge pressure, and a reduced cardiac index (< 2.5 liters/min/m^2). Vasodilator therapy may be valuable both in ventricular septal defects and in mitral insufficiency to support the patient until surgical repair can be done with a reasonable mortality rate after cardiac failure is improved or corrected. Vasodilator therapy with nitroprusside may dramatically reduce the high *v* wave and the pulmonary capillary wedge pressure (Chatterjee, 1977). Results of surgical repair of both of these lesions are gratifying; repair may reverse severe incapacitating cardiac failure and allow restoration of normal activity.

4. Left ventricular aneurysm—

a. Spectrum of left ventricular contraction abnormalities—Acute necrosis of a portion of the left ventricle with resulting healing by fibrosis and scar may lead to a spectrum of disorders of contraction of the left ventricle, varying from hypokinesia or akinesia of a segment which is fully scarred to a definite left ventricular aneurysm with paradoxic outpocketing during systole. This can be established on cineangiography and is often suggested by physical examination and review of plain x-rays of the chest (Figs 8–22 to 8–26).

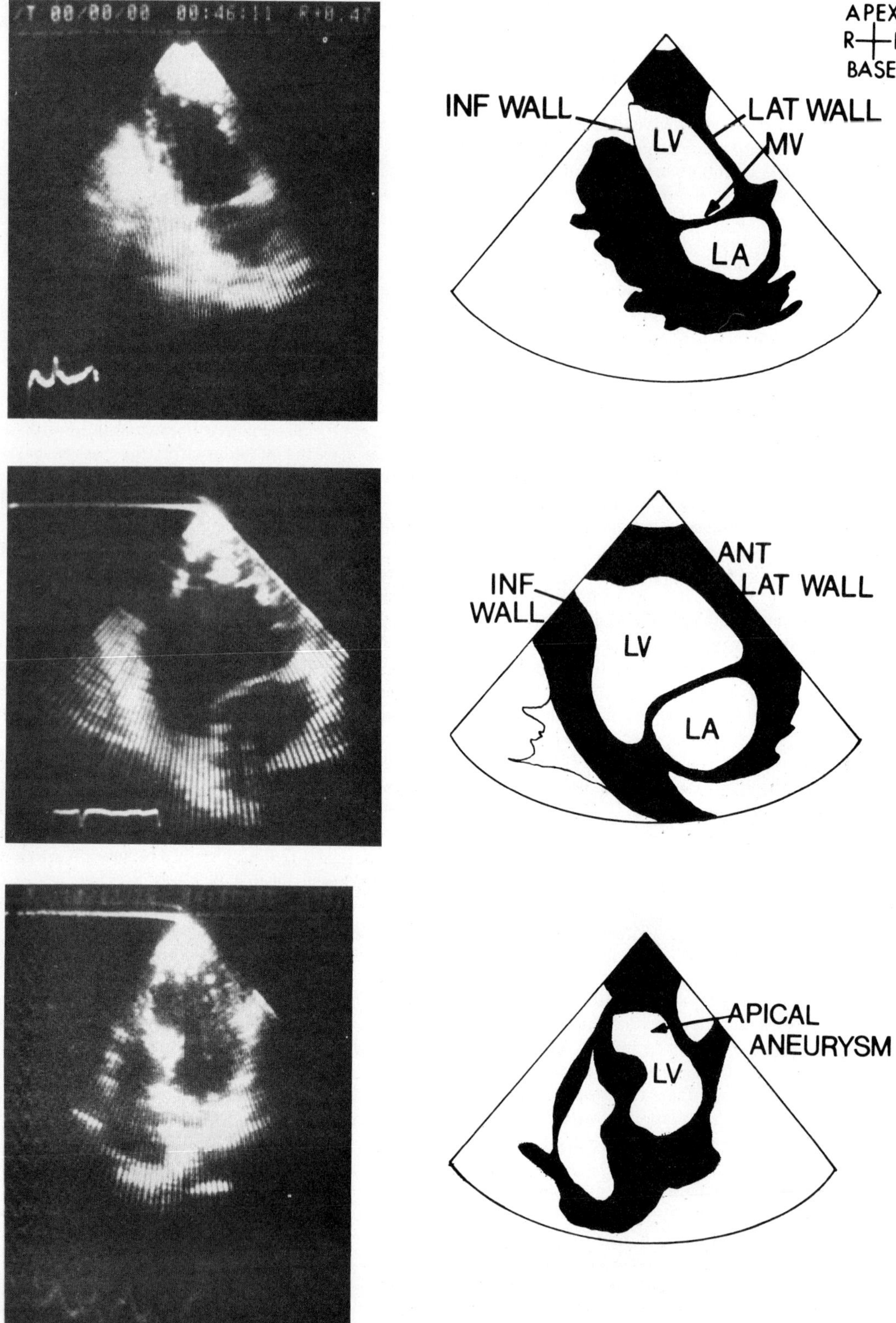

Figure 8–26. Echocardiograms of normal left ventricle and of left ventricular aneurysms. *A:* Normal left ventricle and mitral valve in a modified right anterior oblique position representing a hemiaxial equivalent taken through the apex. *B:* Considerably dilated left ventricle with an aneurysm on the inferior wall. *C:* Apical aneurysm with slightly enlarged left ventricular cavity. (Courtesy of NB Schiller.)

b. Consequences of ventricular aneurysms–The force of left ventricular contraction is wasted by distention of the aneurysm, increasing the work of the left ventricle. This may lead to persistent cardiac failure or ventricular arrhythmias, or both. When persistent left ventricular failure follows the healing of an acute myocardial infarction, the possibility of left ventricular aneurysm should be excluded by left ventricular cineangiograms, and if an aneurysm is found it should be resected surgically if possible. Areas of myocardium receiving minimal perfusion with consequent ischemia on effort may surround the area of the left ventricular aneurysm and result in frequent ventricular arrhythmias which often are disabling.

c. Surgical resection of aneurysms–Surgical resection can abolish the ventricular arrhythmias as well as cardiac failure in many patients. Search for left ventricular aneurysm can be very gratifying; although the mortality rate is about 5%, the surgical results are good in surviving patients. Surgery should be deferred if possible for 4–10 weeks until cardiac failure has stabilized (Donaldson, 1976). Whereas coronary bypass surgery is rarely effective in the presence of severe cardiac failure secondary to ischemic cardiomyopathy, resection of left ventricular aneurysm (as with repair of a perforated intraventricular septum or replacement of the mitral valve in mitral insufficiency from papillary muscle rupture or dysfunction) is often effective in relieving cardiac failure. Resection must not be attempted in patients with only hypokinesia or akinesia with areas of left ventricular contraction abnormalities due to old fibrosis in the absence of a definite paradoxic systolic motion of the area. Surgical treatment is not indicated in patients with irregular or diffuse hypokinesia with cardiac failure, especially when coexisting with a large, flabby left ventricle with increased volume and poor ejection fraction. A minor left ventricular aneurysm in the absence of cardiac failure or severe ventricular arrhythmias is likewise not an indication for surgical resection because it does not influence prognosis.

5. Cardiac rupture–It was once thought that cardiac rupture was an immediately fatal complication of acute myocardial infarction. It is now recognized that the rupture may be subacute and characterized by slight perforation into the pericardium which can be diagnosed on the basis of pericardial pain or effusion. Surgical repair has been successfully accomplished in a few patients.

6. Pericarditis–Although pericarditis occurs in about 15% of patients with acute myocardial infarction, pericardial tamponade is rare. The chief importance of involvement of the pericardium is that it contraindicates anticoagulant therapy, because extensive bleeding in the pericardium may result in tamponade. The diagnosis of pericarditis is important because the differential diagnosis between acute pericarditis and acute myocardial infarction may be difficult, especially if the patient is not seen until the second or third day. ECG abnormalities due to involvement of the epicardium and pericardium may complicate the interpretation of ECG patterns of acute infarction. This is not a problem if the patient has a transmural infarct with diagnostic Q waves but causes difficulty if the patient has a nontransmural infarct.

E. Convalescent Activity and Rehabilitation:

1. Initial period of rest–

a. Rest in bed–The period of rest in bed depends on the severity and size of the infarction. In the average case of acute myocardial infarction, the period of rest in bed is about 2 weeks; shorter in mild uncomplicated cases but extended to about 6 weeks if the patient has had a severe infarction; and even 6 weeks may be too short a time if the patient has residual persistent cardiac failure. After the first week, rest can be in a bed-chair with elastic stockings in place and use of leg exercises. Some authorities would allow use of the bed-chair after the first 1–2 days if there are no complications.

b. Slow ambulation–If the infarction is mild, ambulation may be started slowly after 1 week, and the patient may go home early in the second week if the situation there is favorable to slowly progressive ambulation without stairs or other stress and if the family can provide or perform all required services.

c. Resuming full activity–In general, gradual return to full activity is recommended. How much rest to order initially and later depends upon the initial severity of the infarction and whether activity causes chest pain, hypotension, tachycardia, or the appearance of gallop rhythm or other evidence of left ventricular failure. As a guide, we recommend 2 or 3 weeks of rest, mostly in bed or in a comfortable chair; 2 or 3 weeks of slowly increasing activity, including walking and slow stair climbing; and a third stage of several weeks of restricted but progressive activity before return to part-time work. Even in uncomplicated cases, the average patient requires 2–3 months of convalescence before returning to full preinfarction activity if the patient has been normally active.

d. Usual practice of ambulation–Current practice allows the patient without complications to sit in a comfortable chair after the first few days and by the end of the week to take a few steps about the room. When the patient first begins to walk slowly, the physician should be present to note any deleterious effects that might occur. The patient should not leave the hospital until the activity status has progressed to the stage of relative self-sufficiency. Early ambulation and self-sufficiency improve morale, prevent cardiac invalidism, and restore the patient's confidence in his or her ability to resume a normal life in due course. Progressive increases in ambulatory effort should be possible without chest pain, dyspnea, or undue tachycardia or fatigue. The patient should be assured that restrictions are only temporary and encouraged to increase activity, at first by climbing a few stairs and later by walking out of doors unless the weather is cold and windy. Severe physical exertion should be avoided for at least 2 months. Hills and extensive stair climbing should be avoided in order to prevent left ventricular dilatation and subsequent hypertrophy. A balance must be achieved between excessive exertion too early

Table 8–13. Mobilization program following myocardial infarction. (An adaptation of the program used in the Emory University [Atlanta] practice of Wenger.)*

Step	Exercise
I	Active mobilization of ankles and wrists; respiratory exercises
II	Active mobilization of limbs; partial wash-up care in bed; dangle legs on side of bed (5 minutes)
III	Active mobilization in bed; use of a bedside commode; sitting 15 minutes in armchair twice a day
IV	Active mobilization against resistance; complete care in bed; sitting 30 minutes in armchair twice a day
V	Active mobilization in bed; sitting 1 hour in armchair twice a day; 2 short walks in room
VI–VIII	Active mobilization in bed; light gymnastic exercises; sitting in armchair at will; washing at the washstand; walks in corridor
IX–X	As above plus exercises with footstool
XI	As above plus walking down 1 flight of stairs twice a day
XII–XIV	As above plus walking up 1–3 flights of stairs twice a day

*Reproduced, with permission, from Bloch A & others: Early mobilization after myocardial infarction: A controlled study. Am J Cardiol 34:152, 1974.

and prolonged inactivity and invalidism. A useful mobilization program is presented in Table 8–13.

2. Later rehabilitation–Rehabilitation programs in some centers utilize the services of physical therapists with the object of encouraging the patient to return to normal activity without neurocirculatory asthenia or cardiac neurosis. The physician must balance undue haste in returning the patient to full activity with undue caution that may cause unwarranted anxiety and fear.

a. ECG monitoring during activity–Twelve-hour ECG monitoring (eg, with a Holter monitor) when the patient is first allowed full activity may alert the physician to the presence of residual myocardial ischemia or left ventricular arrhythmias and may require a reduction in activity or the use of antiarrhythmia drugs.

b. Use of graded exercise in postinfarction period–Graded exercise with bicycle ergometers or treadmills up to a ventricular rate of about 130/min provides an estimate of the degree of healing by establishing the presence or absence of ischemia or ventricular arrhythmias and also provides a baseline for assessing the ventilatory and cardiac responses to exercise. The patient is usually greatly encouraged by his ability to perform the exercise tests. At 3 months the patient has regained about 70% of preinfarction exercise tolerance, and recovery is usually complete by 12 months. Sexual activity in both sexes may be resumed after 1–2 months when the patient has shown the ability to tolerate a heart rate of 130/min. Properly supervised rehabilitation exercise programs have been shown to be safe and helpful in that they foster a sense of well-being, decrease anxiety, and induce a healthier emotional response to the life-threatening event; they have not been shown to prolong life or decrease the frequency of recurrence of myocardial infarction.

Prognosis

A. Size of the Infarct: All things being equal, the larger the infarct, the greater the likelihood of complications such as left ventricular failure, cardiogenic shock, Stokes-Adams attacks, and arrhythmias such as ventricular fibrillation.

B. Hemodynamic Abnormalities: Especially if measured serially, hemodynamic abnormalities have been shown to correlate better than clinical findings with the development of "pump" failure. It is important to determine left ventricular filling pressure as well as one or more of the indices of left ventricular performance such as stroke volume, stroke work index, cardiac output, or ejection fraction. A normal cardiac output or stroke work index in the presence of a low left ventricular filling pressure (10–15 mm Hg) is a favorable prognostic sign as far as pump failure is concerned, whereas progressive increase in left ventricular filling pressure with a falling stroke work index is a poor sign. It is valuable to plot progressive changes in these 2 parameters (see Table 4–1, p 65) as a dynamic display of changes in left ventricular function.

C. Arrhythmias: Recurrent tachycardia and ventricular fibrillation are adverse prognostic signs, but they may be temporary, may occur frequently only during the first few days, and may ultimately stop as the infarcted cells heal or undergo fibrosis. Prompt recognition and treatment prevent the development of severe left ventricular dysfunction due to inadequate cardiac output resulting from ventricular tachycardia and fibrillation.

D. Conduction Defects: Conduction defects that develop in the atrioventricular node or in the bundle of His or its branches are associated with a high mortality rate and must be recognized and treated early, especially in anterior infarction. When left anterior hemiblock with or without right bundle branch block or with atrioventricular block appears in anterior infarction, complete atrioventricular block and Stokes-Adams attacks can occur suddenly, and such fatalities can be prevented if an artificial temporary pacemaker is inserted promptly. The prognosis is much better when complete atrioventricular block occurs in inferior infarction, because, as indicated earlier, this is due to ischemia of the atrioventricular node, with the escape pacemaker usually high in the bundle of His, leaving possible secondary and tertiary pacemakers below this area to prevent Stokes-Adams attacks. In anterior infarction there may be necrosis of the entire ventricular conduction system proximal to the Purkinje fibers and very little reserve pacemaker cell activity. Sinus bradycardia is not as ominous a finding as was once thought, although, as indicated previously, ventricular arrhythmias are more common with slow heart rates. If there is borderline left ventricular function, the decreased cardiac output in association with slow heart rates may increase the size of the infarct, depress left ventricular function, and produce impaired cerebral perfusion with adverse clinical results.

E. Overall Mortality Rate: The overall mortality rate during the first month after acute myocardial infarction is in the neighborhood of 30%, with most of the deaths occurring in the first 12 hours and one-fourth of them, due to ventricular fibrillation, in the first 1–2 hours. With mild attacks and no evidence of electrical instability or left ventricular dysfunction or conduction defects, the hospital mortality rate is less than 5%. The hospital mortality rate is 50% higher in recurrent as compared to initial infarctions, but cardiac rupture occurs more frequently with the first infarction. Overall figures are therefore misleading in estimating prognosis. Since the average delay between onset of symptoms and arrival at the hospital is 5–6 hours, arrival of the patient alive at the hospital is itself a favorable prognostic sign with respect to electrical instability but not necessarily pump failure.

F. Prognosis in Patients Who Survive the Infarction: (See Angina Pectoris.) The mortality rate of patients who survive an acute infarction is higher during the first 3–12 months than after that time. Particular care and education of the patient are required to make certain that the development of severe ventricular arrhythmias or a new myocardial infarction will be recognized promptly. Patients with anterior infarction who have had transient complete atrioventricular block are at high risk of sudden death within the year, and permanent pacemakers are being implanted with greater frequency to prevent death caused by a renewed episode of complete atrioventricular block. Patients who have demonstrated severe cardiac failure with a high left ventricular filling pressure and low stroke work index have a higher mortality rate in the 1–2 years following infarction, because the magnitude of left ventricular dysfunction is obviously great. Whether a more aggressive therapeutic approach to this group of patients is indicated has yet to be decided by research efforts.

Since approximately 60% of all patients with coronary heart disease die suddenly and since sudden death is more common in patients who have had a myocardial infarction, the prognosis depends in large part on the presence and degree (complexity) of ventricular arrhythmias during convalescence and afterward and upon the diligence of postinfarction surveillance. Efforts have been made to estimate this risk by determining the number and type of ventricular premature beats following exercise and during prolonged ECG monitoring. The 2 methods are complementary. Attempts to influence the outcome have been inconclusive, chiefly because current antiarrhythmia drugs are inadequate to prevent premature beats and are toxic; the drugs should be tried, however, because they may decrease the complex, prognostically more important beats.

G. Other Factors Influencing Survival: Residual left ventricular dysfunction can be estimated from the size of the heart as shown on x-ray or by echocardiography. There may also be symptoms or signs of left ventricular failure, evidence of high left ventricular filling pressure, or radioisotopic cineangiographic evidence of segmented areas of hypokinesia or akinesia with ischemic cardiomyopathy. If the left ventricle is large or contracts irregularly with or without left ventricular aneurysm, if the ejection fraction is low (less than 30%), and especially if cardiac function cannot be improved with therapy, the prognosis is much worse than in patients with good left ventricular function with equivalent degrees of coronary artery stenosis.

The presence of symptoms of congestive heart failure adversely affects prognosis regardless of the number of diseased vessels, but the mortality rate increases with the number of vessels involved with or without symptoms of congestive heart failure (Table 8–14).

If coronary arteriography is performed, the severity and extent of stenoses in the coronary arteries and the quality of the collateral circulation, combined with angiographic analysis of left ventricular function and volume, are directly related to the mortality rate in various prospective studies. Over a 5-year period, 3-vessel disease with poor left ventricular function has at least 10 times the mortality rate of single-vessel disease with good left ventricular function. The physician must determine which patients are at greatest risk and attempt various educational and therapeutic measures that may improve survival. The role of surgical therapy (see below) is pertinent. At present, prognosis is not influenced by surgical treatment, with the exception of (1) repair of perforated ventricular septum, (2) replacement of the mitral valve when there is gross mitral regurgitation resulting from papillary muscle dysfunction, (3) resection of left ventricular aneurysm associated with left ventricular failure, and (4) bypass procedures when the artery involved is the left main coronary artery. A national study is under way to determine if prognosis can be influenced by surgery in any of the other categories, including unstable angina pectoris.

H. Role of Special Investigations: The role of special investigations in patients who have recovered from an episode of acute myocardial infarction and are

Table 8–14. Mortality rates following coronary arteriography by number of vessels diseased and by symptoms of congestive heart failure (CHF). (Mean duration of follow-up = 21 months.)*

Number of Vessels Diseased	No Symptoms of CHF			Symptoms of CHF		
	Dead (No.)	Alive (No.)	Mortality (Percent)	Dead (No.)	Alive (No.)	Mortality (Percent)
0	2	87	2.2	1	8	11.1
1	1	39	2.5	1	5	16.7
2	4	32	11.1	9	5	64.3
3	8	28	22.2	7	9	43.8
Total	15	186	8.1	18	27	40.0

*Modified from Oberman (1972). Reproduced, with permission of the American Heart Association, Inc., from Kouchoukos NT, Kirklin JW, Oberman A: An appraisal of coronary bypass grafting. Circulation 50:11, 1974.

doing well has not been determined. Noninvasive procedures such as graded exercise with continuous ECG monitoring to determine the presence of residual ischemic ST changes or the development of ventricular arrhythmia are being performed with increasing frequency. Echocardiography to ascertain the degree of residual damage and to estimate left ventricular function, dimensions, wall motion, and ejection fraction is worthwhile when the patient has fully stabilized. Radioisotope perfusion with gated blood pool albumin aggregate scan, thallium 201 (see p 136), or pyrophosphate after exercise can be done with little risk to determine the size of fibrotic or scarred areas, and it allows a measure of the magnitude of irreversible damage. Invasive procedures such as coronary arteriography or cineangiography are best not done unless the patient has disabling residual angina pectoris of effort, chronic left ventricular failure, or recurrent ventricular arrhythmias, which may be due to barely surviving islands of viable myocardium surrounding the scar. In the authors' opinion, until it can be demonstrated that the prognosis for life is improved by surgical treatment in the average case of convalescent acute myocardial infarction, invasive procedures are not indicated. It is an open question whether they should be performed solely to gather general prognostic data such as extent and magnitude of coronary stenosis and left ventricular dysfunction.

ANGINA PECTORIS OF EFFORT

Angina pectoris is usually due to atherosclerotic heart disease, but rare cases occur in the absence of significant coronary disease as a result of severe aortic stenosis or insufficiency, syphilitic aortitis, increased metabolic demands (eg, in hyperthyroidism or after thyroid therapy), marked anemia, or paroxysmal tachycardias with rapid ventricular rates. The underlying mechanism is a discrepancy between myocardial demands for oxygen and substrate and the amount delivered through the coronary arteries. Three groups of variables determine the production of relative or absolute myocardial ischemia:

(1) Limitation of oxygen delivered by the coronary arteries: (a) Vessel factors: atherosclerotic narrowing; inadequate collateral circulation; reflex narrowing in response to emotion, cold, upper gastrointestinal disease, or smoking. (b) Blood factors: anemia, hypoxemia, polycythemia (increased viscosity). (c) Circulatory factors: fall in blood pressure due to arrhythmias, bleeding, and Valsalva's maneuver; decreased filling pressure of or decreased flow to the coronary arteries due to aortic stenosis or insufficiency.

(2) Increased cardiac output: (a) Physiologic factors: exertion, excitement, digestive and metabolic processes following a heavy meal. (b) Pathologic factors (high output states): anemia, thyrotoxicosis, arteriovenous fistula, pheochromocytoma.

(3) Increased myocardial demands for oxygen: Increased work of the heart, as in aortic stenosis, aortic insufficiency, diastolic hypertension; increased oxygen consumption due to thyrotoxicosis or to any state characterized by increased catecholamine excretion (pheochromocytoma, strong emotion, hypoglycemia).

Functional changes in patients who develop exercise-induced angina during cardiac catheterization have shown a rise in arterial pressure and a considerable rise in left ventricular end-diastolic pressure just before the appearance of angina and the ischemic changes in the ECG. Myocardial oxygen consumption increased similarly. The changes indicate that left ventricular failure or decreased compliance often coincides with the appearance of angina.

Clinical Findings

The term angina denotes a specific type of chest discomfort associated with myocardial ischemia and is now used only in that sense. Pain in the chest is one of the most common complaints the physician is called upon to assess, and it is important for the physician to be able to differentiate the various causes of chest pain because of the potential seriousness of the symptom, with its connotation of disability and death.

A. Pain:

1. Interpretation of pain—The interpretation of the symptom must be based on the history alone, because about one-fourth of patients have no objective clinical findings of coronary atherosclerosis to support the history. The diagnosis may be simple or extremely difficult. The diagnosis of angina is more probable if there is ECG evidence of myocardial ischemia, a history of myocardial infarction, or other data establishing the presence of ischemia such as ECG changes induced by exercise, areas of hypoperfusion seen on radioisotopic scans, or abnormalities of left ventricular wall motion seen on echocardiogram. Even the known concurrence of established coronary disease does not rule out other causes of chest pain. However, the likelihood that an uncertain history represents angina is increased by resting or induced myocardial ischemia, the presence of other atherosclerotic manifestations such as intermittent claudication, cerebral ischemic attacks, or bruits over the major arteries. Similarly, a strong family history of early coronary disease or a personal history of hypertension, diabetes, or hypercholesterolemia increases the likelihood of coronary disease in a patient with equivocal chest discomfort. Dyspnea, fatigue, cardiac enlargement, and cardiac failure are not sufficient to establish a diagnosis of angina because they may be due to many other causes.

2. Pain as support for the diagnosis of angina—If the patient's chest discomfort is in fact induced by procedures (such as exercise, rapid atrial pacing, or isoproterenol infusion) that increase myocardial oxygen demand and if production of chest discomfort is associated with ECG evidence of myocardial ischemia, a transiently raised left ventricular end-diastolic pressure with evidence of left ventricular dysfunction, or isotopic demonstration of hypoperfusion in an area of the myocardium, the diagnosis is strongly supported.

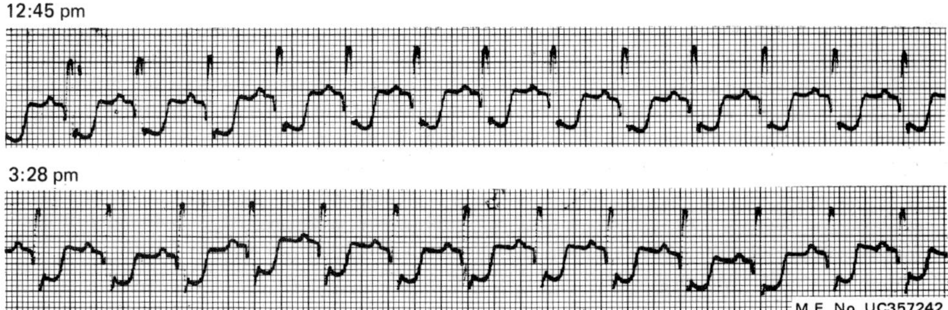

Figure 8–27. Holter monitor ECG of a 65-year-old man showing marked ST depression when the patient carried out his ordinary work routine as a salesperson. There were no symptoms during the time of the ischemic ECG changes, but angina pectoris of effort occurred at other times.

In doubtful cases, 12- to 24-hour continuous ECG tape recordings (Holter) can be used to look for the presence of ischemic ST segments during episodes of pain. Significant ischemic ST segments may be found in patients who have angina pectoris even in the absence of pain (Fig 8–27).

Coronary arteriography is rarely justified for diagnosis alone except in unusual circumstances (see p 167).

3. **Characteristics of anginal pain**–(See also Chapter 2.) The characteristics of anginal pain have been well described in the past by Heberden (1768), Herrick (1912), and Levine (1929). The discomfort is described by most patients as a sensation of tightness or pressure starting in the center of the chest and radiating to the lower jaw and to the inner surface of the left arm and to the lateral 2 fingers.

a. **Precipitating factors**–The pain is induced by anything that increases the oxygen requirements of the myocardium; examples are exercise, emotional stress, cold weather, wind, a large meal, anemia, an increase in blood pressure, tachycardia, high altitude, or decreased oxygen content of the inspired air. The essential features of the history include the circumstances that precipitate or relieve the discomfort and the characteristics of the discomfort itself, including its location, radiation, and duration. The essential feature is that the discomfort is precipitated in circumstances that increase the oxygen demands of the myocardium; the most common circumstance occurs during walking, especially when hurrying or walking up an incline or a flight of stairs.

Prinzmetal (1959) described one type of angina occurring at rest as "variant angina"; it is thought to be due to coronary vasoconstriction. Variant angina occasionally occurs in patients with minimal coronary stenosis or spasms, but most cases have substantial coronary artery lesions.

Usually, however, the discomfort of angina occurs during exertion and subsides promptly if the patient stands or sits quietly. If other factors upset the balance between myocardial oxygen supply and demand, less activity is required to produce angina, especially after meals, during times of emotional excitement, or on exposure to a cold wind. Heavy meals and strong emotion can provoke an attack even with trivial exertion.

The discomfort of angina of effort lasts but a short time if the effort is discontinued–almost always less than 10–15 minutes and usually much less. The discomfort develops and subsides fairly quickly but not abruptly. If the effort is continued unabated, the discomfort increases until the patient must stop. Occasionally a patient learns to decrease his activity until discomfort subsides and thus "walks through" the angina.

b. **Quality of anginal pain**–Patients describe anginal pain as pressing, squeezing, a tightness, a weight on the chest–rarely, as though the chest is in a vise. They may describe it as burning and may have difficulty finding the right word but will convey the type of discomfort by pressing on the chest with both hands, as first noted by Levine (1958). Many patients use the term discomfort or distress rather than pain and will answer "No" to the question, "Do you have or have you had chest pain?" The pain is rarely stabbing, lancinating, pointed, or piercing.

c. **Location of anginal pain**–The pain usually covers a fairly broad area in the central chest and has diffuse, ill-defined edges. Although it may be dominantly left precordial, it almost always involves the central chest and is rarely solely left precordial, lateral, or epigastric. Patients may think that the pain is in the abdomen, but, when asked to define the site on the nude chest and abdomen, will point to the lower mid chest. Nonanginal "abdominal" pain is below the xiphoid and involves only the epigastrium and not the chest. Anginal pain may involve the lower area of the sternum and extend into the epigastrium. Rarely is there localized tenderness during or between attacks–in contrast to patients with musculoskeletal or radicular disease, in whom this is common.

d. **Radiation of anginal pain**–The pain radiates to the lower jaw (almost never to the upper jaw), upper neck, left shoulder, and inner surface of the arm to the ulnar surface of the hand in the fourth and fifth fingers. It may be felt only as a sensation of pressure across the volar surface of the wrist. Rarely, a patient with angina may go to the dentist with a "toothache" or to an orthopedist complaining of upper back pain. Chest discomfort is often the only symptom, but there may be associated dyspnea if there is some element of left ventricular failure during episodes of pain. Angina and left ventricular chest pain are often difficult to distinguish.

The pain or discomfort of angina pectoris is a visceral pain from the heart referred from C8–T4 segmental dermatomes. Small pain fibers run with the autonomic nerves and enter the spinal cord in the T8 and C4 segments. As with all visceral pain, it is poorly localized. The diaphragm is innervated by C4, and neck pain may be related to the cutaneous pattern of this segment. The thumb is innervated by C5 and C6 and is rarely involved in anginal pain.

e. Ease of production of pain–The ease of production of the pain during effort varies on different days, often depending upon how the patient feels emotionally, whether the patient is out of doors or not, how cold and windy it is, and how much time has elapsed since eating. All of these factors increase the work of the heart. When patients with "stable" or chronic angina are exercised in a comfortable laboratory on an empty stomach in a relaxed state of mind, the amount of exercise required to induce pain is fairly constant (within 10%).

f. Patient response to pain–Patients learn to avoid pain by recognizing the earliest manifestations of pressure or tightness in the chest when they are walking or start to get excited. Most patients must slow down or stop walking and stand still, since otherwise the pain worsens until they are forced to stop. A patient may have discomfort hurrying to the bus in the morning but may find that a similar amount of effort later in the morning or in the afternoon causes no discomfort. Similarly, an individual may have discomfort during the first one or 2 holes of golf and then play the rest of the game in comfort. This uncommon "second wind" phenomenon is presumably explicable as local vasodilatation caused by metabolites accumulated during the ischemic pain period.

B. Signs: Examination is often completely negative in patients with angina pectoris who have not had a previous myocardial infarction and who show no evidence of hypertensive or aortic valve disease. The heart may be normal in size, the left ventricular cardiac impulse may be normal, and there may be no abnormal third or fourth sounds. There may, however, be associated evidence of atherosclerosis such as decreased pulsations or bruits over the major arteries. The ocular fundi are usually normal unless the patient has hypertension or diabetes. During an attack, the systolic and diastolic blood pressures are usually significantly elevated, and there may be a third heart sound, pulsus alternans, or transient pulmonary rales.

C. Hemodynamic Observations: The clinical signs mentioned in the foregoing paragraph have been shown in some patients during cardiac catheterization or cardiac pacing to be due to a raised left ventricular end-diastolic pressure caused by the development of transient left ventricular failure or decreased left ventricular compliance, and the signs are often preceded by a rise in arterial pressure of uncertain cause. The pulse rate may be increased, and carotid sinus massage to slow the ventricular rate may abruptly reverse the process. This maneuver (carotid sinus massage) can be used as a diagnostic test.

D. Laboratory Findings: Routine laboratory findings in stable angina pectoris are usually normal. Urinalysis, blood count, and sedimentation rate are normal in the absence of associated conditions that affect them. As discussed in the section on prevention of coronary disease, a search should be made for risk factors that influence the development of coronary disease as well as associated findings that aggravate it. Anemia, hypercholesterolemia, hypertriglyceridemia, diabetes mellitus, hypoglycemia, hyperthyroidism, and upper gastrointestinal tract diseases should be investigated as possible contributing factors. A chest x-ray is valuable to exclude pulmonary or skeletal abnormalities that might be the cause of the pain. The resting ECG is normal in about one-fourth of patients with stable angina. In the remainder, abnormalities include patterns of left ventricular hypertrophy, old myocardial infarction, nonspecific ST–T abnormalities, and atrioventricular or conduction defects.

E. Special Investigations: Table 8–15 indicates the specificity and sensitivity of noninvasive tests in the diagnosis of angina pectoris.

1. Exercise tests–Exercise has been the most common noninvasive technic used for many years to provide objective evidence of myocardial ischemia by inducing the typical chest discomfort. The magnitude of the ischemic changes induced by exercise has also been used to estimate prognosis (see below). Exercise tests have consisted of the Master 2-step method and graded exercise with a bicycle ergometer or treadmill. Whereas in the Master test the ECG was taken immediately after exercise, current exercise studies include continuous ECG during graded exercise. Some physicians merely determine the pulse rate and look for ECG abnormalities; others combine the test with oxygen consumption, hypoxia, and blood pressure determinations, radioisotope perfusion studies of the myocardium, echocardiography, and left ventricular cineangiography.

Exercise testing must not be done in patients with

Table 8–15. Rank order sensitivity and specificity of noninvasive tests in the diagnosis of angina pectoris.

Sensitivity	Specificity
1. Reliable history.	1. Thallium or wall motion studies with induced ischemia.
2. Thallium or wall motion studies with induced ischemia.	2. Ischemia on exercise (ECG).
3. Ischemia on exercise (ECG).	3. Ischemia on Holter monitor.
4. Ischemia on Holter monitor.	4. Reliable history.

acute or subacute myocardial ischemia and pain of recent origin, since acute myocardial infarction can be precipitated. The test must be done under the supervision of a physician, and the patient and the ECG should be continuously observed.

a. ECG changes—(See also p 129.) The criteria for a positive exercise test have varied. Efforts to increase the sensitivity of the test give rise to a high percentage of false-positive results; similarly, a high percentage of false-negatives occurs with the attempt to increase specificity. A reasonable balance between sensitivity and specificity can be achieved if the following conditions constituting the minimal requirements of a positive test are satisfied: the ST segment has a 1.5–2 mm horizontal or downsloping depression at least 0.08 sec in duration that follows the J junction in one or more leads and lasts more than 3 min.

T wave changes alone are not considered diagnostic of myocardial ischemia but do occur in about two-thirds of patients with angina who are given a standardized exercise test. The percentage rises to about 80% if the exercise is continued or increased until chest pain occurs; the ischemic changes may precede the chest pain. The pulse rate during exercise has been used as a measure of the maximal exercise for the patient's age, although most tests use submaximal exercise. In most patients who have sufficient angina pectoris to impel them to consult a physician, a pulse rate during exercise of at least 130/min but preferably 150/min is usually sufficient to elicit ischemic changes and to induce chest pain. If chest pain is not induced by the exercise or if there is little change in the pulse rate, the value of the test is significantly less. In patients who are not taking hypotensive drugs and are not in heart failure, a fall in systolic ventricular pressure accompanying exercise-induced angina is a reliable sign of critical coronary artery narrowing (Thomson, 1975). False-positive interpretations are also common if the resting ECG is abnormal or if the patient has been receiving digitalis.

b. Pulse variations—Under standardized conditions, the pulse rate at which angina is induced is reasonably constant and can be used to evaluate treatment measures such as surgical procedures or drug treatment with vasodilators or beta-adrenergic blocking agents. An ST segment depression of 2 mm or more during exercise is of greater specific diagnostic value because such a response is associated with a higher subsequent mortality rate and significant coronary artery stenosis (Bruce, 1977).

c. Results of exercise tests—Patients with angina and a positive exercise study often have multiple-vessel coronary stenoses and left ventricular wall abnormalities even in the absence of a clinical history of myocardial infarction.

Almost all studies in asymptomatic men have shown a progressive increase in the frequency of ischemic ECG changes with age during exercise. As many as 20–30% of apparently healthy men 50–70 years of age had ischemic changes with maximal exercise. It is possible that ischemic heart disease can be diagnosed at an early age by tests imposing maximal or submaximal effort. Specificity, in terms of significant coronary artery stenosis, is less in asymptomatic men than in men with coronary disease.

d. Prognostic significance—The best studies on the use of stress exercise tests in prognosis are those of Robb and Seltzer (1975), Ellestad (1975), and Bruce (1977), which showed a definite increase in subsequent mortality rates in patients with positive exercise studies (Fig 8–28). (See also Fig 8–8.)

Disorders of rhythm and conduction are major antecedents of sudden death when they occur in the presence of significant myocardial disease but rarely otherwise.

2. Coronary arteriography—(See also p 131.) In some institutions, coronary arteriography is done on almost all patients with definite or suspected angina in order to delineate the anatomy of the coronary vessels, demonstrate the presence and degree of coronary stenoses and collateral flow, and estimate prognosis and determine treatment. The authors take the more conservative view that except in unusual circumstances (see below), coronary arteriography, because of its risk potential, should not be used solely for diagnosis and prognosis until the indications for coronary bypass surgery are established. Experienced workers may find that the procedure involves only a slight risk in their

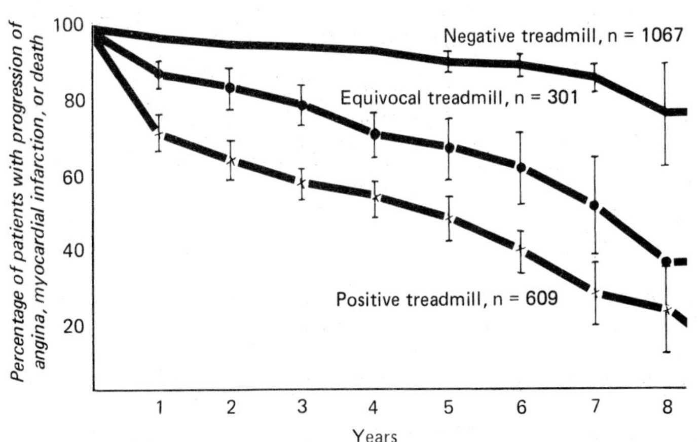

Figure 8–28. Life table display of an 8-year experience in approximately 2000 ambulatory individuals who had a negative, equivocal, or positive (ST depression of 1.5 mm or more) treadmill response (n, number of patients). (Reproduced, with permission of the American Heart Association, Inc., from Ellestad MH, Wan KC: Predictive implications of stress testing: Follow-up of 2700 subjects after maximum treadmill stress testing. Circulation 51:363, 1975.)

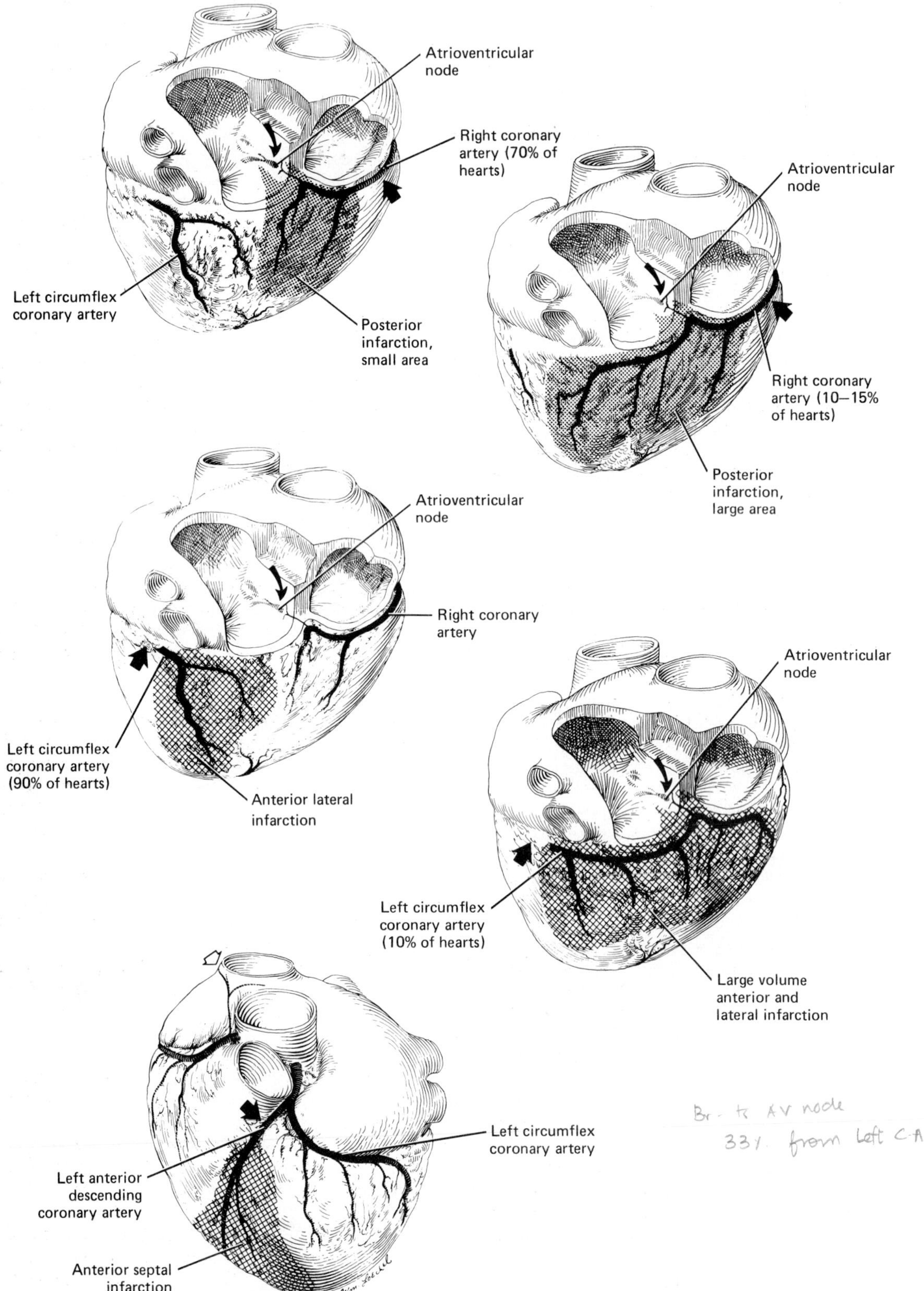

Figure 8–29. Anatomy and distribution of the coronary arteries and the topography of infarction. (Reproduced, with permission, from James TN: Arrhythmias and conduction disturbances in acute myocardial infarction. Am Heart J 64:416, 1962.)

hands and thus reason that extensive use of this technic by other clinicians is justified also. Admittedly, the anatomy of the coronary arteries cannot be predicted from the history of angina and the patient's responses to exercise testing, although it has been shown that a negative exercise test is more likely to be associated with no coronary disease or single-vessel disease, especially of the circumflex or right coronary artery. Patients with stable angina may have one-, 2-, or 3-vessel disease; may have involvement of the left main coronary artery; and may have either normal or severely impaired left ventricular function, as shown by the left ventricular cineangiogram which is done concurrently in practically all cases. Even in mild angina there may be major stenoses of 2 or 3 coronary arteries, although the severity of disease cannot be appreciated clinically. The number of stenotic vessels and the degree of stenosis vary but cannot be determined in advance despite a clinical presentation of angina pectoris or nontransmural or transmural myocardial infarction. Thus, coronary angiograms are required if the physician wishes to know the anatomy of the coronary arteries in any particular case. If the risks of study were truly minimal, the possible benefits might justify more extensive use of invasive technics.

The anatomy and distribution of the coronary arteries and the topography of infarction are illustrated in Fig 8–29. Multiple views and projections are usually necessary to evaluate the coronary angiogram. Fig 8–30 shows examples of branches of the right and left coronary arteries seen in the usual coronary angiograms.

a. Complications—Nationwide surveys have shown that the morbidity and mortality rates associated with coronary arteriography are directly related to the experience of the operator and the frequency with which the procedure is done in the particular hospital. Ventricular fibrillation, acute myocardial infarction, hemorrhage, and thrombosis of the artery are the major problems encountered. Embolism is the least common complication. The mortality rate in various series is about 0.3–0.5%, but Judkins (1974) reports that in his hands it is less than 0.1%. The risk rises with the degree of severity of left main coronary artery disease. Adequate interpretation requires high-quality cineangiograms in at least 2 projections. At institutions doing a few studies a week or less, angiograms of poor quality give inadequate information and at greater risk.

The interpretation of coronary angiograms is hampered by the difficulty of quantitating partial stenosis and the problem of deciding whether arterial spasm or some technical artifacts are present. If the degree of stenosis is less than 80%, different workers offer widely discrepant estimates of extent of narrowing; if the degree of stenosis is greater than 80%, estimates are usually in close agreement. Interpretation of the quality and size of the distal vessels and of the size of collateral channels also depends on the quality of the x-rays and the experience of the observer.

b. Indications for coronary arteriography—A number of studies have shown that survival in patients with angina pectoris depends upon (1) the dominance (whether posterior descending coronary arteries come from right or left systems) of the stenotic artery; (2) the location, severity, and number of coronary stenoses (is there a single severe proximal stenosis or more moderate multiple distal stenoses?); (3) the proximity of the stenosis to the first perforator (left anterior descending); (4) left ventricular function as estimated by the ejection fraction and by left ventricular enlargement; and (5) the presence and adequacy of collateral circulation. If it can be shown either that coronary bypass surgery prevents recurrent myocardial infarction, serious ventricular arrhythmias with sudden death, and the development of ischemic cardiomyopathy, or that it prolongs survival, the indications for coronary arteriography might be broadened to include all patients with angina pectoris and patients recovering from myocardial infarction. This would greatly extend the range of indications for coronary arteriography. However, since prophylactic bypass surgery is rarely indicated at present, routine coronary angiograms are not advised in patients with coronary heart disease.

Coronary arteriography is indicated for the following classes of patients:

(1) Patients being considered for coronary bypass surgery because of disabling stable angina who have failed to improve on an adequate medical regimen.

(2) Patients in whom coronary bypass surgery is being considered because of myocardial infarctions in rapid succession or because of repeated unstable angina causing hospital admissions.

(3) Patients with aortic valve disease who have angina pectoris, especially if the aortic valve gradient is only modest, to determine whether the angina is due to coronary disease or aortic stenosis. Severe angina in the presence of aortic stenosis is commonly though not invariably associated with coronary artery stenosis. About half of patients with significant aortic stenosis have angina pectoris (Hancock, 1977).

(4) Patients who have had coronary bypass surgery with initial improvement and subsequent relapse of symptoms to determine whether or not the bypass graft is patent or occluded.

(5) Patients with coronary disease, ischemic cardiomyopathy, and cardiac failure in whom a left ventricular aneurysm is suspected.

Differential Diagnosis

The differential diagnosis of chest pain requires great skill in history-taking. The physician can usually decide easily enough that the pain is or is not angina, but in some cases even the most careful and thoughtful inquiry may leave the issue in doubt. Chest pain in someone with coronary disease is not necessarily angina.

A. Psychophysiologic Reactions: Psychophysiologic cardiovascular reactions are a loosely defined group of disorders having in common dull aching chest pains often described as "heart pain," lasting hours or days, often aggravated by exertion but not promptly relieved by rest. Darting, knifelike pains of momentary

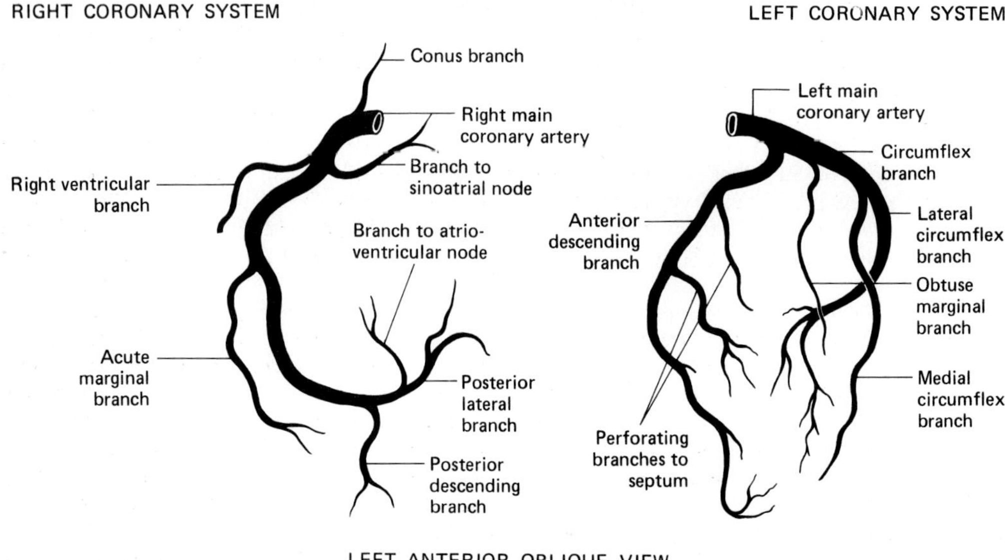

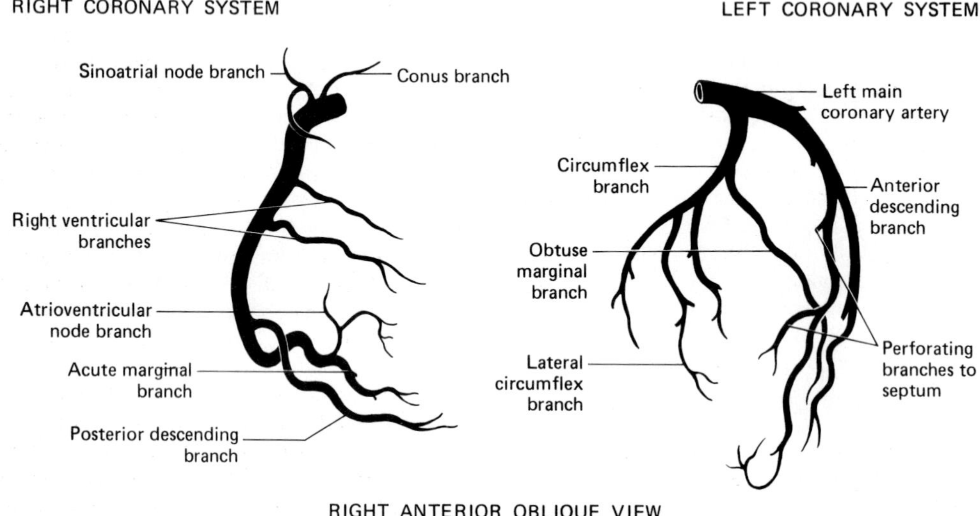

Figure 8–30. Example of branches of the left and right coronary arteries as seen in the usual coronary angiograms, left and right oblique views.

duration at the apex or over the precordium are often present also. Emotional tension and fatigue make the pain worse. Dyspnea of the hyperventilation variety, palpitations, fatigue, and headache are also usually present. Constant exhaustion is a frequent complaint.

B. Anterior Chest Wall Syndrome: This disorder is characterized by sharply localized tenderness of intercostal muscles, and pressure at these sites reproduces the chest pain. Sprain or inflammation of the chondrocostal junctions, which may be warm, swollen, and red (so-called Tietze's syndrome), may result in diffuse chest pain which is also reproduced by local pressure. Intercostal neuritis (herpes zoster, diabetes mellitus) may confuse the diagnosis.

Xiphoid tenderness and lower sternal pain may arise from and be reproduced by pressure on the xiphoid process.

Any of the above may also occur in a patient with angina.

C. Degenerative Thoracic or Cervical Spine Disease: Cervical or thoracic spine disease (degenerative disk disease, postural strain, "arthritis") involving the dorsal roots produces sudden sharp, severe chest pain similar to angina in location and "radiation" but related to specific movements of the neck or spine, recumbency, straining, or lifting, and there are usually sensory changes in the skin. Pain due to cervical thoracic disk disease involves the outer or dorsal aspect of the arm, thumb, and index fingers rather than the ring and little fingers, as in angina pectoris.

D. Gastrointestinal Disorders: Peptic ulcer, chronic cholecystitis, cardiospasm, and functional gastrointestinal disease are often suspected because some patients indisputably obtain relief from angina by belching. In these disorders, symptoms are related to food intake rather than physical exertion. X-ray and fluoroscopic study are helpful in diagnosis. The pain is relieved by appropriate diet and drug therapy.

Hiatal hernia is characterized by lower chest and upper abdominal pain after heavy meals occurring in recumbency, upon bending over, or made worse with the acid or alcohol test. The pain is relieved by bland diet, antacids, the semi-Fowler position, and walking.

E. Shoulder Origin of Pain: Degenerative and inflammatory lesions of the left shoulder or cervical rib and the scalenus anticus syndrome differ from angina in that the pain is precipitated by movement of the arm and shoulder, paresthesias are present in the left arm, and postural exercises and pillow support to the shoulders in bed give relief.

F. Pain of Pulmonary Hypertension: "Tight" mitral stenosis or pulmonary hypertension resulting from chronic pulmonary disease can on occasion produce chest pain which is indistinguishable from that of angina pectoris, including ST segment depression. The clinical findings of mitral stenosis or of lung disease are evident, and the ECG invariably discloses right axis deviation or right ventricular hypertrophy. Pulmonary embolism must also be considered.

G. Spontaneous Pneumothorax: Spontaneous pneumothorax may cause chest pain as well as dyspnea and creat confusion with angina pectoris as well as myocardial infarction.

H. Pericarditis: See Chapter 18.

Complications

The major complications of stable angina are unstable angina, myocardial infarction, arrhythmias, and sudden death.

Treatment

Treatment will be discussed in 3 main categories: (1) overall considerations, (2) treatment of the acute attack of angina pectoris, and (3) management of chronic angina pectoris. See pp 164 and 179 in considering whether the individual case is chronic or acute. In addition, exclude acute myocardial infarction; evaluate the presence of an old infarction or segmental wall motion abnormalities; and evaluate left ventricular function.

A. Overall Considerations:

1. Approach to atherosclerosis in general–One must distinguish between efforts to prevent or relieve anginal pain, efforts to prevent myocardial infarction or arrhythmias, and efforts to avert the fundamental process of atherosclerosis by lowering the blood pressure, reducing fat and carbohydrate intake, losing weight, and giving up cigarettes.

Methods designed to prevent the development of atherosclerosis in patients with angina are at present of doubtful value. Lowering the arterial pressure in the middle-aged (45–64) group of men in the VA Study (1970), while it did reduce the number of hypertensive complications, had no effect on the development of clinical coronary disease. It remains to be seen whether vigorous antihypertensive therapy at a much younger age (20s or early 30s) might prevent coronary disease, and therapeutic trials addressing this specific question are under way in various parts of the world. Similarly, diets low in carbohydrates and cholesterol and other fats may lower the serum cholesterol and plasma glucose but have not been notably successful in preventing angina (but see Leren, 1966). Reducing diets not only lower the serum cholesterol and glucose; substantial weight loss in patients with large protruding abdomens may improve mechanical efficiency during walking and thus lead to fewer anginal attacks. On the other hand, weight loss is often ineffective, and angina may occur in lean, physically fit men or women. Weight reduction with diets that decrease carbohydrate and alcohol intake may produce striking decreases in serum triglyceride and smaller decreases in serum cholesterol. Exogenous type IV hyperlipidemia may therefore appear or disappear depending upon the amount of carbohydrate in the diet and the weight of the patient. Despite the inadequacy of the evidence that lowering serum lipids late in life affects the process of atherosclerosis, the use of hypolipidemic drugs in the hope that reducing the serum lipids may improve the atherosclerotic process is rational if lipid abnormalities are present (Table 8–16). However, prevention of coronary disease should be started in childhood or adolescence, because hypertension and genetic disorders of lipid and carbohydrate metabolism are manifest early in life.

2. Prevention of myocardial infarction–Prevention of myocardial infarction is one of the objectives of treatment of angina; most infarctions, however, come "out of the blue," and close questioning reveals that even the day before the patient had no reason to anticipate any untoward cardiac event. Even cardiologists who have had infarctions have been unable to testify retrospectively to any premonition. Some patients give a history of progressive fatigue, unusual hard work, or long hours, but many patients with angina who do not develop myocardial infarction give the same history. Patients occasionally report unusually severe physical effort which left them breathless and fatigued, although the cardiac pain of infarction was delayed for 24–72 hours. Unusual emotional stress preceding the attack has been described by some patients; tachycardia, raised blood pressure, increased work of the heart, and possible coronary vasoconstriction all contribute to the development of persistent ischemia in these circumstances. Patients with angina who have ventricular premature beats, especially if they occur in runs or are multifocal, may develop ventricular tachycardia which induces prolonged severe

Table 8–16. Hypolipidemic drugs.*

	Nicotinic Acid	Cholestyramine	Dextrothyroxine	Clofibrate (Increases HDL)
Effect on plasma lipoproteins	↓ VLDL, ↓ LDL, ↓ LDL synthesis	↓ LDL, may ↑ VLDL, ↑ LDL catabolism	↓ LDL, little effect on VLDL (?), ↑ LDL catabolism	↓ VLDL, effect on LDL variable
Initial dose	100 mg orally 3 times daily	4 g orally 4 times daily	1 mg orally daily	0.5–1 g twice daily
Maintenance dose	1–2 g orally 3 times daily with meals	4–8 g orally 4 times daily	4–8 mg orally daily	1 g orally twice daily
Adverse effects	Flushing, pruritus, hyperuricemia, ↓ glucose tolerance, hepatotoxicity	Constipation, bloating, nausea, malabsorption of fat at doses exceeding 24–32 g/day	Signs of metabolic overactivity in some patients may increase angina	Nausea, weight gain, myositis, alopecia, agranulocytosis. Abnormal liver function.
Caution	Peptic ulcer in patients. Safe use in pregnancy not established.	Drug binds warfarin, digitalis, thyroxine. Safe use in pregnancy not established.	Warfarin dose may have to be decreased. Avoid in patients with multiple ectopic premature beats. Extreme caution in patients with coronary artery disease. Safe use in pregnancy not established.	Potential effects of warfarin. Safe use in pregnancy not established.
Use	Types III, IV, V, IIb, II	Type IIa, ?IIb	Types II, III	Types III, IV, ?IIb

*Reproduced, with permission, from Levy RI & others: Dietary and drug treatment of primary hyperlipoproteinemia. Ann Intern Med 77:267, 1972. VLDL, very low density lipoproteins; LDL, low density lipoproteins.

ischemia and may thus lead to infarction; treatment of the arrhythmia may prevent infarction.

In the northern USA and in Europe where the weather can be cold in winter with abrupt snowfalls, it is commonplace for middle-aged men to develop acute myocardial infarction while shoveling snow in the cold and wind after a large evening meal or early in the morning. Patients with angina are even more susceptible to this combination of stresses.

The stress of rushing around can be avoided by adequate planning, eg, getting to the airport or train station with time to spare, and arranging social and business engagements with reasonable unscheduled intervals beforehand so that unexpected developments will not necessitate stressful flurries of physical and mental activity.

All of these commonsense methods designed to prevent myocardial infarction in patients with angina are useful to prevent angina also. However, even with the best-organized program of prevention, acute myocardial infarction may develop at any time without apparent reason; it is this unpredictable element and the possibility that sudden death can occur at any time that make the disease so frightening.

3. Risk factors—Management or avoidance of the various risk factors (hypertension, hypercholesterolemia, diabetes, cigarette smoking, emotional stress) that aggravate atherosclerosis is always desirable, but the data are unconvincing that benefit accrues once angina develops except with the treatment of hypertension, avoidance of cigarette smoking, and possibly a regular physical fitness program. Cigarette smoking, which may precipitate ventricular arrhythmias and sudden death in patients with coronary disease, should be stopped permanently. There is no evidence that physical fitness achieved by exercise programs prolongs life. Weight reduction decreases the work of the heart, and a reducing diet low in calories and animal fats is desirable. Sedatives or tranquilizers may reduce the frequency of attacks but are of only marginal benefit except in hyperactive or emotionally stressed individuals. Control of hyperlipidemia is desirable for its possible effect in slowing the progress of atherosclerosis, but the available data are not conclusive that diet or drugs will prevent, reverse, or decrease the pace of the development of atheroma. In order to avoid long-term use of an ineffective regimen, the effects of diets and drugs should be monitored to determine whether lipid values are in fact lowered. In one research study, close monitoring revealed that total cholesterol and betalipoprotein cholesterol were significantly reduced within 2 weeks on a regimen consisting of 81 g of safflower oil per day, substituted for an equicaloric amount of fat (Farquhar, 1958).

A nationwide cooperative randomized study sponsored by the National Heart & Lung Institute (the Coronary Drug Project) has been under way since 1973 to evaluate the effectiveness of a number of drugs and placebo in patients who have survived an acute myocardial infarction. The purpose is to determine whether drugs that lower the serum lipid concentration will decrease the incidence of coronary disease and prolong life. Only a few preliminary data have been published to date.

B. Treatment of Acute Attack of Angina Pectoris: (Table 8–17.)

1. Nitrates and amyl nitrite—Nitroglycerin (must be fresh) taken sublingually or amyl nitrite by inhala-

Table 8–17. General principles of medical treatment of stable angina pectoris of effort.

1. Use sublingual nitroglycerin for acute relief when discomfort starts or sublingual or oral isosorbide dinitrate for prevention of attacks or more prolonged effect.
2. Use nitroglycerin ointment for nocturnal discomfort.
3. Use propranolol to prevent attacks, lower blood pressure, and prevent or treat ventricular arrhythmia.
4. Avoid physical and emotional factors that precipitate the pain.
5. Avoid exercise in the presence of other precipitating factors that increase work of the heart (cold weather, heavy meals, emotional upset).
6. Exercise caution in the face of unusual and unaccustomed effort.
7. Reduce work activity (speed of effort, regulation of time, intermittent rest periods).
8. Treat hypertension if present.
9. Treat arrhythmias if present.
10. Treat cardiac failure if present.
11. Stop cigarette smoking.
12. Reduce weight if overweight.
13. Manage adverse emotional responses.
14. Institute supervised physical fitness program (perhaps beneficial).

tion acts promptly (within a minute), and these are the drugs of choice for terminating acute anginal attacks. The longer-acting nitrates such as isosorbide dinitrate sublingually or orally or nitroglycerin ointment are more valuable when used several times a day or at bedtime for prolonged prophylaxis during the day and to prevent nocturnal angina. Pentaerythritol tetranitrate has been used infrequently recently, and the authors are not aware of recent hemodynamic studies regarding its usefulness.

a. Mechanism of action of nitrates–The nitrates, by causing peripheral pooling of blood, decrease venous return and thereby the ventricular volume and cardiac output. The oxygen demands of the heart are thereby decreased, not only because the volume of the heart is decreased as a result of reduced venous return but also because arterial vasodilatation, which decreases the impedance to left ventricular ejection, lowers intraventricular pressure. The effects are enhanced by standing, but hypotension may occur.

b. Importance of fresh nitroglycerin–Nitroglycerin deteriorates readily and must be fresh and kept in a closed dark container. The larger quantity is best kept in the refrigerator at home and only small quantities kept with the patient. If the patient feels no burning sensation on his tongue or experiences no flushing or headache, a fresh supply should be obtained. A 0.3 mg tablet allowed to dissolve under the tongue is usually sufficient and does not produce unpleasant hypotensive symptoms, but the dose may be increased to 0.4–0.6 mg if the smaller dose is ineffective. Most patients are afraid to use nitroglycerin and must be encouraged to use it freely whenever an attack occurs or to prevent an attack when they embark on an effort that experience has taught them will cause pain.

c. Hemodynamic effects of nitroglycerin–By decreasing venous return and "preload" on the heart, nitroglycerin has been shown (by cineangiography) to decrease cardiac volume and left ventricular filling pressure, to increase the ejection fraction of the left ventricle, and to decrease contraction abnormalities in patients with segmental impairment of wall motion. In the catheterization laboratory, the raised left ventricular end-diastolic pressure that follows the injection of contrast medium is often reversed by nitroglycerin, which constitutes further evidence of that drug's therapeutic benefits. Sublingual isosorbide dinitrate (Isordil), 5–10 mg sublingually or 10–40 mg orally, acts almost as rapidly as nitroglycerin and maintains its benefits for 1–3 hours. Nitroglycerin ointment (paste), 15 mg, has a duration of effect of 3–5 hours.

d. Amyl nitrite inhalation–Amyl nitrite, 1 ampule crushed and inhaled, acts in about 10 sec and is very effective. The drug produces pounding of the pulse, flushing of the face, and sometimes headache and dizziness, and patients must learn how to inhale the drug by rapidly passing the crushed ampule before the nose or from a distance. Patients soon learn how to inhale the amount needed to achieve the desired result. Some dislike amyl nitrite because of its odor and because other people are made aware of what is happening and may become distressed or try to help in an interfering way.

2. Carotid sinus massage–Carotid sinus massage as first recommended by Levine (1958) may relieve the acute anginal attack by decreasing the heart rate and myocardial contractility and thus reducing the oxygen requirements of the myocardium.

3. Need for patient to cease activity inducing angina–During the acute attack the patient should stand still, sit, or lie down as soon as the discomfort begins and remain quiet until the attack has subsided. "Working off" the pain should be discouraged, because myocardial infarction or ventricular arrhythmias may be produced.

C. Management of Chronic Angina Pectoris:

1. Avoidance of precipitating factors–Because avoiding precipitating factors is more effective than treating angina once it has occurred, the patient should be instructed to avoid situations that have produced pain or that the physician knows will increase myocardial oxygen demands. This means walking less and at a slower pace, avoiding hills and stairs–especially after meals, in the cold, or during periods of emotional stress. A useful analogy in explaining all this to the patient is that if all the appliances are plugged in at one time, the circuits will be overloaded and a fuse will blow. Cold is a particularly important precipitating factor. The rapid onset of angina when, for example, a patient opens the front door and is struck by a cold blast of air suggests that coronary vasoconstriction rather than increased cardiac work may be responsible. Coronary vasoconstriction produces myocardial ischemia by decreasing coronary blood flow.

If an activity known to induce angina *cannot* be avoided or the patient believes it must be done (eg, sexual intercourse, walking uphill, carrying a heavy suitcase on a trip), sublingual nitroglycerin 1–2 minutes *before* the activity may prevent the attack. Anginal attacks should be avoided because they may induce ventricular arrhythmias or, if prolonged, myocardial infarction.

Less obvious precipitating factors are paroxysmal arrhythmias, hypotension, hyperthyroidism, anger, left ventricular outflow obstruction, left ventricular failure, anemia, and obesity. Left ventricular failure may be obvious or incipient, and treatment with digitalis or diuretics (or both) may be helpful.

2. Drug prophylaxis–

a. Nitrates and amyl nitrite–Nitroglycerin is not only indicated during the acute attack but may prevent an attack when taken just before an activity that usually causes one. The longer-acting nitrates and nitrites administered sublingually or orally have been shown to increase exercise tolerance for 1–3 hours. Isosorbide dinitrate (Isordil) may be taken in a dosage of 5–10 mg 3 times daily sublingually or 10–20 mg 4 times daily orally. Nitroglycerin ointment (10–15 mg of 2% ointment–determined by inches of ointment as instructed in the package insert–applied to the skin of the chest and covered by plastic) has a longer duration of action than sublingual nitroglycerin and is valuable at bedtime to prevent nocturnal pain. There is no convincing evidence that these agents prolong life, but experimental data support the claim that they increase exercise tolerance. They may be especially effective for coronary spasm with elevated ST segments in the ECG (Prinzmetal's variant).

b. Propranolol–Propranolol (Inderal), 10–40 mg 3–4 times daily, increased to tolerance, has been used prophylactically with benefit to patients. The drug should not be used by patients with a past or present history of ventricular failure or a history of asthma or bronchospasm, diabetics taking insulin, or those who have severe bradycardia or atrioventricular conduction defects. Propranolol is a beta-adrenergic blocking agent that decreases the heart rate at rest and especially after exercise, lowers the blood pressure after exercise, slows left ventricular contraction, decreases the incidence of ventricular arrhythmias, and probably decreases the chances of sudden death (Wilhelmsson, 1974). However, its negative inotropic and chronotropic effects may produce bradycardia or left ventricular failure, and it must be used with caution and under close observation. Propranolol decreases the sympathetic drive to the heart, which may be crucial in maintaining adequate left ventricular performance in patients with poor left ventricular function. In doses of 80–320 mg/day, propranolol significantly reduces the resting heart rate and end-diastolic volume (Winkle, 1976). Most studies have shown that it reduces the frequency of anginal attacks and the need for sublingual nitroglycerin. Propranolol is particularly valuable in patients with unstable angina when full therapy with bed rest, oxygen, nitrites and nitrates, and sedation is advisable before considering surgery. There is evidence that if propranolol is stopped abruptly, angina may rapidly get worse and myocardial infarction may develop; therefore, the drug should be withdrawn gradually under the physician's personal supervision unless the development of left ventricular failure or asthma requires abrupt termination of treatment.

c. Aminophylline–Some patients with incipient left ventricular failure and chronic lung disease with bronchospasm may respond to rectal suppositories of aminophylline, 250–500 mg, and obtain relief of angina and dyspnea as a result of increased cardiac output and bronchodilatation.

3. Control of ventricular premature beats and ventricular arrhythmias–Ventricular arrhythmias are common in patients with coronary heart disease, both those with stable angina pectoris and those recovering from myocardial infarction.

Arrhythmias may precipitate myocardial ischemia and angina pectoris by decreasing the cardiac output and coronary perfusion. Twenty-four-hour ECG monitoring may reveal the onset of salvos of ventricular premature beats or short runs of paroxysmal atrial tachycardia just before the appearance of ischemic ST abnormalities and anginal pain. The arrhythmias may be the cause of nocturnal pain. Prophylactic treatment of the arrhythmia with digitalis, quinidine, procainamide, or propranolol may prevent the attacks of angina. (See Chapter 15.)

Although it is difficult to prove, since most cases of "sudden death syndrome" are due to ventricular fibrillation, often preceded by ventricular premature beats, control of the premature beats may prevent ventricular fibrillation and sudden death. Antiarrhythmia drugs may decrease ventricular premature beats, but, with the exception of the data on beta-blocking agents (see above), it has not been established that they prevent sudden death.

Ventricular premature beats have been classified as single or complex, as frequent to rare, and as induced by exercise, occurring in sleep, or disclosed only by long-term ambulatory ECG monitoring. Tables 8–18 and 8–19 set forth some of the data that have

Table 8–18. Distribution of ventricular premature beats during a 24-hour monitoring session in 184 patients with coronary heart disease. (Each patient is presented once on the basis of maximal grade reached during monitoring.)*

Grade	Description	Percent of Patients
0	No ventricular ectopic beats	12
1	Occasional, isolated ventricular premature beats	17
2	Frequent ventricular premature beats (> 1/min or 30/hour)	6
3	Multiform ventricular premature beats	25
4	Repetitive ventricular premature beats	
4A	Couplets	27
4B	Salvos	14

*Reproduced, with permission of the American Heart Association, Inc., from Lown B & others: Monitoring for serious arrhythmias and high risk of sudden death. Circulation 52 (Suppl 3):189, 1975.

Table 8–19. Serious ventricular arrhythmias in 447 patients during 8-hour monitoring.*

Type of Arrhythmia	Number of Cases
Ventricular fibrillation	1
Ventricular tachycardia	11
Doublets	34
Multiform ventricular premature beats	111
R on T	33
Uniform ventricular premature beats > 4	19
One or more features	139

*Reproduced, with permission of the American Heart Association, Inc., from Ruberman W & others: Ventricular premature beats and mortality of men with coronary heart disease. Circulation 52 (Suppl 3):199, 1975.

been accumulated about ventricular arrhythmias in patients with coronary heart disease.

In most comparative studies, not only are ventricular premature beats more apt to be uncovered by 24-hour ambulatory ECG monitoring of patients with coronary disease than by graded exercise, but the more complex ventricular arrhythmias are also more frequently noted during ECG monitoring. Exceptions occur, however, and both diagnostic procedures should be used in individual patients. Graded exercise induces more frequent and more complex ventricular premature beats in patients with coronary heart disease than in normal subjects even when the duration of the exercise is greater in the latter group. The absence of ventricular premature beats during a standard ECG is no assurance that more prolonged monitoring will not reveal single or complex ventricular premature beats. One-third to one-half of patients with no premature ventricular beats (or only one) on a routine ECG show a variety of ventricular premature beats that are frequent, multifocal, early, or in runs when monitoring is employed. It is important to determine the grade of ventricular premature beats (simple or complex) because the degree of angiographically demonstrated coronary stenosis is greater in patients with more complex premature ventricular beats (Lown, 1973).

4. **Treatment of hypertension**—Episodes of angina are often preceded by rises in blood pressure, and treatment of hypertension may be valuable in these patients (see Chapter 9). The rise in blood pressure that may occur when a patient is riding in a car driven by another person is shown in Fig 8–31.

5. **Treatment of cardiac failure if present**—See Chapter 10.

6. **Social and psychologic factors**—Knowing that one has "a bad heart" is a heavy psychologic burden, and some patients respond by denial, anger, depression, or regression. Sympathetic listening and discussion are an essential part of good management of these emotional responses. The high percentage of patients (50–60%) who report decreased frequency of attacks and decreased need for nitroglycerin when given a placebo attests to the role of emotional factors in increasing the frequency of anginal attacks. Prevention of angina induced by emotional stress, anger, etc is difficult. Mild tranquilizers such as diazepam may be helpful, but use of drugs does not decrease the need for general measures designed to ameliorate the stresses of the patient's life. An attempt should be made to improve the patient's general emotional health and state of mind. Factors that cause unhappiness, resentment, or hostility should be eliminated if possible. Everyone associated with the patient must be considered as a possible source of emotional stress, including the employer, colleagues at work, spouse, and children. The physician who has a good personal relationship with the patient is in the best position to suggest creative solutions to problems of this sort.

Patients with driving personalities who lead hectic lives must learn to moderate their activities, quit smoking, use alcohol only in moderation, take rest periods in the afternoon and frequent short holidays, and avoid all activities shown by experience to bring on attacks. A temporary move to a distant city may break the cycle of frequent anginal attacks by interrupting the stressful habits of work and social engagements. Rest and relaxation in a totally different environment often produce dramatic results when drugs do not.

7. **Anticoagulant therapy**—Anticoagulants have been tried in various parts of the world, both in patients with angina of effort and in patients who have survived an acute infarction, in order to prevent subsequent infarction and death, but the results have shown only minimal benefit if any. The same statement can be made about chronic aspirin usage, now being studied experimentally. Routine anticoagulant therapy of patients with angina of effort is rarely used today except when thromboembolic complications are present or believed to be a substantial risk.

8. **Increased physical activity**—A planned program of daily exercise has been recommended by many as a means of preventing myocardial infarction and death, but the data to support this recommendation are not convincing. It is true that graded physical conditioning has beneficial physiologic and psychologic results.

One must be cautious about recommending exercise programs for another reason. Even if exercises can be tailored to the individual in the laboratory, the circumstances may be different when the patient con-

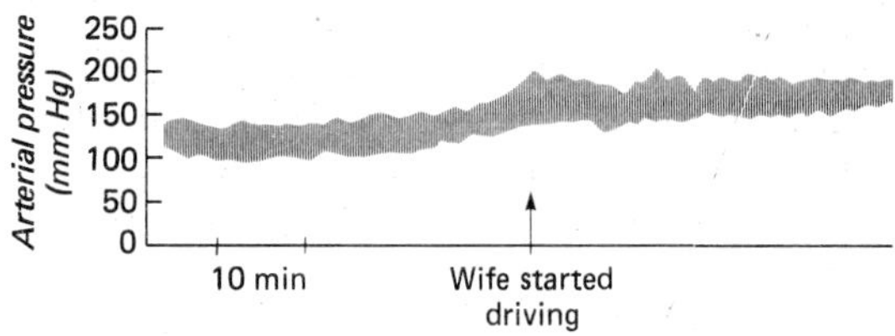

Figure 8–31. Considerable rise in arterial pressure occurred when the patient was driven by his wife, as shown by this direct intra-arterial continuous blood pressure recording. (Reproduced, with permission, from Littler WA, Honour AJ, Sleight P: Direct arterial pressure and electrocardiogram during motor car driving. Br Med J 2:273, 1973.)

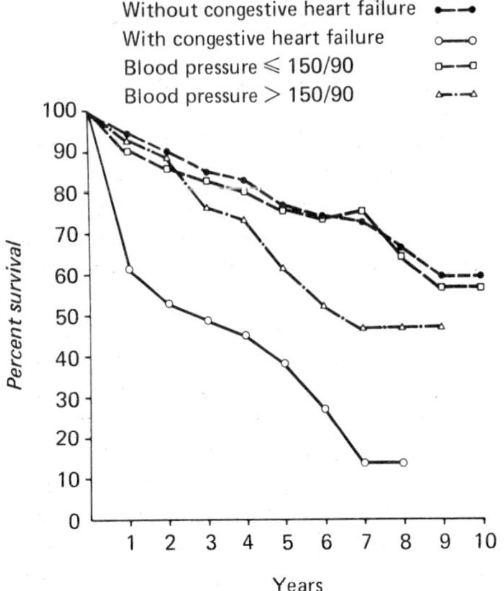

Figure 8–32. Survival with coronary artery disease related to heart failure and blood pressure. (Reproduced, with permission of the American Heart Association, Inc., from Burggraf GW, Parker JO: Prognosis in coronary artery disease: Angiographic, hemodynamic and clinical factors. Circulation 51:146, 1975.)

tinues to exercise later. A patient may have career or family problems, or sodium retention from a respiratory infection, or the weather may turn cold suddenly. The same degree of exercise that is well within the bounds of tolerance in the laboratory or on a pleasant day may not be tolerated under less favorable circumstances.

9. Preparation for survival–

a. Education of family–The patient's family must be taught resuscitation technics and instructed in how to minimize delay in obtaining medical care when needed. Patients with angina are at increased risk of acute myocardial infarction, serious ventricular arrhythmias, or sudden death. When an attack occurs, the patient should be taken promptly to a nearby hospital with good coronary care facilities unless mobile ambulance crews trained in resuscitation are readily available.

2. Education of laymen and ambulance crews–Various communities provide physician and lay educational programs, including use of the media such as newspapers and television, with the simple objective of minimizing the time between onset of symptoms of a coronary event and hospitalization. Emergency medical technicians in specially equipped ambulances and fire department personnel with rescue vehicles have been taught to recognize arrhythmias, to accomplish defibrillation, and to inject drugs such as atropine and lidocaine. Further study is required to determine the precise role of prehospital care of this kind in patients with angina.

Prognosis

A. Overall Mortality Rate: The overall mortality

Table 8–20. Causes of death in patients with stable angina of effort.*

Cause	Number	Percent of Deaths
Noncardiac	8	11
Sudden (outside hospital)	24	34
Chronic congestive heart failure	10	14
Acute myocardial infarction		
Arrhythmia	16	23
Pump failure	13	18
Total	71	100

*Reproduced, with permission of the American Heart Association, Inc., from Burggraf GW, Parker JO: Prognosis in coronary artery disease: Angiographic, hemodynamic, and clinical factors. Circulation 51:146, 1975.

rate of patients with stable angina *as a group* is about 4% per year (Frank, 1973). However, when the group is sorted out into categories based on ECG evidence of left ventricular hypertrophy and hypertension, the annual mortality rate was shown by Frank to be 8% in the former and only 0.3% in the latter. It has been estimated by Kannel (1972), using data from the Framingham Study, that one-fourth of male patients with angina will have a myocardial infarction within 5 years (one-eighth in women); that one-third will die within 8 years; and that half of all deaths will be sudden. Other factors influencing survival include congestive heart failure often due to previous myocardial infarction (Fig 8–32).

The causes of death are listed in Table 8–20.

B. Role of Coronary Artery Anatomy: Angina is often the initial manifestation of coronary disease (Fig 8–33), and the prognosis depends chiefly on the anatomy of the coronary arteries (Fig 8–34) and the left ventricular function. The mortality rate is higher when left ventricular function is impaired–as shown by increase in the left ventricular filling pressure, decrease of the cardiac index, or an ejection fraction of less

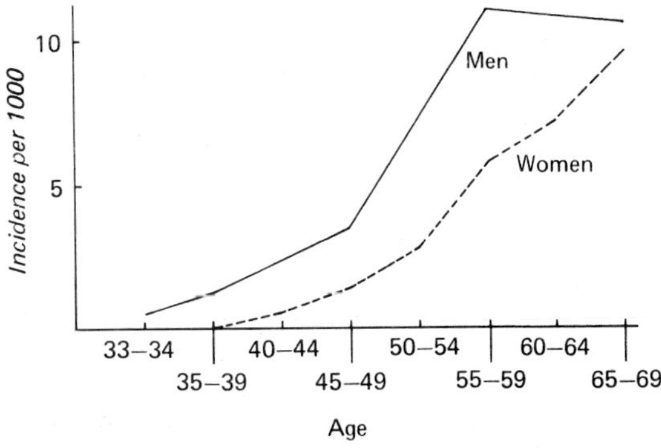

Figure 8–33. Smoothed average annual incidence of angina pectoris as a presenting complaint. Men and women age 33–69, Framingham Study. (Reproduced, with permission, from Kannel WB, Feinleib M: Natural history of angina pectoris in the Framingham Study: Prognosis and treatment. Am J Cardiol 29:154, 1972.)

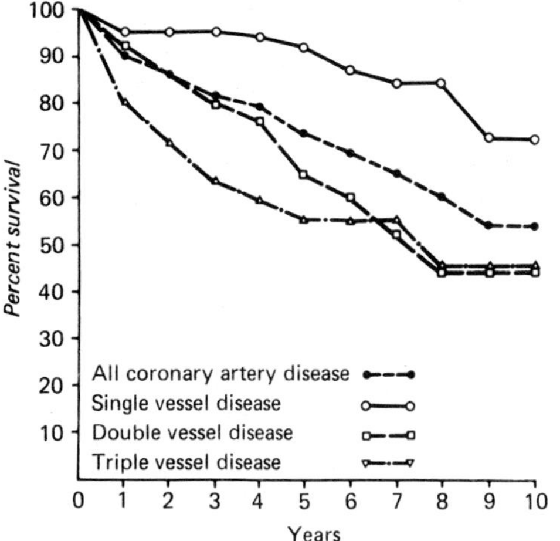

Figure 8–34. Survival related to extent of coronary artery involvement. (Reproduced, with permission of the American Heart Association, Inc., from Burggraf GW, Parker JO: Prognosis in coronary artery disease: Angiographic, hemodynamic and clinical factors. Circulation 51:146, 1975.)

than 0.50 but especially less than 0.30 (Nelson, 1975). When hypertension with ECG evidence of left ventricular hypertrophy is present, the mortality rate increases 5-fold irrespective of the anatomic changes. When both coronary angiograms and left ventricular cineangiograms are available, information about left ventricular ejection fraction and segmental contraction abnormalities and the degree of involvement of the 3 coronary arteries gives a more reliable estimate of prognosis than does the symptom of angina pectoris alone. The 5-year mortality rate in patients with single-vessel disease who have good left ventricular function was only 2.2% in the Johns Hopkins series, where it was 6.8% with 2-vessel disease and 11.4% with 3-vessel disease. Three-vessel disease with diffuse left ventricular functional abnormalities with a low ejection fraction was found by Sheldon (1975) to have an almost 100% 5-year mortality rate, whereas 3-vessel disease with normal left ventricular function had a 35% 5-year mortality rate. Cardiac enlargement and cardiac failure in addition to hypotension and ECG abnormalities greatly worsened the prognosis. Most deaths occur in the year following the onset of angina pectoris or myocardial infarction.

Attempts have been made to devise better systems for "scoring" anatomic lesions not merely in terms of one-, 2-, or 3-vessel disease but also on the basis of number and degree (from trivial to total) of stenoses in each vessel (Humphries, 1974). Among patients with low scores the annual mortality rate is one-tenth that in patients with high scores, who have severe stenoses in multiple vessels. The difficulties in prognosis are emphasized by the fact that the annual mortality rate in left main coronary artery lesions varies from 10–40% (Reeves, 1974).

Another means of estimating the severity of coronary disease involves recognition of the extent of coronary calcification in one, 2, or 3 vessels. As shown in Fig 8–35, the severity of coronary disease increases with the extent of coronary calcification.

C. Importance of Previous Myocardial Infarction: Patients presenting with angina pectoris may have had a previous myocardial infarction which either was silent or coincided with the onset of angina. Some of these patients on cineangiographic study show impaired left ventricular wall motion with segmental contraction abnormalities. The prognosis in this group is that of patients with previous myocardial infarction who also have fibrosis and segmental wall disease, and the mortality rate is higher than that of patients who have not had a previous myocardial infarction. Patients who have had a previous myocardial infarction with diffuse fibrosis from healed ischemic areas have enlarged hearts and ischemic cardiomyopathy and often have evidence of left ventricular failure; in these patients, the 2-year mortality rate is 40–50% regardless of the number of vessels involved. Patients with orthopnea and paroxysmal nocturnal dyspnea have enlarged hearts and an unfavorable prognosis. Even with equivalent vessel disease, large cardiac volumes are associated with a severalfold increase in mortality rate.

The anatomic changes revealed by coronary arteriography have prognostic influence in that the most hazardous lesion is stenosis of the left main coronary artery and then (in decreasing order of risk) the left anterior descending, the left circumflex, and the right coronary artery. Most studies have shown that patients with stenosis of the left main coronary artery have at

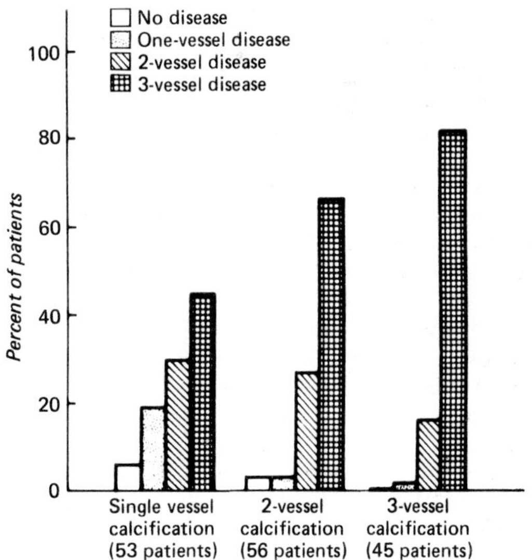

Figure 8–35. The severity of coronary disease increased progressively with the extent of coronary calcification. No "false-positives" were found in patients with 3-vessel calcification. (Reproduced, with permission of the American Heart Association, Inc., from Bartel AG & others: The significance of coronary calcification detected by fluoroscopy: A report of 360 patients. Circulation 49:1247, 1974.)

least twice the mortality rate over a period of 1–3 years of those with equivalent stenoses in the other 2 vessels.

D. Summary of Prognostic Factors: It is clear, therefore, that in estimating prognosis in a patient with stable angina of effort it is necessary to know whether there has been previous myocardial infarction, whether the onset of angina was associated with acute myocardial infarction in the current admission, and whether the patient has already survived 10 or 15 years or is only in the first year of angina. It is also necessary to score the number and degree of stenoses in each of the 3 vessels and to weight them depending on which coronary artery is involved, with greater weight being given to the left main and left anterior descending coronary artery. Left ventricular function and segmental wall abnormalities must be accounted for in the equation chiefly because they reflect previous myocardial ischemia with fibrosis and are often associated with greater cardiac enlargement. Cardiac enlargement or increased cardiac volume adversely influences the score based solely on the anatomy of the stenosed vessels.

E. Prospective Studies of Prognosis: Prospective studies are under way in a number of institutions to attempt to define more precisely the prospective prognosis in individual patients so that decisions regarding surgical treatment can be made. Patients with 3-vessel disease and left ventricular dysfunction may warrant a much more aggressive surgical approach provided the left ventricular dysfunction is not too great; whereas one-vessel disease, especially of the circumflex or right coronary artery, may warrant a more cautious attitude toward surgical treatment because of the relatively good prognosis. Prospective studies are also necessary to determine the impact of the variables influencing prognosis on the mortality rate also on the incidence of new myocardial infarctions, ventricular arrhythmias, cardiac failure, and sudden death. Accurate prognosis is difficult because long-term prospective studies are not available and because angina may be associated with great variability of anatomic disease and left ventricular function, with recognized or unrecognized myocardial infarction, and with other complications if there has been more than one infarction and the patient has ischemic cardiomyopathy. Surgical treatment with coronary bypass surgery is now so frequent that it may be difficult to obtain adequate prospective prognostic studies because medically treated patients may either have refused surgery or have been denied surgery because of inadequate left ventricular function or anatomically unsatisfactory prospects of success.

F. Need for More Precise Delineation and Scoring of Degree of Stenosis: More precise methods of determining the degree of stenosis would be helpful because opinions about the degree of stenosis differ and because it is not now possible to measure accurately the coronary flow across the stenotic vessels. Multiple lesions with 50% stenosis may be more significant than a single lesion with 80% stenosis (assuming that the estimates are accurate). The role of calcification of the coronary arteries is being studied to determine its implications, if any, for diagnosis and prognosis. The relative importance of cardiac volume and of localized areas of hypokinesia has not been sufficiently studied, and the distinction between segmental and diffuse contractile abnormalities must be further defined. The differentiation between localized left ventricular wall abnormalities and aneurysm formation is a matter of degree and opinion, but it is clear that left ventricular aneurysms cause cardiac failure and worsen the prognosis unless they are recognized and surgically resected. If patients with angina have had a previous myocardial infarction and have associated papillary muscle dysfunction with mitral regurgitation, this obviously will affect prognosis adversely. Left ventricular functional abnormalities must take into account a healed fibrotic scar with minimal hypokinesia, a small or large left ventricular aneurysm, and diffuse multifibrotic contraction abnormalities with increased left ventricular volume with or without cardiac failure or decreased ejection fraction. All of these factors must be analyzed, put into subgroups, and matched with the degrees and number of stenoses in the 3 coronary arteries. Useful conclusions cannot be drawn until a large number of patients have been followed prospectively so that the mortality rate in each group can be separately assessed. When all of these data are available, it may be possible to make sense out of all of the material, improve the uncertainties of prognosis, and thereby aid the physician in making a rational decision regarding the prognosis of the patient who has received medical treatment. Data banks, such as at Duke University, may permit computer analysis of the prognosis of individual patients.

G. Supposed Coronary Disease With Normal Coronary Angiograms: In all of the series studied, a small number of individuals who have what their physician considered angina pectoris have had normal coronary angiograms. Because of differences in the quality of the angiograms and the ability of the physician to elicit a reliable history, the frequency of angina occurring with normal coronary angiograms has been variously estimated; nevertheless, when the coronary angiogram is negative, the short-term prognosis (5 years) is very good. Opinion differs about whether these patients have true angina pectoris or pain that resembles angina. In some of the studies, ischemic ST changes were noted with exercise; in others, no abnormality of left ventricular function during stress was found nor were there changes in left ventricular end-diastolic pressure during atrial pacing. No one knows whether the disease in this group of patients represents small vessel disease or some disturbance in cardiac physiology which is not fully understood or whether the history of angina is simply inaccurate. It is also possible that because of some failure of technic, a significant stenosis in a branch of the coronary arteries was unrecognized. The excellent prognosis and the failure to identify left ventricular dysfunction during attacks of pain often make one doubt the validity of the diagnosis of angina pectoris in this group of patients. Another possibility advanced by Roberts (1977) is that coronary emboli which subsequently lyse might explain the subsequent normal coronary angiograms in patients who have had what appears to be either angina pectoris or acute myocardial infarction. He notes that coronary angiograms have not been obtained during the episode of acute myocardial infarction in this group of patients.

One must always exclude vasculitis and arteritis as the cause of angina in patients with normal coronary arteries on angiography. There are many causes of arteritis and vasculitis, eg, rheumatoid arthritis, connective tissue disorders, rheumatic fever, and others as yet unidentified. Syphilis involving the ostia of the coronary arteries may be overlooked, and one should search for clues to the various diagnoses during the course of the general systemic examination.

UNSTABLE ANGINA

The foregoing discussion pertained to the condition known as angina of effort, which is relatively stable. In stable angina, patients can relate frequency of angina to effort expended, emotional state, weather, and meals, and the occurrence of attacks is relatively predictable within a broad range of activities. Intermediate between this stable angina and acute myocardial infarction is a clinical state variously referred to as unstable angina, intermediate coronary syndrome, acute coronary insufficiency, preinfarction angina, and crescendo angina.

Definition of Unstable Angina

Although patients with unstable angina are usually considered as a more or less homogeneous group, they consist of a number of distinguishable subgroups, which may explain the widely differing estimates of prognosis in patients considered to have unstable angina. The usual definition is *crescendo angina,* in which a patient known to have had stable angina of effort (1) develops angina on less exertion, (2) develops angina at rest or during sleep, (3) has pain with a somewhat different duration or radiation, (4) has pain which is not relieved as promptly with nitroglycerin as before, or (5) has angina that gradually worsens over a period of days and in many instances (though not necessarily) develops into acute myocardial infarction. The syndrome was recognized initially because patients with acute myocardial infarction often gave a history of premonitory pain of the crescendo type or pain with a different character prior to the infarct. The term preinfarction angina was chosen because it was thought that this syndrome invariably led to acute myocardial infarction. It has been shown, however, that infarction often does not follow, and so the term preinfarction angina has fallen out of favor. Careful studies utilizing serial serum enzyme determinations, ECGs, and radioisotope perfusion uptake in patients with unstable angina have shown that some of them have already had a small myocardial infarction. If one combines patients who have already had a myocardial infarction with those who have not in a group of patients with unstable angina, the resulting mortality rate will obviously differ from that found in pure subsets of one or the other condition.

Confusing the picture further is the fact that patients who develop angina for the first time are also considered to have unstable angina because of the high frequency with which they develop acute myocardial infarction shortly after onset. On pathologic study, these patients sometimes in fact do have a small unsuspected myocardial infarction or a coronary occlusion which did not result in myocardial infarction because of collateral circulation or other factors. It is clear that when all of the patients are considered as a single group, the experience of different observers will vary depending on how they weight the different groups of patients. In general, angina appearing for the first time has a better prognosis than does angina of effort which progresses to occur at rest, to awaken the patient from sleep, or to last from 15–30 minutes instead of for 1–2 minutes.

Unstable angina also varies considerably with respect to the amount of coronary disease present; most patients have 2- or 3-vessel disease, but 10% have only single-vessel involvement.

Classification & Symptoms of Unstable Angina

It is logical to subdivide unstable angina as follows: (1) initial angina that promptly subsides with bed rest; (2) initial angina that continues despite bed rest and medical treatment; (3) crescendo angina in patients with previous stable angina; (4) angina at rest or during sleep; (5) angina that changes in character and duration; and (6) the occurrence and degree of ECG changes with pain. Categories (3) and (5) can be further subdivided according to whether or not pain subsides promptly with bed rest and medication.

A. Puzzling Diagnosis of Unstable Angina: When unstable angina is the first manifestation of coronary disease, the diagnosis can be very puzzling because there is no history of angina of effort; often the patient states that effort does not induce pain but that pain occurs at unpredictable times when he is at rest. But the quality of the discomfort is typical of ischemic pain, and the change in character of onset of the pain is probably due to occlusion of a small branch of the coronary artery or one of its collaterals, so that an area of myocardium is precariously perfused or actually necrosed, as later demonstrated by serial ECGs and serum enzyme measurements showing evidence of infarction.

B. Possible Presence of Unproved Myocardial Infarction: Radioisotope imaging may help distinguish myocardial necroses in this group of patients. The presence of a small acute myocardial infarction in a patient considered to have unstable angina increases the danger of performing emergency coronary angiography or bypass surgery, which has a higher risk in these patients than in those with stable angina. And finally, invasive diagnostic studies are more hazardous when performed in the presence of even a small myocardial infarction.

C. Hazards of Unstable Angina: The possibility of development of an acute myocardial infarction within the next few hours, days, or weeks after the development of unstable angina makes it one of the most hazardous of all manifestations of ischemic heart disease. As was said in the section on acute myocardial infarction, the mortality rate of acute myocardial infarction is greatest in the first few hours; therefore, it is prudent to monitor all patients with unstable angina in a coronary care unit for 3–5 days both because they might be developing a myocardial infarction which can become obvious at any time and because unstable angina may be associated with serious ventricular arrhythmias requiring immediate care. A further reason for having such patients in the coronary care unit is that restriction of all activity may turn the tide in favor of the myocardium, and infarction may be prevented as the demand for oxygen is reduced over a period of days by bed rest.

Treatment

Because in many patients with unstable angina but without infarction the acute process subsides with bed rest, nitrates, propranolol, and vasodilator therapy, conservative nonsurgical therapy is advised during the acute phase, although 15–30% of patients develop myocardial infarction, usually with multiple plaque hemorrhages (in those seen at autopsy). Patients admitted to a coronary care unit with unstable angina usually do well in the hospital and have many fewer complications than patients with definite myocardial infarction.

A. Aggressive Invasive Bypass Surgery: Most centers report a higher mortality rate when coronary bypass surgery is performed for unstable angina than for stable angina—often because a small myocardial infarction may have occurred. More aggressive therapy during the acute phase may be indicated if the patient has recurrent episodes of angina at bed rest in the hospital despite full therapy, which should include oxygen and anticoagulation (a controversial method of treatment). Under these circumstances, intra-aortic balloon pumping controlled by hemodynamic monitoring may decrease myocardial ischemia and relieve angina. The morbidity rate from insertion of an intra-aortic balloon pump is about 10%, so this method should be used only when it appears that the patient is getting worse despite medical treatment. The balloon pump decreases myocardial oxygen demand and increases coronary blood flow, thus decreasing the work of the left ventricle. Balloon assist can be discontinued in 24–48 hours if the patient is asymptomatic and the hemodynamic status is good. If angina recurs and cannot be controlled, coronary arteriography should be performed with a view to performing coronary bypass surgery if the stenotic lesions are anatomically suitable for the procedure (Gold, 1976).

If the angina subsides and does not recur when the balloon assist device is removed, the physician can continue conservative therapy and consider special investigations about 3 months later on an elective basis after the unstable angina has subsided. Coronary arteriography and left ventricular cineangiography can be done at that time to determine the extent of the disease and the technical likelihood of success of coronary bypass surgery (see below). Bypass surgery is of somewhat greater importance in this group because patients with unstable angina have a higher incidence of acute myocardial infarction, sudden death, and ventricular arrhythmias in the 1–2 years after onset.

B. Conservative Therapy: If one elects conservative treatment during the acute phase, it is important to regard the patient as having had a small myocardial infarction and to avoid early full ambulation and return to work, because the prognosis is less favorable if unstable angina is due to worsening of preexisting angina than when the angina appears for the first time. Earlier investigation may be wise, therefore, if such a patient does not respond promptly to medical treatment. Elective investigation 3 months after the ischemic process has subsided, followed by bypass surgery if the stenotic lesions and the degree of left ventricular dysfunction are appropriate, seems indicated in all patients who have crescendo or progressive angina, nocturnal or rest angina, or angina associated with left ventricular failure. The major advantage of immediate bypass surgery in patients with unstable angina would appear to be prevention of acute myocardial infarction and sudden death, but the published data do not as yet indicate that surgery prevents these complications.

Prognosis

The prognosis of unstable angina is controversial because of the difficulties of definition as stated previously. The outcome is influenced by (1) the extent and nature of the anatomic disease; (2) the presence or absence of a previous myocardial infarction; (3) the possibility that the unstable angina is related to current acute myocardial infarction, which may be indicated by the presence or development of ST segment abnormalities or Q waves; and (4) other factors with adverse prognostic implications even in stable angina, eg, cardiac failure, segmental areas of impaired contraction with asynergy or dyskinesia, ventricular arrhythmias, advanced age, and hypertension or hypotension.

The state of imbalance between supply and demand of oxygen, even at rest, is precarious, and myocardial ischemia is of greater degree, so myocardial necrosis can be imminent. Coronary blood flow to the affected area of the myocardium is barely sufficient, and when its demands are even slightly raised, as after meals or during bathing, showering, or defecating, angina may develop in or outside the hospital. Violent dreams may awaken such patients from sleep and cause angina.

A. Problem of Differentiating Unstable Angina From Myocardial Infarction: The data on prognosis in the literature are hard to interpret because patients in some studies are excluded from the unstable angina group if they develop a myocardial infarction during the first few days in the hospital, whereas in other patients ST–T abnormalities are not considered diagnostic unless they are associated with abnormal Q waves. Absence of ischemic changes in the ST–T segment, absence of serum enzyme elevations, and absence of increased uptake on radioisotopic imaging with technetium Tc 99m pyrophosphate are needed to rule out myocardial infarction in a patient with prolonged or rest pain. Serum enzyme measurements and myocardial imaging have demonstrated that infarction had already occurred in some patients (in one series almost one-third) in whom the ECG failed to show infarction (Willerson, 1975).

B. Need for Prospective Studies to Establish Prognosis: Estimates of prognosis in different series with respect to immediate death as well as the frequency of myocardial infarction or death in the succeeding 1–2 years vary as much as 5-fold, reflecting differences in the characteristics of the patients in groups labeled unstable angina. The differences must be resolved by prospective studies of sharply defined subgroups. Accurate prognosis in this group of patients is particularly important because it influences the choice of therapy.

C. Effect of Treatment on Prognosis: The prognosis of unstable angina is also influenced by the treatment given. In at least one study the patients were allowed out of bed within a few days when the ECG and serial enzymes failed to show a myocardial infarction and thus did not receive optimal treatment; in another, the patients were allowed to remain at work but cautioned to avoid strenuous activity. One cannot compare the prognosis in patients managed in this fashion with that in patients who were hospitalized and given full care as though they had had an acute myocardial infarction.

Accurate prognosis in this group of patients is important not only for its own sake but also because it influences the choice of therapy. A recent review of medical versus surgical treatment of unstable angina concludes that there is no convincing evidence that survival rates are improved by treating unstable angina as an acute surgical emergency and that in most cases the symptoms in unstable angina are relieved by medical treatment. Intensive preliminary medical treatment is advantageous before surgery is considered (Hultgren, 1977).

• • •

CORONARY HEART SURGERY

Over the past 20 years, the relatively poor prognosis of patients with coronary heart disease treated medically has led surgeons who hope to relieve symptoms and prolong life to attempt various surgical procedures aimed at revascularizing the heart. Time after time, initial enthusiasm faded as follow-up surveillance showed that benefits did not accrue to significant numbers of patients. The coronary bypass procedure—in which the obstructed coronary artery is bypassed by inserting the saphenous vein into the aorta proximal to the coronary arteries and beyond the obstruction distally or, alternatively, anastomosing the internal mammary artery to a point distal to the obstructed artery—was at first viewed with widespread skepticism, partly because so many hopes in the recent past had proved to be in vain. Cautious optimism has now replaced the initial doubts, especially in left main coronary artery lesions.

Bypass surgery is now performed extensively for single-, double-, and triple-vessel disease. Although the ultimate results are uncertain with respect to the prevention of myocardial infarction and prolongation of life, sufficient data have accumulated to make it clear that in experienced hands relief of angina of effort occurs in about 85% of patients. The surgical mortality rate of bypass surgery in stable angina is now 1–3%. The mortality rate is higher if patients have unstable angina or require additional procedures such as resection of a myocardial scar, resection of a ventricular aneurysm, replacement of the mitral valve, or closure of an acquired ventricular septal defect.

Many studies, including invasive postoperative observations, indicate that objective improvement occurs in about half of these patients. Electrocardiography shows less evidence of ischemia induced by graded exercise. There is increased left ventricular contractility with improved ejection fraction and improved left ventricular wall motion in patients who preoperatively had impaired segmental left ventricular walls—especially if the graft to the myocardial segment remains patent following surgery. Most patients have sufficient subjective improvement to return to work. Subjective and objective improvement in many patients appears to be genuine, although relapse may occur as a result of occlusion of the previously patent graft when a patient appears to be improving. Prospective randomized clinical trials are now under way to determine the long-term effectiveness of bypass surgery in patients who have had a good technical result and a patent graft.

The one clear indication for surgical treatment about which there is almost unanimous agreement is the presence of severe stenosis of the left main coronary artery in patients with coronary disease, because the survival rate is higher for the surgically treated (85% 2-year survival) as compared to the medically treated group (65%) (Oberman, 1976). In a VA Cooperative Randomized Study of Surgery for Coronary Arterial Occlusive Disease, comparable data reveal that 20% of surgical patients and 36% of medically treated patients with significant left main coronary artery lesions died after an average follow-up of 30 months (Takaro, 1976). There were significant lesions of the other major coronary arteries in about 60% of patients in both groups.

No differences in survival were demonstrated between medically and surgically treated patients with angina when left main coronary lesions were excluded (Hultgren, 1976, 1977).

Problems & Negative Aspects of Coronary Bypass Surgery

The adverse results that have followed bypass surgery include the following:

(1) Intraoperative myocardial infarction in 15–20% of patients, manifested by new Q waves, the development of increased myocardial band creatine phosphokinase, and positive pyrophosphate isotope scans.

(2) A surgical mortality rate of about 1–3%, which rises to 10% if additional procedures such as aortic valve replacement, repair of ventricular septal defect, resection of an aneurysm, or mitral valve replacement are required. It must be understood, of course, that the mortality rate on medical treatment would also be substantially higher in the presence of these associated conditions.

(3) Difficulty in finding a satisfactory distal segment for anastomosis. The quality and availability of the distal segment to which the graft is applied may be difficult to determine with certainty preoperatively by means of coronary arteriography, and at operation the surgeon may not find a distal vessel large enough to permit satisfactory anastomosis of the vein and provide a sufficiently good flow.

(4) Early (within 1 year) occlusion of about 20% of the grafts, often related to a relatively low blood flow at the time of the grafting.

(5) Progression of coronary disease postoperatively. Some patients are worse postoperatively, due in part to the so-called "coronary steal" syndrome and in part to the fact that progression of stenoses is greater in the proximal portion of bypassed arteries than in arteries that have been untouched.

(6) Late occlusion of bypass graft. If, in addition to progression of a partially stenosed artery, the graft applied distally to the stenosis becomes occluded, the patient is then worse off, develops more left ventricular dysfunction and more segmental contraction disorders, and may have more severe angina. In some patients, relief of angina is due to cutting of nerves or to the development of an acute myocardial infarction as a result of the surgery, as shown in patients who no longer have angina despite an occluded graft found on repeat coronary angiogram.

(7) Persistence of exercise-induced ventricular premature beats even when ventricular scars and ventricular aneurysms are resected.

(8) Decrease of collateral circulation which occurs after grafting and deterioration with respect to heart failure and chest pain over a period of years.

Factors Influencing Operative Results

The surgical results, including the operative deaths that occur, are influenced by the presence or absence of acute myocardial necrosis at surgery; by the presence of previous myocardial infarction with segmental abnormalities of left ventricular motion; by increased left ventricular end-diastolic volume and pressure, indicating left ventricular failure or decreased left ventricular compliance; by impaired left ventricular function, as manifested by various parameters of which a decreased ejection fraction is representative; and by the number of procedures performed at one operation (some may be combined). When end-diastolic volume is increased (especially if the patient has cardiac failure) or if the ejection fraction is less than 35%, operative treatment is less likely to result in improvement, and the operative mortality rate is higher. If the bypass procedure is done following a recent acute myocardial infarction, the operative mortality rate is higher than if it is done 2 or 3 months later, when the situation is stable. There is a progressively decreasing mortality rate if the bypass is done within the first week or later. The mortality rate stabilizes at about 30–60 days. As a result, elective surgery is usually delayed at least 2 months following an acute myocardial infarction.

A. Presence of Adverse Factors in Surgical Results: In an unselected group of patients, the greater the number of associated adverse factors, the higher the mortality rate and the less satisfactory the results in those who do not die. If one operates only on patients with excellent left ventricular function and incapacitating angina without a previous myocardial infarction or cardiac failure and if the angina is stable, without evidence of recent myocardial necrosis, the surgical mortality rate will be considerably decreased. If left ventricular wall motion is only slightly depressed, suggesting that it might be due to ischemia and not to an immobile scar, improvement in contractility often follows bypass surgery.

B. Prospective Studies Needed and in Progress: Prospective studies are under way in several centers to determine whether surgical bypass operations prolong life. *At present, there is no convincing evidence that myocardial infarction is prevented or survival prolonged by surgery except in the case of left main coronary artery lesions.* Intraoperative myocardial infarction can undoubtedly be provoked by the surgical procedure.

C. Interpretation of Surgical Results: One must be skeptical of surgical results that report annual mortality rates and incidences of new myocardial infarctions in their control groups which are twice as high as those reported previously from the Framingham and Albany Studies (Frank, 1973) in the days before coronary bypass surgery was being performed. The Framingham data (see p 122) showed an annual incidence of new myocardial infarctions in patients with stable angina of about 2–3% per year, and most of the published data show an average annual mortality rate of about 4% a year in nonoperated patients. The possible combinations of variables that affect results are so intricate that it is difficult to compare different published reports. A larger series—as is now under way in multicenter trials, with longer follow-up periods and with pre- and postoperative coronary angiograms and left ventricular function studies—will be required before the definitive role of coronary surgery can be fully assessed.

The problem is made more acute by the large numbers of patients with coronary disease, the desire of the physician to *do something* for a patient in fear of death at any moment, and the mass of media publicity that is enthusiastic about coronary surgery as a lifesaving procedure.

D. Identification of Anatomic Lesions That Threaten Sudden Death: More recent research has been directed toward identifying the anatomic lesions that are more apt to cause sudden death as a way of selecting patients in whom coronary surgery might be considered more urgent. For example, it is argued that the more proximal the lesion is in the left anterior descending artery in the presence of occlusion of the right coronary system, the greater the need for surgery. The same is said about the presence of severe stenosis of 2 of the 3 arteries, where survival of myocardium depends on patency of the third (remaining) artery. Not everyone agrees that stenosis of the left main coronary artery is an urgent indication for surgery, although intuitively it should be considered a dangerous lesion because of the large area of myocardium that would be jeopardized if the artery were to become completely stenosed—especially if the patient has had a previous inferior infarction. Severe stenosis of the left main coronary artery rarely occurs as an isolated finding and is usually associated with severe 3-vessel coronary disease, and it is probable that it is the severe 3-vessel disease as well as the stenosis of the left main coronary artery that accounts for the adverse clinical course in these patients.

E. Need for Skillful Heart Surgeon and Surgical Team: The availability of a skilled cardiac surgeon with a well-trained, efficient team and adequate diagnostic and therapeutic facilities is assumed in the comments above in which we recommend bypass surgery for incapacitating angina in patients with good left ventricular function. Coronary angiograms of high quality that identify areas of stenosis and give a reliable estimate of the size of the poststenotic distal branches and a clear picture of antegrade or collateral filling are essential in preparation for coronary bypass surgery. The presence of severe disease is not sufficient to justify surgery; the patient must also have vessels that can be bypassed. Similarly, left ventricular function must be good enough so that the patient can survive surgery and handle the depressed left ventricular function that occurs postoperatively. A poor ejection fraction, large left ventricular volume, and cardiac failure secondary to ischemic cardiomyopathy from coronary disease are contraindications to bypass surgery because the surgical mortality rate is high and the benefits almost nil.

Summary

It is generally agreed that coronary bypass surgery using the saphenous vein or the internal mammary artery is a major advance in the treatment of coronary disease and that there is substantial evidence of subjective relief of angina and some evidence of objective improvement following surgery. The surgical mortality rate in skilled hands is less than 3% in stable angina but higher in unstable angina, when associated procedures are performed at the same time, and when surgery is performed soon after an acute myocardial infarction. The operative results are best in stable angina with good left ventricular function and worst when there is ischemic cardiomyopathy with cardiac failure. Morbidity associated with surgery includes intraoperative myocardial infarction in 10–20% of patients and postoperative ventilatory, arrhythmic, infectious, and other complications. The pain and discomfort associated with recovery from surgery and the cost to the patient are also important considerations. The age and general condition of the patient, the presence of extensive vascular disease elsewhere, and the pulmonary, renal, and hepatic function all influence the morbidity and mortality rates of coronary surgery. Cerebrovascular lesions must be treated before bypass surgery is performed. The subsequent course includes closure of grafts in about 20% of patients and increased progression of stenosis in the proximal portion of the bypassed coronary arteries, which may leave the patient worse off if one of the bypass grafts becomes occluded.

The physician should keep an open mind regarding possible broadening of the indications for surgery to include unstable angina, resection of left ventricular aneurysms without bypass surgery, and the role of surgery in patients who have just suffered a myocardial infarction. The prospective clinical trials mentioned above, in conjunction with noninvasive physiologic pre- and postoperative measures such as isotope imaging, induced ischemia, and measurement of segmental "contractility" and left ventricular function, should help clarify the situation within the next few years.

• • •

References

Abbott JA, Tedeschi MA, Cheitlin MD: Graded treadmill stress testing-patterns of physician use and abuse. West J Med 126:173, 1977.

Adgey AAJ, Pantridge JF: The prehospital phase of treatment for myocardial infarction. Geriatrics 27:102, 1972.

Ahlmark G, Saetre H, Korsgren M: Reduction of sudden deaths after myocardial infarction. (Correspondence.) Lancet 2:1563, 1974.

Alderman EL & others: Dose response effectiveness of propranolol for the treatment of angina pectoris. Circulation 51:964, 1975.

Alonso DR & others: Pathophysiology of cardiogenic shock: Quantification of myocardial necrosis, clinical, pathologic and electrocardiographic correlations. Circulation 48:588, 1973.

Anderson WAD: *Pathology*, 6th ed. Mosby, 1971.

Apstein CS & others: Left ventricular performance and graft patency after coronary artery-saphenous vein bypass surgery: Early and late follow-up. Am Heart J 93:547, 1977.

Arbogast R, Solignac A, Bourassa MG: Influence of aortocoronary saphenous vein bypass surgery on left ventricular volumes and ejection fraction: Comparison before and one year after surgery in 51 patients. Am J Med 54:290, 1973.

Aspenstrom G & others: Collaborative analysis of long-term anticoagulant administration after acute myocardial infarction. Lancet 1:203, 1970.

Astrand P: Quantification of exercise capability and evaluation of physical capacity in man. Prog Cardiovasc Dis 19:51, 1976.

Atkins JM & others: Ventricular conduction blocks and sudden death in acute myocardial infarction. N Engl J Med 288:281, 1973.

Auerbach O & others: Smokers' heart. (Editorial.) Arch Intern Med 137:435, 1977.

Bailey IK & others: Thallium-201 myocardial perfusion imaging at rest and during exercise: Comparative sensitivity to electrocardiography in coronary artery disease. Circulation 55:79, 1977.

Barry WH & others: Effects of coronary artery bypass grafting on resting and exercise hemodynamics in patients with stable angina pectoris: A prospective, randomized study. Am J Cardiol 37:823, 1976.

Baxley WA, Reeves TJ: Abnormal regional myocardial performance in coronary artery disease. Prog Cardiovasc Dis 13:405, 1971.

Beller GA & others: Localization of radiolabeled cardiac myosin-specific antibody in myocardial infarcts: Comparison with technetium-99m stannous pyrophosphate. Circulation 55:74, 1977.

Bengtsson C: Ischaemic heart disease in women. Acta Med Scand, Suppl 549, 1973. [Entire issue.]

Biörck G: *Contrasting Concepts of Ischemic Heart Disease: The 1974 Lilly Lectures.* Almquist & Wiksell, 1975.

Bishop SP, White FC, Bloor CM: Regional myocardial blood flow during acute myocardial infarction in the conscious dog. Circ Res 38:429, 1976.

Blum CB, Havlik RJ, Morganroth J: Cholestyramine: An effective, twice-daily regimen. Ann Intern Med 85:287, 1976.

Blumgart HL, Schlesinger MJ, Davis D: Studies on the relation of the clinical manifestations of angina pectoris, coronary thrombosis, and myocardial infarction to the pathologic findings with particular reference to the significance of the collateral circulation. Am Heart J 19:1, 1940.

Blumgart HL, Zoll PM: Clinical pathologic correlations in coronary artery disease. Circulation 47:1139, 1973.

Blumgart HL, Zoll PM: Pathologic physiology of angina pectoris and acute myocardial infarction. Circulation 22:301, 1960.

Bodenheimer MM, Banka VS, Helfant RH: Q waves and ventricular asynergy: Predictive value and hemodynamic significance of anatomic localization. Am J Cardiol 35:615, 1975.

Borer JS & others: Real-time radionuclide cineangiography in the noninvasive evaluation of global and regional left ventricular function at rest and during exercise in patients with coronary-artery disease. N Engl J Med 296:839, 1977.

Botvinick EH & others: Noninvasive diagnosis of a false left ventricular aneurysm with radioisotope gated cardiac blood pool imaging: Differentiation from true aneurysm. Am J Cardiol 37:1089, 1976.

Botvinick EH & others: Noninvasive quantitation of myocardial infarction with technetium 99m pyrophosphate. Circulation 52:909, 1975.

Bourassa MG, Noble J: Complication rate of coronary arteriography: A review of 5250 cases studied by a percutaneous femoral technique. Circulation 53:106, 1976.

Brand RJ & others: Multivariate prediction of coronary heart disease in Western Collaborative Group Study compared to findings of Framingham Study. Circulation 53:348, 1976.

Bristow JD & others: Report of the Ad Hoc Committee on the Indications for Coronary Arteriography. Circulation 55:969A, 1977.

Brown MS, Goldstein JL: Familial hypercholesterolemia: A genetic defect in the low-density lipoprotein receptor. N Engl J Med 294:1386, 1976.

Brown MS, Goldstein JL: Familial hypercholesterolemia: Genetic, biochemical, and pathophysiological aspects. Adv Intern Med 20:273, 1975.

Bruce RA: Exercise testing for evaluation of ventricular function. N Engl J Med 296:671, 1977.

Bruce RA, Hornstein TR: Exercise stress testing in evaluation of patients with ischemic heart disease. Prog Cardiovasc Dis 11:371, 1969.

Bruschke AVG, Proudfit WL, Sones FM Jr: Clinical course of patients with normal, and slightly or moderately abnormal coronary arteriograms. Circulation 47:936, 1973.

Bulkley BH, Roberts WC: Atherosclerotic narrowing of the left main coronary artery: A necropsy analysis of 152 patients with fatal coronary heart disease and varying degrees of left main narrowing. Circulation 53:823, 1976.

Calvert A, Lown B, Gorlin R: Ventricular premature beats and anatomically defined coronary heart disease. Am J Cardiol 39:627, 1977.

Campbell RWF & others: Comparison of procainamide and mexiletine in prevention of ventricular arrhythmias after acute myocardial infarction. Lancet 1:1257, 1975.

Cannom DS, Levy W, Cohen LS: The short- and long-term prognosis of patients with transmural and nontransmural myocardial infarction. Am J Med 61:452, 1976.

Carlson LA, Bottiger LE: Ischaemic heart disease in relation to fasting values of plasma triglycerides and cholesterol: Stockholm prospective study. Lancet 1:865, 1972.

Castelli WP & others: Alcohol and blood lipids: The cooperative lipoprotein phenotyping study. Lancet 2:153, 1977.

Castelli WP & others: HDL cholesterol levels (HDLC) in coronary heart disease: A cooperative lipoprotein phenotyping study. Circulation 52 (Suppl 2):II–97, 1975.

Chaitman BR & others: Clinical, angiographic, and hemodynamic findings in patients with anomalous origin of the coronary arteries. Circulation 53:122, 1976.

Chatterjee K, Parmley WW: The role of vasodilator therapy in heart failure. Prog Cardiovasc Dis 19:301, 1977.

Chatterjee K, Swan HJC: Hemodynamic profile of acute myocardial infarction. Chapter 6 in: *Myocardial Infarction.* Corday E, Swan HJC (editors). Williams & Wilkins, 1973.

Chatterjee K & others: Abnormal regional metabolic and mechanical dysfunction in patients with ischemic heart disease: Improvement after successful regional revascularization by aorto-coronary bypass. Circulation 52:390, 1975.

Chatterjee K & others: Effects of vasodilator therapy for severe pump failure in acute myocardial infarction on short-term and late prognosis. Circulation 53:797, 1976.

Cheitlin MD & others: Correlation of "critical" left coronary artery lesions with positive submaximal exercise tests in patients with chest pain. Am Heart J 89:305, 1975.

Chiang BN & others: Predisposing factors in sudden cardiac death in Tecumseh, Michigan. Circulation 41:31, 1970.

Clausen JP: Circulatory adjustments to dynamic exercise and effect of physical training in normal subjects and in patients with coronary artery disease. Prog Cardiovasc Dis 18:459, 1976.

Cobb LA & others: Resuscitation from out-of-hospital ventricular fibrillation: 4 years follow-up. Circulation 52 (Suppl 3):III–223, 1975.

Coffee and cardiovascular disease. Med Lett Drugs Ther 19:65, 1977.

Cohn JN & others: Chronic vasodilator therapy in the management of cardiogenic shock and intractable left ventricular failure. Ann Intern Med 81:777, 1974.

Conti CR: Coronary arteriography. Circulation 55:227, 1977.

Conti CR & others: Unstable angina pectoris: Morbidity and mortality in 57 consecutive patients evaluated angiographically. Am J Cardiol 32:745, 1973.

Controlled trial of urokinase in myocardial infarction: A European collaborative study. Lancet 2:624, 1975.

Cooperman M & others: Survival and function after left ventricular aneurysmectomy. J Thorac Cardiovasc Surg 69:321, 1975.

Corbalan R, Verrier R, Lown B: Psychological stress and ventricular arrhythmias during myocardial infarction in the conscious dog. Am J Cardiol 34:692, 1974.

Coronary Drug Project Research Group: Clofibrate and niacin in coronary heart disease. JAMA 231:360, 1975.

Coronary Drug Project Research Group: Factors influencing long-term prognosis after recovery from myocardial infarction: Three-year figures of the coronary drug project. J Chronic Dis 27:267, 1974.

Cosby RS & others: Clinicoarteriographic correlations in angina pectoris with and without myocardial infarction. Am J Cardiol 30:472, 1972.

Crawford T, Dexter D, Teare RD: Coronary-artery pathology in sudden death from myocardial ischaemia. Lancet 1:181, 1961.

Cryer PE & others: Smoking, catecholamines, and coronary heart disease. Cardiovasc Med 2:471, 1977.

Dawber TR, Kannel WB: An epidemiologic study of heart disease: The Framingham Study. Nutr Rev 16:1, Jan 1958.

Dawber TR, Kannel WB, Gordon T: Coffee and cardiovascular disease: The Framingham Study. N Engl J Med 291:871, 1974.

Day W: Acute coronary care–A five year report. Am J Cardiol 21:252, 1968.

DeBusk RF, Harrison DC: The clinical spectrum of papillary muscle disease. N Engl J Med 281:1458, 1969.

DeSanctis RW, Block P, Hutter AM Jr: Tachyarrhythmias in myocardial infarction. Circulation 45:681, 1972.

De Soyza N & others: Association of accelerated idioventricular rhythm and paroxysmal ventricular tachycardia in acute myocardial infarction. Am J Cardiol 34:667, 1974.

Dodge HT: Angiographic evaluation of ventricular function. N Engl J Med 296:551, 1977.

Donaldson RM & others: Surgical treatment of postinfarction left ventricular aneurysm in 32 patients. Br Heart J 38:1223, 1976.

Doyle JT & others: Factors related to suddenness of death from coronary disease: Combined Albany-Framingham Studies. Am J Cardiol 37:1073, 1976.

Duguid JB: Thrombosis as a factor in the pathogenesis of coronary atherosclerosis. J Pathol 58:207, 1946.

Ehrich DA & others: The hemodynamic response to intraaortic balloon counterpulsation in patients with cardiogenic shock complicating acute myocardial infarction. Am Heart J 93:274, 1977.

Ekelund LG & others: Effects of the cardioselective beta-adrenergic receptor blocking agent metoprolol in angina pectoris: Subacute study with exercise tests. Br Heart J 38:155, 1976.

Ellestad MH, Wan KC: Predictive implications of stress testing: Follow-up of 2700 subjects after maximum treadmill stress testing. Circulation 51:363, 1975.

Epstein FH: The epidemiology of coronary heart disease: A review. J Chronic Dis 18:735, 1965.

Epstein SE & others: Angina pectoris: Pathophysiology, evaluation and treatment. Ann Intern Med 75:263, 1971.

Epstein SE & others: Early phase of acute myocardial infarction: Pharmacologic aspects of therapy. Ann Intern Med 78:918, 1973.

Erikssen J & others: False positive diagnostic tests and coronary angiographic findings in 105 presumably healthy males. Circulation 54:371, 1976.

Farquhar JW, Sokolow M: Response of serum lipids and lipoproteins of man to beta-sitosterol and safflower oil. Circulation 17:890, 1958.

Favaloro RG & others: Direct myocardial revascularization by saphenous vein graft. Ann Thorac Surg 10:97, 1970.

Folkow B: Role of sympathetic nervous system. Page 68 in: *Coronary Heart Disease and Physical Fitness.* Larson OA, Malmborg O (editors). Munksgaard, 1971.

Forrester JS, Diamond GA, Swan HJC: Correlative classification of clinical and hemodynamic function after acute myocardial infarction. Am J Cardiol 39:137, 1977.

Forrester JS & others: Medical therapy of acute myocardial infarction by application of hemodynamic subsets (2 parts.) N Engl J Med 295:135, 1404, 1976.

Frank CW, Weinblatt E, Shapiro S: Angina pectoris in men: Prognostic significance of selected medical factors. Circulation 47:509, 1973.

Fredrickson DS, Levy RI: Familial hyperlipoproteinemia. Pages 545–614 in: *The Metabolic Basis of Inherited Disease,* 3rd ed. Stanbury JB, Wyngaarten JB, Fredrickson DS (editors). McGraw-Hill, 1972.

Frick MH & others: Changes in native coronary arteries after coronary bypass surgery. Am J Cardiol 36:744, 1975.

Froelicher VF, Oberman A: Analysis of epidemiologic studies of physical inactivity as risk factor for coronary disease. Prog Cardiovasc Dis 15:41, 1972.

Froelicher VF & others: Value of exercise testing for screening man for latent coronary artery disease. Prog Cardiovasc Dis 18:265, 1976.

Fuster V & others: Arteriographic patterns early in the onset of the coronary syndromes. Br Heart J 37:1250, 1975.

Garcia MJ, Gordon T, McNamara PM: Morbidity and mortality in diabetics in a general population: Sixteen year follow-up experience in the Framingham study. Diabetes 19 (Suppl 1):375, 1970.

Gensini G & others: Natural history of coronary disease in patients with or without coronary bypass graft surgery. Circulation 50:11, 1974.

Ginks WR & others: Long-term prognosis after acute anterior infarction with atrioventricular block. Br Heart J 39:186, 1977.

Glass DC: Stress, behavior patterns, and coronary disease: The interaction between psychological and physiological variables indicates that attempts by Type A individuals to master uncontrollable stressful events may be associated with coronary heart disease. Am Sci 65:177, 1977.

Gofman JW, Young W, Tandy R: Ischemic heart disease, atherosclerosis and longevity. Circulation 34:679, 1966.

Gold HK & others: Refractory angina pectoris: Follow-up after intraaortic balloon pumping and surgery. Circulation 54 (Suppl 3):41, 1976.

Goldman MJ: *Principles of Clinical Electrocardiography,* 9th ed. Lange, 1976.

Goldschlager N, Selzer A, Cohn K: Treadmill stress tests as indicators of presence and severity of coronary artery disease. Ann Intern Med 85:277, 1976.

Goldstein JL: Genetic aspects of hyperlipidemia in coronary heart disease. Hosp Pract 8:53, Oct 1973.

Goldstein JL & others: Hyperlipidemia in coronary heart disease: Lipid levels in 500 survivors of myocardial infarction. J Clin Invest 52:1533, 1973.

Goldstein RE & others: Clinical and circulatory effects of isosorbide dinitrate. Circulation 43:629, 1971.

Gordon T & others: High density lipoprotein as a protective factor against coronary heart disease: The Framingham Study. Am J Med 62:707, 1977.

Gott VL: Outlook for patients after coronary artery revascularization. Am J Cardiol 33:431, 1974.

Gould LA & others: Clinical experience with technetium-99m stannous polyphosphate for myocardial imaging. Br Heart J 38:744, 1976.

Green KG & others: Improvement in prognosis of myocardial infarction by long-term beta-adrenoceptor blockade. Am Heart J 92:537, 1976.

Gregg DE: The natural history of coronary collateral development. Circ Res 35:335, 1974.

Hamby RI, Aintablian A, Schwartz A: Reappraisal of the functional significance of the coronary collateral circulation. Am J Cardiol 38:305, 1976.

Hamby RI & others: Left ventricular hemodynamics and contractile pattern after aortocoronary bypass surgery: Factors affecting reversibility of abnormal left ventricular function. Am Heart J 88:149, 1974.

Hamilton GW & others: Myocardial perfusion imaging with ^{99m}Tc or ^{113m}In macroaggregated albumin: Correlation of the perfusion image with clinical, angiographic, surgical, and histologic findings. Am Heart J 89:708, 1975.

Han J: Mechanisms of ventricular arrhythmias associated with myocardial infarction. Am J Cardiol 24:800, 1969.

Hancock EW: Aortic stenosis, angina pectoris, and coronary artery disease. Am Heart J 93:382, 1977.

Harker LA & others: Homocystine-induced arteriosclerosis: The role of endothelial cell injury and platelet response in its genesis. J Clin Invest 58:731, 1976.

Harlan WR & others: Chronic congestive heart failure in coronary artery disease: Clinical criteria. Ann Intern Med 86:133, 1977.

Harrison TR, Reeves TJ: *Principles and Problems of Ischemic Heart Disease.* Year Book, 1968.

Hatle L, Bathen J, Rokseth R: Sinoatrial disease in acute myocardial infarction: Long-term prognosis. Br Heart J 38:410, 1976.

Havel RJ: Classification of the hyperlipidemias. Annu Rev Med 28:195, 1977.

Havel RJ: Pathogenesis, differentiation and management of hypertriglyceridemia. Adv Intern Med 15:117, 1969.

Havel R, Goldstein J, Brown M: Lipoproteins and lipid transport. In: *Duncan's Diseases of Metabolism,* 8th ed. Bondy PK, Rosenberg LE (editors). Saunders, 1978. [In press.]

Heberden W: Some account of a disorder of the heart. Med Trans R Coll Physicians 2:59, 1768.

Heikkilä J: Mitral incompetence as a complication of acute myocardial infarction. Acta Med Scand 182 (Suppl 475):1, 1967. [Entire issue.]

Helfant RH, Banka VS, Bodenheimer MM: Left ventricular dysfunction in coronary heart disease: A dynamic problem. Cardiovasc Med 2:557, 1977.

Henning R, Torbjörn L: Swedish co-operative CCU study: A study of 2008 patients with acute myocardial infarction from twelve Swedish hospitals with coronary care unit. (Part 1.) Acta Med Scand (Suppl 586), 1975.

Herrick JB: Clinical features of sudden obstruction of the coronary arteries. JAMA 59:2015, 1912.

Hillis LD, Braunwald E: Myocardial ischemia. (3 parts.) N Engl J Med 296:971, 1034, 1093, 1977.

Hinkle LE, Carver ST, Argyros DC: The prognostic significance of ventricular premature contractions in healthy people and in people with coronary heart disease. Acta Cardiol (Suppl) 43:5, 1974.

Hoffman JIE, Buckberg GD: The pathophysiology of subendocardial ischemia. Br Med J 1:76, 1975.

Hultgren HN: Medical versus surgical treatment of unstable angina. Am J Cardiol 38:479, 1976.

Hultgren HN: The pathophysiology of subendocardial ischemia. Br Med J 1:76, 1975.

Hultgren HN & others: Unstable angina: Comparison of medical and surgical management. Am J Cardiol 39:734, 1977.

Humphries JO & others: Natural history of ischemic heart disease in relation to arteriographic findings: A twelve year study of 224 patients. Circulation 49:489, 1974.

Hutchins GM & others: Correlation of coronary arteriograms and left ventriculograms with postmortem studies. Circulation 56:32, 1977.

Hutter AM Jr: Early hospital discharge after myocardial infarction. N Engl J Med 288:1141, 1973.

Jackson G & others: Intra-aortic balloon assistance in cardiogenic shock after myocardial infarction or cardiac surgery. Br Heart J 39:598, 1977.

James TN: *Anatomy of the Coronary Arteries.* Hoeber, 1961.

James TN: Arrhythmias and conduction disturbances in acute myocardial infarction. Am Heart J 64:416, 1962.

James TN: The coronary circulation and conduction system in acute myocardial infarction. Prog Cardiovasc Dis 10:410, 1968.

James TN: Sudden death related to myocardial infarction. Circulation 45:205, 1972.

Jelinek MV, Lohrbauer L, Lown B: Antiarrhythmic drug therapy for sporadic ventricular ectopic arrhythmias. Circulation 49:659, 1974.

Jenkins CD: Recent evidence supporting psychologic and social risk factors for coronary disease. (2 parts.) N Engl J Med 294:987, 1033, 1976.

Johnson SA & others: Treatment of cardiogenic shock in myocardial infarction by intraaortic balloon counterpulsation and surgery. Am J Med 62:687, 1977.

Jude JR, Kouwenhoven WB, Knickerbocker GG: Cardiac arrest. JAMA 178:1063, 1961.

Judkins MP, Gander MP: Prevention of complications of coronary arteriography. Circulation 39:599, 1974.

Kannel WB: Some lessons in cardiovascular epidemiology from Framingham. Am J Cardiol 37:269, 1976.

Kannel WB, Feinleib M: Natural history of angina pectoris in the Framingham Study: Prognosis and treatment. Am J Cardiol 29:154, 1972.

Kannel WB, McGee D, Gordon T: A general cardiovascular risk profile: The Framingham Study. Am J Cardiol 38:46, 1976.

Kannel WB & others: Precursors of sudden coronary death: Factors related to the incidence of sudden death. Circulation 51:606, 1975.

Khachadurian AK: The inheritance of essential familial hypercholesterolemia. Am J Med 37:402, 1964.

Khaw BA & others: Localization of cardiac myosin-specific antibody in myocardial infarction. J Clin Invest 58:439, 1976.

Killip T: Arrhythmias in myocardial infarction. Med Clin North Am 60:233, 1976.

Kirklin JW, Rastelli GC: Low cardiac output after open-heart intracardiac operations. Prog Cardiovasc Dis 10:117, 1967.

Knoebel SB & others: Nonparoxysmal junction tachycardia in acute myocardial infarction: Computer-assisted detection. Am J Cardiol 35:824, 1975.

Kosowsky BD & others: Long-term use of procaineamide following acute myocardial infarction. Circulation 47:1204, 1973.

Kostuk W & others: Correlations between the chest film and hemodynamics in acute myocardial infarction. Circulation 48:624, 1973.

Kouchoukos NT, Kirklin JW, Oberman A: An appraisal of coronary bypass grafting: The Sixth Annual George C. Griffith Lecture. Circulation 50:11, 1974.

Lefkowitz RJ: Smoking, catecholamines, and the heart. N Engl J Med 295:615, 1976.

Leren P: The effect of plasma cholesterol lowering diet in male survivors of myocardial infarction: A controlled clinical trial. Acta Med Scand Suppl 466, 1966.

Levine SA: *Clinical Heart Disease,* 5th ed. Saunders, 1958.

Levine SA: Coronary thrombosis: Its various clinical features. Medicine 8:245, 1929.

Levy RI: Drug therapy of hyperlipoproteinemia. JAMA 235:2334, 1976.

Levy RI & others: Dietary and drug treatment of primary hyperlipoproteinemia. Ann Intern Med 77:267, 1972.

Liberthson RR & others: Atrial tachyarrhythmias in acute myocardial infarction. Am J Med 60:956, 1976.

Lie JT, Titus JL: Pathology of the myocardium and the conduction system in sudden coronary death. Circulation 52 (Suppl 3):41, 1975.

Lie KI & others: Factors influencing prognosis of bundle branch block complicating acute antero-septal infarction: The value of His bundle recordings. Circulation 50:935, 1974.

Lie KI & others: Observations on patients with primary ventricular fibrillation complicating acute myocardial infarction. Circulation 52:755, 1975.

Lim JS, Proudfit WL, Sones FM: Left main coronary arterial obstruction: Long-term follow-up of 141 nonsurgical cases. Am J Cardiol 36:131, 1975.

Littler WA, Honour AJ, Sleight P: Direct arterial pressure and electrocardiogram during motor car driving. Br Med J 2:273, 1973.

Lober PH: Pathogenesis of coronary sclerosis. Arch Pathol 55:357, 1953.

Lown B, Graboys TB: Sudden death: An ancient problem newly perceived. Cardiovasc Med 2:219, 1977.

Lown B, Klein MD, Hershberg PI: Coronary and precoronary care. Am J Med 46:705, 1969.

Lown B & others: Basis for recurring ventricular fibrillation in the absence of coronary heart disease and its management. N Engl J Med 294:623, 1976.

Lown B & others: Sleep and ventricular premature beats. Circulation 48:691, 1973.

Madias JE, Gorlin R: The myth of acute "mild" myocardial infarction. Ann Intern Med 86:347, 1977.

Manley JC, Johnson WD: Effects of surgery on angina (pre- and post-infarction) and myocardial function (failure). Circulation 46:1208, 1972.

Mann JI, Thorogood M: Serum lipids in young female survivors of myocardial infarction. Br Heart J 37:790, 1975.

Marx JL: Blood clotting: The role of the prostaglandins. Science 196:1072, 1977.

Master AM: The Master two-step test. Am Heart J 75:809, 1968.

Maurer BJ & others: Changes in grafted and non-grafted coronary arteries following saphenous vein bypass grafting. Circulation 50:293, 1974.

McAlpine WA: *Heart and Coronary Arteries: An Anatomical Atlas for Clinical Diagnosis, Radiological Investigation, and Surgical Treatment.* Springer-Verlag, 1975.

McCans JL, Parker JO: Left ventricular pressure-volume relationships during myocardial ischemia in man. Circulation 48:775, 1973.

McLaughlin PR & others: Reproducibility of thallium-201 myocardial imaging. Circulation 55:497, 1977.

Meister SG & others: Sustained haemodynamic action of nitroglycerin ointment. Br Heart J 38:1031, 1976.

Meyer SL & others: Influence of dobutamine on hemodynamics and coronary blood flow in patients with and without coronary artery disease. Am J Cardiol 38:103, 1976.

Miller GJ, Miller NE: Plasma high density lipoprotein concentration and development of ischemic heart disease. Lancet 1:16, 1975.

Moncada S & others: An enzyme isolated from arteries transforms prostaglandin endoperoxides to an unstable substance that inhibits platelet aggregation. Nature 263:663, 1976.

Moraski RE & others: Left ventricular function in patients with and without myocardial infarction and one, two or three vessel coronary artery disease. Am J Cardiol 35:1, 1975.

Morgan-Jones A: The nature of the coronary problem. Br Heart J 32:583, 1970.

Morris DC, Hurst JW, Logue RB: Myocardial infarction in young women. Am J Cardiol 38:299, 1976.

Moss AJ & others: Clinical significance of ventricular ectopic beats in the early posthospital phase of myocardial infarction. Am J Cardiol 39:635, 1977.

Mudge GH Jr & others: Reflex increase in coronary vascular resistance in patients with ischemic heart disease. N Engl J Med 295:1333, 1976.

Mullins CB, Atkins JM: Prognoses and management of ventricular conduction: Blocks in acute myocardial infarction.

Mod Concepts Cardiovasc Dis 45:129, 1976.

Multicentre International Study: Improvement in prognosis of myocardial infarction by long-term beta-adrenoreceptor blockade using practolol. Br Med J 3:735, 1975.

Murray RG & others: Relation between extent of coronary artery disease and severity of hyperlipoproteinaemia. Br Heart J 37:1205, 1975.

Myerburg RJ, Conde C, Briese FR: Antiarrhythmic therapy in survivors of unexpected cardiac arrest in the community: Initial one-year experience. (Presented at the Association of University Cardiologists, Phoenix, Jan 1977.)

Myers A, Dewar HA: Circumstances attending 100 sudden deaths from coronary artery disease with coroner's necropsies. Br Heart J 37:1133, 1975.

Nelson GR, Cohn PF, Gorlin R: Prognosis in medically treated coronary artery disease: Influence of ejection fraction compared to other parameters. Circulation 52:408, 1975.

Nimetz AA & others: The significance of bundle branch block during acute myocardial infarction. Am Heart J 90:439, 1975.

Noakes TD, Opie LH: The cardiovascular risks and benefits of exercise. Practitioner 216:288, 1976.

Norris RM: Arrhythmias in acute myocardial infarction. In: *Symposium on Cardiac Arrhythmias, Elsinore, Denmark, 1970.* Sandøe E, Flensted-Jensen E, Olesen KH (editors). AB Astra Södertälje, 1971.

Norris RM, Mercer CJ: Significance of idioventricular rhythms in acute myocardial infarction. Prog Cardiovasc Dis 16:455, 1974.

Norris RM & others: Coronary prognostic index for predicting survival after recovery from acute myocardial infarction. Lancet 2:485, 1970.

Norris RM & others: Prognosis after myocardial infarction. Br Heart J 36:786, 1974.

Oberman A & others: Natural history of coronary artery disease. Bull NY Acad Med 48:1109, 1972.

Oberman A & others: Sudden death in patients evaluated for ischemic heart disease. Circulation 52 (Suppl 3):170, 1975.

Oberman A & others: Surgical versus medical treatment in disease of the left main coronary artery. Lancet 2:591, 1976.

Oliver MF: Problems in the presymptomatic diagnosis of ischaemic heart disease. Page 46 in: *Modern Trends in Cardiology–2.* Jones AM (editor). Butterworth, 1969.

Olsson AG: Signs of coronary atherosclerosis in apparently healthy men with different types of hyperlipoproteinemia. Postgrad Med J 51 (Suppl 8):40, 1975.

Pantridge JF & others: *The Acute Coronary Attack.* Pages 27–42. Grune & Stratton, 1975.

Pantridge JF & others: The first hour after the onset of acute myocardial infarction. Page 173 in: *Progress in Cardiology 3.* Yu PN, Goodwin JF (editors). Lea & Febiger, 1974.

Parker JO & others: Effect of nitroglycerin ointment on the clinical and hemodynamic response to exercise. Am J Cardiol 38:162, 1976.

Parkey RW & others: Analysis of ^{99m}Tc stannous pyrophosphate myocardial scintigrams in 242 patients. J Nucl Med 16:556, 1975.

Parmley WW & others: Hemodynamic effects of noninvasive systolic unloading (nitroprusside) and diastolic augmentation (external counterpulsation) in patients with acute myocardial infarction. Am J Cardiol 33:819, 1974.

Patterson D, Slack J: Lipid abnormalities in male and female survivors of myocardial infarction and their first-degree relatives. Lancet 1:393, 1972.

Pedoe HT & others: Coronary heart-attacks in East London. Lancet 2:833, 1975.

Peel AA & others: A coronary prognostic index for grading the severity of infarction. Br Heart J 24:745, 1962.

Pell S, D'Alonzo CA: Immediate mortality and 5-year survival of employed men with first myocardial infarction. N Engl J Med 270:915, 1964.

Perry LW, Scott LP: Anomalous left coronary artery from pulmonary artery: Report of 11 cases; review of indications for and results of surgery. Circulation 41:1043, 1970.

Pitt B, Strauss HW: Evaluation of ventricular function by radioisotopic technics. N Engl J Med 296:1097, 1977.

Powell WJ & others: The protective effect of hyperosmotic mannitol in myocardial ischemia and necrosis. Circulation 54:603, 1976.

Prevention of coronary disease: Summary of the report of a Joint Working Party of the Royal College of Physicians of London and the British Cardiac Society on Prevention of Coronary Disease. Br Med J 1:881, 1976.

Pridie RB & others: Coronary angiography: Review of 1500 consecutive cases. Br Heart J 38:1200, 1976.

Prinzmetal M & others: Angina pectoris. 1. A variant form of angina pectoris. Am J Med 26:375, 1959.

Proger SH, Ayman D: Harmful effects of nitroglycerin: With special reference to coronary thrombosis. Am J Med Sci 184:480, 1932.

Ratshin RA, Massing GK, James TN: The clinical significance of the location of acute myocardial infarction. Chapter 9 in: *Myocardial Infarction.* Corday E, Swan HJC (editors). Williams & Wilkins, 1973.

Reeves TJ & others: Natural history of angina pectoris. Am J Cardiol 33:423, 1974.

Reid DD & others: Smoking and other risk factors for coronary heart-disease in British civil servants. Lancet 2:979, 1976.

Resnekov L: The intermediate coronary care unit: A stage in continued coronary care. Br Heart J 39:357, 1977.

Ridolfi RL, Hutchins GM: The relationship between coronary artery lesions and myocardial infarcts: Ulceration of atherosclerotic plaques precipitating coronary thrombosis. Am Heart J 93:468, 1977.

Rigo P & others: Hemodynamic and prognostic findings in patients with transmural and nontransmural infarction. Circulation 51:1064, 1975.

Riseman JEF: The clinical course of angina pectoris. Am J Med 252:146, 1966.

Ritchie JL & others: Myocardial imaging with thallium-201 at rest and during exercise: Comparison with coronary arteriography and resting and stress electrocardiography. Circulation 56:66, 1977.

Ritter WS & others: Permanent pacing in patients with transient trifascicular block during acute myocardial infarction. Am J Cardiol 38:207, 1976.

Robb GP, Seltzer F: Appraisal of the double two-step exercise test: A long-term follow-up study of 3325 men. JAMA 234:722, 1975.

Robbins SL, Angell M: *Basic Pathology,* 2nd ed. Saunders, 1976.

Robb-Smith AHT: *The Enigma of Coronary Heart Disease.* Lloyd-Luke, 1967.

Roberts WC: Coronary heart disease: A review of abnormalities observed in the coronary arteries. Cardiovasc Med 2:29, 1977.

Roberts WC: Pathology of acute myocardial infarction. Hosp Pract 6:89, Dec 1971.

Roberts WC, Buja LM: The frequency and significance of coronary arterial thrombi and other observations in fatal acute myocardial infarction: A study of 107 necropsy patients. Am J Med 52:425, 1972.

Rokseth R, Hatle L: Sinus arrest in acute myocardial infarction. Br Heart J 33:639, 1971.

Rosenblatt A, Selzer A: The nature and clinical features of myocardial infarction with normal coronary arteriogram. Circulation 55:578, 1977.

Rosenman RH & others: Multivariate prediction of coronary heart disease during 8.5 years follow-up in the Western Collaborative Group Study. Am J Cardiol 37:903, 1976.

Ross J Jr: Hemodynamic changes in acute myocardial infarction. Hosp Pract 7:125, March 1972.

Ross R, Glomset JA: The pathogenesis of atherosclerosis. (Part 1.) N Engl J Med 295:369, 1976.

Ross RS: The case for prevention of coronary heart disease. Circulation 51:1, 1975.

Rotman M, Wagner GS, Wallace AG: Bradyarrhythmias in acute myocardial infarction. Circulation 45:703, 1972.

Ryan M, Lown B, Horn H: Comparison of ventricular ectopic activity during 24-hour monitoring and exercise testing in patients with coronary heart disease. N Engl J Med 292:224, 1975.

Salel AF & others: Accuracy of coronary profile: Correlation of arteriography with risk factors. N Engl J Med 296:1447, 1977.

Sampson JJ, Cheitlin MD: Pathophysiology and differential diagnosis of cardiac pain. Prog Cardiovasc Dis 13:507, 1971.

Sampson JJ, Eliaser M Jr: The diagnosis of impending acute coronary artery occlusion. Am Heart J 13:675, 1937.

Sanders CA & others: Mechanical circulatory assistance: Current status and experience with combining circulatory assistance, emergency coronary angiography, and acute myocardial revascularization. Circulation 43:1292, 1972.

Schaper W: *The Collateral Circulation of the Heart.* North-Holland Publishing Co., 1971.

Scheidt W, Wolk M, Killip T: Unstable angina pectoris: Natural history, hemodynamics, uncertainties of treatment and the ethics of clinical study. Am J Med 60:409, 1976.

Scheinman MM, Abbott JA: Clinical significance of transmural versus nontransmural electrocardiographic changes in patients with acute myocardial infarction. Am J Med 55:602, 1973.

Scheinman MM, Brenman BA: Clinical and anatomical implications of intraventricular conduction blocks in acute myocardial infarction. Circulation 46:753, 1972.

Schelbert HR & others: Serial measurements of left ventricular ejection fraction by radionuclide angiography early and late after myocardial infarction. Am J Cardiol 38:407, 1976.

Schulze RA Jr & others: Left ventricular and coronary angiographic anatomy: Relationship to ventricular irritability in the late hospital phase of acute myocardial infarction. Circulation 55:839, 1977.

Schroeder JS & others: Coronary bypass surgery for unstable angina pectoris: Long-term survival and function. JAMA 237:2609, 1977.

Schwartz JN & others: Comparison of angiographic and postmortem findings in patients with coronary artery disease. Am J Cardiol 36:174, 1975.

Selzer A, Gerbode F, Kerth WJ: Clinical, hemodynamic and surgical considerations of rupture of the ventricular septum after myocardial infarction. Am Heart J 78:598, 1969.

Shapter RK & others: Cardiopulmonary resuscitation: Basic life support. Ciba Clin Symp 26:5, 1974.

Sheffield LT, Roitman D: Stress testing methodology. Prog Cardiovasc Dis 19:33, 1976.

Sheldon WC & others: Surgical treatment of coronary artery disease: Pure graft operations, with a study of 741 patients followed 3–7 years. Prog Cardiovasc Dis 18:237, 1975.

Singh BN, Vaughan Williams EM: The effect of amiodarone, a new antianginal drug, on cardiac muscle. Br J Pharmacol 39:657, 1970.

Slack J: Risk factors in coronary heart disease. Lancet 1:366, 1977.

Slack J: Risks of ischaemic heart-disease in familial hyperlipoproteinaemic states. Lancet 2:1380, 1969.

Slack J, Nevin NC: Hyperlipidaemic xanthomatoses. 1. Increased risk of death from ischaemic heart disease in first degree relatives of 53 patients with essential hyperlipidaemia and xanthomatosis. J Med Genet 5:4, 1968.

Smirk FH: R waves interrupting T waves. Br Heart J 11:23, 1949.

Snow PJ & others: Coronary disease: A pathological study. Br Heart J 17:503, 1955.

Sobel BE & others: Detection of remote myocardial infarction in patients with positron emission transaxial tomography and intravenous ^{11}C-palmitate. Circulation 55:853, 1977.

Solomon H, Edwards A, Killip T: Prodromata in acute myocardial infarction. Circulation 40:463, 1969.

Sones FM Jr: Indications and value of coronary arteriography. Circulation 46:1155, 1972.

Soto B, Russell RO Jr, Moraski RE: *Radiographic Anatomy of the Coronary Arteries: An Atlas.* Futura, 1976.

Sowton E: Pacemaking in acute myocardial infarction. In: *Proceedings of the Symposium on Cardiac Pacing and Cardioversion.* Charles Press, 1967.

Spain DM, Bradess VA, Mohr C: Coronary atherosclerosis as a cause of unexpected and unexplained death. JAMA 174:384, 1960.

Stamler J: Sudden coronary death: Approaches to its prevention. Med Clin North Am 60:245, 1976.

Steele RJ, Burggraf GW, Parker JO: Effects of isosorbide dinitrate on the response to atrial pacing in coronary heart disease. Am J Cardiol 36:206, 1975.

Stephens MR & others: The clinical features and significance of bifascicular block complicating acute myocardial infarction. Eur J Cardiol 3:289, 1975.

Stephenson HE Jr (editor): *Cardiac Arrest and Resuscitation.* Mosby, 1974.

Stiles QR & others: Long-term follow-up of patients with coronary artery bypass grafts. Circulation 54 (Suppl 3):32, 1976.

Stone NJ & others: Coronary artery disease in 116 kindred with familial type II hyperlipoproteinemia. Circulation 49:476, 1974.

Swan HJC & others: Catheterization of the heart in man with use of a flow-directed balloon-tipped catheter. N Engl J Med 283:447, 1970.

Swan HJC & others: Hemodynamic spectrum of myocardial infarction and cardiogenic shock: A conceptual model. Circulation 45:1097, 1972.

Takaro T & others: The Veterans Administration Cooperative Randomized Study of Surgery for Coronary Arterial Occlusive Disease. 2. Subgroup with significant left main lesions. Circulation 54 (Suppl 3):107, 1976.

Talano JV & others: Influence of surgery on survival in 145 patients with left main coronary artery disease. Circulation 51 (Suppl 1):105, 1975.

Tans AC, Lie KI: Clinical setting and prognostic significance of high degree atrioventricular block in acute inferior myocardial infarction. Am J Cardiol 37:176, 1976.

Thomson PD, Kelemen MH: Hypotension accompanying the onset of exertional angina: A sign of severe compromise of left ventricular blood supply. Circulation 52:28, 1975.

Turner R, Ball K: The cardiologist's responsibility for preventing coronary heart disease. Am Heart J 91:139, 1976.

Ullyot DJ & others: Improved survival after coronary artery surgery in patients with extensive coronary artery disease. J Thorac Cardiovasc Surg 70:405, 1975.

Vedin JA, Wilhelmsson C, Werkö L: Chronic alprenolol treatment of patients with acute myocardial infarction after discharge from hospital: Effects on mortality and morbidity. Acta Med Scand Suppl 575, 1975. [Entire issue.]

Veterans Administration Cooperative Group for the Study of Surgery for Coronary Arterial Occlusive Disease: Veterans Administration cooperative study of surgery for coronary arterial occlusive disease. 3. Methods and baseline characteristics, including experience with medical treatment. Am J Cardiol 40:212, 1977.

Veterans Administration Cooperative Study Group on Antihypertensive Agents: Effects of treatment on morbidity in hypertension. 2. Results in patients with diastolic blood pressure averaging 90 through 114 mm Hg. JAMA 213:1143, 1970.

Vlietstra RE & others: Survival predictors in coronary artery artery disease: Medical and surgical comparisons. Mayo Clin Proc 52:85, 1977.

Vlodaver Z & others: *Coronary Heart Disease: Clinical, Angiographic, and Pathologic Profiles.* Springer-Verlag, 1976.

Wackers FJT & others: Location and size of acute transmural myocardial infarction estimated from thallium-201 scintiscans: A clinicopathological study. Circulation 56:72, 1977.

Wallace WA, Napodano RJ, Yu PN: Early care of acute myocardial infarction. Arch Intern Med 136:974, 1976.

Walsh WF & others: Noninvasive evaluation of regional myocardial perfusion in 112 patients using a mobile scintillation camera and intravenous nitrogen-13 labeled ammonia. Circulation 54:266, 1976.

Watson LE, Dickhaus DW, Martin RH: Left ventricular aneurysms: Preoperative hemodynamics, chamber volume, and results of aneurysmectomy. Circulation 52:868, 1975.

Weaver WD & others: Angiographic findings and prognostic indicators in patients resuscitated from sudden cardiac death. Circulation 54:895, 1976.

Weinblatt E & others: Prognostic factors in angina pectoris: A prospective study. J Chronic Dis 21:231, 1968.

Weinsier RL & others: Body fat: Its relationship to coronary heart disease, blood pressure, lipids and other risk factors measured in a large male population. Am J Med 61:815, 1976.

Wellens HJJ, Lie KI, Durrer D: Further observations on ventricular tachycardia as studied by electrical stimulation of the heart: Chronic recurrent ventricular tachycardia and ventricular tachycardia during acute myocardial infarction. Circulation 49:647, 1974.

Wenger NK: Exercise for the coronary patient. Cardiovasc Med 2:69, 1977.

Wenger NK, Bauer S: Coronary embolism: Review of literature and presentation of fifteen cases. Am J Med 25:549, 1958.

Werkö L: Risk factors and coronary heart disease: Facts or fancy? Am Heart J 91:87, 1976.

Whalen RE, Ramo BW, Wallace AG: The value and limitations of coronary care monitoring. Prog Cardiovasc Dis 13:422, 1971.

White PD: The historical background of angina pectoris. Mod Concepts Cardiovasc Dis 43:109, 1974.

Wilhelmsson C & others: Reduction of sudden deaths after myocardial infarction by treatment with alprenolol. Lancet 2:1157, 1974.

Willerson JT & others: Acute subendocardial myocardial infarction in patients: Its detection by Technetium 99-m stannous pyrophosphate myocardial scintigrams. Circulation 51:436, 1975.

Willerson JT & others: Improvement in myocardial function and coronary blood flow in ischemic myocardium after mannitol. J Clin Invest 51:2989, 1972.

Winkle RA & others: Treatment of recurrent symptomatic ventricular tachycardia. Ann Intern Med 85:1, 1976.

Wit AL, Bigger JT Jr: Possible electrophysiological mechanisms for lethal arrhythmias accompanying myocardial ischemia and infarction. Circulation 52:96, 1975.

Wolf S: Psychosocial forces in myocardial infarction and sudden death. Circulation 40 (Suppl 4):IV–74, 1969.

Yatteau RF & others: Ischemic cardiomyopathy: The myopathy of coronary artery disease: Natural history and results of medical versus surgical treatment. Am J Cardiol 34:520, 1974.

Zir LM & others: Interobserver variability in coronary angiography. Circulation 53:627, 1976.

9 . . .
Systemic Hypertension

I. ESSENTIAL HYPERTENSION

INTRODUCTION & BRIEF HISTORY

Measurement of Blood Pressure Before the Modern Era

Hypertension is a 20th century disease only because measurement of the arterial blood pressure became conveniently possible when Scipione Riva-Rocci (1863–1937) perfected an early version of the modern sphygmomanometer in 1896. Stephen Hales, an English clergyman, was the first to measure blood pressure directly—in a mare, in 1733—and investigators utilizing mercury manometers had measured blood pressure in various ways in the 19th century. Richard Bright (1789–1858), during the course of his classic studies of the disease that bears his name, concluded that the thick left ventricle, dilated aorta, and arterial disease could be due to increased resistance to the flow of blood in the blood vessels, but Bright had no method of measuring blood pressure.

Early Sphygmomanometers

At the turn of the century, Recklinghausen noted the falsely high levels of blood pressure (especially in the obese) that could be obtained with narrow cuffs such as those used by Riva-Rocci; the standard 12.5 cm cuff used today owes its origin to Recklinghausen's research. Korotkoff in 1905 described the 5 sounds heard over the brachial artery, distal to the cuff, as the pressure in the sphygmomanometer is reduced: *Phase I,* the abrupt sharp sound as the pressure is reduced to just below systolic pressure. *Phase II,* a prolonged, louder murmuring sound. *Phase III,* a loud clear sound with only a slight murmur. *Phase IV,* an abrupt muffling of sounds, thought by some to represent the diastolic pressure. *Phase V,* the total disappearance of sounds, used usually in the USA to reflect the diastolic pressure.

Mahomed (about 1879) was the first to demonstrate that renal and cardiac diseases were complications of hypertension in some patients (and not the reverse, as had been suggested by Bright and by Allbutt).

Early Investigations Relating Blood Pressure to Organ Changes

In the USA, Janeway in 1913 was one of the first to emphasize the importance of blood pressure in prognosis, particularly with respect to cardiac failure, renal failure, and stroke. Volhard and Fahr in 1914 clearly differentiated benign from malignant hypertension, describing the rapid downhill course and diffuse necrotizing arteriolitis in the malignant phase. The examination of the retina as a "mirror" in which to observe the arteriolar changes in hypertension by Moore in 1916 and Gunn in 1928 was a major development; but the close relationship of fundal changes to prognosis was clarified by Keith, Wagener, and Barker, who in 1939 summarized a decade of work and classified the retinal changes into 4 grades of increasing severity (described in detail on pp 209–210). They sharply distinguished the prognosis of grade I and grade II (benign) from grade III and grade IV (malignant) hypertension. The pathologic studies of Clawson and Bell demonstrated the adverse effects of hypertension on the heart, brain, and kidney. Actuarial studies by life insurance companies, especially the major studies of 1939 and 1959, showed the significance of slight increases in either systolic or diastolic pressure, especially in young people. Many more studies (including those of Stamler, 1967; and Kannel, 1974) in the past 20 or 30 years indicate that hypertension is one of the most important diseases in Western civilization and the single most important risk factor in the pathogenesis of cardiovascular disease.

Etiology & Classification of Hypertension

A. Primary (Essential) Hypertension: Hypertension of undetermined cause.

B. Secondary Hypertension: Hypertension due to—

1. Renal disease—
   a. Renal arterial disease (renal artery stenosis due to atherosclerosis or fibromuscular hyperplasia), aneurysm, embolism, and infarction.
   b. Renal parenchymal disease (acute or chronic glomerulonephritis, pyelonephritis, polycystic kidney, tuberculosis of the kidney, pericapsular hemorrhage, and subsequent scarring from trauma).

c. Renal tumors (Wilms's tumor, renin-producing tumors).
d. Arteritis (polyarteritis nodosa, neurofibromatosis, and nonspecific).
2. Endocrine disorders–
a. Cushing's syndrome.
b. Acromegaly.
c. Primary aldosteronism.
d. Pheochromocytoma.
e. Desoxycorticosterone acetate and salt administration.
3. Coarctation of the aorta.
4. Enzymatic defects–
a. Adrenogenital syndromes–Biglieri's syndrome with enzymatic defects of 11β-hydroxylation and resulting virilism.
b. Enzymatic defect of 17β-hydroxylation leading to amenorrhea from overproduction of cortisol precursors.
5. Neurologic disorders–
a. Increased intracranial pressure from brain tumors or cardiovascular accident.
6. Drug-induced hypertension–
a. Prolonged administration of corticosteroids.
b. Excessive use of desoxycorticosterone and salts of 5α-fluoro compounds in the treatment of postural hypotension.
c. The use of amphetamines or excessive thyroxine.
d. Chronic licorice ingestion, producing pseudoaldosteronism.
e. Oral contraceptive agents.
7. Hypercalcemia from any cause.
8. Neurogenic, possibly psychogenic.
9. Deficiency of vasodilating tissue enzymes (speculative) (prostaglandins, bradykinin, renal medullary tissue).

Antihypertensive Drugs

The introduction of ganglionic blocking agents such as hexamethonium for the treatment of severe hypertension in 1950 was the beginning of a new era in the management of hypertension and showed for the first time that blood pressure could be lowered safely, that the elevated pressure was not essential for adequate perfusion of vital organs (as had been supposed), and that the dire consequences of the hypertension, such as the malignant phase, could be reversed or prevented. Rapid advances in the development and availability of various therapeutic agents have occurred in the last 25 years, and we now have many hypertensive drugs that act in various ways to control raised arterial pressure.

PATHOPHYSIOLOGY OF HYPERTENSION

Mean arterial pressure is the product of the systemic vascular resistance and the mean cardiac output. As a result, either an increase in cardiac output or an increase in systemic vascular resistance—or both—can raise the blood pressure; both factors in this relationship are constantly changing throughout the course of a day. Blood pressure is not a static physiologic feature but a variable one in all individuals, both normal and hypertensive, from one occasion of measurement to another. This variability of the blood pressure must be borne in mind so that a diagnosis of hypertension will not be made on the basis of an isolated reading. (See discussion of ambulatory recording, p 207.)

FACTORS IN MAINTAINING NORMAL BLOOD PRESSURE

Normal blood pressure is maintained by complex mechanisms made up of many interacting regulatory forces acting on cardiac output and peripheral resistance. Hypertension is due to abnormalities of these mechanisms of physiologic regulation.

The Arterial Pressure Drop

As one proceeds along the cardiovascular system from the cardiac "pump" to the capacitance vessels (the veins), the arterial pressure drop is greatest at the precapillary resistance vessels (the arterioles); it is chiefly the caliber of these vessels that controls the systemic vascular resistance (Fig 9–1).

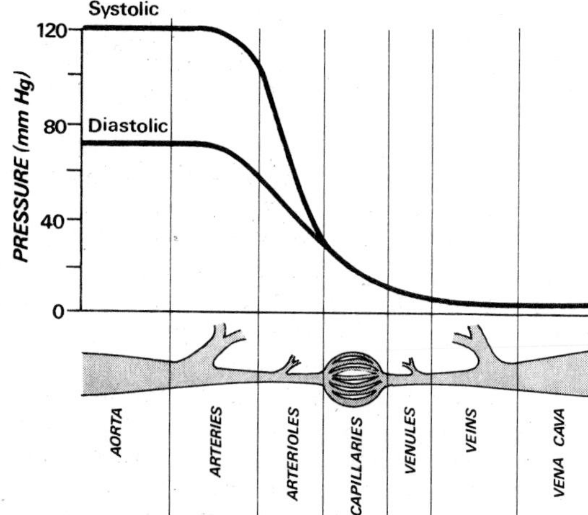

Figure 9–1. Diagram of the changes in pressure as blood flows through the systemic circulation. (Modified and reproduced, with permission, from Ganong WF: *Review of Medical Physiology,* 8th ed. Lange, 1977.)

Table 9–1. Factors contributing to increases in systolic and diastolic blood pressure. Mean arterial pressure = Cardiac output X Systemic arterial resistance.

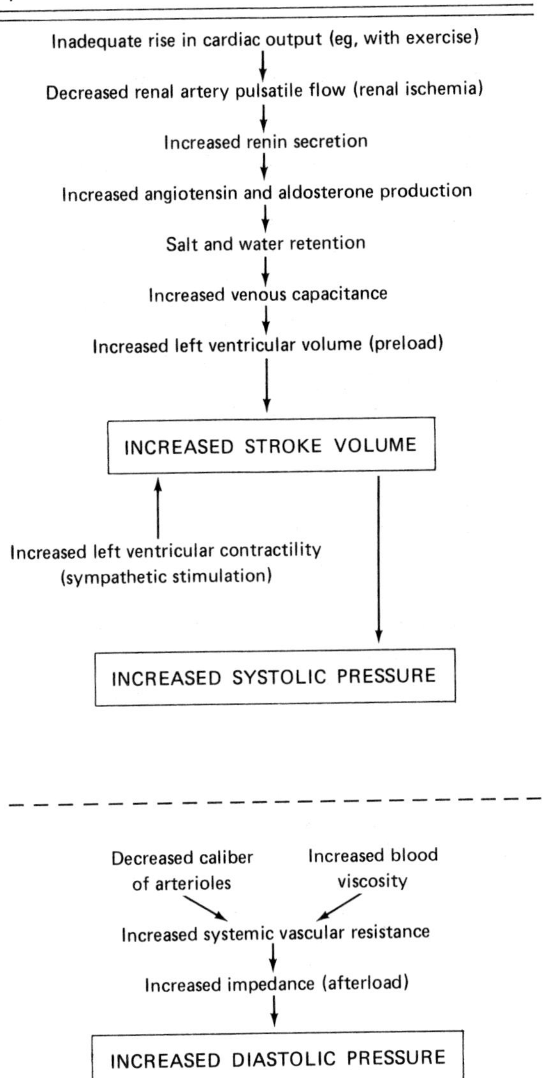

Many homeostatic mechanisms of the body are brought into play to maintain the blood pressure within a normal range (Table 9–1). Functional and structural changes in the resistance vessels (arterioles) are brought about by many influences: increased smooth muscle contraction, baroreceptor reflexes sending afferent impulses to the medulla and hypothalamic centers, other influences on these centers resulting in efferent autonomic discharge, blood volume, humoral and neurogenic influences from the kidneys and endocrine organs, and the renin-angiotensin-aldosterone system. Intrinsic autoregulation also operates to control arteriolar caliber independently of sympathetic adrenergic stimuli (Bayliss, 1902). Transient elevations of blood pressure due to physiologic decrease in the caliber of arterioles should not be confused with sustained or established hypertension. It is apparent, therefore, why such factors as anxiety, emotion, fear, noise, pain, anger, cold, an unfamiliar or threatening environment, exercise, or tachycardia can increase the arterial pressure either by increasing cardiac output or by raising the systemic vascular resistance through arteriolar vasoconstriction. The control systems influencing these various factors have both positive and negative feedback loops. The complex interrelationships of the factors have been subjected to systems analysis by Guyton (1969), have been described by Page as the "mosaic" of hypertension, and have been elaborated by Folkow and Neil (1971).

The Central Nervous System as a Pathophysiologic Mechanism in Hypertension

Although the factors regulating blood pressure are known, the cause of essential hypertension is by definition unestablished. The underlying cause is unknown also in many instances of hypertension associated with the disorders listed above in the section on Etiology and Classification. One theory that has many proponents is that the central nervous system, through its efferent autonomic discharges, increases cardiac output and that this induces contraction of the arteriolar muscle to prevent flooding the capillaries, thus increasing systemic vascular resistance and arterial pressure. Vasoconstrictor autonomic impulses from the central nervous system also constrict the arterioles. Oft-repeated smooth muscle contraction leads ultimately to structural changes in the arterioles, permanently increasing systemic vascular resistance. Fig 9–2 illustrates the effects of the emotional stress of mental arithmetic.

The problem of identification of the mechanisms of primary and secondary hypertension is made more difficult by the fact that no matter what the initial

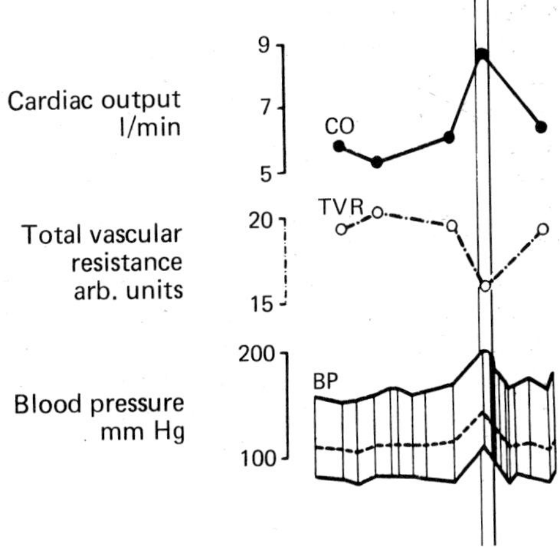

Figure 9–2. Hemodynamic effect of emotional stress (mental arithmetic). (Adapted and reproduced, with permission, from Brod J & others: Circulatory changes underlying blood pressure elevation during acute emotional stress [mental arithmetic] in normotensive and hypertensive subjects. Clin Sci 18:269, 1959.)

mechanisms were that established hypertension, lesions in the arterioles and interlobular arteries in the kidney may lead to small vessel ("Goldblatt") disease with persistent hypertension after the primary cause is removed (eg, renal artery stenosis, aldosteronism, pheochromocytoma, and nephrectomy for unilateral pyelonephritis). The mechanisms responsible for persistence of the hypertension may be different from those responsible for the initiation of hypertension such as secondary vascular changes in the kidney, increased secretion of renin, or other changes.

Mechanisms Involved in Secondary Hypertension

These will be discussed briefly now and amplified in the section dealing with secondary hypertension:

(1) Increased secretion of catecholamines, as in pheochromocytoma (see p 232).

(2) Increased release of renin, as (probably) in renal artery stenosis and acute glomerulonephritis (see also p 13).

(3) Sodium and blood volume play a key role in hypertension, especially when associated with hypertensive renal diseases and renal failure. When sodium intake exceeds the kidneys' ability to excrete sodium, blood pressure rises. Any sodium-retaining agent increases blood volume and makes the hypertension and renal failure worse. Blood pressure regulation depends on the interrelationship of factors that control blood volume and systemic vasoconstriction. Hypertension of chronic renal disease is primarily volume-dependent: either an absolute excess extracellular volume or a relatively reduced plasma volume in relation to the vascular capacity.

In renal failure, if a high-sodium diet is given, patients develop sodium and water retention that worsen the hypertension. The normal diet contains about 3–5 g (130–217 mEq) of sodium.

Hypertension occurs in 80% of patients with chronic renal failure by the time they reach the end stage but may occur early or late. Hypertension accelerates the cardiovascular complications that are the major cause of death in dialysis and transplant patients. The appearance of hypertension in patients with impaired renal function rapidly worsens the renal failure because patients develop sodium retention, especially if they are on a high-sodium diet. All patients with chronic renal disease must be monitored closely for hypertension so that it can be treated promptly, before irreversible renal damage occurs.

(4) Increased extracellular and plasma volume, as in primary aldosteronism, hypertension associated with desoxycorticosterone acetate administration, acute glomerulonephritis, renoprival hypertension (hypertension in the absence of both kidneys), and renal failure.

(5) Reduced perfusion pressure proximal to the kidney, as in coarctation of the aorta, which may initiate increased secretion of renin.

(6) Unknown mechanisms, eg, chronic glomerulonephritis (some patients with uremia have normal blood pressure), chronic pyelonephritis, and vasculitis of the kidney in connective tissue disorders.

FACTORS OPPOSING RISE IN BLOOD PRESSURE

Pathophysiologic influences combating rises in blood pressure include (1) baroreceptor reflexes to the brain via the ninth and tenth cranial nerves from the carotid and aortic bodies, which decrease sympathetic adrenergic vasoconstriction when tension in the carotid body rises; and (2) local tissue factors such as the prostaglandins, which are naturally occurring unsaturated fatty acids that have potent and variable biologic activity. Many prostaglandins are synthesized within the body, but only a few key ones are discussed here. Each prostaglandin is designated by a letter (eg, PGA, PGE). Prostaglandin E (PGE) is synthesized within the walls of blood vessels and decreases vascular tone, producing vasodilatation, which counteracts the vasoconstriction due to neurogenic and humoral influences. PGE_2 is increased whenever angiotensin II production is increased, as by the experimental production of renal ischemia in animals or when angiotensin is infused into the renal artery. Norepinephrine also increases the secretion of PGE_2, which thus influences renal blood flow. When prostaglandin release is inhibited by drugs such as indomethacin, renal blood flow falls and the effects of norepinephrine and angiotensin are enhanced. Despite these effects, indomethacin interferes with renal renin release with decrease in the plasma renin activity (Romero, 1976). The role of prostaglandins in the release of renin therefore requires further research to explain the paradoxic finding.

The role of tissue enzymes, as compared to circulating enzymes or hormones, in counteracting the adrenergic stimuli that increase arteriolar pressure is receiving increasing research study. Prostaglandins are such tissue enzymes, which selectively relax the smooth muscle of blood vessels, including the ductus arteriosus, and have a homeostatic or beneficial effect that prevents a rise in pressure.

Recent studies by Hamberg and Samuelsson (1975) and by Moncada and Vane (1976) (summarized by Marx, 1977) have clarified our knowledge of the conversion of arachidonic acid to prostaglandins (PG) and thromboxanes (TX). It has been known that different prostaglandins have varied biologic action, but the instability of several of them (prostaglandins G_2, H_2, and I_2) made precise study difficult.

Prostaglandins G_2 and H_2 are formed from arachidonic acid, but the conversion is inhibited by aspirin and indomethacin, which therefore inhibit all subsequent steps in the biochemical process. Thromboxane synthetase from platelets is the enzyme that produces thromboxane A_2 (TXA_2) from prostaglandins G_2 and H_2. TXA_2 is a strong platelet aggregator.

Endothelial surfaces of arteries and veins contain an enzyme, prostaglandin I_2 synthetase, that generates an unstable prostaglandin I_2 (PGI_2) from PGG_2 and PGH_2. PGI_2 prevents platelet aggregation and is a vasodilator.

Therefore, control of blood clotting (initiated by

clumping of platelets is influenced by TXA_2 and PGI_2, which have opposite actions on platelets and are formed from platelets and vascular endothelium, respectively.

It has been postulated by Moncada and Vane (1976) that a decreased amount or availability of prostaglandin I_2 synthetase as a result of intimal damage (as in hypertension) tilts the balance of control forces toward the TXA_2 action on platelet clumping which may then foster the development of thrombi and subsequently atherosclerotic plaques.

Bradykinin also increases the production of PGE_2 and so may be involved in control of blood flow in the kidney by altering vascular tone. The antihypertensive effect of the renal medulla may be the result of production of local hormones such as bradykinin and prostaglandin; the interplay between these hormones and vasoconstrictor hormones such as angiotensin and norepinephrine determines the net effect upon arteriolar caliber in the kidney and elsewhere. Imbalance, with decrease in the availability of the vasodilatory hormones, may result in enhanced vasoconstrictor activity and may thus play a role in the development of hypertension. The effect of various antihypertensive agents with respect to prostaglandin synthesis is unclear, although hydralazine, a potent vasodilator, increases the synthesis of PGE_2.

EVOLUTION OF HYPERTENSION

Increased Cardiac Output

Many patients with established hypertension have a record of transiently raised pressures under usual conditions of measurement, sometimes associated with tachycardia and with evidences of emotional lability. Hemodynamic studies in such individuals with so-called early labile hypertension have shown that systemic vascular resistance is normal but cardiac output increased.

Decreased Arteriolar Caliber

It is believed by some (Folkow, Clin Sci, 1971) that increased cardiac output in the presence of normal systemic vascular resistance could, by autoregulation and increased myogenic contractions, decrease arteriolar caliber and thus protect the capillaries in the short term but ultimately induce structural changes in the arterioles. This may explain why, in older people with established hypertension, cardiac output is normal and the hypertension is due to increased systemic vascular resistance. Arteriolar structural changes have been found in the kidneys of patients who have been examined at autopsy or by renal biopsy and are less severe in persons with early mild hypertension than in older people with more advanced disease.

Combined Physiologic Features

In between the above 2 groups of patients are the early middle-aged individuals who may have both increased systemic vascular resistance and increased cardiac output.

SYSTOLIC HYPERTENSION

Systolic hypertension is usually defined as a systolic pressure above 160 mm Hg but a diastolic pressure less than 95 mm Hg. It is most commonly seen in older patients. Various studies (Kannel, 1974) have demonstrated that the mortality rate is as closely related to systolic as to diastolic pressure, which means that the emphasis on diastolic pressure is to be deplored. The mortality rate is probably increased because most cases of purely systolic hypertension (omitting conditions such as complete atrioventricular block, severe bradycardia, arteriovenous fistulas, thyrotoxicosis, and aortic insufficiency) are due to decreased distensibility (increased rigidity) of the central aorta and its branches as a result of atherosclerosis. Atherosclerosis, being a generalized disorder, is apt to be present elsewhere if it occurs in the aorta, and so the mortality rate can be expected to be greater than in persons who do not have aortic atherosclerosis. Furthermore, the correlation coefficient between systolic and diastolic pressures is about 0.7, indicating that both indices usually are elevated together, so that a raised systolic pressure usually is associated with an increased diastolic pressure.

There are few data indicating the prognosis when systolic pressure exceeds 160 mm Hg and the diastolic is not merely below 95 mm Hg but below 70–75 mm Hg, so that the mean pressure is less than 107 mm Hg (upper limits of normal). A diastolic pressure of 90 mm Hg in association with a systolic pressure of 180 mm Hg, for example, would represent a mean pressure of 90 + 90/3, or 120 mm Hg, an elevated mean pressure. A systolic pressure of 180 mm Hg would require a diastolic pressure of 70–75 mm Hg in order to represent a normal mean pressure. Therefore, when the diastolic pressure is about 90 mm Hg, a raised systolic pressure represents a raised systemic vascular resistance as well as decreased elasticity of the aorta. The mean pressure is the best index of the significance of a dominantly or purely systolic elevation of blood pressure with respect to the diagnosis of essential hypertension. If systolic pressure is raised out of proportion to the diastolic pressure, the load on the left ventricle is increased, and cautious therapy with low doses of a diuretic and propranolol may be indicated to decrease the work of the heart if cardiac symptoms are present.

Years ago (1939), Wiggers demonstrated, in an artificial circulation machine, that decreasing the elasticity of the aorta but keeping cardiac output and peripheral resistance constant caused an increased systolic pressure, decreased diastolic pressure, increased pulse pressure, and unchanged mean pressure. Decreasing aortic compliance after arteriolar caliber was decreased caused an increase in all 3 pressures (systolic, diastolic, and pulse). The diastolic pressure increase was less than when peripheral resistance alone was decreased.

The essential effect of aging consists of decreased elasticity and enlargement of the aorta. There are no adequate data describing the benefits or hazards of treating systolic hypertension with a normal mean pressure in an older person. Because the raised systolic pressure "compensates" for the decreased aortic distensibility (compliance), antihypertensive drugs may cause a decreased cardiac output with weakness or faintness resulting from decreased perfusion of the vital organs of the body. If treatment is tried, it should be given cautiously and in low dosage, with careful observation of its effects.

If drugs are to be used, see the section on treatment of mild hypertension on p 240.

RISE OF BLOOD PRESSURE WITH AGE

The mean blood pressure rises with age in most Western populations but not in all individuals in the population groups. In normal subjects, the greatest rise occurs between birth and age 20, when the average systolic pressure may increase from 80 to 120 mm Hg (Fig 9–3). There is then a slow increase in pressure until ages 35–46, when the slope of the rise becomes steeper and many individuals cross over into a range which is arbitrarily defined as high blood pressure (see below) (Figs 9–4 and 9–5). The systolic pressure may then continue to rise more slowly, owing not only to the factor of decreased compliance of the aorta with age but presumably also to familial or genetic factors. The diastolic pressure follows the systolic rise up to about age 40, when the rise with age becomes less steep.

Factors in Blood Pressure Rise With Age

The rise in pressure with age in various epidemiologic studies is greater in persons who gain the most weight (especially black women), in persons who have a family history of hypertension, and in persons who have personality or emotional factors that influence blood pressure. Pickering's studies (1968) show that about 30% of the rise in pressure with age is due to genetic factors and the remainder to environmental factors. The nature of the latter factors has not been precisely determined but could be "factors operating through the mind." The relative roles of genetic and environmental factors vary in different individuals, and Folkow and Neil (personal communication, 1971) suggest that when the genetic factor is strong, environmental factors need be less important. The reverse is also true. The genetically linked factors leading to hypertension may be neurohumoral. It has been noted by Folkow that rats with spontaneous hypertension are more reactive and aggressive and can be distinguished on the basis of these traits by their handlers from nonhypertensive rats.

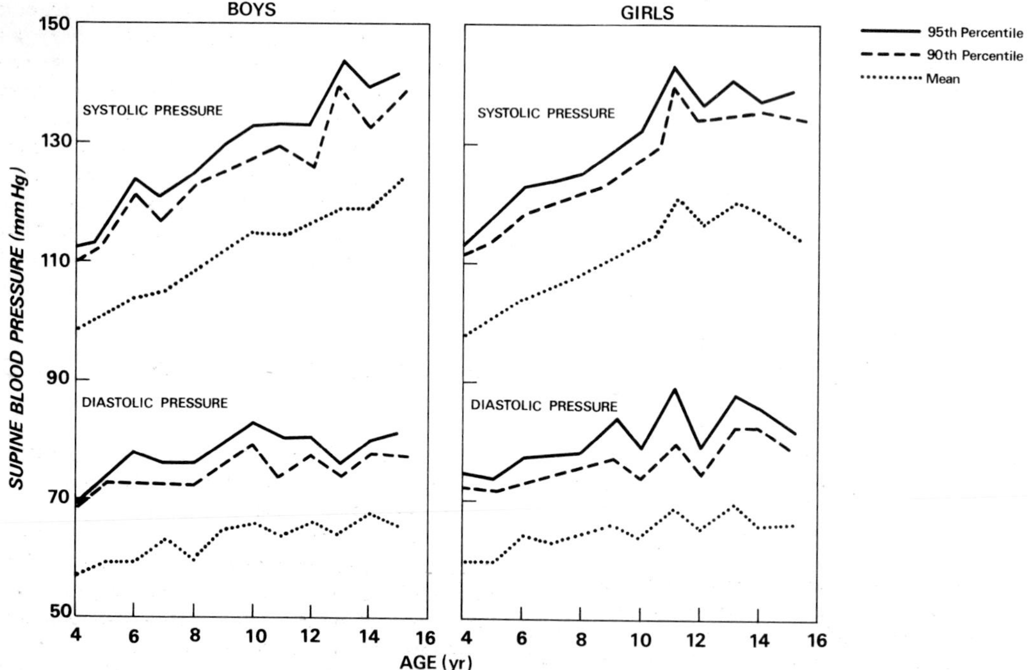

Figure 9–3. Normal blood pressure values for children and adolescents at successive age levels, established in cross-sectional studies by Londe and co-workers, provide a basis for identifying young patients at high risk of later development of sustained hypertension. (Reproduced with permission from Loggie JMH: Hypertension in children and adolescents. Hosp Pract 10:81, June 1975.)

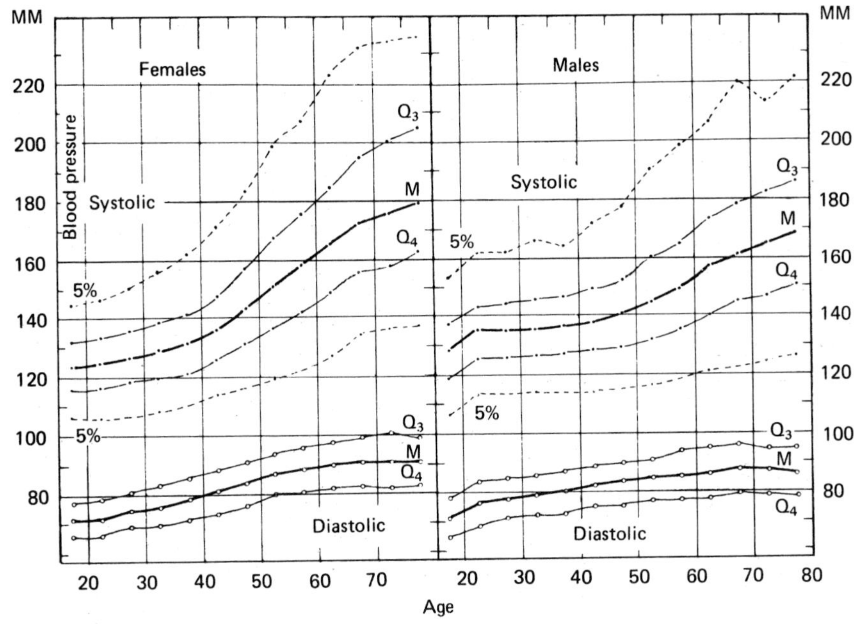

Figure 9–4. The Bergen Series, Group I. The blood pressure distribution according to sex and age in the entire city of Bergen from age 20 on. Half the population has higher and half the population has lower pressure than the median. One-fourth of the population has lower than the lower quartile, and one-fourth has higher pressure than the upper quartile. Q_4, first quartile; M, median or second quartile; Q_3, third quartile; 5%, lowest or highest 5% (5% or 95% of all observations). (Adapted and reproduced, with permission, from Humerfelt S: An epidemiological study of high blood pressure. Acta Med Scand, Suppl 407, 1963.)

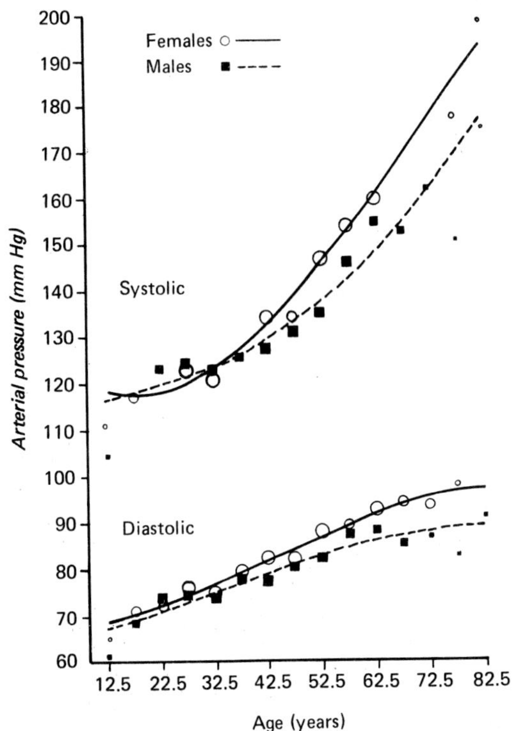

Figure 9–5. Systolic and diastolic pressure for females (open circles) and males (black squares) for each 5-year age group of the population sample, together with the fitted curves. The area of each circle or square is proportionate to the number of subjects in that age group. (Reproduced, with permission, from Hamilton M & others: The aetiology of essential hypertension. 1. The arterial pressure in the general population. Clin Sci 13:11, 1954.)

PULSE PRESSURE

Both systolic and diastolic pressure rise in the usual case of hypertension; the difference between them (the pulse pressure) depends not only upon age but upon whether the major component of the raised pressure is due to an increase in cardiac output or to peripheral resistance. Thus, a wide pulse pressure is most apt to occur in early labile hypertension of young people with a raised output or in the elderly person with perhaps only a slight increase in diastolic pressure but with a greater increase in systolic pressure due to a less distensible aorta. Recent actuarial data indicate that both systolic and diastolic pressures are important with respect to mortality statistics, and it is often difficult to separate their effects because the correlation between them is so high, being of the order of $r = 0.7$.

ROLE OF SYMPATHETIC NERVOUS SYSTEM

The role of the sympathetic nervous system has been extensively studied over the years, and the general conclusion of most workers in the field is that abnormalities of the system are not the cause of primary or essential hypertension. The evidence for this view has been well reviewed by Pickering (1968). The availability of more precise methods of determining catecholamines in the serum may modify our understanding of this relationship, but the observation that drugs that interfere with the sympathetic nervous system inhibit the transmission of adrenergic stimuli and that surgical procedures which interrupt or ablate portions of the sympathetic nervous system can lower the blood pressure does not invalidate the general conclusion. Lowering the blood pressure by inhibiting portions of the sympathetic nervous system does not mean that abnormality of the sympathetic nervous system caused the hypertension.

RENIN-ANGIOTENSIN SYSTEM

Renin, a proteolytic enzyme, is secreted by the juxtaglomerular cells surrounding the afferent arterioles near the vascular pole of the kidney in response to a "signal." It is hypothesized that the signal is related to stretch of the afferent arteriole or to decreased "effective" blood volume or to sodium content of the nearby macula densa of the distal tubule. The renin then acts on a substrate in the plasma (α_2-globulin), producing the decapeptide angiotensin I, which is then acted upon by a converting enzyme in the lung to form the octapeptide angiotensin II, which is a potent pressor substance. Angiotensin II, by an effect on the zona glomerulosa of the adrenal cortex, increases the secretion of aldosterone, which results in sodium and water retention by its characteristic action on the distal renal tubule, thus restoring blood volume. By negative feedback, the secretion of renin is then reduced until equilibrium results (Fig 9–6).

Renin changes in hypertension are probably secondary to pressure changes, because there is no significant difference in renin substrate or plasma renin activity in normal as compared to hypertensive men.

In a random group of hypertensive patients on a normal sodium diet, about 20% will have low, 60% normal, and 20% high plasma renin, defined in different ways by different authorities. Laragh and his group believe the prognosis is better in low renin hypertension than in normal or high renin types, but this conclusion has been disputed by others (see below and Table 9–2).

Low Renin Hypertension; Other Risk Factors

Although Laragh and his associates believe that low renin hypertension is due to increased secretion of a mineralocorticoid that increases the extracellular and plasma blood volume which, by negative feedback, turns off renin production, the mineralocorticoid has not been identified. The Medical Research Council Unit in Glasgow did not find increased extracellular or plasma volume or increased total exchangeable sodium in low renin hypertension. Other investigators find that—when other risk factors are equivalent—complications may occur in low as in normal renin hypertension. Hypertensive patients with normal renin and vascular complications are apt to have, concomitantly, other risk factors, whereas patients whose risk factors are minimal have fewer complications despite the normal renin (Table 9–2).

We believe the evidence does not support Laragh's conclusion that the prognosis of hypertension is better in low renin hypertension when other risk factors, including the height of the blood pressure, electrocardiographic abnormalities, serum cholesterol, age, and plasma volume are taken into consideration (Kaplan,

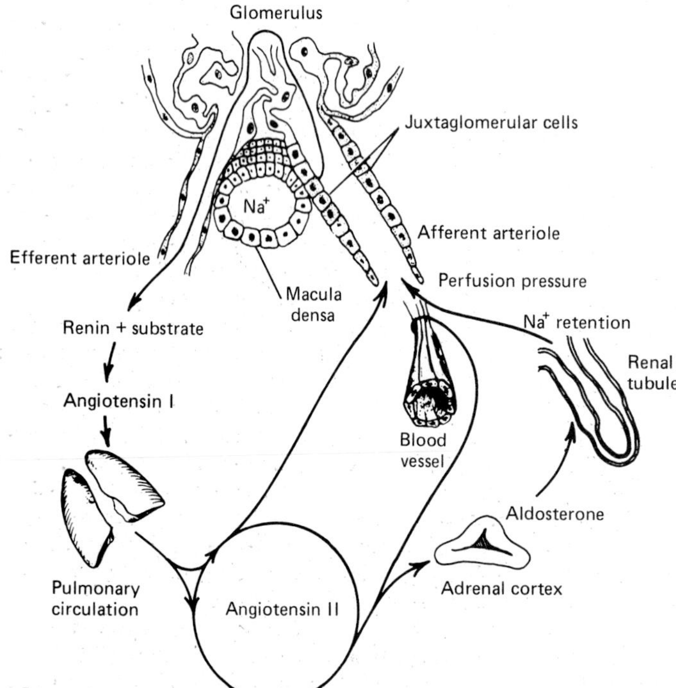

Figure 9–6. Feedback regulation of renin release. Several feedback loops are shown. An increase in angiotensin II concentration results in decreased renin secretion by increased sodium retention resulting in increased extracellular fluid volume; direct negative feedback; increased blood pressure through the central nervous system; increased blood pressure through direct systemic vasoconstriction; and direct sodium effects on the macula densa. (Reproduced, with permission of the American Heart Association, Inc., from Haber E: The role of renin in normal and pathological cardiovascular homeostasis. Circulation 54:849, 1976.)

Table 9–2. Risk factors in 67 hypertensives.*

	Initial Renin Level		
	High or Normal (n = 51)		Low (n = 16)
Number of Patients With Vascular Complications†	13		0
	Complications† (n = 13)	**No Complications† (n = 38)**	
Initial Risk Factors, %			
Mean blood pressure > 130 mm Hg	38	5	6
Abnormal electrocardiogram	77	26	25
Cholesterol level > 260 mg/dl	77	42	29
Duration of hypertension > 10 years	46	45	19

*Reproduced, with permission, from Kaplan NM: The prognostic implications of plasma renin in essential hypertension. JAMA 231:167, 1975. Modified from Christlieb AR & others: Renin, a risk factor for cardiovascular disease? Ann Intern Med 81:7, 1974. Copyright © American Medical Association.

†During 5-year period.

1975; Table 9–2). The question is still controversial, however, as noted below under Prospective Studies. Until the role of renin in prognosis and selection of therapy is established, we think it unwise to stop antihypertensive therapy that is controlling the blood pressure in order to determine the plasma renin unless one is searching for primary aldosteronism. Vigorous antihypertensive therapy is warranted in significant hypertension regardless of the level of the plasma renin.

A further factor confusing the interpretation of the significance of the level of plasma renin concerns the recent discovery of the presence of a prorenin (so-called "big renin") that does not have the physiologic activity of renin itself but is a precursor included in the measurement of plasma activated at a low pH of 3.0–4.0 or by cryoactivation by shaking plasma at –5 °C for 4 days (Sealey, 1977). If an acidification step is used in the assay for renin, or if prorenin is activated by chilling blood, erroneously high values for active renin may be obtained. In Sealey's hypertensive patients, the amount of prorenin averaged 3.4-fold the amount of active renin. The proportion of active to inactive renin is inconstant and altered by various maneuvers that either stimulate or suppress renin secretion. Differences in methodology may therefore explain some of the differences in results by various investigators regarding the pathogenetic significance of renin.

Prospective Studies of Renin

An adequate method of determining the plasma renin prior to the initiation of therapy is to combine 3–4 hours of upright posture with volume depletion utilizing 40–80 mg of oral furosemide.

Prospective studies are under way to clarify the prognostic and therapeutic value of plasma renin determinations in hypertension, and definitive conclusions must await the results of these studies. Subsets of hypertension as determined by plasma renin and its response to inhibitors of the renin-angiotensin system may lead to the use of "preferred" antihypertensive agents. The significance of plasma renin and aldosterone determinations by immunoassay, as well as that of other renin-angiotensin tests, is best evaluated in a specialized center, because of the confounding effects of the circumstances of their measurement (eg, sodium intake, posture, and the possible use of diuretic agents). The availability of agents that either selectively inhibit the enzymatic conversion of angiotensin I to angiotensin II (inhibitor of converting enzymes, SQ 20881; or the new oral agent SQ 14225) (Ferguson, 1977) or that competitively inhibit the action of angiotensin II on the receptor within the kidney (saralasin) suggest that the role of renin and angiotensin in hypertension will be clarified in the near future. It may then be possible to determine whether subsets of primary hypertension can be delineated by their physiologic and biochemical characteristics ("profiled"), which might allow therapeutic agents to be "tailored" to the specific subset. In addition, more effective and safer agents that inhibit either the converting enzyme or angiotensin II may be available in the future. Chemical isolation and synthesis of renin and production of renin antibodies may allow more specific analyses of renin concentration.

The use of specific pharmacologic inhibitors of various components of the renin-angiotensin system may permit clarification not only of the role of the components of the system but also of their interaction with sodium and plasma volume in the pathogenesis of hypertension. New inhibitors of some aspect of the system which may be available in the future, including better analogues of inhibitors of the converting enzyme or the angiotensin II-receptor interaction, or the isolation of plasma renin and the production of renin antibodies await future research.

Haber (1976) has recently summarized the role of angiotensin II in homeostasis and in pathologic states and asserts that angiotensin II has an obligatory role in maintenance of blood pressure in the sodium-depleted but not in the normal state. It is responsible for the initial pressor response of experimental renal vascular hypertension and may be important in causing chronic renal vascular hypertension. Agents that block the conversion of angiotensin I to angiotensin II or that completely inhibit the formation of angiotensin II may identify renin-dependent hypertension.

Caution in the Use of Angiotensin II Inhibitors

The response of the blood pressure and of plasma aldosterone to blockade of development of angiotensin II or blockade of the action of angiotensin II is increased in patients who are in a sodium-depleted state. The fall in pressure may be dramatic and catastrophic, and particular care should be taken before blocking angiotensin II if the patient is sodium-depleted as a result of intensive diuretic therapy. The group from Haber's laboratory in Boston found that angiotensin II was essential for blood pressure maintenance in sodium-depleted individuals because, when sodium-depleted but otherwise normal subjects were tilted upright, all but one of 8 subjects fainted despite a marked rise of plasma renin but not of plasma aldosterone.

A late rise (several hours) in blood pressure to levels that may produce encephalopathy has been reported after infusions of saralasin and indicates the need for caution and careful monitoring of the patient when this inhibiting agent is used, because of this agonist effect.

PHASES IN THE DEVELOPMENT OF HYPERTENSION

Early Labile Phase

In older patients with established hypertension, hemodynamic studies have demonstrated raised systemic vascular resistance and a normal cardiac index.

An early labile phase of hypertension with fluctuating blood pressure is common in younger individuals, often resulting from increased cardiac output with or without increased systemic vascular resistance thought by some investigators (Folkow, Clin Sci, 1971) to be due to excessive sympathetic adrenergic impulses arising in the central nervous system from the cortex, hypothalamus, or medullary cardiovascular centers. Pickering (1968) has suggested that such factors "operate through the mind." There can be no doubt that emotional factors cause neurohumoral discharge from the higher cortical centers and that this in turn increases sympathetic adrenergic excitation impulses and raises arterial pressure by vasoconstriction of the arterioles.

Labile hypertension is clearly related to age, as illustrated in Fig 9–7. Labile hypertension is defined by Moeller and Heyder (1959) as a blood pressure that is elevated (> 140/90 mm Hg) when the patient enters the hospital but which falls to normal (< 140/90 mm Hg) after a few days. Sustained hypertension is that which is present on admission and also after a short hospital stay; normal blood pressure is that which is normal both on admission and after a few days in the hospital. The high frequency of "labile" hypertension as defined by these authors is noteworthy.

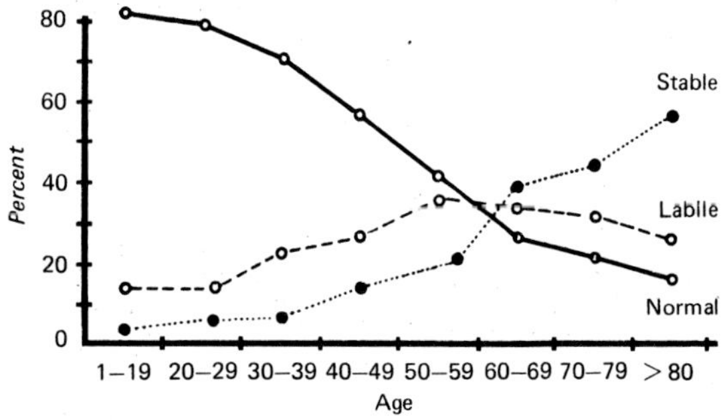

Figure 9–7. Prevalence of labile and stable hypertension and normal blood pressure by age, based on 2405 subjects (486 stable, 663 labile, and 1256 normal) and showing percentage of each type for each decade. The dividing line between normal and abnormal blood pressure is 140/90 mm Hg. (Adapted and reproduced, with permission, from Moeller VJ, Heyder O: Die labile Blutdrucksteigerung. Z Kreislaufforsch 48:413, 1959.)

Established Hypertension

The mechanism of the transition between transiently elevated pressures resulting from emotional factors and established hypertension resulting from structural arteriolar abnormalities is not determined. Folkow (Clin Sci, 1971) believes that periodic distention of smooth muscle by autoregulation may ultimately lead to structural changes. Emotional factors, which superimpose transient further rises of pressure on an individual with established hypertension, could understandably accelerate vascular complications. This hypothesis is supported by studies in spontaneously hypertensive rats which, when exposed to disturbing situations such as noise or vibration, respond with further increases in blood pressure and, ultimately, an increase in vascular complications. One can infer, therefore, that social and psychologic factors operating on an individual who tolerates emotional stress poorly can aggravate an existing elevated blood pressure by superimposing arteriolar vasoconstriction on structural arteriolar changes. There is no conclusive evidence, however, that repetitive functional changes can be the sole cause of such structural abnormalities.

PATHOLOGY OF HYPERTENSION

Hypertension induces arterial and arteriolar disease, predominantly in the arterioles and interlobular arteries of the kidney but also in the larger arteries of the body. Other pathologic changes due to complications of the hypertension will be discussed later.

Thickening of Small Arteries

Early in the course of hypertensive disease, the arterioles and arteries are histologically normal because the rise in pressure is due to functional vasoconstriction with decreased arteriolar caliber and not to structural change. Later on, the renal arterioles demonstrate medial hypertrophy and intimal fibrous thickening, resulting in a lower lumen-to-wall ratio and raising the systemic vascular resistance even at full vasodilatation. Arterioles throughout the body are affected to various degrees, but in almost all cases of established hypertension the renal arterioles show the structural changes known as nephrosclerosis (Fig 9–8).

Changes in the Larger Arteries

The larger arteries are usually spared in established hypertension until atherosclerosis, an independent process accelerated by the hypertension, develops. When this occurs, the arterial lesions show no distinguishing feature that separates atherosclerosis accelerated by hypertension from atherosclerosis that develops independently of hypertension. The lesions may appear in the aorta, the coronary arteries, the arteries to the lower extremities, and the arteries of the neck and brain (Table 9–3).

Atherosclerosis of the aorta aggravates cystic medial necrosis, which is more common in hypertensive atherosclerotic disease, and patients may develop aortic dissection pathologically indistinguishable from cystic medial necrosis in Marfan's syndrome.

Table 9–3. Coronary arteriosclerosis in hypertensive and nonhypertensive patients.*

Grade of Coronary Artery Disease (Left Artery)	Percentage of Patients in Each Grade	
	Hypertensives (152 Cases)	Nonhypertensives (146 Cases)
None	11.2	71.2
Slight to moderate	50.6	26.0
Severe	38.1	2.8
Thrombus	21.0	0

*Modified from Bell ET, Clawson BJ: Primary (essential) hypertension: A study of 420 cases. Arch Pathol 5:939, 1928. Reproduced, with permission, from Heptinstall RH: Relation of hypertension to changes in the arteries. Prog Cardiovasc Dis 17: 25, 1974.

The Kidney in Long-Standing Hypertension

Long-standing hypertension produces progressive renal nephrosclerosis with tubular atrophy, progressive scarring of the glomeruli, and slight shrinkage of the size of the kidney. Unless malignant hypertension supervenes, the clinical findings of renal failure are uncommon; however, the kidneys are somewhat small and granular, with a thin cortex.

Small Arteries of the Kidney

When the hypertension is more severe or occurs rapidly, the interlobular arteries of the kidney become involved, and there may also be focal necrosis of the renal arterioles. This combination of abnormalities impairs renal blood flow and glomerular filtration rate, which in turn increases the secretion of renin and the

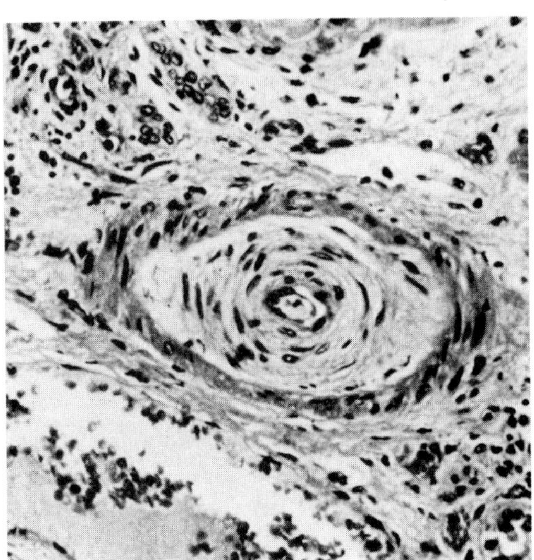

Figure 9–8. Cellular intimal hyperplasia (proliferative endarteritis or endarteritis fibrosa) in an interlobular renal artery (H&E; × 220). (Reproduced, with permission, from Kincaid-Smith P, McMichael J, Murphy EA: The clinical course and pathology of hypertension with papilloedema [malignant hypertension]. Q J Med 27:117, 1958.)

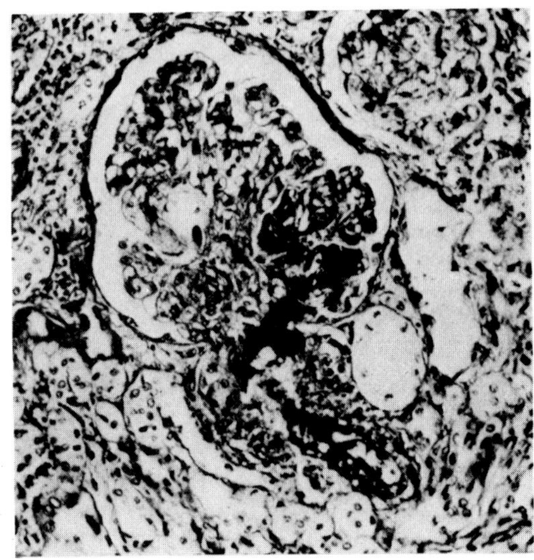

Figure 9–9. Fibrinoid necrosis in an afferent arteriole extending into the glomerular tuft (Mallory's azo carmine; × 180). (Reproduced, with permission, from Kincaid-Smith P, McMichael J, Murphy EA: The clinical course and pathology of hypertension with papilloedema [malignant hypertension]. Q J Med 27:117, 1958.)

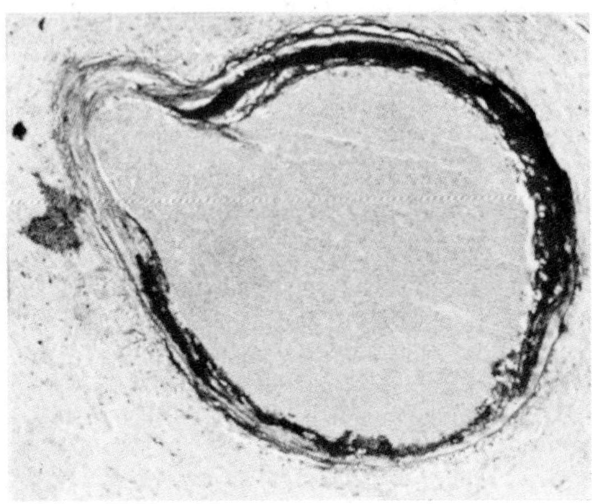

Figure 9–10. Cross section of microaneurysm showing plasma insudation of wall (PTAH; X 90). (Reproduced, with permission, from Ross Russell WR: How does blood-pressure cause stroke? Lancet 2:1283, 1975.)

production of angiotensin, further impairing renal function. This sequence of events is common in accelerated or malignant hypertension in which fibrinoid necrosis of arterioles, especially of the kidney, occurs (Fig 9–9).

Hypertension & the Brain

In long-standing hypertension, so-called Charcot-Boucher microaneurysms (Fig 9–10) may develop in the small arteries of the brain; rupture of these small aneurysms is responsible for cerebral hemorrhage that commonly interrupts the course of long-standing hypertension.

In addition to the microaneurysms, the brain may show atherosclerotic occlusion or thrombosis in the internal carotid, basilar, or vertebral artery system as well as thrombosis in the vessels of the circle of Willis. Cerebral infarction may then occur, although cerebral hemorrhage may result from rupture of microaneurysms into the cerebral hemispheres, which may enter the cerebral ventricles. Cerebral infarction may become hemorrhagic if anticoagulants are used.

Cardiac Hypertrophy & Failure

Raised systemic vascular resistance increases the work of the left ventricle, and, depending upon the stage of the disease, the heart may show concentric hypertrophy or combined hypertrophy and dilatation. The latter indicates inadequacy of compensatory hypertrophy and represents the earliest evidence of left ventricular failure.

Left ventricular wall thickness and left ventricular mass as determined by heart weight are the best signs of left ventricular hypertrophy. The upper limit of normal for left ventricular wall thickness is usually considered to be 1.5 cm, whereas heart weight is related to total body weight and is greater in men than in women. Heart weight exceeding 400 g is abnormal in either sex.

If the patient has been untreated or inadequately treated with antihypertensive agents, there may be evidence of left and right heart failure with chronic passive congestion of the liver. The mechanisms leading to hypertensive heart failure are illustrated in Fig 9–11.

Although left ventricular hypertrophy is initially compensatory and beneficial following the development of hypertension with raised systemic vascular resistance, progressive left ventricular hypertrophy reaches a point at which the increased left ventricular mass no longer is able to compensate for the raised arterial pressure, so its contractile ability deteriorates, leading to the development of left ventricular failure.

Findings in Secondary Hypertension

In secondary hypertension there may be pathologic evidence of primary disease in the kidney, the endocrine glands, or the aorta. Adenoma of the zona glomerulosa of the adrenal cortex is the usual pathologic finding in primary aldosteronism, although bilateral adrenal hyperplasia may be noted in some instances. Cushing's disease is due to a tumor, often

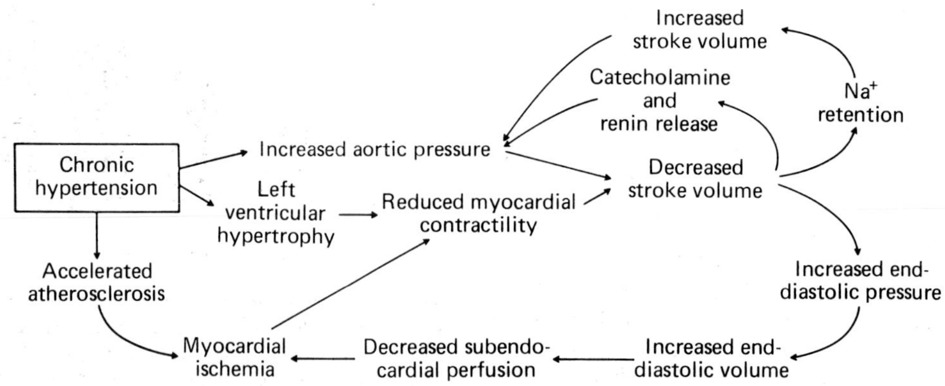

Figure 9–11. Some mechanisms initiated by hypertension that may lead to left ventricular decompensation. Vicious cycles tend to aggravate the problem. (Redrawn and reproduced, with permission, from Cohn JN & others: Hypertension and the heart. Arch Intern Med 133:969, 1974.)

microscopic, of the basophilic or chromophobe cells of the anterior pituitary gland, causing increased secretion of ACTH, which stimulates the adrenal glands to secrete excess cortisol (see p 230). Less commonly, Cushing's syndrome may be due to a benign adenoma of the adrenal gland, an ectopic ACTH-producing tumor, or exogenous corticosteroid or ACTH therapy (see p 230). Unsuspected coarctation of the aorta may be found at autopsy. This is also true of unsuspected pheochromocytoma, which may originate in any part of the chromaffin system. Renal vascular stenosis is rarely overlooked at autopsy today because it is routine to examine the initial portion of the renal artery arising from the aorta. Pathologically, renal vascular stenosis may be due either to atherosclerosis of the proximal part of the renal artery or to fibromuscular hyperplasia with aneurysm formation in the more distal portions of the renal artery. Aneurysm, arteriovenous fistula, and other uncommon vascular anomalies may also be found.

Systemic Disease & Hypertension

A wide variety of systemic diseases may cause vasculitis that results in hypertension. The pathologist, therefore, may find evidence of scleroderma, polyarteritis nodosa, lupus erythematosus, rheumatoid arthritis, or nonspecific arteritis. Disease of the brain (eg, brain tumor) is sometimes an unexpected finding as a cause of raised arterial pressure secondary to increased intracranial pressure or disease of the fourth ventricle.

In summary, the pathologic features may be predominantly in the arterioles, may extend to the small interlobular arteries of the kidney, or may involve the major arteries in the body with atherosclerosis, leading to the consequences that follow all varieties of atherosclerosis. In addition, there may be cardiac hypertrophy, cerebral hemorrhage, aortic dissection, and fundal changes or necrotizing lesions in the kidney following malignant hypertension.

EPIDEMIOLOGIC STUDIES OF THE INCIDENCE OF HYPERTENSION

Epidemiologic studies indicate that about 15–20% of adults in the USA have blood pressures above 160/95, considered by WHO criteria to be the upper limits of normal. Insurance companies consider 140/90 to be the upper limits of normal; the Framingham epidemiologic study, published over the past 10–15 years, classified patients between 140/90 and 160/95 as borderline hypertensives. It should be appreciated that there is no sharp dividing line between normotension and hypertension; when one plots the blood pressure at different ages in a large healthy population, the distribution curve does not demonstrate 2 distinct populations. Hypertension is a quantitative deviation from normal (Pickering, 1968). As a result, the criteria for the diagnosis of hypertension must be regarded as arbitrary; this has caused confusion in the literature because different authors use different numbers to diagnose hypertension.

HYPERTENSION & MORTALITY RATES

Actuarial data gathered during the large insurance study of 1959 dealing with almost 4 million lives and 100,000 deaths—as well as the Framingham Study—show that the mortality rate rises with increasing blood pressure. There is no sharp dividing line below which the mortality rate is unaffected and above which it is increased (Fig 9–12) (Pickering, 1968). There are progressive excessive morbidity and mortality rates as blood pressure rises in the group studied by the insurance companies, especially in younger individuals. (The excess mortality rate is much lower in older subjects.) The physician should think not in terms of hypertension or normotension ("either/or") but of the actual level of the blood pressure, both systolic and diastolic, in relationship to age. Data from many sources show that age is a major factor in determining the importance of the degree of deviation that any pressure represents and is of prognostic significance at any given level of blood pressure. A systolic pressure of 160 mm Hg, for example, would be in the 95th or 98th percentile for a 25-year-old but in the 50th percentile for a 60-year-old. The actuarial data from insurance companies likewise show the importance of age and the much greater likelihood of a fatal outcome over a period of years in younger individuals as compared to older ones with similar pressures. The mortality rate is

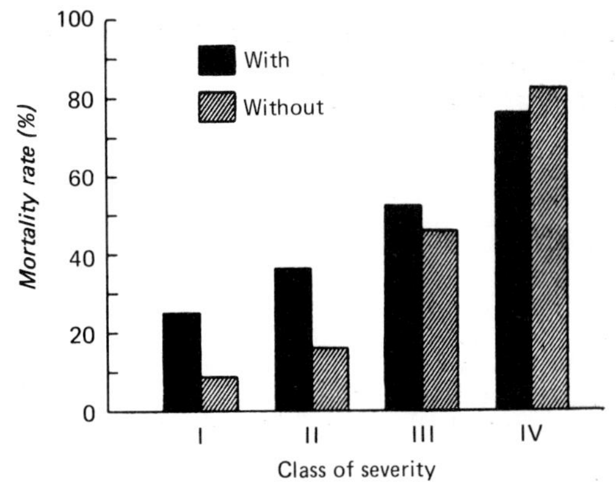

Figure 9–12. Mortality rates of hypertensive patients with and without atherosclerotic complications. Severity classes I–IV are described in the article and indicate progressively increasing severity of vascular complications. (Reproduced, with permission of the American Heart Association, Inc., from Sokolow M, Perloff D: The prognosis of essential hypertension treated conservatively. Circulation 23:697, 1961).

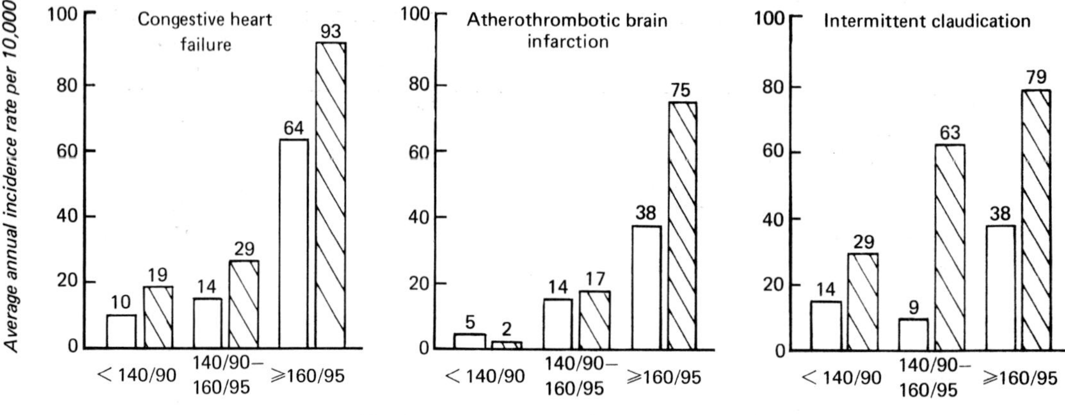

Blood pressure status at each biennial examination

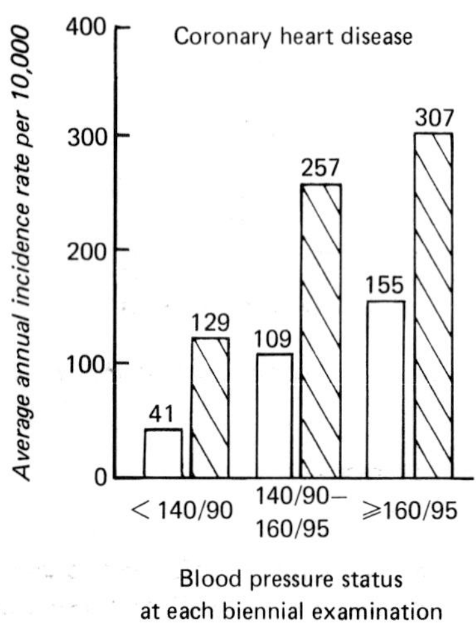

Women

Men

Figure 9–13. Average annual incidence of cardiovascular disease according to blood pressure status at each biennial examination, men and women 55–64, 16-year follow-up: Framingham Study. (Source: Framingham Monograph No. 26.) (Reproduced, with permission, from Kannel WB: Role of blood pressure in cardiovascular morbidity and mortality. Prog Cardiovasc Dis 17:5, 1974.)

higher in males, perhaps because of the increased incidence of coronary disease (Fig 9–13).

Hypertension as Risk Factor

It has been shown that hypertension is the most important of the known risk factors for the development of cardiovascular disease. The American Heart Association and the USPHS are engaged in a major public health effort to educate physicians and patients regarding the disease and its importance. It is well at this point to emphasize that (1) the dividing line between normotension and hypertension is arbitrary and difficult to define, (2) blood pressure varies from one occasion of measurement to another, (3) the circumstances and method of measurement are vital, (4) the level of blood pressure in a healthy population varies with age, and (5) one should think in terms of *probabilities* of vascular complications rather than certainties. Nevertheless, it is well established that the vascular complications of hypertension are the consequences of raised arterial pressure and of the associated atherosclerosis of major arterial circuits (Table 9–4). After a follow-up of 18 years, 105 cerebral infarctions occurred in the Framingham Study, only 10 of which occurred in normotensive persons. Hypertension is the most common and most powerful precursor of cerebral infarction in stroke (Kannel, 1974).

Hypertensive Vascular Disease

Hypertension is classified as hypertensive vascular disease when there is no target organ damage and a raised pressure is the only sign. When left ventricular hypertrophy, left ventricular failure, or associated coronary heart disease is present, hypertensive cardiovascular disease is a more appropriate term.

Transient Versus Established Hypertension

As indicated previously, established hypertension must be differentiated from transient elevation of blood pressure caused by excitement, apprehension, exertion, or the systolic elevation of blood pressure that occurs in elderly people as a result of increased stiffness of the aorta, or at any age from a raised cardiac output, increased cardiac contraction, or increased stroke output from a slow ventricular rate.

Age & Hypertension

Hypertension is regarded as uncommon before

Table 9–4. The frequencies of systemic hypertension and cardiomegaly in various cardiovascular conditions.*

Condition	% With Hypertension†	% With Cardiomegaly at Necropsy‡
Sudden death	50	70
Angina pectoris	50	75
Acute myocardial infarction§	50	75
Complications of acute myocardial infarction		
Rupture of left ventricular free wall	70	85
Rupture of ventricular septum	70	85
Rupture of papillary muscle	70	85
Left ventricular aneurysm (healed)	70	80
Aneurysm of aorta		
Fusiform, saccular, or cylindric	60	80
Dissecting	80	95
Atherothrombotic obstruction of abdominal aorta or of its branches	70	?
Cerebrovascular accident (stroke)		
Atherothrombotic cerebral infarction	50	70
Intracerebral hemorrhage	>90	>90
Lacunar softenings	>90	>95
Charcot-Bouchard aneurysm	>90	>95
Renal failure	>90	>90
Miscellaneous		
Calcific aortic valve disease of the elderly	50	70
Calcification of the mitral annulus	40	60

*Reproduced, with permission, from Roberts WC: The hypertensive diseases: Evidence that systemic hypertension is a greater risk factor to the development of other cardiovascular diseases than previously suspected. Am J Med 59:523, 1975.

†Blood pressure = systolic > 140 mm Hg or diastolic > 90 mm Hg. Limited to persons less than 66 years of age.

‡Heart weight = women > 350 g, men > 400 g.

§Transmural type. Nearly all patients with fatal subendocardial necrosis have cardiomegaly.

age 20, although recent data suggest that this view may not be completely justified because physicians have used adult criteria to determine normality in adolescence. If one uses different criteria for children, secondary hypertension is often found in young hypertensive individuals; coarctation of the aorta, chronic glomerulonephritis, pyelonephritis, renal artery stenosis, endocrine disorders, and raised pressure from oral contraceptive agents must all be considered in this age group.

Identification of Hypertensive Individuals

The importance of early recognition of hypertension cannot be overemphasized since this is the most important preventable cause of cardiovascular disease.

Prospective Studies

Prospective studies have shown that without treatment, hypertension greatly increases the incidence of cardiac failure, coronary heart disease, hemorrhagic and thrombotic stroke, renal failure, dissection of the aorta, and death. The morbid events have a higher incidence with increasing age, even in a treated group (VA Study, 1972). Preventing or reversing hypertensive complications by antihypertensive therapy is a major public health concern. This has led to intensive efforts to screen populations in various ways for the presence of hypertension. One must be cautious in extrapolating pressures under these unnatural conditions because at least half will be found to be "normal" on subsequent examinations. Most "unaware" hypertensive individuals found in screening are of the labile type (Carey, 1976).

Clinical Features of Hypertension

The clinical, laboratory, and radiologic findings relate to (1) the height of the blood pressure; (2) the involvement of "target organs" such as the heart, brain, kidneys, eyes, and peripheral arteries; (3) the presence of vascular complications such as cardiac failure, myocardial infarction, cerebral infarction, cerebral hemorrhage, atherosclerosis elsewhere, and dissection of the aorta; and (4) evidence of secondary "curable" hypertension.

A. Symptoms: Primary hypertension early in its course is usually an asymptomatic disorder and compatible with well-being for many years. Vague symptoms of nonspecific headache, dizziness, fatigue, and pounding of the heart may be present in hypertensive patients (often only after the patient learns that he has the condition) but are no more frequent than in some groups of patients with normotension. The frequency of vague symptoms which resemble those seen in psychoneurotic disorders has led investigators such as Ayman to conclude that these nonspecific symptoms in patients with mild hypertension are functional in origin and not organic. Screening of adult population groups often reveals the blood pressure to be elevated in vigorous subjects who have no symptoms whatever.

1. **Headaches**–When hypertension is more severe, especially if it is the accelerated variety (with rapid rise in pressure and hemorrhages or exudates in the fundi, considered premalignant; see p 217), throbbing suboccipital headaches, worse in the morning and subsiding during the day, are common. In malignant hypertension in association with visual disturbances, the headaches can be severe and most difficult to relieve except by reduction of the blood pressure. In contrast with the typical hypertensive headache, the usual tension headache is more apt to be frontal and nonthrobbing; the differentiation is often difficult.

2. **Heart failure**–When left ventricular dilatation and early left ventricular failure occur in patients with compensatory cardiac hypertrophy, symptoms include progressively more severe dyspnea on exertion, paroxysmal nocturnal dyspnea, and orthopnea (see Chapter 10). If coronary heart disease is also present, as it commonly is, patients may complain of angina pectoris or may develop myocardial infarction. Left ventricular failure resulting from the combination of increased work of the left ventricle due to hypertension and associated coronary heart disease is frequent and makes precise distinction between causative factors difficult. Cardiac failure from modest elevations of blood pressure alone does not usually occur. When the raised blood pressure is greater, and particularly when it occurs abruptly, as in malignant hypertension, cardiac failure may occur in the absence of coronary heart disease and is rapidly reversed when the blood pressure is lowered. Hypertensive patients with cardiac hypertrophy often develop symptoms and signs of cardiac failure if the sodium intake is abruptly increased, as with ingestion of baking soda, Alka-Seltzer, or a high-sodium diet; these patients often respond rapidly to treatment. Cardiac failure is an uncommon cause of death in the well-managed patient unless it follows the complications of myocardial infarction. Typical electrocardiographic examples of left ventricular hypertrophy and its reversal are illustrated in Fig 9–23.

3. **Renal symptoms**–Although nephrosclerosis is a common finding on pathologic examination (either by necropsy or renal biopsy), renal failure is not common unless hypertension is accelerated or malignant. Patients with severe hypertension may develop nocturia or, more rarely, intermittent hematuria. In nonaccelerated cases, renal blood flow and glomerular filtration rate may be somewhat decreased, but renal failure and azotemia are rare. If accelerated or malignant hypertension occurs, however, necrotic lesions in the arterioles and narrowed interlobular arteries may significantly decrease the renal blood flow and glomerular filtration rate; renal function may deteriorate rapidly over a period of weeks or months.

The most common cause of death in malignant hypertension is renal failure; determination of renal function is essential in all patients with hypertension because, as will be discussed in the section on prognosis, it is important to lower the blood pressure before renal failure has occurred.

4. **Central nervous system symptoms**–Older patients with hypertension and associated cerebral and carotid artery sclerosis may develop any of the clinical manifestations of atherosclerosis of the vessels to the head which might be expected from the pathologic findings described above. Patients may develop severe headache, confusion, coma, convulsions, blurred vision, transient neurologic signs, ataxia, or neurologic deficit due to cerebral infarction or hemorrhage. If the blood pressure rises abruptly, patients may develop acute cerebral symptoms such as somnolence, coma, confusion, or convulsions, collectively known as hypertensive encephalopathy–presumably due to cerebral spasm and cerebral edema–and these may be quickly reversed with rapidly acting antihypertensive agents. More commonly, however, when these severe cerebral symptoms develop, a vascular accident has occurred rather than cerebral spasm and edema.

5. **Claudication**–When atherosclerosis involves the aorta and the arteries of the lower extremities, patients may present with intermittent claudication, and hypertension is only noted incidentally.

6. **Chest pain**–Severe chest pain radiating to the back, followed by interruption of the arterial supply to the head, neck, back, and lower extremities, occurs after dissection of the aorta; in type I (see later under discussion of dissection, p 218) involving the ascending aorta, aortic insufficiency may result. Hypertension may be noted only incidentally in patients who present with severe chest pain simulating acute myocardial infarction or acute aortic insufficiency.

As indicated under heart failure above, coronary heart disease frequently complicates hypertension. Patients may develop angina pectoris or myocardial infarction; chest pain may not be due to dissection of the aorta but to angina pectoris and myocardial ischemia.

B. Signs: The physical signs in hypertension are related to the underlying cause of the hypertension, the blood pressure itself, its duration and severity, the presence and degree of involvement of the target organs, and complications resulting from vascular involvement.

1. **Blood pressure**–

a. **Cuff width**–The blood pressure should be taken with a mercury manometer or a well-calibrated aneroid manometer in both arms and in the legs, using a cuff at least 12 cm wide in most persons; a wide leg cuff (14–15 cm) must be used on the arm if the patient is obese or very muscular, with a large upper arm circumference. The cuff should be at least two-thirds as wide as the upper arm is long. Errors are frequently made in diagnosing hypertension if the cuff is too narrow and does not adequately compress the brachial artery. The basic principle is that a cuff which is too narrow for the size of the arm gives readings that are falsely high.

b. **Measuring blood pressure**–The patient should be relaxed, warm, and unhurried, and the physician's routine should include allowing the patient to adjust to the examining room. The pressure must be taken in both arms to avoid discrepancies caused by atherosclerosis of the subclavian artery; the arm in which the pressure is to be taken on subsequent occasions should be noted.

Accurate technic in taking the blood pressure is essential, and nurses, field workers, and others must be carefully instructed in placement of the rubber bag over the artery and the speed of inflation and deflation in measuring the pressure.

c. Home measurement and ambulatory blood pressure recordings—The patient or a member of the patient's family can be taught to take blood pressure readings at home. Systolic and diastolic pressures taken 3 or 4 times a day can be averaged into weekly mean pressures. Mean blood pressures so obtained have been shown to be reliable by Page, Dustan, and their associates at the Cleveland Clinic (Bravo, 1975) not only in establishing the presence of hypertension but also in providing a baseline to evaluate treatment. Ambulatory blood pressure readings can be taken with portable self-recording equipment in order to eliminate the pressor effect of the physician and the medical environment. Mean ambulatory pressures lower than mean office pressures occurred in 85% of 675 untreated hypertensive patients. Mean ambulatory pressures averaged 13% lower than office pressures for the total population, with a wide scatter, even though the correlation coefficient of the 2 methods of measuring pressures is 0.67. These ancillary technics are usually needed only when raised pressures are mild to moderate (~ 180/105 mm Hg) and are necessary when the pressures are considerably raised on 2 or 3 occasions but normal on others. Examples of the use of ambulatory blood pressure monitoring are shown in Figs 9–14 and 9–15. Table 9–5 shows office and ambulatory pressures related to severity of hypertension.

Even when office blood pressures are more than moderately raised, an occasional patient* will have essentially normal readings at home when pressures are taken by someone other than a physician or when pressures are recorded by a portable apparatus. Prolonged recording with intra-arterial or automatic devices, especially during sleep, is valuable in assessing hypertension and may demonstrate a marked decrease in pressures in the early morning hours (Fig 9–16).

Considerable care must be taken to establish the diagnosis of hypertension before instituting treatment, because treatment is usually a lifelong process. Treatment is rarely urgent in the absence of severe or accelerated hypertension.

d. Variations in measurement—The body position of the patient is also important; when the patient sits or stands, the diastolic pressure may increase over recumbent levels because of baroreceptor sympathetic discharge. The systolic pressure may stay the same or occasionally may fall slightly in the standing position, but it may increase in the sitting position. If the patient is hypovolemic as a result of administration of diuretics or has postural hypotension from antihypertensive agents interfering with adrenergic transmission, the systolic and diastolic pressures may be considerably lower in the sitting and standing position than in

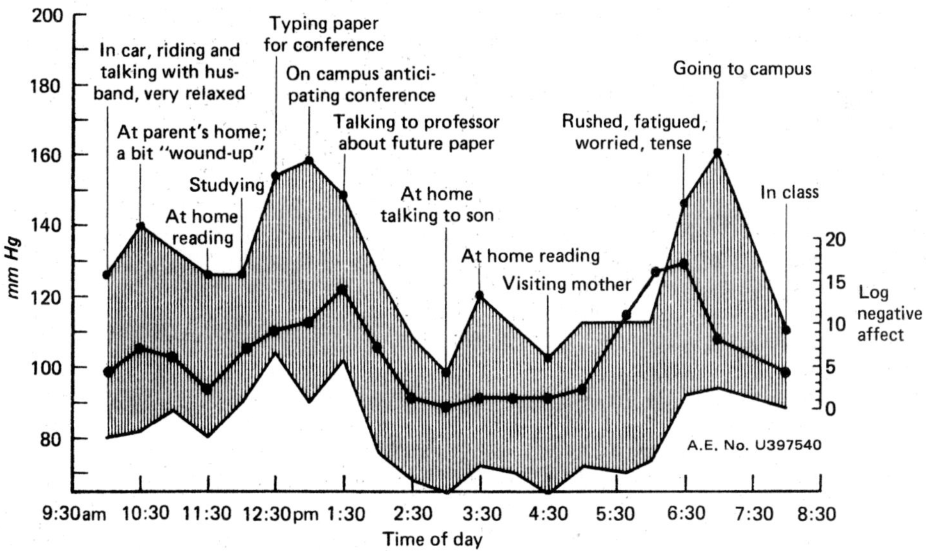

Figure 9–14. Serial blood pressure obtained with ambulatory blood pressure recordings correlated with patient's activities and emotions. The negative affect scale was derived from the patient's serial entries on an adjective check list coincident with each blood pressure recording. The peak blood pressure readings, both systolic and diastolic, occurred when the patient was on the university campus where she returned after a lapse of many years in order to get her PhD. Each time that she was on the campus, the negative affect was greater. She admitted that she really did not want to get her PhD. (Reproduced, with permission, from Sokolow M & others: Preliminary studies relating portably recorded blood pressures to daily life events in patients with essential hypertension. Bibl Psychiatr 144:164, 1970. S. Karger AG, Basel.)

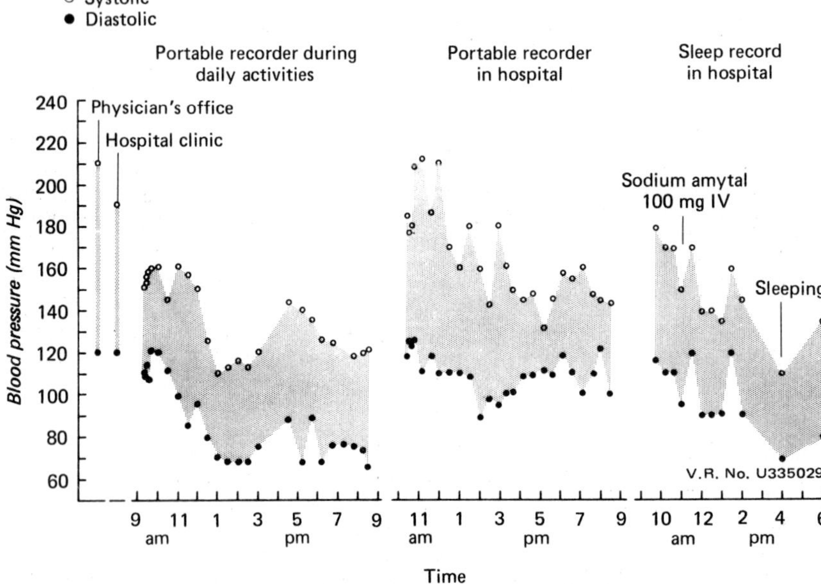

Figure 9–15. Ambulatory blood pressure recordings in a patient who had normal pressures during his daily activities but elevated pressures when in the hospital clinic. When he was put to sleep in the hospital with intravenous sodium amobarbital, his pressures were similar to those during his outside activities.

recumbency. In autonomic insufficiency, postural hypotension is accompanied by little or no tachycardia in contrast to the marked tachycardia that occurs in postural hypotension due to hypovolemia. Because of the transient rise in pressure that occurs with the stress of the examination in the sometimes threatening environment of the doctor's office, a raised pressure must be present on at least 3 different occasions of measurement before one considers the pressure to be representative. Sometimes the pressure is so variable that it is elevated on one occasion but well within the normal range on another; this may occur in 10–20% of individuals during any short period of time. It then becomes necessary to obtain frequent office, home, or ambulatory blood pressure readings over a period of weeks or even months or to have readings taken by a nurse in the office under relaxed circumstances without the doctor being present.

Table 9–5. Ambulatory and office mean systolic and diastolic blood pressures related to degree of severity of hypertensive complications.*

Class or Grade of Severity†	Overall Severity	Severity of Individual Complications		
		Ocular Funduscopic Abnormalities	Left Ventricular Hypertrophy	Cardiac Enlargement
Ambulatory pressures (mm Hg)				
0	137/82	139/83	147/89	155/94
I	150/91	152/92	161/99	
II	165/101	171/105	168/100	162/98
III	192/124	207/128	198/128	171/114
Office pressures (mm Hg)				
0	148/94	154/96	158/99	170/104
I	167/101	167/102	178/108	
II	181/112	183/113	187/111	181/110
III	206/125	237/131	220/129	177/116

*Reproduced, with permission of the American Heart Association, Inc., from Sokolow M & others: Relationship between the level of blood pressure measured casually and by portable recorders and severity of complications in essential hypertension. Circulation **34**:279, 1966.

†Classes of severity are graded 0–III depending on the presence and degree of changes in the fundi, ECG, chest film, and renal function. Class 0 denotes no abnormalities other than a raised blood pressure. (For further details see Sokolow & Perloff, 1961.)

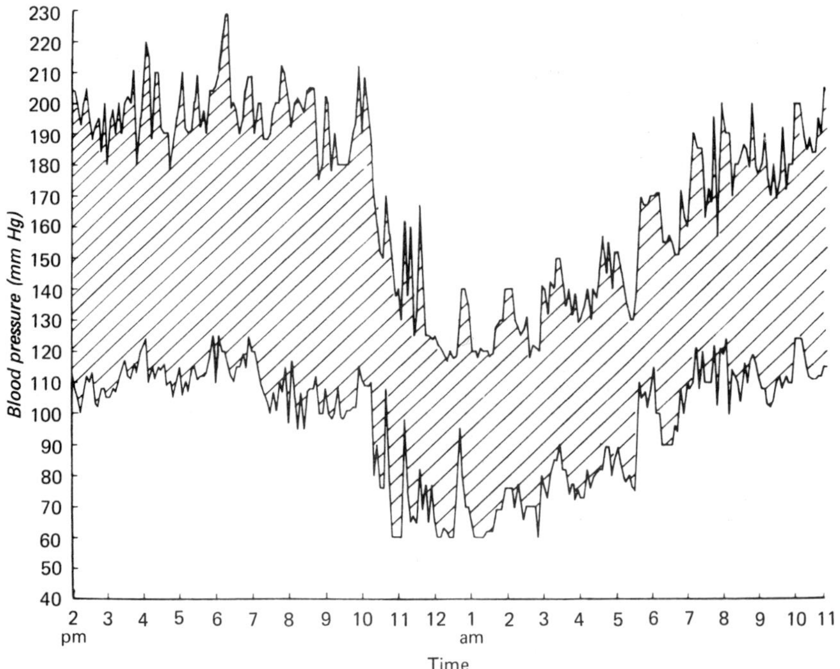

Figure 9–16. Example of prolonged recording of blood pressure in a 47-year-old man with essential hypertension. Pressure recorded at 5-minute intervals throughout. Note the marked fall at about 11 pm, during sleep. (Adapted and reproduced, with permission, from Irving JB & others: Value of prolonged recording of blood pressure in assessment of hypertension. Br Heart J 36:859, 1974.)

2. Signs in target organs—Particular emphasis should be placed on the following signs related to an assessment of the presence and degree of involvement of the target organs affected by hypertension or by the presence or absence of vascular complications of hypertension.

a. Retinas—In examining the retinas one should note particularly the degree of narrowing or irregularity of the arterioles, the presence of arteriovenous defects ("nicking" or "nipping"), the presence of flame-shaped or circular hemorrhages, fluffy cotton wool exudates, or the presence of papilledema with blurring of the temporal edge or elevation of the optic disk (Table 9–6). Keith, Wagener, and Barker (1939) have classified the retinal changes as follows (called Keith-Wagener [KW] changes):

KW I: Minimal arteriolar narrowing, irregularity of the lumen, and increased light reflex.

KW II: More marked narrowing with focal spasm, more marked irregularity, and arteriovenous nicking with changes in course and distention of the vein as it crosses the arteriole. The arteriole and the venule travel in the same sheath, and when there is thickening of the arteriole it compresses the venule.

Table 9–6. The retinal arterioles in hypertension.*
(Figures are in percentages.)

	Irregularity of the Lumen	Narrowing	Pallor of the Blood Column	Nipping at Arteriovenous Crossings	Opacity of the Arteriolar Wall at Arteriovenous Crossings	Light Reflex Broader or More Prominent Than Normal	Hypertensive Retinal Arterioles
Hypertension							
Diastolic pressure 110 or more (45 cases)	76	61	94	36	38	61	89
Control series							
Systolic pressure 155 or less and diastolic pressure 90 or less (103 cases)	0	0	5.4	2	5	12	0

*Reproduced, with permission, from Leatham A: The retinal vessels in hypertension. Q J Med 71:203, 1949.

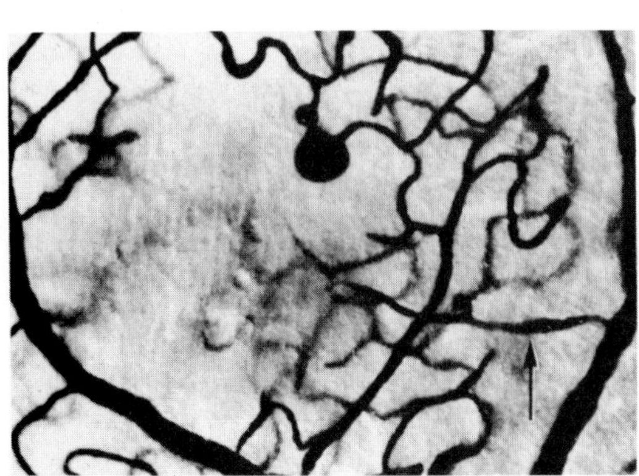

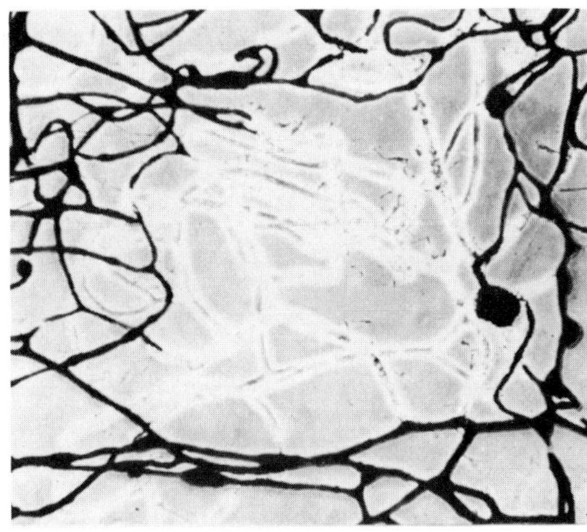

Figure 9–17. *Left:* Retina from a patient with malignant hypertensive retinopathy, showing a cotton wool spot. The capillaries within the affected area have failed to become injected, while the capillaries at the margin are dilated and show aneurysmal formation. Swollen nerve fibers may be seen in the avascular area. The terminal arteriole (arrow) showed hyalin lipid occlusion. (Injected with India ink; stain: oil red O; X 90.) *Right:* Retina from a patient with malignant hypertensive retinopathy, showing a cotton wool spot. The retina has been digested and reveals that capillaries are present within the uninjected zone; they appear patent and consist of simple basement membrane tubes without endothelial cells or pericytes. (Injected with India ink; X 130.) (Reproduced, with permission, from Ashton N: Pathophysiology of retinal cotton-wool spots. Br Med Bull 26:143, 1970.)

KW III: In addition to the arteriolar changes noted previously, multiple flame-shaped hemorrhages and fluffy "cotton wool" exudates are scattered throughout the retinas (Fig 9–17). These are due to localized axon swellings and swollen nerve fibers in avascular areas. Hard, very small, sharply defined, translucent exudates are due to exudation in a different part of the retina, are of lesser significance, and do not indicate acute arteriolar damage.

KW IV: Any of the above with the addition of papilledema with blurring of the temporal side of the optic disk and elevation of the disk.

Caution should be exercised in interpreting blurring of the nasal edge of the disk as being due to papilledema. Old, healed papilledema in the absence of current elevation of the disk margins is often revealed by the presence of small collateral vessels crossing the edge of the disk.

Benign hypertension is the rule when KW I and KW II are present, whereas KW III and KW IV are associated with accelerated or malignant hypertension. When malignant hypertension develops abruptly with only a short history of hypertension, patients may have hemorrhages, exudates, or papilledema in the absence of arteriolar changes or arteriovenous nicking.

The Keith-Wagener classification has some deficiencies, particularly in the differentiation of hypertensive from atherosclerotic changes in KW II and in the interpretation of single hemorrhages and "hard" exudates. The 2 processes, hypertension and atherosclerosis, are independent entities, but hypertension accelerates atherosclerosis. When the arterioles are very narrowed and irregular and compress the venules, the findings are a combination of the 2 pathologic processes and are not due to hypertension alone; therefore, arteriovenous nicking indicates the presence of atherosclerosis and, by inference, a longer duration of the hypertensive process. The fundal changes of accelerated hypertension are an urgent indication for immediate and vigorous antihypertensive therapy.

b. Heart–Examination of the heart and blood vessels may reveal evidence of left ventricular hypertrophy, left ventricular failure, or involvement of the various arteries by atherosclerosis. As shown by Traube in the late 19th century, the best sign of left ventricular hypertrophy is a left ventricular heave, a localized sustained lift of the left ventricular impulse. Because concentric hypertrophy is the rule prior to dilatation and left ventricular failure, the heart is not displaced to the left unless cardiac failure is present. The decreased distensibility of the thick left ventricle commonly produces a presystolic gallop (S_4); this does not indicate cardiac failure but is a sign of decreased left ventricular compliance. The presence of a left ventricular heave and an S_4 indicates established left ventricular hypertrophy and usually long-standing disease.

c. Blood vessels–The jugular venous pulse is usually normal in the absence of right ventricular failure; the carotid pulses are usually normal in volume and upstroke unless the patient has coarctation of the aorta, in which case the carotid pulse is unusually prominent and jerky. The presence of bruits over the carotid should always be sought as a possible clue to the presence of atherosclerotic disease of the internal carotid arteries. The presence or absence of pulmonary rales is valuable in recognizing early left ventricular failure. If the failure is more obvious and more severe, pulsus alternans may be noted. Particular note should be made of the volume and character of all the pulses and their symmetry on the 2 sides. This serves not only to demonstrate coarctation of the aorta if the pulses of the lower extremities are weak and delayed as compared to the radials but also to provide a baseline in the event the patient develops chest pain with variation in the various pulses suggesting aortic dissection. The presence or absence of bruits should be sought, especially over the femoral and popliteal arteries, to determine the presence of atherosclerosis of these vessels. Bruits should be sought in the epigastrium and in the flanks since they may provide clues that suggest renovascular hypertension. Examination of the abdominal aorta may reveal an aneurysm as a complication of concomitant atherosclerosis. Careful palpation below each rib should be done in a search for pulsating intercostal arteries, which are prominent in coarctation of the aorta and serve as collateral vessels to arteries below the coarctated site.

d. Central nervous system signs—Examination for evidence of residual neurologic deficit from previous cerebral infarction may be fruitful. There may be a positive Babinski or Hoffman reflex, hemiparesis, hemiplegia, or hemianopsia. The presence of ataxia may indicate involvement of the posterior inferior cerebellar artery.

e. Endocrine dysfunction—The patient should be examined for signs suggesting any of several types of endocrine abnormalities. *Cushing's syndrome* is suspected if there is central trunk obesity, hirsutism, acne, purple striae, moon facies, and thin skin with ecchymoses. *Primary aldosteronism* is suggested by muscular weakness, hypoactive deep tendon reflexes, and diminished or absent vasomotor circulatory reflexes. *Pheochromocytoma* is suspected if an attack of headache, sweating, palpitations, and a markedly increased blood pressure is induced by an examination over the upper abdomen that presses on a tumor.

f. Coarctation of the aorta—(See Chapter 11.) Coarctation is strongly suggested by the presence of weak or delayed femoral pulses in comparison with the radial arteries, the presence of a basal ejection systolic murmur transmitted to the interscapular area, and palpable collateral intercostal arteries along the inferior rib margins and scapular borders.

g. Polycystic kidneys—Polycystic kidneys are suspected if the kidneys are large and easily palpable, especially in the presence of long-standing hypertension when the kidneys would be expected to be small.

C. Laboratory Findings: Laboratory investigations are designed to determine the involvement of any of the target organs affected by hypertension and to recognize the presence of any evidence of secondary hypertension. (The diagnosis and details of secondary hypertension will be described later.)

1. Urinalysis—

a. Routine urinalysis—Urinalysis is usually normal until renal impairment occurs, when the specific gravity may become low and mild proteinuria may appear. In malignant hypertension there may be substantial proteinuria, approaching values suggesting nephrosis. A low fixed specific gravity suggests advanced renal parenchymal disease or the hypokalemic nephropathy of primary aldosteronism. The presence of granular or red cell casts and hematuria suggests glomerulonephritis. The presence of pyuria favors chronic pylonephritis, but if advanced renal failure is present, the microscopic appearance of the urinary sediment is often not helpful in diagnosis. In connective tissue disorders, such as lupus erythematosus, the so-called "telescopic" urine sediment of Krupp (1943) may be present, with red cells, casts of all sizes, and protein combined.

A fresh, clean voided urine specimen should be examined for bacteria. If organisms are found, the specimen should be cultured and quantitative bacterial counts performed to establish the presence of chronic pyelonephritis. If other features of the history are suggestive of urinary tract infection, cultures should be repeated because the bacilluria in chronic pyelonephritis may be intermittent.

b. Special urine examinations—Quantitative determination of the urinary excretion of 17-hydroxycorticosteroids or serum cortisol in the morning after 1 mg dexamethasone (see below) is indicated if the clinical picture suggests Cushing's disease. Values are significantly elevated in all types of ACTH-dependent Cushing's syndrome.

If pheochromocytoma is suspected, 24-hour excretion of catecholamines or their metabolic products—vanillylmandelic acid (VMA), metanephrine, or normetanephrine—should be determined.

If hypokalemia is present or there are other symptoms suggestive of primary aldosteronism (see below), plasma or urine aldosterone should be determined in specially equipped laboratories, but this need not be done if the serum potassium is consistently normal (ie, above 4 mg/dl).

For further details of the diagnosis of the secondary causes of hypertension, see pp 221 ff.

2. Blood chemistry—In renal parenchymal disease, the serum creatinine and blood urea nitrogen are elevated, and anemia associated with advanced azotemia may be present. In aldosteronism, the blood urea nitrogen and serum creatinine are usually normal; renal function is not severely impaired, but the serum potassium is low and serum sodium and bicarbonate are increased.

It usually is not necessary to do more sensitive renal function studies if the serum creatinine and blood urea nitrogen are normal; however, if the blood urea nitrogen approaches 20 mg/dl or the serum creatinine is 1.3 mg/dl or above, it is wise to determine the creatinine clearance as a measure of the glomerular filtration rate, because the latter may be reduced even though the serum creatinine may be within the normal range.

D. Electrocardiographic Findings:

1. Left ventricular hypertrophy—The ECG is the most sensitive method of establishing the presence of left ventricular hypertrophy and is often abnormal when there is no left ventricular heave and when the chest x-ray shows no left ventricular enlargement. The ECG reflects hypertrophy and not dilatation, whereas the chest x-ray reveals enlargement rather than hypertrophy. The earliest electrocardiographic sign of left ventricular hypertrophy is increased voltage of the QRS complexes in the left ventricular leads. Increased amplitude (> 18 mm) of the R wave in lead X on orthogonal electrocardiography of the Frank lead system may be a better method than conventional electrocardiography in the recognition of early left ventricular hypertrophy. As hypertrophy continues, the T waves become of lower amplitude, and this change is followed by slight depression of the ST segment; later, the ST segment depression is more marked and associated with asymmetrically inverted T waves in the left ventricular leads. In the fully developed pattern, the left ventricular QRS voltage is high and the ST segment in these leads is depressed, with a convex contour followed by an asymmetrically inverted T wave. Table 9–7 gives the criteria for the diagnosis of left ventricular hypertrophy. Examples of the development and regression of the electrocardiographic changes in left ventricular hypertrophy are shown in Figs 9–18 and 9–19.

2. Differentiation from myocardial infarction— The ST segment and T wave changes of left ventricular hypertrophy are in the same direction and are differentiated from myocardial ischemia (see Chapter 8), in which the ST segment when depressed is horizontally

Table 9–7. The criteria for the diagnosis of left ventricular hypertrophy in adults over 30 years of age.*

Standard limb leads

(1) Voltage $R_1 + S_3$ = 25 mm or more.
(2) RS–T_1 depressed 0.5 mm or more.
(3) T_1 flat, diphasic, or inverted, particularly when associated with (2) and a prominent R wave.
(4) T_2 and T_3 diphasic or inverted in the presence of tall R waves and findings in (2), above.
(5) T_3 greater than T_1 in the presence of left axis deviation and high voltage QRS complex in leads I and III.

Precordial leads

(1) Voltage of R wave in V_5 or V_6 exceeds 26 mm.
(2) RS–T segment depressed more than 0.5 mm in V_4, V_5, or V_6.
(3) A flat, diphasic, or inverted T wave in leads V_{4-6} with normal R and small S waves and findings in (2), above.
(4) Ventricular activation time in V_5 or V_6 = 0.06 sec or more, especially when associated with a tall R wave.

Unipolar limb leads

(1) RS–T segment depressed more than 0.5 mm in aVL or aVF.
(2) Flat, diphasic, or inverted T wave, with an R wave of 6 mm or more in aVL or aVF and findings in (1), above.
(3) Voltage of R wave in aVL exceeds 11 mm.
(4) Upright T wave in aVR.

*Reproduced, with permission, from Sokolow M, Lyon TP: The ventricular complex in left ventricular hypertrophy as obtained by unipolar precordial and limb leads. Am Heart J 37:161, 1949.

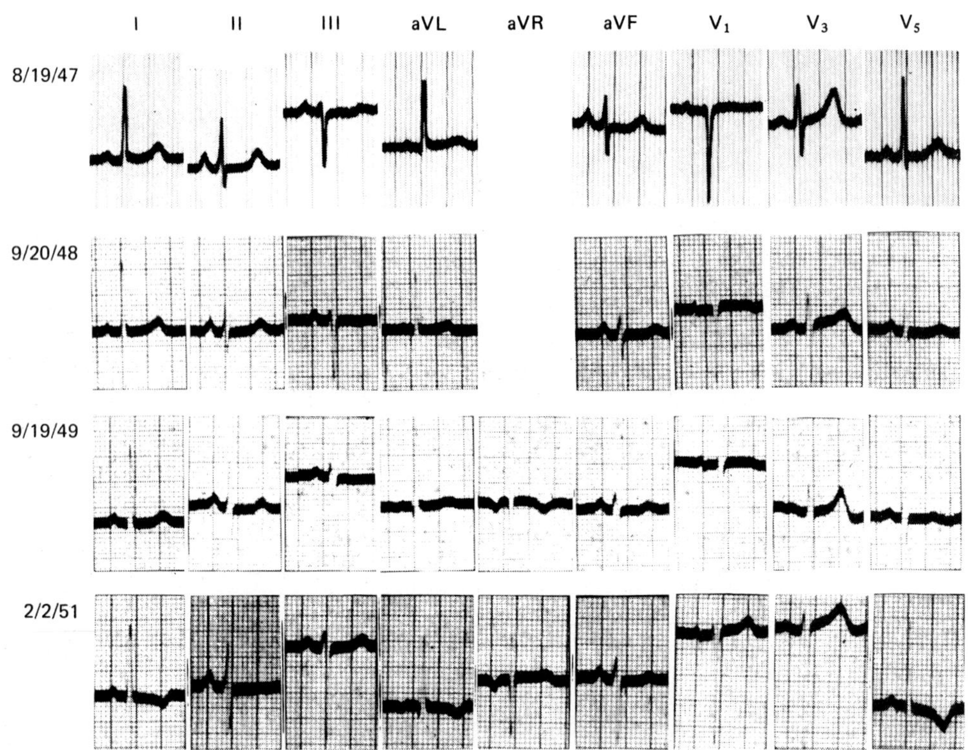

Figure 9–18. Progressive ST–T abnormalities in leads I, aVL, and V_5 between 1947 and 1951 in a 53-year-old woman. Serial chest x-rays showed no change in the size of the heart during this period. (Reproduced, with permission, from Grubschmidt HA, Sokolow M: The reliability of high voltage of the QRS complex as a diagnostic sign of left ventricular hypertrophy in adults. Am Heart J 54:689, 1957.)

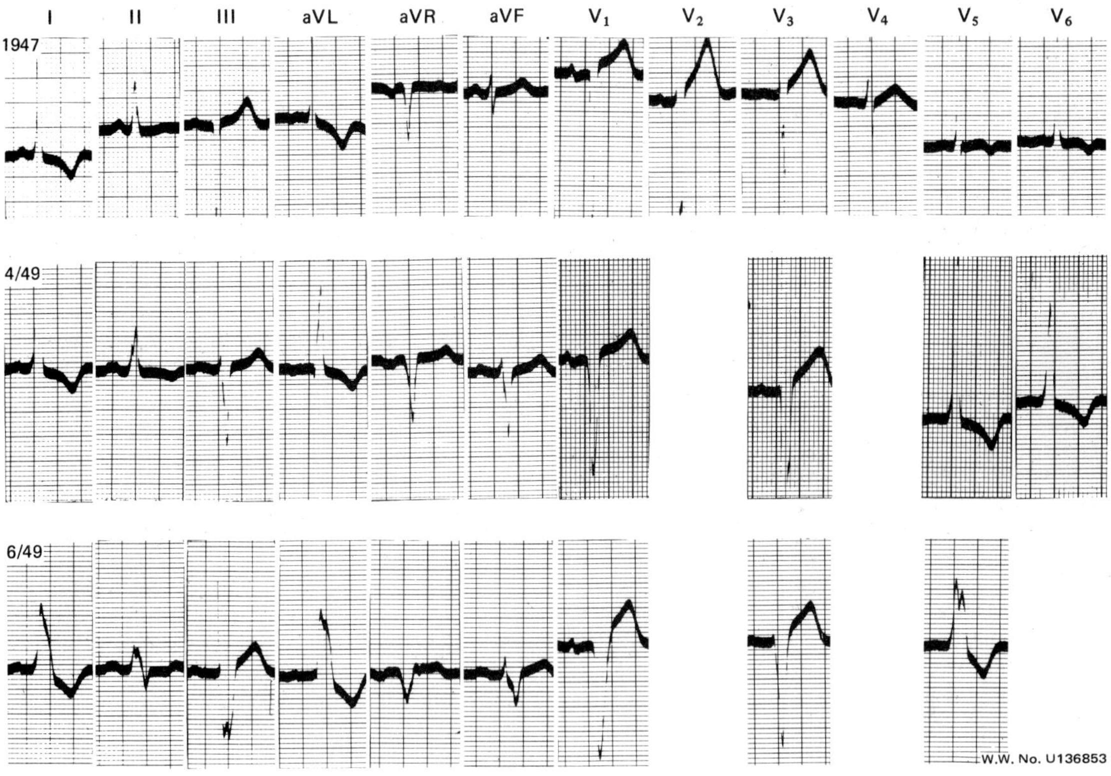

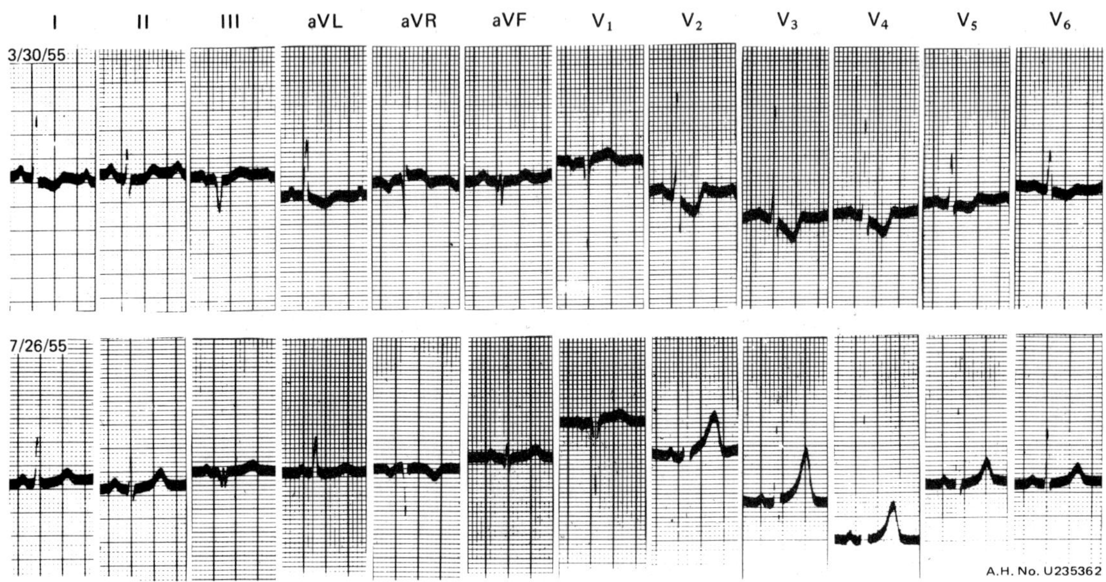

Figure 9–19. *Top:* Hypertensive cardiovascular disease and angina pectoris in a 73-year-old man. Cardiac enlargement +32%. Note progression from left ventricular hypertrophy to incomplete left bundle branch block to complete left bundle branch block with a wide monophasic QRS complex in lead I. *Bottom:* Malignant hypertension reversed to almost normotensive levels following unilateral nephrectomy in a 62-year-old man. Complete return of ST–T changes in lead V_4 to normal in 4 months.

depressed and the T wave when inverted is symmetrically inverted with or without ST depression. The characteristic ST–T changes in left ventricular hypertrophy occur only to the left of the ventricular septum (the transitional zone), and the inverse of this pattern is present in leads to the right of the transitional zone, ie, in the right precordial leads the ST segment is elevated and there is a tall, asymmetrically elevated T wave. This is in contrast to myocardial ischemia (see Chapter 8), in which the ST and T abnormalities seen in the left ventricular leads (V_4-V_6) spread across the transitional zone and may involve V_2 and V_3 as well. The ECG may also reveal evidence of previous myocardial infarction or obvious evidence of myocardial ischemia with classic Q waves or ischemic ST segments. In patients with long-standing hypertension, especially if there have been multiple episodes of myocardial ischemia, peripheral left ventricular conduction defects may be present with slurred QRS complexes, usually with a QRS duration less than 0.12 sec. Even with well-marked left ventricular hypertrophy, the frontal plane axis rarely exceeds –30 degrees; when the axis is farther to the left, in the range of –45 degrees, a left anterior hemiblock is superimposed and the axis change is not due to the left ventricular hypertrophy per se. Progressive abnormalities may include incomplete and complete left bundle branch block.

E. Drugs and Left Ventricular Hypertrophy: It is important to know what medications the patient is receiving in order to evaluate the electrocardiographic pattern in hypertension. In hypertensive patients receiving diuretic agents with resultant hypokalemia, sagging nonspecific ST segments and prominent U waves may be present similar to those found in primary aldosteronism. If the patient has been receiving digitalis, the characteristic sagging ST segments of digitalis and the decreased Q–T interval due to shortening of the action potential may also be present.

F. X-Ray Findings:

1. Plain chest film–The plain chest film may be completely normal despite well-marked hypertension if the concentric hypertrophy has not led to dilatation. The convex rounding of the left ventricle seen especially on the lateral views may allow the radiologist to suspect the presence of concentric hypertrophy, but it is not until left ventricular dilatation has occurred that enlargement of the left ventricle will be confirmed. The chest x-ray may show notching of the ribs in coarctation of the aorta, but this finding is rarely present before the late teen years. If there is left ventricular failure, pulmonary venous engorgement can be seen with or without diversion of blood to the upper lobes and pleural effusion. In the acute pulmonary edema of hypertension, there may be "bat's wing" densities or fluid in the interlobar spaces. The aortic knob may be enlarged and the descending aorta dilated out of proportion to the patient's age, suggesting the presence of associated aortic atherosclerosis. If the widening is excessive, chronic dissection of the aorta may be suspected; this may be confirmed by an aortogram. (For examples of chest x-rays, see Chapters 10 and 11, Cardiac Failure and Congenital Heart Disease.)

2. Intravenous urograms–Excretory urography may provide important evidence of possible renal vascular or renal parenchymal disorders as causes of hypertension. In younger patients with severe hypertension, the presence of unilateral renal artery stenosis may be evidenced by late appearance, hyperconcentration, and late disappearance of the contrast media, and the involved kidney is usually smaller than its mate by more than 1.5 cm (see p 223).

If renal vascular hypertension is suspected on the basis of the clinical picture, the presence of bruits, and the rapid sequence intravenous urographic findings, transfemoral aortography by the Seldinger technic is indicated in combination with differential renal vein renin studies only if renal vascular surgery is contemplated (see p 226 for indications). Selective renal artery angiograms disclose the anatomic features of stenosis, but the functional significance of the stenosis must be determined by still another technic. The method now considered to be most reliable is the relative renal vein renin production on the 2 sides; the difference is considered significant when the renal vein renin concentration on the affected side is at least 1½ times the concentration measured in the opposite (unaffected) side. If differential renal vein renin cannot be determined, renal artery stenosis can be strongly suspected by the decrease in water and sodium, with increased osmolality and creatinine concentration on the affected side. If the selective renal arteriogram shows no lesion of the main renal artery but a suspected lesion in one of the branches, renin from different segments of the kidney may reveal a segmental lesion or renin-producing tumor (Schambelan, 1974).

COURSE OF DISEASE & PROGNOSIS IN HYPERTENSION

Mild Hypertension

The average patient with mild to moderate hypertension is asymptomatic; the only abnormality is the rise in arterial pressure. The patient may complain of nonspecific headache or dizziness, but these have been shown to fluctuate with the emotional state and are unrelated to the height of the blood pressure in benign hypertension. Visual symptoms are absent or unrelated to the blood pressure.

Progression to Moderate Hypertension

Prognostic studies in untreated patients have shown that headaches and dizziness have no adverse prognostic significance unless they are associated with accelerated hypertension or with other evidence of neurologic disorder. When hypertension persists without treatment (as it almost always does), the patient may remain asymptomatic, but examination may reveal evidences of left ventricular hypertrophy as manifested by a left ventricular heave or electrocardio-

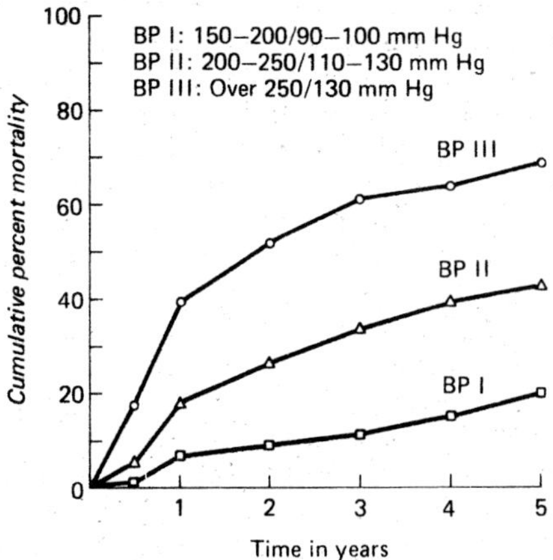

Figure 9–20. Relationship of mortality rate and initial blood pressure. (Reproduced, with permission, from Sokolow M: Some aspects of the natural history of hypertension: Proceedings of the 49th Annual Meeting of the Medical Section of the American Life Convention, 1962.)

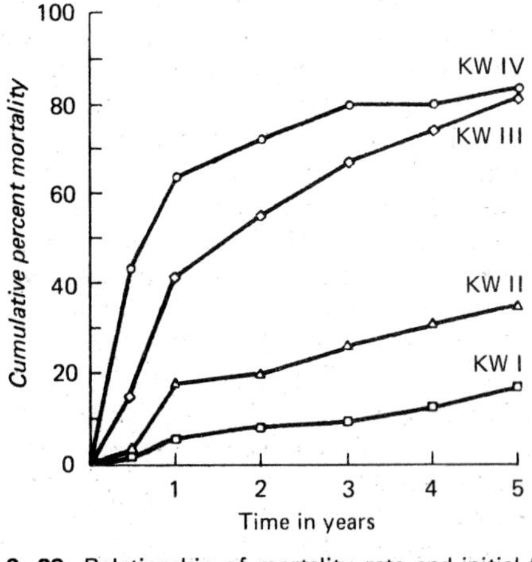

Figure 9–22. Relationship of mortality rate and initial fundal classification in hypertensive patients. (Reproduced, with permission of the American Heart Association, Inc., from Sokolow M, Perloff D: The prognosis of essential hypertension treated conservatively. Circulation 23:697, 1961.)

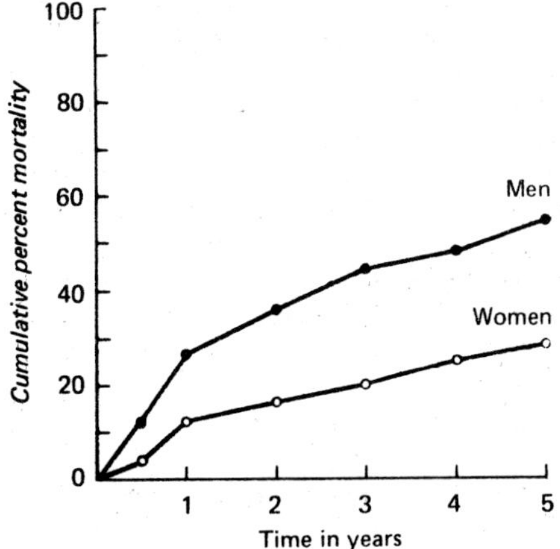

Figure 9–21. Relationship of mortality rate and sex in hypertensive patients. (Reproduced, with permission of the American Heart Association, Inc., from Sokolow M, Perloff D: The prognosis of essential hypertension treated conservatively. Circulation 23:697, 1961.)

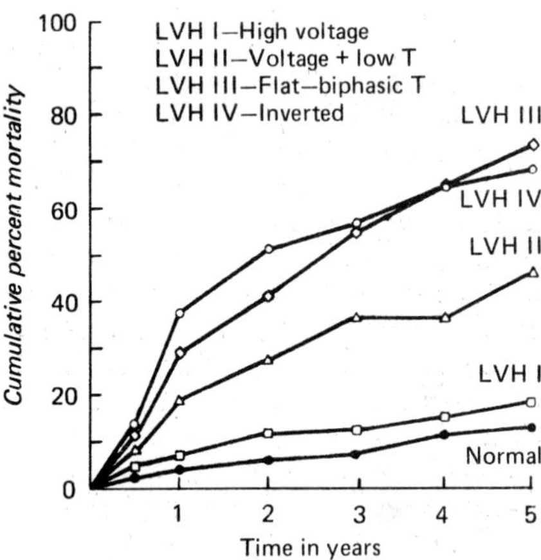

Figure 9–23. Relationship of mortality rate and initial degree of left ventricular hypertrophy (ECG) in hypertensive patients. (Reproduced, with permission of the American Heart Association, Inc., from Sokolow M, Perloff D: The prognosis of essential hypertension treated conservatively. Circulation 23:697, 1961.)

graphic changes (see above). The retinal arterioles may become irregularly narrowed, and arteriovenous nicking with a KW II classification may develop. The development of vascular abnormalities such as left ventricular hypertrophy or retinal arteriolar changes presages the development of clinical events and is an adverse prognostic sign (Sokolow, 1961).

If there is no accelerated phase, the first symptoms may reflect the development of left ventricular failure, with dyspnea, orthopnea, and paroxysmal nocturnal dyspnea associated with pulmonary rales and x-ray evidence of pulmonary congestion.

The prognosis with respect to mortality in hypertension is related to the age, race, and sex, to the height of the blood pressure, to the initial abnormality of the fundi, ECG, and chest x-ray, and to the presence or absence of atherosclerotic complications when the patient is first seen. Figs 9–20 to 9–23 illustrate the relationship of the mortality rate to these various factors.

Development of Clinical Manifestations of Atherosclerosis

The patient may develop a symptom indicating atherosclerotic involvement in one of the major vessels. The most common is the development of angina pectoris or acute myocardial infarction, although the first manifestation may be intermittent claudication, tran-

Table 9–8. Cause of death* in relation to initial severity of hypertension.†

Severity of Hypertension	Total Number Deaths	Cardiac Failure	"Hypertensive" Causes: Uremia	"Hypertensive" Causes: Malignant Hypertension	Coronary Thrombosis	Cerebrovascular Accident	Dissecting Aneurysm	Noncardiovascular Causes
Classes I & II	32	2	0	1	8	11	0	10
Classes III & IV	121	19	9	17	25	41	3	7

*In an additional 8 patients, cause of death was unknown.

†Reproduced, with permission of the American Heart Association, Inc., from Sokolow M, Perloff D: The prognosis of essential hypertension treated conservatively. Circulation 23:697, 1961.

sient ischemic cerebral attacks, or even cerebral infarction or cerebral hemorrhage.

Progression to Severe Hypertension

If the patient develops accelerated or malignant hypertension, the initial symptoms are usually severe suboccipital headaches, weakness, and visual disturbances, and the signs are papilledema, hemorrhages and exudates in the macular area, and gross hematuria. If the malignant hypertension is not recognized and treated promptly, the patient may develop manifestations of rapidly progressive cardiac and renal failure. Table 9–8 shows cause of death in relation to initial severity of hypertension. An abrupt rise of blood pressure often heralds the onset of renal failure in chronic renal disease.

Hypertensive Heart Failure

Before the advent of antihypertensive therapy, heart failure was responsible for death in 25% of patients with hypertension. Because hypertension is the most common cause of heart failure and is the most important risk factor in accelerating coronary atherosclerosis, and because it is responsible for at least half of all deaths from heart failure and for almost all cases of cerebral hemorrhage, epidemiologists participating in the Framingham Study (Kannel, 1974) have stated that the most important means of preventing cardiovascular disease is to identify and treat hypertension before complications develop.

Hypertension as Major Cause of Heart Failure

In a study of left ventricular failure, Bedford (1939) found that 80–85% of patients with paroxysmal dyspnea with or without angina or myocardial infarction had hypertension. Aortic valve disease was the third and least common cause of heart failure in the triad of hypertension, coronary heart disease, and aortic valve disease. The prognosis for life, once left ventricular failure with paroxysmal dyspnea or pulmonary edema occurred, was very poor. The average duration of life was 1 year, and one-third of the patients died within 6 months. In the Framingham Study, 50% of patients with cardiac failure were dead within 5 years even with modern therapy. Goldring and Chasis (1944), in a study of untreated hypertensive patients, found that 85% were dead within 3 years of the development of cardiac failure.

Effect of Antihypertensive Therapy on Prognosis

The introduction of effective antihypertensive therapy has changed the picture dramatically. Table 9–9 from the Veterans Administration Cooperative Study documents the considerable decrease in morbid events in the treated group as compared to the control, untreated group. Morbid events included hypertensive complications such as heart failure, cerebral hemorrhage, accelerated or malignant hypertension, or dissecting aneurysm of the aorta. Not only is heart failure reversed by antihypertensive therapy, but the development of heart failure during adequate therapy is rare, indicating the dominant role played by elevated blood pressure in the development of heart failure. The causes of death in treated hypertension are shown in Table 9–10. At present, no more than 5% of all deaths

Table 9–9. Incidence of morbid events with respect to level of prerandomization blood pressure.*

Prerandomization Blood Pressure (mm Hg)	Control Group: Patients Randomized	Control Group: Patients With "Morbid Event" Number	Control Group: Patients With "Morbid Event" Percent	Treated Group: Patients Randomized	Treated Group: Patients With "Morbid Event" Number	Treated Group: Patients With "Morbid Event" Percent	Percent Effectiveness
Systolic < 165	98	15	15.3	108	10	9.3	40
Systolic 165+	96	41	42.7	78	12	15.4	64
Total	194	56		186	22		
Diastolic 90–104	84	21	25.0	86	14	16.3	35
Diastolic 105–114	110	35	31.8	100	8	8.0	75
Total	194	56		186	22		

*Reproduced, with permission, from Veterans Administration Cooperative Study Group on Antihypertensive Agents: Effects of treatment on morbidity in hypertension. JAMA 213:1143, 1970. Copyright © American Medical Association.

Table 9–10. Causes of death in treated hypertension.*

	1952–59	1960–67	Total
Deaths due to hypertension			
Uremia	38 (44%)	59 (29%)	97
Cerebrovascular disease	24 (28%)	42 (21%)	66
Myocardial infarction	6 (7%)	54 (27%)	60
Sudden cardiac death	. .	3	3
Congestive heart failure	5	11	16
Aneurysm of aorta			
Dissection	5	7	12
Ruptured abdominal aneurysm	. .	3	3
Deaths due to drugs			
Paralytic ileus	4	1	5
Overdose of hypotensive drugs	. .	1	1
Suicide	. .	1	1
Deaths due to other causes			
Carcinoma	. .	12	12
Chronic bronchitis	. .	2	2
Postoperative	1	2	3
Disseminated lupus erythematosus	1	. .	1
Unknown	3	5	8
Total	87	203	290

*Reproduced, with permission, from Breckenridge A, Dollery CT, Parry EH: Prognosis of treated hypertension: Changes in life expectancy and causes of death between 1952 and 1967. Q J Med 39:411, 1970.

in hypertensive patients receiving effective treatment are due to heart failure, although the combination of myocardial infarction and hypertension may lead to ischemic cardiomyopathy and heart failure. Eighty percent of patients with hypertensive heart failure treated by Smirk (1963) were leading productive lives 2–7 years after treatment–in marked contrast to Goldring's (1944) data, which showed that only one-fourth of the patients survived for 3 years. The importance of adequate therapy is shown in Table 9–11.

The rapid response of heart failure in hypertensive patients to antihypertensive therapy is much more striking than the response of heart failure to medical treatment in patients with coronary heart disease without hypertension who develop ischemic cardiomyopathy following myocardial infarction.

Influence of Coronary Disease in Causing Failure

It is difficult to separate the effects of hypertension and coronary heart disease in causing heart failure when they coexist in the same patient. Cardiac failure is frequent, however, in young adults with coarctation of the aorta and hypertension who do not have coronary disease. The importance of treating the elevated blood pressure in such cases, however, should be apparent.

Effect of Hypertension on Coronary Disease

Coronary artery disease associated with hypertension is commonly present without development of hypertensive heart failure. The evidence supporting the role of hypertension in accelerating coronary heart disease has been adduced by the pathologic data of Bell and Clawson and by the prospective studies of the Framingham group (see Chapter 8). Data from Bell and Clawson (1928) indicate that severe coronary disease was 10 times more common in an autopsied group of patients who had hypertension during life than in a normotensive group. Evidence of coronary disease during life was 7 times more common in the hypertensive group. Bell and Clawson also showed a high correlation between the severity of atherosclerosis in the cerebral, carotid, and basilar-vertebral arteries and the systolic blood pressure.

Since the purely hypertensive complications of a raised pressure are prevented or reversed by antihypertensive therapy, the atherosclerotic complications predominate and are the most common cause of disability and death in treated hypertensive patients. Therefore, coronary heart disease in all of its manifestations, cerebral infarction, cerebral hemorrhage, and carotid and extremity atherosclerosis, although particularly prevalent in the hypertensive population, cannot be distinguished from the same manifestations in the nonhypertensive but atherosclerotic population.

Malignant Hypertension

Malignant hypertension is a syndrome characterized by a rapidly rising blood pressure (diastolic pressures usually in excess of 130 mm Hg) from any cause. The symptoms of onset are shown in Table 9–12. Table 9–13 shows cardiac findings. Unless effective antihypertensive therapy is given promptly, there may be severe visual loss associated with hemorrhage, exudates, and papilledema of the ocular fundi, and death due to uremia, heart failure, or cerebral hemorrhage usually occurs in less than 1 year. Pathologic changes are seen in the arterioles and in the small

Table 9–11. Survival of treated hypertensive patients as a function of the adequacy of the control of the elevated blood pressure.*

Number of Patients	Patient Groups	Total Deaths		Causes of Death: Hypertensive Complications		Causes of Death: Atherosclerotic Complications		Causes of Death: Other	
		Percent	Number	Percent	Number	Percent	Number	Percent	Number
38	Uncontrolled	100	38	75	29	14	5	11	4
58	Partially controlled	79	46	36	21	11	6	32	19
220	Controlled	49	108	16	35	13	29	20	44

*Reproduced, with permission, from Perry M, Wessler S, Avioli LV: Survival of treated hypertensive patients. JAMA 210:890, 1969. Copyright © American Medical Association.

Table 9–12. Symptoms marking onset of malignant phase of hypertension in 104 cases.*

Symptom	Number of Cases
Visual impairment	79
Acute headache	6
Gross hematuria	5
Visual impairment and gross hematuria	3
Acute cardiac failure	1
Gastrointestinal upset with nausea, vomiting, and epigastric pain	1
Undetermined due to vagueness of symptoms	9

*Reproduced, with permission, from Schottstaedt MF, Sokolow M: The natural history and course of hypertension with papilledema (malignant hypertension). Am Heart J 45:331, 1953.

interlobular arteries (see Fig 9–9) The kidney is progressively destroyed by ischemic atrophy of the nephrons, with decrease in glomerular filtration rate and renal blood flow because of fibrinoid necrosis of the arterioles and cellular intimal proliferation of the interlobular arteries. Some patients with pathologically proved fibrinoid necrosis do not have papilledema, but they usually have hemorrhages or exudates in the fundi. Prognostic studies have shown that the 3- to 5-year mortality rate is essentially indistinguishable in untreated patients with KW III fundi as compared to those with KW IV fundi; both represent accelerated hypertension.

Table 9–13. Cardiac findings in 104 patients with malignant hypertension.*

Cardiac enlargement (slight or moderate in 67; marked in 14)		
Clinically		81
Radiologically		57
Symptoms of cardiac failure or decreased cardiac reserve		73
Signs of cardiac failure		51
Observed before onset of malignant phase	8	
Observed simultaneously with onset of malignant phase	11	
Developed during first year of illness	28	
Developed during second year of illness	4	
Angina pectoris		20
Murmurs (systolic, except for 5 diastolic)		72
Gallop rhythm (S_3, S_4)		30
Pericardial friction rub		10
Pulsus alternans		9
Arrhythmia		5
Electrocardiographic abnormalities (of 89 patients)		82
Left ventricular hypertrophy:		
"Characteristic of" or "probably"	48	
"Suggestive of"	14	
Myocardial changes secondary to coronary disease	15	
No characteristic pattern	13	
Within normal limits	7	

*Reproduced, with permission, from Schottstaedt MF, Sokolow M: The natural history and course of hypertension with papilledema (malignant hypertension). Am Heart J 45:331, 1953.

The rapid rise in blood pressure may cause cardiac failure within 1–2 weeks and renal failure within a month. Examination of the retinas for evidence of accelerated hypertension is necessary in all hypertensive patients, because the early stages of the malignant phase may be essentially asymptomatic although severe headache, acute visual disturbances, and gross hematuria are the usual presenting manifestations. Cardiac and renal failure may occur with great rapidity, and treatment to lower the blood pressure is urgent. Patients seen early with evidence of accelerated or malignant hypertension may have normal renal function and even absence of proteinuria. This rapidly progresses, however, to malignant hypertension with proteinuria and azotemia and then finally to renal failure. For this reason, treatment is essential before the development of renal failure.

Malignant hypertension is a quantitatively more severe form of hypertension, and prevention is far more effective than treatment of the established or advanced disease. Accelerated or malignant hypertension is rare in properly treated hypertensive patients.

If no treatment is given, the mortality rate in 1 year is 80% and in 2 years approaches 100%.

The importance of prevention of the malignant phase can be outlined as follows:

(1) Malignant hypertension is rare in the properly managed patient with benign hypertension (Smirk, 1963; Kincaid-Smith, 1973; Pickering, 1968; Freis, 1970).

(2) Adequate follow-up and education of patient regarding compliance with therapy is essential. Stopping therapy in severe hypertension is hazardous.

(3) Early symptoms of accelerated disease should trigger therapeutic response (sudden onset of visual disturbances, severe headache, gross hematuria).

(4) Prognosis of malignant hypertension is related to the degree of renal impairment existing when treatment began (Schottstaedt, 1952; Kincaid-Smith, 1958).

(5) Treatment of severe hypertension prevents the malignant phase; early treatment of the malignant phase prevents azotemia; treatment of azotemia without uremia prevents uremia.

(6) Mortality rate in the treatment of severe hypertension is related to the effectiveness with which the blood pressure was lowered (Farmer, 1963; Gifford, 1974; Perry, 1969; Doyle, 1975).

COMPLICATIONS

Dissection of the Aorta

One of the complications of hypertension that often is unrecognized, especially in pregnant women, is dissection of the aorta. Hypertension is the presumed cause in one-third of cases of proximal and two-thirds of cases of distal dissection (Slater, 1976). Cystic medial necrosis and arteriosclerosis are much less common causes. The onset is usually acute (90% of cases), with severe instantaneous chest pain radiating to the back or abdomen combined with evidence of obstruction of the branches of the aorta and diminished or absent pulses from the carotids to the femoral arteries. The diagnosis can be established by supravalvular angiography, although it can be strongly suspected clinically and radiologically (Table 9–14 and Figs 9–24 and 9–25A–D). If one records a widened aorta or a double echo in the aorta in the presence of clinical evidence of aortic root dissection, the diagnosis can also be suspected on the basis of echocardiography. The abrupt development of chest pain, aortic insufficiency, diminished or absent pulses, or the appearance of signs of "sympathectomy" on one side and of neurologic deficit with cerebral symptoms should make one think of dissection of the aorta. The pain may be differentiated from that of acute myocardial infarction by its instantaneous onset, its severity, the absence of central pulses, and the presence of hypertension despite pain or even shock. Aortic dissection has been classified as type I, which involves the proximal ascending aorta and aortic arch, at times extending distally to the iliac arteries; type II, which involves only the ascending aorta and is sometimes combined with type I and called proximal dissection; and type III, which involves only the distal aorta beyond the left subclavian artery. Types I and II may involve the aortic valve, causing aortic insufficiency and heart failure, and are more serious than type III. The pathogenesis of dissection is illustrated in Fig 9–26.

Dissection involving the distal aorta may be treated medically with intensive antihypertensive therapy, and surgical treatment is reserved for the patient who fails to respond. In type I and II dissection the mortality rate is high, aortic insufficiency may occur, and the aorta may rupture into the pericardium or pleura; after immediate lowering of the blood pressure with parenteral antihypertensive agents and establishment of the diagnosis by supravalvular aortography, surgical treatment is recommended. Without treatment the mortality rate is very high, but with modern surgical treatment survival may be as high as 75%.

Table 9–14. Roentgenographic findings in aortic dissection.*

Abnormalities on Chest Roentgenogram	Dissection: Proximal (n = 45) Percent	Dissection: Distal (n = 71) Percent
Definitely abnormal aortic contour	34	64
"Possibly" abnormal aorta	8	5
Normal chest roentgenogram	3	2
"Calcium" sign	0	10
Pleural effusion	2	9

*Reproduced, with permission, from Slater EE, DeSanctis RW: The clinical recognition of dissecting aortic aneurysm. Am J Med 60:625, 1976.

Prognosis of Dissection of the Aorta

Untreated, the prognosis is poor (Fig 9–27). When the dissection is confined to the distal aorta, medical antihypertensive treatment permits most patients to survive without operation. In proximal aortic dissections, the prognosis is poor with medical treatment because of the risks of aortic insufficiency, car-

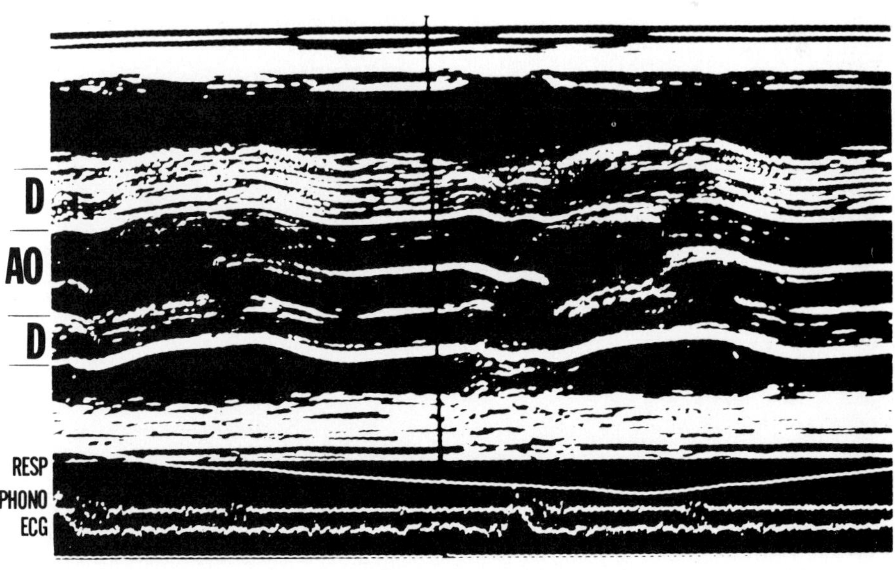

Figure 9–24. Aortic root echogram reveals marked parallel widening of both anterior and posterior walls. Aortic valve cusps are slender and show normal motion pattern. D, width of the dissecting hematoma; AO, aorta; RESP, respirations; PHONO, phonocardiogram; ECG, electrocardiogram. (Reproduced, with permission of the American Heart Association, Inc., from Nanda NC, Gramiak R, Shah PM: Diagnosis of aortic root dissection by echocardiography. Circulation 48:506, 1973.)

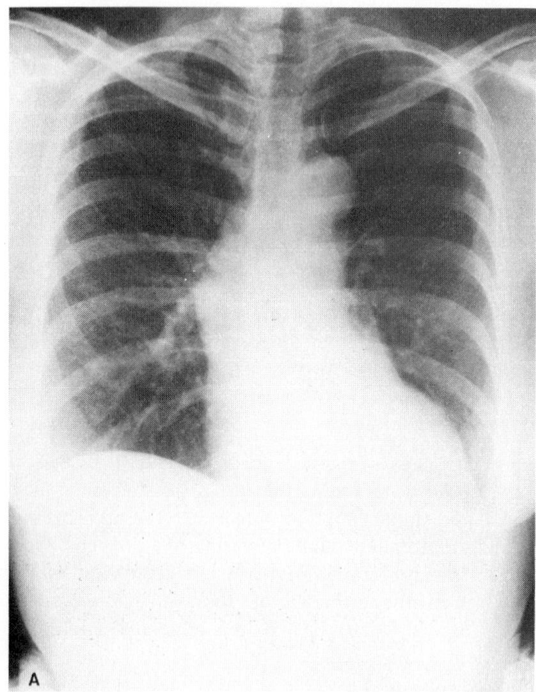

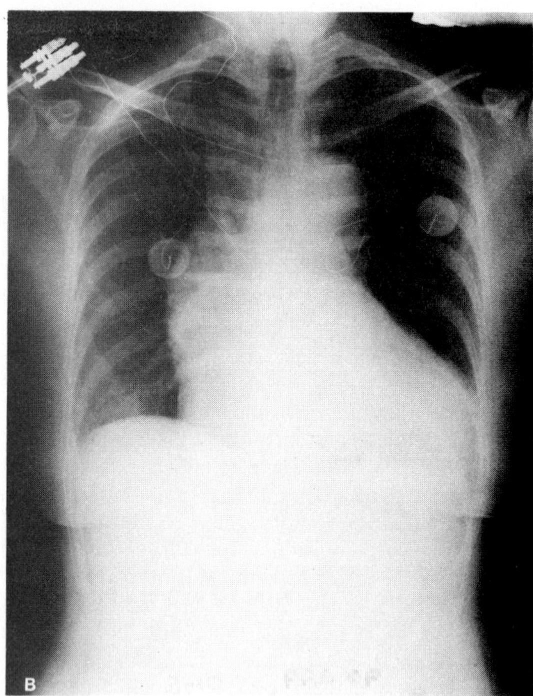

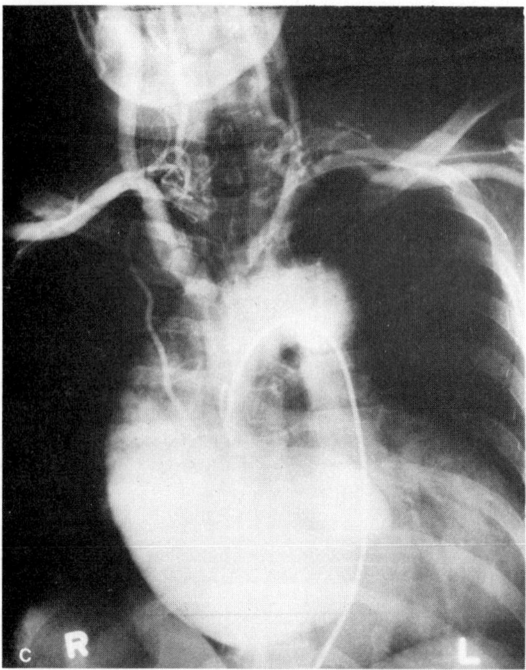

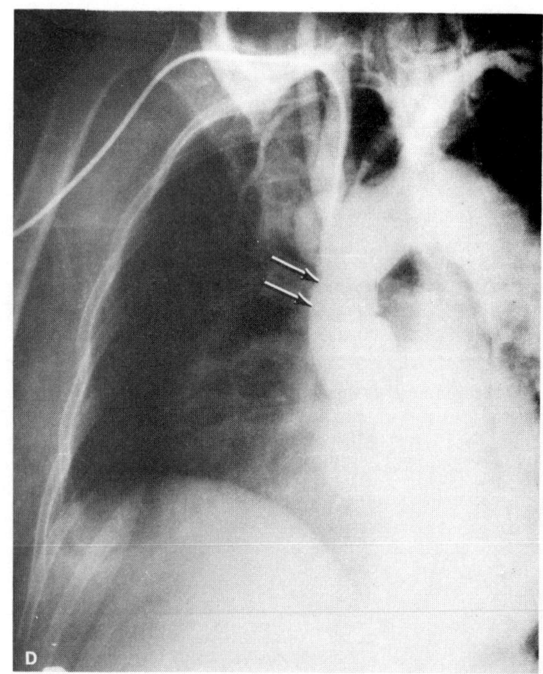

Figure 9–25. Dissection of the aorta in hypertension in a 52-year-old man with severe chest pain. *A:* 3/6/72—Plain chest film predissection showing dilated ascending aorta in asymptomatic patient. *B:* 3/10/72—Preoperative plain chest film postdissection after sudden severe chest pain showing massive dilatation of the ascending and descending aorta with striking changes since *A. C:* 3/7/72—Aortogram showing the true channel (A) and the aneurysmal sac (B), partially filled with contrast medium. The dark line shows the separation between the true and false channels. *D:* 3/28/72—Postoperative angiogram after resection of the ascending aorta and aneurysmal sac and insertion of a Dacron graft (see arrow) from the ascending aorta. Pathologic focal degeneration of media and intimal fibrosis.

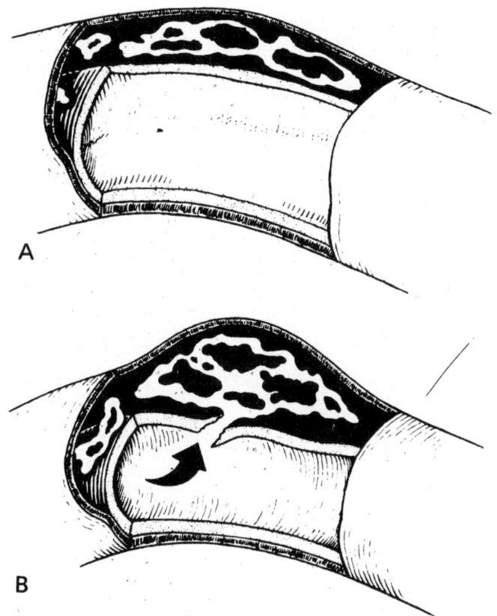

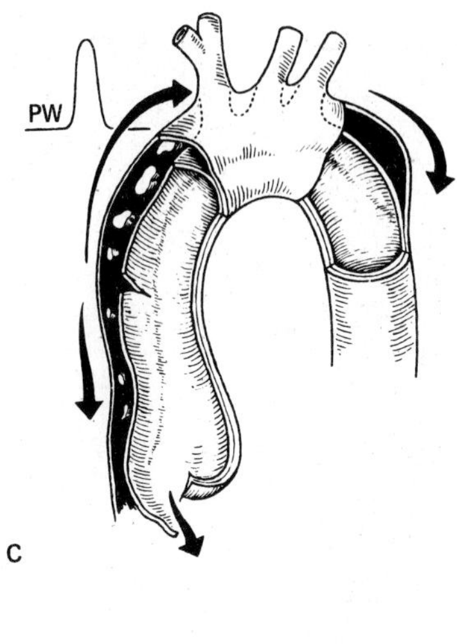

Figure 9–26. Diagrammatic representation of pathogenesis of aortic dissection. *A:* Cystic medial necrosis in the aortic wall sets the stage. *B:* Combined forces acting on the aortic wall result in the intimal tear, directing aortic bloodstream into the diseased media. *C:* Resulting dissecting hematoma is propagated by the pulse wave (PW) produced by each myocardial contraction. (Reproduced, with permission, from Wheat MW: Treatment of dissecting aneurysms of the aorta: Current status. Prog Cardiovasc Dis 16:87, 1973.)

diac failure, rupture of the aneurysm, or progression of the dissection, and surgical treatment is advised. The indications for surgical therapy are summarized in Table 9–15. With surgical treatment of the complications, the mortality rate has decreased from 80% in 2 weeks to 30%.

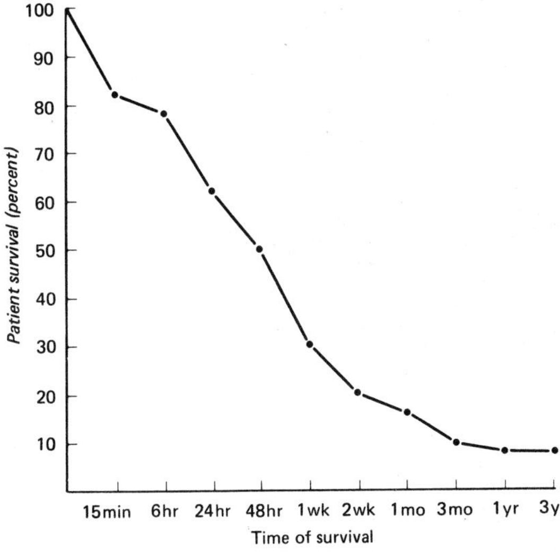

Figure 9–27. Graphic illustration of the length of survival of 963 patients with acute aortic dissection who were not treated. (Reproduced, with permission, from Wheat MW: Treatment of dissecting aneurysms of the aorta: Current status. Prog Cardiovasc Dis 16:87, 1973; as modified from Anagnostopoulos CE, Prabhakar MJS, Kittle CF: Aortic dissections and dissecting aneurysms. Am J Cardiol 30:263, 1972.)

Table 9–15. Specific complications requiring strong consideration for surgical therapy.*

Overwhelming aortic insufficiency
Progressive heart failure
Occlusion of major aortic branches
Progressive symptoms
Continuing dissection
Pain after hypertension is controlled
Uncontrolled bleeding into left side of chest
Hemopericardium and tamponade
Widening of mediastinum on x-ray study
Impending rupture by x-ray study
Shift of left border of descending aorta to the left
Loss of sharpness of border of retrocardiac aortic shadow
Hazy markings in left lower lung field
Left pleural effusion
Enlarging para-aortic mass
Patchy infiltration or "ray"-like infiltration of adjacent lung field

*Modified slightly and reproduced, with permission, from Anagnostopoulos CE, Prabhakar MJS, Kittle CF: Aortic dissections and dissecting aneurysms. Am J Cardiol 30:263, 1972.

II. SECONDARY HYPERTENSION

RENAL ARTERY STENOSIS

Renal artery stenosis is probably the most common cause of curable secondary hypertension, but clinical enthusiasm for seeking out the diagnosis and treating by operation has waned in recent years. This is

Table 9–16. Frequency of major occlusive renal artery disease in relation to clinical indications for arteriography.*

	Patients With Abnormal Arteriogram		Patients With Normal Arteriogram		Total Patients
	Number	Percent	Number	Percent	Cases
Aorto-iliac atherosclerosis	60	73	22	27	82
Onset of hypertension over age 50	33	70	15	30	48
Epigastric bruit	108	64	59	36	167
KW III or IV fundi	28	52	26	48	54
Abnormal intravenous pyelogram	94	41	132	59	226
Recent onset of hypertension	70	40	101	60	171
Recent increase in hypertension	31	37	51	63	82
Onset of hypertension under age 20	7	13	46	87	53
Hypertension without other indications	4	10	35	90	39

*Reproduced, with permission, from Sokolow M & others: Current experiences with renovascular hypertension. Page 341 in: *Proceedings of the International Club on Arterial Hypertension.* Expansion Scientifique Française, 1966.

partly because the vascular complications can often be managed by medical antihypertensive therapy in less severe cases and partly because the operation is associated with significant morbidity and mortality rates in older people with atherosclerotic renal artery stenosis due to clinical atherosclerosis elsewhere in the vascular system. Furthermore, surgical relief of the obstruction does not always cure the hypertension even in patients whose renal artery stenosis has been proved by selective renal angiography and differential renal vein renin concentration. Significant improvement occurs in about 75% of patients with fibromuscular hyperplasia and about 50% of patients with atherosclerotic renal artery stenosis.

When Should a Renal Angiogram Be Done?

It was at one time commonly thought that all persons under age 20–25 as well as older individuals (above age 50–55) who develop hypertension should have a renal angiogram to exclude renal artery stenosis. It is now known that primary hypertension is more common than formerly thought in young people, and the former criterion is no longer used. If a person develops hypertension for the first time after age 50, ie, if there is reliable documentation that blood pressures were normal prior to age 50–55, the indication for renal arteriograms is stronger, especially if the hypertension is severe. Atherosclerotic renal artery stenosis is commonly associated with severe or malignant hypertension, and any patient who develops malignant hypertension who is not known to have primary renal disease should be studied thoroughly, including the use of renal arteriograms, to exclude a surgically treatable lesion. Indications other than onset over age 50 or malignant hypertension are documented in Table 9–16.

Younger individuals (under age 40), especially women, are more apt to have fibromuscular hyperplasia or some unusual renal vascular lesion than atherosclerosis and are apt to have a less severe variety of hypertension. These patients deserve study with invasive technics if they have an epigastric bruit and classic changes on the intravenous urogram, because the surgical mortality rate is low and complete cure of the hypertension is possible.

Clinical Findings of Renal Artery Stenosis

There are no distinctive symptoms that separate primary from secondary hypertension due to renal artery stenosis. Factors that favor a diagnosis of renal vascular hypertension are a negative family history of hypertension, the presence of a systolic or diastolic epigastric bruit transmitted to the flanks, accelerated or malignant hypertension, hypertension appearing for the first time after age 50, or significant x-ray findings (see below). Table 9–17 shows the comparative clini-

Table 9–17. Clinical characteristics of essential hypertension and renovascular hypertension cured by surgery.*†

	Essential Hypertension (Percent)	Renovascular Hypertension (Percent)
Duration of hypertension		
< 1 year	12	24
>10 years	15	6
Age at onset (> 50 years)	9	15
Family history of hypertension	71	46
Fundi, grade 3 or 4	7	15
Bruit		
Abdomen	6	46
Flank	1	12
Abdomen or flank	7	48
Blood urea nitrogen > 20 mg/100 ml	8	15
Serum K < 3.4 mEq/l	8	16
Serum CO_2 > 30 mEq/l	5	17
Urinary casts	9	20
Proteinuria (trace or more)	32	46

*Reproduced, with permission, from Maxwell MH: Cooperative study of renovascular hypertension: Current status. Kidney Int (Suppl 8), pp 153–160, 1975.

†Patients were matched (131 pairs) by age, sex, race, and diastolic blood pressure (from Maxwell).

Table 9–18. Comparison of clinical and radiologic characteristics of patients with renal arterial stenosis due to atherosclerosis or fibromuscular hyperplasia.*

Clinical Data	Atherosclerosis	Fibromuscular Hyperplasia
Total number	95	70
Male/female	56/39	8/62
Bilateral/unilateral stenosis	47/48	36/34
Unilateral stenosis: right/left	30/18	21/13
Severity of hypertension		
Class I	10	26
Class II	40	30
Class III	30	14
Class IV	15	0
Age at time of study (years)		
0–10	0	3
11–20	0	2
21–30	0	14
31–40	6	17
41–50	33	21
51–60	38	10
61–70	16	3
Over 70	2	0
Ocular fundi		
Grade KW–IV	12	0
Grade KW–III	13	3
Renal function impaired	16	0
Extrarenal vascular disease	53	8

*Reproduced, with permission, from Perloff D & others: Renal vascular hypertension: Further experiences. Am Heart J 74:614, 1967.

cal characteristics of essential hypertension versus renovascular hypertension cured by surgery. Table 9–18 compares clinical and radiologic characteristics of the 2 forms of renal artery stenosis—that due to atherosclerosis and that due to fibromuscular hyperplasia.

A. X-Ray and Laboratory Procedures; Intravenous Urogram: Rapid sequence intravenous urogram suggests renal artery stenosis if it shows one kidney to be shorter than the other by 1.5 cm or more, with delayed appearance, hyperconcentration, and delayed emptying of the contrast medium. The most reliable of these signs is delay in appearance of the contrast medium in the calyces on one side. One- and 2-minute films should be obtained to look for the early delay in appearance time; in later films the disparity may be lost. The difference in size of the 2 kidneys is less helpful because occasionally there may be a difference of 1.5–2 cm in size of the 2 kidneys without other abnormality. Hyperconcentration is due to increased reabsorption of water from a proximal tubule with normal reabsorption of sodium. The reduced volume of fluid with a low sodium concentration reaching the distal tubule results in a relatively greater concentration of the contrast medium. Recognition of increased concentration is sometimes difficult because of differences in the anteroposterior depth of the 2 kidneys, and one should examine the 2 ureters for confirmation. Delayed uptake and excretion of radioisotopes on

Table 9–19. Radiologic classification of renal artery abnormalities in 247 hypertensive patients.*

	Number of Patients
Significant renal artery stenosis	
Atherosclerosis	95
Fibromuscular hyperplasia	70
Small renal artery and small kidney	13
Miscellaneous lesions (thrombosis, aneurysm, fibrosis, etc)	17
Total	195
Minor renal artery narrowing	
Atherosclerosis	34
Fibromuscular hyperplasia	14
Miscellaneous	4
Total	52

*Reproduced, with permission, from Sokolow M & others: Current experiences with renovascular hypertension. Page 341 in: *Proceedings of the International Club on Arterial Hypertension.* Expansion Scientifique Française, 1966.

the affected side may be seen also in a triple radioisotope renogram. Notching of the ureters is a helpful sign of increased collateral circulation which, as with arterial stenosis elsewhere, reflects a significant hemodynamic stenosis. Seventy to 80% of patients with renal artery stenosis have positive urologic signs on the rapid sequence intravenous urogram, but both false-positive and false-negative results are reported. A completely negative intravenous urogram suggests the probable absence of renovascular hypertension, but 20–25% of patients with proved renovascular hypertension have a negative intravenous urogram. Table 9–19 reflects the radiologic classification of renal artery abnormalities in 247 hypertensive patients, and Figs 9–28 and 9–29 show typical radiologic findings of renal artery stenosis. Table 9–20 shows radio-

Table 9–20. Age distribution of children and adolescents with nonuremic hypertension (61 patients).*

Site of Abnormality	Age 0–5	6–10	11–15	16–21	Total
Renal parenchyma					
Chronic atrophic pyelonephritis	0	2	1	2	5
Hydronephrosis	0	0	1	4	5
Posttraumatic subcapsular scar	0	0	0	1	1
Tumor	1	0	0	0	1
Small artery supplying a small kidney	0	2	1	3	6
Renal artery and abdominal aorta (stenosis)					
Renal artery	5	5	9	11	30
Abdominal aorta	6	2	1	0	9
Adrenal gland					
Pheochromocytoma	0	1	1	1	3
Aldosteronoma	0	1	0	0	1

*Reproduced, with permission, from Korobkin M & others: Etiologic radiographic findings in children and adolescents with nonuremic hypertension. Pediatr Radiol 110:615, 1974.

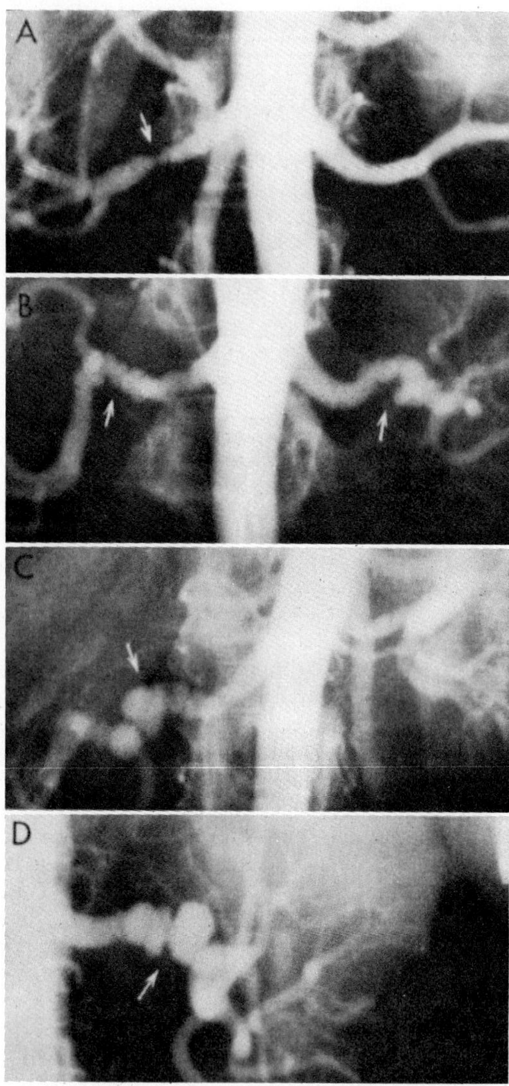

Figure 9–28. Examples of fibromuscular hyperplasia of the renal arteries. *A* and *D*, unilateral; *B* and *C*, bilateral. In *C*, the disease on the left is obscured by the tortuous overlapping vessel; upright arteriograms or studies with the patient in deep inspiration would have better defined the lesion on the left. In *B* the pathologic changes extend into the branches of the main renal arteries, and in *C* and *D* aneurysms are present. (Reproduced, with permission, from Palubinskas AJ, Perloff D, Wylie EJ: Curable hypertension due to renal artery lesions. Radiologia Clinica 33:207, 1964. S. Karger AG, Basel.)

graphic findings of site and age for children and adolescents with nonuremic hypertension.

Atrophic or hypoplastic kidneys shown on the intravenous urogram are a special problem. The small size of a kidney on one side is more apt to be due to a small or stenotic renal artery than to congenital atrophy or chronic pyelonephritis. If the renal vein renin determination indicates a lesion in the atrophic kidney, surgical treatment is indicated.

Despite the value of the rapid sequence intravenous urogram in the recognition of renovascular hypertension, one should not perform the procedure unless one is prepared to go further to establish the diagnosis by renal vein renin determinations and surgery if the studies show definitive abnormalities. The procedure should not be routinely done, because most patients have essential hypertension and not renal artery stenosis and because of the time and great expense of the procedure. These same comments are even more pertinent in the case of determining differential renal vein renin, especially since the total number of patients who have surgically correctable hypertension is a very small percentage of the hypertensive population at large.

B. Assessment of Differential Renal Function (Howard or Stamey Test): Differential renal function measurement by the Howard or Stamey test is not often done today, having been replaced by differential renal vein renin determinations or by the vasodepressor response to angiotensin blockade by a peptide (SQ 20881) which is an inhibitor of the converting enzyme blocking the generation of angiotensin II from angiotensin I. The substantial morbidity rate from catheterization of the ureters and the difficulty of accurate collection of specimens because of the long time involved for the study have made split function tests

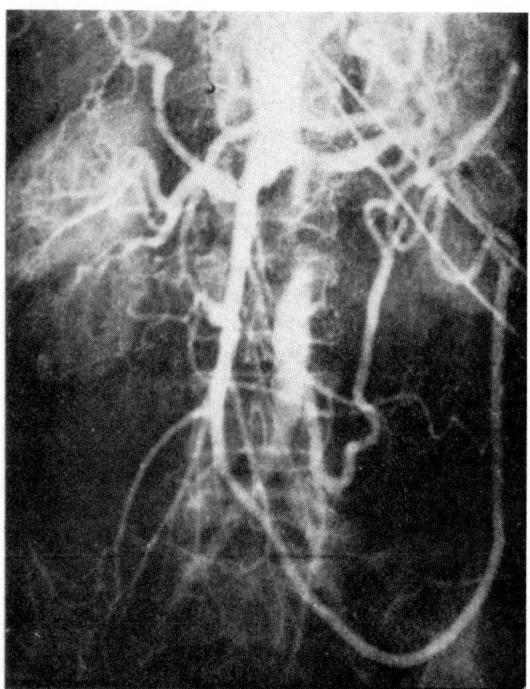

Figure 9–29. Aortogram of a 46-year-old woman; complete obstruction of the abdominal aorta and stenosis of the proximal portion of the left renal artery were found at operation to be due to atherosclerosis. (Reproduced, with permission of the American Heart Association, Inc., from Perloff D & others: Hypertension secondary to renal artery occlusive disease. Circulation 24:1286, 1961.)

relatively uncommon except in hospitals where renal vein renin levels or saralasin (an inhibitor of already formed angiotensin II) responses with or without moderate sodium depletion cannot be obtained, or when the differential renal vein renins are equivocal. Decreased glomerular filtrate and renal blood flow in renal artery stenosis causes a smaller volume of glomerular filtrate to enter the proximal tubule, resulting in the excretion from the affected side of a low volume of urine with a low sodium concentration but a high creatinine concentration and high osmolality.

C. Renal Vein Renin Determination: It has long been postulated that hypertension due to renal ischemia results from increased secretion of renin. What has not been explained is why many patients with renovascular hypertension have normal plasma renin concentration, possibly due to dilution from the normal kidney. Recently it has been shown that when the renal blood pressure was experimentally lowered in dogs, the renal vein renin increased within 1 minute and the arterial pressure rose within 5 minutes, showing the rapid response of the renin-angiotensin system in the regulation of arterial pressure (Haber, 1976). Whether the raised renin is the effect or the cause has not been established. Angiotensin-inhibiting agents also prevent the rise in blood pressure. Various studies have shown that a low plasma renin concentration argues against renovascular hypertension but a normal plasma renin concentration does not; a raised plasma renin level is often absent except in severe hypertension.

1. Differential renal vein renin levels—Much more helpful than single renal vein renins or plasma renin in determining the functional significance of renal artery stenosis is assessment of differential renal vein renin, with a ratio of at least 1.5:1, but preferably 2:1, representing a positive test. Blood from selected tributaries of the renal vein should be obtained to localize an area with an abnormally high renin content when segmental disease or renin-producing tumor is suspected. Schambelan (1974) has found abnormal amounts of renin from branches of the renal vein in segmental disease in which renin from the main renal vein was normal. Differential renal vein renin has been particularly valuable in predicting the results of surgical repair of renal artery stenosis, in contrast to renal arteriography, which displays the anatomic disease. Bookstein (1975), however, has shown that the arteriographic demonstration of collateral circulation, either periureteral collaterals with irregular narrowing of the ureter or tortuous collaterals within the kidney, is a good sign of a hemodynamically significant stenosis. When the renal vein renin concentration on one side is more than 1½–2 times that on the opposite side, 80–90% of patients benefit from surgical repair of the stenosis. About half of patients with equivalent renal vein renins on the 2 sides, in the presence of anatomically proved stenosis, benefit from surgery (Table 9–21). The variable results may be explained in various ways as follows: (1) one-fourth to one-third of patients with renovascular hypertension have bilateral lesions; (2) the methods of determining renal vein renin are not without defects;

Table 9–21. Operative outcome in hypertensive patients with and without lateralizing renal vein renin (RVR) ratios.*

	Summary of Literature Review (Kaufman, 1975)	Present Data	Total
Number of patients	412	56	468
Patients with lateralizing (1.4–2.5) RVR ratios			
Cured or improved	267	24	291
Failed	19	3	22
Patients without lateralizing RVR ratios			
Cured or improved	64	24	88
Failed	62	5	67

*Adapted and reproduced, with permission, from Stamey TA: Unilateral renal disease causing hypertension. JAMA 235:2340, 1976; modified from Kaufman JJ: Progress in the diagnosis and management of renovascular hypertension. Urol Digest 14: 12, 1975.

(3) renal vein renin is sometimes estimated without stimulation of renin release by depletion of sodium or upright posture; or (4) drugs which decrease renin release, such as propranolol or methyldopa, may not be stopped before the study, either because the physician fails to appreciate their importance or because the hypertension is so severe that the physician is reluctant to stop antihypertensive therapy.

2. Technical problems in prognosis—The technical problem of making certain of the location of the catheter may be pertinent in determining segmental disease. It is not known why 20% of operations in patients with a positive 1.5:1 differential renal vein renin ratio are failures nor why 50% of operations in patients with an equivalent or lesser ratio are successful. Nevertheless, the combination of localized anatomic stenosis associated with collateral vessels on renal arteriography and an abnormal differential renal vein renin ratio provides the best means of predicting surgical benefit.

These special invasive technics should not be advised unless the patient's clinical status is such that surgical treatment can be recommended if the structural findings and functional studies are clear-cut. They should not be done in cases where manifestations of atherosclerotic disease elsewhere would be contraindications to operation.

D. Radioisotopic Kidney Studies: Isotopic renograms have been used by many physicians to evaluate the vascularity of each kidney in an effort to determine the presence of regional or localized renal ischemia that might cause renovascular hypertension. Double or triple isotopes have been used (such as the combination of radioactive mercury 203, which shows scars and other renal parenchymal defects; technetium 99m, which allows recognition of reduced renal blood flow by diminished uptake of the isotope by the kidney; and ^{131}I hippurate, which reflects transit time through the kidney and reveals ischemia). Technical difficulties with the method and the frequency of false-positive and false-negative studies have minimized the value of radioactive scans in the diagnosis of renovascular hypertension, but the method is valuable in the follow-up of patients who have had renovascular surgery. Renal scans continue to be important in the diagnosis of renal tumors.

E. Inhibitors of the Renin-Angiotensin System: Agents that either inhibit the generation of angiotensin II from angiotensin I (such as the converting enzyme inhibitor SQ 20881 or SQ 14225) or inhibit already formed angiotensin II (by their affinity for its receptor) are being studied intensively today because the role of the components of the renin-angiotensin system in the pathogenesis of hypertension is still uncertain. Interruption of the system by pharmacologic agents from the release of renin to the generation of angiotensin II may find a useful place in diagnosis. Inhibition of renin release is not yet practical because renin has not been synthesized, but antirenin antibodies have been prepared and used experimentally. Agents that inhibit the conversion of angiotensin I to angiotensin II produce postural hypotension, especially in sodium-depleted individuals, but the effect in normal subjects and the specificity of the vasodepressor response are unclear because the peptide inhibitor also increases the serum bradykinin level, enhancing the hypotensive vasodepressor effect; other tissue enzymes may possibly also be influenced. Recently, in 2 patients, overactivity of the renin-angiotensin system was excluded both by angiotensin blockade with saralasin (an inhibitor of angiotensin II) and by similar renal vein renin from the 2 kidneys. Despite the negative saralasin responses, normal differential renal vein renin determinations, low plasma renin, and low plasma aldosterone, the patients became normotensive after revascularization of the renal artery without the need for antihypertensive drugs for at least 1 year (Marks, 1977). There is considerable interest in determining whether subsets of hypertension can be recognized not only by the relationship between plasma renin and urinary sodium excretion but also by the depressor response to angiotensin inhibitors. A recent study of 65 hypertensive patients indicated that depressor responses to converting enzyme inhibitors (SQ 20881) occurred only when the control plasma renin activity exceeded 2 ng of angiotensin I per ml/hour (Case, 1977). The exact role of converting enzyme inhibitors is unclear, since plasma renin activity failed to rise after they were given to low renin hypertensive patients but did so in patients with normal or high renin (Case, 1977). Saralasin produced a depressor response in all hypertensive patients, including the low renin subgroup, when they were sodium-depleted. There is good evidence that saralasin, which has an affinity for angiotensin receptor and therefore blocks the action of angiotensin II, has a partial agonist action under certain conditions. For this reason, most recent work has dealt with agents that block the conversion of angiotensin I to angiotensin II rather than those that block the action of angiotensin II itself. At present, caution is advised in interpreting the results of renin-angiotensin inhibitors because of their effects on other parts of the circulation and other body systems such as the kallikrein-bradykinin and possibly other as yet unknown systems.

Surgical Treatment of Renovascular Hypertension

Treatment consists of either routine medical management as in essential hypertension (see p 238) or surgery. In the latter case, one must consider the selection of patients, the repair of the artery, the possibility of nephrectomy, and the results of surgical treatment.

A. Selection of Patients: As suggested above, the question how far one should go to search for renal artery stenosis is controversial. Although the number of patients who have surgically correctable renal artery stenosis is small, the benefit to the few is great if they can be identified. Intravenous urography and search for renal artery stenosis by renal angiography, renal vein renin, and possibly angiotensin converting enzyme inhibitor (SQ 20881) or saralasin effects are best confined to younger individuals with severe hypertension and minimal atherosclerosis elsewhere whose hypertension has appeared recently and to those in whom antihypertensive therapy has not been effective.

B. Repair of Distal Artery: As is true of atherosclerosis generally, disease may appear initially in any portion of the arterial circuit and not be demonstrable elsewhere. If the renal arterial lesion is distal, removal of the kidney with its peripheral arteries may allow repair of the distal artery and its branches while the kidney is being perfused, as it is when renal transplantation is undertaken. In this way, it may be possible under direct vision to correct the abnormalities in the distal renal arteries while preserving the function of the kidney. The kidney can then be reanastomosed to the patient. Some brilliant results have followed this procedure. Nephrectomy is inadvisable in the presence of fibromuscular hyperplasia since the disease is often bilateral or, even if not bilateral at the outset, may develop in a few years in the opposite kidney. This consideration is not so important in atherosclerotic disease if the kidney is atrophic and nonfunctioning and the disease unilateral.

Prognosis

A. With Surgical Repair in Patients With Impaired Renal Function: Patients with impaired renal function are a particularly difficult group in which to judge the value of surgery. The results are less good when the creatinine clearance is less than 40 ml/min, but this may be due to accelerated hypertension with vascular necrosis or to bilateral disease. However, the prognosis of accelerated hypertension with impaired renal function is so poor that surgery may be considered if there is a significant stenotic lesion and increased renal vein renin on that side, especially if the patient fails to respond well to medical treatment.

Patients who have angina, a history of myocardial infarction, or extensive cerebral vascular disease have a 5–10% surgical mortality rate following the extensive resection necessary for treatment of atherosclerotic renal artery stenosis; furthermore, the high postopera-

Table 9–22. Surgical and medical treatment of renal artery stenosis compared.*

A. Results of Surgical Treatment for Renal Artery Stenosis With Hypertension (100 Cases)

	Follow-Up Interval for Type of Stenosis Range and Mean (Years)					
	Atheromatous (37 Patients)			Fibromuscular (63 Patients)		
Status of Patients	1–6 (3.6)	5–10 (7.0)	7–12 (8.8)	1–8 (3.0)	5–12 (7.0)	7–14 (8.8)
Surviving	37	29	26	62	60	58
< 90 mm Hg diastolic blood pressure						
No medication	14	13	12	41	39	39
Mild medication	14	14	12	15	16	15
Taking sympatholytic agents	9	2	2	6	5	4

B. Results of Medical Treatment for Renal Artery Stenosis With Hypertension (114 Cases)

	Follow-Up Interval for Type of Stenosis Range and Mean (Years)					
	Atheromatous (44 Patients)			Fibromuscular (70 Patients)		
Status of Patients	1–8 (3.8)	5–12 (7.1)	7–14 (9.0)	1–8 (3.9)	5–12 (7.2)	7–14 (9.1)
Dead	3	16	27	0	5	12
Subjected to surgery	2	7	7	2	9	9
Surviving with medication	39	21	10	68	56	49
Blood pressure control usually < 100 mm Hg diastolic	33	15	9	59	48	43
Unsatisfactory blood pressure control	6	6	1	9	8	6

*Reproduced, with permission, from Hunt JC & others: Renal and renovascular hypertension: A reasoned approach to diagnosis and management. Arch Intern Med 133:988, 1974.

tive incidence of neurologic deficit, myocardial ischemia or infarction, or arrhythmias engenders caution in advocating surgery in people with extensive vascular disease.

B. Results of Surgical Repair in General: The results of surgical treatment vary with the cause—being better when fibromuscular hyperplasia is present. Table 9–22 compares the results of surgical and medical treatment. About half of patients with atherosclerotic renovascular hypertension have diastolic pressures less than 100 mm Hg following surgical repair; the figure is closer to 75% in patients with fibromuscular hyperplasia. One-fourth to one-half of the patients, especially with atherosclerotic disease, require some antihypertensive therapy following surgical treatment.

The National Cooperative Study of Renovascular Hypertension (Maxwell, 1975) indicates that the best results are achieved in patients with the following clinical and historical prognostic indicators: clear-cut lateralization studies, severe hypertension of short duration, secondary aldosteronism, hypokalemia, a negative family history of hypertension, classic urographic findings, and a long systolic or diastolic bruit.

PRIMARY ALDOSTERONISM

Primary aldosteronism was first described by Conn in 1955 in a patient with hypertension who had a low serum potassium of unknown cause and other findings suggesting excess of some mineralocorticoid later found to be aldosterone. An adenoma of the zona glomerulosa of the adrenal cortex was found; following resection, the blood pressure and the serum potassium returned to normal. Further experience has shown that primary aldosteronism is usually due to oversecretion of aldosterone by an adenoma of the adrenal, that it is a relatively uncommon (1–2%) cause of hypertension (Fig 9–30), that some patients (20–25%) have bi-

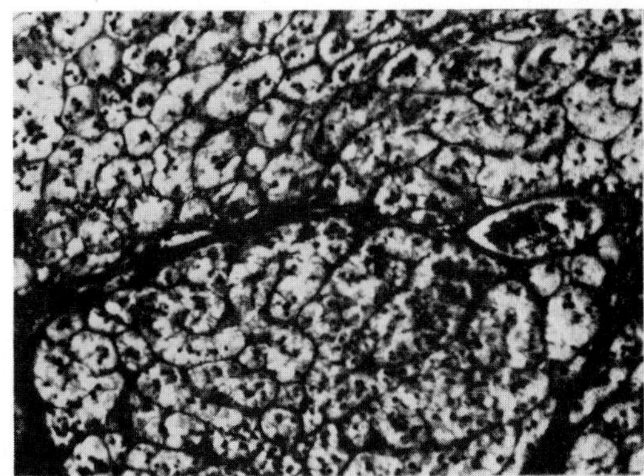

Figure 9–30. Adenoma of the adrenal gland showing clear cells and fibrous trabeculae. (Reproduced, with permission, from Nicholls MG & others: Primary aldosteronism: A study in contrasts. Am J Med 59:334, 1975.)

lateral adrenal hyperplasia rather than adenoma (70–80%), and that these patients have a milder variety of aldosteronism. Patients with primary adenoma excrete greater amounts of aldosterone in the urine and have lower plasma renin and serum potassium levels than do patients with aldosteronism secondary to bilateral adrenal hyperplasia (Biglieri & Lopez, 1976). Aldosteronism itself is not the cause of the hypertension because aldosterone levels may be much higher in conditions in which hypertension is absent, such as normal pregnancy, cirrhosis of the liver, and Addison's disease.

Adenomas may be relatively small (1–2 cm in diameter) and difficult to find at surgery, are golden yellow in appearance, and are associated with normal or hyperplastic adrenal tissue surrounding the tumor. This is in contrast to Cushing's syndrome, in which the gland surrounding a tumor is atrophic and the opposite adrenal may also be hypoplastic.

Clinical Findings

The usual screening test for primary aldosteronism in patients with hypertension is serum potassium determination. The recent availability of radioimmunoassay methods for plasma aldosterone and renin determinations may permit a definite diagnosis if the former is increased and the latter decreased. Interpretation of the plasma renin concentration may be doubtful unless the conditions of testing are rigidly controlled. This is best done in the hospital and consists of control of sodium and potassium intake, avoidance of antihypertensive drugs, ambulation for 4 hours before taking the sample, and sodium depletion with diuretics on the day of the test to make certain that plasma renin does not respond to these maneuvers and remains suppressed (see below).

A. Serum Potassium: If the serum potassium is consistently above 4 mEq/l on a normal sodium intake, the likelihood of a primary aldosterone-producing adenoma is sufficiently remote that no further studies are probably indicated. Patients with aldosterone-producing adenomas of the renal cortex consistently show a fall in serum potassium over the course of 5–10 days when given a high sodium (more than 100 mEq/day) intake. If the serum potassium is less than 4 mEq/l–and especially if it is less than 3.5 mEq/l–the 24-hour urine potassium and serum potassium should be determined on a normal sodium diet of approximately 100–150 mEq/day. In primary aldosterone-producing adenomas, serum potassium falls on a high-sodium diet. If the 24-hour urine potassium exceeds 30 mEq/l in the presence of a serum potassium less than 3.5 mEq/l (especially if the serum potassium falls as a result of the high sodium intake), further biochemical studies such as plasma aldosterone and renin are indicated to exclude aldosteronism because hypokalemia due to other causes such as decreased dietary intake or loss of potassium in the stool from diarrhea usually is associated with a decreased urinary potassium excretion to preserve body potassium stores. If primary aldosteronism accounts for the hypokalemia and increased potassium excretion in the urine, there also should be salt and water retention and increased extracellular and plasma volume, associated with decreased circulatory reflexes (bradycardia) and lack of hypertension overshoot following the Valsalva maneuver.

B. Evaluation of a Low Serum Potassium in Hypertensive Patients: One of the difficult decisions facing the physician is the hypertensive patient who has been receiving antihypertensive therapy, including oral diuretics, who presents with a low serum potassium. Oral diuretics increase the excretion of potassium, so it is common to find a low serum potassium in patients on diuretics, but this does not exclude the possible associated presence of primary aldosteronism. When potassium secretion is increased by diuretics, sodium is excreted as well, producing the combination of a low serum potassium and a low serum sodium between 130 and 135 mEq/l. In addition, mild alkalosis with serum bicarbonate in the range of 25–32 mEq/l is present. If the serum sodium, instead of being decreased, is increased–in the range of 144–149 mEq/l–and if the serum bicarbonate is higher (in the range of 35–39 mEq/l), the possibility of primary aldosteronism is increased in patients in whom the serum potassium is low. To exclude primary aldosteronism, the following procedure is advised (Biglieri & Lopez, 1976).

1. Diuretics should be stopped for at least 2 weeks to allow dissipation of the effects of diuresis and to normalize the serum potassium. Hypertension should be controlled by other measures. Diuretics increase the production of aldosterone and increase the plasma renin activity and so confuse the issue.

2. The diet should be reasonably liberal, with an adequate amount of salt (± 7 g).

3. After 2 weeks, redetermine the serum sodium and potassium. If these are both normal, the need for further investigation for aldosteronism is eliminated.

4. If the serum potassium remains low, additional outpatient studies are indicated in order to determine whether hospitalization is indicated for more definitive diagnostic studies.

5. One should obtain a 24-hour urine sample reading for potassium and aldosterone and obtain a random plasma sample for renin activity. In the normal individual without aldosteronism on a substantial daily salt intake of about 7 g, the urinary 24-hour aldosterone reading varies from 4–17 μg/24 hours, in contrast to primary aldosteronism, in which the values exceed 19 μg/24 hours. Excessive amounts of urinary potassium in the presence of a low serum potassium suggest that the patient has another disease resulting in increased excretion of potassium. If the patient excretes potassium in the order of 100 mEq/l with a low serum potassium, a renal potassium loss is the probable explanation for the low serum potassium. Plasma aldosterone is too variable as an outpatient measurement and is not advised. However, if the urine aldosterone is increased and if the urine potassium excretion is normal, the patient should be hospitalized because the suspicion of aldosteronism is sufficiently strong to warrant it.

In the hospital, the patient is given a normal 7 g salt diet and is kept flat in bed in a supine position for at least 6 hours and preferably overnight. Plasma renin activity and plasma aldosterone are determined at 8:00 am and again at noon, after the patient has been sitting and standing, in order to determine the response of these determinations to posture. If, under these circumstances, the plasma aldosterone is > 20 ng/dl and the plasma renin activity is low (less than 1–2 ng/ml/hour), aldosteronism is diagnosed. Differentiation of adenoma of the adrenal cortex from bilateral adrenal hyperplasia is made by the response to posture. Adenomas fail to reduce plasma aldosterone after the patient has been in the sitting or standing posture, whereas in hyperplasia it usually falls to about 10 ng/dl.

If the conclusion is that the patient has hyperplasia, and hypertension is only mild to moderate, the treatment of choice is with spironolactone, 300 mg/day in divided doses for 1 month followed by smaller doses, because adrenalectomy often does not cure the hypertension. If the patient has chemical findings suggesting adenoma, then other procedures such as adrenal scans to localize the tumor should be done because the surgical results are sufficiently good to warrant the procedure.

C. Plasma Renin: Plasma renin should be decreased to nil or very low values in aldosteronism because the increased blood volume by negative feedback (see negative feedback loop in Fig 9–6) decreases renal renin secretion. If the plasma concentration is normal or high, primary aldosteronism is excluded as a cause of hypokalemia. A low plasma renin level is even more significant if it remains low following upright posture and the use of potent diuretics, which stimulate renin secretion in the normal individual but which may not do so in the presence of the hypervolemia of increased aldosterone production. If the plasma renin level remains low, especially after provocative maneuvers to increase it, plasma and urinary aldosterone values should be determined. These tests are done only in special laboratories that have facilities to measure the hormone accurately.

D. Plasma Aldosterone: It has been reported by Biglieri (1976) and by Melby (1967) that increased plasma aldosterone with clinical and laboratory evidence of excess aldosterone production may be due either to the presence of an isolated adrenal adenoma or to bilateral adrenal hyperplasia. Adenoma is suspected if the plasma aldosterone fails to increase in the upright posture, as it does in hyperplasia, or if an iodine 131 iodocholesterol scintiscan localizes a tumor in one of the adrenals.

Desoxycorticosterone has no effect on adenoma, ie, it does not suppress the production of aldosterone from the tumor, as it does in indeterminate aldosteronism (hyperplasia).

E. Adrenal Scan: Most cases of adrenal adenoma can be identified and localized by an adrenal scintiscan. It is important to attempt to localize the adenoma so the surgeon will know which adrenal is involved. Following intravenously administered radioactive I 131 iodocholesterol, asymmetric uptake of the radioactive compound in the 2 adrenals occurs as a result of adenoma in one of them. In hyperplasia there is symmetric uptake of the radioactive isotope. The test, however, is technically difficult, requiring special equipment, highly trained personnel, and several visits to determine the timing of maximum radioactivity uptake. Hogan (1976) found the average number of visits was 3, and the maximum uptake was usually at some time between 7 and 14 days. Patients require administration of iodide before and 3 weeks after the administration of the isotope to minimize thyroidal uptake. Adrenal imaging with new isotopic compounds with maximum uptake within 24 hours will probably supplant the current compound, but this awaits further research and at present can only be done in research centers. As nuclear medicine centers develop in community hospitals, the procedure will become more readily available.

F. Adrenal Vein Catheterization: If the biochemical studies suggest aldosteronism but an adrenal scan does not reveal the tumor (because it is less than 1 cm in diameter), or if the scan is equivocal, localization should be attempted by percutaneous adrenal vein catheterization via the femoral vein with assays of aldosterone in the venous effluent of blood from both kidneys and from segments of each kidney. The tumor may be small (less than 1 cm), flattened, and difficult to find at surgery. Preoperative localization of the site of the tumor is of considerable help in finding the adenoma and avoiding adrenalectomy.

Adrenal vein catheterization by a skilled team, available now only in research centers (although physicians who perform renal vein catheterization can, with experience, catheterize adrenal veins), not only permits adrenal venous blood to be examined for aldosterone but also allows an adrenal venogram to be done if necessary. This is less desirable, because adrenal hemorrhage has occurred in some cases, and biochemical studies of venous effluent are preferred. In contrast to the 1.5:1 ratio of renal vein renin in the diagnosis of renovascular hypertension, the ratio of aldosterone in the 2 adrenal veins is closer to 5:1 or 10:1 when an adenoma is present in one adrenal (Melby, 1976). Catheterization of the left adrenal vein is easier than catheterization of the right because of the variable origin of the right adrenal vein. The combination of a positive adrenal isotope scan and positive adrenal vein characterization of an adenoma by aldosterone assay permits a positive diagnosis in 85–90% of patients with adenoma. Adrenal arteriography is done infrequently because of the difficulty of the procedure and because it does not allow differential adrenal vein sampling for aldosterone.

Treatment

If bilateral renal hyperplasia rather than adenoma is the cause, the patient should be treated with antihypertensive therapy including spironolactone (the aldosterone antagonist) rather than bilateral adrenalectomy because of the high prevalence of persistent hypertension after surgery and the need for replacement therapy after adrenalectomy. Spironolactone usually corrects both the serum potassium and the hypertension. In adenoma, resection of the adrenal tumor promptly decreases aldosterone production and restores the serum potassium to normal, but hypertension is "cured" in only 60–70% of cases. Because of this relatively low "cure" rate in mild aldosteronism, when the blood pressure, serum potassium, and hypervolemia are corrected by spironolactone, medical rather than surgical treatment can be advised.

Prognosis

Without surgery, even in mild cases, the symptoms of adenoma can only be partially controlled by medical treatment, and surgical removal is required. The serum potassium usually falls to less than 2.5–3 mEq/l after thiazide therapy in unsuspected cases of aldosteronism, leading to hypokalemic symptoms of fatigue, nocturia, arrhythmia, and nephropathy; these are corrected by spironolactone. Failure to control blood pressure leads to cardiac and cerebral complications found in other types of hypertension. Postural hypotension may be a problem because of a defect in circulatory reflexes not due to increased central blood volume.

SECONDARY ALDOSTERONISM

Secondary hyperaldosteronism is much more common than primary and is usually due to accelerated or severe hypertension, which, by reducing renal blood flow, initiates the production of angiotensin which in turn increases the secretion of aldosterone. Patients with secondary aldosteronism are likely to have an elevated plasma renin as well, in contrast to the low plasma renin expected in primary aldosteronism. The serum potassium may be low in both secondary and primary aldosteronism, but the serum sodium is not elevated in secondary as it is in primary aldosteronism. The serum sodium is rarely less than 140 mg/dl in primary cases, and it may be as high as 155 mg/dl. When the blood pressure is reduced by antihypertensive agents such as thiazide diuretics (but not spironolactone), secondary aldosteronism is reduced, and the serum potassium may rise to normal even though the oral diuretics tend to increase the plasma renin. The "effective" blood volume is raised in both types of aldosteronism but is reduced in patients with cirrhosis of the liver or Addison's disease, conditions in which renin levels may be very high. Secondary aldosteronism may also occur in renal artery stenosis because of the increased secretion of renin with resulting increased plasma and urinary aldosterone. The increased plasma renin is critical in separating the 2 varieties.

Treatment

Treatment is by vigorous antihypertensive therapy to lower the blood pressure, which then causes the secondary aldosteronism to disappear.

CUSHING'S DISEASE & SYNDROME

Cushing's syndrome is probably a more common cause of hypertension than primary aldosteronism. Although the terms Cushing's disease and Cushing's syndrome have been used loosely and often interchangeably, they should be distinguished by careful writers. The term Cushing's disease originally described a primary tumor of the anterior pituitary causing bilateral adrenal hyperplasia and hypercortisolism, and it is properly used in this sense. Because the pituitary tumor often could not be identified, the oversecretion of cortisol and the bilateral adrenal hyperplasia were called Cushing's syndrome. It was subsequently learned that a benign adenoma of the adrenal could cause hypercortisolism, also termed Cushing's syndrome. Furthermore, when ectopic ACTH-producing tumors (eg, bronchogenic carcinoma) were recognized, Cushing's syndrome embraced the ectopic hypercortisolism as well. Complicating the terminology even more is the cushingoid syndrome induced by exogenous administration of corticosteroids or ACTH for a wide variety of diseases—iatrogenic Cushing's syndrome.

The advent of microsurgery of the anterior pituitary has clarified the picture. It now appears that Cushing was right—that most cases of overproduction of cortisol are due to a tumor (often microscopic) of the basophilic or chromophobic cells of the anterior pituitary or to an adenoma of the adrenal gland; idiopathic bilateral adrenal hyperplasia is now considered rare. It is speculated that some cases of Cushing's syndrome are hypothalamic in origin, with the anterior pituitary stimulated by excess hypothalamic releasing factor.

The mechanism by which there is an increased production of ACTH from the pituitary gland is not known, but a current theory suggests that increased serotonin may be present in the hypothalamus and may increase the release of CRH (hypothalamic corticotropin-releasing hormone). This theory has been supported by observation of the beneficial effect of the serotonin antagonist cyproheptadine (see below), which has induced remission in some patients with Cushing's syndrome.

Cushing's syndrome may be iatrogenic in patients who receive corticosteroids that have salt-retaining properties, as sometimes is the case in arthritis; the relationship between corticosteroid administration and the hypertension is often not appreciated. In one patient with long-standing mild primary hypertension, abrupt worsening of the hypertension was due to monthly intramuscular injections of a corticosteroid that caused retention of salt and water, produced a cushingoid appearance, and made the hypertension more difficult to control.

Hypertension is a common accompaniment of

Cushing's syndrome, although most patients present primarily to an endocrinologist because of a characteristic appearance with "moon" facies, central truncal obesity, muscular weakness, ecchymosis with thin skin, purple striae, increased acne, hirsutism, and perhaps osteoporosis. Although hypertension may be mild, it is not uncommonly severe, although malignant hypertension is rare. In older patients, cardiac failure and other cardiovascular complications may occur if the diastolic pressure rises abruptly or above 120 mm Hg.

Clinical Findings

A. Symptoms and Signs: The diagnosis of Cushing's syndrome is suspected from the clinical features, but most patients with obesity, hirsutism, and cushingoid facies do not have Cushing's disease (Table 9–23).

B. Laboratory Findings: Because cortisol is increased several times above normal values, retention of sodium and water with increased extracellular fluid volume may occur. The pathogenesis of hypertension in Cushing's syndrome is not established but is probably due to increased salt and water retention associated with excess cortisol production, increased vascular responsiveness to pressor agents, or increased plasma renin substrate. The last may contribute to increased aldosterone production and superimpose a mineralocorticoid excess on the glucocorticoid excess. In pure cortisol excess, plasma renin and aldosterone are normal, as is the serum potassium.

The diagnosis of pituitary hypercortisolism (Cushing's disease) is most reliably made by determining morning plasma 17-hydroxycorticosteroid (17-OHCS) levels after suppression of ACTH by giving the patient 1 mg of dexamethasone and a sedative (phenobarbital, 100 mg, or flurazepam [Dalmane], 15–30 mg) at bedtime the night before. Normal individuals usually suppress the plasma 17-OHCS from the normal value of 10–20 μg/dl to less than 5 μg/dl, whereas patients with Cushing's syndrome rarely suppress from elevated values of 15–40 μg/dl to less than 10 μg/dl (Melby, 1976). Values of 5–10 μg/dl are borderline. Suppression of plasma cortisol by dexamethasone implies that the hypercortisolism is primary in the pituitary or in an ectopic ACTH-producing tumor and is not due to autonomous adrenal secretion. If plasma cortisol is not suppressible by dexamethasone, an adrenal tumor or hyperplasia is usually the cause of the excess secretion of cortisol. The overnight suppression test following 1 mg of dexamethasone is the screening test of choice (Biglieri, 1976).

Urinary corticosteroids usually fall to 50% or more below normal levels. Larger doses of dexamethasone have also been used to suppress ACTH secretion; a common procedure is to give 0.5 mg of dexamethasone every 6 hours and obtain a 24-hour urinary 17-OHCS determination. In the presence of Cushing's syndrome, there will be at least 4 mg in a 24-hour specimen. Because Cushing's syndrome may be due to hyperplasia or tumor, larger doses of dexamethasone (2 mg every 6 hours for 2–3 days) are used to distinguish the two. In the presence of adrenal tumor, patients fail to suppress to less than half of the basal level, whereas those with bilateral adrenal hyperplasia almost always do.

The adrenal tumors are usually large and associated with atrophy of the surrounding as well as the contralateral adrenal. Preoperative lateralization of the tumor is not always successful, so it is always necessary to expose and explore both adrenal glands. Sampling of blood from both adrenal veins and adrenal venography may be helpful in identifying the tumor, but the adrenal scan is simpler and should be employed first. If a carcinoma of the adrenal is suspected, arteriography may be helpful because the tumor is vascular.

Table 9–23. Common initial signs and differential diagnoses in Cushing's disease.*

Common Initial Signs	Differential Diagnoses
Rapid onset	
Facial edema	Hypothyroidism
Rapid weight gain	Nephritis or nephrosis
Renal colic	Allergic or cardiac edema
Amenorrhea with facial edema or rapid weight gain	Simple obesity; Idiopathic renal calculi
Physical weakness	Psychoses
Mental disturbance	Collagen disease
Gradual onset	
Gradual weight gain	Simple obesity
Oligomenorrhea and hirsutism	Familial hirsutism; psychogenic amenorrhea
Diabetes mellitus	Diabetes mellitus
Hypertension	Essential hypertension
Mental or emotional changes	Psychosomatic conditions
Osteoporosis	Postmenopausal osteoporosis

Other differential diagnoses: hyperthyroidism, Guillain-Barré syndrome or diabetic neuropathy, hyperparathyroidism, peptic ulcer, polycythemia, purpuras, ovarian tumors.

*Reproduced, with permission, from Hurxthal LM, O'Sullivan JB: Cushing's syndrome: Clinical differential diagnosis and complications. Ann Intern Med 51:1, 1959.

Treatment

Once the diagnosis of Cushing's syndrome is made and exogenous administration of corticosteroids or ACTH excluded, a search should be made for ectopic ACTH-producing tumors or an adrenal adenoma. If either of these tumors is identified (see diagnosis above), surgical resection is the treatment of choice. If neither is present and Cushing's disease is diagnosed, microresection of the tumor of the pituitary under microscopic visualization is now the preferred treatment. Irradiation of the anterior pituitary or cryosurgery, formerly used in treatment, has been superseded by microsurgery of the pituitary.

Chemotherapy with cyproheptadine has been reported to have achieved favorable results in a few cases.

If ectopic ACTH-producing tumors cannot be resected, metyrapone can be tried in order to inhibit the synthesis of cortisol.

Prognosis

Without treatment, patients have progressive abnormalities of the syndrome, although the hypertension may be controlled by antihypertensive therapy. If hypertension is overlooked because other findings dominate the clinical picture, complications of hypertension such as cardiac failure and cerebral or renal vascular disease may develop and may be the cause of death.

PHEOCHROMOCYTOMA

This is a dramatic but rare condition, only one or 2 a year being seen in the usual large general hospital. Pheochromocytoma is due to a tumor arising anywhere in the chromaffin system (the remnant of the fetal neural crest) which synthesizes epinephrine and norepinephrine. The overwhelming majority occur in the adrenal medulla, but these tumors may occur in chromaffin cells in the abdomen, the periaortic area, the organ of Zuckerkandl, and rarely in the thorax and bladder wall (Fig 9–31). They are often multiple and familial and rarely may be associated with other endocrinopathies such as Sipple's disease (multiple parathyroid adenomas) or Recklinghausen's disease (neurofibromatosis); most patients have no associated endocrinopathy. The tumor is usually benign, but about 10% are malignant.

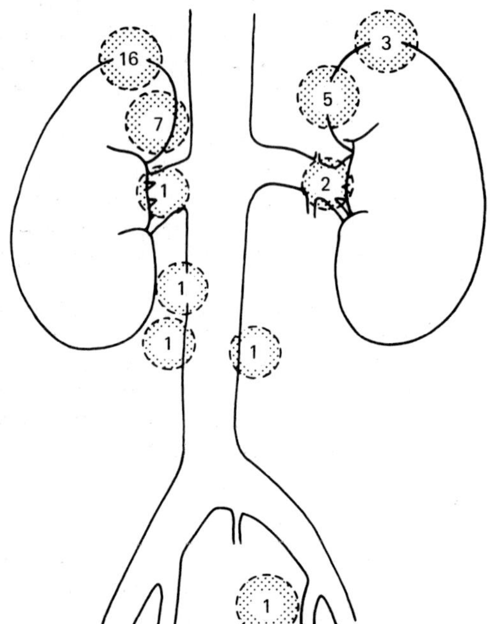

Figure 9–31. Illustration of the sites of occurrence of pheochromocytoma in 34 patients, with the number of tumors found at various locations indicated in the circles. (Adapted and reproduced, with permission, from Zelch JV, Meaney TF, Belhobek GH: Radiologic approach to the patient with suspected pheochromocytoma. Radiology 111:279, 1974.)

Table 9–24. Symptoms in 100 patients with pheochromocytoma.*

Symptom	No.	Symptom	No.
Headache	80	Dizziness or faintness	8
Perspiration	71	Convulsions	5
Palpitation (with or without tachycardia)	64	Neck-shoulder pain	5
		Extremity pain	4
Pallor	42	Flank pain	4
Nausea (with or without vomiting)	42	Tinnitus	3
		Dysarthria	3
Tremor or trembling	31	Gagging	3
Weakness or exhaustion	28	Bradycardia (noted by patient)	3
Nervousness or anxiety	22		
Epigastric pain	22	Back pain	3
Chest pain	19	Coughing	1
Dyspnea	19	Yawning	1
Flushing or warmth	18	Syncope	1
Numbness or paresthesia	11	Unsteadiness	1
Blurring of vision	11	Hunger	1
Tightness in throat	8		

*Reproduced, with permission, from Thomas JE, Rooke ED, Kvale WF: The neurologist's experience with pheochromocytoma: A review of 100 cases. JAMA 197:754, 1966. Copyright © American Medical Association.

Tumors vary in the relative amounts of norepinephrine and epinephrine that they secrete, and the clinical signs may vary depending on which catecholamine is secreted.

Clinical Findings

A. Symptoms and Signs: The most typical clinical features are those associated with an abrupt surge of catecholamine secretion, causing pallor, sweating, palpitations, headache, and anxiety, usually all occurring together in association with an abrupt rise in systolic and diastolic pressure (Table 9–24).

1. Cause of attacks—The attacks may be spontaneous or precipitated by changes in posture, pressure on the abdomen, or procedures such as intravenous urograms. (*Note:* Intravenous phentolamine must be available for emergency use.) One or another of these symptoms may be present in anxiety attacks, and most patients referred with a diagnosis of possible pheochromocytoma have transient rises in pressure associated with anxiety. If epinephrine is the amine secreted, flushing rather than pallor is characteristic, and the patient is more tremulous. In rare instances, precursors of norepinephrine may be secreted, and hypotension has occasionally been found when dopamine is secreted in large amounts. The hypertension may be sustained or intermittent. In most cases it is sustained, with intermittent superimposed rises in conjunction with paroxysmal symptoms. Malignant hypertension may occur with papilledema, and this is seen relatively more frequently than in Cushing's syndrome or aldosteronism.

2. Symptoms during attack—The rise in blood pressure may be severe, and, during attacks in young people, diastolic pressures of 150 mm Hg are not un-

Table 9–25. Normal range of catecholamine and metabolite concentrations.*†

Urine
Catecholamines‡
Norepinephrine: 10–70 μg/24 hours
Epinephrine: 0–20 μg/24 hours
Normetanephrine and metanephrine: < 1.3 mg/24 hours
Vanilmandelic acid: 1.8–9.0 mg/24 hours
Dopamine: < 200 μg/24 hours
Blood
Catecholamines: < 1 μg/l
Adrenal medulla
Norepinephrine: 0.04–0.16 mg/g
Epinephrine: 0.22–0.84 mg/g

*Since the values obtained in different laboratories vary considerably, only a general range can be given.

†Reproduced, with permission, from Melmon KL: Catecholamines and the adrenal medulla. Part 2, pages 283–322, in: *Textbook of Endocrinology,* 5th ed. Williams RH (editor). Saunders, 1974.

‡In most patients with pheochromocytomas, total catecholamine excretion is > 300 μg/day.

usual. The high, abrupt rises in pressure may cause myocardial ischemia or infarction, ventricular arrhythmias, or cardiac failure; patients may present with one or more of these complications.

B. Laboratory Findings: The laboratory diagnosis of pheochromocytoma in patients who have a characteristic history usually can be accomplished by assay of catecholamine excretion in the 24-hour urine specimen. Table 9–25 shows the normal range of catecholamine and metabolite concentrations in the urine and blood.

1. VMA determination—The spectrophotometric determination of vanillylmandelic acid (VMA), one of the products of catecholamine metabolism, is a screening test that is available in most laboratories. Clofibrate (Atromid-S) gives false-negative results, but the spectrophotometric assay is not affected by common foods such as bananas, coffee, or vanilla desserts which do affect the less precise and commonly used simple colorimetric test. Normal VMA excretion is less than 7 mg/24 hours but may be 5–10 times this amount in pheochromocytoma. Methyldopa does not interfere with assay for VMA, but it does interfere with assay for total urinary catecholamine excretion.

2. Metanephrine and normetanephrine—More recently, determination of other metabolites, notably the combination of metanephrine and normetanephrine, on a single voided specimen has been shown to be simple and highly reliable, with the distinct advantage of not requiring a 24-hour specimen. The upper limits of normal for the assay are 1 μg/mg of creatinine in the urine. Single voided urine specimens from 500 hypertensive patients contained 0.351± 0.356 μg of metanephrine per mg of creatinine, whereas in pheochromocytoma, spot specimens were almost always 5–10 μg/mg and sometimes many times more than this (Kaplan, Arch Intern Med, 1977). Chlorpromazine produces falsely high readings, but no diet or obesity drugs or antihypertensive drugs interfere with the test. This assay may be positive when the VMA assay is negative, but the reverse is rarely true.

3. Urine tests—Urinary assay of the free catecholamines norepinephrine and epinephrine is rarely used in screening, because these substances are technically more difficult to measure and may be increased in the urine, causing false-positive results if the patient has been receiving bronchodilators, nasal sprays, or drugs that produce urinary fluorescence such as tetracycline or chlorpromazine. Methyldopa also interferes with the catecholamine test but not the VMA test.

4. Pharmacologic tests—Tests based on administration of drugs are rarely used today because they may cause both false-positive and false-negative results. *Histamine,* by inducing outpouring of catecholamines from the tumor, *may produce a hypertensive crisis* with arrhythmia, myocardial ischemia, or even death (Fig 9–32).

5. Other tests—The availability of the more specific chemical tests makes the provocative tests with histamine or glucagon unnecessary today except in those individuals with an otherwise suspicious history whose pressures are completely normal and in whom no attacks are observed over a period of weeks. In these patients, 0.01 mg of histamine may be used as a provocative measure to induce an attack.

Plasma Norepinephrine

Newer methods of determining plasma norepinephrine concentrations indicate that in patients with pheochromocytoma, levels of 2.5–5 μg/l occur, in contrast to the normal 0.25–1 μg/l. Most of the norepinephrine released at the adrenergic nerve ending is reabsorbed, metabolized, or taken up again by the axon terminal. That which escapes into the circulation, while much higher than normal, is only a small fraction of the amount that is released. The sudden release of norepinephrine into the circulation in hypertensive crises in patients with pheochromocytoma produces dramatic effects. Patients with pheochromocytoma constitute less than 1% of all hypertensive subjects and can be diagnosed by measuring the amount of catecholamines or their metabolites in the urine or by measuring plasma norepinephrine concentration. Not only is measurement of the latter a most useful diagnostic test, but plasma measurements at different venous sites may help localize the tumor.

Treatment

Because the increased secretion of catecholamines results in hypertension and reduction of the plasma volume in many instances, alpha-adrenergic blocking drugs combined with beta-adrenergic blocking agents in order to inhibit the peripheral actions of the catecholamines must be used regardless of the ultimate method of treatment (medical or surgical).

A. Medical Treatment: Give phentolamine (Regitine), 10–30 mg orally every 4–6 hours, or phenoxybenzamine (Dibenzyline), 10–50 mg orally twice

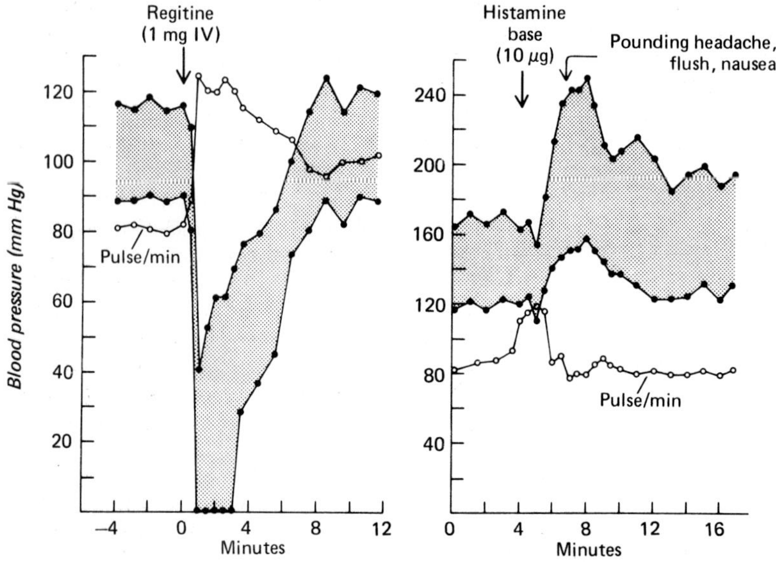

Figure 9–32. Responses to administration of phentolamine (Regitine) (1 mg) and histamine (10 μg) in patients with pheochromocytoma, showing that even small amounts of these agents (20% of the doses usually recommended for pharmacologic testing) can cause profound changes in blood pressure. (Reproduced, with permission, from Melmon KL: Part II—Catecholamines and the adrenal medulla. Pages 283–322 in: *Textbook of Endocrinology,* 5th ed. Williams RH [editor]. Saunders, 1974.)

daily, to control both blood pressure and blood volume before technical procedures which may cause marked rise or fall in pressure are done to localize the tumor (Fig 9–33).

Treatment of acute episodes. During such acute hypertensive episodes, patients should be given phentolamine, 1–5 mg intravenously every 5–10 minutes, until the pressure falls and is stabilized in order to avoid myocardial ischemia or arrhythmias. If the latter occurs or if there is severe tachycardia, 1–2 mg of propranolol can be given intravenously over a 10-minute period followed by 20 mg orally every 6 hours. When intravenous phentolamine is given, the patient is best placed in the semi-Fowler position so that if excessive fall of pressure occurs a shift to the supine position can be swiftly made. Dramatic abortion of attacks occurs with intravenous phentolamine, and the drug should be available for all diagnostic procedures that might liberate catecholamines and induce an attack.

B. Surgical Treatment: After the diagnosis of pheochromocytoma is made and surgery is contemplated, careful examination of the head and neck, chest fluoroscopy, chest x-rays, and intravenous urograms with tomography should be carried out. Inferior vena cava and adrenal venous venography with multiple venous sampling for catecholamine concentration are also used to determine the site of the tumor. Adrenal arteriography may be necessary, especially if the tumor is extrarenal; adrenal scans are less helpful when this is so.

After suitable preparation with alpha-adrenergic blocking agents (see above) to restore the blood volume and lower the blood pressure, as well as daily

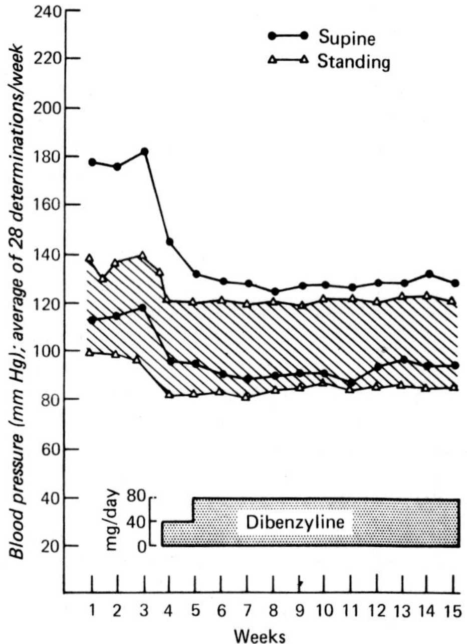

Figure 9–33. Response of the supine and standing blood pressure to treatment with phenoxybenzamine in a patient with malignant pheochromocytoma. Note that the marked orthostatic fall in blood pressure present in the pretreatment period is reduced after therapy is begun. (Reproduced, with permission, from Engelman K, Sjoerdsma A: Chronic medical therapy for pheochromocytoma: A report of 4 cases. Ann Intern Med 61:231, 1964.)

propranolol (10–40 mg 3 times daily) to control tachycardia and arrhythmias, surgical excision of the tumor is the treatment of choice. Before it was recognized that it was important to control the blood volume preoperatively, the intraoperative course was characterized by marked rises in pressure due to surgical manipulation, and a fall to hypotensive levels when the tumor was excised. Phentolamine (Regitine) should be available for immediate intravenous use for the former and norepinephrine and volume expanders for the latter.

Prognosis

As indicated above, acute hypertensive crises may precipitate ventricular arrhythmias and myocardial or cerebral ischemia or infarction. These are not prevented by the usual antihypertensive therapy, and patients with acute crises are therefore at considerable risk from these complications.

In patients with sustained hypertension without acute severe hypertensive episodes, conventional antihypertensive therapy may lower the blood pressure without affecting the basic mechanism of increased secretion of catecholamine.

CONGENITAL ADRENAL HYPERPLASIA

17-Hydroxylase Deficiency

These rare conditions were not considered to be hypertensive disorders until recently. They are due to enzymatic defects in the synthesis of cortisol and have the virtue of being effectively treated with cortisol. Biglieri (1966) demonstrated in some patients with amenorrhea and hypertension a 17-hydroxylase deficiency that blocked the synthesis not only of cortisol from cholesterol and pregnenolone but also of androgens (androsterone) and estrogens (17-hydroxyprogesterone) from the adrenal gland. As a result, failure of development of secondary sex characteristics at puberty occurred and women presented themselves with amenorrhea. The decreased synthesis of cortisol, by positive feedback, stimulates the pituitary gland to secrete excessive amounts of ACTH, which in turn stimulates the adrenal to produce increased deoxycorticosterone, causing mineralocorticoid excess with hypertension and hypokalemia.

Treatment with moderate doses of cortisol corrects the abnormality and diminishes the excessive ACTH secretion and consequently the amount of deoxycorticosterone secreted, correcting the hypokalemia and hypertension.

11-Hydroxylase Deficiency

The only other known enzymatic defect in the synthesis of cortisol is 11-hydroxylase deficiency in congenital adrenal hyperplasia associated with virilism. Deficiency of this enzyme blocks the formation of cortisol from the precursors 11-deoxycortisol and 17-hydroxyprogesterone as well as the conversion of deoxycorticosterone to corticosterone. The adrenal androgens, however, are not blocked; the increased secretion of ACTH resulting from decreased cortisol therefore stimulates the adrenal androgens, causing infant virilization, which is the presenting symptom. The excessive deoxycorticosterone causes hypertension and hypokalemia.

Therefore, 17-hydroxylase deficiency presents with hypertension, hypokalemia, and amenorrhea at puberty, whereas the 11-hydroxylase deficiency presents with hypertension, hypokalemia, and virilism in infancy.

Treatment consists of oral cortisol, which, by negative feedback, turns off the increased ACTH secretion, resulting in less androgen secretion and decreased virilism; the decreased deoxycorticosterone corrects the hypokalemia and hypertension.

COARCTATION OF THE AORTA

(See also Chapter 11.)

The adult variety of coarctation usually is a localized narrowing or constriction in the region of the ligamentum arteriosum and is often associated with a bicuspid aortic valve. The patient may present with hypertension or with a basal ejection systolic murmur which is crescendo-decrescendo when due to the bicuspid aortic valve or late systolic when it occurs at the coarcted site. Rarely, patients present with intermittent claudication of the legs. The patient is usually male, and coarctation can be suspected from the elevated blood pressure, the increased pulsations of the carotid arteries, and the delayed weak pulsations in the femoral arteries and in the arteries distal to them. If there is doubt about whether the pulses are weak and delayed in the legs, the blood pressure should be taken in the legs; if there is still doubt, direct intra-arterial pressures can be obtained in the brachial and in the femoral arteries before and after exercise. Exercise aggravates the disparity between the pressures in the upper and lower extremities. If the patient is postpuberal, pulsating collateral intercostal arteries below the margins of the ribs may be found. Coarctation varies in severity, but by early adult life the patient almost always has signs of left ventricular hypertrophy, both clinically and electrocardiographically, and the chest x-ray may show scalloping of the ribs as a result of the enlarged collateral intercostal arteries (see Chapter 11).

Surgical correction is required for all but the mildest cases of coarctation, and repair can usually be carried out safely in early childhood and even in infancy. The surgical mortality rate of repair of coarctation is less than 3%. The risk is higher if surgery is delayed until the 40s, when coronary heart disease may be superimposed and the sclerotic aorta is hard to repair.

Prognosis

Without treatment, coarctation usually leads to

death by the 40s and the patient dies of cardiac failure, ruptured cerebral aneurysm, or aortic dissection.

The incidence of persistent hypertension following repair of a coarctation has been considered in the past to be about 40%, but this was before grafts were used to bypass the coarctated segment and recoarctation thus prevented. The incidence after surgery is now 5–10%. If surgery is delayed until late adult life, complications of the hypertension may still follow. It is therefore desirable to identify and operate on patients with coarctation early in life.

RENAL PARENCHYMAL LESIONS

Acute and chronic glomerulonephritis, chronic pyelonephritis, lupus erythematosus, polycystic kidney, and scarring from old trauma probably are the most common causes of secondary hypertension due to renal factors. Prior to the phase of renal failure, the diagnosis of acute glomerulonephritis can be strongly suspected from the history of poststreptococcal proteinuria, edema, or hypertension with associated hematuria and red cell casts. It can also be discovered by accidentally finding hematuria or proteinuria in a healthy young adult from a history of pyelonephritis or lupus erythematosus, or finding bacteria and white cells in the urine; by finding evidence of renal or ureteral stone; or by uncovering a family history of early death from uremia and hypertension due to polycystic kidneys. The presence of polycystic kidneys can be established by an intravenous urogram to demonstrate polycystic or large cystic kidneys. Urinalysis, urine culture, renal function studies, and serologic studies to rule out hyperparathyroidism, lupus erythematosus, or diabetes are helpful ancillary measures. Additional studies may include a retrograde urogram with determination of ureteral reflux during cystoscopy in patients with pyelonephritis, renal arteriograms, and renal biopsy. When renal failure has occurred, the urinary sediment and the degree of proteinuria may be similar in primary hypertension in the malignant phase and in chronic renal parenchymal disease.

The accelerated form of hypertension that occurs in the late stages of renal disease further aggravates renal function, and efforts to lower the blood pressure are essential regardless of the cause. Control of the high blood pressure prolongs life and delays the onset of renal failure; when the latter occurs, dialysis or renal transplantation (or both) is indicated.

HYPERTENSION DUE TO ORAL CONTRACEPTIVE AGENTS

It is becoming increasingly apparent that there is an association between the use of oral contraceptive agents and the development of hypertension. In many instances the rise in pressure is slight, but in a few patients severe or even malignant hypertension has resulted. There is some evidence that the individuals who develop hypertension have either a family history of hypertension or a history of preeclampsia-eclampsia. The rise in pressure is often gradual, and the incidence of hypertension is greater over a period of years than during the first 6 months of use of the agent.

The mechanism by which the oral contraceptive agents produce hypertension is not certain. The most generally accepted hypothesis is that it is caused by the considerable rise in renin substrate that follows the use of the estrogen-progesterone agents. Renin substrate is the plasma globulin (α_2-globulin) upon which renin acts to produce angiotensin I, which is then cleaved to angiotensin II during passage through the lung. There has been no consistent increase in angiotensin II in patients receiving oral contraceptive agents, so this mechanism should be considered doubtful at the moment.

Oral contraceptive agents increase plasma renin and aldosterone as well as renin substrate. When hypertension is associated with a raised plasma aldosterone as well as a raised plasma renin, primary aldosteronism is excluded, but oral contraceptive agents must be considered in females. The combination of a low plasma renin, a high plasma aldosterone, and normal serum potassium in a hypertensive patient taking oral contraceptive agents virtually excludes the latter as likely causative agents. Screening of female hypertensives by determining plasma renin and aldosterone levels may make it unnecessary to stop the oral contraceptive agents for several months, as is otherwise necessary in order to determine this possible etiologic role in the hypertension.

A *rising* blood pressure, however, calls for cessation of the oral contraceptives and the use of an alternative method of contraception.

CONNECTIVE TISSUE DISORDERS (Polyarteritis Nodosa, Lupus Erythematosus)

(See also Chapter 20)

Connective tissue disorders such as polyarteritis nodosa are often associated with vasculitis of the interlobular arteries and of the arterioles and are associated with hypertension in about half of cases. The hypertension may be severe and rarely may present with the malignant phase. The disease is often generalized, involving many body systems, and the hypertension may merely be part of a total systemic disease (Table 9–26).

Renovascular lesions are common in lupus erythematosus, but hypertension is much less common than in polyarteritis nodosa. Other forms of arteritis of nonspecific cause may also induce hypertension and subsequent renal failure when the lesions involve the kidney.

Treatment is with corticosteroids and convention-

Table 9–26. Incidence of polyarteritis in various organs at necropsy.*

	Incidence of Polyarteritis	
	Group With Lung Involvement (30 Cases) (%)	Group Without Lung Involvement (54 Cases) (%)
Lungs (pulmonary arteries)	47	0
Heart	60	35
Kidneys: Glomerulitis	57	30
Renal polyarteritis	60	65
Stomach and intestines	40	30
Liver	37	54
Pancreas	17	39
Spleen	43	35
Brain	3	4
Peri-adrenal connective tissue	40	41
Voluntary muscle	33	20

*Reproduced, with permission, from Rose GA, Spencer H: Polyarteritis nodosa. Q J Med, New Series 26, 101:43, 1957.

al drug treatment for hypertension. Immunosuppressive drugs may be of value.

ACROMEGALY

Acromegaly is caused by excessive production of growth hormone by specific cells of the anterior pituitary gland. The disorder may be associated with hypertension, although other clinical and metabolic consequences are more common. These include progressive mandibular enlargement, as shown by serial photographs, large tongue, increase in the soft tissue over the heels, hands, and feet, enlargement and ballooning of the sella turcica, and widening of the space between the teeth. Patients describe increasing size of the hat, gloves, and shoes; arthralgia; headaches; and visual disturbances developing insidiously over a period of years. The hypertension is rarely severe, and treatment is directed at the acromegaly per se (Table 9–27).

The diagnosis can be established by finding a high serum growth hormone by immunoassay which falls below 5 mg/ml 1–2 hours after administration of 100 g of oral glucose. This is a useful screening test. About 10% of patients have a lower than expected serum growth hormone concentration, and in these patients abnormal growth hormone regulation by the hypothalamus is thought to be the cause. It is still not certain how many cases of acromegaly are due to an independent pituitary tumor and how many are due to abnormality of the hypothalamic growth hormone releasing factor, which then induces pituitary hyperfunction.

Treatment

Treatment now consists of microsurgery of the pituitary tumor, as in Cushing's disease. However, if the tumor is large, encroaching on the optic chiasm and the third ventricle, open surgical resection may be indicated. Irradiation of the pituitary is disappointing as judged by the fall in serum growth hormone, perhaps because the disease is far advanced before surgery. Serum concentrations above 15 mg/ml may persist for several years, and reoperation may be necessary. Chemotherapy with agents such as bromocriptine, a semisynthetic ergot alkaloid which activates dopamine receptors in the brain, reducing growth hormone, is under investigation, but the effects are only transient.

Table 9–27. Symptoms and signs in acromegaly.*

	Percent
A. Symptoms	
Earliest	
Fatigue or lethargy	82
Paresthesias	62
Amenorrhea	32
Headache	64
Later	
Excessive perspiration	88
Weight gain	76
Photophobia	46
Acral enlargement	96
Voice change	50
Decreased libido	27
Late	
Joint pain	76
Cardiac symptoms	12
B. Signs	
Acral changes	96
Warm, moist, fleshy handshake	96
Hypertension	23
Goiter	18
Lactation	8
C. Dermal changes	
Fibromata mollusca	38
Acanthosis nigricans	26

*Adapted and reproduced, with permission, from Medical Staff Conference, University of California, San Francisco: Manifestations and treatment of acromegaly. Calif Med 116:57, March 1972.

RECKLINGHAUSEN'S DISEASE (Neurofibromatosis)

The frequency of pheochromocytoma in this condition has been stressed in the literature, based on the frequency of Recklinghausen's disease in patients with pheochromocytoma. However, vascular lesions of the small to medium-sized arteries with decreased or obliterated lumen, microaneurysm formation, and intimal proliferation are more common. The vascular lesions of neurofibromatosis are different from those of polyarteritis nodosa and do not show perivascular infiltration or necrosis. Differential renal vein renin may demonstrate increased renin production by a unilaterally involved kidney, especially one with aneurysms. Arteriography may demonstrate small aneurysms in various larger tributaries of the gastrointestinal tract, as can also be seen in polyarteritis. Hypertension can occur, as it may in any condition associated with renal arteritis, and the mechanism probably involves the renin-angiotensin system.

III. TREATMENT OF ESSENTIAL OR PRIMARY HYPERTENSION

INTRODUCTION

One of the major advances in cardiology in the past 20 years has been the development and widespread use of effective antihypertensive agents. Before 1950, the only means of lowering blood pressure in patients with hypertension were a strict low-sodium diet, such as the rice-fruit diet of Kempner (1948) (Fig 9–34), and sympathectomy. The diet was extremely difficult for most patients to follow, and sympathectomy was a major surgical procedure associated with a substantial morbidity rate and some deaths. The long-term benefits of sympathectomy were controversial; on balance, it was considered helpful in severe or malignant hypertension, but the operation was promptly abandoned when the ganglionic blocking agents became available.

Since 1950, when agents such as hexamethonium were introduced, a succession of effective compounds with different mechanisms of action have been developed which usually can be taken without seriously interfering with the patient's accustomed mode of life. The dramatic decrease in mortality rate—about 40% in the past 20 years—was most strikingly evident in the more severe varieties of hypertension and its complications. The effectiveness of the available drugs has made hypertension important by emphasizing the need to find the large numbers of people with unrecognized hypertension so that they can receive the benefit of therapy.

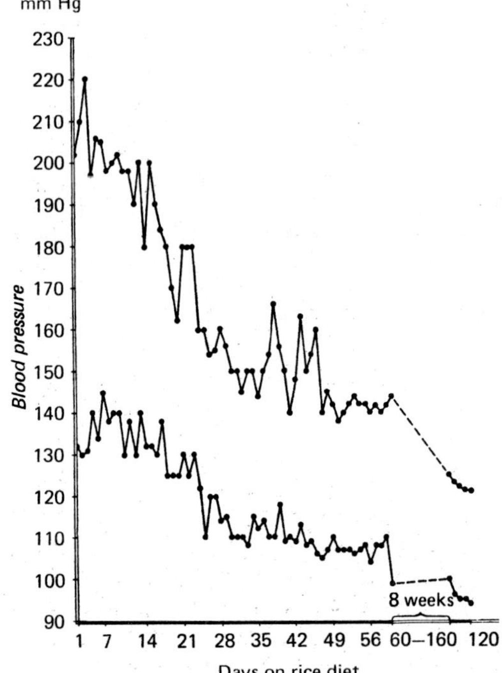

Figure 9–34. Thirty-five-year-old woman with hypertensive vascular disease of 11 years' duration beginning during the eighth month of her second pregnancy. Of 2 brothers with hypertensive vascular disease, one had died at the age of 37 (stroke). The patient had 2 retinal hemorrhages. Total PSP excretion in 2 hours was 64%; serum cholesterol was 250 mg/dl. Rice diet was started April 23, 1947, and strictly followed (7–14 mg Cl/dl of urine). No medication was given. A decrease in blood pressure began in the third week on the rice diet. (Reproduced, with permission, from Kempner W: Treatment of hypertensive vascular disease with rice diet. Arch Intern Med 133:758, 1974.)

Hypertension per se should be treated because vascular abnormalities and their complications occur no matter whether raised blood pressure is primary or secondary. Any drug regimen that brings the blood pressure down into the normal range will prevent and reverse the malignant phase of hypertension, improve cardiac failure, decrease the mortality rate from dissection of the aorta, prevent hemorrhagic stroke, and prolong life (Tables 9–28 and 9–29). Many studies have shown that malignant hypertension, cardiac failure, and hemorrhagic stroke are rare in the properly treated hypertensive patient and that when malignant hypertension and cardiac failure develop in an untreated or inadequately treated hypertensive patient, lowering the blood pressure with effective agents will reverse these complications. Whether lowering the blood pressure will prevent late atherosclerotic complications such as cerebral infarction, coronary heart disease, or atherosclerosis of the peripheral vessels is still an unanswered question. Atherosclerosis develops over a period of years, and most of the therapeutic trials have been too short to demonstrate the effectiveness of therapy. The

Table 9–28. Percentages of hypertensive patients surviving 5 years according to the presence and severity of various complications.*

Complication of Hypertension	Grade of Severity of Complication			
	1	2	3	4
Retinopathy (all cases)	82	65	20	18
Retinopathy plus renal failure	43	24	23	11
Radiologic cardiac enlargement	79	51	35	0
Electrocardiographic abnormalities	82	55	34	28

*Reproduced, with permission of the American Heart Association, Inc., from Nagle R: The prognosis of hypertension. Practitioner 207:52, July 1971. Modified from Sokolow M, Perloff D: The prognosis of essential hypertension treated conservatively. Circulation 23:697, 1961.

age of the patient when therapy has begun also influences the incidence of morbid events. In the VA Study (1972), 15% of the control group developed morbid events if under age 50, but 43% developed morbid events if they were over age 50. In the treated group, there was still a distinct disadvantage in the older group, but the incidence of morbid events was less than in the untreated group. Seven percent of those under age 50 and 18% of those 50 or over developed morbid events during the period of observation. Therapeutic trials are now under way in various parts of the world to test the hypothesis that effective antihypertensive therapy begun at a younger age and in milder hypertensive patients will decrease, delay, or prevent atherosclerosis, which is the leading cause of death in mild to moderate hypertension.

Basic Principles of Treatment of Essential Hypertension

(1) Establish that persistent and not transient hypertension is present.

(2) Institute appropriate treatment of "curable" secondary causes of hypertension, if present.

(3) Evaluate the functional integrity or the degree and speed of involvement of target organs to estimate prognosis.

(4) Assess the need for treatment by the height of the arterial pressures taken in the office or home or while ambulatory and by the associated vascular complications.

(5) Assess the need for treatment in borderline or mild hypertension (diastolic pressure 90–104 mm Hg) in the light of adverse prognostic factors such as youth, male sex, positive family history, black race, and the presence of target organ damage. Also determine the presence of other risk factors known to influence atherosclerosis, eg, hypercholesterolemia, hypertriglyceridemia, cigarette smoking, diabetes, family history of atherosclerosis, personality disturbances, obesity. Decisions about therapeutic options such as the potency and mode of administration of drugs and whether to use one agent or a combination of agents are based upon the height of the arterial pressure and the urgency of the hypertensive complications, eg, cardiac failure, hypertensive encephalopathy and progression to malignant hypertension, aortic dissection, or hemorrhagic stroke.

(6) Begin treatment in mild to moderate hypertensive disease with an agent of moderate potency that is known to cause minimal side-effects. Gradually increase the dose until the desired therapeutic effect is achieved or unpleasant side-effects occur. If necessary, add another and then perhaps another agent until a combination of drugs is arrived at that gives an acceptable pressure with the fewest possible or least disturbing side-effects.

(7) The aim is to achieve a standing office diastolic pressure less than 90 mm Hg or a systolic pressure less than 140 mm Hg. However, a pressure of 150/100 mm Hg is acceptable if untoward side-effects make a lower pressure difficult to achieve, especially in patients with severe hypertension at the outset or in patients over age 70.

(8) Assess the patient's social, emotional, economic, and environmental problems in all cases, especially if the response to treatment is poor.

(9) Educate the patient and make treatment as convenient as possible to ensure compliance with long-term treatment.

(10) Treatment should be individualized, with minimal doses in frail, elderly people.

Principles of Management of Malignant Hypertension

(1) Prevent progression into the malignant phase by adequate treatment of underlying hypertension due to any cause.

(2) Treat as an emergency. Hospitalization and vigorous treatment are mandatory.

(3) Choose a mode of parenteral treatment appropriate to the speed of the desired effects: (a) seconds (sodium nitroprusside), (b) a few minutes (diazoxide,

Table 9–29. Effect of treatment on mortality rate and major cardiovascular complications. (After Veterans Administration Cooperative Study Group, 1970.)*

Diastolic Blood Pressure (mm Hg)	Placebo				Treated				
			Complications				Complications		Follow-Up Period (Years)
	No.	Deaths	No.	%	No.	Deaths	No.	%	
115–129	70	4	27	38.6	73	0	1	1.4	1.6
90–114	194	19	56	29	186	8	22	11.8	3.3

*Reproduced, with permission, from Nagle R: The prognosis of hypertension. Practitioner 207:52, July 1971.

trimethaphan), (c) 20–40 minutes (hydralazine), (d) hours (reserpine, methyldopa, minoxidil).

(4) Observe the patient closely, preferably in the coronary or intensive care unit; titrate the dosage of parenteral drugs carefully.

(5) Start with small doses if the patient is hypovolemic, over age 60, or has vascular disease (angina, cerebral or extremity ischemic attacks).

(6) If one drug proves ineffective, add another rather than attempting massive doses of any one drug. Combined therapy is usually more effective and causes fewer side-effects.

(7) Avoid dehydration and hypervolemia. The former causes extrarenal azotemia; the latter interferes with effective treatment, raises the blood pressure further, and causes heart failure.

(8) Start vigorous treatment at the first manifestation of accelerated hypertension, such as a diastolic pressure exceeding 130 mm Hg or hemorrhages or exudates in the fundi.

(9) Lower the blood pressure despite impaired renal function; use dialysis if necessary for relief of uremic symptoms or complications while acute arterial lesions heal as the blood pressure is lowered.

(10) Use vigorous antihypertensive treatment both orally and intravenously in combination with intermittent hemodialysis to control the blood pressure, even if the plasma renin level is high. Bilateral nephrectomy is rarely indicated.

(11) If the patient is overloaded with fluid, oliguric, and dyspneic, with pulmonary edema, dialyze to remove excess fluid and permit the antihypertensive agents to lower the blood pressure.

(12) Institute oral therapy as soon as possible—usually on the first or second day.

WHEN TO TREAT HYPERTENSION

The physician's decision to start treatment is in many instances based on the individual's philosophic perception of the consequences of inaction. The premise underlying antihypertensive therapy is that lowering the blood pressure will decrease the likelihood of disability and death from vascular complications. There is no single point at which all physicians will agree that treatment is required.

Hypertension As a Continuum

Hypertension can be considered a continuum, progressing from (1) the earliest manifestations of transient occasional rises of blood pressure to (2) asymptomatic established hypertension without vascular abnormalities or complications through (3) the presence of vascular abnormalities alone without complications to (4) the presence of vascular complications and finally to (5) death. At what point along the continuum one decides to institute treatment depends on the philosophy and conviction of the physician that the benefits warrant the difficulties of lifelong treatment with antihypertensive agents.

Early Treatment

Some physicians are sufficiently concerned about the potential hazards of hypertension, for example, that they will begin treatment in a black male teenager if his blood pressure exceeds the 95th percentile for age, sex, and race—especially if he has a family history of hypertension. Others wait until hypertension is established and even then do not treat unless the diastolic pressure consistently exceeds 105 mm Hg in the office unless other circumstances suggest that the risk of vascular complications is great. This majority view is based on the Veterans Administration Study, a randomized study of approximately 400 hypertensive patients whose blood pressure elevation persisted in the hospital and who were found to be compliant to therapy in an outpatient trial following hospitalization, half of whom were treated, half untreated (VA Study, 1970). The results (Table 9–30) unequivocally demonstrated the benefit of antihypertensive therapy in patients whose average office diastolic pressures equalled or exceeded 105 mm Hg. Vascular complications were 3 times as great in untreated as in treated patients. Other physicians treat patients whose diastolic blood pressures vary between 90 and 105 mm Hg if they are under 35, male, black, and have a positive family history or other risk factors for atherosclerosis. Although individuals in this so-called borderline zone develop established higher blood pressures with a greater frequency than the population at large, the majority do not; it is nonetheless safe to observe such patients twice a year unless there is a more compelling reason to begin therapy such as noted above.

The younger the individual, the more significant is any given level of blood pressure, so that a pressure that might be in the 50th percentile in the sixth decade would be in the 90th or 95th percentile in an individual in the third decade, with a corresponding doubled or tripled mortality rate over a period of 20–30 years. Although it has not been proved that treating borderline hypertension prevents the development of atherosclerosis, the Framingham Study showed that the development of coronary disease is more frequent in borderline hypertensive than in normotensive individuals (Fig 9–13). The problem is further complicated by the fact that some investigators use the term borderline hypertension to mean diastolic pressures between 90 and 104 mm Hg; others to mean pressures less than 160/95 but more than 140/90 mm Hg (90–95 systolic is still borderline) (Kannel, 1974); and still others to denote diastolic pressures that are sometimes 90–100 mm Hg and sometimes < 90 mm Hg. The term borderline hypertension is most commonly used when average pressures are less than 160/100 mm Hg, associated with occasional normal readings; the term "mild hypertension" is used to mean average diastolic pressures between 90 and 104 mm Hg.

Table 9–30. Incidence of assessable events by age and diagnostic category in the VA Study.*

	Age (Years)						Total Events	
	< 50		50–59		60+			
Diagnostic Category	C	T	C	T	C	T	C	T
Cerebrovascular accident	5	1	5	1	10	3	20	5
Congestive heart failure	1	0	1	0	9	0	11	0
Accelerated hypertension or renal damage	5	0	2	0	0	0	7	0
Coronary artery disease†	4	4	4	2	5	5	13	11
Atrial fibrillation	0	2	0	1	2	0	2	3
Dissecting aneurysm	0	0	1	0	1	0	2	0
Other‡	0	0	1	0	0	3	1	3
Total morbid events	15	7	14	4	27	11	56	22
Diastolic > 124 mm Hg	15	0	3	0	2	0	20	0

Abbreviations: C = control group; T = treated group.

*Reproduced, with permission of the American Heart Association, Inc., from Veterans Administration Cooperative Study Group on Antihypertensive Agents: Effects of treatment on morbidity in hypertension. 3. Influence of age, diastolic pressure, and prior cardiovascular disease; further analysis of side-effects. Circulation 45:991, 1972.

†Myocardial infarction or sudden death.

‡Includes in treated group one patient terminated because of hypotensive reactions, one death from ruptured atherosclerotic aneurysm, and one patient with second degree heart block. Control group includes one patient with left bundle branch block.

Blacks Versus Whites

Among the factors that induce many physicians to treat mild hypertension are age, family history, the presence of other risk factors for atherosclerosis, and target organ involvement. It is clear from a number of studies that the death rate from hypertension in blacks is considerably greater than that in whites, but this may be a function of access to treatment rather than an inherent susceptibility to hypertension, because in the VA Study (1967) black and white patients did equally well with treatment and equally badly in the untreated group. There are few data to indicate that the prognosis is worse in blacks than whites with mild hypertension; the higher mortality rate from hypertension in blacks is to a great extent due to their greater likelihood of having severe hypertension with cardiac failure or malignant hypertension.

Vascular Complications

The development of vascular complications ("clinical events") is clearly related to the presence of prior vascular abnormalities (fundal or electrocardiographic abnormalities), even when comparable degrees of elevation of blood pressure are present. For example, in the VA Study (1972), vascular complications developed 2–3 times more frequently in patients who had initial vascular abnormalities irrespective of whether they were in the control or treated group. Insurance data and recordings of blood pressure have shown that for any given elevation of blood pressure the likelihood of cardiac failure and death is much greater when either left ventricular hypertrophy or abnormalities of the arterioles of the retina are present. For this reason, the presence of target organ damage warrants therapy in mild hypertension because the measured blood pressure at any given time may not be representative of the average value, which may be higher.

Treatment With Onset of Symptoms

Conservative physicians wait to begin treatment until vascular complications have appeared, but this is often unwise because the first complication may be one that carries a high mortality rate, eg, cardiac failure, malignant hypertension, aortic dissection, or hemorrhagic stroke. These complications, unfortunately, are commonly seen in untreated hypertensives, especially in black patients who have not had access to medical therapy or who have discontinued therapy.

Six Months' Observation

Patients with transient temporary elevations of pressure (most diastolic readings < 90 mm Hg) or patients with borderline hypertension (some diastolic readings of 90–100 mm Hg but others < 90 mm Hg) should be observed twice a year and instructed to return sooner if new or progressive symptoms appear. Treatment may be initiated in the mild hypertensive group if any of the associated factors indicating an adverse prognosis (youth, black race, male sex, positive family history, evidence of target organ damage, or presence of hypercholesterolemia or hyperglycemia) are present. The decision whether 90, 95, or 100 mm Hg should be the starting point for treatment is at the discretion of the individual and is based on personal therapeutic philosophy and recognition of other adverse factors. The weight of opinion is that almost all patients whose average diastolic pressure is 105 mm Hg or higher should receive antihypertensive therapy. The physician's discretion is exercised when the diastolic pressure is between 90–104 mm Hg. Prospective studies currently under way should provide prognostic data which will help the physician to determine whether antihypertensive treatment is better than no treatment in milder cases. Studies on spontaneously hypertensive rats of the Okamoto strain suggest that the earlier the blood pressure is lowered, the more likely are structural arteriolar changes in the kidney to be prevented. There is no reason why the same should not be true in humans. One should not withhold treatment until irreversible damage to the vascular system (or a complication) has already occurred.

IMPORTANCE OF EARLY IDENTIFICATION & TREATMENT OF HYPERTENSION

Evaluation of Blood Pressure

From the above, it follows that one should identify hypertension early in its course because it is often asymptomatic, because the first manifestation may be a complication, and because, if it is not recognized until later, damage to the arterioles and arteries may have already occurred. For these reasons, vigorous efforts are now being made to make certain that the blood pressure is measured and recorded in every patient who enters the health care system for any reason. Patients who attend skin, orthopedic, dental, eye, or even general medical clinics commonly do not have their blood pressure taken unless there is a complaint calling for a general medical examination and work-up. Public and voluntary health agencies have been encouraging widespread screening to identify asymptomatic hypertensive individuals. As is true also of other types of screening (eg, glaucoma, diabetes), the purpose of this effort is not to make the diagnosis but to find people who need further evaluation. As discussed earlier, single pressures may be misleading even in the doctor's office; pressures obtained in unfamiliar surroundings, sometimes without privacy and without the customary period of rest, and pressures obtained in patients who are coerced or fearful may merely represent transient increases of no clinical significance. A high percentage of patients with elevated blood pressure in screened populations have normal pressures in the doctor's office. At least one-third of patients with initial diastolic pressures over 105–110 mm Hg will have pressures less than 90 mm Hg when readings are taken later. The current standards of what constitutes normal blood pressure are based on resting office pressures.

Number of Readings Required

Even if the pressure is raised in the doctor's office, one must be certain that the elevated pressure is not transient. For example, one needs measurements on at least 3 separate occasions even if the diastolic pressure varies between 100 and 120 mm Hg. If diastolic pressures are so variable that they are 90–100 mm Hg on one occasion but less than 90 mm Hg on another occasion, it may be necessary to take 10, 20, or even 30 readings over a period of months before concluding that the patient is indeed an established hypertensive who needs lifelong therapy. Ten to 20% of patients at any given time may have variable pressures above or below whatever arbitrary line the physician regards as the upper limit of normal, above which he will initiate treatment; it is then necessary to use ancillary methods to try to obtain blood pressures under ordinary circumstances of the patient's life. As discussed previously, pressures can be taken by the patient or a family member at home, or by a nurse in the office in nonthreatening situations. Near basal pressures utilizing sedation can be measured, as recommended by Smirk (1959) in New Zealand, and ambulatory pressures can be obtained semiautomatically by utilizing a portable blood pressure recorder. In almost 30% of cases, even patients with consistently elevated office pressures will have normal pressures after several days of hospitalization. The average drop in blood pressure is about 20–30 mm Hg depending on the age of the patient and the height of the pressure, but the significance of this difference is not known.

Decision to Begin Treatment

When the physician has taken an adequate number of readings under appropriate conditions and is convinced that this particular patient will benefit from treatment even after the potential side-effects of the drug regimen have been considered, the patient must then be educated regarding the duration of treatment, and every responsible effort must be made to see to it that the patient continues in treatment indefinitely. In the VA Study (1975), hypertension returned, usually by 6 months, in 85% of patients in whom treatment was deliberately stopped (Fig 9–35).

The decision to begin antihypertensive therapy requires careful judgment and thorough discussion with the patient and should never be undertaken light-

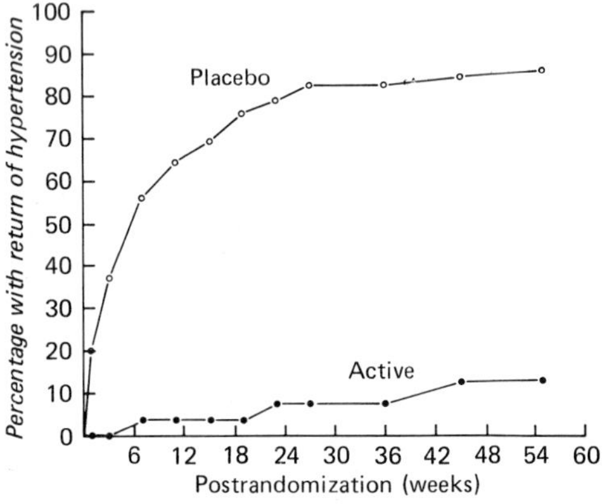

Figure 9–35. Cumulative percent of patients attaining diastolic blood pressure of 95 mm Hg or higher on 2 successive clinic visits is shown on the ordinate. Time after randomization is shown on the abscissa. At 6 weeks after randomization, 51% of the placebo group demonstrated 95 mm Hg, and at 6 months 82% of the placebo group had reached this level. (Reproduced, with permission of the American Heart Association, Inc., from Veterans Administration Cooperative Study Group on Antihypertensive Agents: Return of elevated blood pressure after withdrawal of antihypertensive drugs. Circulation 51:1107, 1975.)

ly. Antihypertensive therapy is a cooperative venture between the patient and the doctor, and agreement on a mutual objective at the outset increases the likelihood of patient compliance. Once begun, treatment should be continued without interruption, modified if necessary, along with treatment of other risk factors of atherosclerosis.

Treat According to Severity

In the average patient with mild or moderate hypertension, it is preferable to begin slowly and gradually increase the dosage and potency of the therapeutic agents used; however, this is not adequate when the patient has accelerated hypertension, encephalopathy, cardiac failure, or similar urgent situations. The physician must estimate the urgency of the role of the elevated blood pressure and match the choice of drugs with the necessities of the situation. Even when it is urgent to lower the pressure quickly, one must not act precipitously and then have to retreat if the fall in pressure is excessive or if side-effects occur.

In mild to moderate disease, one should begin with drugs of modest potency in low dosage given once or twice daily in order to avoid toxic side-effects that might discourage the patient. The objective of treatment is to use as few agents as possible with the fewest possible side-effects and to bring down the blood pressure and keep it down without interfering too much with the patient's life-style. Each drug must be used until the desired effect is achieved or until side-effects prevent increased dosage. In the latter event, a new agent is added. The availability of a number of drugs with different mechanisms of action allows the physician to use trial and error to obtain an effective combination of agents with which the patient can live comfortably. Forcing the patient to accept unpleasant side-effects usually leads to discouragement and noncompliance, especially if the patient is asymptomatic. The drugs are used orally except in compelling situations, when parenteral therapy is used in combination with oral therapy. (See below for details.)

GENERAL THERAPEUTIC MEASURES

General measures such as diet, exercise, loss of weight in obesity, and attention to other risk factors should not be neglected in the care of the hypertensive patient.

Although the use of diuretic agents makes strict sodium restriction less important, a high sodium intake, either by the use of salt in the diet or by sodium-containing agents such as Alka-Seltzer, reduces the effectiveness of diuretic agents. The patient's sodium intake should be limited. There should be no added salt in the diet, and the patient should be advised to avoid very salty foods such as potato chips, bacon, soy sauce, etc. If the patient has carbohydrate intolerance, a prudent diet of modest carbohydrate and caloric restriction is advised; we encourage the patient to stay on this diet permanently. If the patient has hypercholesterolemia or hypertriglyceridemia, and especially if type IV hyperlipidemia is present as a result of increased carbohydrate or alcohol intake, reduced intake of these substances should be encouraged in order to reduce the serum triglycerides that may favor the development of coronary heart disease. In the presence of type II hypercholesterolemia, a reduced cholesterol intake is encouraged, and the patient is given drugs (clofibrate or cholestyramine), as indicated in Chapter 8.

Weight reduction is recommended, not only because this may rarely reduce the blood pressure to normal but also because obesity aggravates and increases the likelihood of diabetes, marginally increases the likelihood of coronary heart disease, and interferes with the patient's sense of well-being.

Moderate physical activity is encouraged not only for its effect on weight loss and general sense of well-being but also because moderate exercise decreases the systemic vascular resistance and seems beneficial, although there are scarce data to substantiate this. Advocates of physical exercise as a preventive measure against the development of acute myocardial infarction believe that physical conditioning increases the collateral circulation and decreases the likelihood of fatality if the patient does develop acute myocardial infarction.

Cigarette smoking may not only increase the likelihood of coronary heart disease but may also increase the likelihood of ventricular fibrillation and sudden death if the patient has concomitant coronary disease, as most hypertensives do. Hypertensive patients should stop smoking if possible.

There is no evidence that moderate amounts of alcohol, coffee, or tea are harmful to hypertensive patients; in fact, they may be helpful by virtue of their relaxant effects. Excessive use of alcohol, however, is undesirable because it increases the serum triglyceride concentration and because prolonged excessive use of alcohol may produce alcoholic cardiomyopathy. In a patient whose cardiac load is already increased by raised blood pressure, alcohol may favor the development of cardiac failure. The combination of hypertensive heart disease, coronary heart disease, and alcoholic cardiomyopathy is particularly ominous.

Mental tranquility is always desirable. Over the years a variety of methods have been used to relax patients. Prior to the days of antihypertensive therapy, sedation, progressive relaxation, psychotherapy, frequent vacations, and attention to the environment were all used, but with only marginal benefit in the reduction of blood pressure. More recently, transcendental meditation, biofeedback, yoga, and other methods of relaxation have been explored in an effort to combat the environmental increase in systemic vascular resistance and cardiac output that occurs with the stresses of modern life. A recent study, however, reported that in a group of 20 hypertensive patients who received a professionally supervised program of

Table 9–31. Oral treatment of hypertension (adult dosages).

	Tablet Size (mg)	Initial and Incremental Dose (mg)	Doses Per Day	Usual Oral Daily Dose (mg)	Interval Between Increment of Doses
Commonly used mild diuretics					
Hydrochlorothiazide (Hydrodiuril, Esidrix, Oretic)	25, 50, 100	25, 50	1–2	25–100	2 weeks
Chlorothiazide (Diuril)	250, 500	250, 500	1–2	250–1000	2 weeks
Bendroflumethiazide (Naturetin, Benuron)	2.5, 5.0, 10	2.5	1–2	2.5–10	2 weeks
Chlorthalidone (Hygroton)	50, 100	50	1	50–100	2 weeks
Metolazone (Zaroxolyn)	2.5, 5.0, 10	2.5	1	2.5–10	2 weeks
Potassium-sparing diuretics					
Triamterene (Dyrenium)	50, 100	50	1–2	50–200	2 weeks
Spironolactone (Aldactone)	25	25	1–3	25–150	2 weeks
Potent diuretics					
Furosemide (Lasix)	20, 40	20–80	1–3	20–300	1 week
Ethacrynic acid (Edecrin)	25, 50	25, 50	1–3	25–200	1 week
Adrenergic inhibitors					
Reserpine (Serpasil)	0.1, 0.25, 0.5, 1	0.1	1	0.1–0.25	4 weeks
Methyldopa (Aldomet)	125, 250, 500	250	2–4	500–2000	1 week
Guanethidine (Ismelin)	10, 25	10	1	10–200	1 week
Mecamylamine (Inversine)	2.5, 10	2.5	1–4	10–100	1 week
Pentolinium (Ansolysen)	20, 40, 100	20	1–4	80–200	1 week
Propranolol (Inderal)	10, 40, 80	10	2–4	20–320	1 week
Clonidine (Catapres)	0.1, 0.2	0.1	1–2	0.1–0.6	1 week
Vasodilators					
Prazosin (Minipress)	1, 2, 5 caps	0.5–1.0	2–4	10–15	1 week
Hydralazine (Apresoline)	10, 25, 50, 100	10	2–4	100–200	1 week
Minoxidil*	1, 5, 10	2.5	2–4	5–20	1 week

*Not approved by the US Food & Drug Administration.

Table 9–32. Parenteral treatment of hypertension (adult dosages).

	How Supplied	Initial Dose and Route	Onset of Action	Duration of Action (Before Repeat Dose)
Adrenergic inhibitors				
Methyldopa (Aldomet)	250 mg/5 ml ampule	250–500 mg IV	2–4 hours	4–12 hours
Trimethaphan camsylate† (Arfonad)	500 mg/10 ml ampule	1–4 mg/minute IV infusion	Seconds to minutes	As long as infused
Reserpine (Serpasil)	5 mg/2 ml (also 10 ml)	0.5–1 mg IM or IV bolus, slowly	2–6 hours	6–12 hours
Propranolol (Inderal)	1 mg/ml ampule	1 mg bolus, slowly	Minutes	4–6 hours
Pentolinium (Ansolysen)	100 mg/10 ml	1–2.5 mg bolus, slowly	10–30 minutes	2–6 hours
Vasodilators				
Diazoxide† (Hyperstat)	300 mg/20 ml ampule	75–300 mg rapidly IV	1–5 minutes	5–12 hours
Hydralazine (Apresoline)	20 mg/ml ampule	10–20 mg bolus slowly, IV or IM	15–30 minutes	1–4 hours
Sodium nitroprusside‡ (Nipride)	50 mg/5 ml vial	0.5–8 μg/kg/minute IV by infusion of 5% dextrose and water, not by direct injection	Immediate; can increase infusion rate every 5–10 minutes as needed	As long as infused
Diuretics				
Furosemide (Lasix)	20 mg/2 ml ampule	40–80 mg IV bolus	15–30 minutes	8–12 hours
Ethacrynate sodium (Edecrin)	50 mg/50 ml vial	50 mg IV bolus	15–30 minutes	8–12 hours

*Information regarding products, precautions, and methods of administration of all agents being given parenterally should be reviewed in the *Physicians' Desk Reference* prior to use in patients if the physician is not using the drugs frequently.

†Requires closely monitored supervision and titration for proper dose.

‡Photosensitive—should be protected from light.

transcendental meditation, no significant change in blood pressure occurred after 6 months (Pollack, 1977), although some subjects had a greater sense of well-being. There have been some reports that meditation lowered the blood pressure in a few patients. On the other hand, it should be appreciated that some forms of meditation in fact produce violent increases in blood pressure, such that one patient had "private thoughts" during meditation that raised his diastolic pressure to 170 mm Hg for several hours. We have been unimpressed by the reports of beneficial effects of biofeedback, and in the absence of data solidly demonstrating its value we rely on antihypertensive agents rather than on psychologic methods as the primary therapy in treating hypertension. Psychologic methods such as relaxation therapy can be considered as auxiliary therapy.

DRUGS AVAILABLE FOR TREATMENT

These vary in dosage, potency, side-effects, mechanism of action, and route of administration (oral or parenteral). The antihypertensive drugs available are summarized in Tables 9–31 and 9–32, and Table 9–33 reviews the adverse effects of these various agents.

Oral Diuretic Agents

The thiazides are the prototype of this group of drugs, which act initially by depleting the body of sodium, potassium, and fluid volume and later by decreasing the systemic vascular resistance.

The sodium, potassium, chloride, and water losses may be substantial over the first few days and then tend to diminish. The 24-hour excretion after a standard dose of a thiazide diuretic is almost 100–200 mEq of Na^+, 40–50 mEq of K^+, 200 mEq of Cl^-, and 1000–1500 ml of water. Early in the course of treatment, hypovolemia may be associated with dizziness, weakness, nausea, cramps, and postural hypotension; later, the plasma volume and extracellular volume return almost to normal (reduced by about 3–5%), and postural hypotension is uncommon. The dose-response curve of a given drug is such that maximum diuretic effects of the drugs occur with about 100 mg of hydrochlorothiazide or 500 mg of the more potent furosemide, given as single doses. Continued hypovolemia can be inferred from the slight increases in serum creatinine and uric acid that occur in most patients. A major problem associated with the use of diuretics is hypokalemia, which tends to occur with many of the diuretic agents and is due to impaired reabsorption at the sodium-potassium exchange site, where aldosterone causes increased secretion of potassium and reabsorption of sodium.

The magnitude of the decrease in serum K^+ is variable but averages about 0.6 mEq/l (10–15%) in patients receiving the usual daily dose of hydrochlorothiazide in 2 divided doses. It requires 60–80 mEq/day of a 10% elixir of potassium chloride to raise the serum potassium to the pretreatment value (Schwartz, 1974). Total potassium in the body is usually low when the serum potassium is reduced, but many patients have a substantial loss of total body potassium with a normal serum potassium because the correlation between serum potassium and total exchangeable potassium is only 0.4 (Liebman, 1959). Acid-base equilibrium influences the intra- and extracellular balance of potassium, and if there is a tendency to alkalosis, the serum potassium may fall. Table 9–34 shows the average serum electrolytes after 6–8 weeks of treatment with diuretics. In the VA Study (1967), the serum potassium levels on the initial and first and second annual examinations showed that most patients after 1–2 years had serum K^+ levels exceeding 3.5 mEq/l but that 20% were between 2.5 and 3.5 mEq/l. The electrolyte response to a diuretic is enhanced by bed rest; the urine volume and sodium excretion in normal individuals when they are in bed is of the same order of magnitude as when they are up and about receiving a diuretic. During bed rest, water and sodium excretion doubles, but K^+ excretion does not change. The decreased absorption of uric acid in the proximal tubule leads to raised serum uric acid, which in individuals

Table 9–33. Adverse effects of antihypertensive agents.

Diuretics	Nausea, muscle cramps, hypovolemia, hypokalemia, hyponatremia, hyperuricemia, hyperglycemia, rash
Potassium-sparing diuretics	Hyperkalemia, gynecomastia
Adrenergic inhibitors	
Methyldopa	Drowsiness, dry mouth, impotence, hepatitis, postural hypotension, hemolytic anemia, fever
Reserpine	Somnolence, nasal congestion, nightmares, mental depression
Guanethidine	Postural hypotension, diarrhea, retrograde ejaculation, weakness on exertion
Propranolol	Bradycardia, left ventricular failure, asthma, Raynaud's syndrome, central nervous system symptoms, sodium retention
Mecamylamine and trimethaphan	Postural hypotension, parasympathetic blockade with constipation and paralytic ileus, loss of visual accommodation
Clonidine	Dry mouth, drowsiness, rebound hypertension if drug stopped abruptly
Vasodilator agents	
Prazosin	Tachycardia, headache, postural weakness and hypotension
Hydralazine	Lupuslike syndrome, headache, tachycardia, angina
Minoxidil	Tachycardia, hirsutism, headache, sodium retention
Diazoxide	Hyperglycemia, tachycardia, angina, sodium retention
Sodium nitroprusside	Excess hypotension, acute tubular necrosis, thiocyanate toxicity

Table 9–34. Average serum electrolytes after 6–8 weeks' treatment with 50 mg hydrochlorothiazide or 100 mg ethacrynic acid daily.*

Treatment Group	Sodium (mEq/l)	Potassium (mEq/l)	Chloride (mEq/l)	Bicarbonate (mEq/l)	Urea (mg/dl)	Uric Acid (mg/dl)
Control	143.9	4.3	103.3	27.5	29.8	5.3
Hydrochlorothiazide	137.8	3.7	95.4	29.0	32.0	7.2
Ethacrynic acid	139.4	3.8	98.0	27.9	41.1 (31.8)†	7.0

*Reproduced, with permission, from Dollery CT, Parry EHO, Young DS: Diuretic and hypotensive properties of ethacrynic acid: A comparison with hydrochlorothiazide. Lancet 1:947, 1964.

†This figure is the average after eliminating the results on one patient whose blood urea rose to 155 mg/dl on ethacrynic acid.

with a history of gout may cause acute gout that can be prevented by the use of probenecid or allopurinol. Infrequently, glucose reabsorption in the proximal tubule is also impaired, and patients with a susceptibility to diabetes may develop hyperglycemia. If the dosage of diuretics is excessive, the patient may develop severe hyponatremia and dehydration with hypovolemia, but this is uncommon if the thiazides and not the "loop" diuretics (eg, furosemide) are used in moderate doses. The potassium loss makes digitalis toxicity more likely, so that particular care must be taken to avoid hypokalemia if digitalis is used. Hypokalemia is more common when dietary potassium is low, sodium intake is high, and laxatives are used frequently. If the serum potassium falls below 3.5 mEq/l on ordinary doses of thiazides, the possibility of primary hyperaldosteronism should be considered. If symptoms of hypokalemia develop or if digitalis is prescribed, potassium-sparing diuretics such as spironolactone or triamterene should be added to the thiazides or other diuretics such as chlorthalidone, furosemide, and metolazone, provided renal function is adequate and the patients do not take oral potassium supplements (see below). Alternatively, patients should be placed on a high-potassium diet (as suggested in Table 9–35), including fruits, vegetables, and a preparation in tablet form that releases potassium slowly and does not produce ulceration of the small bowel. (Enteric-coated potassium supplements should be avoided because of their propensity for producing ulceration of the small intestine.) Liquid potassium preparations are unpleasant to take. If hypokalemia occurs at levels of 3–3.5 mEq/l, oral potassium supplements of 40–80 mEq/day should be prescribed.

Oral diuretic agents should be considered basic treatment of most hypertensive patients because they suffice in many cases to lower the pressure satisfactorily when used alone. The average reduction in blood pressure with hydrochlorothiazide is about 30 mm Hg systolic and 15 mm Hg diastolic. There is a minimal postural effect. This is approximately the magnitude of the fall following the use of methyldopa, but the diuretics diminish the required dosage of other agents added to a therapeutic regimen or are additive to other drugs. For example, when hydrochlorothiazide is added to methyldopa, the average fall in blood pressure is greater than with either drug used alone and averages about 40 mm Hg systolic and 20 mm Hg diastolic (Table 9–36). Furthermore, they counteract the sodium retention that occurs with other drugs such as the vasodilator agents and methyldopa. If oral diuretics are added to an already stabilized regimen because of sodium retention or excessive hypotension, the dose of the basic drug should be reduced about 50% before the diuretic is added to avoid excessive fall in pressure. When methyldopa is added after the full effect of a thiazide diuretic is achieved, not only are the systolic and diastolic pressures lower, but the reduction of the glomerular filtration rate and the renal blood flow are reversed toward normal. Plasma renin activity, which is increased by a diuretic, is increased only half as much when methyldopa is added. If the diuretic is added after the full effect of methyldopa is obtained, the

Table 9–35. Foods that are helpful to take in addition to the normal diet to supplement potassium (K^+) intake.*

Quantities of foods to supply approximately 0.5 g (500 mg) (13 mEq) of potassium (K^+)

1 cup tomato juice†
1 cup low sodium tomato juice, prune juice
1¼ cups orange juice, tangerine juice, orange-grapefruit juice, grapefruit juice

1 medium-sized banana
7–8 dates
4 figs
7 large prunes
½ cup raisins (dark)
6 apricots (fresh)
½ cantaloupe

1 cup broccoli
¾ cup winter squash
10 brussels sprouts, cooked
1 large white potato
1 large sweet potato
1/3 cup lentils (dry)
1½ cups raw cauliflower

4 tbsp nonfat milk powder†
1½ cups nonfat milk†

*Reproduced, with permission, from the California Heart Association.

†High in potassium but also high in sodium.

Table 9–36. Combined antihypertensive effect of methyldopa and hydrochlorothiazide. Arithmetic mean arterial blood pressure before and after 4 weeks of treatment.*

	Methyldopa (n = 22)		Hydrochlorothiazide (n = 20)		Methyldopa With Hydrochlorothiazide (n = 21)		Placebo (n = 21)	
	Before	After	Before	After	Before	After	Before	After
Erect blood pressures (mm Hg)								
Systolic	169.0	154.3†	170.2	146.3‡	169.6	133.2‡§	169.6	173.6
Diastolic	116.1	104.9¶	115.9	106.0¶	115.8	94.8‡**††	115.8	117.0
Mean	133.7	121.4†	134.0	119.4†	133.7	107.6‡**§	133.7	135.9
Supine blood pressures (mm Hg)								
Systolic	177.0	167.4	177.3	152.7‡	177.4	145.3‡§	177.4	181.1
Diastolic	111.3	104.8	110.6	101.1¶	110.4	95.9‡††	110.4	112.0
Mean	133.2	125.7	132.8	118.3†	132.7	112.4‡§	132.7	133.4

*Reproduced, with permission, from McMahon FG: Efficacy of an antihypertensive agent: Comparison of methyldopa and hydrochlorothiazide in combination and singly. JAMA 231:155, 1975. Copyright © American Medical Association.
†Significantly less than corresponding mean placebo values ($P < .01$).
‡Significantly less than corresponding mean placebo values ($P < .001$).
§Significantly less than corresponding mean methyldopa values ($P < .01$).
¶Significantly less than corresponding mean placebo values ($P < .05$).
**Significantly less than corresponding mean hydrochlorothiazide values ($P < .05$).
††Significantly less than corresponding mean methyldopa values ($P < .05$).

glomerular filtration rate is reduced by about 15 ml/min, renal blood flow is reduced by about 20 ml/min, and the plasma renin activity doubles or triples.

Reserpine

Reserpine can be given orally, intramuscularly, or intravenously. It inhibits sympathetic nervous transmission by depleting the peripheral nerve endings of norepinephrine as well as by depleting the central stores in the cardiovascular centers in the medulla. Because of its central action, its main side-effects are lethargy, fatigue, and, especially with larger doses, nightmares and depression. If depression is severe and the patient is suicidal, however, an alternative drug to reserpine should be employed. The last is rare when the daily dose does not exceed 0.1–0.2 mg/day. When combined with the oral diuretics or with hydralazine, it is an effective hypotensive agent. Another unpleasant side-effect is stuffy nose, which is difficult to control although nose drops may be helpful. (Avoid those that are strong vasoconstrictors.) Reserpine increases gastric acidity, but this is rarely significant with the small oral doses that are used, and peptic ulcer is rare. A reported association between the use of reserpine and carcinoma of the breast in women was not confirmed by later investigations, and the FDA did not remove reserpine from the market as was briefly expected. Intramuscular or intravenous reserpine is reserved for hypertensive emergencies when the pressure must be reduced within hours, and therapy is most effective when combined with hydralazine in acute glomerulonephritis. Reserpine may cause somnolence and thus is not the drug of choice in patients with hypertensive encephalopathy or cerebral symptoms, because the action of the drug makes interpretation of the patient's progress more difficult. Nevertheless, it is a valuable drug and has the advantage of not requiring minute-to-minute titration as do some of the other parenteral agents (see below).

Methyldopa

Methyldopa can be given orally, intramuscularly, or intravenously. The magnitude of the effect of methyldopa alone and with diuretics is discussed above under Diuretics and illustrated in Table 9–36.

Methyldopa acts by interfering with sympathetic transmission by a central action. To a much lesser degree, it acts by replacing norepinephrine in the granules at the peripheral nerve endings with one of its metabolites, α-methylnorepinephrine, which is then released upon nerve stimulation instead of norepinephrine. Because α-methylnorepinephrine is a weaker vasoconstrictor than norepinephrine, the blood pressure is lowered. The central action is responsible for its major side-effects of drowsiness and fatigue, so that individuals whose work involves mental activity may find the drug unsatisfactory (Table 9–37). Systemic vascular resistance is decreased with time, but cardiac output and renal blood flow are not affected; thus, the drug is valuable in the presence of impaired renal function.

Methyldopa is considered by many nephrologists to be the one drug of choice when hypertension complicates renal dialysis or renal failure. It decreases renin secretion and does not interfere with tests of the renin-angiotensin-aldosterone system, which is an advantage when investigators are reluctant to stop all antihypertensive therapy to determine the status of the renin-angiotensin system. Raised renin production that follows hypovolemia with oral diuretics can be neutralized by the use of methyldopa. The drug may cause fever (infrequently), a direct positive Coombs test, hemolytic anemia (rarely), hepatitis with jaundice (rarely), and impotence—the commonest cause of pa-

Table 9–37. Side-effects of antihypertensive treatment with methyldopa in 100 cases.*

	No. of Cases
Temporary drowsiness	22
Persistent listlessness	19
Dryness of mouth and nasal congestion	16
Edema	10
Dizziness (nonpostural)	9
Nausea	8
Postural hypotension	7
Diarrhea	4
Nightmares	4
Depression	4
Muscular weakness	2
Impotence	2
Miscellaneous†	4
Nil	28

*Reproduced, with permission, from Johnson P & others: Treatment of hypertension with methyldopa. Br Med J 1:133, 1966.

†Includes one each of paresthesia, shivering attacks, malaise, and headaches.

tient noncompliance with treatment. All of these adverse effects are reversible when the drug is stopped.

Methyldopa can be used intramuscularly or intravenously in severe hypertension, when hours or 1–2 days are sufficient to achieve satisfactory lowering of the pressure without the necessity for minute-to-minute monitoring. It is not as effective as some of the other parenteral agents (see below) but is a valuable adjunct in severe but not accelerated or malignant hypertension.

Table 9–38. Adverse reactions to propranolol among 25 patients.*

Life-threatening reactions	
Bradycardia and shock	3
Pulmonary edema	3
Complete heart block	1
Bradycardia and angina	1
Total	8
Non-life-threatening reactions	
Asymptomatic bradycardia	5
Neurologic disturbances	4
Hypotension and syncope	3
Asymptomatic hypotension	2
2:1 heart block	1
Fluid retention	1
Epigastric pain	1
Total	17
Total with adverse reactions	25

*Reproduced, with permission, from Greenblatt DJ, Koch-Weser J: Adverse reactions to propranolol in hospitalized medical patients: A report from the Boston Collaborative Drug Surveillance Program. Am Heart J 86:478, 1973.

Propranolol

This beta-adrenergic blocking agent acts in part through its beta-blocking activities but also by decreasing renin release and by a quinidinelike action. The last 2 effects usually occur with larger doses, after beta blockade has already been achieved. Because of the effect of propranolol in decreasing renin release and plasma renin, it has been recommended particularly for patients with hypertension who have high peripheral plasma renin. Because propranolol neutralizes the reflex tachycardia and increase in cardiac output that follow vasodilator drugs, it is particularly effective when combined with diuretic and vasodilator drugs (Fig 9–36). It rarely may mask the tachycardia and sweating and other warning signs of hypoglycemia in diabetics receiving insulin, especially while they are fasting. Suitable precautions should be taken. Propranolol may cause Raynaud's phenomenon in cold weather, bradycardia, asthma, left ventricular failure, and occasionally central nervous system symptoms. Table 9–38 lists adverse reactions to propranolol.

The absorption of propranolol from the gastrointestinal tract is highly variable, ranging from 10–80%. The plasma half-life is 4–5 hours. Therapeutic plasma levels are usually achieved with 160 mg/day, but there is marked variation among patients. Following administration of propranolol, there is a rapid fall of plasma renin but a relatively slow fall in blood pressure, with no time relationship between the two. Furthermore, there has been no correlation between the efficacy of particular beta-blockers in lowering plasma renin and their effect on blood pressure, thus

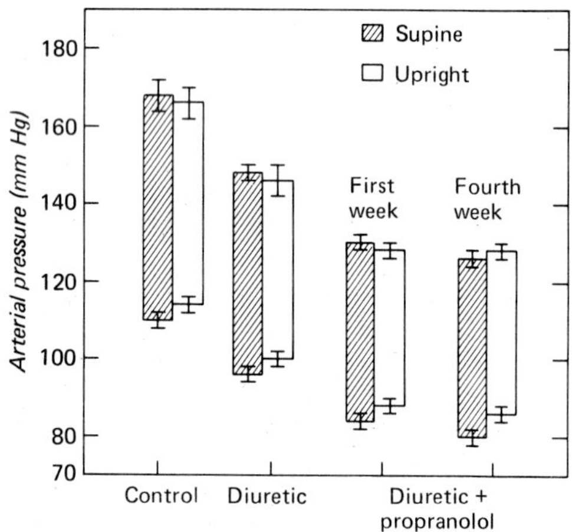

Figure 9–36. Time course of the fall in pressure and the magnitude of the hypotensive effect with addition of propranolol in 20 diuretic-treated patients with essential hypertension. Each paired column represents weekly averages of blood pressures with subjects supine and upright, measured at home twice daily (expressed as mean ± SE). Values attained with addition of propranolol are significantly different ($P < 0.001$) from control levels and from those during diuretic therapy alone. (Reproduced, with permission, from Bravo EL, Tarazi RC, Dustan HP: β-Adrenergic blockade in diuretic-treated patients with essential hypertension. N Engl J Med 292:66, 1975.)

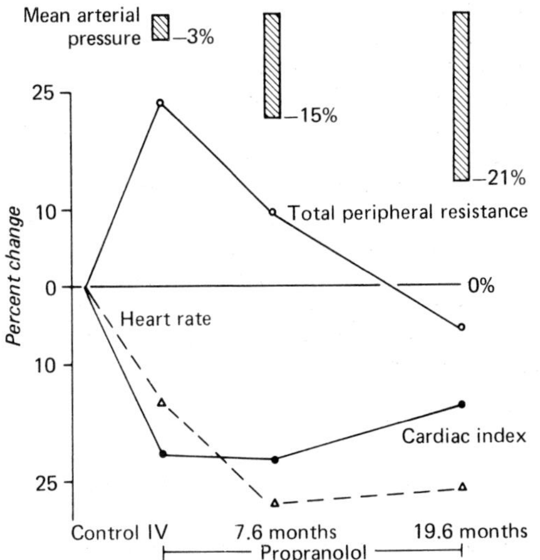

Figure 9–37. Sequential changes with intravenous and long-term (7.6 and 19.6 months) propranolol therapy in 10 hypertensive patients; changes in cardiac index, total peripheral resistance, and heart rate as well as reduction of mean arterial pressure are all expressed as percent of value before treatment. (Adapted and reproduced, with permission, from Tarazi RC, Dustan HP: β-Adrenergic blockade in hypertension: Practical and theoretical implications of long-term hemodynamic variations. Am J Cardiol 29:633, 1972.)

throwing doubt on the concept that propranolol reduces hypertension by decreasing renin release, despite the fact that propranolol does, in fact, reduce plasma renin. Propranolol has a progressive action that may increase over a period of months. Its reduction of cardiac index, heart rate, and mean blood pressure is illustrated in Fig 9–37.

Because propranolol alone in the usual doses of 80–160 mg/day orally has only a slight antihypertensive effect, preliminary results suggest that combining propranolol with dibenzyline is more effective than propranolol alone because dibenzyline reverses the unopposed alpha-adrenergic receptor-mediated systemic vasoconstriction. Combined alpha and beta blockade is therefore valuable when the latter is ineffective. Dibenzyline is given initially in doses of 10–20 mg/day and increased by small increments every 2 weeks up to about 50 mg/day divided into 2–4 doses. Propranolol is also titrated, beginning with 10–20 mg every 4 hours up to 160–320 mg/day. The major side-effects of dibenzyline are dryness of the mouth, nasal stuffiness, dizziness, and fatigue. Tachycardia results when dibenzyline is given alone, so it has not been successful except when counteracting beta-blockers have been added.

Hydralazine

Hydralazine can be used orally, intramuscularly, or intravenously and acts directly on the smooth muscle of the arteriole, decreasing its contractility and thus decreasing systemic vascular resistance. The vasodilator effect with fall in pressure stimulates the baroreceptors to reflexly increase sympathetic discharge, with resulting tachycardia and raised cardiac output, which may cause side-effects of palpitations, angina pectoris, and headache. These side-effects can be prevented when propranolol is given first or, less effectively, when reserpine, methyldopa, or guanethidine is used. Hydralazine fell out of favor in the early days of its use when it was given as the sole agent in doses of 600–800 mg/day; side-effects were prominent, including a syndrome of arthritis, fever, positive LE cell preparations, and antinuclear antibody in the serum. These lupus erythematosus-like findings were usually temporary and only occurred with large doses. They rarely occur today with doses of 200 mg/day or less, and hydralazine was part of the combination of drugs that was so beneficial in the VA Study (Tables 9–29 and 9–30) (VA Study, 1970). Hydralazine can be used intramuscularly when a fall in blood pressure within 20–40 minutes is desired, especially when combined with parenteral reserpine in acute nephritis in children. It can also be given intermittently by injection to keep the pressure under control in severe hypertension until combined oral drug therapy has become effective.

Guanethidine

Guanethidine is a potent agent that produces selective sympathetic blockade and inhibits transmission of adrenergic stimuli across peripheral nerve endings by impairing the release, and possibly the storage, of norepinephrine. Because it does not cross the blood-brain barrier, central nervous system symptoms such as occur with reserpine, methyldopa, and clonidine do not occur. It increases renin production. Its major side-effects are postural and exercise hypotension, diarrhea, and retrograde ejaculation into the bladder (Table 9–39). Postural hypotension results from interruption of the normal reflex autonomic vasoconstriction that occurs on standing, causing a fall in blood pressure; decreased venous return and cardiac

Table 9–39. Guanethidine: Side-effects in 70 cases.*

Symptoms	Number of Cases	Percent
Orthostatic symptoms	48	70
Diarrhea	43	61
Muscle weakness	28	40
Nasal congestion	24	34
Headache	21	30
Frequency of micturition	21	30
Dyspnea	13	18
Constriction in chest	10	14
Paresthesia	6	9
Tinnitus	6	9
Sweating	5	7
Sexual difficulties	4	6
Sciatica	4	6

*Reproduced, with permission, from Turner RWD: Choice of drug in the treatment of hypertension. Proc R Soc Med 55:280, 1962.

output are due to unopposed parasympathetic action. The effectiveness of the drug should be determined with the patient in the standing position, especially after exercise, to avoid the syndrome of elevated pressures in the doctor's office and symptoms of fainting at home in the morning. The diarrhea can be distressing and is helped by small doses of ganglionic blocking agents such as mecamylamine or by cholinergic blocking drugs. Because of its potency, guanethidine is used when other combinations of agents have given unsatisfactory control of blood pressure. It is not often used by itself because of the resulting increased blood volume; its effectiveness is enhanced by combination with oral diuretics (Fig 9–38).

An unsatisfactory aspect of guanethidine therapy is its half-life of 5 days, the 3- to 5-day delay in the onset of its therapeutic effect, and the delay in subsidence of its hypotensive effect if too large a dose is given. On the other hand, its long duration of action allows the drug to be used once daily, which is helpful in securing patient compliance. The dose of the drug can be changed every 1–2 weeks. Tricyclic antidepressants and chlorpromazine compete with guanethidine for neuronal uptake and so diminish the hypotensive effect of guanethidine, which can be a serious clinical disadvantage (Fig 9–39).

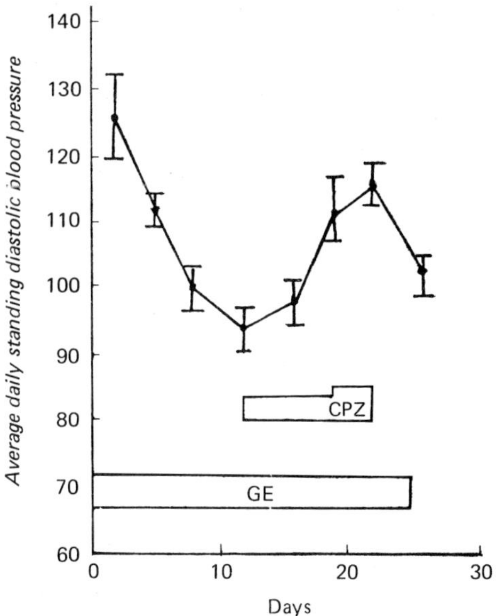

Figure 9–39. Antagonism by chlorpromazine of the hypotensive properties of guanethidine. Each point represents a mean ± SEM over a period of days. GE, guanethidine in mg/day; CPZ, chlorpromazine in mg/day. (Reproduced, with permission, from Fann WE & others: Chlorpromazine reversal of the antihypertensive action of guanethidine. Lancet 2:436, 1971.)

Clonidine

Clonidine acts by stimulating the alpha-adrenergic receptors in the medulla, decreasing sympathetic discharge to the arterioles, and lowering the blood pressure by decreasing systemic vascular resistance. The drug crosses the blood-brain barrier, and patients may have fatigue and lethargy and also complain of dry mouth and hypotension. The drug also decreases renin release from the kidney, suggesting that the activation of an alpha-adrenergic receptor is also occurring in the kidney and perhaps other peripheral sites. More than other antihypertensive compounds, it appears to cause a rebound vasoconstriction with hypertensive crises if it is stopped abruptly, so that patients must be warned against this eventuality. If the drug is to be stopped, it should be withdrawn gradually over a period of 3–5 days.

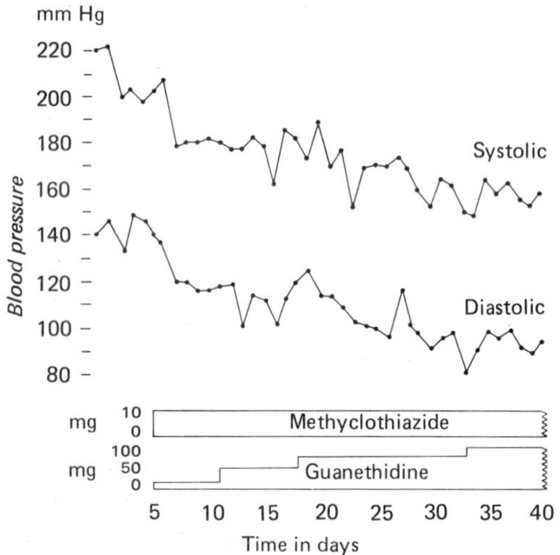

Figure 9–38. Daily averages of home blood pressure recordings of a 43-year-old man with severe uncomplicated group 2 hypertension. Because the pretreatment diastolic pressure was in the range of 130–150 mm Hg, treatment was started with methyclothiazide and guanethidine simultaneously. The dosage of guanethidine was increased gradually until the desired response was obtained. Blood pressure in the sitting position is shown; the standing pressure was considerably lower. This regimen continued to be effective after 8 months. (Reproduced, with permission, from Fairbairn JF II & others: Newer treatment of hypertension. Postgrad Med 34:546, Dec 1963.)

Minoxidil

Minoxidil is a potent oral agent that is not yet approved by the FDA but which, because of its potency and effectiveness in the presence of impaired renal function, should soon be approved. It acts as a pure vasodilator, decreasing smooth muscle contractility of the arterioles and hence systemic vascular resistance. In common with other potent vasodilators, it causes reflex tachycardia and increased cardiac output, which then cause palpitations, headache, and angina. It also produces sodium retention. For all of these reasons, diuretics and propranolol are used whenever minoxidil is prescribed. Table 9–40 describes the adverse effects of vasodilators. About half of patients receiving minoxidil over a period of weeks develop hirsutism, which is particularly disturbing to women. Vigorous use of

Table 9–40. Adverse effects with vasodilators.*

Common to all
(1) Reflex tachycardia, increased cardiac output
(2) Angina, palpitations
(3) Increased renin
(4) Contraindicated in dissecting aneurysm
(5) Sodium and water retention
Hydralazine
(1) Drug-induced lupus erythematosus
Diazoxide
(1) Local burning
(2) Hyperglycemia
(3) Nausea and vomiting

*Reproduced, with permission, from Nies AS: Adverse reactions and interactions limiting the use of antihypertensive drugs. Am J Med 58:495, 1975.

minoxidil in combination with large doses of furosemide and propranolol has proved very effective in the treatment of severe hypertension, especially in the presence of renal failure, and when patients have failed to respond adequately to conventional antihypertensive medication. A typical chart showing the striking benefit of the addition of minoxidil to the regimen of a patient whose blood pressure was poorly controlled despite a combination of hydrochlorothiazide, methyldopa, propranolol, and hydralazine is shown in Fig

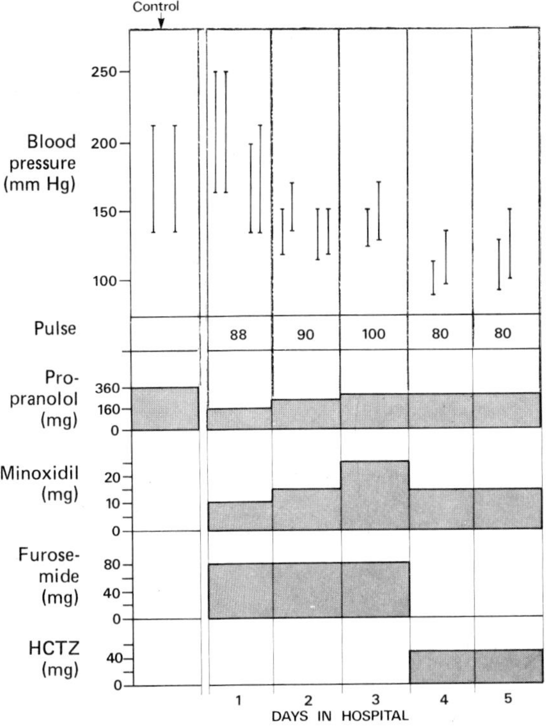

Figure 9–40. Successful treatment of hypertension with minoxidil following unsuccessful prehospital treatment with combined hydrochlorothiazide (HCTZ), methyldopa, propranolol, and hydralazine. (Courtesy of JA McChesney.)

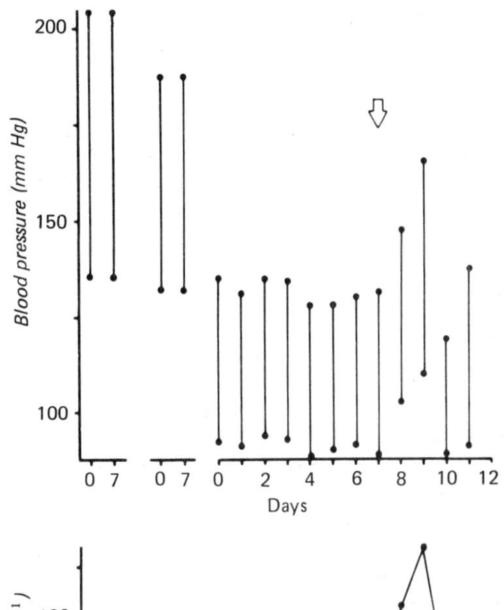

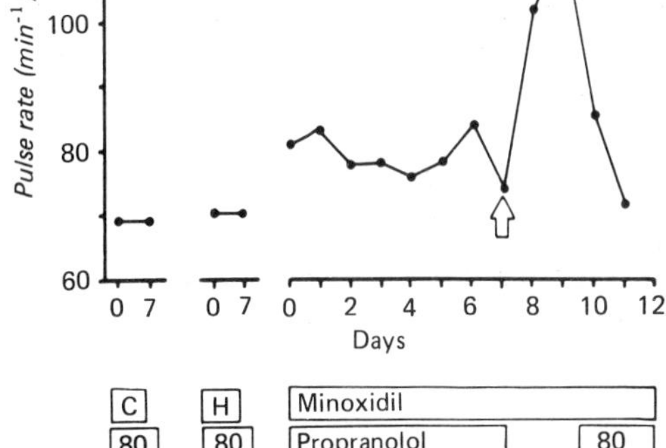

Figure 9–41. Blood pressure and heart rate data are summarized from one patient during the control period (C), the hydralazine period (H), and the minoxidil period. The effect of withdrawing propranolol (arrows) is shown by the increase in blood pressure and heart rate. HCTZ, hydrochlorothiazide. (Reproduced, with permission of the American Heart Association, Inc., from Gottlieb TB, Katz FH, Chidsey CA III: Combined therapy with vasodilator drugs and beta-adrenergic blockage in hypertension. Circulation 45:571, 1972.)

9–40. Fig 9–41 shows the dramatic effect of the addition of minoxidil to the medications of a patient receiving hydrochlorothiazide, propranolol, and hydralazine and the rapid increase in pulse rate when propranolol was stopped. As with other vasodilators, therefore, propranolol should be added to the regimen when potent drugs such as minoxidil are used to prevent the subsequent reflex tachycardia. Another reason for adding propranolol is to reverse the increase of plasma renin activity that follows the use of minoxidil.

Peak plasma levels occur rapidly within an hour after an oral dose, and the serum half-life, although said to be only 4 hours, allows a longer duration of action because the drug is bound in the vascular wall.

Prazosin (Minipress)

Prazosin is a moderately effective vasodilator recently approved by the FDA. It acts predominantly as a smooth muscle relaxing agent and does not block alpha-adrenergic receptors. It is supplied as 1 mg capsules for oral administration. The plasma concentration reaches a peak in about 3 hours, and the plasma half-life is 2–3 hours. Experience with the drug is limited, but it has approximately the same potency as methyldopa or hydralazine plus the advantage of not increasing the cardiac output or plasma renin or decreasing the renal blood flow or glomerular filtration rate. The precise place of prazosin in the management of hypertension will depend upon the results of further trials. It may cause postural hypotension and collapse; the initial dose should be small, such as 0.5–1.0 mg at bedtime, gradually increased to tolerance depending upon the response of the patient. Plasma volume is increased, and fluid retention may occur; so the drug should be used in combination with a diuretic.

Diazoxide

Diazoxide is a recently approved parenteral vasodilator that acts directly on the smooth muscle of the arterioles. When given in a bolus intravenously, it lowers the blood pressure within minutes and lowers systemic vascular resistance about 25%, and the fall in pressure persists for many hours (Fig 9–42). The hemodynamic effects also include an increase in heart rate of about 30 beats/min, increased cardiac index of 30–40%, and an increase in the left ventricular ejection rate of about 15%. Hypotension occurs infrequently, but if the situation is less urgent one can use a smaller dose such as 75 mg instead of 300 mg and repeat the dose at intervals of 5–10 minutes until the desired antihypertensive effect is achieved. If diazoxide is used repeatedly, intravenous furosemide should be added to combat sodium and water retention.

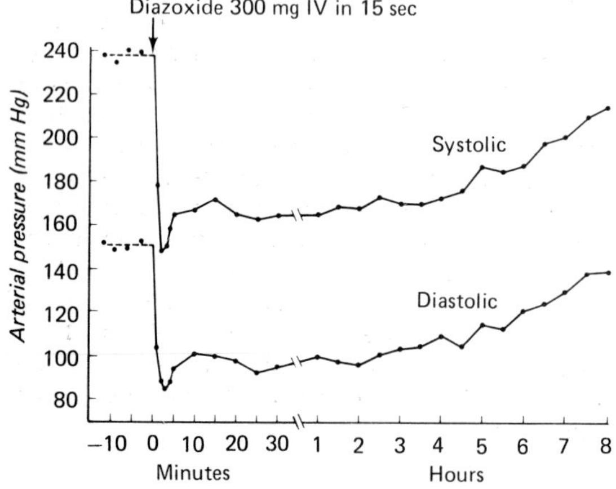

Figure 9–42. Time course of antihypertensive action of diazoxide in a patient with accelerated primary hypertension. (Reproduced, with permission, from Koch-Weser J: Drug therapy: Diazoxide. N Engl J Med 294:1271, 1976.)

Diazoxide is valuable in hypertensive emergencies because of its effectiveness, because of its rapid onset and long duration of action, and because monitoring usually is required only for the first 15 or 20 minutes to make certain that excess hypotension has not occurred. Like hydralazine, it can be given intermittently in severe hypertension when potent oral therapy is being titrated. The major side-effect, other than the possibility of excess hypotension, is hyperglycemia, and, like other vasodilators, including hydralazine and minoxidil, it increases renin secretion. Despite this fact, all of the antihypertensive agents that increase renin secretion reverse the complications of hypertension, and increased renin production should not be considered a contraindication to the use of the drug. In some parts of the world, diazoxide is used orally in large doses with good effect on the blood pressure, but hyperglycemia prevents its continued use. It may be used for short periods to bring the pressure under control.

Ganglionic Blocking Agents

Ganglionic blocking agents such as trimethaphan camsylate (Arfonad), hexamethonium, pentolinium, and mecamylamine (Inversine) act by competing with acetylcholine at sympathetic ganglia and by blocking both parasympathetic and sympathetic outflow. As a result, their use has been sharply curtailed and superseded by other potent parenteral agents. An exception to this is the use of trimethaphan for short periods (1–2 days) in the treatment of malignant or accelerated hypertension or aortic dissection when it is desired to bring blood pressure under control in a matter of minutes. Hemodynamic observations in severe hypertension following the use of trimethaphan camsylate show a marked fall in arterial pressure, peripheral resistance, cardiac index, and left ventricular ejection rate, but a rise in heart rate (Bhatia, 1973). Unlike nitroprusside sodium, it acts in minutes rather than seconds. The drug should be given by continuous intravenous infusion under close monitoring in the coronary care or intensive care unit with the patient in the sitting position so that if excess hypotension occurs the patient can lie down to counteract the hypotension.

Nitroprusside Sodium

This potent vasodilator, recently approved by the FDA, is used almost exclusively in acute hypertensive emergencies or in acute cardiac failure with abnormal or elevated blood pressure. It acts directly on the smooth muscle of the arterioles and lowers the pressure within seconds. The drug is given by continuous dilute intravenous infusion by a constant infusion pump, and the dose is titrated to produce the desired effect (see Chapter 10 and Fig 10–22). As with trimethaphan, its use should be monitored by specially trained personnel to avoid excessive hypotension, which may lead to acute tubular necrosis of the kidney.

Experience with nitroprusside is still limited, but

it may prove to be the treatment of choice in acute left ventricular failure with pulmonary edema and severe hypertension because, unlike other vasodilators such as hydralazine and minoxidil, reflex tachycardia occurs much less often and to a lesser degree. Why this is so with such a potent vasodilator is unclear, but the associated venodilating effect may be the explanation.

PRACTICAL ASPECTS OF TREATMENT OF HYPERTENSION WITH SUGGESTED PROTOCOLS

As indicated in the introductory paragraphs, the physician must first determine how urgent it is to lower the blood pressure and choose accordingly oral or parenteral treatment, the drugs and doses to be initiated, the frequency with which they should be repeated, and the speed with which the blood pressure should be brought under control. The physician must also balance the beneficial response of the blood pressure to treatment against side-effects that may interfere with treatment and may require adjustment of dosage or change to a different therapeutic agent. Clinical judgment is required to decide when to be content with a moderate therapeutic response if side-effects (such as lethargy or impotence with methyldopa) are disabling or when frequent medications cause difficulties in patient compliance. The costs of medications, visits to the physician, and laboratory tests to determine the effect on potassium, glucose, uric acid, or creatinine must also be considered. Treatment is empiric. By trial and error one arrives at the drug or combination of drugs that will lower the blood pressure while interfering as little as possible with the patient's life and work. Outpatient treatment is usually not urgent, so that therapy can be started slowly, utilizing one drug in low dosage, with a gradual increase to higher dosage or to additional more potent drugs.

The object of hypotensive therapy is to lower the blood pressure to 140/90 mm Hg or below for as much of the day as possible, consistent with the patient's cooperation and the absence of disabling side-effects. With the exception of mild disease, good control is rarely achieved with a single drug. In older patients with impaired cerebral or coronary circulation in whom it is important to avoid excess hypotension or rapid changes in pressure, one should accept a diastolic pressure of 100 mm Hg if lowering the pressure produces further cerebral symptoms. In uncooperative patients with a poor compliance record, or in patients who find it difficult to take medication more than once or twice a day, the physician should accept partial control of the blood pressure if insisting on more frequent medication would cause the patient to abandon therapy altogether. The response to therapy should be determined not only by office pressure readings but by some variety of basal, home, or ambulatory recordings to obtain more representative pressures.

Steps in the Progressive Approach to Treatment of Hypertension

It is best to consider antihypertensive regimens as various steps depending upon the responses of the patient.

Step 1:

In almost all mildly to moderately hypertensive patients except those who have a history of sensitivity to diuretics or a history of repeated attacks of gout from prior thiazide therapy, or diabetics who would require a change to insulin therapy, initial therapy should be with one of the oral diuretics, either the short-acting mild diuretics (the thiazides), or the longer-acting mild diuretics (chlorthalidone or metolazone). Approximately 40% of patients with borderline or mild hypertension with diastolic pressures between 90 and 110 mm Hg will respond satisfactorily to diuretics alone. Since the need to lower the pressure is not urgent, thiazides should be begun in low dosage, such as 25–50 mg of hydrochlorothiazide once daily, the lower amount being used in patients who are elderly or are receiving digitalis or in those who have a clinical condition in which an unexpectedly large diuresis of water, sodium, and potassium would be precarious. The response to the thiazides begins to be evident within a few days, and by 2 weeks one can be fairly certain whether the dosage used is adequate. If not, it can be increased by increments of 25 mg up to a maximum single dose of 100 mg. Usually 50 mg once or twice a day is sufficient if diuretics alone are going to be effective in lowering the blood pressure. If the patient responds well to 50 mg of hydrochlorothiazide once or twice a day, for example, the dose can then be decreased to 25 mg once daily and perhaps to 25 mg every other day. The smaller doses may maintain the beneficial effects initially obtained by larger doses and decrease the urinary potassium loss. Since the average decrease in serum potassium with 50 mg of hydrochlorothiazide twice a day is about 0.6 mEq/l, the loss can often be offset by increased oral intake of potassium with potassium-rich foods such as fruits and vegetables (see Table 9–35); or, if the serum potassium falls below 3.5 mEq/l and if the patient has symptoms from the hypokalemia, the physician can prescribe oral potassium supplements of at least 60 mEq/day in the absence of renal failure. Liquid potassium preparations are preferred but are sometimes poorly tolerated. One can use the matrix potassium Slow-K (Ciba); enteric-coated potassium tablets should not be used because of the frequency of ulcerations in the small bowel. If a month of oral diuretics does not lower the blood pressure to the desired level, one can then proceed to step 2 in treatment.

Step 2:

A variety of drugs are available that can be added to the thiazides. The second drug can be propranolol, methyldopa, reserpine, clonidine, prazosin, or hydralazine—each has its supporters. The choice often depends on the familiarity of the physician with the various drugs, but there are situations in which one drug or another drug is particularly desirable.

Propranolol is considered by many to be the best second drug because it not only effectively lowers the blood pressure but also decreases the plasma renin, the pulse rate, and the likelihood of arrhythmias or angina if the patient is receiving vasodilators or has concomitant coronary heart disease. However, propranolol cannot be used if the patient has a history of asthma, incipient left ventricular failure, bradycardia, ventricular conduction defects, or a history of Raynaud's phenomenon.

Propranolol should be begun in low dosage—10–20 mg once or twice a day—primarily to determine if any adverse effects will occur with its use. Propranolol may induce an attack of asthma or pulmonary edema; may cause bradycardia; may mask hypoglycemia in a diabetic patient taking insulin; and may produce central nervous system symptoms with excitement. Although the usual prescription calls for the drug to be taken 4 times daily, since the half-life is short (a matter of hours), the biologic effect may be more persistent. Many patients respond satisfactorily to twice-daily dosage. Infrequently, it is necessary to give more than 320 mg/day; however, some authors have prescribed 800–1000 mg/day in patients who fail to respond to the lower dosage. Propranolol is the only beta-receptor blocking agent that is approved by the FDA, but a variety of other beta-blocking drugs, some of which are cardio-selective and do not produce bronchial constriction, are used elsewhere in the world. Future research will determine whether these other compounds are more effective; particularly promising from initial reports are timolol and atenolol.

Methyldopa is moderately effective, but it produces lethargy and decreased mental acuity as well as impotence in men. There are very few data regarding the effect of methyldopa on sexual function in women. It is important to obtain accurate information regarding sexual function and activity in men prior to institution of therapy, because impotence, as well as other side-effects, may occur with placebo medication and may not be due to the antihypertensive drug. An accurate history prior to starting therapy is helpful in interpreting the possible role of antihypertensive drugs in causing symptoms. Patients who require a high order of mental alertness at their jobs or patients in whom lethargy is a particularly unpleasant effect do poorly with methyldopa. On the other hand, if the patient is hyperactive, the sedative action of methyldopa is often beneficial. Postural hypotension is usually not too prominent with methyldopa, but it may be so in some cases. Methyldopa is begun in a dose of 250 mg once or twice daily; often this is sufficient to lower the pressure. As with propranolol, it is usually supposed to be taken 4 times daily, but patients often comply poorly with such frequent dosage, and many respond satisfactorily to 2 or 3 doses daily if they are going to respond to the drug at all. Although some patients respond to an increase of dosage to 2 g/day, this may produce more side-effects and no more benefits than 1–1.5 g/day.

Reserpine, 0.1 mg once a day, is often effective as a second drug. It has the advantage of relaxing the patient and slowing the heart rate, but the disadvantage that it may cause mental depression in susceptible individuals. Patients with a history of mental depression should not be given reserpine. The daily dose of reserpine should not exceed 0.25 mg/day and preferably not more than 0.1 mg/day. Reserpine is effective in once-daily dosage. When reserpine was discontinued because of reports of an association with carcinoma of the breast, it often took weeks to stabilize the patient equally well on methyldopa, propranolol, or even guanethidine. A combination of thiazides and reserpine is often effective, and when this is so, a total daily consumption of only 2–3 tablets is sufficient to control the hypertension.

Prazosin is a mild vasodilator that can be used if the patient is unable to take propranolol, reserpine, or methyldopa because of the side-effects mentioned above, and it can be substituted for hydralazine if this drug is ineffective or causes tachycardia (see below). It should be started in small doses, usually 0.5 mg or at most 1 mg at bedtime. A marked fall in pressure and collapse have been described when the drug is first begun. The first dose response can occur with doses of less than 2 mg, so the patient should be observed closely for this event. The patient is titrated with progressively increasing doses, as with all antihypertensive agents, and usually requires 2–5 mg 2 or 3 times daily for an effective response. Experience is still limited, so caution should be exercised until more data are available.

Clonidine is a recently approved drug that as yet has few enthusiastic supporters because it produces an unpleasantly dry mouth and lethargy. It can be started with 0.1 mg and increased to 0.2–0.4 mg 2 or 3 times a day, depending upon the response.

Hydralazine is an effective antihypertensive agent, especially when combined with propranolol, which neutralizes the headache and tachycardia that often follow the vasodilating action of hydralazine used alone. If propranolol, methyldopa, or reserpine is not used first, and hydralazine is used alone in full doses, patients often complain of severe headache and tachycardia, and if they have coronary heart disease they may develop angina pectoris. Reserpine and methyldopa are not as effective as propranolol in preventing the reflex tachycardia and palpitations, but they should be considered effective substitutes. In the VA Study (1967, 1970), a combination of thiazide, reserpine, and hydralazine showed convincing benefit to patients whose average diastolic pressure was 105 mm Hg or more.

Hydralazine has a plasma half-life of only a few hours, but its biologic action is longer because the drug becomes bound to smooth muscle of the blood vessels; twice-daily dosage is usually effective. It is begun with

10–25 mg once or twice a day, gradually increased at weekly intervals to 100 mg twice daily. Two hundred mg/day is usually the maximum dose that is used because larger doses are associated with a lupus erythematosus-like syndrome with arthritis and a positive serum LE preparation. Hydralazine is metabolized by acetylation; the rate of acetylation is genetically determined, and patients vary in the rate of inactivation of the drug, with the rapid ones having a lower plasma concentration. Another reason for rarely exceeding 100 mg/dose is that hemodynamic studies in patients with chronic cardiac failure have shown that 50–75 mg of hydralazine effectively increases the cardiac output; therefore, this size dose is hemodynamically effective. A dose of 5–10 mg of hydralazine intramuscularly is effective in acute glomerulonephritis and in severe hypertension.

Step 3: Guanethidine

If the combination of drugs listed above fails to reduce the blood pressure to a satisfactory level, or if side-effects prevent their effective use, guanethidine may be introduced. Guanethidine is a potent adrenergic blocking agent which can be used in increasing dosage but which requires close supervision because of frequent side-effects. Postural hypotension is greater with guanethidine than with any of the other drugs. The patient may have the unpleasant experience of marked postural hypotension in the morning after he is vasodilated from being warm in bed, yet in the afternoon and evening have a blood pressure that is high and out of control. Guanethidine also produces unpredictable diarrhea, retrograde ejaculation into the bladder, and dizziness on exertion, especially in the morning. The postural hypotension and dizziness after exertion are not rapidly relieved by rest, especially if the exercise has been vigorous. Guanethidine is a very potent drug and has proved beneficial in many patients. It is begun in a dose of 10–20 mg orally which can be adjusted at weekly intervals because of its long half-life. This is convenient for outpatient therapy but is a disadvantage if overdosage occurs, because it takes 3–5 days for the drug effect to be eliminated when the drug is stopped. If guanethidine is used, reserpine and methyldopa usually add nothing to the therapeutic protocol except in unusual circumstances, because they all are adrenergic-depleting agents. However, diuretic therapy is a useful and important additive to guanethidine. It counteracts the sodium retention and allows a smaller daily dose of guanethidine.

Step 4: Minoxidil

At present this is an experimental drug not yet approved by the FDA. It is the most potent vasodilator and may reduce the blood pressure strikingly when all of the conventional drugs mentioned above fail to do so (Fig 9–40 and 9–41). It has the adverse effects shared by all vasodilator drugs, and in addition has the unusual side-effect of hirsutism which limits its use in females. The drug is an extremely useful addition to the oral therapeutic protocol in severe hypertension, especially if there is beginning impairment of renal function. Minoxidil is begun in small dosage of 2.5–5 mg/day and may be given 2–3 times daily with gradually increasing titration to a maximum dosage of 20 mg/day. As seen in Fig 9–40, 10 mg/day lowered the diastolic blood pressure in a patient from 150 mm Hg to 115 mm Hg; 20 mg of minoxidil lowered the diastolic pressure to close to normal from a pretreatment value which persisted at 150 mm Hg despite full conventional therapy.

Step 5:

About 90–95% of all patients with mild to moderately severe hypertension will be controlled by the drugs listed above. If the blood pressure is not controlled, one should suspect that the patient is not taking the medication, that the malignant phase has supervened, or that a new process such as pyelonephritis has occurred. A patient with renal impairment, cardiac failure, or hypertensive encephalopathy should be hospitalized. This removes the patient from the surrounding social and work environment, which may be contributing pressor influences interfering with the antihypertensive drugs, and also allows close monitoring of treatment of the blood pressure and, if necessary, the use of parenteral medication. Patients who have failed to respond to the full therapeutic regimen listed above, as well as patients who have acute hypertensive encephalopathy, malignant hypertension, acute pulmonary edema or severe cardiac failure, aortic dissection, hemorrhagic stroke with a markedly raised blood pressure, or episodic rises in pressure suggesting pheochromocytoma, should be hospitalized and given parenteral therapy (see Table 9–32).

TREATMENT OF MALIGNANT HYPERTENSION: COMPLICATIONS & EMERGENCIES

The hallmark of malignant hypertension, as noted earlier, is papilledema; after the patient is hospitalized, the blood pressure should be lowered within hours or days depending upon the physician's estimate of the urgency of the clinical situation. Some patients with malignant hypertension are critically ill, with diastolic pressures exceeding 150 mm Hg; their blood pressure should be lowered within hours. Other patients, early in the course of the malignant phase, may have much less commanding symptoms; therapy can then be given orally or parenterally but intermittently, with the objective of lowering the pressure within a few days.

The importance of prompt reduction of the pressure in patients with malignant hypertension is shown

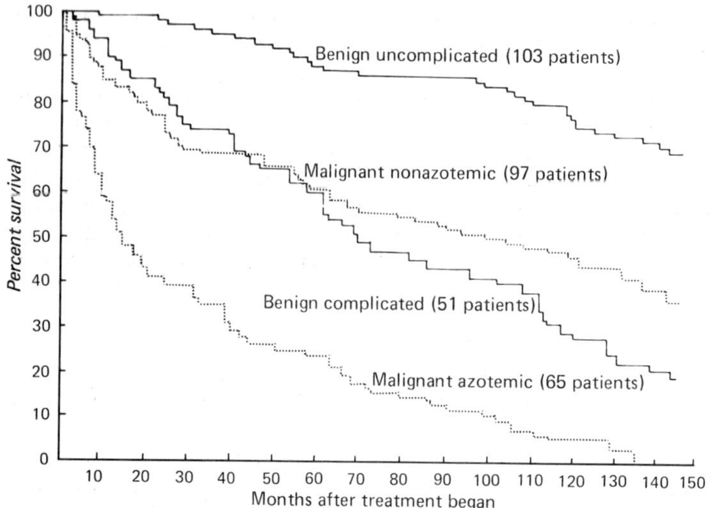

Figure 9–43. Percentage of surviving patients in each group for every month after inception of therapy. (Reproduced, with permission of the American Heart Association, Inc., from Perry HM Jr & others: Studies on the control of hypertension. 8. Mortality, morbidity, and remission during 12 years of intensive therapy. Circulation 33:958, 1966.)

in Fig 9–43. Not only do the data demonstrate the great improvement in survival of patients with malignant hypertension given modern therapy (40% survival after 10 years, as compared to nil in the days before treatment was available), but they show that the improved survival occurs only in the cases of nonazotemic malignant hypertension in which the blood pressure is lowered before renal failure occurs. In patients with malignant hypertension in whom renal failure and azotemia were present when the patient was first treated, the 10-year survival was nil, although the 5-year survival was still 20%, in contrast to the average survival of 8 months in the days before modern therapy was possible. Dialysis treatment will probably improve the figures. One of our early cases, treated in 1951, is shown in Fig 9–44. This young man presented with severe headache uncontrolled by morphine, inability to read the headlines of the newspaper, marked vomiting associated with papilledema, and a diastolic pressure of 150 mm Hg. He failed to respond to symptomatic therapy in the hospital. He was then given hexamethonium subcutaneously in increasing doses, which lowered his blood pressure. The decrease in his headache, vomiting, and visual symptoms was dramatic and occurred in a matter of days. Papilledema, hemorrhages, and exudates disappeared within weeks, and he was seen in 1976 after a follow-up of 25 years with a normal blood pressure and normal renal function without antihypertensive therapy. This long remission is unique in our experience and was one of the early demonstrations of the importance of lowering blood pressure in malignant hypertension.

It should be appreciated that when the more potent drugs such as nitroprusside sodium and diazoxide are used, the blood pressure may be lowered in a matter of seconds or minutes, but the hazard of over-

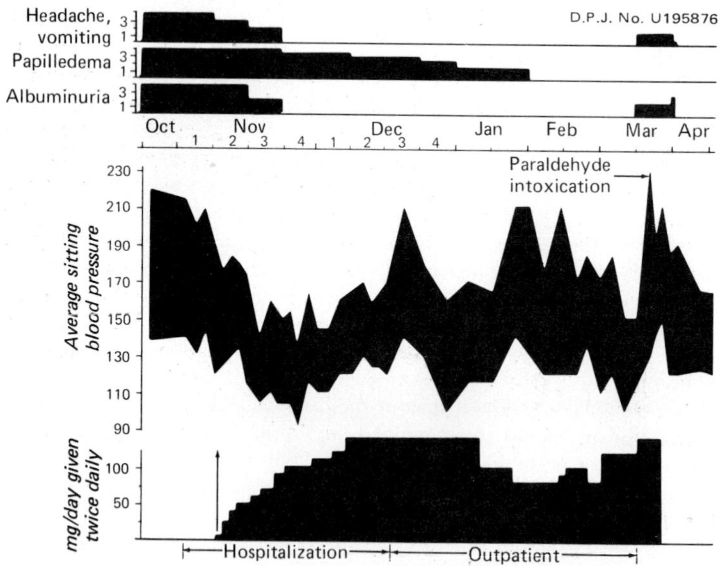

Figure 9–44. Essential hypertension with papilledema in a 23-year-old man. Hexamethonium treatment of malignant hypertension, 1951. (Reproduced, with permission, from Sokolow M, Schottstaedt MF: The management of malignant hypertension. Ann Intern Med 38:647, 1953.)

stepping the mark and producing severe hypotension is also greater. Drugs that can be used in malignant hypertension and other hypertensive emergencies are listed in Table 9–32 along with route of administration, initial dose, time of onset, and duration of action. Which of the drugs a physician uses depends upon the individual's own experience and the availability of second-to-second surveillance, as is necessary with infusions of nitroprusside sodium or trimethaphan. Both of these drugs should be given under the closest supervision, so that the patient can be placed in the recumbent position if hypotension develops. The rate of infusion must be carefully titrated to avoid excessive hypotension and should be decreased as soon as possible after the blood pressure falls. One can then give intermittent intramuscular hydralazine or bolus injections of diazoxide. As soon as practicable, oral therapy should be given. If the clinical care facilities do not permit careful, moment-to-moment titration of the infusion in a coronary care or intensive care unit, it is safer to give boluses of diazoxide, 75–300 mg rapidly intravenously, which lowers the pressure in minutes but may last for hours. If the situation is less urgent, 5–20 mg hydralazine intramuscularly or 1–5 mg reserpine intramuscularly or intravenously can also be given intermittently and does not require as close supervision. Intramuscular hydralazine acts in 15–30 minutes and may persist for hours. Reserpine acts more slowly and may take several hours to lower blood pressure. As with all parenteral antihypertensive drugs, hypotension may occur. For this reason, 1 mg rather than the previously recommended 2.5–5 mg is advised as the initial dose. Reserpine has the disadvantage of producing drowsiness and makes interpretation of cerebral symptoms more difficult. Methyldopa, 250–500 mg, can be given intramuscularly or intravenously, but this drug also takes 2–6 hours before its effect becomes obvious; and although it is effective in some patients, it may not lower the pressure in severe hypertensive emergencies.

In dissecting aorta, hemorrhagic stroke with high arterial pressure, and severe acute left ventricular failure, either sodium nitroprusside or trimethaphan is the drug of choice at the beginning, after which potent oral drugs can be substituted.

One should not lower the pressure to normal immediately because this may produce neurologic deficit or oliguria; it is wiser to give smaller doses to lower the diastolic pressure to about 120 mm Hg and observe whether this pressure is tolerated without neurologic symptoms or evidence of decreased cardiac output with oliguria. The therapy can then be continued or increased to lower the pressure to 110 mm Hg diastolic for a day or 2 before gradually bringing it down to 100 mm Hg. It should be reemphasized that the great potency of the parenteral drugs is a distinct hazard. One should start with the smallest possible dose and increase the rate of infusion if needed. A modest fall in pressure is satisfactory at first; a greater fall can be achieved later after it is demonstrated that this can be tolerated without untoward symptoms.

The presence of impaired renal function should not deter the physician from lowering the pressure, although drugs such as guanethidine that decrease the cardiac output should be avoided if possible. In the presence of impaired renal function, thiazide diuretics are less effective, and furosemide should be used instead. Propranolol and either hydralazine or minoxidil are effective in the presence of impaired renal function and can be used alone or in combination after the blood pressure is brought under control with the parenteral therapy.

Renal Failure & Dialysis

If renal failure is present and the patient is receiving intermittent renal dialysis, therapy should include rigorous use of furosemide, propranolol, and minoxidil or hydralazine with intermittent injections of diazoxide if needed to lower the pressure without decreasing the renal blood flow. If the patient's serum creatinine is less than 3 or 4 mg/dl, indicating moderate renal failure, and if the patient is not on dialysis and is not oliguric, vigorous oral therapy combined with diazoxide may prevent the need for hemodialysis. If the patient is receiving hemodialysis, lowering the pressure will often gradually reduce the required frequency of hemodialysis, so that patients who were having dialysis several times a week might need it only once every few weeks to several months. Renal dysfunction is greatly aggravated by severe hypertension, and lowering the blood pressure is an essential aspect of the treatment of renal failure, utilizing renal dialysis if necessary to control blood volume until the renal interlobular and arteriolar lesions can heal.

Follow-Up Evaluation

After the blood pressure is brought under control with potent parenteral medication, the beneficial antihypertensive effect can usually be maintained with more moderate oral therapy. Once the malignant phase is reversed by antihypertensive therapy, the patient often reverts to benign hypertension and can be controlled for years with a rather modest regimen of antihypertensive drugs. The serum creatinine, which may rise modestly during the first 2–3 weeks after antihypertensive therapy is begun, gradually falls, and 6 months later it is usually lower than when the patient was first seen with malignant hypertension. The impaired renal function persists, however, although the serum creatinine and creatinine clearance may stabilize at a low or moderately high level. The inability to completely restore renal function to normal, once it has reached a certain point of impairment, is the main reason why vigorous antihypertensive therapy should be given to patients with accelerated hypertension.

FOLLOW-UP THERAPY

The patient being treated with oral therapy of mild to moderate disease as well as the patient discharged from the hospital under treatment for severe or malignant hypertension should be seen approximately once a week as an outpatient until the situation is stabilized and an acceptable therapeutic program has been achieved. The frequency of visits can gradually be decreased, but in all but the mildest cases patients should be seen at intervals of 3–6 months even after they are well controlled to be certain that they are taking their medication and that the response to therapy is maintained. Circumstances in the patient's life, acute pyelonephritis, or unknown factors may worsen the hypertension even when the patient is on therapy. The patient must be encouraged to communicate with the physician whenever new or untoward symptoms appear and should be warned frequently against stopping medication without consulting the physician because of the danger of uncontrolled hypertension as well as the rebound effect that may occur when any antihypertensive agent is abruptly stopped. It is common for patients to run out of medication, and they often do not renew the prescription because they are free of symptoms and the drugs are not inexpensive. This problem should be anticipated and prevented by full discussion with frequent reinforcements. Failure of compliance with the physician's instructions is a persistent problem that must never be overlooked if the response to therapy seems not to be adequate (see p 259). Before assuming that antihypertensive therapy is inadequate—especially if the patient has previously been well controlled on the same medication—the possibility of noncompliance should be carefully considered. In some cases hospitalization may allow a more adequate estimate of the effectiveness of treatment and has the added advantage of removing the patient from a perhaps stressful environment that may be raising the blood pressure.

At each visit, the blood pressure should be determined and the patient questioned regarding medication, life events, and the appearance of new or untoward symptoms that may suggest a change in the course of the disease. Specific search should be made for any evidence of involvement or worsening of the target organs; in particular, examination of the fundi, heart, and peripheral vessels should be made at each visit. At approximately yearly intervals, repeat ECG, renal function studies, and chest x-rays are desirable. If the patient is taking oral diuretic agents, serum potassium, uric acid, plasma glucose, and serum creatinine should be measured every year. The effect of upright posture should be noted at each visit, not only with drugs that interfere with sympathetic transmission but also with oral diuretic agents, because postural hypotension may occur if hypovolemia is excessive. If the patient is receiving spironolactone or triamterene, serum potassium should be checked more frequently, and the ECG should be repeated frequently to exclude hyperkalemia; the patient must be repeatedly admonished not to take oral potassium agents. If renal function is impaired, these potassium-sparing drugs should not be used.

THE USE OF NURSE ASSISTANTS IN LARGE CLINICS

As more and more hypertensive patients are identified and started in treatment, the load on the physician may become excessive, especially in large clinics. It appears to be well established now that nurse assistants, supervised closely by physicians, can see the routine follow-up patients who are adequately controlled. The nurse should not initiate therapy or regulate therapy in patients who have severe hypertension or those who have complications; however, once the patient is stabilized on a good program, it is possible to train nurse assistants to take an appropriate history to detect the presence of new complications, particularly transient ischemic attacks, angina pectoris, intermittent claudication, or symptoms that herald the development of left ventricular failure. The nurse assistant can be taught to examine the fundi, listen to the heart for gallop rhythm, and examine for rales in the lungs and changes in the arterial pulses. More and more reports are appearing in the literature indicating that well-trained nurse assistants are successfully fulfilling their role in the follow-up care of patients with hypertension in a clinic setting. The nurse assistant must communicate with the physician, who must always be readily available, and discuss the progress of each patient during each clinic visit.

Industrial nurses have also been used effectively in hypertension clinics in large factories. Preliminary data indicate that worker acceptance is good; that compliance may be even better than in the usual clinic; and that control of hypertension is relatively easily accomplished. It should be remembered, of course, that factory workers are generally healthy people whose hypertension is usually mild to moderate and not severe and that the union and employers have cooperated to provide free drugs, free use of union secretaries to remind patients about their appointments, and easy access to the medical facility in the plant. Expansion of this approach to the general population of patients with mild hypertension seems warranted, although problems related to the role of the private physician and possible failures in communication between the nurse assistant, the plant physician, and the private physician may cause some difficulty.

The use of nurse assistants in private practice has not been studied in sufficient detail to conclude whether this is desirable.

MANAGEMENT OF PATIENT COMPLIANCE

Studies on patients' compliance with the treatment program have shown that this is a difficult problem not entirely eliminated by free drugs, easy access to the physician, education of the patient regarding his disease, and education of the physician to fortify his understanding of the need for antihypertensive drug therapy. Frequent follow-up visits are a nuisance and an expense, take time away from work, and are often emotionally disturbing, so that patients tend to find excuses not to make or keep appointments.When patients are asked why they have not complied as urged and directed to do, common answers are, "I forgot," or "I feel all right," or "I ran out of pills and I don't like to be scolded." Perhaps more important and less well articulated is the attitude of the patient toward the physician or the clinic, especially in institutions in which physicians change frequently. In large clinics, a patient often has to wait several hours to see the physician, must then wait longer at the pharmacy to get the prescription filled or renewed, and then—all too often—has only a few minutes with the physician. Nurse assistants may help with this problem by making more time available for the patient, including a discussion of personal problems. A social worker can function in somewhat the same way by developing a relationship in which the patient feels free to discuss personal and socioeconomic problems, and clinical volunteers can often assist with the less severe or complicated cases. Every large clinic should provide some means whereby patients can get clear answers to questions about their disease, the drugs, and their concerns. If the physician does not see the patient, an experienced clinical pharmacist should make a point of doing so and discussing the mechanism of action and problems concerning drugs, including possible interactions with drugs prescribed for other disorders. The physician, of course, should supervise this process and should know, for example, that tricyclic antidepressants neutralize the effect of guanethidine because both drugs compete for the same receptor sites.

A concerned physician who makes the patient an acknowledged partner in the therapeutic enterprise will have minimal problems with patient compliance.

MANAGEMENT OF COMPLICATIONS

Complications such as cardiac failure, malignant hypertension, aortic dissection, hemorrhagic stroke or myocardial infarction, transient ischemic attacks, or cerebral infarction are discussed in appropriate sections elsewhere in this book. In general, the presence of a significant complication warrants hospitalization so that patients can be given appropriate treatment for severe hypertension. Ancillary methods of treatment should not be neglected, such as digitalis in cardiac failure, anticoagulants and surgical correction of the carotid artery lesion in transient ischemic attacks, and, if necessary, surgery in aortic dissection. Treatment of the elevated blood pressure is usually of less importance than other approaches in patients with angina pectoris, myocardial infarction, or atherosclerosis of the legs with intermittent claudication. The pressure may be high in hemorrhagic stroke and hypertensive encephalopathy with neurologic deficit; these patients should have their pressures lowered cautiously, as described under malignant hypertension.

SHOULD THERAPY BE STOPPED IF THE BLOOD PRESSURE HAS REMAINED NORMAL FOR MONTHS OR YEARS?

This question has been studied by a number of investigators, and the general conclusion is that with infrequent exceptions, moderate to severe hypertension requires antihypertensive therapy for life because hypertension returns when the drugs are stopped. In cases of mild hypertension, on the other hand, after the blood pressure has been normal for several years, about 5–20% of patients remain normotensive when antihypertensive therapy is discontinued. A recent Veterans Administration Study (1975) has indicated that there is a gradual recurrence of hypertension over a period of 3–9 months in 85% of patients with mild to moderate disease when antihypertensive therapy is stopped. More rarely, the pressure may begin to rise within the first month, especially if the patient has had severe disease before therapy is begun. If the pressure remains normal for 18 months to 2 years, the recurrence rate is very low.

The hazard of stopping therapy is that there may be a rebound phenomenon with intense vasoconstriction, which may then be more difficult to reverse even if the same regimen used for successful control is restarted. Research groups who interrupt therapy for several weeks in order to perform renin, angiotensin, or steroid studies report that problems rarely occur when the drug is stopped for this short amount of time.

With the exception of stopping therapy for a short time to do specialized studies to exclude secondary hypertension, we ordinarily do not stop therapy. Once a diagnosis of hypertension has been established, patients require antihypertensive treatment for life. An attempt can be made to decrease dosage, but rarely should therapy be stopped—even though 5–10% of patients remain normotensive for 1–2 years after all therapy is stopped. If the blood pressure is controlled at a low normal level for 1 or 2 years, the size of the dose of the most potent agent that the patient is receiving can be decreased, especially if the patient has side-effects which, while tolerated, are undesirable. This is done in slow, stepwise fashion. If the patient's pressure stays low for 6 months, we stop the most potent drug and then decrease the dose of the next most potent agent in similar fashion. If the blood pressure again remains normal for 6 months, we repeat the procedure with the remaining therapeutic agents. The likelihood of the blood pressure remaining normal is sufficiently small so that if one attempts to stop therapy, close observation should be maintained to make certain that the patient does not have a high pressure rebound. Patients should be informed about what is being done so that they will maintain close contact with the physician and not be lost to follow-up, only to return after months or years with severe complications of hypertension such as cardiac failure, malignant hypertension, or aortic dissection.

SOCIAL & PSYCHOLOGIC FACTORS

Adverse social and psychologic factors in hypertensive patients may set off adrenergic impulses from the central nervous system and cause increased vasoconstriction, superimposing further transient rises in pressure on established hypertension and gradually worsening the structural changes in the arterioles and the interlobular arteries of the kidney. This leads to higher blood pressures and consequent vascular abnormalities and complications.

There is no clear evidence that social or psychologic factors *cause* hypertension. Folkow's hypothesis—that emotional factors operating through the central nervous system cause smooth muscle contraction, arteriolar structural changes, and thus hypertension—has not been fully accepted. Adverse social and psychologic factors might accelerate hypertension by inducing substantial recurrent rises in pressure, thus increasing the load on the heart and precipitating left ventricular failure. In the presence of coronary disease, transient blood pressure elevations may precipitate cardiac arrhythmias and angina pectoris or may rupture a Charcot microaneurysm in one of the small penetrating arteries in the brain.

For this reason, attention to the social and psychologic aspects of the patient's life is an integral part of management of the hypertensive patient. One could say the same thing about every patient with heart disease, but the principle seems particularly applicable to the hypertensive patient.

• • •

References

Abrams DG, Wilson C: Effect of hypotensive drugs on renal function in chronic renal disease. Lancet 1:68, 1957.

Anderson BG, Beierwaltes WH: Adrenal imaging with radioiodocholesterol in the diagnosis of adrenal disorders. Adv Intern Med 19:327, 1974.

Aoki VS, Wilson WR: Hydralazine and methyldopa in thiazide-treated hypertensive patients. Am Heart J 79:798, 1970.

Atkinson RL & others: Acromegaly: Treatment by transsphenoidal microsurgery. JAMA 233:1279, 1975.

Bayliss WM: On the local reactions of the arterial wall to changes of internal pressure. J Physiol (Lond) 28:220, 1902.

Bech K, Hilden T: The frequency of secondary hypertension. Acta Med Scand 197:65, 1975.

Bechgaard P: The natural history of benign hypertension: 1000 hypertensive patients followed from 26–32 years. Page 357 in: *The Epidemiology of Hypertension.* Stamler J, Stamler R, Pullman TN (editors). Grune & Stratton, 1967.

Bedford DE: Left ventricular failure. Lancet 1:1303, 1939.

Beilin IJ, Juel-Jensen BE: Alpha- and beta-adrenergic blockage in hypertension. Lancet 1:979, 1972.

Bell ET, Clawson BJ: Primary (essential) hypertension: A study of 420 cases. Arch Pathol 5:939, 1928.

Bevan AT, Honour AJ, Stott FH: Direct arterial pressure recording in unrestricted man. Br Heart J 31:387, 1969.

Bhatia SK, Frohlich ED: Hemodynamic comparison of agents useful in hypertensive emergencies. Am Heart J 85:367, 1973.

Biglieri EG: A perspective on aldosterone abnormalities. Clin Endocrinol 5:399, 1976.

Biglieri EG, Herron M, Brust N: 17-hydroxylation deficiency in man. J Clin Invest 45:1946, 1966.

Biglieri EG, Lopez JM: Clinical and laboratory diagnosis of adrenocortical hypertension. Cardiovasc Med 1:335, 1976.

Biglieri EG & others: Plasma aldosterone concentration: Further characterization of aldosterone-producing adenomas. Circ Res 34-35 (Suppl 1):183, 1974.

Bøe J, Humerfelt S, Werdevang F: The blood pressure in a population: Blood pressure readings and height and weight determinations in the adult population of the city of Bergen. Acta Med Scand, Suppl 321, 1957.

Bookstein JJ, Walter JF: The role of abdominal radiography in hypertension secondary to renal or adrenal disease. Med Clin North Am 59:169, 1975.

Bookstein JJ & others: Cooperative study of radiologic aspects of renovascular hypertension: Bilateral renovascular disease. JAMA 237:1706, 1977.

Bravo EL, Tarazi RC, Dustan HP: β-Adrenergic blockade in diuretic-treated patients with essential hypertension. N Engl J Med 292:66, 1975.

Bryan RK & others: Effect of minoxidil on blood pressure and hemodynamics in severe hypertension. Am J Cardiol 39:796, 1977.

Build and Blood Pressure Study. Vol 1. Chicago: Society of Actuaries, 1959.

Byrom FB: Pathogenesis of hypertensive encephalopathy and its relation to the malignant phase of hypertension: Experimental evidence in the hypertensive rat. Lancet 2:201, 1954.

Caldwell JR & others: The dropout problem in antihypertensive treatment: A pilot study of social and emotional factors influencing a patient's ability to follow antihypertensive treatment. J Chronic Dis 22:579, 1970.

Carey RM & others: The Charlottesville Blood-Pressure Survey: Value of repeated blood-pressure measurements. Blood-Pressure Survey. JAMA 236:847, 1976.

Case DB & others: Possible role of renin in hypertension as suggested by renin-sodium profiling and inhibition of converting enzyme. N Engl J Med 296:641, 1977.

Case D & others: Usefulness and limitations of saralasin, a partial competitive agonist of angiotensin II, for evaluating the renin and sodium factors in hypertensive patients. Am J Med 60:825, 1976.

Chalmers J & others: Effects of timolol and hydrochlorothiazide on blood-pressure and plasma renin activity: Double-blind factorial trial. Lancet 2:328, 1976.

Clark AB, Dunn M: A nurse clinician's role in the management of hypertension. Arch Intern Med 136:903, 1976.

Clarke E, Murphy EA: Neurological manifestations of malignant hypertension. Br Med J 2:1319, 1956.

Cole FM, Yates PO: Comparative incidence of cerebrovascular lesions in normotensive and hypertensive patients. Neurology 18:255, 1968.

Colwill JM & others: Alpha-methyldopa and hydrochlorothiazide: A controlled study of their comparative effectiveness as antihypertensive agents. N Engl J Med 271:696, 1964.

Committee on Hypertension: Drug treatment of ambulatory patients with hypertension. JAMA 225:1647, 1973.

Conn JW: Primary aldosteronism and primary reninism. Hosp Pract 9:131, Oct 1974.

Connolly ME, Kersting F, Dollery CT: The clinical pharmacology of beta-adrenoceptor-blocking drugs. Prog Cardiovasc Dis 19:203, 1976.

Conway J: Labile hypertension: The problem. Circ Res 27:43, 1970.

Couch NP, Sullivan J, Crane C: Predictive accuracy of renal vein renin activity in surgery of renovascular hypertension. Surgery 79:70, 1976.

Dalen JE & others: Dissection of the thoracic aorta: Medical or surgical therapy? Am J Cardiol 34:803, 1974.

Davidson C & others: Effects of long-term diuretic treatment on body-potassium in heart-disease. Lancet 2:1044, 1976.

Davis JO: The pathogenesis of chronic renovascular hypertension. Circ Res 40:439, 1977.

Day RP, Luetscher JA: Biochemical properties of big renin extracted from human plasma. J Clin Endocrinol Metabol 40:1085, 1975.

Deming QB: Blood pressure: Its relation to atherosclerotic disease of the coronaries. Bull NY Acad Med 44:968, 1968.

Dissecting aneurysm: Medical Staff Conference, University of California, San Francisco. West J Med 121:482, 1974.

Dollery CT, Harrington M: Methyldopa in hypertension: Clinical and pharmacological studies. Lancet 1:759, 1962.

Dollery CT, Emslie-Smith D, Milne MD: Clinical and pharmacological studies with guanethidine in the treatment of hypertension. Lancet 1:381, 1960.

Dollery CT, Lewis G, Myers MG: Clinical evaluation of a new beta-adrenoceptor antagonist ICI 66082 in essential hypertension. Br J Clin Pharmacol 2:185P, 1975.

Douglas JG, Hollifield JW, Liddle GW: Treatment of low-renin essential hypertension: Comparison of spironolactone and a hydrochlorothiazide-triamterene combination. JAMA 227:518, 1974.

Doyle AE: In: Berglund G, Hansson L, Werkö L (editors): *The Pathophysiology and Management of Arterial Hypertension.* Astra Int Ltd, 1975.

Dustan HP: Atherosclerosis complicating chronic hypertension.

Circulation 50:871, 1974.

Dustan HP (editor): *Hypertension.* Clinician, Searle, 1973.

Eddy RL & others: Cushing's syndrome: A prospective study of diagnostic methods. Am J Med 55:621, 1973.

Farmer RG, Gifford RW, Hines EA Jr: Effect of medical treatment on severe hypertension: Follow-up study of 161 patients with group three or group four hypertension. Arch Intern Med 112:118, 1963.

Ferguson RK & others: A specific orally active inhibitor of angiotensin-converting enzyme in man. Lancet 2:775, 1977.

Finnerty FA, Davidov M, Kakariatos N: Hypertensive vascular disease: The long-term effect of rapid repeated reductions of arterial pressures with diazoxide. Am J Cardiol 19:377, 1967.

Finnerty FA Jr, Mattie EC, Finnerty FA III: Hypertension in the inner city: 1. Analysis of clinical dropouts. Circulation 47:73, 1973.

Folkow B: The haemodynamic consequences of adaptive structural changes of the resistance vessels in hypertension. Clin Science 41:1, 1971.

Folkow B: Nervous control of blood vessels. Physiol Rev 35:629, 1955.

Folkow B, Neil E: *Circulation.* Oxford Univ Press, 1971.

Foster JH & others: Renovascular occlusive diseases: Results of operative treatment. JAMA 231:1043, 1975.

Fregly MJ, Fregly MS (editors): *Oral Contraceptives and High Blood Pressure.* Dolphin Press, 1974.

Freis ED: The clinical spectrum of essential hypertension. Arch Intern Med 133:982, 1974.

Freis ED: Salt, volume, and the prevention of hypertension. Circulation 53:589, 1976.

Frohlich ED: Hemodynamic concepts in hypertension. Hosp Pract 9:59, Nov 1974.

Ganong W: Sympathetic effects of renin secretion: Mechanism and physiological role. Pages 17–32 in: *Control of Renin Secretion.* Assaykeen TA (editor). Plenum Press, 1972.

Genest J, Koiw E, Kuchel O (editors): *Hypertension: Physiopathology and Treatment.* McGraw-Hill, 1977.

Genest J & others: The adrenal cortex and essential hypertension. Recent Prog Horm Res 32:377, 1976.

Gifford RW Jr: Drug combinations as rational antihypertensive therapy. Arch Intern Med 133:1053, 1974.

Gifford RW & others: Clinical features, diagnosis and treatment of pheochromocytoma: A review of 76 cases. Mayo Clin Proc 39:281, 1964.

Goldberg LI Jr: Current therapy of hypertension: A pharmacologic approach. Am J Med 58:489, 1975.

Goldblatt H, Lynch J, Hanzai R: Studies on experimental hypertension. 1. The production of persistent elevation of systolic blood pressure by means of renal ischemia. J Exp Med 59:347, 1934.

Goldfien A: Treatment of pheochromocytoma. Mod Treat 3:1360, 1966.

Goldring W, Chasis H: *Hypertension and Hypertensive Disease.* Commonwealth Fund, 1944.

Gordon DA, Hill FM, Ezrin C: Acromegaly: A review of 100 cases. Can Med Assoc J 87:1106, 1962.

Gore I, Hirst AE Jr: Dissecting aneurysm of the aorta. Prog Cardiovasc Dis 16:103, 1973.

Graham JDP: High blood pressure after battle. Lancet 1:239, 1945.

Gross F (editor): *Antihypertensive Therapy: Principles and Practice.* Springer, 1966.

Gross RE: Hypertension from coarctation of the aorta. Am J Surg 107:14, 1964.

Guiha NH & others: Treatment of refractory heart failure with infusion of nitroprusside. N Engl J Med 291:587, 1974.

Guyton AC, Coleman TG: A quantitative analysis of the pathophysiology of hypertension. Circ Res 24:1, 1969.

Guyton AC & others: Arterial pressure regulation: Overriding dominance of the kidneys in long-term regulation and in hypertension. Am J Med 52:584, 1972.

Haber E: The role of renin in normal and pathological cardiovascular homeostasis. Circulation 54:849, 1976.

Hallbäck M: Interaction between central neurogenic mechanisms and changes in cardiovascular design in primary hypertension: Experimental studies in spontaneously hypertensive rats. Acta Physiol Scand (Suppl 424):5, 1975.

Hallbäck M, Folkow B: Cardiovascular responses to acute mental "stress" in spontaneously hypertensive rats. Acta Physiol Scand 90:684, 1974.

Hamberg M, Svensson J, Samuelsson B: Thromboxanes: A new group of biologically active compounds derived from prostaglandin endoperoxides. Proc Natl Acad Sci USA 72:2994, 1975.

Hansson L, Werkö L: Beta-adrenergic blockade in hypertension. Am Heart J 93:394, 1977.

Harington M, Kincaid-Smith P, McMichael J: Results of treatment in malignant hypertension. Br Med J 2:969, 1959.

Harris RE & others: Response to psychologic stress in persons who are potentially hypertensive. Circulation 7:874, 1953.

Havel RJ: Classification of the hyperlipidemias. Annu Rev Med 28:195, 1977.

Henry JP: Understanding the early pathophysiology of essential hypertension. Geriatrics 31:59, 1976.

Heptinstall RH: Renal biopsies in hypertension. Br Heart J 16:133, 1954.

Hodge JV, Dollery CT: Retinal soft exudates. Q J Med 33:117, 1964.

Hogan MJ & others: Location of aldosterone-producing adenomas with ^{131}I-19-iodocholesterol. N Engl J Med 294:410, 1976.

Hollifield JW & others: Proposed mechanisms of propranolol's antihypertensive effect in essential hypertension. N Engl J Med 295:68, 1976.

Hurxthal IM, O'Sullivan JB: Cushing's syndrome: Clinical differential diagnosis and complications. Ann Intern Med 51:1, 1959.

Hypertension Detection and Follow-Up Program Cooperative Group: The hypertension detection and follow-up program. Circ Res 40 (Suppl 1):106, 1977.

Inter-Society Commission for Heart Disease Resources: Guidelines for detection, diagnosis and management of hypertensive populations. Circulation 44:A263, 1971.

Joint National Committee on Detection, Evaluation and Treatment of High Blood Pressure: A cooperative study. JAMA 237:255, 1977.

Julius S: Borderline hypertension: Definitions and treatment. Cardiovasc Med 1:77, 1976.

Kain HK, Hinman AT, Sokolow M: Arterial blood pressure measurements with a portable recorder in hypertensive patients. 1. Variability and correlation with "casual" pressures. Circulation 30:882, 1964.

Kalis BL & others: Response to psychological stress in patients with essential hypertension. Am Heart J 53:572, 1957.

Kannel WB: Role of blood pressure in cardiovascular morbidity and mortality. Prog Cardiovasc Dis 17:5, 1974.

Kannel WB: Role of blood pressure in the development of congestive heart failure. N Engl J Med 287:782, 1972.

Kannel WB, McGee D, Gordon T: A general cardiovascular risk

profile: The Framingham Study. Am J Cardiol 38:46, 1976.

Kaplan NM: Adrenal causes of hypertension. Arch Intern Med 133:1001, 1974.

Kaplan NM: Low-renin hypertension. Pages 272–287 in: *Clinical Hypertension.* Kaplan NM (editor). Medcom Press, 1973.

Kaplan NM: The prognostic implications of plasma renin in essential hypertension. JAMA 231:167, 1975.

Kaplan NM: Renin profiles: The unfulfilled promises. JAMA 238:611, 1977.

Kaplan NM & others: Single-voided urine metanephrine assays in screening for pheochromocytoma. Arch Intern Med 137:190, 1977.

Kaufman JJ: Progress in the diagnosis and management of renovascular hypertension. Urol Digest 14:12, 1975.

Keith NM, Wagener HP, Barker ND: Some different types of essential hypertension: Their course and prognosis. Am J Med Sci 197:332, 1939.

Kempner W: Treatment of hypertensive vascular disease with rice diet. Am J Med 4:545, 1948.

Kilcoyne MM, Richter RW, Alsup PA: Adolescent hypertension. 1. Detection and prevalence. Circulation 50:758, 1974.

Kincaid-Smith P: Management of severe hypertension. Am J Cardiol 32:575, 1973.

Kincaid-Smith P, Bulles M, Millis V: Prolonged use of methyldopa on severe hypertension of pregnancy. Br Med J 1:274, 1966.

Kincaid-Smith P, McMichael J, Murphy EA: The clinical course and pathology of hypertension with papilledema (malignant hypertension). Q J Med 27:117, 1958.

Kirkendall WM & others: Recommendation for human blood pressure determination by sphygmomanometer. Circulation 36:981, 1967.

Koch G: Acute hemodynamic effects of an alpha- and beta-receptor blocking agent (AH 5158) on the systemic and pulmonary circulation at rest and during exercise in hypertensive patients. Am Heart J 93:585, 1977.

Koch-Weser J: Correlation of pathophysiology and pharmacotherapy in primary hypertension. Am J Cardiol 32:499, 1973.

Koch-Weser J: Hydralazine. N Engl J Med 295:320, 1976.

Koch-Weser J: Vasodilator drugs in the treatment of hypertension. Arch Intern Med 133:1017, 1974.

Koshy MC & others: Physiologic evaluation of a new antihypertensive agent: Prazosin HCl. Circulation 55:533, 1977.

Kosman ME: Management of potassium problems during long-term diuretic therapy. JAMA 230:743, 1974.

Krieger DT, Amorosa L, Linick F: Cyproheptadine-induced remission of Cushing's disease. N Engl J Med 293:893, 1975.

Krupp MA: Urinary sediment in visceral angiitis (periarteritis nodosa, lupus erythematosus, Libman-Sachs disease): Quantitative study. Arch Intern Med 71:54, 1943.

Laragh JH (editor): *Laragh's Hypertension Manual.* Yorke Medical Books, 1974.

Laragh JH (editor): Symposium on hypertension. (2 parts.) Am J Med 60:733; 61:721, 1976.

Leatham A: The retinal vessels in hypertension. Q J Med (New Series) 18:203, 1949.

Leckie BJ & others: An inactive renin in human plasma. Circ Res 40 (Suppl 1):46, 1977.

Lee JB, Mookerjee BK: The renal prostaglandins as etiologic factors in human essential hypertension: Fact or fantasy? Cardiovasc Med 1:302, 1976.

Lefkowitz RJ: Biochemical properties of alpha- and beta-adrenergic receptors and their relevance to the clinician. Cardiovasc Med 2:573, 1977.

Lew EA: High blood pressure, other risk factors and longevity: The insurance viewpoint. Am J Med 55:281, 1973.

Liddle GW, Shute AM: The evolution of Cushing's syndrome. Adv Intern Med 15:41, 1969.

Lieberman E: Childhood hypertension: Evaluation and management. Cardiovasc Med 1:24, 1976.

Liebman J, Edelman IS: Interrelations of plasma potassium concentrations, plasma sodium, arterial pH, and total exchangeable potassium. J Clin Invest 38:2176, 1959.

Limas CJ, Freis ED: Minoxidil in severe hypertension with renal failure. Effect of its addition to conventional antihypertensive drugs. Am J Cardiol 31:355, 1973.

Lindsay J Jr, Hurst JW: Clinical features and prognosis in dissecting aneurysm of the aorta. Circulation 35:880, 1967.

Littler WA, Honour AJ, Sleight P: Direct arterial pressure, pulse rate, and electrocardiogram during micturition and defecation in unrestricted man. Am Heart J 88:205, 1973.

Londe S, Goldring D: High blood pressure in children: Problems and guidelines for evaluation and treatment. Am J Cardiol 37:650, 1976.

Low J, Oparil S: Oral contraceptive pill hypertension. J Reprod Med 15:201, 1975.

Lund-Johansen P: Hemodynamic changes in longterm diuretic therapy of essential hypertension. Acta Med Scand 187:509, 1970.

Manifestations and treatment of acromegaly: Medical Staff Conference, University of California, San Francisco. Calif Med 116:57, March 1972.

Marks LS, Maxwell MH, Kaufman JJ: Non-renin-mediated renovascular hypertension: A new syndrome? Lancet 1:615, 1977.

Marks LS & others: Detection of renovascular hypertension: Saralasin test versus renin determinations. J Urol 116:406, 1976.

Maron BJ & others: Prognosis of surgical corrected coarctation of the aorta: Twenty-year postoperative appraisal. Circulation 47:119, 1973.

Marshall AJ & others: Evaluation of beta blockade, bendrofluazide, and prazosin in severe hypertension. Lancet 1:271, 1977.

Marx JL: Blood clotting: The role of the prostaglandins. Science 196:1072, 1977.

Masson GMC & others: Hypertensive vascular disease as a consequence of increased arterial pressure. Am J Pathol 34:817, 1958.

Maxwell MH: Cooperative study of renovascular hypertension: Current status. Kidney Int 8 (Suppl):153, 1975.

McCormack LJ & others: Effects of antihypertensive treatment in the evolution of renal lesions in malignant nephrosclerosis. Am J Pathol 34:1011, 1958.

McGiff JC & others: Release of a prostaglandin-like substance into renal venous blood in response to angiotensin II. Circ Res 27 (Suppl 1):121, 1970.

McMichael J: Reorientations in hypertensive disorders. (2 parts.) Br Med J 2:1239, 1310, 1961.

Melby JC: Assessment of adrenocortical function. N Engl J Med 285:735, 1971.

Melby JC: Solving the adrenal lesions of primary aldosteronism. N Engl J Med 294:441, 1976.

Melby JC & others: Diagnosis and localization of aldosterone-producing adenomas by adrenal-vein catheterization. N Engl J Med 277:1050, 1967.

Mellander S, Johansson B: Control of resistance, exchange, and capacitance functions in the peripheral circulation. Pharmacol Rev 20:117, 1968.

Melmon KL: The clinical pharmacology of commonly used antihypertensive drugs. Cardiovasc Clin 6(2):175, 1974.

Mersey JH & others: Relationship between aldosterone and bradykinin. Circ Res 40 (Suppl 1):84, 1977.

Mitchell JRA: Hypertension and arterial disease. Br Heart J 33:122, 1971.

Mitchell JR, Arias L, Oates JA: Antagonism of the antihypertensive action of guanethidine sulfate by desipramine hydrochloride. JAMA 202:149, 1967.

Moeller VJ, Heyder O: Die labile Blutdrucksteigerung. Z Kreislaufforsch 48:413, 1959.

Moncada S & others: An enzyme isolated from arteries transforms prostaglandin endoperoxides to an unstable substance that inhibits platelet aggregation. Nature 263:663, 1976.

Moyer JH & others: The effect of treatment on the vascular deterioration associated with hypertension, with particular emphasis on renal function. Am J Med 24:177, 1958.

Mroczek WJ & others: The value of aggressive therapy in the hypertensive patient with azotemia. Circulation 40:893, 1969.

Muirhead EE: The antihypertensive function of the renal medulla. Hosp Pract 10:99, Jan 1975.

National Heart, Lung and Blood Institute's Task Force on Blood Pressure Control in Children: Report of the task force on blood pressure control in children. Pediatrics 59:797, 1977.

Okamoto K (editor): *Spontaneous Hypertension: Its Pathogenesis and Complications.* Igaku Shoin, Ltd, 1972.

Onesti G, Fernandes M, Kim KE (editors): *Regulation of Blood Pressure by the Central Nervous System.* Grune & Stratton, 1976.

Oparil S, Haber E: The renin-angiotensin system. (2 parts.) N Engl J Med 291:389, 446, 1974.

Peart WS: Renin-angiotensin system. N Engl J Med 292:302, 1975.

Perera GA: Hypertensive vascular disease: Description and natural history. J Chronic Dis 1:33, 1955.

Perloff D: Diagnostic assessment of the patient with hypertension. Geriatrics 31:77, 1976.

Perloff D & others: The value of portable blood pressure recording in guiding the treatment of hypertension. Page 181 in: *Biotelemetrie: Symposium am 29./30. November 1968 in Erlangen.* Demling L, Bachmann K (editors). Georg Theime Verlag, 1970.

Perry HM Jr: The management of malignant hypertension. Drug Ther 1:33, Oct 1971.

Perry M, Wessler S, Avioli LV: Survival of treated hypertensive patients. JAMA 210:890, 1969.

Pickering G: *High Blood Pressure,* 2nd ed. Churchill, 1968.

Pickering G: Hyperpiesia: High blood pressure without evident cause: Essential hypertension. Br Med J 2:959, 1965.

Pickering G: Hypertension. Am J Med 52:570, 1972.

Pickering G: Hypertension: Definitions, natural histories, and consequences. Am J Med 52:570, 1972.

Pickering G: Reversibility of malignant hypertension. Lancet 1:413, 1971.

Poblete PF & others: Effect of treatment on morbidity in hypertension. Veterans Administration Cooperative Study on Antihypertensive Agents: Effect on the electrocardiogram. Circulation 48:481, 1973.

Pollack AA & others: Limitations of transcendental meditation in the treatment of essential hypertension. Lancet 1:71, 1977.

Prichard BNC, Gillam PMC: Use of propranolol in treatment of hypertension. Br Med J 2:725, 1964.

Proceedings of the Fourth Meeting of the International Society of Hypertension, Sydney, 24–26 February, 1976. Clin Sci Mol Med 51 (Suppl 3), Dec 1976.

Proger S: Antihypertensive drugs: Praise and restraint. N Engl J Med 286:155, 1972.

Ramalho PS, Dollery CT: Hypertensive retinopathy: Caliber changes in retinal blood vessels following blood pressure reduction and inhalation of oxygen. Circulation 37:580, 1968.

Ramirez EA & others: Veterans Administration Cooperative Study Group on Antihypertensive Agents: Multiclinic controlled trial of bethanidine and guanethidine in severe hypertension. Circulation 55:519, 1977.

Reid IA & others: Studies concerning the mechanism of suppression of renin secretion by clonidine. J Pharmacol Exp Ther 192:713, 1975.

Remine WH & others: Current management of pheochromocytoma. Ann Surg 179:740, 1974.

Richards DA & others: Pharmacological basis for antihypertensive effects of intravenous labetalol. Br Heart J 39:99, 1977.

Richardson DW & others: Variation in arterial pressure throughout the day and night. Clin Sci 26: 445, 1964.

Rockson SG & others: Plasma dopamine-β hydroxylase activity in oral contraceptive hypertension. Circulation 51:916, 1975.

Romero JC, Strong CG: Hypertension and the interrelated renal circulatory effects of prostaglandins and the renin-angiotensin system. Mayo Clin Proc 52:462, 1977.

Romero JC, Dunlap CL, Strong CG: The effect of indomethacin and other anti-inflammatory drugs on the renin-angiotensin system. J Clin Invest 58:282, 1976.

Romhilt DW, Estes EH Jr: A point score system for the ECG diagnosis of left ventricular hypertrophy. Am Heart J 75:752, 1968.

Ross Russell RW: How does blood pressure cause stroke? Lancet 2:1283, 1975.

Ruskin A, Beard OW, Schaffer RL: "Blast hypertension": Elevated arterial pressures in the victims of the Texas City disaster. Am J Med 4:228, 1948.

Safar ME & others: Control of cardiac output in essential hypertension. Am J Cardiol 38:332, 1976.

Safar ME & others: Overhydration and renin in hypertensive patients with terminal renal failure: A hemodynamic study. Clin Nephrol 4:183, 1975.

Sancho J & others: The role of the renin-angiotensin-aldosterone system in cardiovascular homeostasis in normal human subjects. Circulation, 53:400, 1976.

Sandok BA, Whisman JP: Hypertension and the brain. Arch Intern Med 133:947, 1974.

Sannerstedt R: Hemodynamic response to exercise in patients with arterial hypertension. Acta Med Scand (Suppl 458):1, 1966.

Schambelan M & others: Role of renin and aldosterone in hypertension due to renin-secreting tumor. Am J Med 55:86, 1973.

Schambelan M & others: Selective renal-vein sampling in hypertensive patients with segmental renal lesions. N Engl J Med 290:1153, 1974.

Schirger A, Sheps SG: Prazosin: New hypertensive agent: A double-blind crossover study in the treatment of hypertension. JAMA 237:989, 1977.

Schottstaedt MF, Sokolow M: The natural history and course of hypertension with papilledema (malignant hypertension).

Am Heart J 45:331, 1952.

Schwartz AB, Swartz CD: Dosage of potassium chloride elixir to correct thiazide-induced hypokalemia. JAMA 230:702, 1974.

Scotch NA: Sociocultural factors in epidemiology of Zulu hypertension. Am J Public Health 53:1205, 1963.

Sealey JE & others: Plasma prorenin in normal, hypertensive, and anephric subjects and its effect on renin measurements. Circ Res 40 (Suppl 1):41, 1977.

Sevitt LH, Evans DJ, Wrong OM: Acute oliguric renal failure due to accelerated (malignant) hypertension. Q J Med 40:127, 1971.

Shand DG: Propranolol. N Engl J Med 293:280, 1975.

Sheps SG, Kincaid OW, Hunt JC: Serial renal function and angiographic observations in idiopathic fibrous and fibromuscular stenoses of the renal arteries. Am J Cardiol 30:55, 1972.

Sheps SG, Kirkpatrick RA: Hypertension. Mayo Clin Proc 50:709, 1975.

Simpson FO, Gilchrist AR: Prognosis in untreated hypertensive vascular disease. Scott Med J 3:1, 1958.

Skeggs LT & others: The biochemistry of the renin-angiotensin system and its role in hypertension. Am J Med 60:737, 1976.

Slater EE, DeSanctis RW: The clinical recognition of dissecting aortic aneurysm. Am J Med 60:625, 1976.

Smirk FH: *High Arterial Pressure.* Blackwell, 1957.

Smirk FH, Veale AMO, Alstad K: Basal and supplemental blood pressures in relationship to life expectancy and hypertension symptomatology. NZ Med J 58:711, 1959.

Smirk H, Hodge JV: Causes of death in treated hypertensive patients: Based on 82 deaths during 1959–61 among an average hypertensive population at risk of 518 persons. Br Med J 2:1221, 1963.

Smith WM: Treatment of mild hypertension: Results of a 10-year intervention trial. Circ Res 40 (Suppl 1):1, 1977.

Smith WM & others: Cooperative clinical trial of alpha-methyldopa III: Double-blind control comparison of alpha-methyldopa and chlorothiazide and chlorothiazide and rauwolfia. Ann Intern Med 65:657, 1966.

Smith WM & others: The evaluation of antihypertensive therapy: Cooperative clinical trial method. 1. Double blind control comparison of chlorothiazide, rauwolfia, serpentine, and hydralazine. Ann Intern Med 61:829, 1964.

Sokolow M, Lyon TP: The ventricular complex in left ventricular hypertrophy as obtained by unipolar precordial and limb leads. Am Heart J 37:161, 1949.

Sokolow M, Perloff D: The choice of drugs and the management of essential hypertension. Prog Cardiovasc Dis 8:253, 1965.

Sokolow M, Perloff D: Five year survival of consecutive patients with malignant hypertension treated with antihypertensive agents. Am J Cardiol 6:858, 1960.

Sokolow M, Perloff D: The prognosis of essential hypertension treated conservatively. Circulation 23:697, 1961.

Stamler J: Page 67: On the natural history of hypertension and hypertensive disease. Page 107: On the epidemiology of hypertension and hypertensive disease. Page 392: On renal factors in the pathogenesis of essential hypertension. In: *The Pathogenesis of Essential Hypertension: Proceedings of the WHO Prague Symposium, 1960.*

Stamler J, Stamler R, Pullman TN (editors): *The Epidemiology of Hypertension.* Grune & Stratton, 1967.

Steptoe A: Psychological methods in treatment of hypertension: A review. Br Heart J 39:587, 1977.

Streeten DHP, Anderson GH Jr: Angiotensin blockade in hypertension. Ann Intern Med 86:353, 1977.

Taguchi J, Freis ED: Partial reduction of blood pressure and prevention of complications in hypertension. N Engl J Med 291:239, 1974.

Tarazi RC & others: Plasma volume and chronic hypertension: Relationship to arterial pressure levels in different hypertensive diseases. Arch Intern Med 125:835, 1970.

Thomas CB: Developmental patterns in hypertensive cardiovascular disease: Fact or fiction? Bull NY Acad Med 45:831, 1969.

Thomas JE, Rooke ED, Kvale WF: The neurologist's experience with pheochromocytoma: A review of 100 cases. JAMA 197:100, 1966.

Tobian LJ Jr: The clinical approach to essential hypertension. Hosp Pract 10:33, July 1975.

United States National Center for Health Statistics: Vital and Health Statistics. Blood Pressure Levels of Persons 6–74 Years of Age in the United States. Government Printing Office, Series 11, No. 203 (in press), April 1977.

US Department of Health, Education and Welfare, National Institutes of Health: *The National High Blood Pressure Education Program.* Department of Health, Education and Welfare Publication No. (NIH) 74–593, 1973.

US Public Health Service Hospitals Cooperative Study Group: Treatment of mild hypertension: Results of a ten-year intervention trial. Circ Res 40 (Suppl 1):98, 1977.

Uvila JM & others: Blood pressure in chronic renal failure: Effect of sodium intake and furosemide. JAMA 220:233, 1972.

Vane JR, McGiff JC: Possible contributions of endogenous prostaglandins to the control of blood pressure. Circ Res 36 (Suppl 1):68, 1975.

VanZwieten PA: The central action of antihypertensive drugs, mediated via central α-receptors. J Pharm Pharmacol 25:89, 1973.

Veterans Administration Cooperative Study Group on Antihypertensive Agents: Effects of treatment on morbidity in hypertension. 1. Results in patients with diastolic blood pressures averaging 115 through 129 mm Hg. JAMA 202:1028, 1967.

Veterans Administration Cooperative Study Group on Antihypertensive Agents: Effects of treatment on morbidity in hypertension. 2. Results in patients with diastolic blood pressure averaging 90 through 114 mm Hg. JAMA 213:1143, 1970.

Veterans Administration Cooperative Study Group on Antihypertensive Agents: Effects of treatment on morbidity in hypertension. 3. Influence of age, diastolic pressure, and prior cardiovascular disease; further analysis of side-

Veterans Administration Cooperative Study Group on Antihypertensive Agents: Propranolol in the treatment of essential hypertension. JAMA 237:2303, 1977.

effects. Circulation 45:991, 1972.

Veterans Administration Cooperative Study Group on Antihypertensive Agents: Return of elevated blood pressure after withdrawal of antihypertensive drugs. Circulation 51:1107, 1975.

Voors AW & others: Studies of blood pressures in children, ages 5–14 years, in a total biracial community: The Bogalusa Heart Study. Circulation 54:319, 1976.

Weber MA, Drayer JI, Laragh JH: Beta-blockade, renin and blood-pressure. Lancet 1:367, 1977.

Weidmann P & others: Interrelations among blood pressure, blood volume, plasma renin activity and urinary catecholamines in benign essential hypertension. Am J Med 62:209, 1977.

Weir RJ & others: Blood pressure in women after one year of oral contraception. Lancet 1:467, 1971.

Weiss L, Hallbäck M: Time course and extent of structural vascular adaptation to regional hypotension in adult spontaneously hypertensive rats (SHR). Acta Physiol Scand 91:365, 1974.

Wiggers CJ: *Physiology in Health and Disease,* 3rd ed. Lea & Febiger, 1939.

Wilber JA, Barrow JG: Hypertension: A community problem. Am J Med 52:653, 1972.

Wilburn RL, Blaufuss A, Bennett CM: Long-term treatment of severe hypertension with minoxidil, propranolol and furosemide. Circulation 52:706, 1975.

Williams GH: Angiotensin-dependent hypertension–Potential pitfalls in definition. N Engl J Med 296:684, 1977.

Wilson GM: Diuretics. Practitioner 200:39, 1968.

Wilson HM & others: Saralasin infusion in the recognition of renovascular hypertension. Ann Intern Med 87:36, 1977.

Woods JW, Blythe WB, Huffines WD: Management of malignant hypertension complicated by renal insufficiency. N Engl J Med 291:10, 1974.

Woosley RL, Nies AS: Guanethidine. N Engl J Med 295:1053, 1976.

Yun J & others: Role of prostaglandins in the control of renin secretion in the dog. Circ Res 40:459, 1977.

Zacest R, Gilmore E, Koch-Weser J: Treatment of essential hypertension with combined vasodilation and beta-adrenergic blockade. N Engl J Med 286:617, 1972.

Zinner SH, Levy PS, Kass EH: Familial aggregation of blood pressure in childhood. N Engl J Med 284:401, 1971.

10 . . .
Cardiac Failure

DEFINITIONS

Cardiac failure can be broadly defined as a state in which the heart fails to meet the varying oxygen and metabolic needs of the body under differing circumstances, or a state in which cardiac output (the ability of the heart to pump blood) is reduced relative to the metabolic demands of the body, assuming the existence of adequate venous return. The definition is arbitrary and controversial, because the phenomena of heart failure are complex and incompletely understood. If one uses a symptom such as dyspnea on exertion appearing for the first time as the manifestation signaling the onset of cardiac failure in left ventricular disease, this criterion may be deceptive because physically active patients will demonstrate dyspnea earlier than patients who are sedentary and because a sedentary person with no heart disease may experience dyspnea on unaccustomed exertion.

Cardiac failure may be present in the resting state or may appear only with excessive stress. It is easily recognized in its later stages, when symptoms and signs due to pulmonary or systemic venous congestion, increased ventricular volume and diastolic pressure, and decreased cardiac output are present.

Cardiac failure may occur as a manifestation or complication of many types of heart disease. Not all patients with heart disease develop cardiac failure, however, and it is not known why some patients whose hearts have worked against increased loads for many years ultimately develop cardiac failure.

Cardiac failure may be "forward" failure, as after myocardial infarction, in which the cardiac output is sharply reduced; or "backward failure," when right ventricular failure follows left ventricular failure because of raised left atrial pressure and right ventricular dilatation. Congestive heart failure is diagnosed when systemic congestive phenomena (edema, enlarged and tender liver, raised venous pressure with pulsating neck veins) occur as a result of right ventricular failure, usually with tricuspid insufficiency. Left ventricular failure is diagnosed when pulmonary venous congestion follows left ventricular dilatation and increased left atrial pressure, manifested by dyspnea, orthopnea, paroxysmal nocturnal dyspnea, and pulmonary edema. It is seen on chest x-ray as pulmonary congestion.

In patients with heart disease, transient cardiac failure may be induced by any of the acute precipitating events (arrhythmias, respiratory infection, etc) listed on p 268. When the precipitating event subsides with time or is cured by appropriate treatment, the patient's cardiac status may return to its previous asymptomatic state. In these instances, it is more proper to speak of precipitation of reversible cardiac failure than spontaneous development of failure.

A definition of cardiac failure based not on symptoms but on objectively measured hemodynamic indices would be a useful clinical and research tool. One may, for example, decide that cardiac failure is present when there is increased ventricular volume and ventricular end-diastolic pressure and decreased cardiac output at rest or on exercise in patients with left ventricular disease due to any cause.

It should be obvious that the diagnosis of cardiac failure, like that of any other disease, depends upon its definition, which varies with different authorities. The distinction must be maintained between the presence of heart disease and the presence of cardiac failure, and the latter should be perceived as a continuum from (1) recognition of the presence of cardiac disease, to (2) a preclinical phase in which hemodynamic abnormalities but not symptoms may be present, and finally to (3) an overt clinical phase in which it is obvious to all that cardiac failure is present.

The heart fails ("decompensates") when various compensatory mechanisms (cardiac hypertrophy, raised atrial pressure, ventricular dilatation, increased force of contraction; see p 268) are inadequate to maintain the function of a diseased heart whose work load has been increased. As the compensatory mechanisms begin to falter, symptoms or hemodynamic indices of cardiac failure may not be obvious at rest but may be produced when the demands on the heart are increased by exercise, emotion, or precipitating factors. Depending upon what is being demanded, therefore, cardiac failure may be present when cardiac output is normal, increased (high output failure), or decreased.

Initially, either the left or, less commonly, the right ventricle may fail; ultimately, however, especially after salt and water retention occurs, combined left and right failure is the rule (congestive failure).

CAUSES OF HEART FAILURE

Left ventricular failure is most commonly due to hypertension, coronary heart disease, or valvular heart disease, usually aortic valvular disease; less common causes are mitral valve disease, congestive cardiomyopathies, hypertrophic cardiomyopathy, left-to-right shunts, and congenital heart lesions. Infective endocarditis may occur in a normal heart or may complicate other valvular disease, and left ventricular failure may also occur. Cardiac failure may also occur in various connective tissue disorders, thyrotoxicosis, severe anemia, arteriovenous fistula, myocarditis, beriberi, and myocardial involvement by tumors or granulomas.

Isolated right ventricular failure is most commonly due to mitral stenosis with raised pulmonary vascular resistance, pulmonary parenchymal or vascular disease, or pulmonary valvular stenosis; less commonly, to tricuspid valvular disease or infective endocarditis involving the right side of the heart. Carcinoid involving the pulmonary or tricuspid valves is a rare cause. Systemic venous congestion follows, leading to congestive heart failure.

Factors precipitating failure. In at least half of cases, demonstrable precipitating disease or factors that increase the work load of the heart are present, and these factors should be sought in every patient with cardiac failure. They include arrhythmias, respiratory infection, myocardial infarction, pulmonary embolism, rheumatic carditis, thyrotoxicosis, anemia, excessive salt intake, corticosteroid administration, pregnancy, and excessive or rapid administration of parenteral fluids. Fever may aggravate failure (as in acute myocardial infarction) but does not cause it de novo.

Heart failure may occur in patients with normally functioning hearts that are subjected to excessive loads. The clearest example of this is systemic arteriovenous fistula. Even in otherwise healthy young people, a large fistula can produce heart failure; in older people, thyrotoxicosis, severe anemia, beriberi, or Paget's disease of bone may cause heart failure even though cardiac output is high.

Summary

The causes of ventricular failure can be summarized as follows:

(1) Intrinsic myocardial disease: Coronary heart disease, cardiomyopathy, infiltrative diseases such as hemochromatosis, amyloidosis, sarcoidosis, and myocarditis.

(2) Excess work load:

   (a) Increased resistance to ejection (pressure load): Hypertension, stenosis of aortic or pulmonary valves, hypertrophic cardiomyopathy.

   (b) Increased stroke volume (volume load): Aortic insufficiency, mitral insufficiency, tricuspid insufficiency, congenital left-to-right shunts.

   (c) Increased body demands ("high output failure"): Thyrotoxicosis, anemia, pregnancy, arteriovenous fistula.

HEMODYNAMIC & PATHOPHYSIOLOGIC FEATURES OF HEART FAILURE

Compensatory Mechanisms

The compensatory mechanisms by which the heart responds to an increased load include the following: (1) concentric hypertrophy (hypertrophy without dilatation), which provides larger contractile cells; (2) increased fiber length or dilatation, which increases the force of contraction, as shown by the Frank-Starling law (Fig 10–1); and (3) increased sympathetic nervous system activity, by which the force of contraction is increased at any fiber length without increasing the filling pressure.

A. Hypertrophy and Compliance: Concentric hypertrophy is most apt to occur when the load placed on the heart is due to increased resistance to ejection with increased impedance, characteristically seen in aortic stenosis and hypertension. Early in the course of the disease, the only cardiac abnormality that can be identified is left ventricular hypertrophy, recognized both clinically and by electrocardiography (Fig 10–2). The increased thickness causes a decrease in the distensibility or compliance of the left ventricle, so that the

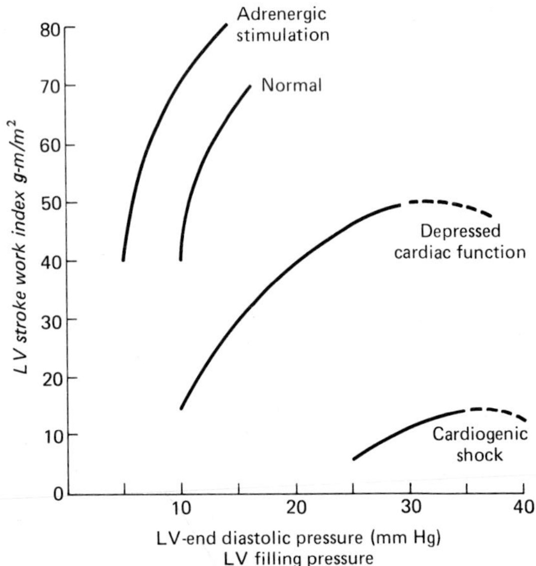

Figure 10–1. Family of Frank-Starling curves showing relation of force of contraction (left ventricular stroke work index) to fiber length or pressure (left ventricular end-diastolic pressure or filling pressure). (Modified and reproduced, with permission, from Swan HJC, Parmley WW: Congestive heart failure. Chapter 10 in: *Pathologic Physiology: Mechanisms of Disease,* 5th ed. Sodeman WA Jr, Sodeman WA [editors]. Saunders, 1974.)

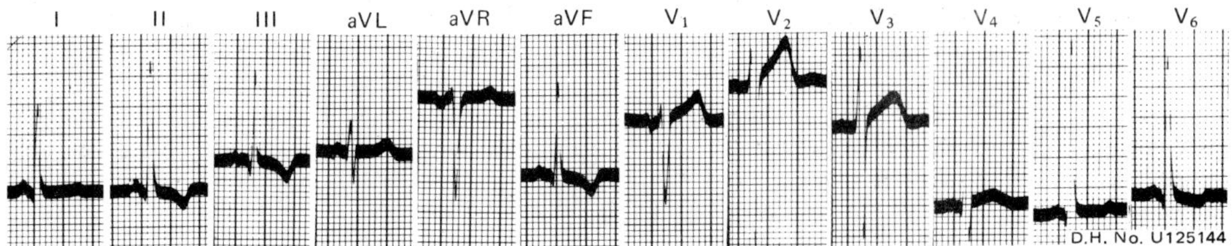

Figure 10–2. An example of moderate left ventricular hypertrophy in a vertically placed heart in a 28-year-old man with coarctation of the aorta.

left ventricular end-diastolic pressure is raised, with a normal left ventricular volume; the raised filling pressure is required to augment left ventricular output in accordance with the Frank-Starling principle. The raised left ventricular end-diastolic pressure does not necessarily imply ventricular failure but occurs whenever compliance is decreased, as in the cardiac states noted above or in hypertrophic or infiltrative cardiomyopathy. It also occurs early in acute myocardial infarction, when the infarcted area becomes stiff and less distensible. Later—eg, in patients with hypertension or aortic stenosis—when left ventricular volume increases (because cardiac hypertrophy and more forceful contraction alone are insufficient to compensate), the left ventricular end-diastolic pressure rises even further and left ventricular failure occurs.

B. Increased Stroke Volume and Failure: When the increased cardiac load is due to increased stroke volume, typically represented by aortic insufficiency, the increased stretch increases fiber length and so increases the force of left ventricular contraction as demonstrated by the Frank-Starling principle. As the stretch increases, left ventricular volume increases, as can be demonstrated by enlargement of the heart on the plain film of the chest or the echocardiogram or by left ventricular angiography. In these circumstances, distensibility is not decreased, and it is common to find an increased left ventricular volume with normal left ventricular end-diastolic pressure and normal or increased cardiac output. When left ventricular performance declines in the later stages of this type of lesion (as well as in so-called congestive cardiomyopathy), the ejection fraction falls from its normal value of 60–70% as left ventricular failure occurs and may be as low as 10–20% in very severe failure. The ejection fraction correlates positively with the cardiac index: the greater the ejection fraction, the higher the cardiac index. It is best determined by left ventricular angiography, although echocardiography provides an estimate. In general, patients tolerate increased volume load better than increased resistance load even though left ventricular wall tension and myocardial oxygen consumption increase when the heart is dilated and enlarged (law of Laplace). (See p 17 and Fig 1–24 for definition and details.)

C. Increased Sympathetic Stimulation: Increased sympathetic stimulation can be demonstrated in patients with cardiac failure by increased levels of catecholamines in blood and urine and by depletion of norepinephrine in cardiac tissue, notably atrial appendages removed at operation. Sarnoff (1954) and Braunwald (1970), as well as other investigators, have demonstrated the importance of the sympathetic nervous system in improving cardiac contractility in cardiac failure and have noted its exhaustion in failure (first curve in Fig 10–1). Beta-adrenergic blocking agents such as propranolol, by decreasing the sympathetic drive to the heart, may worsen or precipitate ventricular failure.

Hemodynamic Indices

The derived indices used in this chapter are discussed in Chapter 4.

Pathophysiology of Decompensation

Early in the course of various cardiac diseases, the compensatory mechanisms are adequate to maintain a normal cardiac output and normal intracardiac pressures at rest and after exercise. Hypertrophy may be recognized on the ECG or plain chest film. Compensated heart disease becomes "decompensated" as ventricular volume and filling pressures of the respective ventricles increase, although, as stated earlier, a raised filling pressure may be due to decreased compliance rather than to ventricular failure early in the course of the disease. As the filling pressure increases, pulmonary venous congestion occurs as the raised left atrial pressure is transmitted backward. This leads to interstitial and then alveolar edema of the lungs, resulting in symptoms of left ventricular failure, with dyspnea, exertional cough, orthopnea, paroxysmal nocturnal dyspnea, and pulmonary edema when the disease involves the left ventricle. Raised venous pressure, hepatomegaly, dependent edema, and ascites occur when failure involves the right ventricle (congestive or right ventricular failure). Cardiac output may be normal at this phase, especially at rest, but may be decreased on exercise; as the cardiac output on exercise diminishes, tachycardia occurs and thus increases the minute cardiac output when the stroke volume cannot increase adequately. The arteriovenous oxygen difference widens as blood flow to nonessential vascular systems decreases. When the ventricular filling pressure is increased—especially when compliance is decreased—atrial hypertrophy increases the force of atrial systole and so aids filling; loss of this "atrial kick" can decrease the cardiac output when atrial fibrillation occurs.

High Output Failure

The mechanisms involved in high output failure are best illustrated by the example of a large arteriovenous fistula. The fistula acts as a low-resistance pathway through which large amounts of blood pass from the arteries to the veins back to the right heart, increasing the venous return and hence the cardiac output in accordance with the Frank-Starling mechanism. The baroreceptor mechanism has no control over the shunt pathway, and a normal blood pressure must be maintained by a combination of increased cardiac output and vasoconstriction in some other portion of the systemic circulation.

In anemia, the systemic vascular resistance is decreased as cardiac output is increased. The vasodilatation may allow a greater runoff from artery to vein (as in arteriovenous fistula), permitting a decrease in arterial blood volume and setting off the signal that results in increased renin release and the sequence of events leading to increased aldosterone production. The role of tissue hypoxia in causing an increase in catecholamine secretion is unknown. The high cardiac output in thyrotoxicosis is probably due to a combination of the effects of thyroxine and catecholamines on the heart.

A. Compensation: Even when there is no evidence of cardiac failure in such patients, there is a compensatory increase in circulating blood volume. The patient withstands exercise relatively well, because the lowered resistance in the muscular circulation diverts blood away from the fistula and tends to provide an increased blood flow to the muscle without a significant further increase in cardiac output. Conversely, anything that tends to increase the peripheral resistance, eg, exposure to cold, upright posture, dehydration, or salt deprivation, tends to divert more blood to the fistula and starve the rest of the circulatory system of blood flow.

B. Decompensation: The kidneys respond to inadequate perfusion (relative or absolute) by increased salt and water retention, and blood volume expansion occurs. This tends to cause pulmonary and systemic venous congestion and the clinical syndrome of heart failure. The extra work performed by the heart in high output states also plays a part in accelerating degenerative changes in the myocardium (eg, fibrosis).

C. Hypertrophy and Compensation: Cardiac hypertrophy results from dilatation in response to the chronic "flow load" of an arteriovenous fistula. Such changes do not occur in response to muscular exercise because the load of exercise is not continuous and because the period of reduced output during sleep presumably permits appropriate compensatory repair mechanisms to function.

D. Other Factors: The hemodynamic effects of high output states vary considerably with the underlying state of the myocardium. Thus, a relatively minor "high output" factor such as anemia may be of much greater importance in an older patient with degenerative heart disease than in a younger person. In addition, the "high output" load may increase the demand of oxygen by the myocardium relative to supply and cause anginal pain rather than heart failure.

PATHOPHYSIOLOGIC MECHANISMS OF SALT & WATER RETENTION

Apart from the changes in pressure, volume, compliance, and contractility just described, excessive and detrimental retention of salt and water is responsible for many of the symptoms and signs of cardiac failure and may be the dominant clinical feature of heart failure. It occurs as the kidneys attempt to restore the status quo in response to a fall in renal perfusion pressure.

When cardiac output fails to increase normally with exercise in cardiac failure, the renal perfusion pressure and glomerular filtration rate fall; this is detected by the macula densa between the afferent and efferent arterioles or by the juxtaglomerular cells surrounding the afferent arteriole of the kidney, resulting in increased secretion of renin.

Renin acts on renin substrate in the plasma to form angiotensin I, which is converted to angiotensin II in one passage through the lungs. The converting enzymes also deactivate bradykinin. Angiotensin II increases the secretion of aldosterone from the adrenal cortex, which in turn acts on the distal renal tubule to increase the reabsorption of sodium from the renal tubule (see Fig 9–6).

Increased sodium reabsorption leads to increased osmolality of the serum, which decreases the secretion of antidiuretic hormone from the pituitary, causing retention of an equivalent amount of water until osmolality is restored. The increased sodium and water retention leads to an increase in blood volume, which, by raising the hydrostatic pressure in the capillaries, leads first to interstitial edema and then to transudation of fluid into tissues which have decreased tissue pressure, such as the subcutaneous tissues. As a result, edema of the ankles and lower extremities occurs when the patient is ambulatory and edema of the sacrum when the patient is recumbent. Symptoms such as dyspnea and edema are aggravated by salt and water retention and are reversed by the use of diuretics and low-sodium diets.

The precise mechanisms of salt and water retention in the development of cardiac failure are not known. In response to reduced renal blood flow and glomerular filtration rate, the kidney initiates the biochemical changes described above which increase the secretion of aldosterone and thus cause salt and water retention. The result is that blood volume is maintained for a time, and the overall mechanism is similar to that whereby the kidney responds to decreased blood volume due to hemorrhage or dehydration. As is

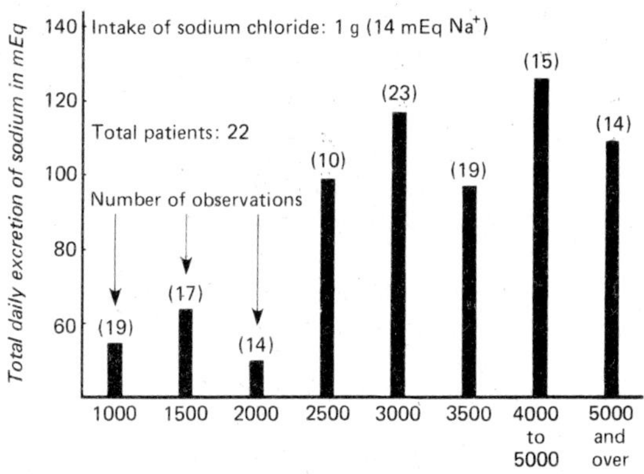

Figure 10–3. When sodium intake is low (approximately 14 mEq), the total daily excretion increases when daily fluid intake increases. (Reproduced, with permission, from Gorham LW & others: The relative importance of dietary sodium chloride and water intake in cardiac edema. Ann Intern Med 27:575, 1947.)

the case with many compensatory mechanisms, salt and water retention in cardiac failure occurs at great physiologic expense since it results in pulmonary and systemic venous congestion with dyspnea and edema. Other vasoactive amines are involved in the angiotensin-aldosterone combination, and it is possible that prostaglandins, bradykinin, and perhaps as yet undiscovered mineralocorticoids secreted by the adrenal glands interact to affect salt and water retention in heart failure.

If sodium is restricted, moderate water intake does not add to sodium retention, as it does with free sodium intake. Water need not be restricted if sodium intake is (Gorham, 1947; Fig 10–3) unless dilutional hyponatremia is present.

CLINICAL FINDINGS

When a patient with any type of heart disease—congenital, valvular, hypertensive, coronary, metabolic, etc—develops symptoms and signs of cardiac failure, the findings are usually not specific for any particular category. Symptoms and signs of pulmonary or systemic venous congestion, increased cardiac volume, and diastolic pressure combined with decreased cardiac output, raised venous pressure, and evidences of salt and water retention clearly indicate that cardiac failure has occurred. In patients with congenital heart disease, pulmonary heart disease, endocarditis involving the valves on the right side, primary pulmonary hypertension, or obstructive diseases of the lungs, raised venous pressure, enlarged tender liver, and systemic edema indicate that cardiac disease has progressed to right-sided congestive failure. This is also true when pulmonary hypertension complicates mitral stenosis and right heart failure and tricuspid regurgitation follow. Right heart failure occurs most commonly as a sequel to left heart failure. Right heart failure is the rule in congenital heart disease, although there are a variety of congenital lesions such as patent ductus arteriosus, coarctation of the aorta, ventricular septal defect, and tricuspid atresia in which the excess load is on the left ventricle, which may ultimately fail. These conditions are all discussed in greater detail elsewhere in this book.

The manifestations of congestive heart failure vary depending on the cause, on the nature of the failure (acute or chronic), and on the location of primary load (left ventricle, right ventricle, or both). The criteria for congestive heart failure are listed in Table 10–1.

Left Ventricular Failure

Before symptoms of left ventricular failure develop, the patient will show evidences of the primary disease (unless failure follows acute myocardial infarction), such as hypertension or aortic stenosis, as well as physical signs of left ventricular hypertrophy and other compensatory changes in the left ventricle (see below). When the compensatory mechanisms fail, the left ventricular end-diastolic pressure rises, and this increased pressure is transmitted to the left atrium and to the pulmonary veins, resulting in pulmonary venous congestion which is recognized hemodynamically by a rise in pulmonary capillary wedge pressure. Depending upon the acuteness and magnitude of the rise in pressure in the pulmonary capillaries, transudation of fluid into the tissue spaces occurs when the pulmonary cap-

Table 10–1. Criteria of diagnosis of congestive heart failure (left and right).*

Major criteria
Paroxysmal nocturnal dyspnea or orthopnea
Neck vein distention
Rales
Cardiomegaly
Acute pulmonary edema
S_3 gallop
Increased venous pressure > 16 cm water
Hydrothorax
Minor criteria
Ankle edema
Night cough
Dyspnea and cough on exertion
Hepatomegaly
Pleural effusion
Vital capacity reduced by one-third from maximum
Tachycardia (rate of ⩾ 120/min)
Major or minor criterion
Weight loss ⩾ 4.5 kg in 5 days in response to treatment

*For establishing a definite diagnosis of congestive heart failure, 2 major or one major and 2 minor criteria must be present concurrently. (Adapted and reproduced, with permission, from McKee PA & others: The natural history of congestive heart failure: The Framingham Study. N Engl J Med 285:1441, 1971.)

illary wedge pressure exceeds the combination of the oncotic pressure of serum and tissue pressure. If the removal of fluid from the tissue spaces via the lymphatics is incomplete, fluid appears in the alveoli, causing more acute symptoms.

A. Symptoms:

1. Dyspnea–Both by reflex action and by increased work of breathing, the increased fluid in the tissue spaces causes dyspnea, at first on effort and then at rest. The work of breathing is greater because of the increased stiffness of the lungs, and the patient is aware of difficulty in breathing. Transudation of fluid into the alveoli superimposes cough on dyspnea of effort, and this combination is suggestive of left ventricular failure. The symptoms are usually progressive, and the earliest manifestation is shortness of breath on exertion that previously caused no difficulty. As pulmonary engorgement progresses, less and less activity brings on dyspnea and cough, until both are present even when the patient is at rest.

2. Orthopnea–Shortness of breath in recumbency which is promptly relieved by propping up the head or trunk is precipitated by the increase in pulmonary engorgement that occurs in the recumbent position. When the pulmonary blood volume is thus increased, the patient characteristically goes to sleep without difficulty but awakens several hours later with dyspnea (paroxysmal nocturnal dyspnea). The mechanism is believed to be increased pulmonary blood volume associated with recumbency and the "autotransfusion" of fluid accumulated in the lower half of the body during upright posture when the blood is returned to the heart. The enhanced venous return (Frank-Starling mechanism) results in greater force of contraction to restore the status quo; when ventricular performance is on or near the descending limb of the Frank-Starling curve, increased contractility cannot compensate for the greater venous return.

3. Paroxysmal nocturnal dyspnea–Paroxysmal nocturnal dyspnea with cough usually develops in a setting of progressive dyspnea on exertion and orthopnea but it may appear at any time and may be the first manifestation of left ventricular failure in severe hypertension, aortic stenosis or insufficiency, or myocardial infarction. It also occurs in patients with tight mitral stenosis, but in this condition it is due to pulmonary venous congestion from obstruction at the mitral valve rather than left ventricular failure. Paroxysmal nocturnal dyspnea or cough is an exaggerated form of orthopnea and may be associated with inspiratory and expiratory wheezing from bronchospasm (so-called cardiac asthma). Depending upon the amount of fluid that accumulates in the lungs, the patient with paroxysmal nocturnal dyspnea may awaken with dyspnea that lasts only a few minutes and is relieved by sitting or standing, or it may progress rapidly into an alarming episode of pulmonary edema.

4. Acute pulmonary edema–Acute pulmonary edema resulting from gross transudation of fluid into the alveoli from the rapidly rising pulmonary capillary pressure causes the patient to sit up in bed gasping for breath; the patient is also cold, pale, anxious, sweating profusely, and prevented by air hunger from finishing a sentence. The patient may become cyanotic, cough up frothy white or pink sputum, and be fearful of imminent death. Patients may ignore progressive dyspnea on exertion, but they rarely ignore acute pulmonary edema. Most attacks subside gradually in 1–3 hours, possibly because of the upright position as well as the progressive decrease in cardiac output. In some instances the left ventricle rapidly weakens, leading to shock and death. Left atrial pressure has been shown to rise to 50 or 60 mm Hg when measured during episodes of pulmonary edema.

Heroin administration is one of the common causes of pulmonary edema; the mechanism of action is presumably the increased capillary permeability. This results in arterial hypoxemia and acidosis, which can be quite marked. The arterial P_{O_2} is usually less than 40 mm Hg in the presence of pulmonary edema, and the pH hovers around 7.15.

5. Interpretation of dyspnea–When dyspnea on exertion is the only symptom, its interpretation is often difficult, especially when the patient is obese and in poor physical condition (see Chapter 2).

a. Patients in poor physical condition almost never have orthopnea or paroxysmal nocturnal dyspnea, and the dyspnea is rarely progressive over a short period of time as it is when left ventricular failure develops in aortic stenosis or coronary disease.

b. Pulmonary causes of dyspnea such as chronic bronchitis, pulmonary fibrosis, and asthmatic bronchitis are more difficult to differentiate because the wheezing of left ventricular failure due to bronchospasm may simulate that of asthma. However, the patient with chronic lung disease usually gives a history of smoking, long-standing cough, or sputum production and frequent episodes of purulent bronchitis in winter. Cough is often present in the absence of dyspnea.

c. Moderate to severe anemia may also produce exertional dyspnea.

d. Advanced age, debility, extreme obesity, ascites from any cause, abdominal distention from gastrointestinal disease, or advanced stages of pregnancy may produce orthopnea in the absence of heart disease.

e. Neurocirculatory asthenia–Patients with neurocirculatory asthenia or anxiety states with psychophysiologic cardiovascular reactions may suffer from sighing respirations simulating dyspnea. This syndrome is more frequent in wartime, though it also occurs in civilian life. So-called soldier's heart is associated with fatigue, chest pain, and palpitations and is induced by activities related to being a member of the armed forces unwillingly and under unpleasant circumstances.

6. Fatigue–Exertional fatigue and weakness due to reduced cardiac output are late symptoms and disappear promptly with rest. Severe fatigue rather than dyspnea is the chief complaint of patients with mitral stenosis who have developed pulmonary hypertension and low cardiac output.

7. **Nocturia as a symptom of edema**–Nocturia may represent excretion of edema fluid accumulated during the day and increased renal perfusion in the recumbent position; it reflects the decreased work of the heart at rest and often the effects of diuretics given during the day. It may also be due to noncardiac causes.

B. Signs: Evidence of the primary disease responsible for the failure, eg, hypertension or aortic stenosis, is almost always present. In some instances of severe failure due to aortic stenosis, the murmur may be absent or difficult to hear because of the decreased velocity of ejection and reduced cardiac output.

Evidence of so-called primary disease is at times misleading. For example, because of the compensatory systemic vasoconstriction that occurs in any condition with reduced cardiac output via the baroreceptor mechanism, blood pressure may be modestly raised in patients with cardiac failure due to any cause; one should therefore be cautious in defining the disease as hypertensive heart failure unless the blood pressure remains elevated after the failure is relieved by treatment.

Left ventricular failure may occur acutely with fluid overload, as may happen with too rapid infusion of large amounts of blood or saline in patients with minimal evidence of left ventricular failure prior to the infusion. Ventricular or atrial arrhythmias associated with a rapid ventricular rate, severe anemia, acute leukemia, or abrupt slowing of the ventricular rate as in atrioventricular block may abruptly result in left ventricular failure. Unaccustomed severe exertion, as in severe aortic stenosis, may cause acute left ventricular failure and may be the first manifestation of failure in patients with aortic stenosis. Drugs such as propranolol that have a negative inotropic effect may rapidly cause left ventricular failure by removing sympathetic drive to the heart and should be used with caution in patients with incipient left ventricular failure.

1. **Enlargement of heart**–In the presence of symptoms of cardiac failure, hypertrophy or dilatation of the left ventricle is usually found on examination and confirmed by evidence of left ventricular hypertrophy on the ECG and left ventricular enlargement on the x-ray or echocardiogram.

2. **Ventricular heave**–The best clinical sign of left ventricular hypertrophy is a left ventricular heave at the apex of the heart. The heave is a localized, sustained, systolic outward motion of the left ventricular impulse that differs from the hyperdynamic left ventricular impulse of exertion, anxiety, or regurgitant valve disease and from the right ventricular heave of right ventricular hypertrophy. The latter is more diffuse, is felt over the center of the chest, and causes apical retraction rather than a lift during systole.

3. **Third heart sound**–(See Chapter 3.) When there is increased left ventricular volume, an exaggerated third heart sound is often heard as ventricular filling occurs during the rapid inflow phase.

4. **Fourth heart sound**–Decreased compliance of the left ventricle with resultant hypertrophy of the left atrium causes a fourth heart sound or atrial gallop which may be felt or seen and is also manifested by a large *a* wave in the jugular venous pulse or in the apexcardiogram.

5. **Rales**–Rales in the lungs may be absent at rest and even early in the episode of nocturnal dyspnea, when transudation occurs into the tissue spaces and not into the alveoli. Later, however, when alveolar fluid appears, the rales are loud and generalized; forthy, bubbling fluid may be obvious all over the lungs. Pleural effusion may occur (see p 297).

6. **Cheyne-Stokes respiration**–Cheyne-Stokes respiration is commonly seen in advanced cardiac failure (see Chapter 3). A typical illustration of the beneficial effects of aminophylline can be seen in Fig 10–4. Following intravenous aminophylline, there is a fall in P_{CO_2}, progressive decrease in the duration of the apneic period until the respirations are normal, and an increase in minute volume respiration.

7. **Tachycardia**–As the stroke volume decreases, tachycardia compensates to increase the minute cardiac output; it is usually present in cardiac failure.

8. **Pulsus alternans**–(See Chapter 3.)

C. Electrocardiography: The ECG is usually much more sensitive than the chest x-ray in demonstrating chamber hypertrophy but may be normal or minimally abnormal when the chest x-ray shows concentric left ventricular hypertrophy and dilatation of the proximal aorta in aortic stenosis. When dilatation predominates over hypertrophy, the chest x-ray may show enlargement, whereas the ECG may show little or no abnormality. The ECG also may be confusing, with nonspecific manifestations of associated effects of treatment

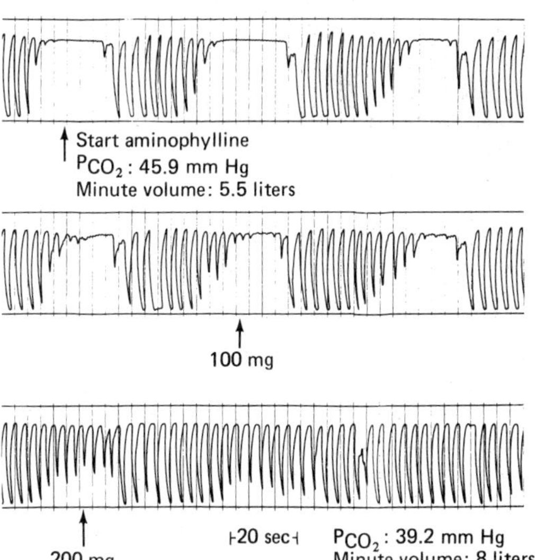

Figure 10–4. Effect of aminophylline on Cheyne-Stokes respiration in a 71-year-old man. Note the progressive decrease in the duration of the apneic period during administration of the agent. (Reproduced, with permission, from Dowell AR & others: Effect of aminophylline on respiratory-center sensitivity in Cheyne-Stokes respiration and in pulmonary emphysema. N Engl J Med 273:1447, 1965.)

with digitalis or diuretics (hypokalemia) or with superimposed coronary disease. An apparent discrepancy in the specific chamber that is hypertrophied or enlarged on the chest x-ray as compared to the ECG usually means that both chambers are involved, although the ECG is less likely to give an erroneous picture when the abnormality is clear-cut.

Echocardiography

A valuable sign of left ventricular failure is a wide E point separation between excursion of the anterior mitral valve leaflet and the ventricular septum (Massie, Am J Cardiol 39, 1977). Fig 10–5 illustrates the normal case, in which there is no separation at all. Fig 10–6 shows a 10 mm separation in a patient with a low ejection fraction but no increase in left ventricular end-diastolic volume. This is to be distinguished from the case in Fig 10–7, in which, although there is an acute volume overload from ruptured chordae and a large end-diastolic volume, the ejection fraction remains normal and there is no E point separation.

Right Ventricular Failure

Right ventricular failure is secondary to chronic left ventricular failure but may occur alone. The most common causes of right ventricular failure are tight mitral stenosis with pulmonary hypertension, pulmonary valve stenosis, cor pulmonale from chronic lung disease, primary pulmonary hypertension with tricuspid insufficiency and other congenital diseases such as Eisenmenger's complex, and pulmonary hypertensive ventricular or atrial septal defects. Tricuspid valve disease may produce the same systemic venous congestion, but, like mitral stenosis, the congestion is due to obstruction at the tricuspid valve and not to right ventricular failure unless there is an associated obstruction higher up such as mitral stenosis. Rare causes are involvement of the pulmonary and tricuspid valves from carcinoid or infective endocarditis. Right ventricular infarction is a somewhat more common cause.

A. Symptoms: The dominant symptoms of right ventricular failure are those of systemic venous congestion—in contrast to left ventricular failure, in which symptoms of pulmonary venous congestion predominate. Pulmonary symptoms are rare unless there is associated left ventricular failure or unless right ventricular failure is due to chronic lung disease. Paroxysmal nocturnal dyspnea is uncommon.

1. Fatigue—The patient may complain of fatigue as cardiac output is reduced.

2. Dependent edema—Edema of the ankles may occur when the patient is up and about; edema of the sacrum, flanks, and thighs when in bed.

3. Liver engorgement—If right ventricular failure occurs rapidly, as when atrial fibrillation develops in tight mitral stenosis, congestion of the liver with distention of its capsule may result, causing right upper quadrant pain which has often been confused with cholecystitis or other abdominal disease.

4. Anorexia and bloating—Hepatic and visceral engorgement secondary to the raised venous pressure may cause anorexia, bloating, and other nonspecific gastrointestinal symptoms.

B. Signs: Evidence of the underlying disease is usually found when specifically sought, although special investigations may be necessary.

1. Right ventricular hypertrophy—In primary right ventricular failure, right ventricular hypertrophy can be diagnosed on the basis of right ventricular heave and right atrial gallop rhythm by auscultation.

2. Right ventricular heave—A right ventricular heave over the lower central chest, pulsation of the pulmonary arteries if there is increased pulmonary blood flow, right atrial gallop rhythm, a loud pulmonary second sound at the base of the heart, and increased jugular venous pressure with systolic pulsations of tricuspid insufficiency are usually present.

3. Right atrial gallop—A right S_3 is often heard, especially when right ventricular failure is due to increased resistance to right ventricular outflow, as in

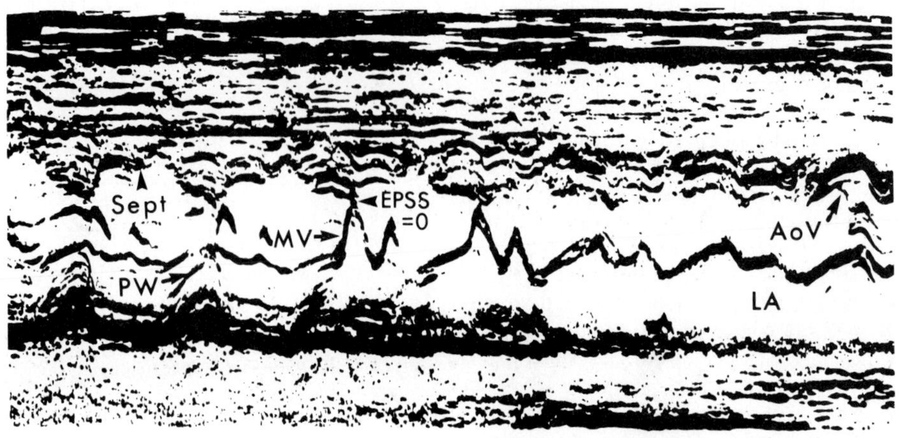

Figure 10–5. Normal echocardiogram showing E point separation (EPSS) = 0. Sept, septum; PW, posterior wall; MV, mitral valve; AoV, aortic valve; LA, left atrium; EPSS, E point separation. (Reproduced, with permission, from Massie BM & others: Mitral-septal separation: A new echocardiographic index of left ventricular function. Am J Cardiol 39:1008, 1977.)

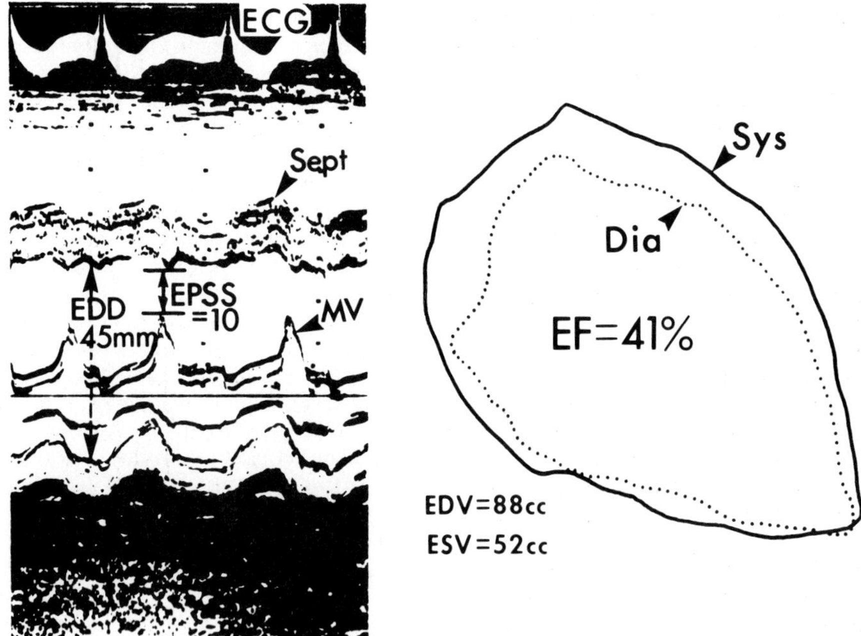

Figure 10–6. Ten mm E point separation (EPSS) in a patient with low ejection fraction and no increase in left ventricular end-diastolic volume as determined by left ventricular angiography. EDD, end-diastolic dimensions; EDV, end-diastolic volume; ESV, end-systolic volume; Sys, systole; Dia, diastole; EF, ejection fraction; MV, mitral valve. (Reproduced, with permission, from Massie BM & others: Mitral-septal separation: A new echocardiographic index of left ventricular function. Am J Cardiol 39:1008, 1977.)

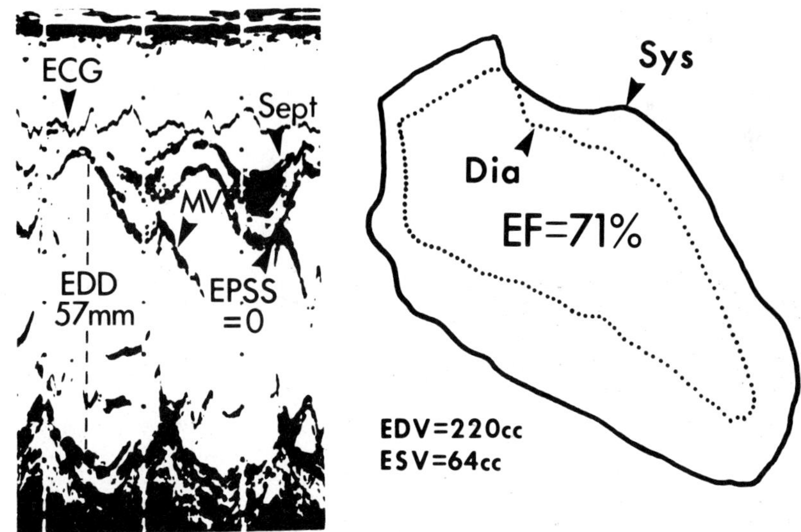

Figure 10–7. Echocardiogram showing no E point separation (EPSS) and normal ejection fraction in spite of acute volume overload from ruptured chordae and a large end-diastolic volume as determined by left ventricular angiography. EDD, end-diastolic dimensions; EDV, end-diastolic volume; ESV, end-systolic volume; Sys, systole; Dia, diastole; EF, ejection fraction; MV, mitral valve. (Reproduced, with permission from Massie BM & others: Mitral-septal separation: A new echocardiographic index of left ventricular function. Am J Cardiol 39:1008, 1977.)

pulmonary stenosis or pulmonary hypertension.

4. Murmurs–If the underlying disease is congenital or valvular, characteristic murmurs will be heard, although in some patients with Eisenmenger's syndrome with severe pulmonary hypertension and a balanced shunt flow no murmurs may be heard–as is true also of primary pulmonary hypertension and chronic lung disease.

5. Chronic pulmonary signs–If right ventricular failure is secondary to chronic lung disease, there will be evidence of decreased distensibility of the lungs, rales, rhonchi, wheezes, and signs of chronic bronchitis.

6. Jugular pulse–Careful inspection of the jugular venous pulse will not only demonstrate the pulsating systolic wave of tricuspid insufficiency (which may also be palpated over the liver, with systolic expansion of the liver); there may also be prominent presystolic *a* waves when there is decreased compliance of the right ventricle and raised right atrial pressure. *a* waves are also prominent in pulmonary stenosis with right ventricular failure and in tricuspid stenosis. The venous pressure rises further when right upper quadrant pressure is exerted by the physician, and the right atrial pressure may be raised as much as 5 mm Hg by this maneuver (hepatojugular reflux). The systolic jugular venous pulse of tricuspid insufficiency is often associated with a pansystolic murmur over the xiphoid, often accentuated by inspiration and associated with a right atrial gallop which is also louder on inspiration.

7. Pulmonary second sound–The pulmonary second sound is accentuated if there is pulmonary hypertension but may be absent in severe pulmonary stenosis and fainter, with a wider split from A_2, if pulmonary stenosis is mild to moderate.

8. Pitting edema–Pitting edema of the ankles, lower extremities, and back is found in established right ventricular failure.

9. Ascites–Initially, the dependent edema caused by right heart failure usually subsides overnight. Eventually, it fails to subside with initial bed rest and may even increase during recumbency. Ascites is rarely prominent unless right ventricular failure has been neglected or if obstructive lesions such as constrictive pericarditis, tricuspid stenosis, or cardiac tamponade are present. In these instances, the jugular venous pressure is raised but there is no clinical evidence of tricuspid insufficiency; in fact, the dominant wave seen in the neck may be a prominent *y* descent.

10. Hydrothorax (pleural effusion)–Hydrothorax is common in congestive heart failure, occurring in about a third of severe cases. It is more common in right than in left ventricular failure and more apt to occur in the right pleural space than in the left; bilateral hydrothorax is less common. Some authorities believe that isolated left hydrothorax should make one consider other conditions such as pulmonary infarction, but well-documented isolated left hydrothorax has often been reported. Fluid may accumulate in any serous cavity (eg, the pericardial and peritoneal cavities–the latter more apt to result from tricuspid stenosis or constrictive pericarditis). Rapid changes in the heart shadow should make one think of pericardial effusion rather than shrinkage of cardiac enlargement.

The mechanism of hydrothorax is not clearly understood. It is a result of systemic venous hypertension but is rare in acute pulmonary edema. Another possible cause is leakage from engorged lymphatics from a swollen liver that penetrate the diaphragm en route to the thoracic duct.

C. Electrocardiography:

1. Left ventricular pattern–If the ECG shows dominant left ventricular hypertrophy (Fig 10–2), the likelihood is that right ventricular failure is not the primary disorder but is secondary to left-sided failure.

2. Right ventricular pattern–Right ventricular hypertrophy is almost always found in congenital heart disease (eg, pulmonary stenosis) (Fig 10–8), although combined hypertrophy may be found when ventricular septal defect produces cardiac failure. Right ventricular hypertrophy is also marked in primary pulmonary hypertension or pulmonary hypertensive mitral stenosis (Fig 10–9), but the pattern of right ventricular hypertrophy is usually slight in clinically significant chronic cor pulmonale.

3. Right axis deviation and right ventricular hypertrophy–See Figs 11–23 and 11–28.

4. P waves–Prominent P waves in leads II and III and a dominant peaked anterior P wave in V_1 and V_2 indicate right atrial hypertrophy, which is often a clue to the presence of chronic cor pulmonale–in contrast to mitral stenosis, in which the P waves are wide and slurred and posteriorly (negatively) directed in V_1, indicating left atrial hypertrophy.

High Output Failure

Arteriovenous fistula is an uncommon cause of heart failure and may be congenital or acquired. The congenital variety may be due to congenital arteriovenous angioma, often involving a limb. Acquired fistulas are due to trauma (including surgical trauma), usually involving the larger arteries of the limbs. They may be visceral (eg, following nephrectomy) or musculoskeletal (eg, after laminectomy). The condition may be insidious, and the fistula may not be clinically obvious.

Arteriovenous fistulas are created surgically in patients with renal disease in order to facilitate hemodialysis. Although such arteriovenous shunts are well tolerated by patients with normal hearts, they may cause heart failure in older patients with associated heart lesions. In high output failure due to other causes such as severe anemia, Paget's disease of bone, thyrotoxicosis, or beriberi, the factor responsible for the failure is usually less obvious.

A. Symptoms: Dyspnea on exertion, edema of the ankles, and fatigue are indistinguishable from the same symptoms occurring in other patients with heart failure.

B. Signs: It is the physical signs of high output failure that provide the clue to diagnosis. The cardinal sign is tachycardia, which is disproportionate to the degree of failure and associated with a hyperdynamic

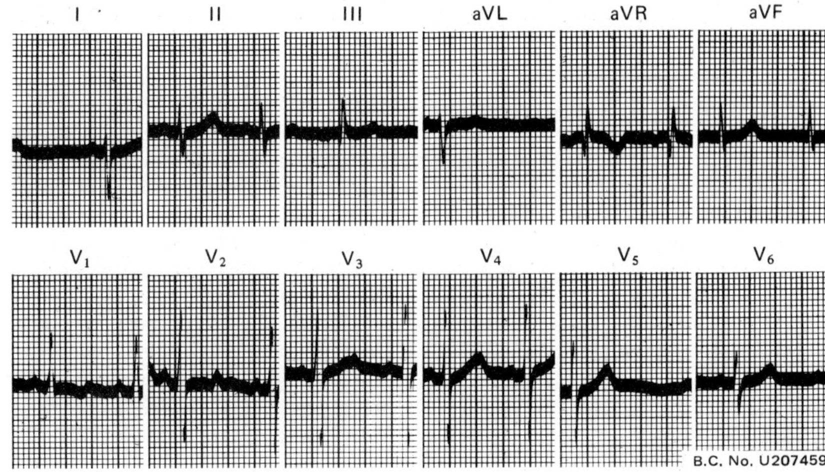

Figure 10–8. Pulmonary stenosis in a 7-year-old girl with right ventricular pressure of 43/0 mm Hg and pulmonary artery pressure 15/5 mm Hg. The ECG shows typical marked right ventricular hypertrophy despite the moderate rise in right ventricular pressure.

cardiac impulse and clinical evidence of cardiac enlargement. Venous pressure is often elevated, and the pulse pressure is widened. A systolic ejection murmur may be heard at the base, resulting from increased stroke volume. If the patient has an arteriovenous aneurysm in a limb, where it can be occluded, it is useful to determine whether occlusion of the fistula has any effect on heart rate. In large fistulas, occlusion increases peripheral resistance, raises systemic arterial pressure, and causes a reflex bradycardia via the baroreceptor reflexes (Branham's sign). If this sign is positive, the fistula is large enough to be a potential cause of heart failure. The fact that this sign is not positive does not exclude arteriovenous fistula as a cause of failure. The presence of a hidden fistula should be sought in any patient with unexplained heart failure with a large heart and tachycardia. Examination of the patient should include listening for bruits over the abdomen, extremities, and back. If the fistula is in a limb, the extremity may be larger than normal, warm, and show marked varicosities. Infection of the fistula may lead to infective endocarditis.

When cardiac failure is acute, the clinical picture is different in different disorders and will be described in the respective sections dealing with specific causes of acute failure. For example, when the chordae of the

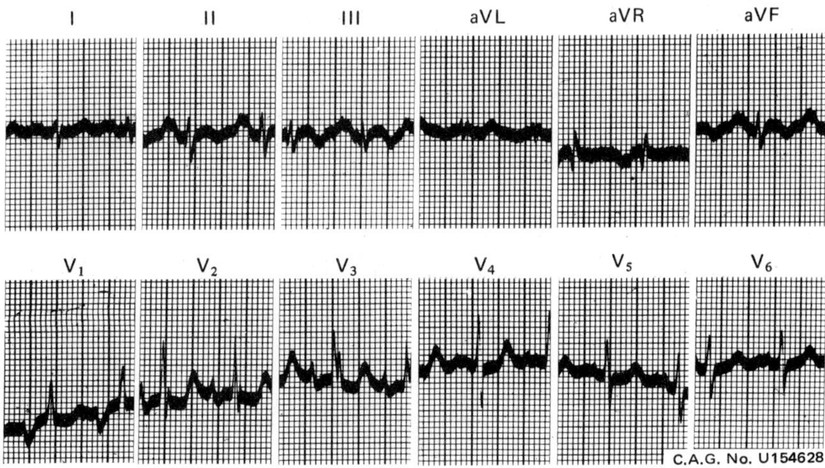

Figure 10–9. Progressive pulmonary venous congestion of 7 years' duration in a 39-year-old man with mitral stenosis and a recent femoral embolus. The ECG shows marked left atrial hypertrophy in association with right ventricular hypertrophy, indicating that the patient has mitral stenosis rather than congenital heart disease, in which right atrial hypertrophy would be expected with anteriorly rather than posteriorly directed P waves.

mitral valve rupture, acute to subacute pulmonary venous congestion occurs, with rapid development of mitral regurgitation and left ventricular failure. However, the left atrium is smaller, sinus rhythm is the rule, and the clinical picture differs from that of chronic mitral regurgitation.

C. Radiology and Electrocardiography: Cardiac enlargement is usually seen on the chest x-ray, and the ECG may show evidence of left ventricular hypertrophy.

RADIOLOGIC EXAMINATION IN HEART FAILURE

X-Ray Changes in Chronic Cardiac Failure

The chest x-ray may reveal right ventricular enlargement, but the reliability of right chamber identification is less than is the case with left ventricular enlargement, especially when the 2 are combined. In the presence of pulmonary hypertension, the pulmonary artery is dilated; and in severe pulmonary hypertension, especially primary pulmonary hypertension, there may be enlargement of the main and central pulmonary arteries with abrupt cutoff in the caliber of the more peripheral pulmonary arteries. The pulmonary venous engorgement that occurs in left ventricular failure is absent, and there is no evidence of redistribution of blood, with widening of the pulmonary arteries of the upper lobes as compared to the lower, such as occurs in left ventricular failure. Attention to the pulmonary pattern, therefore, may be helpful in confirming chamber enlargement and in distinguishing left and right ventricular failure.

Plain Film

Posteroanterior and lateral views of the chest may provide the first evidence of cardiac failure.

A. Heart Shadow: The film is usually abnormal, with hypertrophy and enlargement of the involved chamber, although the heart may not be enlarged if the patient has concentric hypertrophy (as in aortic stenosis or hypertension) or coronary heart disease.

B. Pulmonary Congestion: As the resistance of the lower lobe pulmonary arteries increases in left ventricular failure or in the pulmonary venous congestion of mitral stenosis, blood flows to the arteries with lower resistance, resulting in redistribution of fluid to the upper lobes (Figs 10–10 and 10–11), as can be seen on the plain film when the left atrial pressure rises to 20–25 mm Hg.

When fluid accumulates in the interlobular septa, horizontal Kerley B lines at the angles of the lateral lower lobes can be seen which reflect such fluid.

Attempts have been made to estimate left atrial pressure on the basis of signs of pulmonary venous congestion on the plain film, but the reliability of this method is only about 60%, chiefly because of the lag in appearance and disappearance of the findings in the chest film.

C. Pleural Effusion: In chronic left ventricular failure, there may be right- or left-sided pleural effusion, usually the former.

D. Calcification: Calcification of the mitral or

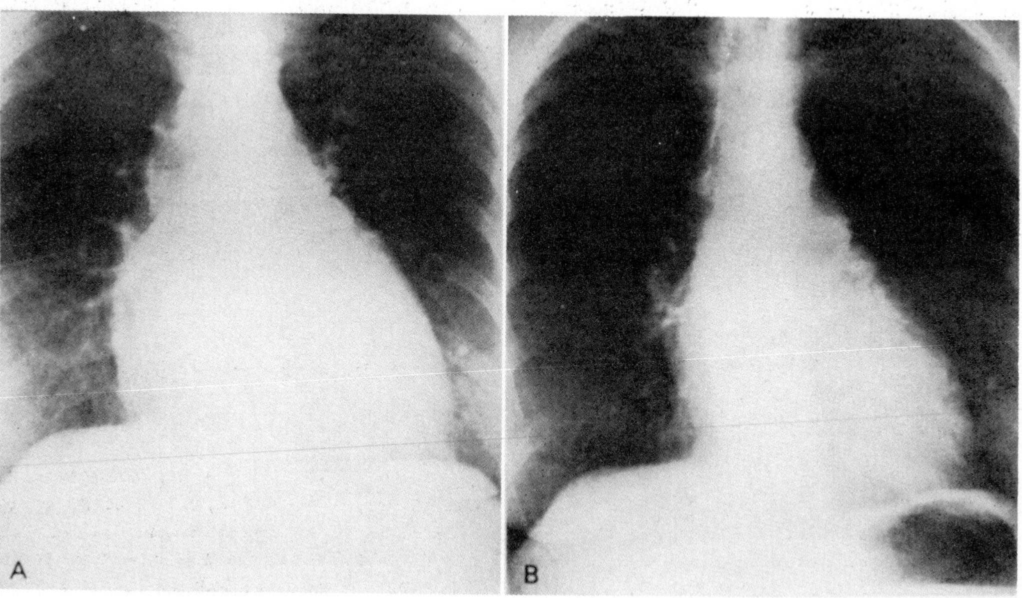

Figure 10–10. Enlarged heart and pulmonary venous congestion in a patient with high output cardiac failure due to an end-to-side cephalic vein– radial artery fistula *(A)* before and *(B)* after banding of the vein. One month after banding, the heart has become smaller and pulmonary venous congestion has improved. (Reproduced, with permission, from Anderson CB & others: Cardiac failure and upper extremity arteriovenous dialysis fistulas. Arch Intern Med 136:292, 1976.)

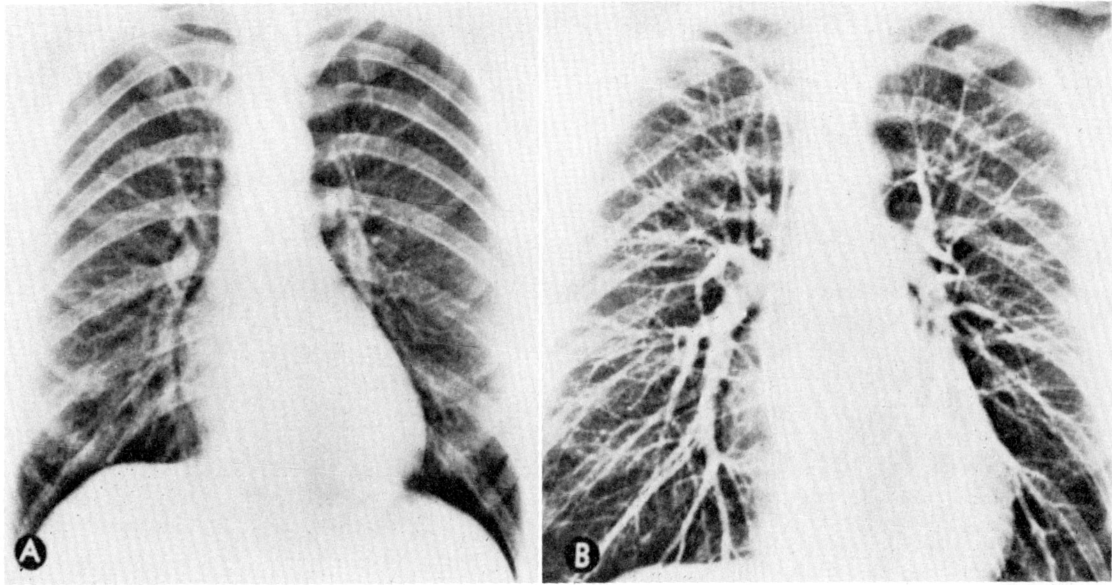

Figure 10–11. Chest x-rays and pulmonary arterial angiograms demonstrating that the vessels to the upper lobes are larger and more numerous than those to the lower lobes with hilar indistinction. *A:* Chest x-ray. *B:* Pulmonary arterial angiogram. (Reproduced, with permission, from Turner AF, Lau FYK, Jacobson G: A method for the estimation of pulmonary venous and arterial pressures from the routine chest roentgenogram. Am J Roentgenol Radium Ther Nucl Med 116:1, 1972.)

aortic valve or in the pericardium or coronary arteries may be the clue to diagnosis.

E. The Aorta: Examination of the aorta is often rewarding. If it is diffusely dilated, it suggests hypertensive disease; but if only the proximal aorta is dilated, especially if it can be seen within the heart shadow, it strongly suggests aortic stenosis. Fine egg-shell calcification of the proximal aorta suggests syphilis (see Chapter 20); if the aorta is widely dilated proximally and in the arch but not distally, the question of dissection must be resolved by further studies. A localized aneurysm may also be demonstrated. The aorta may be small, with atrial septal defect or mitral stenosis because of decreased left ventricular flow. All of the congenital anomalies that may affect the aorta or its branches may be seen.

F. Rib Notching: Notching of the ribs may be the first sign of coarctation of the aorta in a patient with hypertension (see Chapter 11).

G. Left Atrial Study: Careful study of the left atrium is often helpful. Disproportionate left atrial enlargement, as in mitral stenosis or mitral regurgitation, may lead to a search for calcification of the mitral valve, echocardiographic studies, and careful physical examination. With left ventricular enlargement, the left atrium may be enlarged proportionately.

H. Other Findings: Chest films often show unexpected findings such as acute inflammatory disease of the lungs, pneumothorax, malignancy, or hilar nodes of lymphoma or sarcoidosis. In patients presenting with severe dyspnea, carcinomatous lymphatic spread in the lungs may occasionally lead to the diagnosis of carcinoma of the stomach or other organs.

LABORATORY FINDINGS

Red and white cell counts, hemoglobin, packed cell volume, and sedimentation rate are normal in uncomplicated heart failure. Polycythemia may occur in chronic cor pulmonale (see Chapter 19). Urinalysis often discloses significant proteinuria and granular casts. The BUN may be elevated because of reduced renal blood flow, but the urine specific gravity is high in the absence of primary renal disease. Serum sodium, potassium, chloride, and HCO_3^- are within normal limits in the usual case of congestive heart failure before diuretics are used. Specific tests should be made for any suspected unusual causes of heart failure such as thyrotoxicosis, infective endocarditis, syphilis, connective tissue disease, and pheochromocytoma.

DIFFERENTIAL DIAGNOSIS

Cardiac failure must be distinguished from all conditions associated with dyspnea, cough, pulmonary venous congestion, venous pressure elevation, decreased cardiac output, cardiac enlargement, or peripheral edema. These clinical findings occur in a wide variety of conditions that can be conveniently discussed in groups as in the following paragraphs.

Noncardiac & Nonthoracic Conditions Simulating Cardiac Failure

Examples include the dyspnea and fatigue of obesity, of sedentary individuals, and of emotional states with hyperventilation, and the edema that occurs as a result of thrombophlebitis or prolonged sitting in people with varicose veins. In these conditions, there are usually no objective signs of heart disease such as significant murmurs, friction rub, gallop rhythm, cardiac enlargement, or raised venous pressure. Cardiac diagnostic procedures–noninvasive or invasive–reveal no abnormalities of the cardiovascular system. At times these symptoms and signs from noncardiac causes occur in patients with known cardiac disease. As indicated in the introductory paragraphs, the presence of cardiac disease does not imply that all of the patient's symptoms and signs are due to cardiac failure.

Cardiac failure must be diagnosed on the basis of symptoms and signs combined with noninvasive and invasive technics discussed in this chapter.

Lung Disease & Acute Respiratory Tract Infections Presenting With Respiratory Symptoms

These entities are discussed in Chapter 19. Right heart failure may occur in chronic lung disease (cor pulmonale), but many patients with chronic lung disease with chronic bronchitis, emphysema, etc have dyspnea and cough for many years without abnormality of the heart. Patients with acute respiratory symptoms may have acute infections of the bronchi or lungs associated with fever and other symptoms and signs of acute illness. The differential diagnosis, including clinical and pulmonary function studies, is discussed in Chapter 19. Most helpful in chronic lung disease is the long history of chronic cough and sputum production, dyspnea, and wheezing combined with clinical findings of poor lung expansion and chronic wheezes and rales. A history of cigarette smoking or of repeated respiratory infections in the absence of cardiac enlargement, gallop rhythm, ventricular heaves, or raised venous pressure is most helpful. Venous pressure becomes elevated when cardiac failure complicates chronic lung disease, but pulmonary symptoms are present for many years without this objective finding. Pulmonary function studies aid in the diagnosis of specific chronic lung diseases, and hemodynamic studies reveal increases of pressure in the pulmonary artery and the right heart with no abnormality in the left heart. When the 2 conditions coexist, the differentiation may be difficult.

Massive Pulmonary Embolism

Pulmonary embolism may produce symptoms similar to those of cardiac failure, or acute right ventricular failure may follow (1) massive pulmonary embolism with the development of acute pulmonary infarction as noted on chest x-ray or (2) pulmonary hypertension associated with signs of acute right ventricular overload, with physical signs of pulmonary hypertension and ECG evidence of right ventricular dilatation rather than systemic venous congestion (Sokolow, 1940). More precise diagnosis is provided by the combination of chest film, pulmonary radioisotope scan, and pulmonary angiography (see Pulmonary Embolism, p 296).

Diseases of the Pericardium & Myocardium

Pericarditis and myocarditis due to various causes are discussed at length in Chapters 18 and 17, respectively. The most important distinguishing feature is raised left ventricular filling pressure relative to the right side, indicating that the disease is due to congestive cardiomyopathy with cardiac failure. Echocardiography is helpful in recognizing and quantifying the presence of pericardial effusion, which may not be suspected clinically, although findings of pericarditis such as pericardial friction rub can be diagnostic.

TREATMENT OF CARDIAC FAILURE

Cardiac failure may be of any degree of severity ranging from mild to moderate evidence of left ventricular failure with increasing dyspnea on accustomed effort to an emergency characterized by severe pulmonary edema, markedly reduced cardiac output, and an urgent threat to life (as in acute myocardial infarction or infective endocarditis with acute valvular insufficiency). Treatment therefore varies from a calm, conservative approach with nonurgent methods to urgent emergency measures depending upon the judgment of the physician.

The objectives of treatment are to remove the cause, increase the force and efficiency of myocardial contraction, and reduce the abnormal retention of sodium and water. The patient shares a significant responsibility in the management of his disease, because treatment is long-term and involves restriction in diet and activity and the reliable use of cardiac drugs.

Identify, treat, and if possible eliminate the factor precipitating the cardiac failure, eg, infection (especially respiratory), pulmonary infarction, overexertion, increased sodium intake, medication (especially digitalis), arrhythmias, particularly with rapid ventricular rates (eg, atrial fibrillation), myocardial infarction, and anemia.

The principles governing the treatment of cardiac failure are outlined in Table 10–2 and will be elaborated below.

1. VERIFY THE DIAGNOSIS & ESTIMATE THE URGENCY OF TREATMENT

Dyspnea, edema, fatigue, and other findings may not be due to cardiac failure even in patients with known heart disease. Careful questioning, taking into

Table 10–2. Principles of treatment of cardiac failure. Discussed in sequence in the text that follows.

1. Make certain the diagnosis is correct and estimate the urgency of the need for therapeutic measures.
2. Reduce the energy requirement of the heart.
3. Reduce sodium intake unless diuretics have been given.
4. Consider and treat disturbances of rhythm.
5. Provide adequate but not excessive diuresis.
6. Identify and treat unsuspected acute myocardial processes.
7. Determine the presence of surgically treatable conditions that increase the mechanical load on the heart or interfere with left ventricular function.
8. Identify and treat precipitating factors in cardiac failure.
9. Digitalize adequately.
10. Treat systemic diseases that affect the heart.
11. Obtain a history of the use of cardiac depressant or damaging drugs and adjust or stop.
12. Mechanically remove fluid accumulations.
13. Treat with vasodilators in severe or refractory cardiac failure.

account the patient's intelligence, cooperation, understanding of language, and the possible effects of statements or diagnoses made by previous physicians, is always required.

The urgent treatment of pulmonary edema is discussed on p 301.

2. REDUCE THE ENERGY REQUIREMENT OF THE HEART

This is achieved by restricting physical and psychologic activity. Even modest activity induces sodium retention, tachycardia, and increased oxygen demands.

Rest

Physical and mental rest may be the most important aspect of treatment of early cardiac failure when cardiac reserves are reduced because compensatory mechanisms are beginning to falter and compensated heart disease is starting to "decompensate." The patient may be asymptomatic and have sufficient cardiac reserve to supply tissue oxygen needs at rest but not when stress is imposed. Many patients with mild cardiac failure improve dramatically with no treatment other than rest in bed, although if failure is more severe other forms of therapy may be required. Rest not only decreases the work of the heart; recumbency decreases the stimulus to aldosterone production induced by erect posture, and sodium diuresis may result. About one-third of patients with left ventricular failure will respond with sodium and water diuresis and recover from cardiac failure with bed rest alone.

The duration of the period of physical and mental rest depends upon the severity of the heart failure, the age of the patient, and the cause of the underlying heart disease leading to failure, but even in the mildest cases the physician usually errs in allowing the patient to resume activity too early. For example, the patient in unequivocal left ventricular failure should be treated as though a small myocardial infarction has occurred and should have at least 2 or 3 weeks of rest with gradual return to ambulatory status. Rest is preferably in the hospital but can be at home if failure is not severe, because the danger of ventricular arrhythmia is less than in acute myocardial infarction. In older patients, prolonged rest is associated with an increased risk of other problems (eg, thromboses, weakness, postural hypotension), and one should provide rest but not necessarily in bed. The use of a comfortable chair is equally effective, and short periods of walking decrease the likelihood of phlebothrombosis. Attention to the domestic, economic, and social situation of the patient is important; it obviously does no good to prescribe bed rest or rest in a chair if the patient has to do the marketing, cook and clean house, and care for other members of the family. Social service agencies, home care assistance programs, and mobilization of all family resources for the patient's benefit are often helpful. A major flaw in treatment is an insufficient period of rest before the patient returns to the accustomed routine of stressful activities.

Reassurance

Dyspnea due to cardiac failure is a frightening experience. A reassuring and realistically optimistic attitude on the part of the physician and the judicious use of sedatives are important features of management.

3. DECREASE SODIUM INTAKE (Unless Diuretics Have Been Given)

Sodium in any form aggravates the peripheral manifestations of cardiac failure. Decreased cardiac output or failure of cardiac output to rise with emotion—or especially with exertion—and decreased renal perfusion pressure, associated with cardiac failure, result in redistribution of blood through the body, preserving the flow to the brain and heart and diminishing the flow to the kidneys and skin. This (and perhaps other unappreciated signals) sets in motion the renin-angiotensin-aldosterone mechanism, resulting in salt and water retention aggravated by the upright posture. The exact mechanisms are not completely understood. Sodium excretion in patients with cardiac failure is usually decreased, and if the failure is severe it may be markedly decreased. In the days before oral diuretic agents came into use, strict sodium restriction was often difficult to achieve. When diuretics are used in adequate doses, strict sodium restriction is usually not necessary unless cardiac failure is severe or the patient has severe sodium retention such as occurs in chronic constrictive pericarditis. It is usually sufficient to avoid added salt in the diet, but patients must be warned about the sodium content of medications such as Alka-Seltzer or baking soda and foods high in sodium such as potato chips, pretzels, salted nuts, etc. Severe cardiac failure has occurred in patients ingesting large amounts of "baking soda" who thought they were taking a low-sodium diet, and also in patients who drink "softened" water. Booklets made available by local chapters of The American Heart Association give the sodium contents of common foods and should be distributed to patients at risk. Restriction of sodium is especially important in patients whose normal diet is salty (potato chips, pretzels, bacon, ham, packaged soups), and reeducation may be difficult. However, it has been said in this context that "the punishment should fit the crime," ie, the severity of sodium restriction should be adjusted according to the severity of cardiac failure and the effectiveness of diuretic therapy.

4. CORRECT ARRHYTHMIAS

Intermittent disturbances of rhythm may include paroxysmal atrial fibrillation or flutter, frequent ventricular premature beats or ventricular tachycardia, complete atrioventricular block, junctional rhythms from digitalis toxicity, and "sick sinus" syndrome. Either rapid or slow heart rates may be deleterious. Rapid heart rates decrease diastolic filling time and impair coronary perfusion and may produce myocardial ischemia, decreasing the total cardiac output when stroke volume cannot be increased. An irregular rapid ventricular rate is more harmful than a regular rate, because systolic ejection is more profoundly disturbed by the irregular ventricular filling and subsequent response. When the ventricular rate is slow and the stroke output cannot be increased sufficiently to maintain an adequate minute volume output, patients may develop cardiac failure as well as impaired cerebral perfusion independently of episodes of syncope or Stokes-Adams attack.

The prevention and treatment of arrhythmias and of heart block may be crucial in the management of cardiac failure and are discussed at length in Chapters 14 and 15. Disturbances in rhythm and conduction may not be fully appreciated because they may be paroxysmal or nocturnal. In patients with paroxysmal nocturnal dyspnea, the precipitating role of the arrhythmia may not be recognized without continuous ECG monitoring. With slow ventricular rates, artificial endocardial pacemakers may be required to induce a more rapid rate.

5. DIURETIC THERAPY

Physiology & Pharmacology

One of the spectacular advances in the past 40 years in the treatment of cardiac failure has been the development of diuretic agents, culminating in the introduction of the oral thiazide diuretics in 1957. About 40% of patients with cardiac failure will fail to respond to bed rest and digitalis and will require diuretic therapy to overcome the hypervolemia of cardiac failure.

A. Sodium Reabsorption in Cardiac Failure: Although the major pathologic event in cardiac failure is loss of the pumping action of the heart, failure of this function leads to hemodynamic changes in the kidneys, resulting in secondary retention of salt and water from increased aldosterone secretion and other less well defined causes, which in turn leads to the congestive phenomena of the lungs and extremities that we call left and right heart failure, respectively. Although cardiac output is maintained adequately at rest in many patients as cardiac disease progresses, there comes a time when additional stresses such as exercise, emotional stress, or tachycardia fail to elicit an adequate increase in cardiac output, resulting in renal hemodynamic changes leading to increased renal tubular reabsorption of sodium. Renal tubular reabsorption of sodium is an important mechanism in regulation of isotonicity and volume of the extracellular fluids. The kidney responds to decreased cardiac output, especially with stress, by requiring increased sodium and water retention to preserve extracellular water and isotonicity. This may be life-saving in the event of hemorrhage but is deleterious in the presence of cardiac failure, causing pulmonary and systemic venous congestion and many of the more distressing clinical symptoms and signs of cardiac failure.

B. Treatment With Low-Sodium Diets: Prior to the advent of diuretic agents which interfere with sodium reabsorption in the renal tubule, the mainstay of treatment to eliminate salt and water in cardiac failure was the low-sodium diet, which reduced sodium reabsorption by presenting less sodium to the renal tubules. In the latter part of the 19th century, Philip Karell, a dietary enthusiast, advocated a skimmed milk diet for the treatment of cardiac failure as well as for other diseases; his regimen (the Karell diet), which consisted solely of 200 ml of skimmed milk 4 times a day given until cardiac failure was improved, was commonly recommended in the USA in the mid 1930s. The diet was low in sodium, fat, and calories and was simpler than a regular diet low in sodium, which required the use of low-sodium bread (which was not readily available) as well as avoidance of other sodium-containing foods. Pfeiffer in 1911 (Fig 10–12) demonstrated that it was the sodium in salt that was harmful because a variety of sodium salts increased weight, decreased urine output, and increased dyspnea in patients with cardiac failure, whereas potassium, calcium, or ammonium salts did not; this set the stage for the rational modern appreciation of the role of sodium in cardiac failure. Widal advocated salt restriction in 1903 but thought it was the chloride and not the sodium ion that was important.

C. Mercurial Diuretics: For many years, mercurial diuretics were the physician's major resource in the

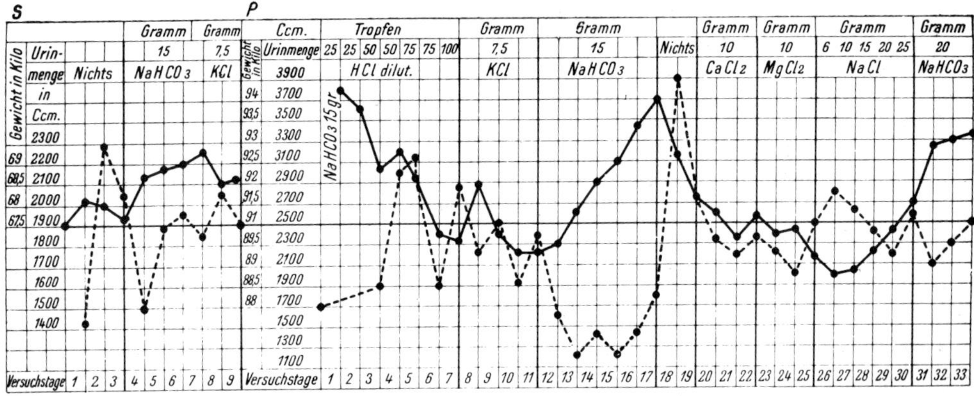

Figure 10–12. This early work from Pfeiffer (1911) showed that a gain in weight and a decrease in urine volume occurred whenever sodium salts such as sodium bicarbonate or sodium chloride were given but that weight gain did not occur when a variety of chloride compounds such as hydrochloric acid, potassium chloride, calcium chloride, and magnesium chloride were used. This demonstrated that it was the sodium ion and not the chloride ion in NaCl that caused the deleterious weight gain and worsening of cardiac failure noted by previous observers. (Reproduced, with permission, from Pfeiffer E: Wasser-Retention durch Natriumsalze. Verhandlungen des Deutschen Kongresses für innere Medizin K27-28:506, 1910–1911.)

diuretic treatment of left ventricular failure, but they had to be given parenterally, usually intravenously. The need for parenteral injection limited the usefulness of this form of treatment, especially in chronic cardiac failure, and the mercurials were used chiefly in hospitals. Oral mercurial therapy never became widely used. Mercurial diuretics act on the proximal tubule and are ineffective when there is impaired renal function and in the presence of hypochloremic alkalosis, which often followed the diuresis. The introduction of the thiazide diuretics in 1957 was a huge step forward and marked the beginning of the modern era of oral diuretic therapy.

D. Rational Use of Diuretic Therapy: The rational use of diuretic therapy (the increased excretion of sodium and water) requires a knowledge of the physiology of the nephron and of the sites in the nephron where sodium is filtered, reabsorbed, and exchanged for potassium (Fig 10–13). Sodium is filtered at the glomerulus, where it enters the proximal renal tubule as part of the protein-free ultrafiltrate fluid that begins its passage down the renal tubule. Drugs such as aminophylline and digoxin that increase the glomerular filtration rate may promote sodium excretion in the urine by increasing the amount of sodium filtered at the glomerulus. Mercurial diuretics act primarily on the proximal tubule (where 70% of the filtered sodium is normally reabsorbed), decreasing the reabsorption of sodium, but may also act on the distal tubule. The more potent, newer "loop" diuretics, such as furosemide and ethacrynic acid, act on the ascending limb of the loop of Henle, where sodium without water is reabsorbed. These so-called loop diuretics prevent reabsorption of sodium in the loop of Henle, with the result that the tubular fluid proceeding distally contains almost all of the sodium filtered at the glomerulus (except for that reabsorbed in the proximal tubule), thus causing diuresis of sodium and water. The thiazide diuretics have their site of action at the beginning of the distal convoluted tubule following the end of the ascending limb of the loop of Henle (see Fig 10–13) and decrease the reabsorption of sodium, thus increasing the excretion of sodium and water (diuresis). However, because the amount of sodium reabsorbed at this site is less than that reabsorbed more proximally in the ascending limb of the loop of Henle, the thiazide diuretics are less potent than the loop diuretics. The tubular fluid containing sodium then proceeds down the distal convoluted tubule to the so-called sodium-potassium exchange site at the end of the tubule, which is under the influence of aldosterone. The amount of potassium exchanged for sodium depends upon the amount of sodium in the tubular fluid delivered to this distal tubular site; it is greater when the sodium in the diet is high or when decreased reabsorption of sodium follows the use of thiazide or loop diuretics. As a result, a drug that prevents reabsorption of sodium as it passes along the tubule increases the excretion of potassium as well as sodium, and loss of both ions is the physiologic result of the diuretic agents. Increased diuresis of sodium is what is desired; increased diuresis of potassium is not desired and may produce hypokalemia–usually mild, with serum potassium rarely below 3 mEq/l.

E. Excessive Sodium Loss With Diuresis: The increased sodium and water retention resulting from decreased cardiac output and consequently decreased glomerular filtration rate in cardiac failure can be counteracted by the diuretic agents. However, with large doses of diuretic agents (especially the potent loop diuretics), when the amount of generalized edema from salt and water retention is great, diuresis may be excessive, ie, the patient may lose such large quantities of salt and water in a matter of days that sodium depletion and hypovolemia replace sodium retention and hypervolemia. The patient may then become lethargic

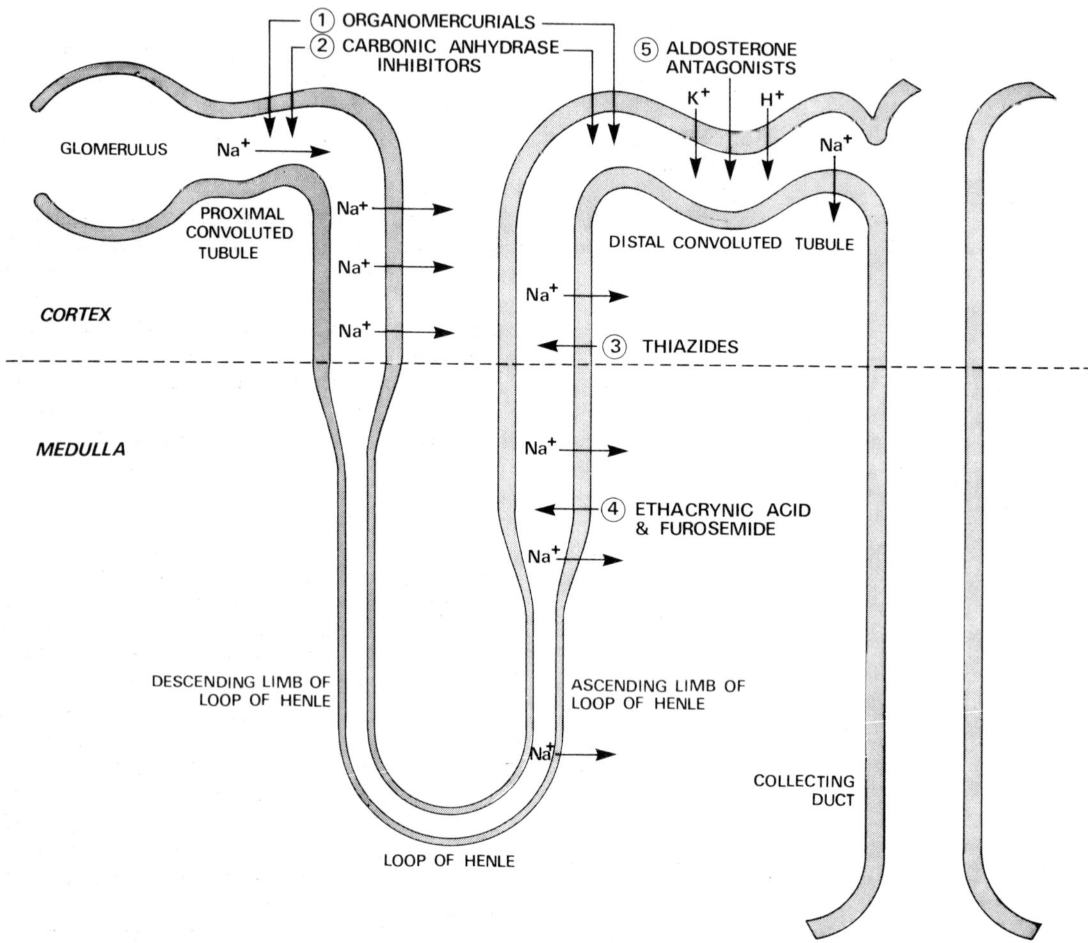

Figure 10–13. Sites of sodium reabsorption in the nephron and of action of different diuretics and carbonic anhydrase inhibitors. The mercurials (1) and carbonic anhydrase inhibitors (2) act in the proximal or distal tubule to inhibit sodium reabsorption. Thiazides (3) act in the ascending limb of the loop of Henle, preventing sodium reabsorption and interfering with dilution. Ethacrynic acid and furosemide (4) also block sodium reabsorption. Aldosterone antagonists (5) prevent potassium excretion and increase sodium excretion. (Adapted and reproduced, with permission, from Laragh JH: Diuretics in the management of congestive heart failure. Hosp Pract 5:43, Nov 1970; and Wilson GM: Diuretics. Practitioner 200:39, 1968.)

and sleepy, have postural hypotension and muscle cramps, and become severely ill. The physician must then liberalize the sodium intake and stop the diuretics until balance has been restored. To prevent excessive hypovolemia, diuresis should be started with milder diuretics in small doses–eg, hydrochlorothiazide, 50 mg daily (or 25 mg in an older patient)–and the dose increased only when it is certain that diuresis is not adequate with the smaller dose.

F. Counteracting Potassium Loss: In patients in whom significant hypokalemia results from the diuretic therapy, a high-potassium diet containing fresh fruits and vegetables, especially oranges, tomato juice, and other foods shown in Table 9–35, is helpful. The average fall in serum potassium in patients receiving 50 mg hydrochlorothiazide twice daily was 0.62 mEq/l. A daily potassium supplement of 60 mEq 10% KCl elixir was required to restore the original level in most patients (Schwartz, 1974). If the serum potassium is still low, agents such as spironolactone, which is a competitive antagonist of aldosterone, or triamterene, which is not, can be used to decrease the amount of potassium exchanged for sodium at the distal sodium-potassium exchange site. Spironolactone by itself is a weak sodium diuretic, but when given in combination with other diuretics it decreases the loss of potassium and so prevents hypokalemia. If, however, the patient has impaired renal function with oliguria or is receiving potassium supplements, serum potassium may rise progressively and hyperkalemia, with resulting severe cardiac conduction defects, may follow. In the presence of normal urine output and normal renal function, spironolactone rarely produces hyperkalemia because of the built-in defense system whereby an increase in serum potassium decreases the secretion of aldosterone. However, if spironolactone or triamterene is used, serum potassium must be monitored frequently and frequent ECGs obtained so that an early rise in serum potassium or the appearance of high peaked T waves will not be missed. When the serum potassium increases to 5 or 6 mg/dl, the drugs should be stopped; levels over 8 mg/dl are extremely dangerous and must be avoided because of the cardiac effects. Because oral potassium supplements are unpleasant to take and only marginally improve the low serum potassium resulting from use of diuretics, spironolactone or triamterene administration in combination with other diuretics to prevent hypokalemia is becoming more widespread with the precautions specified.

Clinical Use of Diuretics

The prototype class of oral diuretic agents is the thiazide group of drugs typified by chlorothiazide and hydrochlorothiazide (see Chapter 9 for additional details about drugs and dosages).

A. Action of Oral Diuretics:

1. Treatment of mild edema—When edema is minimal or the evidence of left ventricular failure is slight, bed rest and sodium restriction may be adequate to effect diuresis.

2. Treatment of more severe failure—When cardiac failure is more severe, diuretic therapy is needed unless absolute bed rest and restriction of sodium intake to 200–300 mg/day are ordered. These restrictions on activity and diet are undesirable, and most patients with cardiac failure are not given strict low-sodium diets. Moderate restriction of sodium (no added salt in the diet) and small doses of a diuretic will usually reverse the salt and water retention that occurs with moderate cardiac failure.

B. Drugs and Dosages:

1. Thiazide diuretics—The initial dose of the thiazide diuretics is 25–50 mg of hydrochlorothiazide once daily, increased to 50 mg twice daily or to 100 mg once or twice daily if the diuresis is inadequate. The dose-response characteristics of the thiazides are such that the maximum response occurs at a dosage of 100 mg, so this dosage should not be exceeded in a single dose. The drug should be given intermittently (every other day or 2–3 times a week if possible) to allow restoration of losses of potassium and sodium; if the patient can be held at a steady dry weight without symptoms with a diuretic given twice a week, side-effects are rare. Long-acting diuretics (chlorthalidone, metolazone) are discussed in Chapter 9.

2. Furosemide and ethacrynic acid—If cardiac failure is severe or renal failure is present, and diuresis does not occur with use of drugs of moderate potency such as the thiazides, more potent drugs such as furosemide or ethacrynic acid can be used which act on the ascending loop of Henle and have a dose-response curve that results in continued excretion of sodium up to a dose of 500 mg. It is the size of the individual dose rather than the daily dose that matters. The more potent diuretics may be started in a dosage of 40 mg daily, but this can be gradually quadrupled and then given twice daily if necessary, depending upon the severity of the heart failure and the presence of renal failure. When given orally, both the thiazides and the loop diuretics begin to act in about an hour, reach a peak in about 4 hours, and have varying durations of action sometimes extending into the next 24-hour period. When the more potent diuretics are given intravenously, as is done in the management of acute pulmonary edema, there may be significant diuresis within 15–30 minutes.

3. Spironolactone and triamterene—These diuretics counteract the action of aldosterone at the distal tubule Na^+-K^+ exchange site (spironolactone by competitive antagonism). They rarely are used alone but are combined with thiazide or "loop" diuretics to diminish potassium loss. They should not be used in the presence of oliguria or renal failure because of the hazard of hyperkalemia (see Chapter 9). Acetazolamide, acidifying drugs, aminophylline, and osmotic diuretics are rarely useful in cardiac failure.

Toxicity of Diuretics

In addition to sodium depletion and hypokalemia (discussed above), chronic hypovolemia produced by the diuretics as well as by direct action of the diuretics on the renal tubule may result in 20–30% increases of serum creatinine and uric acid and occasionally of plasma or serum glucose. Patients with a history of gout may develop acute gouty arthritis, and the dosage of thiazides must be reduced or the patient be given a uricosuric drug such as probenecid. Diabetes mellitus is rarely induced in individuals with no history of the disease, but in patients with diabetes, hyperglycemia induced by diuretics may require increasing doses of insulin. The slight increases in serum creatinine and uric acid and plasma or serum glucose and the associated hypokalemia usually cause no symptoms and are reversible when the agents are discontinued. The long-term hazards of these biochemical changes are not known, but there have been no reports of their deleterious effects on the kidney or other organs despite the fact that the thiazides have been used for almost 20 years.

Metabolic Alkalosis

Additional electrolyte and water disturbances that may occur in patients with cardiac failure treated with diuretic agents include hypokalemic and hypochloremic alkalosis. An increase in serum bicarbonate compensates for the loss of chloride and hydrogen ions, because both hydrogen and potassium are exchanged in the distal tubule for sodium. Chloride replacement is necessary, and correction of hypokalemia corrects the hypokalemic alkalosis; this requires the use of potassium chloride.

Dilutional Hyponatremia

Dilutional hyponatremia may occur in treated cardiac failure, especially when water intake is increased. In contrast to patients who develop depletional hyponatremia due to sodium depletion resulting from excessive diuresis, patients with dilutional hyponatremia (although they may have equivalent degrees of hyponatremia, sometimes to as low as 110 mEq/l) continue to have generalized edema despite low serum sodium. Edelman (1958) and Maffly (1961) clarified this picture in a series of experiments showing that the edema almost always occurred in association with an increase in total body sodium and that edema in the presence of hyponatremia indicated an excess of body water rather than a depletion of body sodium. Edelman concluded that the serum sodium concentration served as a means of estimating the osmolality of the body fluids and reflected the total body solute/body water ratio. The use of hypertonic saline, which is valuable in depletional hyponatremia, may worsen cardiac failure in dilutional hyponatremia because the total body sodium is already increased. The patient may be very ill, thirsty, and weak, and treatment consists of decreasing the water intake to about 500–700 ml/day and giving furosemide if necessary. As excess body water is lost through the skin and lungs, the balance between sodium and water is restored and the serum sodium gradually rises.

There is some evidence that the syndrome can be treated also with the potent loop diuretics combined with diminished water intake, thereby increasing sodium excretion and decreasing fluid intake.

In depletional hyponatremia, the specific gravity of the urine is usually high; in dilutional hyponatremia it is low because of decreased solute excretion.

Caution With Diuretic Therapy

Diuretic therapy should be used with caution in patients who are receiving digitalis because hypokalemia increases the hazard of digitalis toxicity. Diuretics should be used intermittently whenever possible and in the smallest effective dose, and digitalis should be given cautiously, with frequent observations including determinations of serum digitalis levels. Not only may hypokalemia and digitalis interact to increase digitalis toxicity, but the sicker cardiac patients may have decreased appetite and take less potassium in their diet, aggravating the situation. In these circumstances, small doses of spironolactone can be added if oliguria or renal failure is not present. In addition to the hyperkalemia which may then result, patients should be observed for hirsutism and enlarged breasts, which can be very painful. In the presence of renal failure, the loop diuretics are effective, whereas the thiazides are not; spironolactone should be avoided, especially if there is oliguria with renal failure. The loop diuretics are not recommended for the treatment of moderate cardiac failure if adequate diuresis can be achieved with the milder diuretics such as the thiazides, but one should not hesitate to use them if the thiazides fail.

6. IDENTIFY & TREAT UNSUSPECTED OR UNRECOGNIZED ACUTE MYOCARDIAL DISORDERS

The principal examples are listed in Chapter 17. The cause of cardiac failure is often unsuspected unless one specifically seeks it out by using appropriate investigative technics. Acute dyspnea may mask the chest discomfort of acute myocardial infarction. The fever of infective endocarditis may be low-grade and intermittent. Murmurs may be minimal, and preexisting cardiac disease may be unsuspected, especially in drug addicts. Acute nephritis with salt and water retention may be entirely unsuspected unless one examines the urine, takes the blood pressure, and *thinks* of the possibility. Acute pericardial effusion must be distinguished from cardiac dilatation not only because unrecognized tamponade may be life-threatening but also because the cause of the effusion must be determined and specific therapy given as needed. (For further details see Chapters 9, 15, 16, 17, and 20.)

7. TREAT OPERABLE CONDITIONS THAT INCREASE THE LOAD ON THE HEART OR INTERFERE WITH LEFT VENTRICULAR FUNCTION

This should be done after maximal improvement has been achieved on medical treatment. Obviously, emergency situations must always be dealt with first, but the ideal management of cardiac failure is to identify and remove the cause of ventricular dysfunction if that is possible. Medical treatment is a temporizing measure that does not reach the underlying cause. Operative procedures may also be palliative but in many instances can be semicurative and result in dramatic improvement.

Conditions potentially treatable by means of operation should be evaluated while the patient is responding to bed rest and medical treatment. (See other chapters for surgical treatment of individual diseases.)

8. TREAT EXTRACARDIAC FACTORS

Extracardiac factors that increase the work of the heart include fever, anemia, acid-base, electrolyte, and endocrine abnormalities, hypoxia, and obesity, among many others. These factors increase the heart rate and myocardial oxygen demand; may decrease coronary blood flow and produce myocardial ischemia; may lead to the development of cardiac arrhythmias, with resulting impairment of coronary perfusion and production of myocardial ischemia; and may aggravate or induce toxicity from therapeutic agents such as digitalis when hypokalemia is present. Cardiac failure induced by such extracardiac factors should be treated in accordance with the principles outlined in this chapter. At the same time, the underlying extracardiac factors should also be treated with appropriate measures.

9. DIGITALIS

In addition to rest, diuretics, management of arrhythmias, and the other approaches discussed above, treatment with digitalis should be started.

Digitalis has been one of the major medical resources in the treatment of cardiac failure ever since William Withering, in 1785, described the use of aqueous extracts of the leaves of the foxglove plant in the treatment of that disorder. There are a wide variety of digitalislike preparations, but digitalis is the generic term for any compound containing a steroid glycoside ring, a lactone ring, and a sugar residue. Differences in the sugar residues of various compounds influence their absorption, potency, and duration of action (see Tables 10–3 and 10–4). In recent years, digitalis leaf and digitoxin have been used less frequently than digoxin, the former because it is poorly absorbed and the latter because of its long duration of action. The purified glycosides with shorter duration of action, such as digoxin, are overwhelmingly the most frequent digitalis preparations used in the USA, and the same applies to similar preparations, perhaps with different names, used in other parts of the world. In Table 10–4 are listed the dosages and methods of administration of

Table 10–3. Average adult dosages of digitalis drugs given orally to digitalize and then to maintain digitalization, according to degree of urgency. Maintenance dosages are only averages and may be varied according to individual patient response.

Urgency	Drug	Dosage
Moderate	Digitalis leaf	0.4 g every 8 hours for 3 doses, then 0.1 g/day.
	Digitoxin	0.4 mg every 8 hours for 3 doses, then 0.1 mg/day.
	Digoxin	0.5 mg every 8 hours for 3 doses, then 0.25 mg once daily.
Intermediate	Digitalis leaf	0.2 g 3 times daily for 2 days or 0.1 g 4 times daily for 3 days, then 0.1 g/day.
	Digitoxin	0.2 mg 3 times daily for 2 days, then 0.1 mg/day.
	Digoxin	0.5 mg twice daily for 2 days or 0.25 mg 3 times daily for 3 days, then 0.25 mg once daily.
Least	Digitalis leaf	0.1 g 3 times daily for 4–5 days, then 0.1 g/day.
	Digitoxin	0.1 mg 3 times daily for 4–6 days, then 0.1 mg/day.
	Digoxin	0.25 mg twice daily for 4–6 days, then 0.25 mg once daily.

Table 10–4. Cardiac glycoside preparations: Average adult doses and routes of administration.*

Glycoside and Preparations Available	Dose		Rapid Method of Administration	Speed; Maximum Action and Duration
	Digitalizing	Maintenance		
Parenteral preparations				
Ouabain, 1 and 2 ml ampules, 0.25 mg	0.25–0.5 mg	Not used for maintenance	0.25–0.5 mg (1–2 ml) diluted in 10 ml saline slowly IV; follow with another drug (see below).	3–10 min; 30–90 min; duration, 12–36 hours.
Deslanoside (Cedilanid-D), 2 and 4 ml ampules, 0.4 and 0.8 mg	8 ml (1.6 mg)	0.2–0.4 mg (1–2 ml)	1.2 mg (6 ml) IV or IM and follow with 0.2–0.4 mg (1–2 ml) IV or IM every 3–4 hours until effect is obtained.	1–2 hours; duration, 3–6 days.
Digitoxin (dilute before use), 1 and 2 ml ampules, 0.2 and 0.4 mg	1.2 mg (6 ml)	0.05–0.2 mg	0.6 mg (3 ml) IV or IM followed by 0.2–0.4 mg every 4–6 hours until 1.2 mg has been given.	3–8 hours; duration, 14–21 days.
Digoxin (Lanoxin), 2 ml ampules, 0.25 mg/ml	1.5 mg (6 ml)	0.125–0.75 mg (1–3 ml)	0.5–1 mg (2–4 ml) IV and 0.25–0.5 mg (1–2 ml) in 3–4 hours; then 0.25 mg (1 ml) every 3–4 hours until effect is obtained.	1–2 hours; duration, 3–6 days.
Oral preparations				
Digitalis, 0.03, 0.06, and 0.1 g tablets	1–1.5 g	0.05–0.2 g	0.6 g stat; 0.4 g in 6–8 hours; 0.2 g every 6 hours for 2–3 doses; then 0.1 g twice daily until effect is obtained.	6–8 hours; duration, 18–21 days.
Digitoxin, 0.1, 0.15, and 0.2 mg tablets	1.2 mg	0.05–0.2 mg	0.6 mg stat and repeat in 12 hours and then 0.2 mg twice daily until effect is obtained.	6–8 hours; duration, 14–21 days.
Digoxin, 0.25 and 0.5 mg tablets	1.5–3 mg	0.125–0.5 mg	1 mg stat and then 0.25–0.5 mg every 6 hours until effect is obtained.	4–6 hours; duration, 2–6 days.
Lanatoside C (Cedilanid), 0.5 mg tablets	7.5 mg	0.5–1.5 mg	2 mg stat and then 0.5–0.75 mg every 6 hours until effect is obtained.	
Acetyldigitoxin (Acylanid), 0.1 and 0.2 mg tablets	1.6–2.4 mg	0.1–0.2 mg	1.6 mg in 24 hours or 0.6–1 mg daily until effect is obtained.	4–6 hours; duration, 14–21 days.
Gitalin (Gitaligin), 0.5 mg tablets	4–6 mg	0.5 mg	1 mg 3 times on first day followed by 0.5 mg every 6 hours until effect is obtained.	4–6 hours; duration, 8–14 days.

*Check manufacturers' descriptive literature. Dosage sizes of tablets and ampules change from time to time.

Table 10–5. Digoxin and digitoxin serum levels.*†

	Serum Levels (ng/ml)	
	Therapeutic	**Toxic**
Digoxin	0.5–2.5	3+
Digitoxin	20–35	45+

*Reproduced, with permission, from Doherty JE: Digitalis glycosides: Pharmacokinetics and their clinical implications. Ann Intern Med 79:229, 1973.

†Significant overlap may occur in electrolyte (K^+, Mg^{2+}) imbalance, thyroid disease, myocardial infarction, and hypoxia.

glycoside preparations (both oral and parenteral) that are available for clinical use. Table 10–3 lists the average doses of digitalis drugs given orally for digitalization and maintenance, according to degree of urgency. Effective maintenance dosage may differ as much as 5-fold from patient to patient because of individual variation in response.

Indications for Administration (See also Chapter 15.)

(1) Cardiac failure with sinus rhythm or atrial fibrillation.

(2) Atrial fibrillation or flutter with a rapid ventricular rate.

(3) Supraventricular paroxysmal tachycardia.

(4) Prevention of paroxysmal atrial or junctional arrhythmias in patients in whom quinidine has failed or is not tolerated.

(5) As maintenance therapy to prevent recurrence of cardiac failure in patients who have received digitalis initially for cardiac failure (Fig 10–14).

Mechanism of Action

The exact mechanisms by which digitalis preparations increase the inotropic properties of the heart are not universally agreed on, but there is no doubt that digitalis increases the force and velocity of cardiac contraction whether or not the heart is failing. Digitalis apparently has no direct action on the metabolism of heart muscle except as it affects excitation-contraction coupling by affecting the movement of calcium ions and electrolytes. The use of beta-adrenergic blocking agents does not interfere with the inotropic action of digitalis, and this apparently rules out the sympathetic nervous system as the mediator of its inotropic effect.

Table 10–6. Frequency of various digitalis-induced arrhythmias in 10 series with a total of 631 patients.*

	Number of Series	Number of Arrhythmias		
Ventricular arrhythmias		470 (71%)		
Ventricular premature beats			420	
Bigeminy	9			150
Multifocal	4			121
Not specified	4			79
Other (frequent, unifocal, occasional, etc)	3			70
Ventricular tachycardia	7		50	
Atrioventricular block		194 (29%)		
First degree	7		87	
Second degree	10		58	
Wenckebach	3			4
Third degree	6		37	
Unspecified	2		12	
Atrial arrhythmias		177 (26%)		
Atrial fibrillation	9		80	
With slow rate	2			21
Paroxysmal atrial tachycardia with block	7		59	
Atrial premature beats	4		27	
Atrial flutter	4		11	
Sinoatrial arrhythmias		85 (13%)		
Sinus tachycardia	3		29	
Sinus bradycardia	4		27	
With nodal escape	1			11
Sinus arrest	2		11	
Sinoatrial block	3		7	
Wandering pacemaker	3		11	
Atrioventricular dissociation	4	65 (9.8%)		
Atrioventricular nodal arrhythmias		47 (7%)		
Nodal tachycardia	4		32	
Nodal rhythm	2		11	
Nodal premature beats	1		4	

*Reproduced, with permission, from Fisch C: Treatment of arrhythmias due to digitalis. J Indiana State Med Assoc 60:146, 1967.

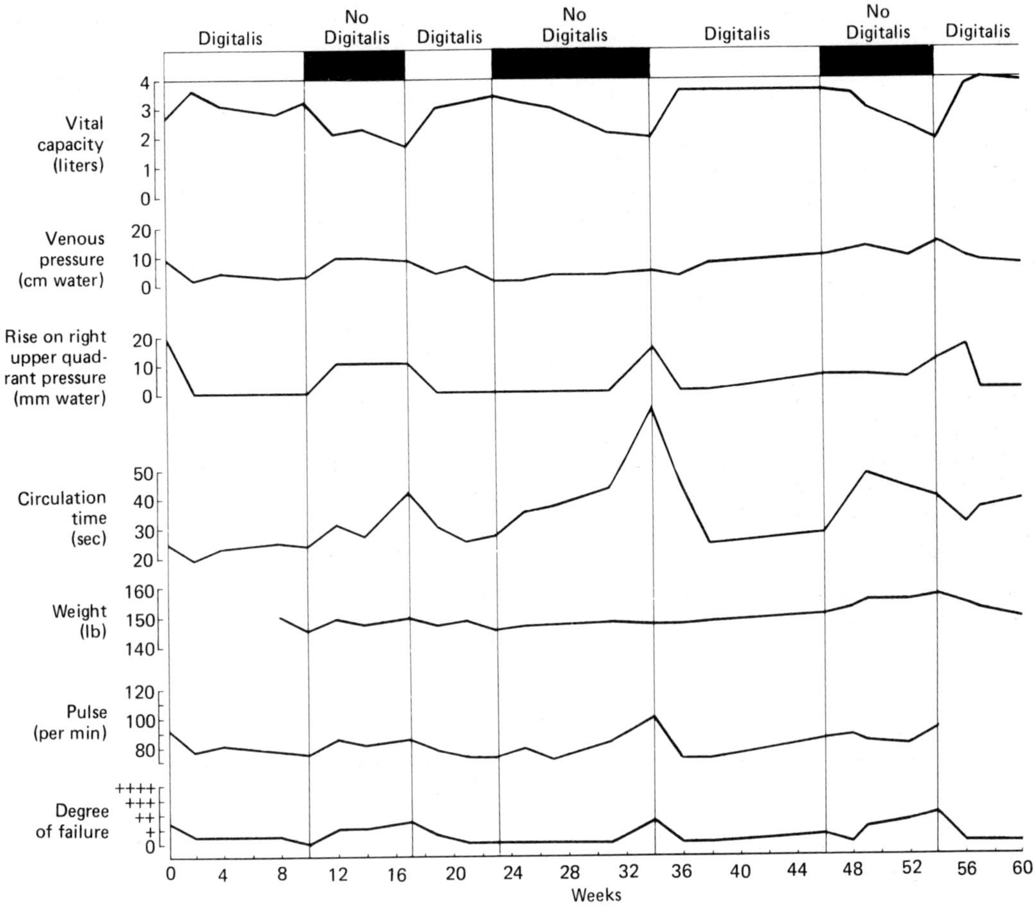

Figure 10–14. Note the decrease in vital capacity, increase in venous pressure (at rest and after right upper quadrant pressure), increase in circulation time, and increase in degree of cardiac failure with minimal change in weight when digitalis was stopped, and the improvement when digitalis was restarted in a patient who previously had cardiac failure. The only change in treatment was omission of digitalis. (Reproduced, with permission, from Sokolow M & others: Digitalis in the prevention of recurrent cardiac failure in patients with sinus rhythm. Ann Intern Med 16:427, 1942.)

Digitalis is bound to sites on the membrane of heart muscle cells, where it may affect the net uptake of potassium, sodium, and calcium. Increased availability of calcium ions, enhancing cardiac contraction, is thought by many to be the basic mechanism by which digitalis acts to increase the force and velocity of contraction.

Digitalis has a potent electrophysiologic action that results in increased automaticity of the secondary pacemakers in the atrial-atrioventricular nodal junction, in the atrioventricular nodal-His bundle junction, and in secondary pacemakers throughout the Purkinje system responsible for the ectopic rhythms which are a sign of digitalis toxicity. In addition, digitalis decreases impulse conduction in the heart, which is desirable when conduction is delayed through the atrioventricular node in patients with atrial fibrillation but undesirable when it leads to reentry phenomena and paroxysmal atrial arrhythmias. Its electrophysiologic action is thought to be due to its inhibiting effect on the active sodium-potassium pump mechanism, which affects the flow of sodium and potassium across the membranes of cardiac cells and, in toxic doses, markedly alters the action potential of both ordinary and automatic cells. Digitalis slows conduction velocity by increasing the refractory period of both specialized and ordinary cells, and when this occurs in the atrioventricular node it is of special benefit to patients with atrial fibrillation because it slows the ventricular rate. Digitalis increases the automaticity of cells by increasing the rate of spontaneous diastolic depolarization (phase 4; see Chapter 14), and in larger doses it decreases the slope of initial rapid depolarization (phase 0) and decreases the magnitude and shortens the duration of the action potential.

Pathophysiologic & Hemodynamic Effects

One must distinguish the effects of digitalis described above on the isolated cardiac muscle fiber in vitro from the clinical effects in the patient with cardiac failure or myocardial ischemia. Hemodynamic studies in patients who are in manifest heart failure have shown that digitalis increases cardiac output, decreases right atrial and peripheral venous pressure, decreases the filling pressure of the left ventricle, and increases the urinary excretion of sodium and water, thereby correcting some of the hemodynamic and metabolic abnormalities in cardiac failure. These clinical effects are not uniform, however, and digitalis is less effective in the presence of acute myocarditis, myocardial ischemia, high output cardiac failure, pulmonary or systemic venous congestion resulting from mechanical defects, and some cases of diffuse extensive primary cardiomyopathy or ischemic cardiomyopathy. It is possible that the stage of hemodynamic alteration in cardiac failure affects the response to digitalis and that this may explain the minimal hemodynamic benefit seen in some patients. Digitalis is more effective in the presence of atrial fibrillation with a rapid ventricular rate because its ability to block conduction through the atrioventricular node decreases the ventricular rate and improves coronary perfusion and results in better ventricular filling during diastole, decreasing left atrial pressure and pulmonary venous congestion. The effect of slowing the ventricular rate is particularly advantageous in the presence of obstructive lesions such as mitral stenosis. The increased myocardial oxygen demand resulting from the increased force of cardiac contraction from the inotropic action of digitalis may be deleterious if the oxygen supply cannot be increased because of severe coronary disease. For this reason, digitalis infrequently shows consistent hemodynamic benefit in patients with acute myocardial infarction with cardiac failure, although in some studies the stroke work index has improved even when cardiac output has not.

Pharmacokinetics

A. Effect of Drug: As is true of all drugs, the various digitalis preparations may have different clinical effects depending upon the rate of absorption, the amount of body fluid in which the drug is distributed, its bioavailability, the renal function, the rate of metabolic degradation, thyroid function, and the mode of excretion—all of which may differ in different patients, so that no one dosage schedule is suitable for all patients. The bioavailability of digitalis—or the amount absorbed and available to the body—became a matter of concern to the FDA after it was found that giving apparently equivalent doses of a number of digoxin preparations resulted in widely different serum digoxin levels. This could be of clinical importance if patients stabilized on one manufacturer's preparation shifted to a similar drug from a different manufacturer. Some patients developed symptoms of toxicity and had higher blood levels, whereas in others the therapeutic effect disappeared because impaired absorption of the new preparation decreased its availability. The result has been that FDA now includes dissolution rates as a part of the criteria for acceptance of all digoxin and other preparations. All digoxin and other preparations must now meet these requirements, and it is anticipated that bioavailability will not be a problem in the future.

B. Effects of Body Physiology: A number of studies have been published on the kinetics of digoxin and other digitalis preparations (Doherty, 1973). In addition to the speed of dissolution of the tablets, absorption is enhanced by sluggish gastrointestinal motility and hypothyroidism, decreased by the concomitant use of nonabsorbable drugs or antacids; it is increased by hyperthyroidism and the use of elixir as compared to tablet digoxin preparations. In patients with normal renal function, the mean half-life of digoxin is about 36 hours, but the range is wide and the standard deviation is about 8 hours. In contrast, the half-life of digitoxin is 4–6 days. (The half-life is the time required for the digoxin in the body to decrease by 50%.) The renal excretion of digoxin depends on the glomerular filtration rate and not on the volume of urine; the dose of drug must be decreased in patients with impaired renal function and reduced glomerular filtration rate to prevent accumulation with high serum levels and toxicity. Fig 10–15 relates the BUN to the dose of digoxin, reflecting the delayed clearance in the presence of poor renal function.

Radioisotope studies have shown that when digoxin is given to patients who have not received digitalis in the past few days, a daily dose leads to a steady-state serum digoxin level in 6–9 days. If renal function is normal, a loading or saturation dose—once thought to be essential—is now considered unnecessary unless rapid digitalization is desired. A daily dose of digoxin given for 4–5 "half-lives" of digoxin results in a steady-state plateau of serum digoxin even if the dose is continued indefinitely. The drug is bound tightly to the tissues and so is not removed by dialysis or by open heart bypass procedures.

The half-life of other digitalis preparations varies from about 21 hours for ouabain to 4–6 days for digitalis leaf or digitoxin.

C. Digoxin Levels Affected by Dosage: About three-fourths of an oral dose of digoxin is absorbed from the gastrointestinal tract, and patients who have reached a steady state with daily maintenance doses of the drug achieve a new peak within 3 hours of administration of the next oral dose of digoxin, with the level beginning to rise within an hour. Because about one-third of the body stores of digoxin is excreted daily (assuming normal renal function) and because the half-life of digoxin is about 1½ days, the effects of digoxin will be dissipated in 4–5 days (4–5 half-lives) after the drug is stopped. The serum levels fall to zero in a week, but this may not adequately reflect the total loss of digoxin from the body since ST–T abnormalities caused by digitalis may persist for as long as 3 weeks after the drug has been stopped.

Serum Digoxin Levels

Recent technologic developments, including radio-

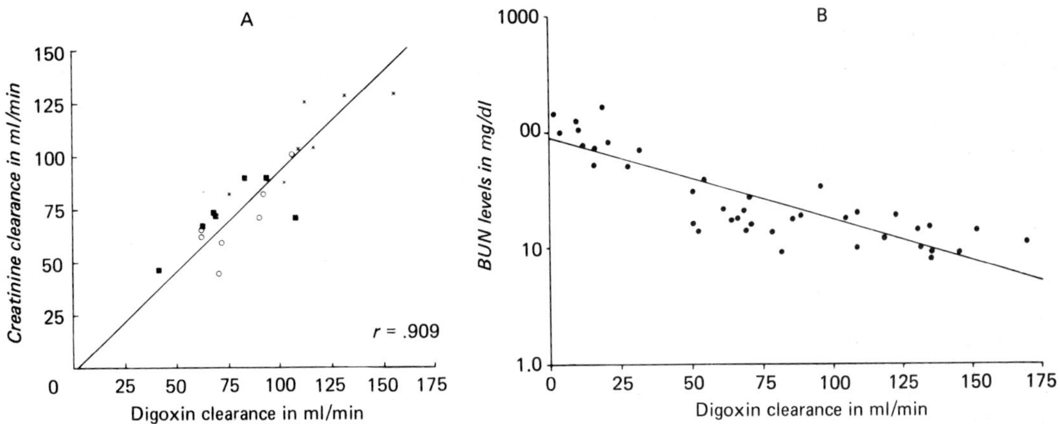

Figure 10–15. *A:* Relationship of creatinine clearance to digoxin clearance in donors before (x) and after (○) unilateral nephrectomy and in recipients (■) of these kidneys. The correlation coefficient, $r = .909$, is highly significant. (Reproduced, with permission, from Doherty JE, Flanigan WJ, Dalrymple GV: Tritiated digoxin. 17. Excretion and turnover times in normal donors before and after nephrectomy and in the paired recipient of the kidney after transplantation. Am J Cardiol 29:470, 1972.) *B:* Relationship of the blood urea nitrogen (BUN) to the clearance of digoxin. The higher the BUN level, the lower the digoxin clearance. (Reproduced, with permission, from Doherty JE: Digitalis glycosides: Pharmacokinetics and their clinical implications. Ann Intern Med 79:229, 1973.)

immunoassay technics, have permitted accurate and reliable measurement of serum digoxin and digitoxin levels (Table 10–5) which can be correlated with the dose of the drug and the clinical effects (Smith, 1969). Age, renal function, thyroid status, and interference with absorption by noncardiac drugs have all been shown to influence the serum digoxin level. The average serum digoxin levels 7–10 days following a daily dose average approximately 0.8, 1, and 1.4 ng/ml as the daily dose is increased from 0.125 mg to 0.25 mg and 0.5 mg/day (Marcus, 1975). The average levels in each group of patients receiving the respective maintenance dose are associated with a large standard deviation, indicating a considerable overlap between daily dose and blood level in different patients. In general, levels under 2 ng/ml are not likely to be associated with digitalis toxicity, whereas levels greater than 3 ng/ml are quite likely to be associated with toxic effects. Careful judgment is required in attempting to use the serum level as an isolated indication of toxicity (Smith, 1975). The factor most often neglected in patients receiving digitalis who develop digitalis toxicity is renal function. In patients with renal failure the half-life of digoxin is prolonged, resulting in toxic serum levels unless smaller doses of the drug are given. Thyroid abnormalities, electrolyte and acid-base balance, the severity and nature of the underlying heart disease, the patient's age and renal function, and the patient's compliance with therapy are other important factors. Serum levels must be interpreted in the light of all of the factors that might influence toxicity, including interactions with other drugs the patient may be taking. Serum levels are particularly helpful in patients who are unable to give a clear clinical history, especially of preceding digitalis administration, and whenever patients fail to respond to the drug or seem to become toxic with only average doses of digoxin (Smith, 1975).

Administration of Digoxin

(See also Tables 10–3 and 10–4.)

A. Average Situation: As noted above, in the average patient with mild to moderate cardiac failure in whom digitalization is not urgent, digoxin can be given orally in an average maintenance dose of 0.25 mg/day. If the patient is old or has impaired renal function, hypothyroidism, or hypokalemia, the dose should be halved, eg, 0.125 mg/day. No saturation or loading dose is required. If after 7–10 days a therapeutic effect has not been obtained (relief of cardiac failure, slowing of the ventricular rate, diuresis and weight loss), serum digoxin levels should be measured to be certain that the patient is absorbing or taking the drug and that an adequate serum level has been achieved. If the serum level is low (< 0.8–1.2 ng/ml) and clinical improvement has not occurred, the daily dose can be increased to 0.375 mg/day for 7–10 days and the serum digoxin level again determined. If the level is still low, the maintenance dose can be increased to 0.5 mg/day. Some patients require 0.75 mg/day to produce clinical benefit without toxicity. In rare instances, even larger doses have been given, but these reports are suspect in the light of recent data on bioavailability (see above). In general, when digitalis is given, all other factors that might have a bearing on digitalis toxicity should be stabilized so that a maintenance dose can be established that will be safe over a prolonged period. Serum levels measured when renal function is fluctuating, with varying degrees of hypoxia or acid-base imbalance, varying degrees of hypokalemia resulting from diuretic therapy, and unstable clinical manifestations such as ischemia cannot be used to determine the proper maintenance dose for a patient in the steady state.

B. Urgent Situation: If the clinical situation is more urgent, with increasing dyspnea and orthopnea, give 0.25 or 0.5 mg of digoxin every 6 hours until 1.5 mg has been given and then maintain the level with 0.25 mg every 8–12 hours until the appearance of evidence of therapeutic benefit or toxicity or until serum digoxin levels exceed 2.5–3 ng/ml. If satisfactory blood levels following a proper dose are not accompanied by adequate therapeutic effect, the dose should not be increased but the situation reassessed and other forms of treatment used (see below). As already noted, the clinical response to digitalis is not uniformly good, especially in severe cardiac failure or when failure is due to extracardiac, mechanical, or inflammatory causes. About 20% of patients given digoxin in general hospitals develop signs of toxicity, perhaps because they continue to receive progressive increments of digoxin after failing to respond to usually adequate doses.

C. More Urgent Situation: When it is necessary to obtain a digitalis effect within hours, as in pulmonary edema, or when symptomatic atrial fibrillation occurs postoperatively, or in the presence of mitral stenosis, or when the rapid ventricular rate produces dyspnea, angina, or cerebral impairment, intravenous therapy can be given, eg, deslanoside (Cedilanid-D), 0.2–0.4 mg intravenously every 2–4 hours to a total of 0.8 mg; or digoxin, one-third to one-half of the total (1–1.5 mg) digitalizing dose every 2–4 hours, decreasing the dose by half when the ventricular rate begins to slow. Oral digoxin therapy should then be started to avoid toxicity, which is more likely to occur when frequent doses of digoxin are given intravenously.

Criteria of Adequate Digitalization

Digitalis is administered until a therapeutic effect is achieved (eg, relief of cardiac failure or slowing of the ventricular rate in atrial fibrillation) or until anorexia or arrhythmia appears (the earliest toxic effect). In congestive failure with normal sinus rhythm, digitalization is adequate (1) if further diuresis with weight loss and loss of edema fluid occurs; (2) if cardiac size is decreased as the increased force and velocity of contraction improve the cardiac output and decrease cardiac dilatation; (3) if the jugular venous pressure and circulation time return toward normal; (4) if sinus tachycardia decreases (if the increase was due to cardiac failure); (5) if an engorged, tender liver becomes smaller and nontender; and (6) if symptoms of congestive failure subside or disappear. In atrial fibrillation, slowing of the ventricular rate to less than 80/min after mild exercise such as 5 or 6 sit-ups is usually sufficient evidence that digitalis is blocking atrial impulses in the atrioventricular node.

The most characteristic ECG. changes following administration of digitalis are sagging, depressed ST segments in a direction opposite to that of the major QRS deflection in the lead involved. This causes depressed sagging ST segments in the left ventricular leads and reciprocal elevated "reversed sagging" ST changes in the right arm lead (Figs 10–16 and 10–17). Later, especially if the serum levels are higher, the P–R interval may be prolonged as partial atrioventricular block develops and the Q–T interval shortens as the duration of the action potential decreases. ST–T changes cannot be used as criteria of digitalis toxicity but merely of digitalis effect because they do not correlate positively with toxic symptoms or other manifestations such as arrhythmia; furthermore, they may

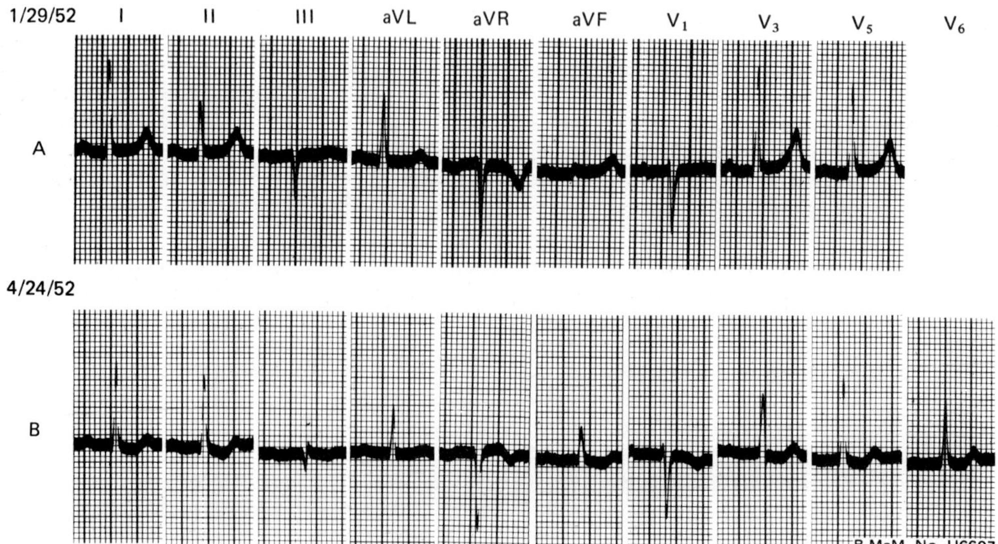

Figure 10–16. Typical sagging ST–T changes resulting from digitalis administration in a 52-year-old woman. Tracing A on 1/29/52 shows slight left ventricular hypertrophy and no ST abnormalities. The patient was digitalized on 2/12/52 and given digitalis leaf, 0.1 g 3 times daily. Tracing B on 4/24/52 shows typical ST sagging.

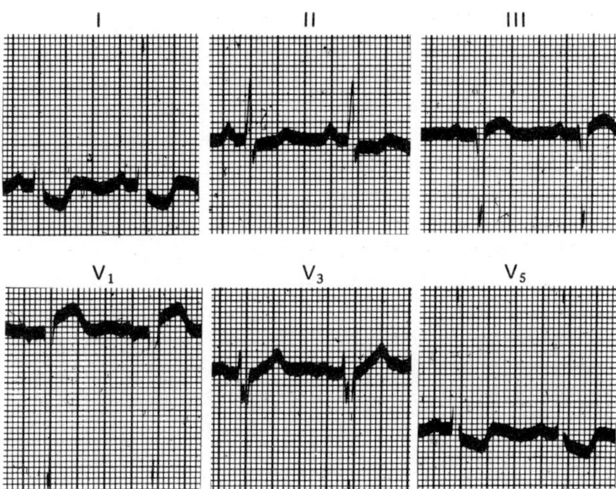

Figure 10–17. ST changes in a 56-year-old woman with left ventricular hypertrophy given digitalis. The patient had hypertensive cardiac failure and was digitalized. The sagging ST segments are superimposed on left ventricular hypertrophy.

persist after the serum levels fall to zero. Typical ST–T changes are helpful, however, in alerting the physician to the possibility that the patient has been receiving digitalis without knowing it.

Digitalis Toxicity

A. Symptoms and Signs; ECG Changes: In patients with cardiac failure who are otherwise in a relatively stable state, the first manifestation of digitalis toxicity is usually anorexia or mild nausea. To detect this change one must obtain a clear history of appetite before beginning digitalis therapy. If the patient is seen before each dose and the drug stopped when anorexia or mild nausea develops, more important manifestations of toxicity can be avoided, and the gastrointestinal symptoms will subside in 24 hours.

The most common important myocardial manifestation of digitalis toxicity is cardiac arrhythmia which results from enhanced automaticity and decreased conduction in the specialized automatic cells in the atria and ventricles and in the atrioventricular node. The combination leads to reentry as well as ectopic rhythms (Table 10–6). Ventricular premature beats are the most common arrhythmia occurring as a result of digitalis overdosage, but they do not usually progress to ventricular tachycardia or fibrillation unless early warnings are ignored, large doses are used, or high serum levels result from impaired renal function or other factors previously discussed.

Paroxysmal atrial tachycardia with block is probably the next most common arrhythmia; the pacemaker focus of the atrial arrhythmia is often the junctional tissue at the atrial-atrioventricular nodal junction. This arrhythmia is rarely seen in the absence of associated diuretic therapy with hypokalemia–in contrast to the ventricular arrhythmias and atrioventricular block that occur even when diuretics are not used (Fig 15–7).

Atrioventricular block is the third most common disturbance in rhythm in digitalis toxicity, and this is directly related to decreased conduction in the atrioventricular node, which is a cardinal electrophysiologic effect of digitalis. The atrioventricular block is usually slight, consisting only of prolongation of the P–R in-

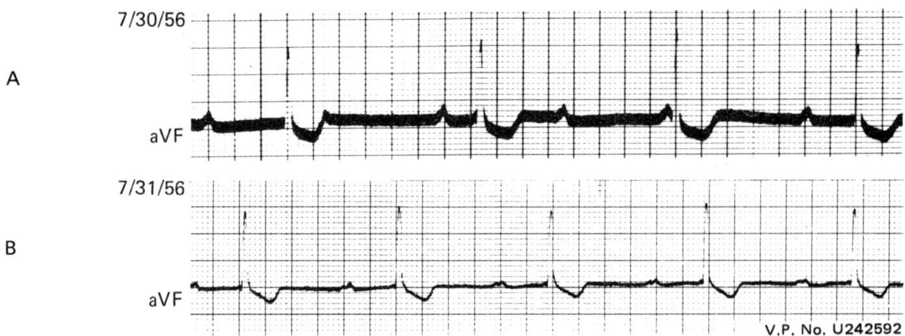

Figure 10–18. *A:* Complete atrioventricular block due to digitalis toxicity in a 60-year-old man given potassium chloride, 10 g orally daily. *B:* Partial atrioventricular block with P–R interval of 0.4 sec in 24 hours.

terval, but in more severe toxicity complete atrioventricular block may occur (Figs 10–18A and 18B). Digitalis also slows conduction in the sinoatrial node, and sinoatrial block with a shift in the pacemaker to the atrioventricular junction or to the lower atrium may result; digitalis excess must always be considered when sinoatrial abnormalities are present. Atrioventricular dissociation (see Chapter 14), with the atria and ventricles beating independently, is most commonly the result of digitalis excess and is due to a combination of atrioventricular block and enhanced pacemaker activity in the junctional regions proximal or distal to the atrioventricular node. The atrioventricular dissociation may be intermittent, owing to a combination of only a partial defect in conduction and the fortuitous occurrence of P waves when the ventricles are not refractory. Atrioventricular dissociation may be due to acceleration of a subsidiary pacemaker in the junctional region even when the dominant sinus pacemaker is not unduly depressed or atrioventricular block present. So-called nonparoxysmal atrioventricular junctional tachycardia due to enhanced acceleration of the junctional pacemaker can occur with or without complete atrioventricular dissociation by chance capture of the ventricles, since atrioventricular block is not present.

B. Influence of Cardiac Disease on Arrhythmias: The extent and type of the underlying cardiac disease influence the likelihood of development of toxicity from digitalis. A person with no heart disease may ingest large doses of digitalis in a suicide attempt without dying or developing severe ventricular arrhythmias, yet patients with severe cardiomyopathy and cardiac failure may develop ventricular arrhythmias with only average doses of digoxin, especially if the drug is given intravenously. Changing conditions during the course of the cardiac illness may precipitate digitalis toxicity even if the dose of the drug is unchanged. These include hypokalemia resulting from diuretic therapy, hypoxia, and decreases in renal function which may follow hypovolemia or decreased cardiac output. Toxicity may therefore occur not because the drug is given incorrectly or in excessive doses but because there are other factors that must be recognized and managed.

C. Cardiac Disease Producing Arrhythmias: Cardiac arrhythmias in patients with cardiac failure do not always imply digitalis toxicity but may occur even when digitalis is not given. This is particularly true in heart failure associated with coronary heart disease, when ventricular arrhythmias may be the composite result of (1) localized ischemia, (2) variable and disproportionate duration of action potentials in adjacent fibers, with disparate refractory periods, and (3) variable conduction because of patchy myocardial fibrosis, leading to reentry or ectopic arrhythmias. The presence of arrhythmia, therefore, must not be assumed to be due to digitalis toxicity, especially at the onset of digitalis administration or if the patient is first seen on a stable maintenance dose.

Cardiac arrhythmias often disappear when cardiac failure is appropriately treated. Clinical judgment based on experience and careful analysis of all of the clinical findings, including serum digoxin levels, may warrant the conclusion that cardiac failure and not digitalis excess is the cause of the arrhythmia. If the reverse is the case and digitalis toxicity is strongly suspected and confirmed by serum digoxin levels, digitalis and diuretics must be stopped and the patient observed closely. If renal function is adequate and serum potassium normal, digitalis-induced arrhythmias usually subside in 2–3 days.

Treatment of Digitalis Toxicity

A. Initial Measures: The obvious initial step is to stop digitalis and diuretics and identify and treat conditions that increase the likelihood of digitalis toxicity: hypokalemia, hypoxia, myocardial ischemia, hypovolemia, and impaired renal function. It is usually sufficient to stop the digitalis and diuretics and observe the patient closely if there are no life-threatening arrhythmias with rapid ventricular rates, such as ventricular tachycardia or multifocal ventricular premature beats occurring early in diastole, or if these arrhythmias do not induce myocardial ischemia or hypotension or make the cardiac failure worse. If rapid ventricular arrhythmias induce severe hemodynamic abnormalities or threaten ventricular fibrillation, intravenous potassium should be infused at a rate of 10–20 mEq/hour unless the patient has hyperkalemia or severely impaired renal function. A common method is to give 50–100 mEq/l of potassium chloride in 5% dextrose or saline at a slow rate of 0.25–0.35 mEq/min. If the situation is less urgent, potassium can be given orally in a dosage not to exceed 100 mEq in 4–6 hours.

B. Alternative Measures: If potassium is ineffective or cannot be used, the most effective drug is phenytoin or propranolol, with quinidine or lidocaine in reserve. The dosages are phenytoin, 3–5 mg/kg intravenously; or propranolol, 0.5–2 mg, at a rate of 0.5 mg/min repeated in 1–2 hours intravenously; or quinidine gluconate, 0.8 g in 500 ml dextrose, 1 ml/min; or lidocaine, 1 mg/kg every 1–5 min followed by an infusion of 0.5–2 mg/min.

C. Monitoring of ECG With Potassium: When potassium is given by infusion, the ECG should be monitored continuously and serum potassium levels determined. Oral therapy should be given when the infusion is stopped. The need for potassium is less urgent in the presence of atrioventricular block, and in such circumstances the drug should be used intravenously with considerable caution. An example of the ECG in hyperkalemia is shown in Fig 10–19.

D. Temporary Pacemaker: If complete atrioventricular block is present with a slow ventricular rate—and especially if it is associated with an accelerated junctional tachycardia—a temporary endocardial pacemaker should be introduced prior to the use of drugs that depress escape pacemakers to avoid ventricular standstill and a Stokes-Adams attack.

E. Electric Cardioversion: Great caution must be exercised in the use of electric cardioversion in the presence of ectopic rhythms which may be due to digitalis toxicity, whether atrial or ventricular. Digitalis

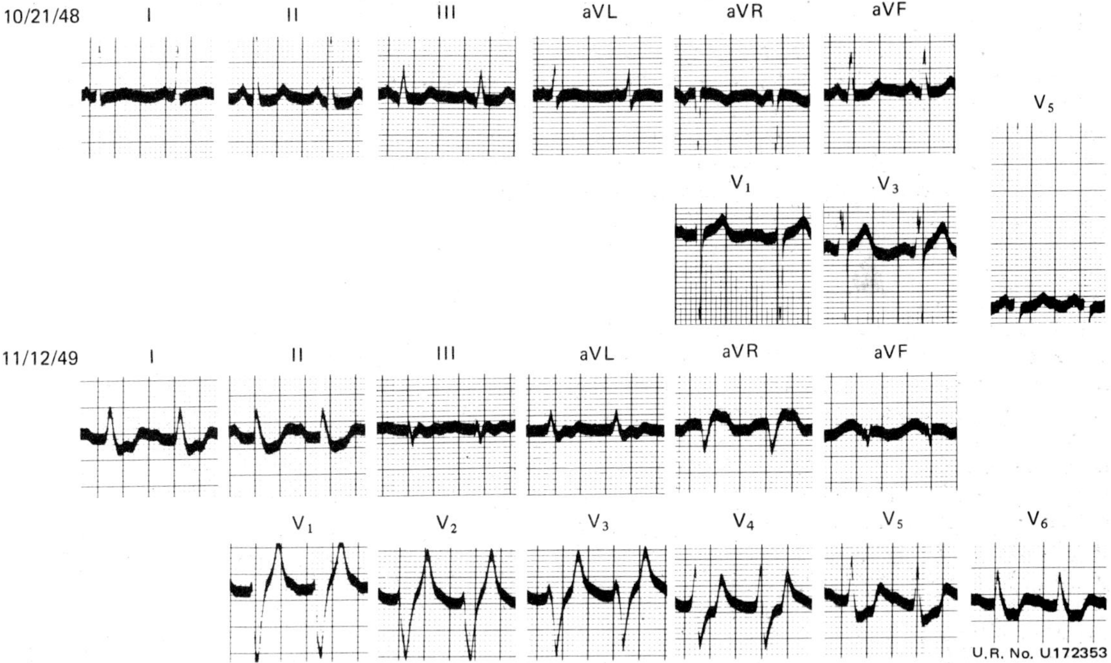

Figure 10–19, ECG showing wide QRS intraventricular conduction defect and idioventricular rhythm in a hyperkalemic patient with a serum potassium of 9 mEq/l.

enhances the susceptibility of the myocardium to electric shock, and ventricular fibrillation may result. If the arrhythmia is life-threatening, atrial pacing with overdrive suppression of the ectopic foci is probably the treatment of choice if intravenous drug therapy as outlined above is ineffective.

F. Digitalis Antibodies: Recent work with purified antibodies to digitalis suggests that they may be of value in reversing severe digitalis toxicity (Smith, 1976).

G. Prevention of Toxicity: Digitalis toxicity would not be so frequent, especially in the presence of sinus rhythm, if the physician had better clinical methods of measuring the adequacy of digitalization and was aware of the subtle signs of early digitalis toxicity (anorexia, nausea, ventricular premature beats), or if it were possible at the outset of therapy to better predict a safe effective dose of the drug. Prevention of toxicity is obviously superior to treatment of toxicity. Digitalis toxicity is *least* in the following circumstances: (1) when the drug is used in patients in whom hypokalemia, hypoxia, and other factors influencing the half-life of the drug and hence its serum level are known and treated before the drug is used; (2) when digoxin is used in the smallest maintenance dose likely to be effective in the light of the total clinical picture; (3) when the patient during digitalization is seen daily prior to the next dose and early manifestations of toxicity are carefully sought; (4) when rapid digitalization and rapid diuretic therapy are avoided unless the clinical situation is urgent; and (5) when oral rather than parenteral preparations are used unless the indications for parenteral therapy are clear.

10. TREAT SYSTEMIC DISEASES AFFECTING THE HEART

Myxedema

Myxedema may result in a large "quiet" heart (poor pulsations) with myocardial dilatation and edema between the fibers or pericardial effusion or a mixture of both. Myxedema is a slowly progressive disease with subtle signs that may be missed such as slow speech, hoarse voice, and cold dry skin. Specific treatment with thyroxine is curative (See Chapter 17). In older patients, it is best to begin with very small doses and then gradually increase the dosage.

Hyperthyroidism

Hyperthyroidism may not be obvious, especially in the apathetic form in older people, but can be suspected from the "salmon skin" of increased blood flow, alert movements despite cardiac disability, and rapid sinus tachycardia or paroxysmal atrial fibrillation. Diagnosis is not difficult, and treatment with radioiodine or antithyroid drugs (eg, propylthiouracil) is usually effective.

Cardiac failure is uncommon in younger people with thyrotoxicosis; more commonly, the increased secretion of thyroxine unmasks preexisting cardiac disease, usually coronary heart disease, and is more common in patients over 40 years of age. As a result, the response to treatment with radioiodine or thyroidectomy is not as dramatic as the treatment of myxedema heart with thyroxine; nevertheless, substantial benefits accrue from treatment of the hyperthyroidism (see Chapter 17).

Connective Tissue Disorders

Lupus erythematosus and other disorders in this group should be specifically sought because the acute vasculitis and hypertension often respond to corticosteroid therapy.

Pericardial Effusion

This must be considered because tamponade may occur, although it is not common.

Thiamin Deficiency

Beriberi heart disease is uncommon except in chronic alcoholics who eat poorly and in areas where famine is severe. In patients with borderline thiamin nutritional status, cardiac failure may develop when food intake is abruptly reduced or if an increased requirement for thiamin develops, such as in a febrile illness. In this situation, the patient may become abruptly breathless, and cardiac dilatation may develop, with warm extremities and evidence of high output failure. Large doses of thiamin abruptly reverse the process; within 1–2 weeks the patient may be asymptomatic, with a heart of normal size.

When chronic thiamin deficiency has resulted in chronic cardiac failure, cardiac output is reduced rather than increased, and there is no evidence of increased flow to the extremities; the clinical picture resembles that of the low output state that occurs in congestive cardiomyopathy due to alcohol. Thiamin deficiency is diagnosed by a history of inadequate thiamin intake, increased demand for thiamin (eg, fever), or a long history of high alcohol intake and confirmed by decreased urinary excretion of thiamin before and after intravenous injection of the vitamin. The response to thiamin and conventional cardiac therapy (rest, digitalis, diuretics) at this stage is slow and incomplete.

Anemia

Severe anemia, whether from blood loss, blood dyscrasias, or acute leukemia, may result in cardiac dilatation, with evidence of generalized cardiac failure such as systemic and pulmonary venous congestion, functional regurgitation of the mitral and tricuspid valves, and rarely, if the anemia is quite severe, dilatation of the aortic ring associated with an aortic diastolic murmur. Less severe anemia can produce or aggravate cardiac failure if the patient has underlying heart disease of any kind–coronary, hypertensive, or rheumatic; the decreased oxygen-carrying capacity of the hemoglobin and the increased cardiac output demanded by the anemia may precipitate cardiac failure. When anemia develops slowly, as in untreated pernicious anemia, it may be quite severe before dyspnea or other evidence of cardiac failure develops. It is of interest that when Minot was doing his pioneer work on the use of liver (orally or by crude extract) in pernicious anemia, he found dyspnea to be the cardinal indication for stopping the experiment and giving blood transfusions.

When blood is given for severe anemia, especially in the presence of cardiac failure, the patient should be closely monitored by inspection of the venous pulse, examination of the lung bases for rales, and auscultation for the development of gallop rhythm. The patient should be recumbent during the infusion of blood so that if fluid overload results in pulmonary edema with acute dyspnea, the patient can sit up, abruptly decreasing the pulmonary blood volume. Blood should be given slowly. If the patient needs only red cells and not plasma, then red cell mass rather than whole blood should be given if possible.

Inadvertent Rapid Administration of Sodium

The principles outlined above pertaining to administration of blood apply as well to infusions containing sodium. Acute pulmonary venous congestion and left ventricular failure may develop postoperatively in patients without intrinsic cardiac disease if intravenous saline is given too rapidly, as may happen in patients with borderline compensation or chronic cardiac disease in whom intravenous saline is given for any reason. Saline solution should be given slowly and with the same precautions as when blood is given, and the physician should consider whether dextrose and water or 0.5 N saline would serve as well.

Diseases Being Treated With Adrenal Corticosteroids

Corticosteroid therapy, especially with sodium-retaining steroids such as 9α-fluorinated compounds for postural hypotension due to autonomic insufficiency, may lead to salt retention and hypertension, increasing both the load on the heart and the extracellular volume, which may in turn lead to cardiac failure. Parenteral corticosteroids sometimes given for arthritis may unobtrusively cause iatrogenic Cushing's syndrome with hypertension, salt and water retention, and left ventricular failure, especially in patients with underlying heart disease.

Polycythemia Vera

This is an uncommon cause of cardiac failure. The increased circulating red cell mass increases blood viscosity and impairs coronary perfusion. The diagnosis is suggested by the high red blood count and confirmed by the finding of a high total red cell mass with normal oxygen saturation, thus excluding chronic lung disease and secondary polycythemia.

Pulmonary Embolism

Pulmonary emboli often precipitate congestive heart failure in patients with heart disease, and the abrupt development of cardiac failure in a patient with known heart disease should prompt a search for unsuspected pulmonary emboli. Recurrent pulmonary emboli—even very small ones—may over a period of months or years cause diffuse obstructive pulmonary arterial disease and severe pulmonary hypertension. The episodes may not have been recognized, and the presenting picture is of primary pulmonary hypertension with right ventricular hypertrophy and right ventricular failure. If recurrent pulmonary emboli are recognized, anticoagulant therapy or appropriate venous ligation may prevent recurrent episodes and pulmonary hypertension.

11. WITHDRAW OFFENDING DRUGS AFFECTING THE HEART

Obtain a history of the use of medications that may cause cardiac damage or depression (see Chapter 17). Excessive sedation may not be obvious in patients taking several drugs, and some may not even know what drugs they are receiving.

Propranolol

Propranolol is probably the most important offender because it is given for a wide variety of disorders such as arrhythmias, angina, hypertension, and hypertrophic cardiomyopathy; when given to patients with incipient left ventricular failure, it may produce florid ventricular failure in hours or days. Inappropriate use of propranolol must be considered in every patient with cardiac failure, particularly when the onset is abrupt.

Quinidine

Quinidine has a negative inotropic action, but cardiac failure is likely to be induced only in patients with chronic cardiac disease and atrial fibrillation who are not given digitalis before quinidine. In this circumstance, the ventricular rate may rise to 150/min or more, resulting in cardiac failure as decreased diastolic filling impairs coronary perfusion. Cardiac failure was the most common manifestation of quinidine "toxicity" in the early days of its use, when digitalis was not given first, but it is now quite rare. Quinidine in toxic doses may produce ventricular arrhythmias, especially when combined with rapidly acting digitalis preparations in combination with a diuretic agent, but this is not cardiac failure per se.

Antileukemic Agents

Daunorubicin or doxorubicin (Adriamycin) may produce cardiomyopathy and cardiac failure, especially when given in combination with other cytotoxic agents. This toxic effect is dose-related (± 500 mg) and associated with manifestations of cardiac toxicity such as ECG changes prior to the development of cardiac failure (see Chapter 17).

Emetine

Emetine given for amebiasis may produce ECG evidence of myocardial toxicity, but cardiac failure is rare.

Corticosteroids

See Chapter 17.

Spironolactone

In patients with impaired renal function who are receiving spironolactone, especially those who are taking potassium salts as well, hyperkalemia may develop with resulting cardiac conduction defects and idioventricular rhythms that may induce cardiac failure (Fig 10–20). Conduction defects, however, are more common.

Digitalis

Digitalis may produce ectopic rhythms by increasing automaticity and favoring reentry arrhythmias, which may lead to cardiac failure. Similarly, it may uncommonly produce complete atrioventricular block, and the slow ventricular rate in patients with borderline compensation may result in cardiac failure.

Phenothiazines & Tricyclic Antidepressants That Have a "Quinidinelike" Action

These drugs may cause arrhythmias but have not been reported to cause cardiac failure unless underlying heart disease is present and failure is precipitated by the arrhythmias.

12. CONTROL ASCITES & EFFUSIONS

Thoracocentesis and abdominal paracentesis are not often required today because of the potency of the newer diuretics such as furosemide. However, large amounts of fluid in the pleural and abdominal cavities may cause severe distress, and fluid retained in cavities under increased pressure may itself, by uncertain mechanisms, trigger retention of salt and water. Removing the fluid mechanically not only makes the patient more comfortable by relieving dyspnea and abdominal distress but may also induce sodium diuresis.

The problem is more complex when cardiac and renal failure coexist. In renal failure, sodium loss is exaggerated if the patient is abruptly given a low-sodium diet; the patient may rapidly become hypovolemic and dehydrated, with nausea and vomiting and more severe renal failure. Restricting sodium or giving diuretics is beneficial for cardiac failure but makes renal failure worse. Conversely, if patients with combined renal and cardiac failure are given increased amounts of sodium and water to combat dehydration, overcome spontaneous sodium loss, and restore blood volume, the manifestations of cardiac failure may increase, and the patient may develop acute dyspnea with left ventricular failure or exaggerated systemic venous congestion with edema. If a middle course of modest sodium restriction is insufficient either to prevent exacerbation of renal failure or to ameliorate the cardiac failure, peritoneal dialysis utilizing hypertonic dextrose may dramatically dehydrate the patient with no ill effect on the renal failure. Large amounts of excess fluid can be removed in this manner, with relief of symptoms and reduction of jugular venous pressure, so that the patient can again respond favorably to conventional treatment. Hemodynamic evidence of improvement such as increase in cardiac output is seldom obtainable, but the secondary manifestations of salt and water retention and fluid overload are relieved.

13. VASODILATORS IN THE TREATMENT OF CARDIAC FAILURE

An important advance in the treatment of heart disease has been the use of vasodilators in the treatment of severe cardiac failure that responds inadequately to conventional therapy as outlined above.

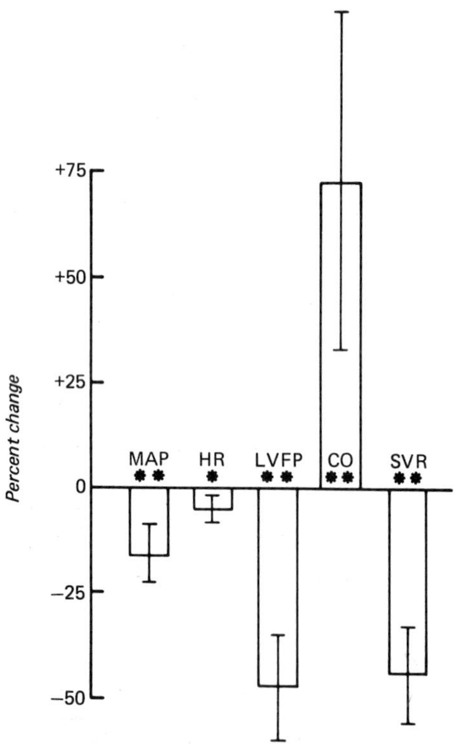

Figure 10–20. Average percentage change from control values during intravenous infusion of sodium nitroprusside in 18 patients with intractable heart failure. Vertical lines represent the standard error of the mean. MAP, mean arterial pressure; HR, heart rate; LVFP, left ventricular filling pressure; CO, cardiac output; SVR, systemic vascular resistance. $^{**}P < 0.001$; $^{*}P < 0.01$. (Reproduced, with permission, from Guiha NH & others: Treatment of refractory heart failure with infusion of nitroprusside. N Engl J Med 291:587, 1974.)

Patients with severe chronic failure require repeated hospitalizations and vigorous diuresis, leading to chronic weakness and electrolyte abnormality. The use of vasodilators has not been extensive or of long duration, but the results to date have been impressive and at times dramatic.

Vasodilators were first used in severe heart failure during acute myocardial infarction or cardiomyopathy, with the response monitored in the coronary care unit (see Chapter 8). Patients with left ventricular failure and cardiogenic shock who have low cardiac output and a high left ventricular filling pressure (> 20 mm Hg) often improve when impedance to left ventricular output (afterload) is reduced by vasodilator therapy. The striking benefit from intravenous nitroprusside, illustrated in Fig 10–20, led to the use of oral nitrates and nitrites to determine whether the acute short-term benefits (decreased left ventricular filling pressure and increased cardiac output) followed by diuresis and clinical improvement could be extended to chronic oral therapy. Fig 10–21 demonstrates that this is so. Hemodynamic measurements show a substantial fall after treatment with isosorbide dinitrate in the pulmonary artery end-diastolic pressure and wedge pressure ($\overline{PCW}$), reflecting the filling pressure of the left ventricle. A more moderate rise in cardiac index and a marked rise in venous capacitance followed the sublingual therapy, indicating that reduced venous return (decreased preload) and lessened systemic vascular resistance decreased the left ventricular outflow impedance and so improved left ventricular performance. Decrease in cardiac size demonstrated by x-ray (Fig 10–22) sub-

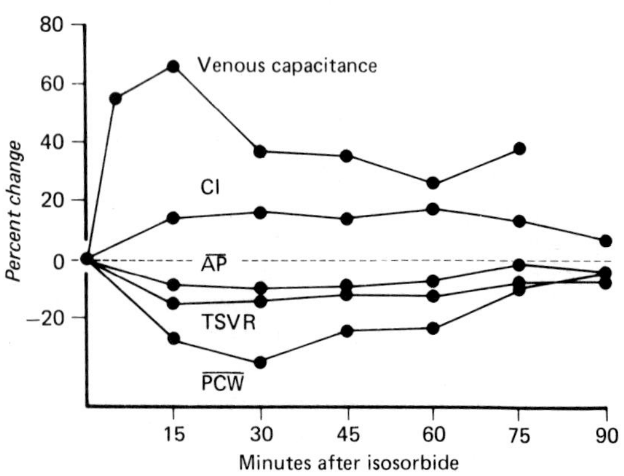

Figure 10–21. Effect of isosorbide dinitrate on 5 hemodynamic parameters over the course of 90 minutes. These data represent the mean percentage change from control values in 12 patients. A substantial increase in venous capacitance is seen at 5 min, with peak effect at 15 min. All other hemodynamic parameters have peak effect at 15–30 min. After 75 min, these effects are markedly reduced. $\overline{AP}$, mean arterial blood pressure; CI, cardiac index; $\overline{PCW}$, mean pulmonary capillary wedge pressure; TSVR, total systemic vascular resistance. (Reproduced, with permission, from Gray R & others: Hemodynamic and metabolic effects of isosorbide dinitrate in chronic congestive heart failure. Am Heart J 90:346, 1975.)

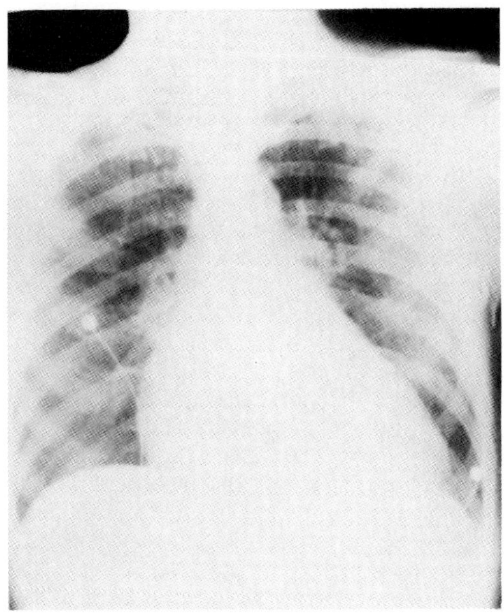
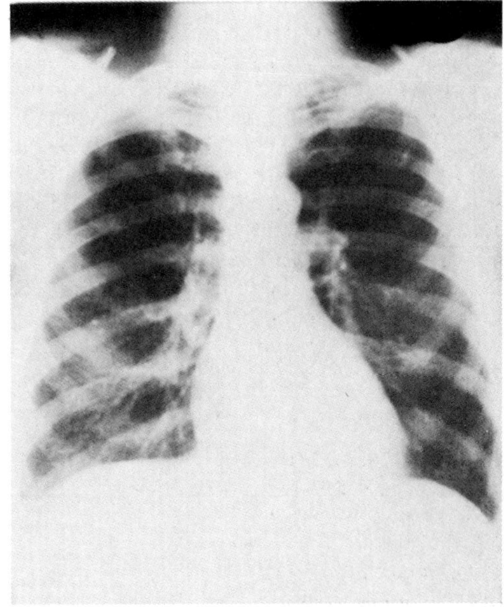

Figure 10–22. Marked decrease in size of the cardiac shadow followed 8 months of oral nitrate therapy in a patient with severe left ventricular failure. (Reproduced, with permission, from Cohn JN & others: Chronic vasodilator therapy in the management of cardiogenic shock and intractable left ventricular failure. Ann Intern Med 81:777, 1974.)

stantiates further the long-term benefit of oral nitrate therapy in severe cardiac failure. Fig 10–23 indicates that nitroglycerin ointment is also effective.

Patients with congestive or ischemic cardiomyopathy often respond inadequately to digitalis; vigorous diuretic therapy, while causing improvement of symptoms, induces weakness, hypokalemia, and hypovolemia. Furthermore, cardiac failure rapidly recurs when patients become ambulatory, so that the usual treatment is unsatisfactory. However, if vasodilators are given, these patients may remain ambulatory without recurrence of cardiac failure.

Because the principal effect of the nitrites and nitrates is venous dilatation, it was a natural extension to determine the effects of arteriolar vasodilators. Such agents, which relax arteriolar smooth muscle and decrease systemic vascular resistance, include hydralazine, prazosin, minoxidil, and phentolamine. Oral nitrates chiefly decrease the ventricular filling pressure, whereas hydralazine increases the cardiac index and the stroke work index. In Fig 10–24, the effects of vasodilator drugs are projected onto the family of Frank-Starling curves after adrenergic stimulation and in shock. It can be seen that the combination of nitrates and hydralazine is more effective than either alone in decreasing the left ventricular filling pressure and increasing the cardiac index and stroke work index (Massie, Am J Cardiol [in press]).

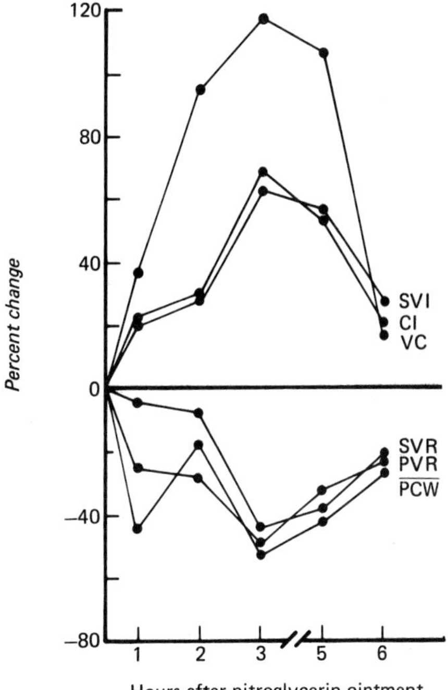

Figure 10–23. Hemodynamic changes after administration of nitroglycerin ointment in a patient with severe mitral regurgitation. CI, cardiac index; $\overline{\text{PCW}}$, mean pulmonary capillary wedge pressure; PVR, pulmonary vascular resistance; SVI, stroke volume index; SVR, systemic vascular resistance; VC, venous capacitance. (Reproduced, with permission, from Taylor WR & others: Hemodynamic effects of nitroglycerin ointment in congestive heart failure. Am J Cardiol 38:469, 1976.)

Drugs, Dosages, & Routes of Administration

A. Sodium Nitroprusside (Nipride): Administration of sodium nitroprusside is begun at a rate of 16 μg/min and the infusion rate increased at intervals of

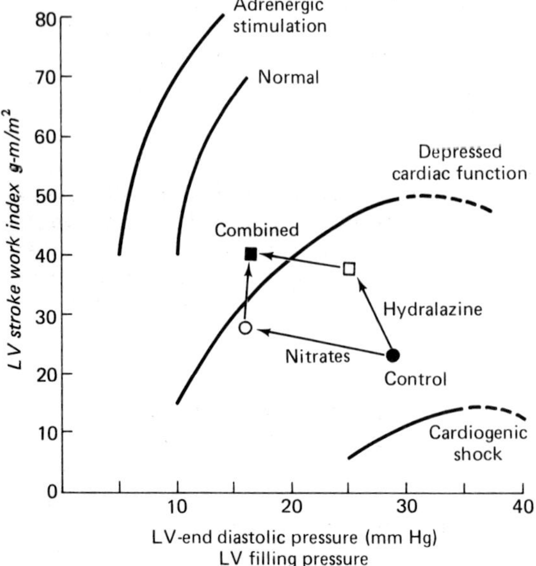

Figure 10–24. Effect of nitrates and hydralazine, alone and combined, on left ventricular performance in 12 patients with severe chronic cardiac failure projected onto the family of Frank-Starling left ventricular performance curves of Fig 10–1. (Reproduced, with permission, from Massie B & others: Hemodynamic advantage of combined oral hydralazine and nonparenteral nitrates in the vasodilator therapy of chronic heart failure. Am J Cardiol, 1977. [In press.]

3–5 minutes until the pulmonary capillary wedge pressure is reduced to normal or becomes stable–provided the systolic blood pressure remains above 100 mm Hg. Chatterjee (1977) found that vasodilator therapy in mitral regurgitation reduced the regurgitant flow, improved the systolic emptying of the left ventricle, and thus increased the forward ejection fraction. Left ventricular wall tension was reduced by the decreased impedance because of the decreased left ventricular chamber size. The resulting improved left ventricular performance may have important therapeutic benefits in patients with mitral and aortic regurgitation and cardiac failure.

Acute intravenous vasodilator therapy has had relatively limited use and should only be given when patients can be monitored closely, as in the coronary care unit; when hypotension can be avoided; and when serum thiocyanate levels can be monitored to avoid toxicity if sodium nitroprusside is used for prolonged periods.

Sodium nitroprusside is supplied as a powder in vials containing 50 mg for intravenous use. Solutions with 500–1000 ml of dextrose in water must be prepared immediately before administration, should not be given after 4 hours, and should be given alone without other medication. The intravenous solution should be wrapped in aluminum foil to protect it from light and given by microdrip regulator to allow precise measurement of the rate of flow. Some patients respond much more sensitively over a wide range of flow (16–200 μg/min), and the drip rate must be individualized accordingly. Side-effects of nausea and sweating occur if blood pressure is lowered too rapidly, because the drug works in seconds.

B. Isosorbide Dinitrate: 10–40 mg orally or 5–15 mg sublingually every 4–6 hours.

C. Nitroglycerin Ointment (Nitrol): Nitroglycerin ointment as used in mitral regurgitation and heart failure (Fig 10–23) is usually applied to the skin of the abdomen, and the dose is determined by the size of the ointment strip applied to the skin. The beginning dose is usually 15 mg, or about 3.8 cm (1½ inches) of the ointment strip. This is particularly valuable in patients with nocturnal angina or dyspnea because the duration of action is 3–6 hours. Left ventricular filling pressure decreases by about one-third and cardiac index increases by about one-fourth in patients with heart failure managed in this way. Sublingual or oral isosorbide dinitrate, as with nitroglycerin, has a predominant effect on venous pooling, thus decreasing venous capacitance, and therefore has a greater effect on venous return than on systemic vascular resistance, as have the smooth muscle relaxers (hydralazine, minoxidil [not approved by FDA], and prazosin).

D. Hydralazine, Prazosin, and Minoxidil: (See Chapter 9.) Begin with 25 mg, 0.5–1 mg, and 2.5 mg, respectively, and gradually increase the dose, depending on the patient's response, to 25–75 mg, 2.5–10 mg, and 5–20 mg, 3 times daily, respectively.

NEWER INOTROPIC AGENTS IN THE TREATMENT OF CARDIAC FAILURE WITH LOW OUTPUT STATE

Experience in coronary care units and intensive care units has shown that patients with acute myocardial infarction in cardiac failure with low output states as well as patients recovering from open heart surgery with low output states often benefit from inotropic agents other than digitalis. Norepinephrine, isoproterenol, and dopamine have been used and are discussed in Chapter 8. The choice of drugs depends upon the status of the hemodynamic variables at the time, and, as with the vasodilator agents, it is desirable to monitor these variables prior to treatment. Arterial pressure, left ventricular filling pressure, and cardiac output are the essential parameters to be monitored.

Norepinephrine & Isoproterenol

If the left ventricular filling pressure and cardiac index are within the normal range (LVFP, 12–15 mm Hg; CI [CO/m^2] 2.5–3.5 liters/min/m^2) and hypotension is the dominant presenting clinical feature, a drug such as norepinephrine, which acts chiefly as a peripheral vasoconstrictor, can be used. If the left ventricular filling pressure is on the high side (> 15 mm Hg), norepinephrine may further increase the filling pressure and lead to pulmonary edema. Similarly, if the patient has moderate hypovolemia, continued use of vasopressor drugs such as norepinephrine will aggravate hypovolemia by disproportionate increase in venous constriction as compared to arteriolar constriction, with subsequent loss of fluid into the interstitial tissues. Isoproterenol, by producing vasodilatation, may aggravate hypotension, although it has a positive inotropic action; and, if hypotension is not present, it may simultaneously decrease left ventricular filling pressure and increase cardiac output. On the other hand, it may induce ventricular premature beats and increase heart rate and myocardial oxygen consumption. As a result, coronary perfusion may be decreased following stimulation of the heart by isoproterenol.

Dopamine & Dobutamine

The most recent additions to the inotropic agents which are useful in cardiac failure are dopamine hydrochloride (Intropin) and dobutamine (a relatively cardiospecific beta-adrenergic agent). Dopamine is the immediate precursor in the synthesis of norepinephrine and has the advantage that while it may increase cardiac output and decrease left ventricular filling pressure in low output cardiac failure, it does so without decreasing renal blood flow. Sodium and water diuresis, therefore, may be enhanced, and when dopamine is used in conjunction with diuretics the patient with cardiac failure may improve. The effects of dopamine depend upon its dose; because it is a beta-adrenergic agonist, it may produce tachycardia and ventricular arrhythmia as the dose is increased. In larger doses it also stimulates alpha-adrenergic receptors, and a raised blood pressure may result, whereas dobutamine does not have this effect. In the smaller range of dosage ($<$ 10 μg/kg/min), dopamine usually does not cause tachycardia or raise the arterial pressure. As with vasodilator agents, dopamine should be started at a low rate of infusion, eg, 2–4 μg/kg/min, while the hemodynamic parameters are being monitored. The flow should be adjusted as with vasodilator agents, depending upon the hemodynamic response.

Derivatives of dopamine have advantages over the parent drug. Dobutamine is one such derivative and is a selective inotropic drug. In preliminary reports (Stoner, 1977; Sakamoto, 1977), it had a striking effect on increasing the cardiac output with only a slight increase in the heart rate and a moderate increase in the mean blood pressure and without important side-effects. This and similar drugs deserve greater therapeutic trials in low output cardiac failure.

Experience with dopamine and dobutamine is limited, and while they seem to have definite advantages over norepinephrine and isoproterenol under certain circumstances, further studies are required regarding not only their benefits but also their possible harmful effects. Digital ischemia with cyanosis and pain may occur as a result of vasoconstriction due to alpha-adrenergic stimulation from dopamine. Treatment consists of alpha-adrenergic blockade, such as the use of chlorpromazine intravenously. In a typical case of cardiac failure, a 10 mg intravenous loading dose followed by an infusion at a rate of 0.6 mg/min (7.3 μg/kg/min) was given by Valdes (1976) with reversal of the digital ischemia within minutes. Other alpha-adrenergic blockers (eg, phentolamine, 50 mg) may be used alternatively.

Glucagon

Glucagon, which has a variable and limited inotropic effect in therapeutic doses, has been largely superseded by the other inotropic agents. For further details, see the sections on treatment of cardiac failure, cardiogenic shock, and acute myocardial infarction.

INTRA-AORTIC BALLOON COUNTERPULSATION

This is discussed in Chapter 7.

EMERGENCY TREATMENT OF SEVERE HEART FAILURE OR ACUTE PULMONARY EDEMA

These are often grave emergencies, and treatment varies depending upon the cause and severity. For example, in a mild attack, morphine and rest in bed in the sitting position alone may suffice, although intravenous diuretics (see below) may also be required. If the attack is due to ventricular tachycardia or to atrial fibrillation with a rapid ventricular rate and the patient has severe dyspnea or pulmonary edema, cardioversion should be instituted without delay.

The 3 most common causes of severe heart failure–acute myocardial infarction, acute hypertensive heart failure, and acute valvular insufficiency secondary to infective endocarditis–are discussed in Chapters 8, 9, and 12, respectively.

A patient who fails to respond to bed rest, digitalis, and diuretics in the hospital–and antihypertensive therapy if hypertensive–should be monitored in a critical care unit. Continuous monitoring of ECG and intra-arterial blood pressures is required, and a flow-directed catheter should be introduced to allow intracardiac pressures and cardiac output to be intermittently observed, ie, pulmonary artery diastolic pressure or preferably pulmonary capillary wedge pressure, cardiac output by the thermodilution method, and arterial blood gases. Special nursing care is required for continuous close observation.

The patient is sedated with morphine, 5–10 mg intravenously, and placed in the sitting position, which decreases the venous return to the heart–the equivalent of venesection–and may allow an increase in cardiac output. Intravenous furosemide is given in a dosage of 40–80 mg, and oxygen with a face mask in high concentration (40–60%) and a high flow rate

(6–8 liters/min). Improvement should occur within an hour. Morphine relieves anxiety, depresses pulmonary reflexes, and induces sleep. Relief from forceful respiration decreases the negative intrathoracic pressure and the venous return to the heart. Oxygen relieves hypoxia and dyspnea and decreases pulmonary capillary permeability. Positive pressure breathing for short periods may be of great value, especially if there is respiratory acidosis with impaired ventilation. Positive pressure breathing improves ventilation, removes CO_2, and decreases venous return to the heart. If the patient has severe impairment of cardiac output, positive pressure breathing should be used with caution because the cardiac output may fall further. If the patient has acute bronchospasm, aminophylline, 0.25–0.5 g infused slowly intravenously, is often helpful. In addition to decreasing the bronchospasm, it may increase the glomerular filtration rate, renal blood flow, and cardiac output as well as the urinary excretion of sodium and water.

If the patient is still dyspneic or has episodic increases in dyspnea and fails to respond to the treatment given above, vasodilator agents should be added. If the situation is critical and systolic pressure exceeds 100 mm Hg, an infusion of sodium nitroprusside titrated to the response of the patient, beginning with 16 μg/min, can be started (see above and Chapter 8). If the situation is less critical, isosorbide dinitrate, 5–15 mg sublingually or 10–40 mg orally, can be used, and if the systolic pressure is not decreased below 100 mm Hg one can give sublingual nitroglycerin, 0.3–0.6 mg. This is often of considerable value in acute pulmonary edema associated with hypertension. If the vasodilators just mentioned are not effective in relieving the dyspnea, one should add hydralazine, 50–75 mg orally or 2.5–10 mg intramuscularly, to dilate the arteriolar bed. The combination of nitrates *and* hydralazine produces both venous and arteriolar dilatation and is more effective than either drug used alone (Fig 10–24). If the patient has acute hypertensive heart failure, minoxidil, 2.5 mg, should be started, repeated in 6 hours, and the patient then reevaluated in the sitting or standing position—and the drug repeated, if necessary and if tolerated without hypotension. Rotating soft rubber tourniquets are rarely used today because the agents mentioned previously are sufficient to reduce the venous flow to the heart and improve the stroke volume. If tourniquets are used, they should be applied with sufficient pressure to obstruct the venous but not the arterial flow and should be rotated every 15 minutes. The tourniquets should be removed gradually as the attack subsides. Venesection is also infrequently used today unless the patient has acute pulmonary edema secondary to rapid intravenous infusion of sodium-containing fluids. Removal of 300–500 ml of blood is the most direct way of reducing the venous return to the heart and may strikingly increase cardiac output and decrease right atrial and peripheral venous pressure in low output cardiac failure. It should not be used if anemia is present.

If the patient remains critically ill, intra-aortic balloon counterpulsation may be added to decrease the work of the heart, as discussed in Chapter 7.

If ventilation is impaired and acidosis is present, tracheal intubation may be helpful and further decrease the work of the heart.

If the patient does not promptly respond to the aggressive therapy described above, one should consider potentially curable causes of congestive heart failure which may require specific treatment directed at the cause, such as severe aortic stenosis, acute valvular insufficiency from infective endocarditis, severe mitral or pulmonary stenosis, severe thyrotoxicosis or myxedema heart disease, pericardial effusion, and the other conditions mentioned earlier in this chapter.

CARDIAC TRANSPLANTATION

Enthusiasm for cardiac transplantation has waned in most cardiac centers since it was first performed in 1967. At present, Shumway and his associates at Stanford are compiling the largest experience in the USA, transplanting about one heart per month. Other cardiac surgeons have largely abandoned the effort, probably because of the complexity of the ancillary procedures ie, the problem of determining death of the donor so as to obtain a heart quickly; the intensive immunosuppressive therapy required indefinitely to prevent rejection; the high frequency of serious infections, which often are fatal; the large investment in manpower, space, biochemical procedures, and tissue typing; the need for intensive follow-up; and the relatively high mortality rate in the first 3 years. In the most recent report of the Stanford experience in 90 patients (Schroeder, 1976), the 1-year survival rate was 47%, the 2-year survival rate 37%, and the 3-year survival rate 27%. It is very difficult to accurately predict that a patient has irremediable heart disease, especially with the availability of newer medical and surgical methods of treatment (ie, more potent loop diuretics, vasodilator therapy, more potent isotropic agents, intra-aortic balloon assist devices, and left ventricular aneurysmectomy). Bedside monitoring with Swan-Ganz catheters allows more rigorous therapy than was previously safe.

The selection of patients suitable for cardiac transplantation has been narrowed to *exclude* patients over 50 with a history of recent pulmonary embolism, pulmonary hypertension, or sepsis or with preformed antibodies against tissues of the prospective donor (Lower, 1976).

Some patients have survived 5 years, and most of these have been successfully rehabilitated socially.

The effort required is massive for a relatively small number of patients, but continued research by the Stanford group may find simpler methods of management of patients who have undergone transplantations until a better method of treatment can be devised for the patient with otherwise unmanageable far-advanced disease.

PROGNOSIS

The overall prognosis of congestive or cardiac failure, while considerably improved in recent years because of the therapeutic advances discussed in the foregoing pages—especially the availability of oral diuretics, vasodilators, inotropic agents, and surgical and medical treatment of underlying causes—remains poor because treatment is often delayed until cardiac failure is far-advanced, ie, because treatable conditions such as hypertensive heart failure and valvular heart disease with heart failure are not recognized and treated early. At times, however, the basic cause (eg, ischemic cardiomyopathy) cannot be reversed, and treatment is therefore only palliative. Fig 10–25 shows the Framingham data, indicating the poor 5- and 10-year survival rates in cardiac failure.

The pessimistic prognosis of cardiac failure indicated from the McKee data (Fig 10–25) may well be excessively gloomy because many of the most dramatic recent therapeutic advances were not fully exploited during the period covered by the Framingham Study. The use of the more potent loop diuretics such as furosemide and ethacrynic acid in full dosage, especially in the presence of renal failure, has reversed cardiac failure even in far-advanced disease. The introduction of oral vasodilators such as prazosin, hydralazine, and minoxidil (not yet approved by the FDA) as well as the longer-acting nitrates such as oral isosorbide dinitrate and rapidly acting nitrites such as intravenous sodium nitroprusside has not yet had an effect on mortality statistics. The newer inotropic agents such as dopamine and dobutamine have been in use only in the past few years, and their inotropic action, additive to that of digitalis, has resulted in significant hemodynamic benefit which may decrease the mortality rate in cardiac failure. The surgical treatment of congenital and acquired rheumatic valvular heart disease, nonrheumatic mitral and aortic mitral insufficiency, and valvular disruption in infective endocarditis, as well as resection and grafting of dissecting aorta and resection of atrial myxomas, may improve the prognosis of cardiac failure in general.

Improved diagnostic methods utilizing echocardiography, and isotope scanning, better biochemical technics (serum enzymes, serum digoxin levels, immunologic determination, and renin-angiotensin-aldosterone determinations), and more precise invasive procedures are now available in many medical centers and community hospitals. Better diagnosis and classification into subsets of myocardial infarction lead to better therapeutic decisions, both medical and surgical. Circulatory assist devices such as intra-aortic balloon counterpulsation have been employed only in recent years, and technologic advances may make this method of treatment more generally available in severe cases.

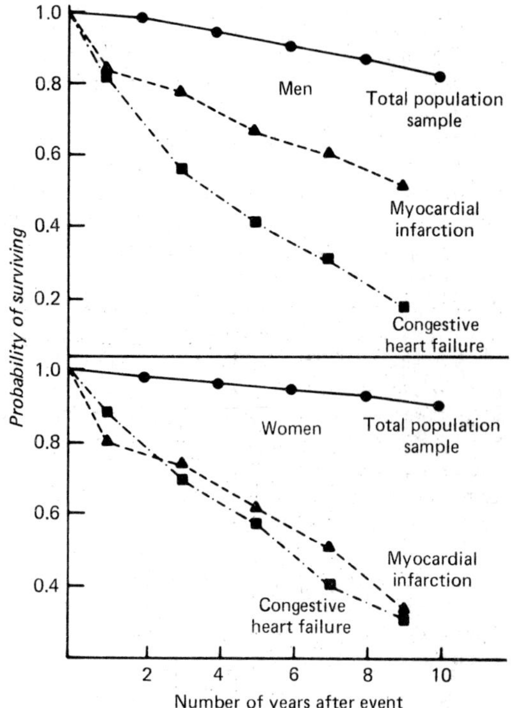

Figure 10–25. Probability of survival for subjects 45 years of age and older and after the development of congestive heart failure or myocardial infarction as compared to the survival of the total Framingham Heart Study population (16-year follow-up results). (Reproduced, with permission, from McKee PA & others: The natural history of congestive heart failure: The Framingham Study. N Engl J Med 285:1441, 1971.)

The role of alcohol and tobacco in causing cardiac disease has been recently reemphasized, and educational efforts designed to decrease the use of these toxic substances in the general population may decrease the incidence of cardiac failure. The extensive public health effort aimed at identifying and treating hypertension should lead to earlier and more intensive treatment of hypertension with resulting prevention of cardiac failure, the most common cause of death in untreated hypertension.

Once extensive cardiac enlargement with increased cardiac volume and congestive cardiomyopathy has developed, treatment is less effective than if cardiac failure is prevented by appropriate early treatment, before the reserve capacity of the heart is exhausted.

• • •

References

Aberman A, Fulop M: The metabolic and respiratory acidosis of acute pulmonary edema. Ann Intern Med 76:173, 1972.

Ablad B: A study of the mechanism of the hemodynamic effects of hydralazine in man. Acta Pharmacol Toxicol [Suppl] (Kbh) 20:1, 1963.

Ahearn DJ, Maher JF: Heart failure as a complication of hemodialysis arteriovenous fistula. Ann Intern Med 77:201, 1972.

Akhtar N & others: Hemodynamic effect of dobutamine in patients with severe heart failure. Am J Cardiol 36:202, 1975.

Bank N: Physiological basis of diuretic action. Annu Rev Med 19:103, 1968.

Bedford DE: Left ventricular failure. Lancet 1:1303, 1939.

Beller GA & others: Digitalis intoxication: A prospective clinical study with serum level correlations. N Engl J Med 284:989, 1971.

Bolen JL, Alderman EL: Hemodynamic consequences of afterload reduction in patients with chronic aortic regurgitation. Circulation 53:879, 1976.

Braunwald E: Control of myocardial oxygen consumption: Physiologic and clinical considerations. Am J Cardiol 27:418, 1971.

Braunwald E: Determinants and assessment of cardiac function. N Engl J Med 296:86, 1977.

Braunwald E: The sympathetic nervous system in heart failure. Hosp Pract 5:31, Dec 1970.

Cagin NA & others: Digitalis: New knowledge about an old drug. Cardiovasc Med 2:183, 1977.

Cairns KB & others: Clinical and hemodynamic results of peritoneal dialysis for severe cardiac failure. Am Heart J 76:227, 1968.

Cannon PJ: The kidney in heart failure. N Engl J Med 296:26, 1977.

Cannon PJ & others: Ethacrynic acid: Effectiveness and mode of diuretic action in man. Circulation 31:5, 1965.

Chatterjee K, Parmley WW: The role of vasodilator therapy in heart failure. Prog Cardiovasc Dis 19:301, 1976.

Chatterjee K & others: Beneficial effects of vasodilator agents in severe mitral regurgitation due to dysfunction of subvalvular apparatus. Circulation 48:684, 1973.

Cohn JN, Franciosa JA: Vasodilator therapy of cardiac failure. (2 parts.) N Engl J Med 297:27, 254, 1977.

Cohn JN & others: Chronic vasodilator therapy in the management of cardiogenic shock and intractable left ventricular failure. Ann Intern Med 81:777, 1974.

Cohn K & others: Variability of hemodynamic responses to acute digitalization in chronic cardiac failure due to cardiomyopathy and coronary artery disease. Am J Cardiol 35:461, 1975.

Davis JO: The mechanisms of salt and water retention in cardiac failure. Hosp Pract 5:63, Oct 1970.

Dodge HT: Hemodynamic aspects of cardiac failure. Hosp Pract 6:91, Jan 1971.

Dodge HT, Lord JD, Sandler H: Cardiovascular effects of isoproterenol in normal subjects and subjects with congestive heart failure. Am Heart J 60:94, 1960.

Doherty JE: Digitalis glycosides: Pharmacokinetics and their clinical implications. Ann Intern Med 79:229, 1973.

Dowell AR & others: Effect of aminophylline on respiratory-center sensitivity in Cheyne-Stokes respiration and in pulmonary emphysema. N Engl J Med 273:1447, 1965.

Duberstein JL, Kaufman DM: A clinical study of an epidemic of heroin intoxication and heroin-induced pulmonary edema. Am J Med 51:704, 1971.

Earley LE: Diuretics. (2 parts.) N Engl J Med 276:966, 1023, 1967.

Edelman IS & others: Interrelations between serum sodium concentration, serum osmolarity and total exchangeable sodium, total exchangeable potassium and total body water. J Clin Invest 37:1236, 1958.

Eichna LW: The George E. Brown Memorial Lecture: Circulatory congestion and heart failure. Circulation 22:864, 1960.

Fisch C: Digitalis intoxication. JAMA 216:1770, 1971.

Fisch C: Treatment of arrhythmias due to digitalis. J Indiana State Med Assoc 60:146, 1967.

Franciosa JA, Pierpont G, Cohn JN: Hemodynamic improvement after oral hydralazine in left ventricular failure: A comparison with nitroprusside infusion in 16 patients. Ann Intern Med 86:388, 1977.

Franciosa JA & others: Hemodynamic effects of orally administered isosorbide dinitrate in patients with congestive heart failure. Circulation 50:1020, 1974.

Frand UI, Shim CS, Williams MH Jr: Heroin-induced pulmonary edema: Sequential studies of pulmonary function. Ann Intern Med 77:29, 1972.

Friedberg CK: Prevention of heart failure. Am J Cardiol 22:190, 1968.

Goldberg LI, Hsieh YY, Resnekov L: Newer catecholamines for treatment of heart failure and shock: An update on dopamine and a first look at dobutamine. Prog Cardiovasc Dis 19:327, 1977.

Gorham LW & others: The relative importance of dietary sodium chloride and water intake in cardiac edema. Ann Intern Med 27:575, 1947.

Gottlieb TB, Thomas RC, Chidsey CA: Pharmacokinetic studies of minoxidil. Clin Pharmacol Ther 13:436, 1972.

Gould L, Lyon AF: Pulsus alternans: An early manifestation of left ventricular dysfunction. Angiology 19:103, 1968.

Graettinger JS, Parsons RL, Campbell JA: Correlation of clinical and hemodynamic studies in patients with mild and severe anemia with and without congestive failure. Ann Intern Med 58:617, 1963.

Grainger RG: Interstitial pulmonary edema and its radiological diagnosis. Br J Radiol 31:201, 1958.

Gray R & others: Hemodynamic and metabolic effects of isosorbide dinitrate in chronic congestive heart failure. Am Heart J 90:346, 1975.

Greenberg H & others: Effects of nitroglycerin on the major determinants of myocardial oxygen consumption: An angiographic and hemodynamic assessment. Am J Cardiol 36:426, 1975.

Guiha NH & others: Treatment of refractory heart failure with infusion of nitroprusside. N Engl J Med 291:587, 1974.

Güllner HG & others: Correlation of serum concentrations with heart concentrations of digoxin in human subjects. Circulation 50:653, 1974.

Guyton AC, Jones CE, Coleman TG: *Circulatory Physiology: Cardiac Output and Its Regulation,* 2nd ed. Saunders, 1973.

Helfant RH, Scherlag BJ, Damato AM: The electrophysiologic properties of diphenylhydantoin sodium as compared to procainamide in the normal and digitalis-intoxicated heart. Circulation 36:108, 1967.

Hesse B & others: Hemodynamics, compartments and the renin-aldosterone system in chronic heart failure. Eur J Cardiol 3:107, 1975.

Hesse B & others: Transcapillary escape rate of albumin and right atrial pressure in chronic congestive heart failure before and after treatment. Circ Res 39:358, 1976.

Howarth S, McMichael J, Sharpey-Schafer EP: Effects of venesection in low output heart failure. Clin Sci 6:41, 1946.

Hultgren HN, Flamm MD: Pulmonary edema. Mod Concepts Cardiovasc Dis 38:1, 1969.

Ingelfinger JA, Goldman P: The serum digitalis concentration: Does it diagnose digitalis toxicity? N Engl J Med 294:867, 1976.

Jelliffe RW & others: An improved method of digitoxin therapy. Ann Intern Med 72:453, 1970.

Jewitt D & others: Clinical cardiovascular pharmacology of dobutamine: A selective inotropic catecholamine. Lancet 2:363, 1974.

Kannel WB & others: Role of blood pressure in the development of congestive heart failure: The Framingham Study. N Engl J Med 287:781, 1972.

Kastor JA: Digitalis intoxication in patient with atrial fibrillation. Circulation 47:888, 1973.

Katz AM: Congestive heart failure: Role of altered myocardial cellular control. N Engl J Med 293:1184, 1975.

Kirkendall WM, Wilson CB: Treatment of the patient with refractory heart failure. Med Clin North Am 52:1157, 1968.

Kovick RB & others: Vasodilator therapy for chronic left ventricular failure. Circulation 53:322, 1976.

Laragh JH: Diuretics in the management of congestive heart failure. Hosp Pract 5:43, Nov 1970.

Laragh JH: Ethacrynic acid and furosemide. Am Heart J 75:564, 1968.

Laragh JH: The proper use of newer diuretics. Ann Intern Med 67:606, 1967.

Lee KS, Klaus W: The subcellular basis for the mechanism of inotropic action of cardiac glycosides. Pharmacol Rev 23:193, 1971.

Leonard JJ, deGroot WJ: The thyroid state and the cardiovascular system. Mod Concepts Cardiovasc Dis 38:23, 1969.

Lower RR & others: Clinical observations on cardiac transplantation. Transplant Proc 8:9, 1976.

Lown B, Levine SA: *Current Concepts in Digitalis Therapy.* Little, Brown, 1954.

Lutch JS, Murray JF: Continuous positive-pressure ventilation: Effects on systemic oxygen transport and tissue oxygenation. Ann Intern Med 76:193, 1972.

Mackenzie J: *Diseases of the Heart.* Oxford Univ Press, 1908.

Maffly RH, Edelman IS: The role of sodium, potassium, and water in the hypo-osmotic states of heart failure. Prog Cardiovasc Dis 4:88, 1961.

Mailloux LU & others: Peritoneal dialysis for refractory congestive heart failure. JAMA 199:873, 1967.

Majid PA, Sharma B, Taylor SH: Phentolamine for vasodilator treatment of severe heart failure. Lancet 2:719, 1971.

Mantle JA & others: Isosorbide dinitrate for the relief of severe heart failure after myocardial infarction. Am J Cardiol 37:263, 1976.

Marcus FI: Current concepts of digoxin therapy. Mod Concepts Cardiovasc Dis 45:77, 1976.

Marcus FI: Digitalis pharmacokinetics and metabolism. Am J Med 58:452, 1975.

Marriott HJL, Menendez MM: A-V dissociation revisited. Prog Cardiovasc Dis 8:522, 1966.

Massie B & others: Hemodynamic advantage of combined oral hydralazine and nonparenteral nitrates in the vasodilator therapy of chronic heart failure. Am J Cardiol, Nov 1977. [In press.]

Massie B & others: Mitral-septal separation: A new echocardiographic index of left ventricular function. Am J Cardiol 39:1008, 1977.

McGuire LB, O'Brien WM, Nolan SP: Patient survival and instrument performance with permanent cardiac pacing. JAMA 237:558, 1977.

McIntosh HD, Morris JJ Jr: Problems in the use of digitalis in the management of congestive heart failure. Prog Cardiovasc Dis 7:360, 1965.

McKee PA & others: The natural history of congestive heart failure: The Framingham Study. N Engl J Med 285:1441, 1971.

Meister SG & others: Sustained hemodynamic effects of nitroglycerin ointment. Am J Cardiol 37:155, 1976.

Mikulic E, Franciosa JA, Cohn JN: Comparative hemodynamic effects of chewable isosorbide dinitrate and nitroglycerin in patients with congestive heart failure. Circulation 52: 477, 1975.

Mikulic E, Franciosa JA, Cohn JN: Comparative hemodynamic effects of nitroglycerin forms in heart failure. Circulation 51, 52 (Suppl 2):36, 1975.

Miller RR & others: Afterload reduction therapy with nitroprusside in severe aortic regurgitation: Improved cardiac performance and reduced regurgitant volume. Am J Cardiol 38:564, 1976.

Miller RR & others: Combined dopamine and nitroprusside therapy in congestive heart failure: Greater augmentation of cardiac performance by addition of inotropic stimulation to afterload reduction. Circulation 55:881, 1977.

Miller RR & others: Pharmacological mechanisms for left ventricular unloading in clinical congestive heart failure: Differential effects of nitroprusside, phentolamine, and nitroglycerin on cardiac function and peripheral circulation. Circ Res 39:127, 1976.

Mitchell JH, Wallace AG, Skinner NS Jr: Intrinsic effects of heart rate on left ventricular performance. Am J Physiol 205:41, 1963.

Parmley WW, Chatterjee K: Vasodilator therapy for chronic heart failure. Cardiovasc Med 1:17, 1976.

Paulk EA Jr, Hurst JW: Intractable heart failure and its management. Med Clin North Am 54:309, 1970.

Perloff JK: The clinical manifestations of cardiac failure in adults. Hosp Pract 5:43, Sept 1970.

Pfeiffer E: Wasser-Retention durch Natriumsalze. Verhandlungen des Deutschen Kongresses für innere Medizin K27–28:506, 1910–1911.

Pool PE, Braunwald E: Fundamental mechanisms in congestive heart failure. Am J Cardiol 22:7, 1968.

Popp RL: Echocardiographic evaluation of left ventricular function. N Engl J Med 296:856, 1977.

Pratt JH: Cardiac asthma. JAMA 87:809, 1927.

Proger S, Ginsburg E, Magendantz H: The effects of the ingestion of excessive amounts of sodium chloride and water on patients with heart disease. Am Heart J 23:555, 1942.

Rader B & others: Comparison of the hemodynamic effects of mercurial diuretics and digitalis in congestive heart failure. Circulation 29:328, 1964.

Rapaport E: Congestive heart failure. Page 1 in: *Tice's Practice of Medicine.* Vol 6. Conn H (editor). Hoeber-Harper, 1970.

Robie NW, Goldberg LI: Comparative systemic and regional hemodynamic effects of dopamine and dobutamine. Am Heart J 90:340, 1975.

Sakamoto T, Yamada T: Hemodynamic effects of dobutamine in patients following open heart surgery. Circulation 55:525, 1977.

Salmon SE, Schrier RW: Congestive heart failure after acute myocardial infarction. Calif Med 114:23, Feb 1971.

Sarnoff SJ, Berglund E: Ventricular function. 1. Starling's law of the heart studied by means of simultaneous right and left ventricular function curves in the dog. Circulation 9:706, 1954.

Scheinman M, Brown M, Rapaport E: Hemodynamic effects of ethacrynic acid in patients with refractory acute left ventricular failure. Am J Med 50:291, 1971.

Scheinman M, Rapaport E: Critical assessment of the use of central venous O_2 saturation as a mirror of mixed venous oxygen in severely ill cardiac patients. Circulation 40:165, 1969.

Schick D, Scheuer J: Appraisal and reappraisal of cardiac therapy: Current concepts of therapy with digitalis glycosides. (Part 1.) Am Heart J 87:253, 1974.

Schmidt DH, Butler VP Jr: Reversal of digoxin toxicity with specific antibodies. J Clin Invest 50:1738, 1971.

Schreiner BF Jr & others: The pathophysiology of pulmonary congestion. Prog Cardiovasc Dis 14:47, 1971.

Schroeder JS & others: Cardiac transplantation: Review of seven years' experience. Transplant Proc 8:5, 1976.

Schwartz A: Is the cell membrane Na^+-K^+ ATPase enzyme system the pharmacological receptor for digitalis? Circ Res 39:2, 1976.

Schwartz AB, Swartz CD: Dosage of potassium chloride elixir to correct thiazide-induced hypokalemia. JAMA 230:702, 1974.

Sheiner LB: Digitalis blood levels and toxicity. N Engl J Med 295:226, 1976.

Smirk FH & others: The treatment of hypertensive heart failure and of hypertensive cardiac overload by blood pressure reduction. Am J Cardiol 1:143, 1958.

Smith TW: Digitalis toxicity: Epidemiology and clinical use of serum concentration measurements. Am J Med 58:470, 1975.

Smith TW, Butler VP, Haber E: Determination of therapeutic and toxic serum digoxin concentrations by radioimmunoassay. N Engl J Med 281:1212, 1969.

Smith TW, Haber E: Digitalis. (4 parts.) N Engl J Med 289:945, 1010, 1063, 1125, 1973.

Smith TW, Haber E: Digoxin intoxication: The relationship of clinical presentation to serum digoxin concentration. J Clin Invest 49:2377, 1970.

Smith TW & others: Reversal of advanced digoxin intoxication with Fab fragments of digoxin-specific antibodies. N Engl J Med 294:797, 1976.

Sokolow M: The importance of the sodium intake in the management of cardiac failure. Am Practitioner 3:353, 1949.

Sokolow M, Chamberlain FL: Clinical evaluation of Cedilanid. Ann Intern Med 18:204, 1943.

Sokolow M, Katz LN, Muscovitz AN: The electrocardiogram in pulmonary embolism. Am Heart J 19:166, 1940.

Sokolow M & others: Digitalis in the prevention of recurrent cardiac failure in patients with sinus rhythm. Ann Intern Med 16:427, 1942.

Staub NC: Pathogenesis of pulmonary edema. Am Rev Respir Dis 109:358, 1974.

Stein L & others: Pulmonary edema during volume infusion. Circulation 52:483, 1975.

Stoner JD III, Bolen JL, Harrison DC: Comparison of dobutamine and dopamine in treatment of severe heart failure. Br Heart J 39:536, 1977.

Swan HJC, Parmley WW: Congestive heart failure. Chapter 10 in: *Pathologic Physiology: Mechanisms of Disease,* 5th ed. Sodeman WA Jr, Sodeman WA. Saunders, 1974.

Taylor WR & others: Hemodynamic effects of nitroglycerin ointment in congestive heart failure. Am J Cardiol 38: 469, 1976.

Turner AF, Lau FYK, Jacobson G: A method for the estimation of pulmonary venous and arterial pressures from the routine chest roentgenogram. Am J Roentgenol Radium Ther Nucl Med 116:1, 1972.

Valdes ME: Post-dopamine ischemia treated with chlorpromazine. N Engl J Med 295:1081, 1976.

Walker WG: Indications and contraindications for diuretic therapy. Ann NY Acad Sci 139:481, 1966.

Walker WG & others: Topics in clinical medicine: A symposium on uses and complications of diuretic therapy. Johns Hopkins Med J 121:194, 1967.

Wayne KS: Positive end-expiratory pressure (PEEP) ventilation: A review of mechanisms and actions. JAMA 236:1394, 1976.

Williams DO & others: Hemodynamic assessment of oral peripheral vasodilator therapy in chronic congestive heart failure: Prolonged effectiveness of isosorbide dinitrate. Am J Cardiol 39:84, 1977.

Wilson GM: Diuretics. Practitioner 200:39, 1968.

11...
Congenital Heart Disease

Congenital heart disease represents the largest share of pediatric cardiologic practice. Increasing emphasis has been placed on investigation and treatment of younger patients with congenital heart lesions. Neonatal cardiology, which differs significantly from adult cardiology, is a subject of great current interest. Although it is reasonable to equate congenital heart disease in older children (6 years and over) with that seen in adults, it is not possible to devise a single description of the characteristics of congenital heart disease encompassing neonatal, infant, and adult disease. This chapter is confined to the clinical picture of congenital lesions as seen in patients over 6 years of age.

Surgically Modified Disease

Because of increasing longevity, more patients with congenital lesions are being seen in adult life who have had corrective or palliative surgery in infancy or childhood. In many of these patients the disease has been surgically modified, creating new unnatural conditions that merit clinical description. The best example is the effect on congenital disease of an earlier palliative surgical procedure (Blalock's operation) for relief of Fallot's tetralogy. Many patients with Fallot's tetralogy now seen as adults have had a palliative operation, and the long-term effects of the procedure on the clinical status of the patient are clearly important.

Causes of Congenital Heart Disease

The causes of congenital heart disease are basically unknown. A number of factors can be identified in about 10% of cases, but in the majority no obvious cause can be pinpointed. The complex embryologic pattern of cardiac development can be disturbed at different stages of fetal life with varying results. In general, congenital lesions can be considered either as a failure of some structure to form (eg, a septum, as in ventricular or atrial septal defect) or as a failure of some structure to disappear (eg, double aortic arch, right-sided aorta, or persistent ductus arteriosus). In most lesions, the anatomic picture is determined at an early stage of gestation (about the seventh week of pregnancy), but in persistent patent ductus arteriosus, patent foramen ovale, and some cases of pulmonary atresia, the causative factor appears at the end of pregnancy or in the neonatal period, eg, when the ductus arteriosus remains patent in infants with respiratory distress syndrome.

The commonest identifiable cause of congenital heart disease is maternal viral infection, usually rubella but occasionally mumps or influenza. An infection of this type can be identified in only about 5% of cases of congenital heart disease. The resulting clinical picture includes congenital deafness and cataract, and patent ductus arteriosus is the commonest cardiac lesion.

Genetic disturbances involving the sex chromosomes are particularly likely to cause congenital heart lesions. Thus, trisomy 21 (Down's syndrome), in which there is an extra (47th) chromosome, and Turner's syndrome, in which there are only 45 chromosomes, are associated with congenital heart lesions in about 20% of cases. Patients with Down's syndrome are particularly likely to have endocardial cushion (atrioventricular canal) defects, but ventricular septal defects and pulmonary stenosis are also seen. Turner's syndrome, which is characterized by female infantilism, hypertelorism, web neck, dwarfism, and cubitus valgus, is associated with coarctation of the aorta and also with pulmonary stenosis.

The incidence of congenital heart lesions in spontaneously aborted fetuses is high, and some mechanism clearly exists which detects severe congenital abnormalities and leads to spontaneous termination of pregnancy. Some drugs such as thalidomide are thought to increase the incidence of congenital heart disease by exercising an antiabortifacient action.

Metabolic changes in maternal and placental circulation are thought to play an important part in some types of congenital heart lesions. If a toxic substance reaches the fetus from the mother, it is most likely to affect the left side of the heart because umbilical venous blood passes across the atrial septum into the left atrium, left ventricle, and ascending aorta. The lesions associated with this type of injury include underdeveloped left heart syndromes, with mitral atresia, aortic stenosis or atresia, endomyocardial fibrosis, and coarctation of the aorta.

Musculoskeletal defects are the congenital anomalies most commonly associated with congenital heart lesions. They include thoracic deformities with kyphoscoliosis, syndactyly, polydactyly, absent fingers or toes, phocomelia (vestigial flipperlike arms), and long

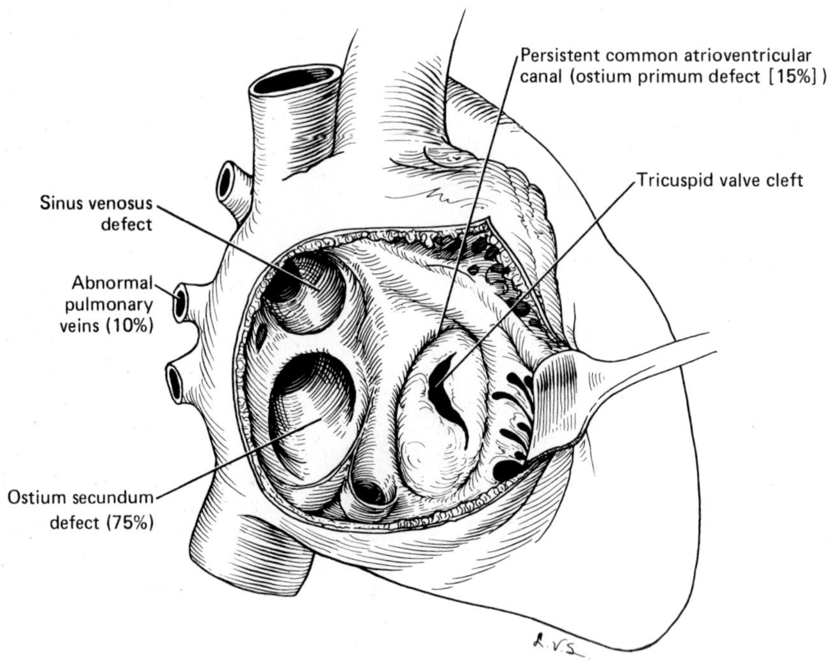

Anatomic features of atrial septal defects.

Cardinal features: *Left-to-right shunt into right atrium; high tricuspid flow; increased pulmonary blood flow; normal pulmonary arterial pressure.*

Variable factors: *Size of defect; size of shunt; anomalous venous drainage with sinus venosus defect; valve clefts with ostium primum defect.*

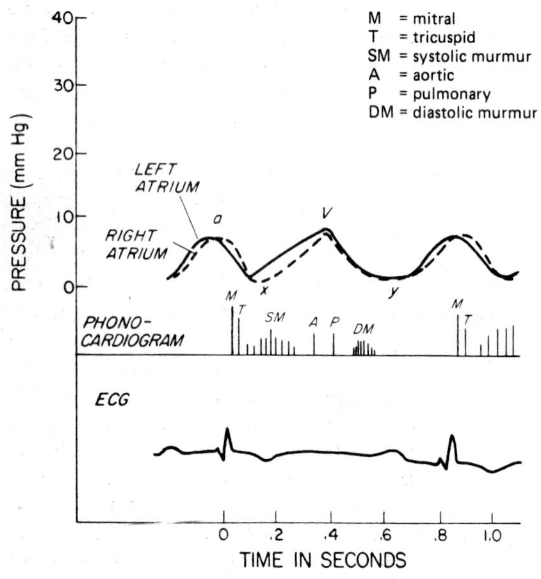

Diagram showing auscultatory and hemodynamic features of atrial septal defect.

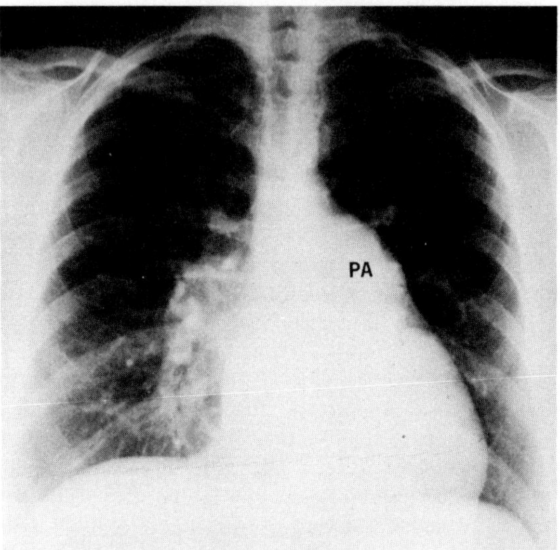

Chest x-ray of a patient with an ostium secundum atrial septal defect. The heart is large, with a prominent pulmonary artery (PA) and a small aorta.

Figure 11–1. Atrial septal defect. Structures enlarged: Right atrium, right ventricle, pulmonary artery, and left atrium; small left ventricle and aorta.

spidery fingers (arachnodactyly). Marfan's syndrome is a mesodermal abnormality in which the cardiac defect is cystic medial necrosis of the aorta. This results in aortic dilatation that may lead to rupture of the aorta in early adult life. Aortic incompetence develops as the aortic valve ring stretches, and there may be associated intracardiac lesions, especially mitral valve prolapse. Dislocation of the lens, gigantism, with large hands and feet, arachnodactyly, and kyphoscoliosis are also seen.

Classification of Congenital Heart Disease

There is no satisfactory classification of congenital heart disease. A classification based on embryologic studies is too comprehensive for use in adult patients because most individuals with extensive defects do not survive. The following clinical classification, based on that of Wood, gives an indication of the relative frequency with which the various lesions are encountered after puberty.

Without shunt	
1. Right-sided	
Pulmonary stenosis	25%
Ebstein's malformation	Rare
2. Left-sided–Coarctation of the aorta	5%
With shunt	
1. Acyanotic	
Atrial septal defect	30%
Patent ductus arteriosus	7%
Ventricular septal defect	9%
2. Cyanotic	
Tetralogy of Fallot	10%
Eisenmenger's syndrome	7%
Ebstein's malformation	Rare
Transposition of great vessels	Rare
Truncus arteriosus	Rare
Tricuspid atresia	Rare

This classification omits isolated valvular lesions such as aortic stenosis and congenital mitral lesions in which the cause cannot always be identified with certainty. The various lesions in combination, eg, atrial septal defect with pulmonary stenosis and atrial plus ventricular septal defect, will be mentioned only in passing. The various forms of valvular disease that occur both as congenital and as acquired lesions are discussed under the various valvular diseases.

ATRIAL SEPTAL DEFECT

Anatomic Types

The clinical syndrome of atrial septal defect covers a wide range of lesions that are often clinically indistinguishable. The anatomic sites of the different types of defects are shown in diagrammatic form in Fig 11–1. The commonest form–ostium secundum defect–involves the center of the atrial septum in the area of the fossa ovalis. The next most common–ostium primum defect–involves the lower part of the septum above the atrioventricular valves. The valves themselves are not infrequently cleft, giving rise to incompetence of the mitral or tricuspid valves. An even more extensive form of the defect results in a complete endocardial cushion defect, in which there is also a ventricular septal defect and a common atrioventricular canal. This defect is seen in about 20% of persons with Down's syndrome, a common form of mental deficiency associated with chromosomal abnormalities. A third form of defect involves the upper part of the septum and is known as sinus venosus defect. It is often associated with partial anomalous pulmonary venous drainage, usually drainage of the right upper lobe into the superior vena cava. A persistent left-sided superior vena cava and anomalous venous drainage into the coronary sinus or right atrium may occur. Rarely, a patient presenting with signs of an atrial septal defect may have partial anomalous venous drainage as the sole abnormality, without an atrial defect, but in most cases with anomalous venous drainage there is also an atrial defect.

Cardinal Features & Pathogenesis

The essential feature of atrial septal defect is a left-to-right shunt of arterialized blood into the right atrium that produces a high tricuspid flow and increased blood flow to the lungs with a normal pulmonary arterial pressure. The severity of the lesion depends primarily on the size of the defect, which in turn limits the size of the shunt. The size of the defect is not the sole determinant of the severity of the lesion, however, as can be seen from the natural history of the condition. Atrial septal defect is often not diagnosed in infancy or childhood. At birth, the right and left ventricles are equal in size and thickness in normal infants, and right-to-left shunt via a patent foramen ovale can normally occur. Whenever an atrial septal defect is present, however, left-to-right shunting is minimal at birth. With the normal decrease in pulmonary vascular resistance that follows birth, the right ventricle becomes more compliant. It then fills more readily than the left ventricle, and, as a result, left-to-right shunting becomes apparent. Most atrial septal defects are large enough (2 × 2 cm or more) to equalize pressures between the right and the left atrium. Thus, the magnitude of the left-to-right shunt depends mainly on the filling characteristics of the right and left ventricles. In most cases (85%) in which the diagnosis can be made, the left-to-right shunt is at least equal to the left ventricular output, so that pulmonary flow is more than twice systemic flow. The increased pulmonary flow is readily accepted by the pulmonary circulation so that pulmonary arterial pressure is usually low. The presence of anomalous venous drainage does not affect the clinical picture, but the presence of associated mitral or tricuspid incompetence or a complete endocardial cushion defect makes the lesion more severe.

The increase in flow involves both atria, the right ventricle, and the pulmonary circulation, but not the left ventricle or the aorta in uncomplicated cases. The extra load on the heart is a pure "flow load" and is well tolerated for many years. Since the magnitude of the left-to-right shunt depends on the relative diastolic compliances of the 2 ventricles, the shunt is not fixed. Any factor that increases the load on the left ventricle tends to decrease its compliance and increase the left-to-right shunt. Conversely, anything that increases the resistance to right ventricular emptying decreases the shunt and tends to reverse it.

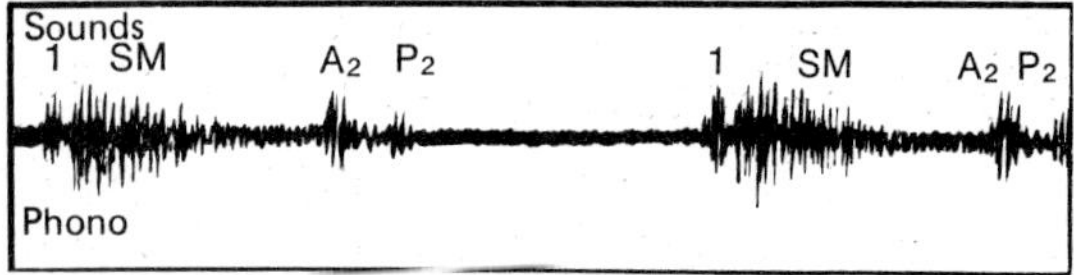

Figure 11–2. Ejection murmur (SM) and widely split second sound recorded at the upper left sternal border in a patient with atrial septal defect. (Courtesy of Roche Laboratories Division of Hoffman-La Roche, Inc.)

Clinical Findings

A. Symptoms and Signs: Atrial septal defect is difficult to diagnose, and the examiner must maintain a high index of suspicion if all cases are to be recognized and treated surgically.

About half of patients with atrial septal defect are asymptomatic when the diagnosis is made. Symptoms develop in 60% of patients by age 30. This indicates that the lesion is often noted in early adult life, either on routine physical examination or (more often) on a chest x-ray. The commonest presenting symptom is dyspnea on exertion (65%), followed by palpitations (20%) due to atrial arrhythmia, and chest pain, which is usually not anginal in nature. A spurious past history of rheumatic fever may be present (5%). Children with left-to-right shunts are prone to develop bronchitis and other lung infections. In about 20% of adult cases the diagnosis of atrial septal defect presents some difficulty, either because the patient is middle-aged and the possibility of a congenital lesion is not considered or because the clinical picture is atypical. In about half of these cases, the patient is in right heart failure when first seen; in such cases, edema and ascites tend to be more prominent than dyspnea.

Patients with Marfan's syndrome, a congenital mesodermal abnormality associated with cystic medial necrosis of the aorta and ectopia lentis, may have atrial septal defect. Patients with other skeletal abnormalities may also have the lesion (eg, Ehlers-Danlos syndrome), and atrial septal defect is said to occur in tall, thin persons with long spidery fingers (arachnodactyly) and a high-arched palate, but these appearances are not of diagnostic value.

1. Cardiac signs—The physical signs depend on the magnitude of pulmonary blood flow. Increased right ventricular stroke volume produces a hyperdynamic right ventricular impulse with a visible and palpable pulse over the pulmonary artery in the second or third left intercostal space. A pulmonary ejection systolic murmur is almost always present because of increased flow through the pulmonary valve, but the murmur is often slight. The first heart sound is often loud because the tricuspid valve closes from a wide open position with right ventricular systole. There is relative tricuspid stenosis in patients with atrial septal defect because the diastolic flow across the tricuspid valve is usually twice the normal value or more. In addition to the loud tricuspid first sound, there is often a right-sided third sound and a tricuspid diastolic murmur that becomes louder during inspiration.

2. Second heart sound—The second heart sound is widely split in patients with atrial septal defect. The normal widening of the split with inspiration does not occur, and the failure of the second sound to become single on expiration (fixed split) is an important clue to the presence of the lesion (Fig 11–2). These findings are caused by the combination of delayed activation of the right ventricle and prolonged ejection time, associated with increased right ventricular stroke volume. Inspiration has little effect on the condition because only a relatively small increase in the already large flow occurs through the pulmonary valve upon inspiration.

3. Ostium primum defects—In patients with ostium primum defects there may also be a hyperdynamic left ventricular impulse and a pansystolic apical murmur if mitral incompetence is present. Tricuspid incompetence is a defect that also occurs with ostium primum defects, giving a pansystolic murmur that is best heard at the left lower sternal border. Incompetence of the atrioventricular valves can also occur in ostium secundum defects, especially when heart failure develops.

4. Pulse—The pulse is of small amplitude, and the venous pressure is normal. Atrial fibrillation commonly develops after age 40, and other varieties of atrial arrhythmia are also seen.

B. Electrocardiographic Findings: The ECG demonstrates a right ventricular conduction defect in 90% of individuals with an atrial septal defect (Fig 11–3). Because of late depolarization of the hypertrophied right ventricular outflow tract, the terminal portion of the QRS complex will be oriented anteriorly (producing an rsR' in V_1) and rightward (producing a permanent S in lead I). In 80% of patients the duration of the QRS complex is less than 0.12 sec; in 10% of cases it equals or exceeds 0.12 sec. Although the ECG tracing has the appearance of an incomplete or complete right bundle branch block, it must be understood that the conduction delay is not in the main right bundle system but rather peripherally in the myocardium.

In the 10% of patients in whom the ECG is normal, the diagnosis is more difficult. Prolongation of the P–R interval is more common in older patients with

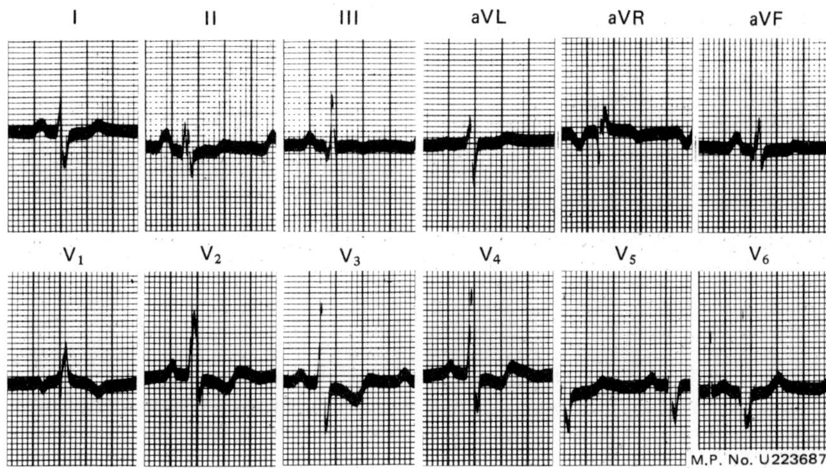

Figure 11–3. ECG from a 23-year-old woman with atrial septal defect proved by catheter. Widely split second sound and short systolic murmur at the base on phonocardiogram. Incomplete right bundle branch block with rsR′ in lead V_1. Right ventricular pressure 35/0.

large atria and often precedes the development of atrial fibrillation in middle life. Left axis deviation in a patient with a right ventricular conduction defect (Fig 11–4) is strongly suggestive of ostium primum defect, but a normal or rightward axis does not rule out such a defect. If pulmonary hypertension develops, there will almost certainly be evidence of progressive right ventricular hypertrophy on the ECG. The presence, rather than the development, of a tall secondary R wave in patients with conduction defects (Fig 11–5) has been taken as evidence of right ventricular hypertrophy, but this ECG sign is far from pathognomonic of increased right ventricular pressure and may be due solely to the conduction defect.

C. **X-Ray Findings**: The chest x-ray is of great importance in the diagnosis of atrial septal defect. The heart is usually enlarged in proportion to the pulmonary blood flow, and the main pulmonary artery and its branches are dilated and stand out in contrast to the aorta, which is small (Fig 11–1). The right atrium is more prominent in this lesion than in any other except Ebstein's malformation, and the right ventricle is also enlarged. It is notoriously difficult to distinguish between right and left ventricular enlargement in atrial septal defect. The left atrium is less prominent than it is in patients with mitral valve disease because left atrial pressure is not markedly increased, but the left atrium tends to be large in older patients. Anomalous

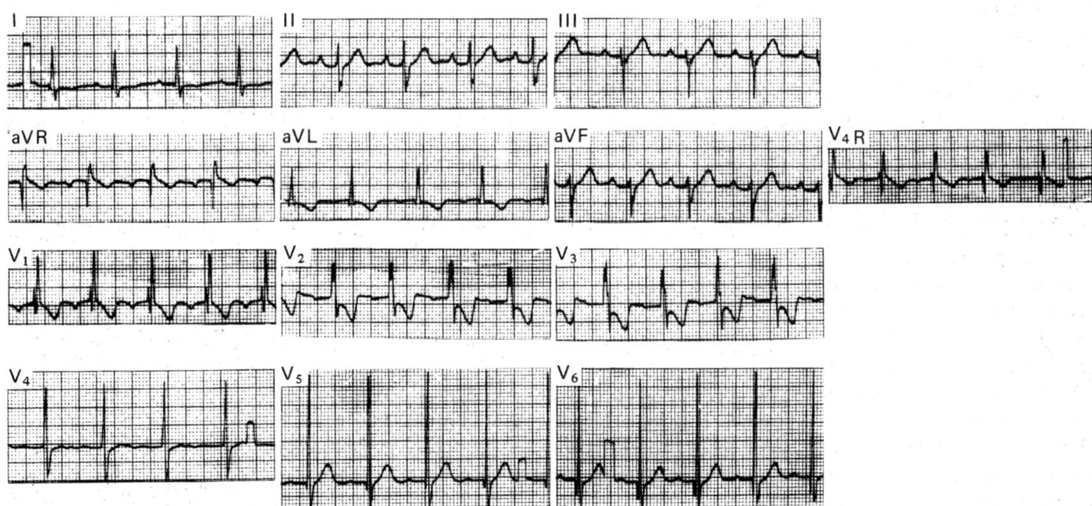

Figure 11–4. ECG of a patient with ostium primum defect showing left axis deviation and right bundle branch block. (Reproduced, with permission, from Chung EK: *Electrocardiography.* Harper & Row, 1974.)

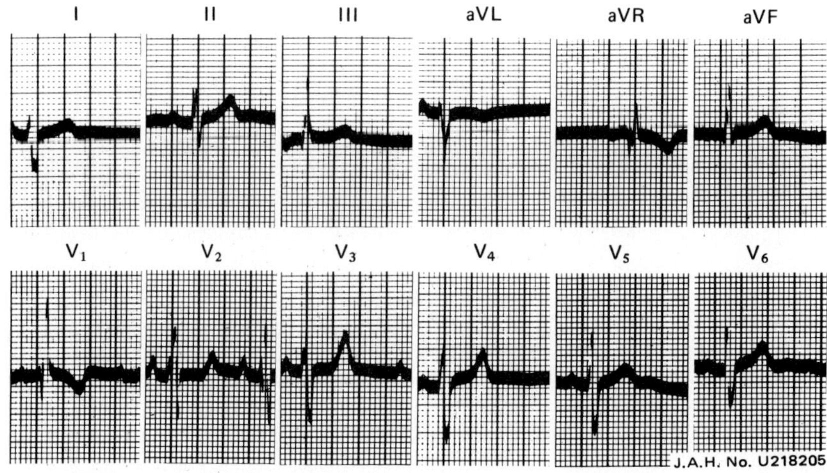

Figure 11–5. ECG of a 7-year-old girl with atrial septal defect proved by catheter; right ventricular pressure 40/2. Tall secondary R wave with rsR′ in V_1.

venous drainage may cause abnormal radiologic findings, but angiocardiography is ordinarily needed to define them. A persistent left-sided superior vena cava is common in sinus venosus defects and can be detected on the chest x-ray (Fig 11–6).

Pulmonary plethora with increased lung markings due to enlarged pulmonary arteries and veins is common, and increased pulsation of the main branches of the pulmonary artery (hilar dance) is a prominent sign on fluoroscopy. These signs are due to increased pulmonary blood flow and are nonspecific. They are more common in atrial septal defect than in other types of left-to-right shunt because the pulmonary blood flow is so often large in this lesion. The most specific radiologic sign of an atrial defect is right atrial enlargement because this does not occur in ventricular septal defect or patent ductus arteriosus. Unfortunately, this sign is difficult to evaluate and is therefore unreliable.

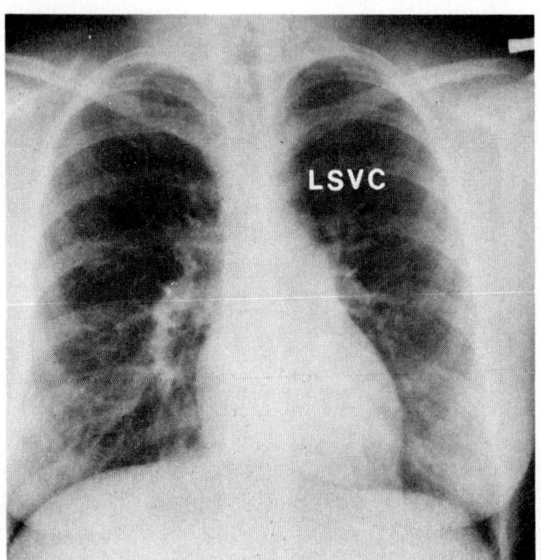

Figure 11–6. Chest x-ray of a 19-year-old woman with sinus venosus atrial septal defect with anomalous pulmonary venous drainage and a persistent left-sided superior vena cava (LSVC).

D. Special Investigations: Although echocardiography, phonocardiography, and ear oximetry are often useful in the diagnosis of atrial septal defect, cardiac catheterization is essential for confirmation of the diagnosis.

1. Noninvasive technics–

a. Echocardiography can be used to detect reduced or paradoxic movement of the ventricular septum (Fig 11–7) as well as increased right ventricular size. These signs are indicative of increased right ventricular stroke volume, which suggests but does not specifically establish a diagnosis of atrial septal defect. Tricuspid or pulmonary incompetence can also cause this sign. Echocardiography is also helpful in comparing and detecting mitral and tricuspid valve motion (Fig 11–8). In atrial septal defect, the increased tricuspid flow causes increased excursion of valve leaflets. Echocardiography can distinguish between left and right ventricular enlargement in patients with large hearts.

b. Phonocardiography has been extremely helpful in defining the auscultatory signs in patients with atrial septal defects. It is used now mainly to confirm the findings noted on physical examination and to show that the split of the second heart sound remains fixed during respiration.

c. Ear oximetry can be used to detect the temporary shunt reversal which can be induced in many patients who have a small atrial septal defect. If the patient performs Valsalva's maneuver and shuts off the venous return for 10 sec by raising the intrathoracic pressure to 40 mm Hg, the right heart becomes relatively empty. When intrathoracic pressure is released at the end of the maneuver, systemic venous blood rushes

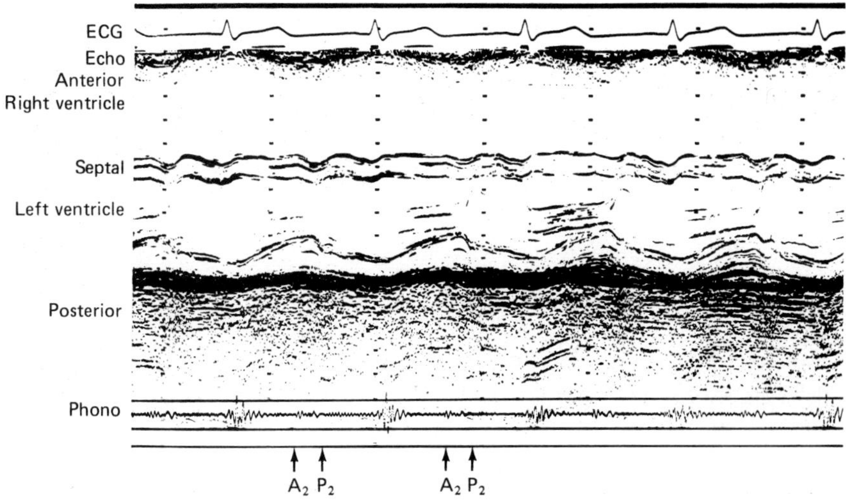

Figure 11–7. Echocardiogram showing large right ventricle, reduced septal motion, and smaller left ventricle in a patient with atrial septal defect. Phonocardiogram shows split S_2. Aortic (A_2) precedes pulmonary (P_2) closure sound. (Courtesy of NB Schiller.)

into the right atrium, raising the right atrial pressure above that of the left and causing a temporary shunt reversal, which is detected at the ear by means of an oximeter as a short drop in arterial saturation (Fig 11–9). A sudden increase in systemic venous return caused by suddenly squatting down will also produce temporary shunt reversal (Fig 11–10). In patients with large left-to-right shunts, the large volume of blood passing through the right heart may cause an abnormal (square wave) response to Valsalva's maneuver (Fig 11–11). In this case, altering the venous return has a negligible effect on intracardiac pressure and shunt. In patients with ventricular septal defect or patent ductus arteriosus, there is such a large pressure difference between the right and left heart that the increase in right heart pressure following the release of pressure in Valsalva's maneuver does not affect the shunt, and no fall in arterial saturation occurs. Shunt reversal following squatting or the release of pressure following Valsalva's maneuver is thus seen only in small atrial defects.

2. **Invasive technics**–

a. **Cardiac catheterization** is used in atrial septal defect to measure pulmonary and systemic blood pressure and flow and to pass the catheter through the atrial septal defect into the left atrium and ventricle.

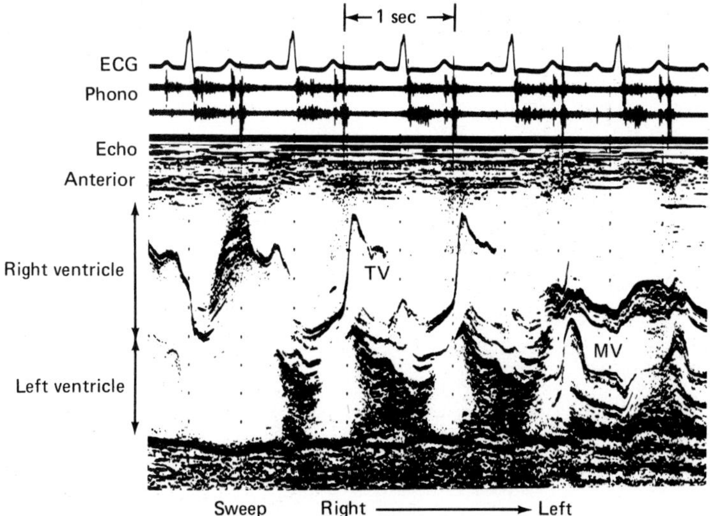

Figure 11–8. Echocardiogram showing sweep from tricuspid valve (TV) to mitral valve (MV) in a patient with atrial septal defect. The right ventricular chamber is larger than the left ventricular chamber. (Courtesy of NB Schiller.)

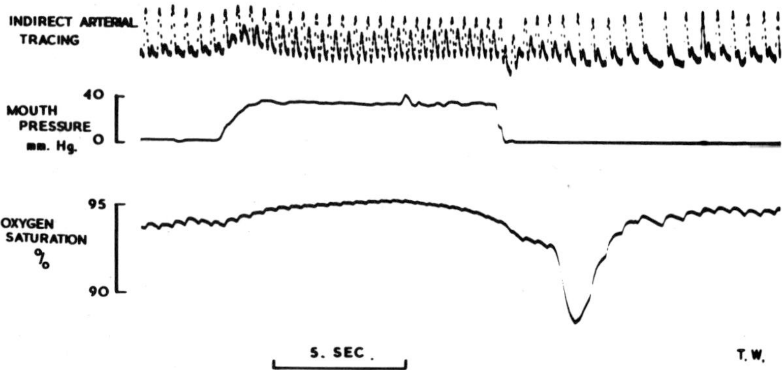

Figure 11–9. Ear oximeter tracing from a patient with small atrial septal defect showing fall in arterial oxygen saturation due to right-to-left shunt following release of pressure in Valsalva's maneuver.

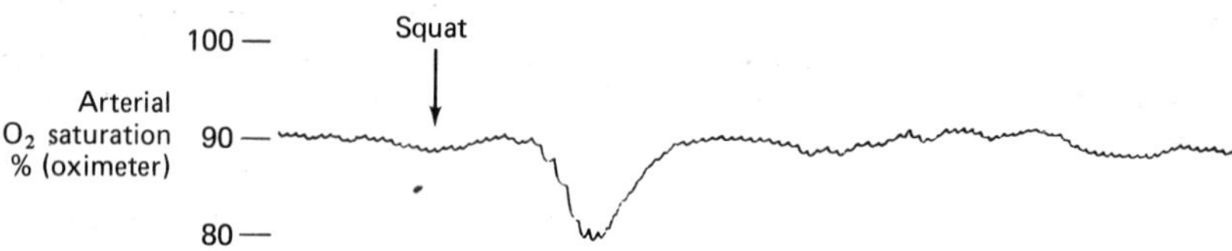

Figure 11–10. Ear oximeter tracing from a patient with atrial septal defect showing a fall in arterial oxygen saturation due to right-to-left shunt caused by suddenly squatting down.

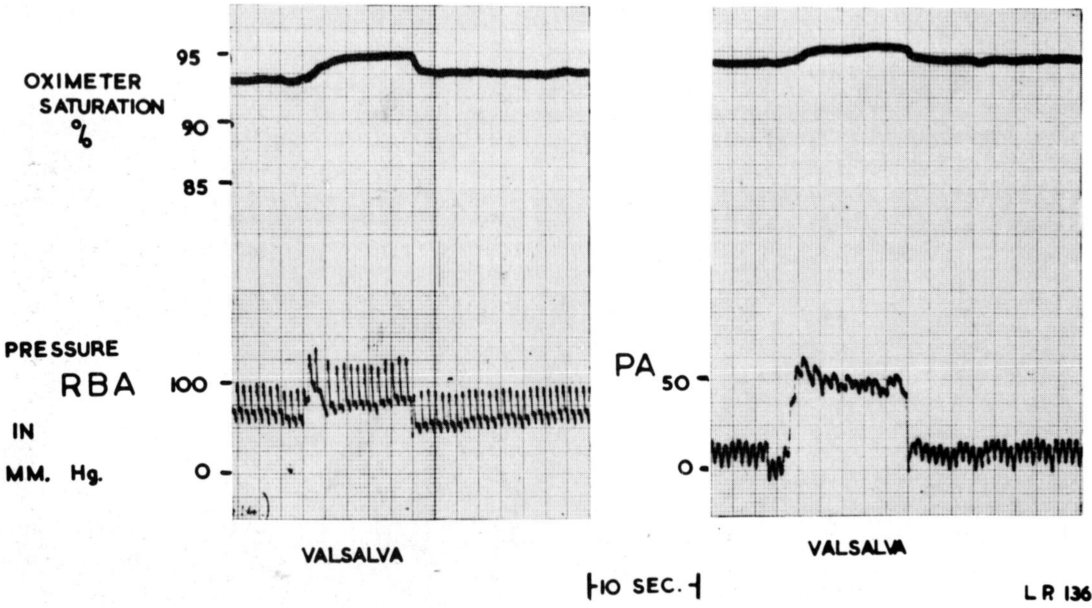

Figure 11–11. Brachial (RBA) and pulmonary arterial (PA) pressure tracings showing a square wave response to Valsalva's maneuver in a patient with large atrial septal defect and increased pulmonary blood flow. No fall in arterial oxygen saturation is seen after the release of strain.

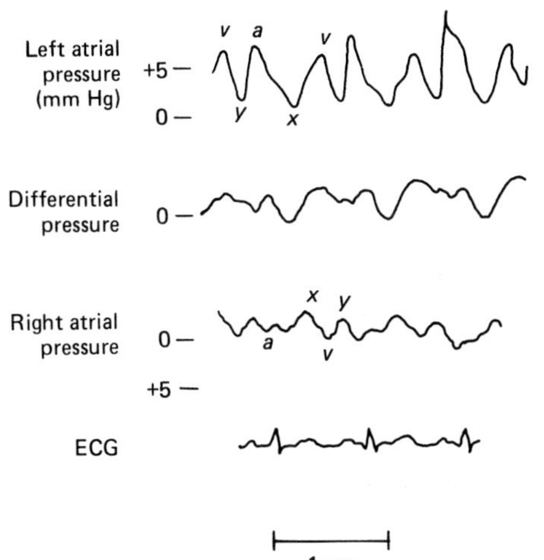

Figure 11–12. Simultaneous left and right atrial and differential pressure across an atrial septal defect. The pressure difference across the defect is greatest before the *v* wave. The right atrial pressure tracing is inverted because it is recorded by a differential manometer.

The left atrium should be entered in about 85% of cases in which the catheterization is performed using an arm vein and the left ventricle in about 60%. The chances of passing the catheter across an atrial defect are better if the study is performed using a leg vein, but the pulmonary artery is more difficult to enter using the leg approach. The left and right atrial mean pressures usually appear to be equal, and the pressure difference across the defect is small and occurs mainly late in systole, before the *v* wave, as shown in Fig 11–12.

b. **Pulmonary flow measurement** as strictly defined involves simultaneous pulmonary venous and arterial blood samples, but, in general, pulmonary venous oxygen content is assumed to equal either left atrial content or 97% of the oxygen capacity. Pulmonary arterial oxygen saturation gives a rough indication of the size of pulmonary blood flow. Values between 80 and 85% indicate slightly increased flow; 85–90%, moderate increase; and over 90%, a large flow. The accuracy of pulmonary flow measurements falls as the size of the left-to-right shunt increases. The pulmonary arteriovenous oxygen difference becomes smaller, with the result that small errors in the measurement of oxygen content have a large effect on the calculated pulmonary flow. Values for pulmonary flow in excess of 20 liters/min indicate the presence of artifacts.

c. **Systemic flow measurement.** Systemic output cannot be accurately measured in atrial septal defect because mixed venous oxygen content is difficult to measure. Some appropriately adjusted average value for superior and inferior vena caval oxygen contents must be selected to use as a value for a mixed venous sample. It is conventionally assumed that the inferior vena caval flow is twice that of the superior vena cava, and mixed venous oxygen content is considered to be one-third of the superior vena caval content plus two-thirds of the inferior vena caval content. Systemic blood flow tends to vary with age in patients with atrial septal defect. It is normal in young persons and decreases with age as atrial fibrillation and heart failure become more prevalent. The increase in pulmonary to systemic flow ratio with age is due as much to a decrease in systemic flow as to an increase in pulmonary flow. The ratio of pulmonary to systemic flow is generally considered to be the best overall indication of the hemodynamic significance of an atrial septal defect. A value of 2:1 or more is usually considered to indicate a significant defect, but in borderline cases other methods of assessing severity are required, such as heart size, atrial pressure, and pulmonary blood flow.

d. **Complete anatomic diagnosis** of atrial septal defect cannot be established with certainty in all cases. Unexpected anomalies of pulmonary venous return may be overlooked, but since cardiac defects are now surgically closed under direct vision, such deficiencies in diagnosis are now less important than they were before. In contrast, recognition of ostium primum defects is still important, since mitral valve surgery may be needed in addition to surgical closure of the defect. Left ventricular angiography is the best means of diagnosing this lesion. A "gooseneck" deformity of the left ventricular outflow tract is seen on a posteroanterior view of the ventricle (Fig 11–13).

e. **Selective indicator dilution curves** have in the past been used to detect abnormal venous drainage, but selective angiocardiography has been more widely used for this purpose in recent years. The functional route of venous return is all that can be determined by indicator dilution technics, whereas selective angiocar-

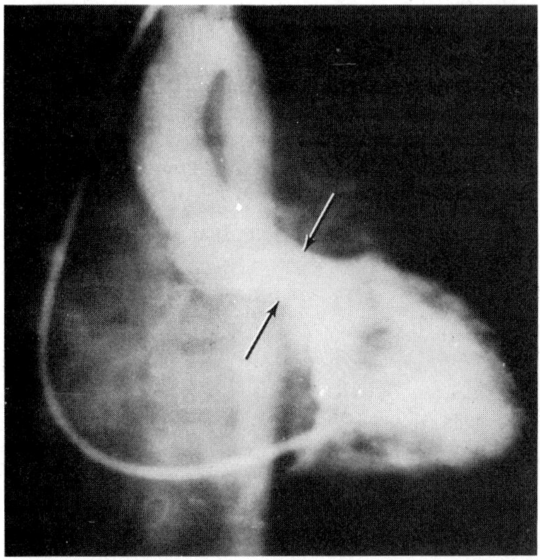

Figure 11–13. Left ventricular angiogram in a patient with ostium primum defect showing "gooseneck" deformity of the left ventricular outflow tract. (Courtesy of E Carlsson.)

diography gives both functional and anatomic information.

f. Intracardiac pressure measurements in atrial septal defect are an important procedure, but the accuracy of tracings is poor because the hyperdynamic right ventricular contractions associated with the high flow tend to cause marked catheter fling. Right-sided pressures are usually lower than expected. Pressure differences between the right ventricle and the pulmonary artery are found in patients with markedly increased flow and in patients with associated pulmonary stenosis. If the patient presents with signs of an atrial defect, the gradient across the pulmonary valve is almost always less than 50 mm Hg, and surgically important pulmonary stenosis is not present. The pressure difference is due to the increased flow and falls dramatically when the defect is closed.

g. Pulmonary vascular resistance should be measured in all patients with atrial septal defect. It is normally less than 2 mm Hg /l/min. It tends to be slightly raised (up to 3.5 mm Hg /l/min) in older patients with large shunts. A marked increase in resistance (7.5 mm Hg /l/min or more) constitutes a possible contraindication to surgery, and the decision whether or not to close the defect may be difficult. Right and left atrial pressures may be raised in older patients in whom heart failure has occurred, but values over 15 mm Hg are uncommon when the 2 atria are in free communication. In small defects there may be a detectable mean pressure difference between the 2 atria. A raised left atrial pressure with a significant pressure difference between the 2 atria indicates associated mitral disease. This may be either congenital, as in ostium primum lesions, or acquired, as in Lutembacher's syndrome, where it is presumably rheumatic in origin.

Differential Diagnosis

A. Rheumatic Heart Disease: Atrial septal defect is likely to be misdiagnosed as rheumatic mitral valve disease with mixed mitral stenosis and incompetence. The combination of cardiac enlargement, systolic and diastolic murmurs arising at the atrioventricular valves, and atrial fibrillation in a middle-aged woman can easily be mistaken for a rheumatic lesion, and pulmonary plethora due to increased blood flow can be confused in the chest x-ray with pulmonary congestion. If there is no rsR′ pattern on the ECG, the possibility of a congenital lesion may not be considered until cardiac catheterization reveals a high pulmonary arterial oxygen saturation. The presence of a large heart with only mild symptoms and the patient's ability to easily tolerate the onset of atrial fibrillation should suggest the possibility of an atrial defect. A large pulmonary artery and right atrium, combined with a small aorta and small left atrium on the chest x-ray, should suggest a possible diagnosis of atrial septal defect.

B. Other Lesions: Small atrial septal defects may be confused with a normal heart picture especially in the presence of pectus excavatum, which tends to cause systolic and even diastolic murmurs and to make the heart look large on posteroanterior view. Idiopathic dilatation of the pulmonary artery may also lead to confusion. It causes a systolic ejection murmur, a widely split second heart sound, and a large main

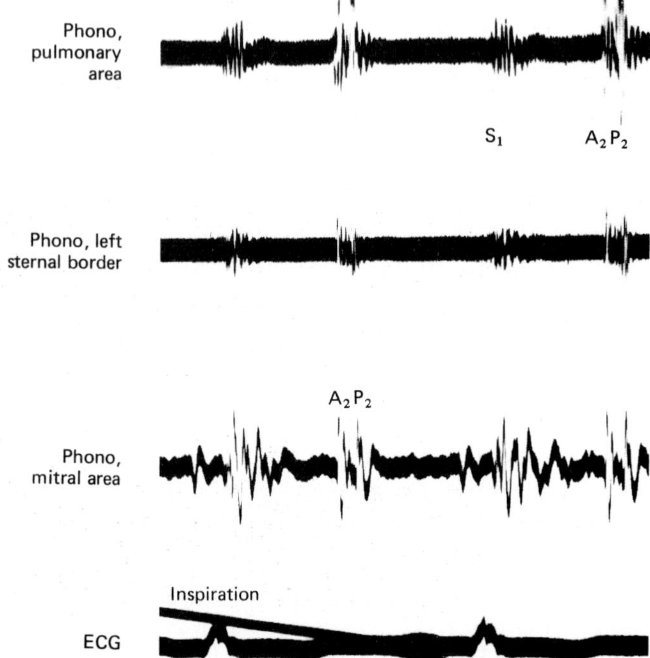

Figure 11–14. Phonocardiogram from a patient with atrial septal defect and pulmonary hypertension (mean pulmonary arterial pressure 40 mm Hg, pulmonary vascular resistance 9 mm Hg/l/min) showing fixed splitting (0.05 sec) of the second sound with pulmonary component (P_2) greater than aortic component (A_2) in the pulmonary area and P_2 transmitted to the mitral area. There is neither an ejection systolic murmur nor a tricuspid flow murmur. (Reproduced, with permission, from Leatham A: *Auscultation of the Heart & Phonocardiography*, 2nd ed. Churchill-Livingstone, 1975.)

pulmonary artery on the chest x-ray, and it is often associated with an rsR′ pattern in lead V_1 of the ECG. Cardiac catheterization must always be accurate enough to provide a correct diagnosis.

Complications

A. Pulmonary Vascular Disease: Pulmonary vascular disease is the most important complication of atrial septal defect. In patients with ostium secundum defects, it is always acquired rather than congenital. In patients with ostium primum or sinus venosus defects with anomalous venous drainage, the congenital form of pulmonary hypertension (Eisenmenger's syndrome) occurs, in which a raised pulmonary vascular resistance is present in infancy or childhood but does not develop in later life (see p 337). In patients with acquired pulmonary hypertension, the heart is large, the patient is usually over age 20, and pulmonary hypertension is progressive. Acquired pulmonary hypertension is due to the long-term effects of increased pulmonary blood flow on the pulmonary vascular bed, and pulmonary thromboembolism may initiate or aggravate the condition, especially in pregnancy. The incidence of this form of pulmonary hypertension, sometimes called acquired Eisenmenger's syndrome, is decreasing with earlier and more accurate diagnosis of congenital heart disease, but it still occurs in about 10% of cases. This complication is not inevitable, and patients with atrial septal defect who have been recatheterized after an interval of up to 20 years usually show no significant increase in pulmonary vascular resistance.

1. Symptoms and signs of pulmonary vascular disease—Increased dyspnea or cyanosis on exertion and intolerance of altitude are the commonest presenting symptoms. The patient may develop cyanosis and clubbing of the fingers, and polycythemia and increase in hematocrit are almost invariably found. There is usually a large *a* wave in the jugular venous pulse, and the heart is almost always greatly enlarged, with a prominent right ventricular heave. A pulmonary ejection click and a loud pulmonary valve closure sound are heard (Fig 11–14), and the second sound is closely split. ECG shows right ventricular hypertrophy and often atrial fibrillation (Fig 11–15). Chest x-ray confirms cardiac enlargement and usually shows marked enlargement of the central pulmonary arteries. There is a progressive increase in the heart size and also in the size of the pulmonary arteries (Fig 11–16).

2. Cardiac catheterization—Cardiac catheterization shows pulmonary arterial hypertension and a pulmonary blood flow that is normal or only slightly increased. Right-to-left shunting may be present at rest, with an arterial saturation of 85–95%, or desaturation may develop during exercise. Accurate measurement of pulmonary vascular resistance, plus study of the effects of vasodilator drugs such as tolazoline (Priscoline) or acetylcholine plus oxygen breathing, is needed to decide whether surgery is warranted. Closure of the defect is likely to be successful when the upper level of pulmonary vascular resistance does not exceed 7.5 mm Hg/l/min. The magnitude of the left-to-right shunt is a factor of almost equal importance. If the pulmonary blood flow is increased, closing the defect can reduce the load on pulmonary circulation and reverse or halt the progress of pulmonary vascular disease. Surgery in advanced cases has a high mortality rate, and the results are poor because the "safety valve" of an actual or potential right-to-left shunt is removed.

B. Heart Failure: Heart failure is the other, almost equally important complication of atrial septal defect (Fig 11–17). It is usually seen in association with atrial fibrillation and is directly related to the age of the patient and the presence of a lesion interfering with filling of the left ventricle. In the natural course of atrial septal defect that is not surgically treated, heart failure probably occurs with almost the same frequency as shunt reversal due to pulmonary hyperten-

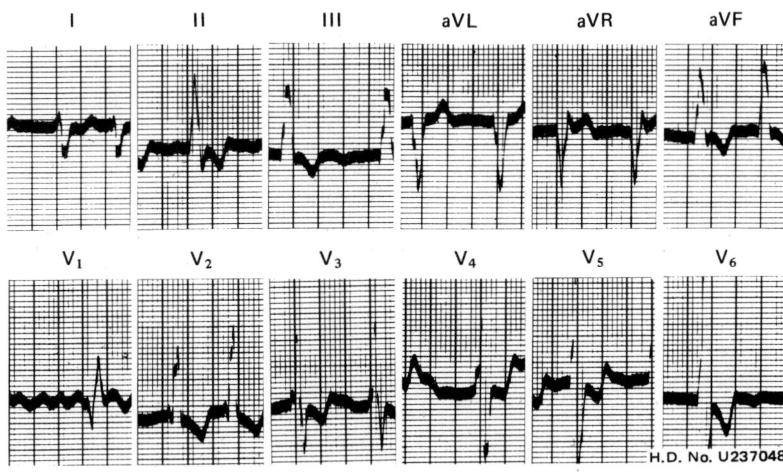

Figure 11–15. ECG of a 56-year-old woman with severe cardiac failure, pulmonary hypertension, and large atrial septal defect proved at autopsy. Tracing shows atrial fibrillation, right ventricular hypertrophy, and right ventricular conduction delay.

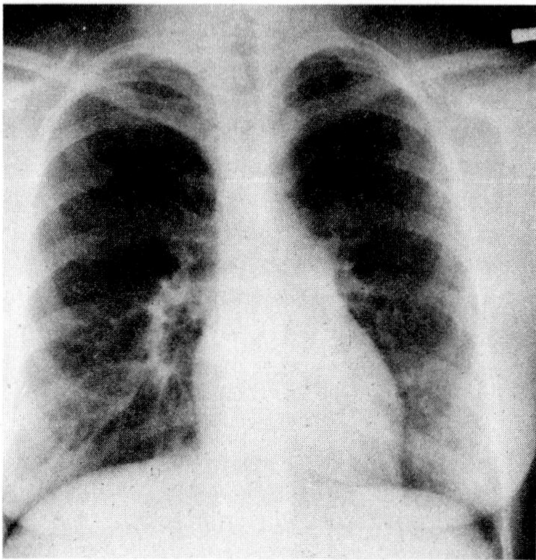

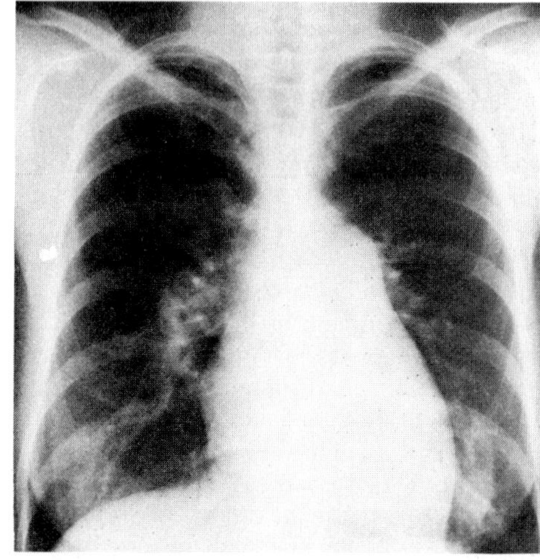

Figure 11–16. Serial chest x-rays taken 4 years apart in a 19-year-old patient with an atrial septal defect (sinus venosus) and systemic lupus erythematosus in whom severe pulmonary vascular disease developed. Heart size increased, and pulmonary arterial enlargement became more prominent.

sion. The exact mechanism of the congestive heart failure is not clear.

It is possible that mechanical factors play a part, because the enlarged right ventricle displaces the left ventricle posteriorly. This abnormal position of the left ventricle, shown in Fig 11–18, suggests that bulging of the right ventricle into the left interferes with filling. Left ventricular filling is apparently compromised by deterioration in left ventricular function secondary to systemic hypertension, coronary arterial disease, or advancing age. When the left ventricle does not fill properly, its compliance decreases and its diastolic pressure rises. As left atrial pressure tends to increase, the magnitude of the left-to-right shunt increases and loads the right heart. Atrial fibrillation and tricuspid incompetence tend to aggravate the situation, and right heart failure with edema, hepatomegaly, and raised jugular pressure follows. The right and left atrial pressures are the same if the defect is large, and values as high as 15–20 mm Hg are common. These levels are not sufficient to cause serious pulmonary congestion but are enough to produce significant right-sided congestion. The response to treatment with digitalis and diuretics is good, and the prognosis for surgical closure

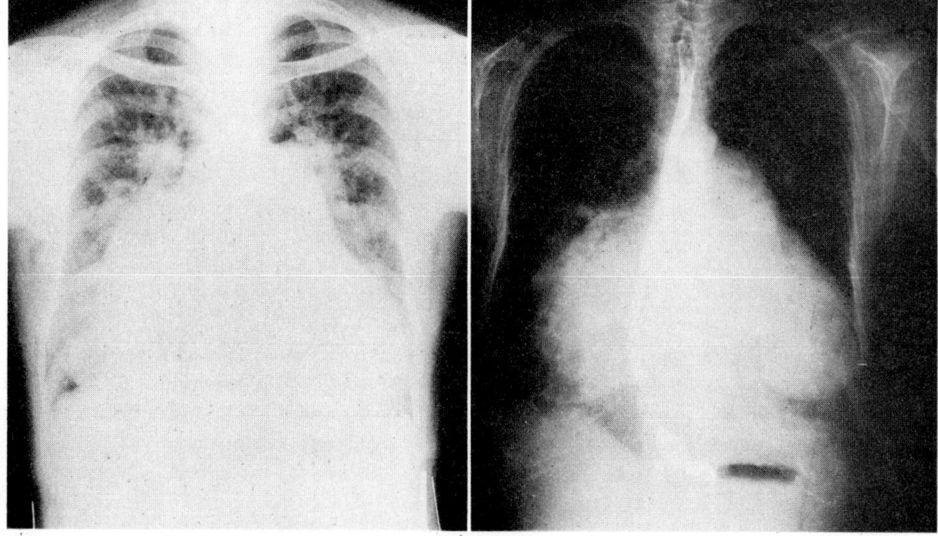

Figure 11–17. Chest x-ray with overpenetrated view and barium-filled esophagus in a patient with atrial septal defect in heart failure.

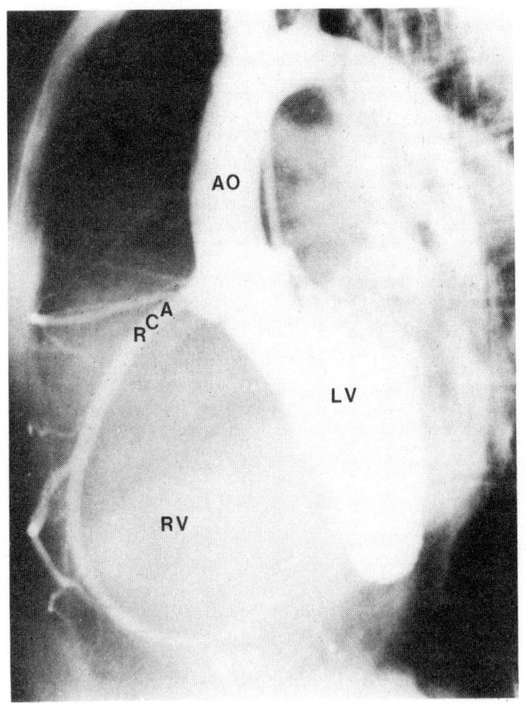

Figure 11–18. Angiocardiogram in left anterior oblique position showing distortion and posterior displacement of the left ventricle (LV) in a patient with atrial septal defect and heart failure. The anterior margin of the large right ventricle can be inferred from the position of the right coronary artery (RCA). AO, aorta; RV, right ventricle; LV, left ventricle.

of the defect is much better than was formerly thought.

C. **Atrial Arrhythmias**: Atrial fibrillation and other atrial arrhythmias are almost inevitable, especially atrial fibrillation after age 40 in the absence of surgical treatment. These arrhythmias are also related to the severity of the lesion and are less common in patients with small shunts. Restoration of sinus rhythm should be postponed until after surgery in most cases, since the arrhythmia is well tolerated.

D. **Other Complications**: Infective endocarditis is rare in atrial septal defect. Patients with ostium primum defects are more prone to develop this complication than are those with other atrial septal defects, presumably because of valvular involvement. Mitral valve disease is an associated lesion rather than a complication of atrial septal defect. The mitral lesion is usually mild, but it tends to readily produce congestive heart failure by reducing systemic flow and increasing the left-to-right shunt.

Treatment

Surgery is the treatment of choice in patients with atrial septal defect. Timing of the operation, the technic involved, and possible contraindications must be discussed by the surgeon and the patient.

A. **Closure of Defect**: Closure of atrial defects is now always carried out under direct vision during cardiopulmonary bypass. Ostium secundum defects can usually be sutured directly; the insertion of patches and baffles is likely to be needed only in ostium primum and sinus venosus defects. Although surgery almost always reduces the size of an atrial defect, residual holes may be overlooked, or the lesion may recur if stitches tear out postoperatively. Such complications are rare with open repair, and incorrect closure, such as directing the inferior vena cava into the left atrium, is less likely with cardiopulmonary bypass than with hypothermia.

B. **Relocation of Pulmonary Veins**: Relocation of pulmonary veins is needed in patients with partial anomalous venous drainage. The defect can often be sutured in such a way as to provide a tunnel through which the anomalous venous flow can be redirected without actually transecting the anomalous vein.

C. **Mitral Incompetence**: Suture of valve clefts, especially in the mitral valve, is the treatment of choice in younger patients. Mitral valve replacement is reserved for older patients.

Indications & Contraindications to Surgery

Surgery is indicated in all patients with a pulmonary to systemic flow ratio of 2:1 or more. Smaller defects can safely be left as is, especially when there is a significant pressure difference across the defect. Age is no bar to surgery. Since the operation "cures" the patient, it is recommended for asymptomatic persons as well. If heart failure develops, the patient should receive medical treatment with digitalis and diuretics, and surgical correction should be undertaken when the patient's condition has stabilized. A good response to medical therapy does not eliminate the need for operation. Severe pulmonary vascular disease with shunt reversal is the principal contraindication to surgery. The results of operation and the mortality rate (around 10%) are significantly worse than in patients with low resistance, in whom the mortality rate should be less than 1%. An attempt to restore sinus rhythm should be made about 6 weeks after operation in any patient with atrial fibrillation or flutter in whom arrhythmia persists.

Prognosis

The prognosis in atrial septal defect is good even without surgical treatment, and if operation is performed before symptoms develop, the patient should have a normal life expectancy. Patients with small defects who do not develop associated degenerative or atherosclerotic lesions in middle life may live long enough to die of another cause. The possibility of increasing left-to-right shunting with increasing age, the development of atrial fibrillation, and left ventricular disease are generally sufficient causes to advise surgery without waiting for signs of deteriorating cardiac function. The prognosis in ostium secundum lesions is better than that in ostium primum defects, and the development of pulmonary hypertension greatly worsens the prognosis.

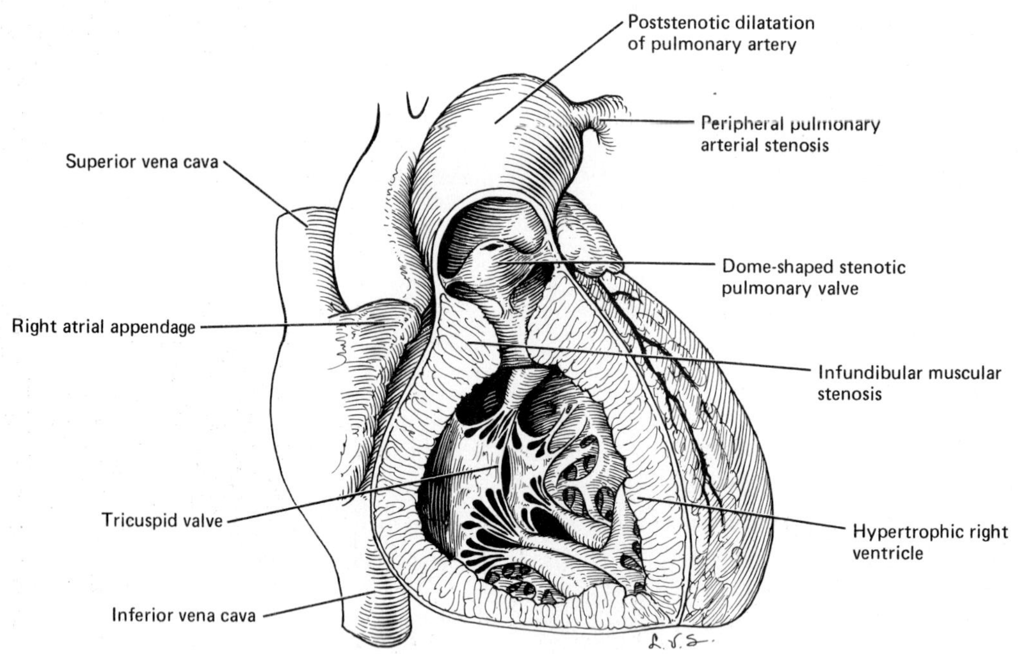

Anatomic features of pulmonary stenosis.

Cardinal features: *Reduction in pulmonary blood flow; right ventricular hypertrophy; murmur at the site of obstruction.*

Variable factors: *Severity of obstruction; site of obstruction: valvular, infundibular, or in pulmonary artery; patency of foramen ovale determines reversed interatrial shunt.*

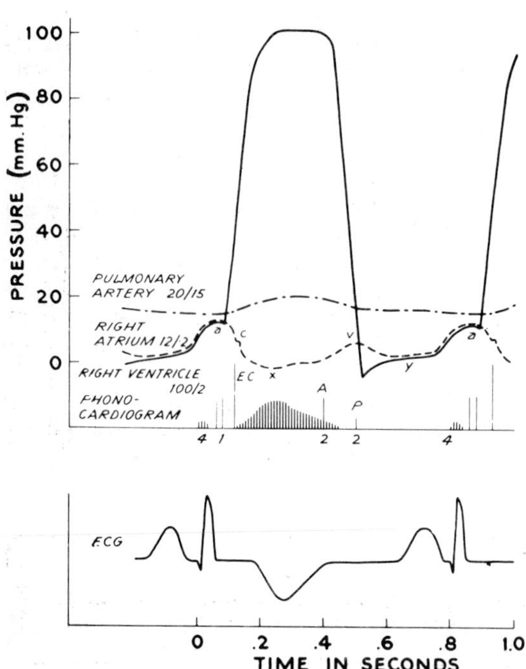

Diagram showing auscultatory and hemodynamic features of pulmonary stenosis.

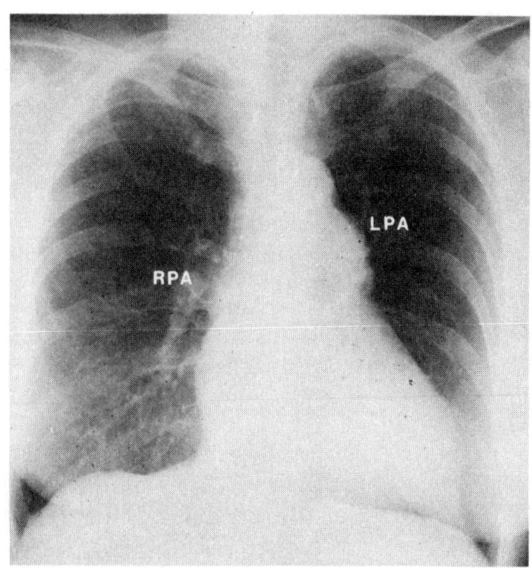

Chest x-ray of a patient with severe pulmonary stenosis showing large left pulmonary artery.

Figure 11–19. Pulmonary stenosis. Structures enlarged: Right ventricle and sometimes pulmonary artery (poststenotic dilatation).

PULMONARY STENOSIS

Cardinal Features & Pathogenesis

Pulmonary stenosis includes a number of conditions in which blood flow from the right heart to the lungs is obstructed.

The cardinal features include reduction in pulmonary blood flow, right ventricular hypertrophy, and a murmur at the site of obstruction. Among the variable factors that may be operating, the severity of obstruction influences the pulmonary blood flow and the extent of hypertrophy. Other factors are the site of obstruction (valvular, infundibular, or in the pulmonary artery) and the patency of the foramen ovale, which determines the presence of reversed interatrial shunt.

Various combinations of obstructive lesions are possible, and the severity of the obstruction varies. The principal load is on the right ventricle. The pulmonary artery is often dilated at the point at which the jet of blood passing through the narrowed valve impinges on the artery (poststenotic dilatation). In severe cases, a patent foramen ovale may permit right-to-left shunting at the atrial level. Pulmonary stenosis is the second most common form of congenital heart disease in adults mainly because this category includes patients with hemodynamically insignificant lesions. Two-thirds of adult cases are mild, and many could be classified as examples of idiopathic dilatation of the pulmonary artery. The spectrum of cases as shown in Fig 11–19 is wide, both because of differences in severity and because of varying sites of obstruction.

Pulmonary stenosis is more common in women than in men and is well tolerated in all but its severest forms. In mild cases the right ventricular systolic pressure is less than 50 mm Hg, and the gradient across the stenosis is 20 or 30 mm Hg at rest. In moderate cases the right ventricular systolic pressure is in the range of 50–100 mm Hg, with a gradient of up to 80 mm Hg. In severe cases the diagnosis is usually made in childhood, and severe cases with right ventricular pressures at or above systemic level are rarely seen in adults.

Clinical Findings

A. Symptoms and Signs: Hemodynamically insignificant or mild pulmonary stenosis does not cause significant symptoms. If a murmur has been detected, the patient may be abnormally aware of the heart and develop noncardiac pain.

1. Dyspnea–Dyspnea is the commonest presenting symptom in patients with moderate or severe pulmonary stenosis. Its origin is obscure, and the conventional explanation of cardiac dyspnea–pulmonary congestion and reduced lung compliance–is not applicable. Patients with pulmonary stenosis tend to hyperventilate during exercise, and inadequate perfusion of the exercising muscles is thought to provoke reflex ventilatory stimulation.

2. Dizziness and faintness on exertion, palpitations, and chest pain–These may rarely be the presenting symptoms in severe cases of pulmonary stenosis. The chest pain may be indistinguishable from that of angina of effort, and the fainting attacks are similar to the syncope on unaccustomed effort that occurs in patients with severe aortic stenosis.

3. Right heart failure–Right heart failure often occurs in early adult life in severe cases, and if the patient has not been seen previously, the diagnosis may be difficult when the patient presents in right heart failure with an extremely low cardiac output and little or no murmur.

The pulse is of small amplitude, and there is a giant *a* wave in the jugular venous pulse in severe cases. A right ventricular substernal heave is felt in moderate and severe cases.

A systolic murmur is always present except in moribund patients. In cases of valvular stenosis, the duration of the murmur is a function of the severity of the lesion. In mild cases of valvular stenosis, the murmur is short and diamond-shaped on the tracing. It is preceded by an ejection click (Fig 11–20). If the obstruction is infundibular, the murmur is longer and more like the pansystolic murmur of ventricular septal defect. In pulmonary artery stenosis, the murmur peaks later and resembles the murmur of coarctation of the aorta. The loudness and timing of the pulmonary valve closure sound are valuable clues to the severity of valvular stenotic lesions. In mild cases the second sound is normally or widely split, and the split moves normally with respiration. In moderately severe lesions the pulmonary closure sound is delayed, occurring up to 0.1 sec after aortic closure. It is also diminished in intensity because pulmonary blood flow tends to be low, but it still moves with inspiration (Fig 11–21). In severe cases the pulmonary valve closure sound is inaudible, and even aortic closure may not be heard because the sound is buried in the long pulmonary systolic murmur (Fig 11–22) which results from prolonged contraction of the overloaded right ventricle. Pulmonary diastolic murmurs are uncommon before surgery, but pulmonary incompetence not infrequently follows valvotomy. In pulmonary artery stenosis the auscultatory findings can be confused with those of pulmonary hypertension because pulmonary valve closure is usually loud and often palpable and the second sound is often split.

Patients with Turner's syndrome–characterized by 45 rather than 46 chromosomes, amenorrhea, hypertelorism, webbing of the neck, and short stature–

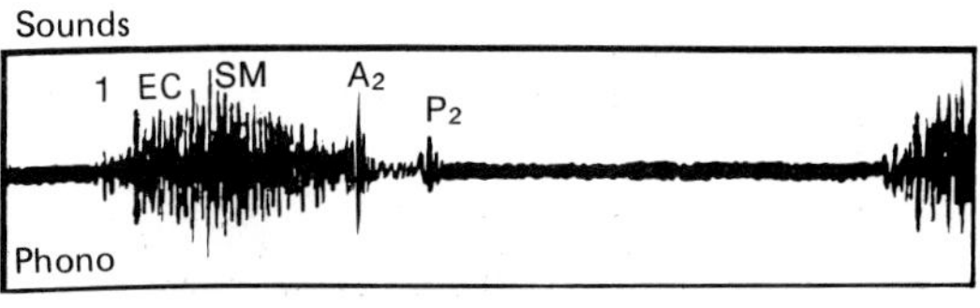

Figure 11–20. Typical phonocardiogram (recorded in third left interspace) in valvular pulmonary stenosis showing ejection click (EC), ejection murmur (SM) and late soft P_2. (Courtesy of Roche Laboratories Division of Hoffman-La Roche, Inc.)

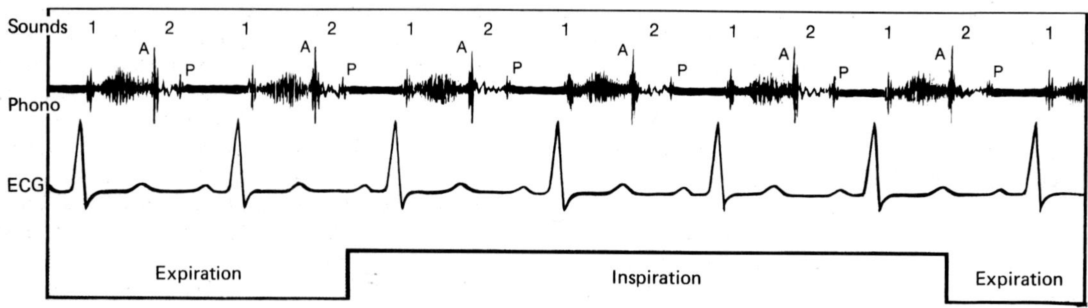

Figure 11–21. Phonocardiogram showing ejection murmur and soft late P_2—later still on inspiration—in pulmonary stenosis. (Courtesy of Roche Laboratories Division of Hoffman-La Roche, Inc.)

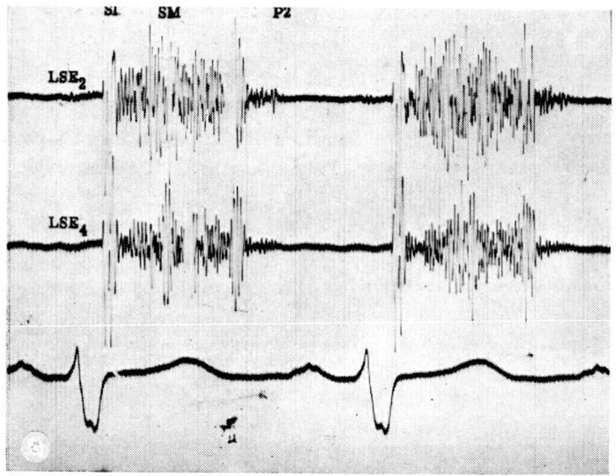

Figure 11–22. Phonocardiograms recorded at the left sternal edge in the second and fourth interspaces (LSE_2 and LSE_4) and ECG in a 14-year-old girl with severe pulmonary stenosis (right ventricular pressure 190/10 mm Hg). The systolic murmur continues through aortic valve closure, and P_2 is hardly detectable. (Reproduced, with permission, from Auerback ML, Sokolow M: Phonocardiography in acyanotic heart disease. Pediatrics 24:1026, 1959.)

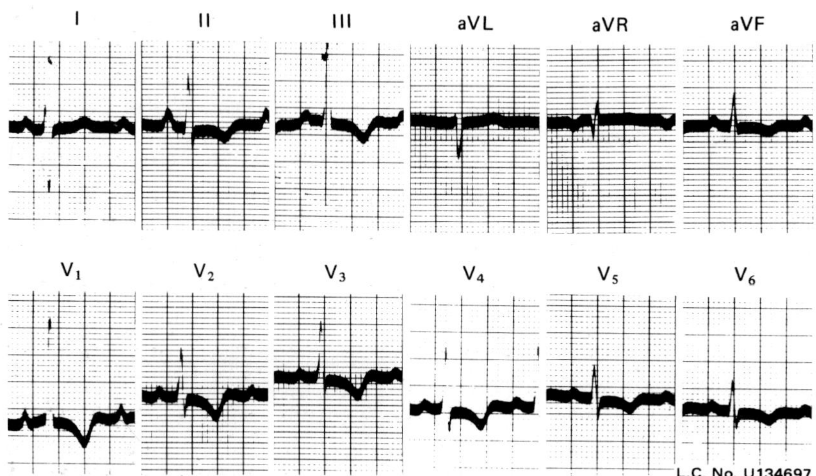

Figure 11–23. ECG of 25-year-old woman with pulmonary stenosis, patent interatrial septum, and cyanosis. Right ventricle 1.5 cm; left ventricle 1.1 cm. Normal coronary arteries. The tracing shows severe right ventricular hypertrophy.

may have pulmonary stenosis, and a moon-shaped face has also been described in patients with this lesion. Cyanosis is seen only in severe cases. It may be peripheral and due to low cardiac output, or central, due to arterial desaturation as a result of reversed interatrial shunt through a patent foramen ovale. In this case, it is associated with clubbing of the fingers and polycythemia.

B. Electrocardiographic Findings: Right ventricular hypertrophy in pulmonary stenosis is proportionate to the severity of the obstruction to right ventricular outflow. In mild cases the ECG shows only slight right ventricular dominance, whereas at the other end of the spectrum, severe pulmonary stenosis produces some of the most striking examples of right ventricular hypertrophy (Fig 11–23). Tall peaked P waves seen in severe cases are evidence of right atrial enlargement, and right bundle branch block sometimes occurs.

C. X-Ray Findings: The heart is of normal size in mild cases. Even in moderate to severe cases, cardiac enlargement may be absent because hypertrophy of the right ventricle occurs at the expense of the cavity of the ventricle. If the patient develops right ventricular failure, however, cardiac enlargement involving the right ventricle and right atrium always occurs. The main pulmonary artery and left pulmonary artery are commonly enlarged when the lesion is valvular. Poststenotic dilatation does not involve the right pulmonary artery, which is smaller and lies lower in the chest than the left pulmonary artery, as shown in Fig 11–19. Pulmonary arterial dilatation is unrelated to the severity of stenosis, and in cases with insignificant lesions, the main pulmonary artery may be markedly dilated. In such cases a diagnosis of idiopathic dilatation of the pulmonary artery is sometimes made, and it is not clear if a distinction can or should be made between hemodynamically insignificant pulmonary stenosis and idiopathic dilatation of the pulmonary artery. Both lesions are equally benign and are seldom if ever associated with symptoms. In infundibular lesions the pulmonary artery is not dilated. If the lesion is severe, the configuration of the heart resembles that seen in Fallot's tetralogy with infundibular obstruction (see p 325). If the lesion is in the pulmonary arteries, the main pulmonary artery is usually dilated. In any severe obstructive lesion the pulmonary blood flow is reduced, and the lung markings are abnormally sparse.

D. Special Investigations:

1. Noninvasive technics–Phonocardiography can be useful in establishing the timing and intensity of the pulmonary valve closure sound and demonstrating the length of the murmur. In severe cases, phonocardiography often makes it easier to detect that aortic valve closure is buried in a long systolic murmur.

Echocardiography can be helpful in identifying the site of obstruction when it is infundibular or valvular or both. The thickness of the pulmonary valve does not always indicate the severity of the obstruction, but it makes it possible to assess the degree of right ventricular hypertrophy. The distinction between pulmonary stenosis and other lesions such as Fallot's tetralogy and ventricular septal defect can also be made by echocardiography.

2. Invasive technics–The definitive technic for diagnosis and assessment of severity of pulmonary stenosis is cardiac catheterization. Measurement of pulmonary arterial and right ventricular pressures and pulmonary blood flow is needed to establish the diagnosis and severity of the stenosis. The anatomic site of the stenosis can usually be established by drawing the catheter from the pulmonary artery to the right atrium through the right ventricle and closely following the pressure changes. A sample tracing of pulmonary arterial and right ventricular pressures is shown in Fig 11–24; and right ventricular and right atrial pressures in Fig 11–25. In patients with high infundibular le-

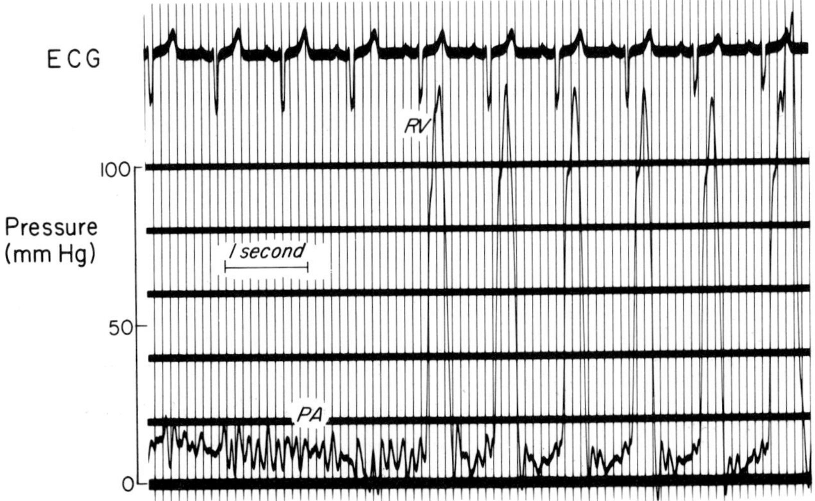

Figure 11–24. Pressure tracing showing withdrawal of the catheter across a stenotic pulmonary valve.

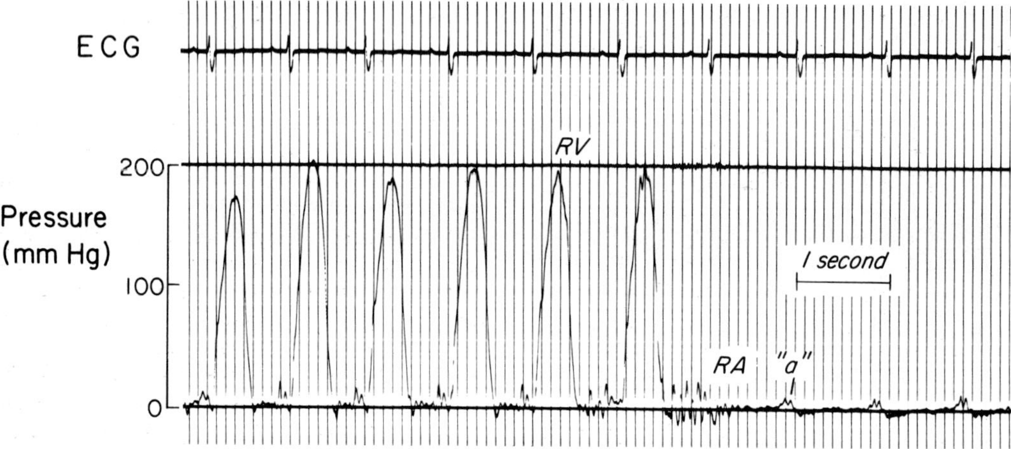

Figure 11–25. Pressure tracing showing withdrawal of a catheter across the tricuspid valve in a patient with severe pulmonary stenosis.

sions and those with both valvular and infundibular stenosis, angiography may be needed to establish the site of obstruction. Angiography is also valuable in differentiating pulmonary stenosis from Fallot's tetralogy.

Differential Diagnosis

The differential diagnosis of pulmonary stenosis depends on the severity of the lesion and on the anatomical level of the stenosis.

A. Atrial Septal Defect: Mild valvular lesions can resemble or be associated with an atrial septal defect. The systolic murmur and widely split second sound are common to both lesions.

B. Ventricular Septal Defect: Infundibular stenosis may be confused with a small ventricular septal defect because both lesions have a loud, long systolic murmur, best heard to the left of the sternum.

C. Pulmonary Hypertension: Pulmonary artery stenosis tends to be confused with primary pulmonary hypertension or with Eisenmenger's syndrome. The pressure in the main pulmonary artery is raised in these conditions, and the loud second heart sound and evidence of right ventricular overload are common to all of them. Cardiac catheterization is necessary to confirm the diagnosis.

D. Fallot's Tetralogy: When the pulmonary stenosis is moderate or severe and at the valvular or infundibular level, Fallot's tetralogy is the most important differential diagnosis. The ready fall in arterial oxygen saturation with exercise or amyl nitrite inhalation is perhaps the clearest point suggesting a diagnosis of Fallot's tetralogy.

Complications

A. Right Heart Failure: Right heart failure is an important late complication of moderate or severe pulmonary stenosis. It almost inevitably occurs immediately after surgical treatment of the lesion, and the postoperative course in adult patients is often difficult.

B. Infective Endocarditis: Infective endocarditis occurs in under 5% of cases of pulmonary stenosis and has a good prognosis because valvular damage is seldom severe and is well tolerated.

C. Valvular Calcification and Incompetence: Valvular calcification and incompetence can occur with advancing age and are more likely after valvotomy.

D. Pulmonary Thrombosis and Embolism: Pulmonary thrombosis and embolism tend to occur in severe cases in which pulmonary blood flow is reduced. They may cause an increase in pulmonary vascular resistance in old patients. If this is the case, surgical relief of the stenosis does not bring complete relief.

Treatment

Insignificant and mild lesions run a benign course. An example of a chest x-ray that was indistinguishable from another taken 30 years later is shown in Fig 11–26. No treatment is needed, but the patient should be followed and seen at intervals. Antibiotic prophylaxis (see Chapter 16) for the prevention of endocarditis is necessary in both idiopathic dilatation of the pulmonary artery and mild pulmonary stenosis, even though this complication is rare.

Surgery is recommended when the pressure difference between the right ventricle and the pulmonary artery is more than 60 mm Hg, with a normal pulmonary blood flow. With pressure differences in the 40–60 mm Hg range, other considerations such as heart size, age, and associated lesions influence the decision for or against surgery.

Valvular lesions are more amenable to surgical treatment than infundibular or supravalvular lesions. Pulmonary artery stenoses may be multiple and so far distal that they are inaccessible. Surgical treatment of valvular stenosis may not relieve the obstruction to right ventricular outflow because bands of hypertrophied muscle in the outflow tract may form a secondary obstruction, which persists when the primary valvular lesion is relieved. It may be difficult to decide

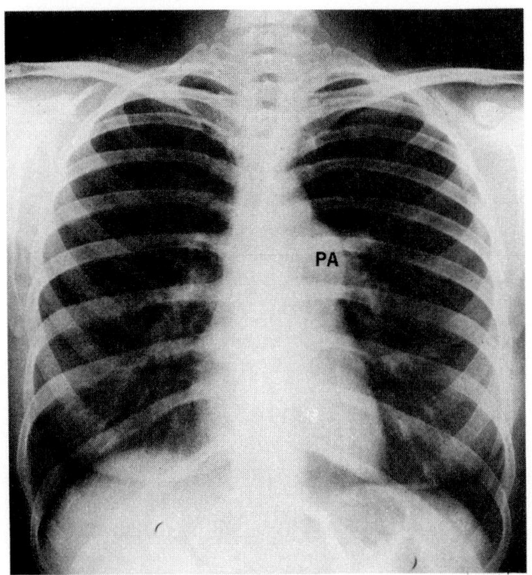

Figure 11–26. Chest x-ray of a 28-year-old woman with a dilated pulmonary artery. Another chest x-ray taken 30 years later showed no change in the size of the heart or the pulmonary artery.

whether to perform only a simple valvotomy or proceed with a resection of the hypertrophied muscle bands.

The decision to operate is the most problematic in mild and moderate cases because the long-term effects of the disease are not known. It is not clear whether the lesion becomes more severe with age or whether apparent progression stems from age-related changes in the right ventricular muscle. Surgical treatment is palliative rather than curative, and problems may arise later, either from pulmonary valve calcification or from the effects of surgically induced pulmonary incompetence.

The technic consists of opening up a dome-shaped diaphragm that bears no cusps. Pulmonary incompetence almost inevitably results, and if the analogy of congenital aortic stenosis is appropriate, it is likely that pulmonary valve replacement may be needed later, especially when valvular calcification occurs. The operation for the relief of infundibular obstruction involves resection of hypertrophic muscle.

Prognosis

The prognosis in pulmonary stenosis is directly related to the severity of the lesion. The surgical mortality rate is negligibly low in moderate lesions but rises to about 10% when right ventricular pressure is at or above systemic level. The truly long-term (30- to 40-year) prognosis of patients operated on in infancy and childhood has yet to be determined.

FALLOT'S TETRALOGY

Cardinal Features & Pathogenesis

The cardinal features of Fallot's tetralogy (Fig 11–27) are right ventricular hypertrophy, large ventricular septal defect, right ventricular outflow obstruction, and overriding aorta.

The ventricular septal defect is high in the membranous portion of the septum and large enough to equalize the pressures in the right and left ventricles. The right ventricular obstruction can be either valvular or infundibular or both, and the overriding of the aorta results in ejection of some right ventricular blood directly into the aorta. In some forms of the condition, both great vessels arise from the right ventricle, a condition termed double outlet right ventricle. The principal variable determining the severity of Fallot's tetralogy is the degree of right ventricular outflow obstruction. The site (valvular, infundibular, or both) of obstruction and the degree of overriding of the aorta play little part in determining the size of the pulmonary blood flow (the principal variable is outflow obstruction) because the right and left ventricular pressures are kept equal by the large ventricular defect.

The spectrum of cases of Fallot's tetralogy ranges from cases of pulmonary atresia in which no blood passes through the pulmonary valve to patients with low, moderate, and high pulmonary blood flow. In the mildest cases of pulmonary stenosis there is even a left-to-right shunt through the ventricular defect and a pulmonary to systemic blood flow of more than 2:1. Physicians disagree about the appropriateness of the term Fallot's tetralogy for patients with mild pulmonary stenosis, who are said to have acyanotic Fallot's tetralogy. However, the hemodynamic picture in patients with ventricular septal defect large enough to equalize pressures in the 2 ventricles conforms sufficiently to the definition to make the use of the term Fallot's tetralogy acceptable. The most characteristic feature of the condition is the marked drop in arterial oxygen saturation which occurs with exercise. This is not seen in patients with smaller ventricular defects; for these patients the term ventricular septal defect with pulmonary stenosis is appropriate.

The overall heart size in Fallot's tetralogy varies with the severity of the lesion. In the severest cases the heart is not enlarged; in fact, it may be smaller than normal. The aorta is usually large and may be right-sided. The right ventricle, although hypertrophied, is not large unless there is a left-to-right shunt. There may be poststenotic dilatation of the pulmonary artery if the right ventricular obstruction is at the valve. The left pulmonary artery may be absent in Fallot's tetralogy, but this abnormality, like a right-sided aortic arch, may occur independently (see Chapter 21).

Clinical Findings

A. Symptoms and Signs:

1. Cyanosis at birth–In all but its mildest forms Fallot's tetralogy is detectable at birth when cyanosis

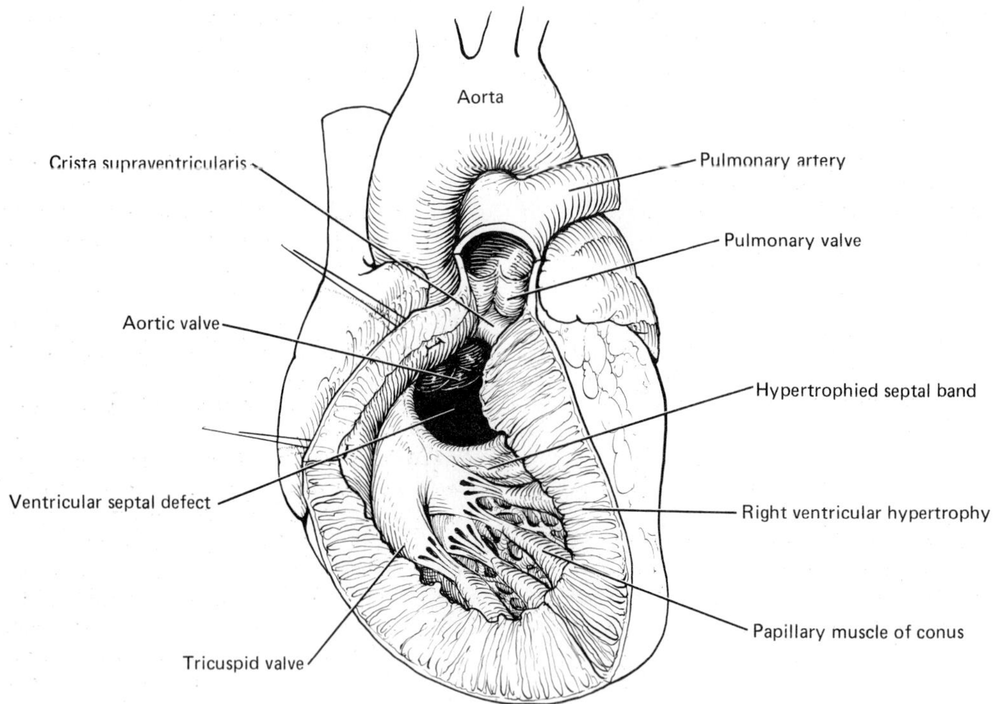

Anatomic features of Fallot's tetralogy. (Reproduced, with permission, from Dunphy JE, Way LW [editors] : *Current Surgical Diagnosis & Treatment,* 3rd ed. Lange, 1977.)

Cardinal features: *Right ventricular hypertrophy; large ventricular septal defect; right ventricular outflow obstruction; overriding aorta.*

Variable factors: *Severity of right ventricular outflow obstruction determines size of shunt and pulmonary blood flow; site of obstruction: valvular or infundibular or both.*

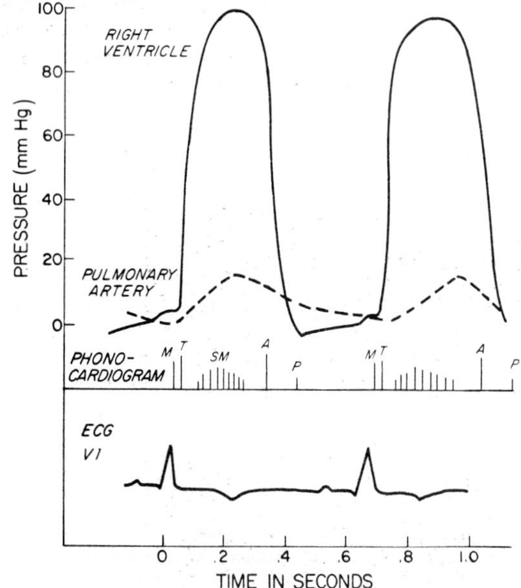

Diagram showing auscultatory and hemodynamic features of Fallot's tetralogy. SM, systolic murmur.

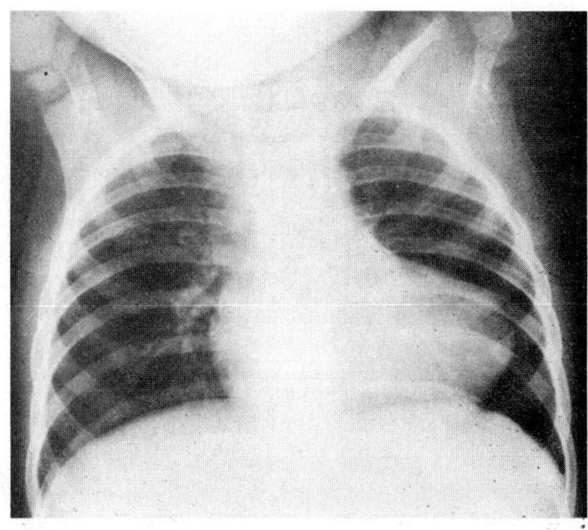

Chest x-ray of a child with Fallot's tetralogy showing a boot-shaped heart (coeur en sabot). (Courtesy of G. Gamsu.)

Figure 11–27. Fallot's tetralogy. Structures enlarged: None in severe cases. Large aorta. Large right ventricle in mild cases.

(blue baby) is noted. Cyanosis on exercise always occurs, but clubbing of the fingers is not seen in milder cases.

2. Dyspnea–Patients with Fallot's tetralogy are always disabled by dyspnea. Some patients say that they are not short of breath, perhaps because they have never experienced normal exercise tolerance, and sometimes it is not until after the lesion has been treated surgically that they realize how short of breath they actually were.

3. Squatting–Adopting the squatting position for relief of dyspnea after exercise is almost pathognomonic of Fallot's tetralogy in children. It is seldom seen in adults, who prefer to relieve dyspnea by sitting down and putting their feet up or by lying down. The mechanisms underlying the relief obtained from squatting are described in Chapter 2.

4. Other symptoms–Chest pain, arrhythmia, and congestive heart failure are rare in Fallot's tetralogy but are more commonly seen in adults than in children. Because the right ventricle never generates a systolic pressure higher than the systemic arterial pressure, the clinical picture is different from that of severe pulmonary stenosis, in which a right ventricular pressure above systemic level can cause chest pain and right heart failure.

B. Attacks of Faintness: In some severe cases, especially with infundibular stenosis, the patient is subject to attacks of faintness and cyanosis. The patient seldom presents with these features initially, but they tend to occur later in the course of the disease. The mechanism of these attacks is infundibular muscular spasm, which reduces pulmonary blood flow. The right-to-left shunt increases, and the patient becomes progressively more hypoxic. Death may occur in the attack, but more commonly the right ventricular muscle itself becomes hypoxic and dilates, relieving the condition. These attacks rarely persist into adult life and respond to treatment with propranolol or the administration of general anesthetics.

C. Hemodynamic Findings: The characteristic hemodynamic feature of Fallot's tetralogy is the shunting of blood across the ventricular septal defect dependent on the relative resistance of the systemic and pulmonary circulation. Because the resistance to blood flow to the lungs–the pulmonary stenosis–is usually fixed, the systemic resistance is of great importance. Systemic vasodilatation due to muscular exercise, arterial hypoxia, fever, pregnancy, and increased environmental temperature tends to increase or produce right-to-left shunting. As a result, the clinical status of patients with Fallot's tetralogy tends to be unstable and varies from day to day with the weather and the patient's activity and environment.

D. Other Physical and Cardiac Signs: The physical signs of Fallot's tetralogy vary widely according to the severity of the lesion. Growth is retarded in the most severe cases, and cyanosis and clubbing of the fingers and toes are seen in all but the mildest.

The pulse is of normal volume because the systemic output is well maintained. The venous pressure is normal with at most a small *a* wave visible in the neck.

The heart is quiet, with little right ventricular heave in severe cases. In milder cases with left-to-right shunts, there is a larger, more hyperdynamic right ventricle. The intensity and length of the murmur arising from right ventricular outflow obstruction vary with the severity of the lesion. In pulmonary atresia or with severe pulmonary stenosis, the pulmonary blood flow may be so small that there is no pulmonary ejection systolic murmur. In such cases an almost continuous murmur due to collateral bronchial blood flow may be heard, especially over the back. In mild acyanotic cases the murmur is long and loud. It may be pansystolic and arise from the ventricular septal defect in patients with a left-to-right shunt. Since the outflow obstruction is always severe enough to raise the right ventricular pressure to systemic levels, the pulmonary valve

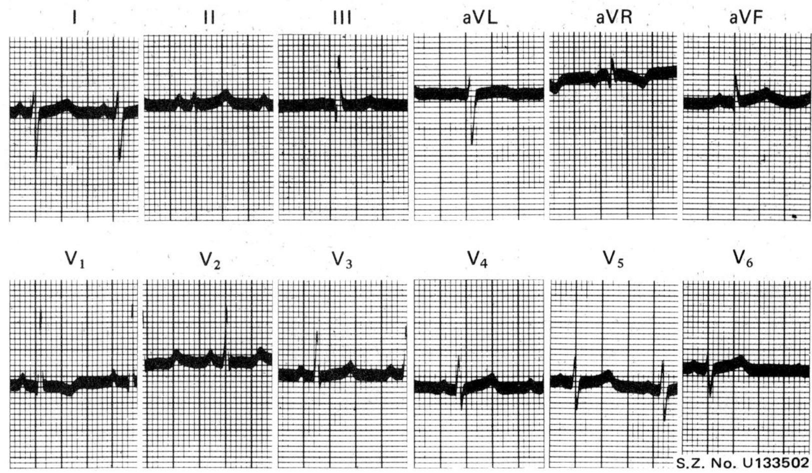

Figure 11–28. ECG of 7-year-old boy with tetralogy of Fallot showing right ventricular hypertrophy.

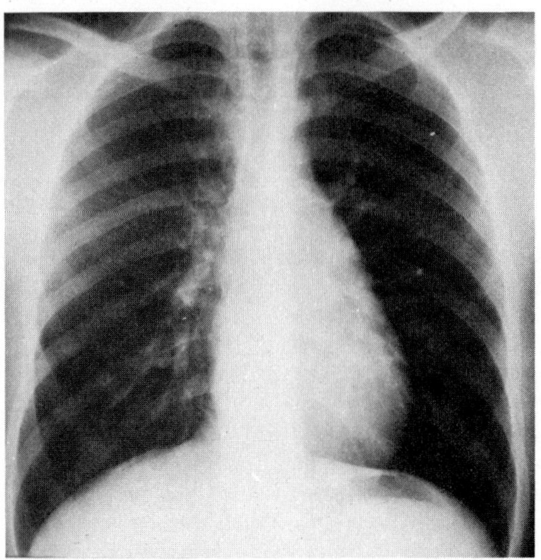

Figure 11–29. Chest x-ray of a 16-year-old boy with mild Fallot's tetralogy. The cardiac silhouette is almost normal in size and shape.

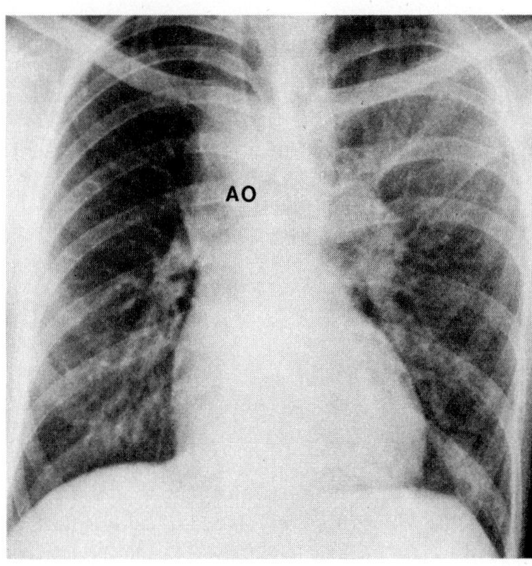

Figure 11–30. Chest x-ray of a man with Fallot's tetralogy with a Blalock anastomosis. The aorta (AO) is right-sided.

closure sound is usually inaudible. However, it can be detected by phonocardiography.

During cyanotic attacks the pulmonary systolic ejection murmur may become fainter as pulmonary blood flow falls, and relief of the attack may be first detected by hearing an increase in the intensity of the murmur.

E. Electrocardiographic Findings: The ECG always shows some evidence of right ventricular hypertrophy in Fallot's tetralogy (Fig 11–28), but the changes may be surprisingly mild. In milder cases with a left-to-right shunt, there may be evidence of biventricular hypertrophy. P waves are seldom abnormal, and gross right ventricular hypertrophy of the type found in severe pulmonary stenosis is not seen. Left ventricular hypertrophy only occurs in patients with a large, palliative, surgically produced left-to-right shunt.

F. X-Ray Findings: The size of the heart on the chest x-ray is inversely related to the severity of the lesion.

1. Severe lesions–With severe pulmonary stenosis and reduced pulmonary blood flow, the left atrium and left ventricle are small; as a consequence, the overall heart size is reduced. The combination of right ventricular hypertrophy and infundibular stenosis gives the classical "coeur en sabot" (boot-shaped heart) radiologic picture, with the apex pointing upward and to the left (Fig 11–27). In severe cases, especially those with pulmonary atresia, increased bronchial collateral blood flow may give rise to a reticulated pattern of blood vessels in the lungs. Underfilled lungs with sparse pulmonary vessels are seen in cyanotic cases.

2. Milder lesions–In milder, acyanotic cases and those with valvular stenosis, the heart shadow is larger, and poststenotic dilatation of the pulmonary artery is seen. In some cases with infundibular stenosis, the heart shadow may appear surprisingly normal, as shown in Fig 11–29. Normal lung fields or even pulmonary plethora is seen in the milder cases.

The finding of a right-sided aortic arch (Fig 11–30) is independent of the severity of the lesion.

G. Special Investigations:

1. Noninvasive technics–

a. Hematocrit–The degree of polycythemia, as shown by the hematocrit, varies with the degree of arterial hypoxia and thus with the severity of the lesion. Hematocrit levels as high as 75–80% are seen, especially in adults.

b. Echocardiography–Echocardiographic examination of the heart is of particular value in establishing the diagnosis of Fallot's tetralogy. By starting at a site intersecting the ventricular septum and pointing the ultrasound beam progressively upward toward the root of the aorta, it is possible to determine the presence and extent of overriding of the aorta and to see the break in continuity of the echoes that represent the ventricular septal defect (Fig 11–31). This noninvasive examination can thus distinguish between Fallot's tetralogy and pulmonary stenosis with intact ventricular septum. However, the actual diagnosis of Fallot's tetralogy by echocardiography cannot be made with absolute certainty because a similar form of overriding of the aorta is seen in Eisenmenger's complex (see p 337), in which pulmonary hypertension rather than pulmonary stenosis is present.

2. Invasive technics–Cardiac catheterization is always indicated before any surgical operation in patients with Fallot's tetralogy. The aim of the study is to measure the pulmonary arterial pressure and show that the right ventricular and aortic pressures are the same. In more than half of cases, these aims can be accomplished by right heart catheterization that passes

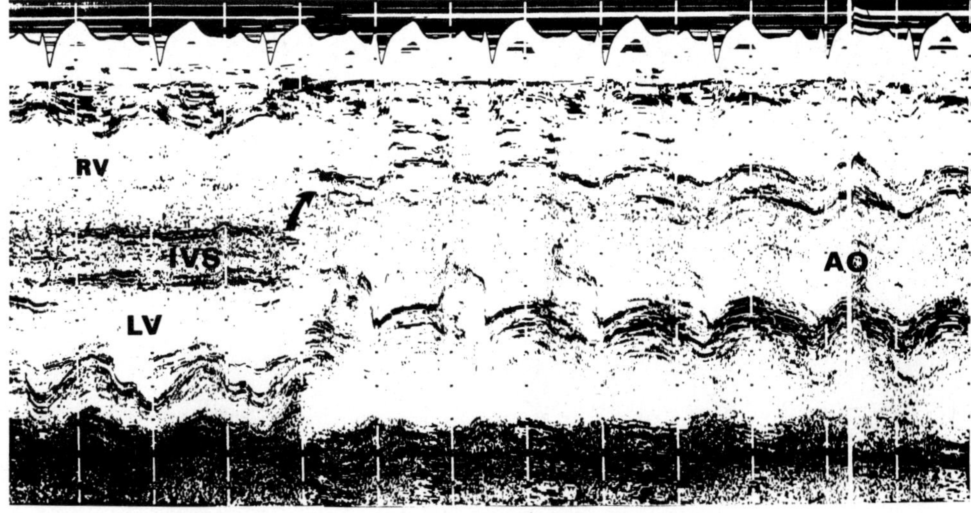

Figure 11–31. Echocardiogram showing aorta overriding ventricular septum in a patient with Fallot's tetralogy. RV, right ventricle; IVS, interventricular septum; LV, left ventricle; AO, aorta. (Courtesy of NB Schiller.)

the catheter through the ventricular septal defect into the aorta as well as into the pulmonary artery. In patients who have had palliative shunt operations, it is also important to determine the patency of the anastomosis that was produced. This may require retrograde arterial catheterization.

Angiographic demonstration of right ventricular outflow obstruction, aortic anatomy, and the ventricular defect should also be carried out routinely. Angiography shows that the right-to-left shunt in Fallot's tetralogy is actually from the right ventricle into the aorta, so it is not surprising that the left ventricle is seldom entered during right heart catheterization.

The average mean right atrial pressure was 6 mm Hg in 20 patients with Fallot's tetralogy age 15–53 (mean age, 33). The arterial oxygen saturation at rest averaged 90%, and the hematocrit was 55%. The systemic cardiac output was normal, and the pulmonary blood flow and pulmonary arterial pressure were inversely related to the severity of the lesion.

Differential Diagnosis

Fallot's tetralogy must be distinguished from pulmonary stenosis with reversed interatrial shunt. It is not always possible to make the distinction on clinical grounds, and cardiac catheterization is often necessary to make the correct diagnosis. It may sometimes be difficult to distinguish Fallot's tetralogy from Eisenmenger's complex (ventricular septal defect with pulmonary hypertension), especially when Fallot's tetralogy is mild and there is a bidirectional shunt. Adequate cardiac catheterization studies are mandatory before surgery in such cases because exploratory thoracotomy is often fatal in patients with pulmonary hypertension.

Complications

Progressive polycythemia may lead to cerebral or pulmonary thrombosis. Cerebral embolism or abscess formation is sometimes seen as a result of paradoxic embolization from the right heart through the shunt. Infective endocarditis can occur at the site of the ventricular septal defect in mild cases, or on the pulmonary valve, or in both places. It is occasionally seen both before and after palliative surgery. Right heart failure with edema and raised venous pressure is extremely rare, except after surgery.

Prevention

Antibiotic prophylaxis (see Chapter 16) for the prevention of endocarditis is necessary both before and after the operation.

Treatment

A. Medical Treatment: The fainting attacks seen in patients with Fallot's tetralogy respond to propranolol, either intravenously in the acute stage, or orally as a preventive measure. Morphine has been used in the past, and inhalational anesthetics, especially cyclopropane, are also known to be effective.

B. Surgical Treatment:

1. Palliative surgery—Palliative surgery to increase the blood flow to the lungs by producing an anastomosis between the subclavian and pulmonary arteries (Blalock-Taussig operation) or the aorta and the pulmonary artery (Potts operation) was introduced over 25 years ago with dramatic results. Patients with severe forms of Fallot's tetralogy benefited greatly from these operations, which resulted in lessening of cyanosis and marked improvement in exercise tolerance. However, the operations were only palliative, and the basic defect was not corrected. Palliative surgery is still occasionally indicated in infants, but curative surgery, with complete repair of the defect, is now the treatment of choice.

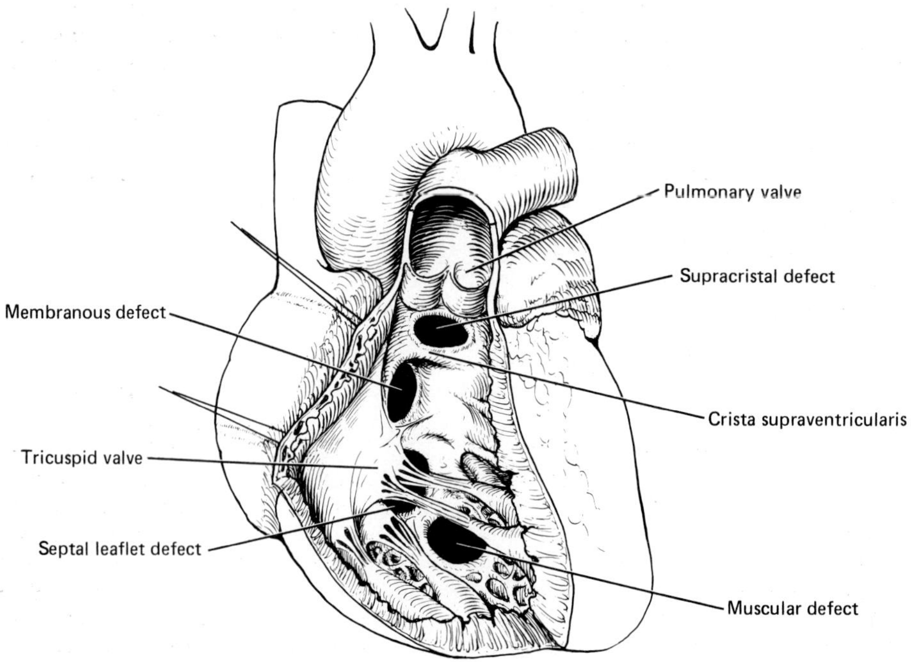

Anatomic location of ventricular septal defects.

Cardinal features: *Left-to-right shunt into right ventricle; increased pulmonary blood flow; pulmonary arterial pressure usually low.*

Variable factors: *Size of defect; site of defect: membranous or muscular; associated aortic incompetence.*

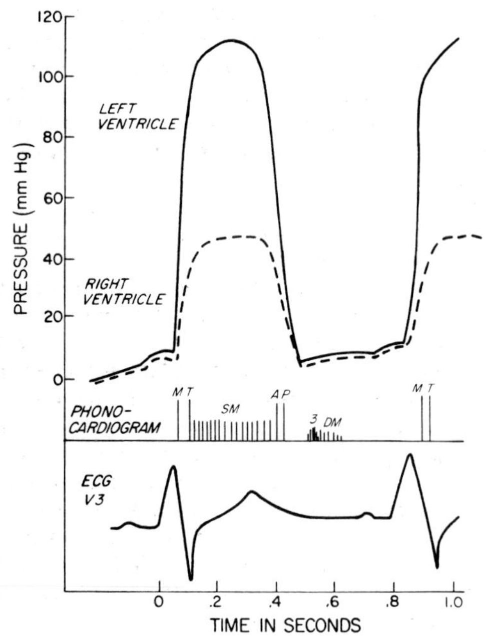

Diagram showing auscultatory and hemodynamic features of ventricular septal defect. SM, systolic murmur, DM, diastolic murmur.

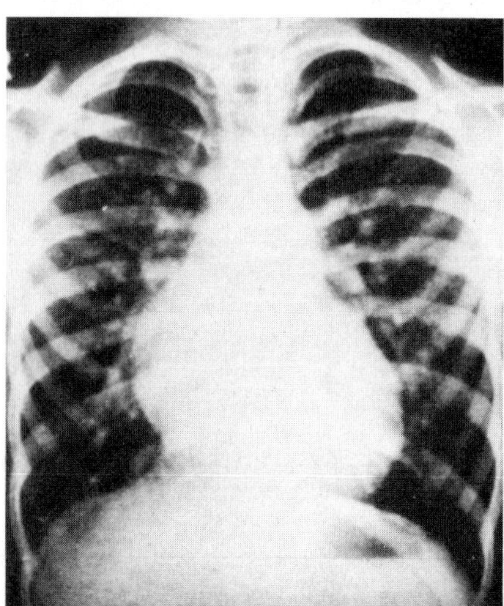

Dilatation of the pulmonary artery and pulmonary plethora in a case of ventricular septal defect. (Reproduced, with permission, from Wood P: *Diseases of the Heart and Circulation,* 3rd ed. Lippincott, 1968.)

Figure 11–32. Ventricular septal defect. Structures enlarged: Left atrium, left ventricle, and right ventricle.

2. Complete repair–Complete repair is always indicated in adult patients. If the patient has reached adult life without surgery, the lesion is likely to be relatively mild, and complete correction should be comparatively easy since the pulmonary vascular bed, left atrium, and ventricle are probably capable of accepting a normal right ventricular output. The mortality rate of complete repair in adult patients is about 10–15%, and some residual pressure difference between the right ventricle and pulmonary artery is usually present after operation. If an attempt at complete correction is only partially successful, recatheterization and reoperation are indicated because pulmonary hypertension with a large left-to-right shunt through an open ventricular defect may develop rapidly and lead to right heart failure.

3. Complete repair following palliative surgery–If the patient has previously had a Blalock or Potts operation, complete repair is still indicated. The operation may be more difficult because the shunt must be identified and closed, and the right ventricular outflow tract may be hypoplastic. Any patient with symptoms severe enough to have warranted palliative surgery in childhood would probably not have survived to adulthood without operation. These patients represent a new form of heart disease, which did not exist until palliative surgery was introduced. A decision about the timing of complete operative repair is difficult because the patient may be reasonably stable, leading a sheltered life, and unwilling to submit to a second life-threatening cardiac operation. It is important to follow such patients closely and to be alert to the possible development of pulmonary vascular disease, even though this is quite uncommon. Recatheterization does not always provide an adequate answer because pulmonary arterial pressure may be difficult to obtain.

It is not yet clear whether iatrogenic problems in patients with Fallot's tetralogy will be less common in the future. The modern trend toward attempting complete repair at earlier stages before the patient is fully grown may possibly reduce the number of patients reaching adult life with palliative shunts.

Prognosis

The prognosis in untreated Fallot's tetralogy is poor, and only patients with mild lesions survive to adult life without surgery. Fallot's tetralogy is a severe condition, and even in its mild form the pulmonary stenosis must be considered severe because right ventricular pressure equals systemic pressure. The prognosis is also poor in patients who have had a palliative shunt operation in childhood. Infective endarteritis may develop in the shunt. Blalock shunts between the subclavian and pulmonary arteries may close off with time, or the patient may "outgrow" the shunt, and cyanosis may recur. In patients with Pott's shunt from the aorta to the pulmonary artery, the pulmonary blood flow is more likely to be too large than too small. Left ventricular enlargement, increased pulmonary blood flow, aortic incompetence, pulmonary hypertension, and right heart failure may occur. Although the risks of complete correction may be high, the benefits of successful surgery are great, and it is important to routinely advise complete correction. In unoperated cases, progressively increasing pulmonary vascular resistance may occur in the fourth or fifth decade, presumably because of thrombosis and embolism. In these patients, the prognosis is dismal, and complete correction inadvisable.

VENTRICULAR SEPTAL DEFECT

Ventricular septal defect without other associated anomalies constitutes about 10% of cases of congenital heart disease seen in adults. The anatomic but clinically irrelevant presence of a ventricular defect is much more common, being found in Fallot's tetralogy, Eisenmenger's complex, and a number of complex congenital lesions. The cardinal features of ventricular septal defect (Fig 11–32) are left-to-right shunt into the right ventricle, increased pulmonary blood flow, and a usually low pulmonary artery pressure. Variable features are the size of the defect (large or small), the site of the defect (membranous or muscular), and the presence or absence of associated aortic incompetence. Only a small number of ventricular defects occur in the muscular part of the septum, and these may be multiple. The acquired form of the lesion, seen with rupture of a necrotic area in the septum after myocardial infarction, also involves the muscular part of the septum. This lesion is described in Chapter 8. The size and site of the ventricular defect determines the size of the left-to-right shunt, which in turn determines the clinical picture. Associated aortic incompetence causes further left ventricular enlargement. A left-to-right shunt at the ventricular level produces an increased flow through the left atrium, left ventricle, and right ventricle. The right atrium is the only chamber through which flow is normal.

The clinical spectrum of cases is wide, varying from maladie de Roger, in which a loud murmur and thrill are the only detectable abnormalities, to defects large enough to cause moderate pulmonary hypertension and large left-to-right shunts. Ventricular septal defect is more important in infants and children than in adults. The defect may become smaller or even close spontaneously as the child grows. A significant percentage of the patients seen in infancy with large ventricular septal defects develop pulmonary hypertension or infundibular stenosis, and some die in infancy. This leaves a relatively small number (usually those with milder defects) to grow to adult life.

Clinical Findings

A. Symptoms and Signs: Symptoms in patients with ventricular septal defect depend on the size of the defect and the age of the patient. Small shunts cause no significant hemodynamic effects and are compatible with a normal life expectancy. Larger defects, with

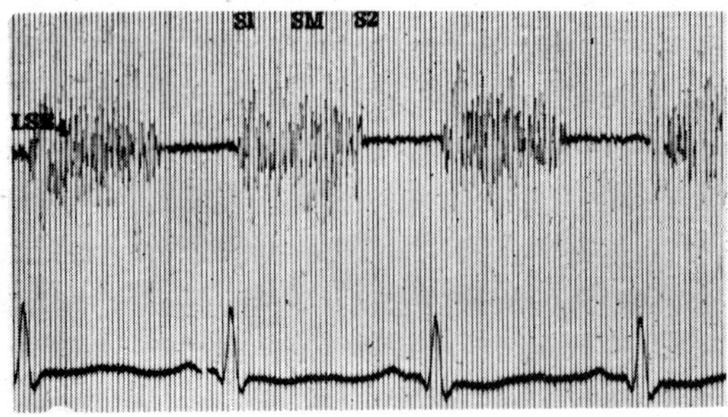

Figure 11–33. Phonocardiogram showing pansystolic murmur (SM) in a patient with a small ventricular septal defect. Recorded at the fourth left intercostal space (LSE_4). (Reproduced, with permission, from Auerback ML, Sokolow M: Phonocardiography in acyanotic congenital heart disease. Pediatrics 24: 1026, 1959.)

pulmonary to systemic flow ratios of 1.5:1 or more, may cause dyspnea after age 30, and large defects with flow ratios of 3:1 or more are rare but are usually associated with dyspnea on exertion. There is usually a history of a heart murmur present since birth.

The physical signs of ventricular septal defect are dominated by the loud pansystolic murmur and thrill which are present in the third and fourth left intercostal space inside the apex (Fig 11–33). In more than half of adult cases, these are the only abnormal physical signs. In patients with larger shunts, the pulse is jerky, resembling a miniature water-hammer pulse, and the cardiac impulse is hyperdynamic. The increased force of left ventricular contraction, which is associated with ejection of an increased stroke volume out through the aorta and into the low pressure right ventricle, causes a hemodynamic pattern similar to that seen in mitral incompetence.

The increased pulmonary blood flow causes increased flow through the mitral valve, which produces a third heart sound and a short diastolic flow murmur resulting from relative mitral stenosis.

B. Electrocardiographic Findings: The ECG is normal in more than half of adult cases. In patients with large left-to-right shunts there is evidence of mild biventricular overload, with both tall R waves and deep S waves over the transitional zone leads, together with Q waves in the left ventricular leads. These findings are illustrated in Fig 11–34.

C. X-Ray Findings: The chest x-ray shows a normal cardiac configuration if the shunt is small. Cardiac enlargement is proportionate to the size of the shunt. Since large left-to-right shunts are rare in adults, increased heart size, which typically involves the left atrium, both ventricles, and the pulmonary artery, is not often seen. Left atrial appendage enlargement is not seen in ventricular septal defect, even when the left atrium is enlarged.

D. Special Investigations:

1. Noninvasive technics–Echocardiography is particularly helpful in differential diagnosis. Although ventricular septal defect may be confused with certain conditions on physical examination, echocardiography reveals distinguishing features of these disorders, which include mitral incompetence, hypertrophic cardiomyopathy, infundibular stenosis, and ostium primum defects with mitral incompetence. The differential diagnosis can thus be made by exclusion when the defect itself cannot be detected and the paradoxic motion of the interventricular septum is not marked.

2. Invasive technics–Cardiac catheterization is in-

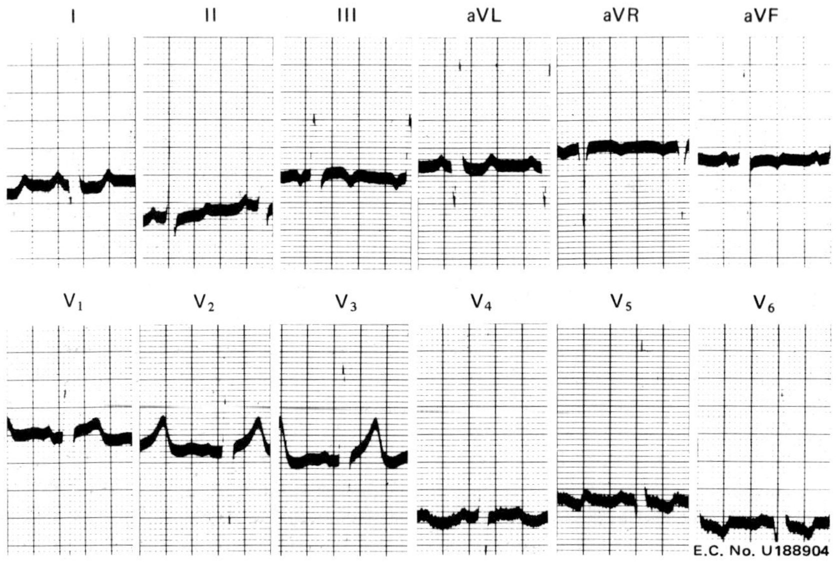

Figure 11–34. ECG of a 21-year-old man with ventricular septal defect proved by catheter; right ventricular pressure is 39/6. (Reproduced, with permission, from Auerback ML, Sokolow M: Phonocardiography in acyanotic heart disease. Pediatrics 24:1026, 1959.)

dicated to confirm the diagnosis, especially if surgical treatment is contemplated. In patients with small defects, a left-to-right shunt may not be detectable from blood samples taken from the right heart chambers, and right-sided pressures are usually normal. The absence of the large *v* wave of mitral incompetence in the wedge pressure tracings and the results of angiography, either with pulmonary arterial injection or with left ventricular injection of contrast material, will almost always establish the diagnosis. In some centers, qualitative detection of small left-to-right shunts of the type encountered in ventricular septal defect is performed using indicator gases such as hydrogen introduced via the lungs. The early appearance of hydrogen in the right ventricle following the start of inhalation of the gas is detected with a platinum catheter tip electrode. The practical value of such methods is not great, because a shunt that cannot be discovered from oxygen content differences and which needs a hydrogen electrode for its detection is of no surgical significance, and even the smallest defect needs antibiotic cover to prevent infective endocarditis. In patients with larger shunts, the wedge pressure and pulmonary arterial pressure may be increased. Measurement of pulmonary vascular resistance is always important; values of more than 7.5 mm Hg/l/min are seldom seen in patients with large shunts.

Differential Diagnosis

Ventricular septal defect is readily confused on physical examination with mitral incompetence, infundibular stenosis, ostium primum defects with cleft mitral valves, and hypertrophic obstructive cardiomyopathy. All these lesions can cause a loud pansystolic murmur and thrill in the left chest. Although the differential diagnosis is relatively easy in cases of severe defect, it is more difficult in patients with milder lesions, especially those in whom the murmur is the only abnormality. The almost inevitably severe left ventricular hypertrophy seen on the ECG in obstructive cardiomyopathy should serve to distinguish that lesion, but cardiac catheterization is generally indicated to confirm the diagnosis, even though echocardiography, which displays the ventricular septum and the mitral valve so readily, can be most helpful.

Complications

Infective endocarditis is the principal complication of ventricular septal defect. It occurs on the right ventricular wall at the point at which the jet stream of the shunt impinges on the endocardium. Since the infection is initially confined to the right heart and no valve is involved, the prognosis with treatment is good. Endocarditis occurs in about 15% of cases of uncomplicated ventricular septal defects and may recur.

Aortic incompetence occasionally occurs as an associated lesion. It is usually due to prolapse of an aortic valve cusp. It gives rise to a long diastolic murmur which, in conjunction with the pansystolic murmur of the ventricular defect, gives an almost continuous murmur. The aortic incompetence is usually moderate or severe and may develop as the patient grows up.

Heart failure, acquired pulmonary hypertension, and atrial arrhythmias are all much less common than in atrial septal defect, because so few patients with large ventricular defects are seen in adult life. Systemic hypertension and coronary atherosclerosis may occur in older patients but do not cause the severe problems seen in patients with atrial septal defects, because the size of the left-to-right shunt is limited by the size of the defect and is relatively uninfluenced by the compliance of either ventricle.

Treatment

A. Medical Treatment: The need for antibiotic prophylaxis (see Chapter 16) and acute awareness of the possibility of infective endocarditis are important points to remember in treating patients with ventricular septal defect.

B. Surgical Treatment: Closure of the defect is indicated if the pulmonary/systemic flow ratio is 2:1 or greater. In patients with smaller shunts, closure of the defect is sometimes advised in order to prevent the occurrence or recurrence of endocarditis and to "cure" the patient. The hazards of not operating on a ventricular defect are much less than those involved in leaving an atrial defect unclosed, but since the mortality rate is almost negligible in uncomplicated cases, more of the smaller defects are now surgically treated after it has become apparent that the defect is not going to close spontaneously. Spontaneous closure usually occurs before puberty.

Prognosis

The prognosis in uncomplicated ventricular septal defect in adults is good. Few patients have defects large enough to cause serious hemodynamic problems, and those few who have been recatheterized after 10 years of follow-up have shown no significant change in their status. The incidence of endocarditis has been negligible in those patients who have been followed.

PATENT DUCTUS ARTERIOSUS

Cardinal Features

Patent ductus arteriosus is the commonest form of aortopulmonary communication. The shunt is from the aorta at a point just distal to the left subclavian artery into the left pulmonary artery, as shown in Fig 11–35. Aortopulmonary window, in which there is a large communication between the proximal aorta and the main pulmonary artery, is a much rarer lesion that is clinically indistinguishable. The size of the aortopulmonary communication determines the size of the left-to-right shunt, which in turn determines pulmonary arterial pressure, which is usually low.

Patent ductus arteriosus results in an increased

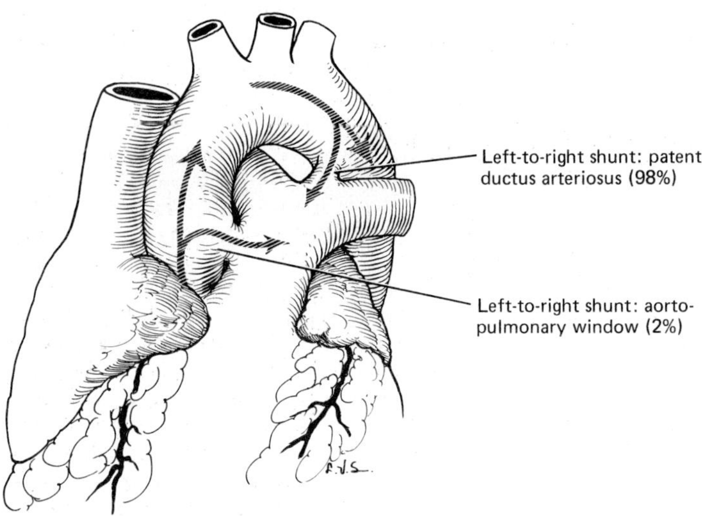

Anatomic sites of aortopulmonary defects.

Cardinal features: *Ductus distal to left subclavian; aortopulmonary window near root of aorta; left-to-right shunt; pulmonary arterial pressure usually low in patent ductus arteriosus.*

Variable factors: *Size of communication; size of left-to-right shunt.*

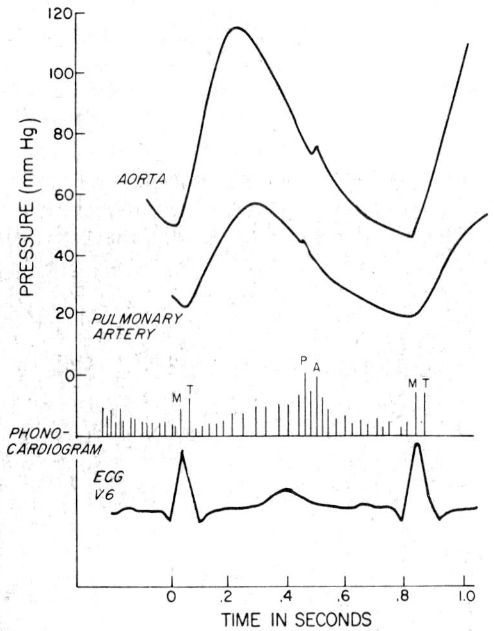

Diagram showing auscultatory and hemodynamic features of patent ductus arteriosus. The continuous murmur is loudest at the time of the second heart sound.

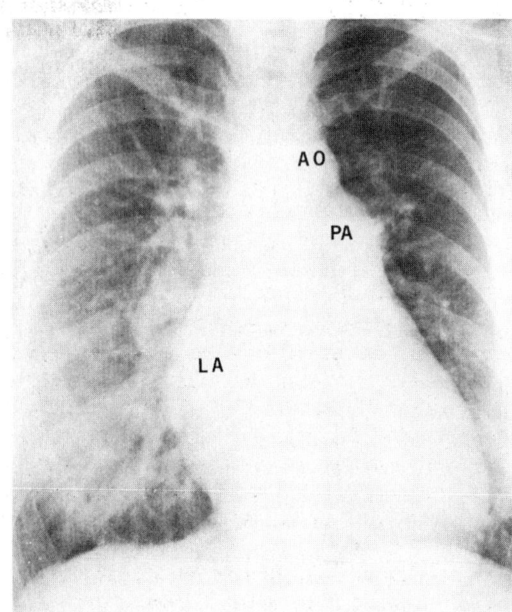

Chest x-ray of a patient with a large patent ductus arteriosus. The aorta (AO), pulmonary artery (PA), and left atrium (LA) are enlarged.

Figure 11–35. Patent ductus arteriosus and aortopulmonary window. Structures enlarged: Left atrium and ventricle, aorta, and pulmonary artery.

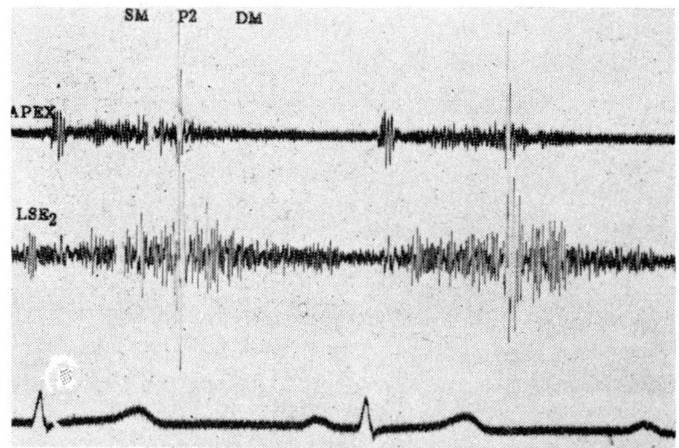

Figure 11–36. Phonocardiograms recorded at the apex and second left intercostal space (LSE_2) in a patient with patent ductus arteriosus. The murmur is accentuated at the time of the second heart sound and is heard best at the base of the heart. (Reproduced, with permission, from Auerback ML, Sokolow M: Phonocardiography in acyanotic congenital heart disease. Pediatrics 24:1026, 1959.)

flow through the left atrium and left ventricle and also through the aorta and pulmonary artery. Since there is not an increased flow through the right heart, the lesion loads only the left heart.

Patent ductus arteriosus is more than twice as common in females as in males, and the diagnosis is now usually made in infancy or childhood.

Clinical Features

A. Symptoms and Signs: Symptoms in patients with patent ductus vary with the size of the left-to-right shunt. In hemodynamically insignificant lesions, which constitute more than half of adult cases, the patient is asymptomatic. A murmur has sometimes been present since birth, but more commonly the diagnosis is made later in childhood. A false history of rheumatic fever is present in about 10% of cases. The principal symptom is dyspnea on exertion, with palpitation and chest pain much less frequently seen.

The only abnormality in more than half of cases is the typical "machinery" murmur, heard high in the left chest below the clavicle. It is loudest at the time of the second heart sound, as shown in Fig 11–36. The murmur is not necessarily continuous in infancy and may be mainly systolic up to age 5, perhaps because the pressure difference between the aorta and pulmonary artery is less at this time. In patients with large left-to-right shunts, cardiac enlargement and a prominent hyperdynamic left ventricular impulse are found. In patients with the largest shunts, a wide pulse pressure and a collapsing pulse are seen because of the large left ventricular stroke volume and the rapid runoff of aortic blood into the low-pressure pulmonary circulation. Palpable pulmonary valve closure, reversed splitting of the second heart sound, and a diastolic murmur of relative mitral stenosis are found in patients with large shunts. All of these features are seen in aortopulmonary window; the only distinguishing feature—a murmur heard low down in the third or fourth left interspace—is not a reliable indication of the diagnosis.

B. Electrocardiographic Findings: Left ventricular hypertrophy in patent ductus arteriosus is related to the size of the shunt. It is absent in hemodynamically insignificant lesions and may be severe with large shunts.

C. X-Ray Findings: The heart is of normal size when the shunt is small. A prominent pulmonary artery shadow running up to a large aortic knob is the most distinguishing radiologic sign of patent ductus arteriosus. Pulmonary plethora with left atrial and left ventricular enlargement and a large ascending aorta are seen in patients with large shunts (Fig 11–35). The ductus may calcify in later life.

D. Special Investigations:

1. **Noninvasive technics**—Phonocardiography may be helpful in establishing the characteristic timing of the murmur, but auscultation by an experienced observer is usually sufficient to establish the diagnosis.

2. **Invasive technics**—Cardiac catheterization is indicated to confirm the presence of a left-to-right shunt at pulmonary arterial level and to measure the pulmonary and systemic pressure and flow. In right heart catheterization the aorta can occasionally be entered via the ductus in patients with large shunts. The characteristic position of the catheter is shown in Fig 11–37, and its passage down the descending aorta leaves no doubt about the diagnosis. Measurement of the pulmonary/systemic flow ratio is the best means of establishing the hemodynamic severity of the lesion. Ratios of 2:1 or more are found in moderate and severe lesions.

Because of the increasing availability of left heart catheterization, it has become customary to make absolutely certain of the site of the shunt by retrograde aortography. An injection of contrast material into the aortic arch with the patient in the left anterior oblique

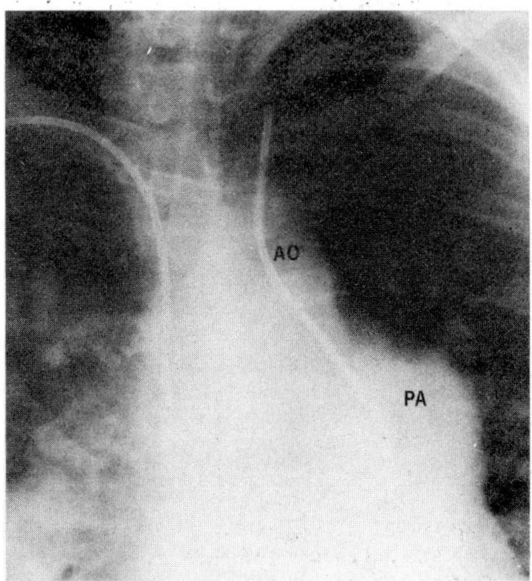

Figure 11–37. Chest x-ray showing the position of a cardiac catheter passing through a patent ductus arteriosus from the pulmonary artery (PA) to the aorta.

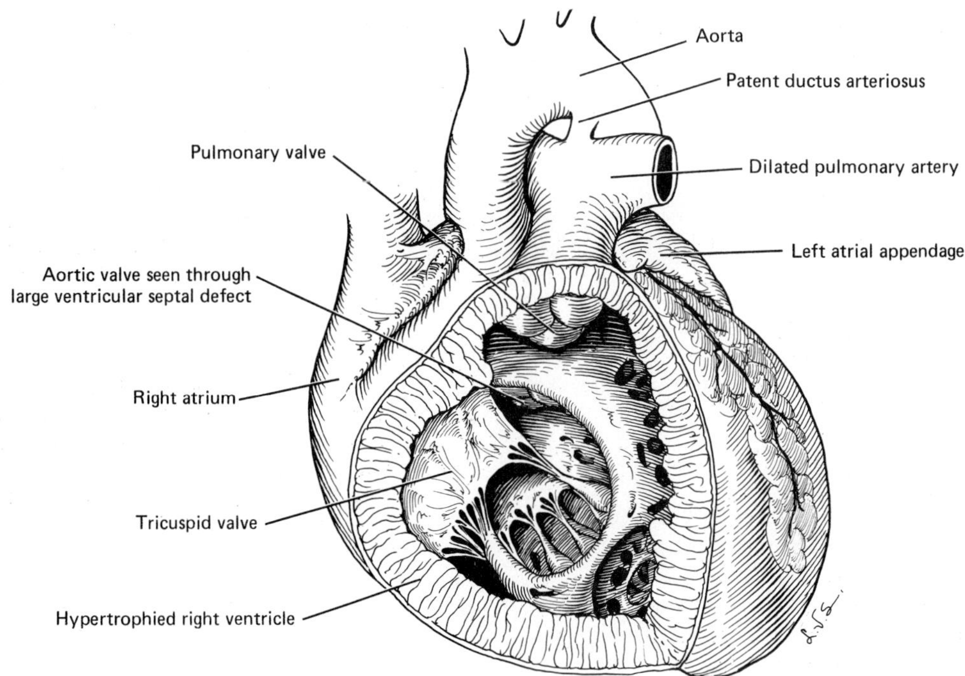

Anatomic features of Eisenmenger's complex.

Cardinal features: *Pulmonary hypertension at systemic level; communication(s) between right and left heart; bidirectional or right-to-left shunt; raised pulmonary vascular resistance.*

Variable factors: *Site of communication: Ventricle (Eisenmenger's complex), patent ductus arteriosus, aortopulmonary window, ostium primum defect, atrioventricular canal, truncus arteriosus transposition, single atrium, single ventricle, total anomalous venous drainage.* Not *present in ostium secundum defect.*

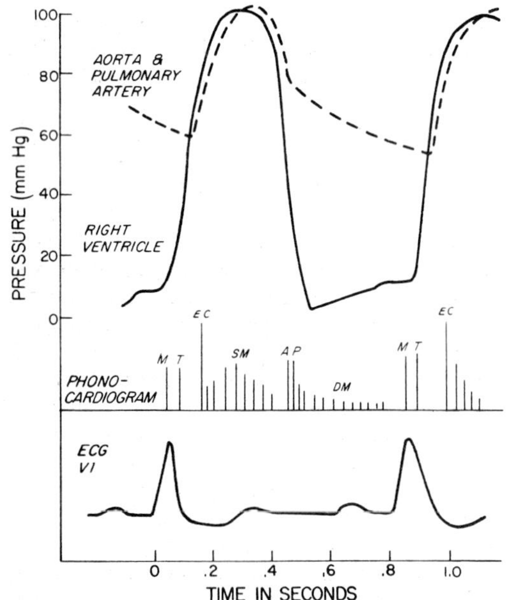

Diagram showing auscultatory and hemodynamic features of Eisenmenger's complex. EC, ejection click; SM, systolic murmur; DM, diastolic murmur.

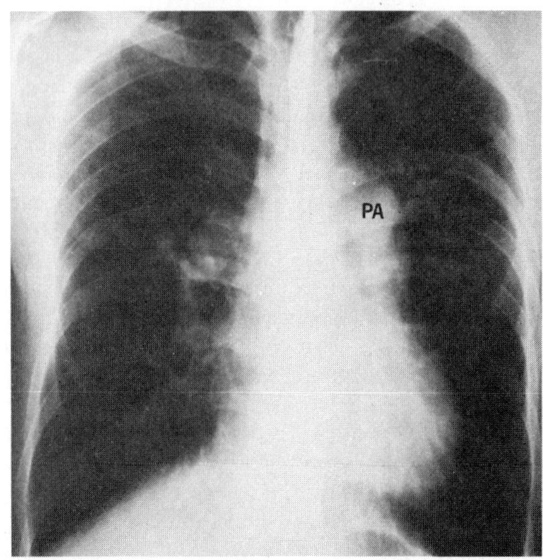

Chest x-ray of a patient with Eisenmenger's syndrome showing small heart and large pulmonary artery (PA) with oligemic lungs.

Figure 11–38. Eisenmenger's syndrome. Structures enlarged: Right ventricle, right atrium, and pulmonary artery.

position will fill the pulmonary artery and outline the ductus. Aortopulmonary windows can also be demonstrated by aortography, thus pointing out the difference between these 2 otherwise similar lesions.

Differential Diagnosis

Patent ductus arteriosus can only be differentiated from aortopulmonary window by cardiac catheterization and angiography. The other lesions that have to be distinguished are those causing continuous or near continuous murmurs. A venous hum gives a continuous bruit heard above the clavicle and is abolished by pressing on the veins at the root of the neck to interfere with blood flow. The bruit is caused by local narrowing of the vein and is often influenced by posture. Aortic valve disease and ventricular septal defect with aortic incompetence cause murmurs that may be continuous but show 2 peaks, one in mid systole and the other in early diastole. The murmurs of pulmonary artery stenosis and increased collateral bronchial blood flow start late in systole and peak before the second sound. The murmur of coronary arteriovenous fistula is probably the one most readily confused with patent ductus. It is truly continuous, and the fact that it is best heard at the left lower sternal border rather than in the second left interspace may be the only distinguishing feature.

Complications

Infective endarteritis is an important but infrequent complication. The infection occurs where the jet of aortic blood impinges on the wall of the pulmonary artery. Since no valve is involved and the infection is usually confined to the pulmonary circulation, endarteritis is not a serious complication in cases in which the causative organism responds to antibiotic therapy.

The left recurrent laryngeal nerve runs in close proximity to the ductus. It may be subjected to pressure or cut at surgery, causing hoarseness.

Acquired pulmonary hypertension with increase in pulmonary vascular resistance can rarely occur in patients with large left-to-right shunts. In most patients with pulmonary hypertension, the raised resistance is present from birth or early infancy (see Eisenmenger's syndrome).

Heart failure can occur in older patients with large left-to-right shunts. Cardiac enlargement, pulmonary congestion, and finally right heart failure occur.

Treatment

Surgical ligation and division of a patent ductus arteriosus is recommended in all patients with left-to-right shunt in whom the diagnosis is confirmed. The operative mortality rate is negligible if the shunt is small. In patients with small shunts, the operation is the simplest type of cardiac surgery and does not require cardiopulmonary bypass. In older patients and those with large left-to-right shunts, the aortopulmonary communication is short and friable and may be calcified. The aortic wall may tear easily, and surgical closure can be extremely difficult, even with cardiopulmonary bypass. In such cases the mortality rate rises to about 10%. It is important to divide the ductus at surgery rather than simply tie it. Recurrence of left-to-right shunt is not uncommon; it occurs in about 10% of cases in which division is not performed. If left-to-right shunt recurs several years after ligation, the acquired shunt lesion is much less well tolerated than the congenital shunt. Patients with such lesions readily develop left heart failure, and the disease runs a more rapidly progressive course than in those who have never had surgical treatment.

Prognosis

The prognosis is good in mild cases. Surgery is performed to make the patient "normal" and is usually purely prophylactic in hemodynamically insignificant lesions. Endarteritis seldom threatens life, and it is only in the rare patient with a huge left-to-right shunt that life expectancy is less than normal.

EISENMENGER'S SYNDROME

Cardinal Features & Pathogenesis

The term Eisenmenger's syndrome is used to describe pulmonary hypertension with reversed shunt. By definition, the pulmonary hypertension does not develop in the course of the disease but is seen on initial examination and has been present from birth or early infancy or childhood. The pathogenesis of the pulmonary vascular obstruction is poorly understood. The pulmonary arterial pressure is at or near systemic level, and the shunt is either bidirectional or right-to-left. The pulmonary vascular resistance is raised to more than 7.5 mm Hg/l/min and is often in the same range as the systemic vascular resistance. The principal variable is the level at which the shunt takes place. In Eisenmenger's complex, which is the prototype of the lesion, the location is the ventricle, as shown in Fig 11–38. Because Eisenmenger's original patient had a ventricular defect, the term Eisenmenger's complex is used to indicate the ventricular nature of the defect, as opposed to the more general term Eisenmenger's syndrome, in which the defect may be at any level. The shunt may be at the aortopulmonary, atrioventricular, atrial, or ostium primum level, but it is never solely at the level of an ostium secundum atrial defect. Complex congenital lesions such as truncus arteriosus, transposition of the great arteries, single atrium or ventricle, or total anomalous venous drainage may be associated with the pulmonary hypertension.

It is thought that the Eisenmenger reaction, which is the development of severe pulmonary vascular disease, may occur in any form of congenital heart disease in which a large pulmonary blood flow or raised left atrial pressure is present in fetal, neonatal, or infant life. Clues to the mechanism of development of this form of pulmonary hypertension must be sought in the neonatal period. In adult patients, the pulmonary vascular disease of Eisenmenger's syndrome is severe enough to rule out closure of the defect or defects.

The right ventricle and pulmonary artery are almost always enlarged in Eisenmenger's syndrome. The other chambers which may be enlarged depend on the site of the associated lesion or lesions.

Acquired Pulmonary Hypertension (Eisenmenger Reaction)

Pulmonary hypertension develops in postpuberal life in some patients, usually those with large left-to-right shunts due to ostium secundum atrial septal defects. In these cases the term "atrial septal defect with pulmonary hypertension" or "acquired Eisenmenger syndrome" has been used. In extremely rare cases, pulmonary hypertension develops in postpuberal patients with other lesions, eg, ventricular septal defect or patent ductus arteriosus. Acquired pulmonary hypertension tends to progress more rapidly than the pulmonary vascular lesions seen in the Eisenmenger complex. Acquired pulmonary hypertension is almost entirely restricted to patients with atrial septal defect (see p 317).

Use of the Term Eisenmenger's Syndrome

Because the clinical features vary little with the site of lesions and the signs of pulmonary hypertension are dominant, it is convenient to group together under the heading Eisenmenger's syndrome all patients with cardiac defects associated with pulmonary hypertension that has been present since early life. The clinical course of the patient is also independent of the exact anatomic nature of the defect and depends instead on the pulmonary hypertension. In practice, the exact anatomic nature of the lesion in adults with Eisenmenger's syndrome remains unproved until autopsy, and associated lesions such as a ventricular defect in addition to a patent ductus arteriosus and an ostium secundum atrial defect can be present without changing the clinical picture.

Eisenmenger's syndrome accounts for about 7% of cases of adult congenital heart disease and is more common in females than in males. In about one-third of cases, ventricular septal defect is the only lesion associated with the pulmonary hypertension.

Clinical Findings

A. Symptoms and Signs: Patients with Eisenmenger's syndrome are invariably disabled by dyspnea. A murmur or cyanosis is often said to have been present from infancy, and the absence of any history of severe illness in infancy or childhood is striking. Pneumonia, heart failure, feeding problems, and susceptibility to infection, which are common manifestations of large left-to-right shunts in infancy, are not encountered in retrospective reviews of the history of adults with Eisenmenger's syndrome. It appears that pulmonary vascular resistance is raised at or before birth and that the patient has not passed through a phase of high pulmonary blood flow. Whereas dyspnea is invariably present regardless of age, hemoptysis, palpitation, chest pain and fainting attacks may be seen in adolescence and young adult life. Pregnancy is poorly tolerated, and spontaneous abortion is common.

The physical signs are those of pulmonary hypertension. Cyanosis and clubbing of the fingers may be present, and there is often a prominent *a* wave in the jugular venous pulse. There may be "differential" cyanosis in patients with a reversed shunt through a patent ductus arteriosus. The shunted blood passes preferentially to the lower part of the body via the ductus and descending aorta. Thus, there may be cyanosis and clubbing of the toes when the hands—especially the right hand—are pink and show no clubbing of the fingers. The difference is best seen when the systemic circulation has been subject to vasodilatation, eg, after a hot shower or bath. These clinical findings can be confirmed by finding a difference in the oxygen content (or saturation) between right brachial and femoral blood samples.

The heart is usually not much enlarged and is often quiet. A right ventricular heave may be present, and pulmonary valve closure is often palpable. There is usually a systolic ejection click, followed by a short systolic ejection murmur over the pulmonary artery and a loud single second heart sound (Fig 11–39). An early diastolic murmur of pulmonary incompetence is common, and the clearest examples of this murmur (Graham Steell murmur) are encountered in Eisenmenger's syndrome. Signs of congestive heart failure are seldom seen, but progressive cyanosis and polycythemia are common.

B. Electrocardiographic Findings: The ECG in patients with Eisenmenger's syndrome always shows right ventricular hypertrophy (Fig 11–40). In patients with atrioventricular canal defects, left axis deviation may be present even when pulmonary vascular resistance is markedly raised.

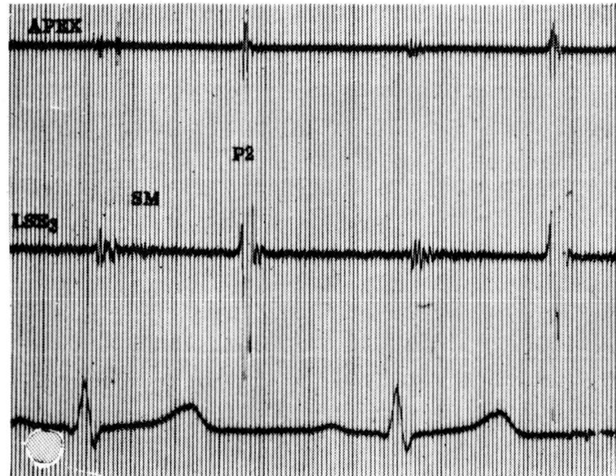

Figure 11–39. Phonocardiogram showing loud single second heart sound (P_2) and short systolic murmur (SM) in a patient with Eisenmenger's syndrome (ventricular septal defect with pulmonary hypertension). (Reproduced, with permission, from Auerback ML, Sokolow M: Phonocardiography in acyanotic congenital heart disease. Pediatrics 24:1026, 1959.)

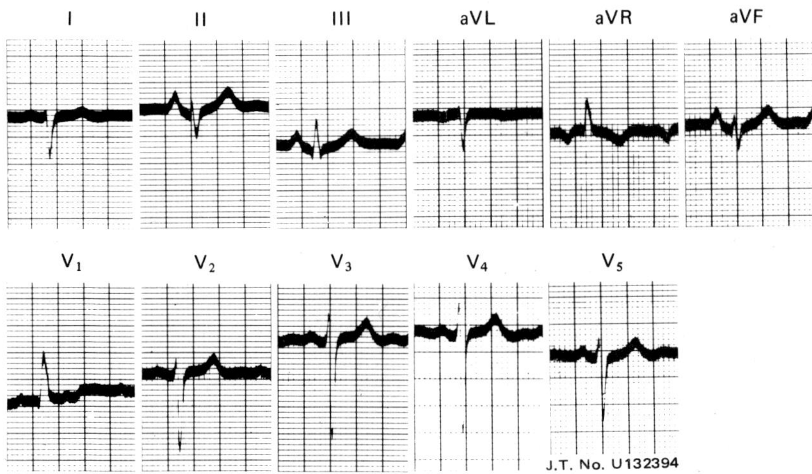

Figure 11–40. ECG of a 30-year-old man with Eisenmenger's syndrome showing right ventricular hypertrophy.

C. X-Ray Findings: The main trunk and branches of the pulmonary artery are large, but the heart is usually only slightly enlarged (Fig 11–38). Evidence of slight pulmonary plethora may be present, and the sparseness of the peripheral pulmonary vessels may be difficult to recognize.

D. Special Investigations:

1. Noninvasive technics—Following the level of the hematocrit is useful in assessing the progress of the disease. Echocardiography may be helpful in determining the site of the shunt lesion.

2. Invasive technics—

a. Cardiac catheterization is always required to establish the diagnosis and show that pulmonary arterial pressure is raised and that pulmonary vascular resistance is at about the same level as systemic resistance. A left-to-right shunt may be detectable from analysis of the oxygen content of samples of blood obtained from the right heart chambers, and the catheter may cross a septal defect at catheterization. When the defect is at the atrioventricular level, pulmonary arterial pressure may be less than systemic pressure.

Angiocardiography is now more frequently used than indicator dilution curves to demonstrate the intracardiac defects.

b. Wedge pressure measurement is of great importance since it is always possible that the patient has a curable lesion that can be identified in this way. The abruptly tapering peripheral pulmonary arteries of patients with Eisenmenger's syndrome may not permit the wedging of a conventional cardiac catheter. In such cases, a Swan-Ganz balloon catheter should be used, and the pressure in the pulmonary artery distal to the inflated balloon should be taken as an indirect measure of the pulmonary venous pressure.

Differential Diagnosis

Eisenmenger's syndrome must be distinguished from pulmonary hypertension due to acquired lesions that raise left atrial pressure. Tight mitral stenosis is by far the commonest of these lesions, but rare lesions such as left atrial myxoma, cor triatriatum, and sclerosing mediastinitis with pulmonary venous obstruction may occur. Primary (idiopathic) and thromboembolic pulmonary hypertension should also be excluded because such conditions carry a worse prognosis than Eisenmenger's syndrome. The history of a murmur and cyanosis dating back to infancy is of great help in identifying congenital lesions but is not always available. In some patients with severe acquired pulmonary hypertension, opening of the foramen ovale may cause right-to-left shunting and lead to an erroneous diagnosis of a congenital lesion. Complete cardiac catheterization studies may be needed, including measurements of the effects of oxygen and vasodilator drugs on pulmonary vascular resistance. Pulmonary artery stenosis may also be a possible cause of the physical signs of increased pressure in the main pulmonary artery.

Complications

When patients with Eisenmenger's syndrome are recatheterized after 10–20 years, it is remarkable how few changes are found in the hemodynamic status of the patient. Similarly, clinical findings show little change occurring between adolescence and the third and fourth decades. Complications of progressive polycythemia, pulmonary thromboembolism, and pulmonary infarction tend to become more frequent with the passage of time. Infective endocarditis is rare and atrial arrhythmias uncommon.

Treatment

A. Medical Treatment: Anticoagulant therapy and phlebotomy are recommended but have not been shown to have any significant effects on the course of the disease.

B. Surgical Treatment: The surgical closure of intracardiac or extracardiac (ductus or aortopulmonary

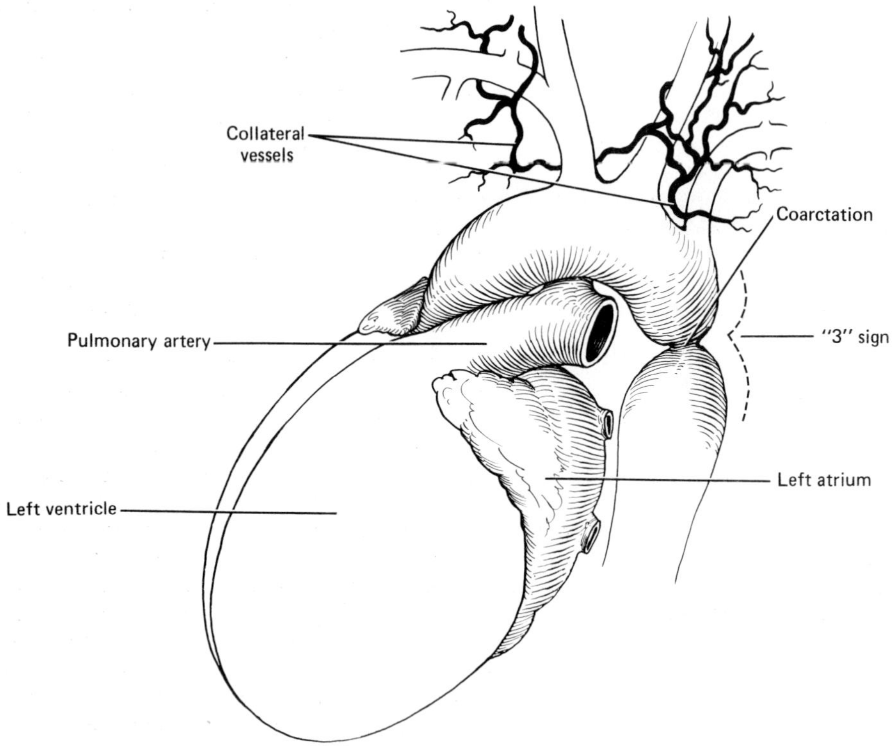

Anatomic features of coarctation of the aorta.

Cardinal features: *Obstruction distal to left subclavian artery; high pressure in proximal aorta; pressure drop across obstruction; poststenotic dilatation.*

Variable factors: *Severity of obstruction; size of collateral vessels; site in acquired lesions.*

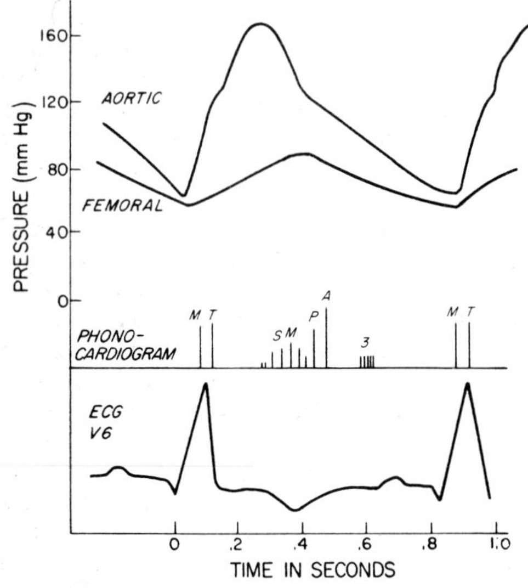

Diagram showing auscultatory and hemodynamic features of coarctation of the aorta. SM, systolic murmur; 3, 3rd heart sound.

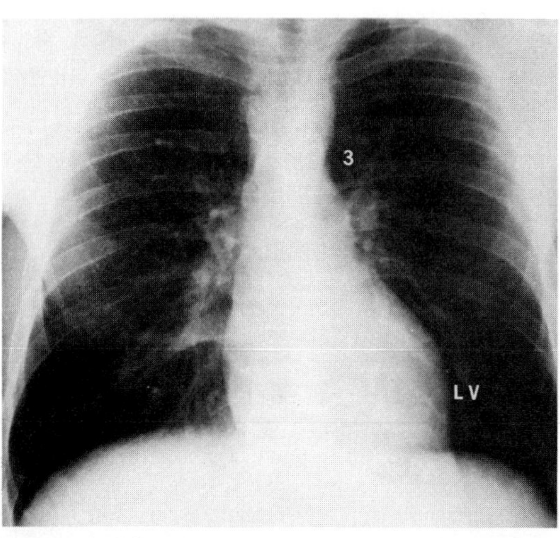

Chest x-ray of 19-year-old man with coarctation of the aorta showing "3" sign and slight left ventricular (LV) prominence.

Figure 11–41. Coarctation of the aorta. Structures enlarged: Left ventricle, proximal aorta. Distal aorta: poststenotic dilatation.

window) defects in patients with Eisenmenger's syndrome is contraindicated. It removes the "safety valve" of a right-to-left shunt and tends to convert the patient's status to that associated with primary pulmonary hypertension. If the patient survives the operation, right heart failure and early death are likely to follow.

In some cases it is difficult to be sure that the pulmonary vascular resistance is indeed so high that surgical correction of the defect is out of the question. The decision against surgery effectively shuts off all hope of cure and condemns the patient to a shortened life of invalidism. In patients with obvious cyanosis and pulmonary vascular resistance at or near the level of systemic resistance, there is no question of surgical correction, but in some cases there is still some left-to-right shunt, the pulmonary arterial pressure may not be as high as the systemic (as in a patient with an atrioventricular defect), and the possibility exists that surgery might be feasible. There is no substitute for obtaining full studies, including the response to exercise, vasodilator drugs, oxygen, and possibly also temporary obliteration of the defect. The outlook is best in patients with aortopulmonary defects, especially patent ductus arteriosus, and worst in cases with ventricular septal defect. In some cases with patent ductus, the defect has been clamped at thoracotomy and pulmonary and aortic pressures measured to see whether pulmonary arterial pressure will fall sharply, but even this is not completely satisfactory since it is the long-term reversibility of the pulmonary vascular changes that is the key factor affecting the outcome.

Prognosis

Life expectancy is significantly reduced in patients with Eisenmenger's syndrome, and few patients in their 40s and 50s are seen by physicians. The course of the disease is not one of steady progression, as in primary pulmonary hypertension, and in a sheltered environment patients can live for 20 years or more with surprisingly little disability or evidence of progression. Since the diagnosis was not made with certainty in many patients until the early 1950s, lifetime follow-up is not yet available in proved cases.

COARCTATION OF THE AORTA

Cardinal Features & Pathogenesis

This obstructive aortic lesion, which is characteristically associated with hypertension in the upper half of the body, with lower pressure in the legs, is usually diagnosed in childhood. The obstruction almost invariably is in the aortic isthmus just distal to the origin of the left subclavian artery and at the level where the ductus arteriosus joins the descending aorta, as shown in Fig 11–41. The obstruction may rarely be at other sites in the aorta. There is usually poststenotic dilatation of the aorta distal to the site of obstruction. Collateral vessels develop that tend to bypass the obstruction. The principal variables in the lesion are the severity of the obstruction, which varies from complete aortic atresia to slight narrowing, and the size of the collateral vessels. These can be so large that a minimal pressure difference is present between the ascending and descending aorta in a patient with complete aortic obstruction at the site of coarctation.

In coarctation of the aorta, the left ventricle is hypertrophied and enlarged in proportion to the severity of the lesion. The proximal aorta is distended, and there is poststenotic dilatation of the aorta distal to the obstruction.

Coarctation of the aorta is associated with a number of other left-sided congenital lesions, namely bicuspid aortic valve, patent ductus arteriosus, aortic stenosis, ventricular septal defect, mitral stenosis, aortic or mitral atresia, and other hypoplastic left heart syndromes. One theory of the cause of coarctation is that the specialized tissue in the ductus arteriosus near the area of the isthmus of the aorta (which constricts with the rise in aortic oxygen tension at birth), spills over into the aorta and causes constriction at this site in addition to or instead of that at the ductus. Coarctation of the aorta represents about 5% of cases of adult congenital heart disease and is more common in males than in females by a factor of more than 3:1. Some clinically insignificant narrowing of the aorta at the isthmus of the aorta is common, even in the absence of hypertension. This should not be emphasized, however, and the use of the term pseudocoarctation to describe such a condition is not endorsed.

Clinical Findings

A. Symptoms and Signs: Coarctation of the aorta produces few symptoms. The lesion is usually discovered by finding an abnormally high blood pressure or a systolic murmur. Dyspnea on exertion, headache, and throbbing in the head are sometimes seen. In older, untreated cases, intermittent claudication may occur. Left heart failure, with pulmonary congestion and edema, occurs late in the disease, even in cases presenting in adult life.

The diagnosis of coarctation of the aorta can be readily made on physical examination. The carotid arteries show well-marked, bounding pulsations due to the forceful ejection of the left ventricular stroke volume into the reduced capacity of the arterial bed. There is usually a prominent pulsation in the suprasternal notch. The level of arterial pressure varies considerably with the age of the patient, being higher in older persons. The pulse pressure in the arms is wide, whereas that in the legs is reduced. The femoral pulses may be absent in severe cases; if they are present, the characteristic sign of delay between the timing of the upstrokes of the radial and femoral pulses should be sought. The examiner should first locate the femoral pulse with one hand and then palpate the radial pulse to detect and time the difference between the arrival of the 2 waves. The pulses are synchronous in normal subjects, and delays of 0.1 sec are readily discernible.

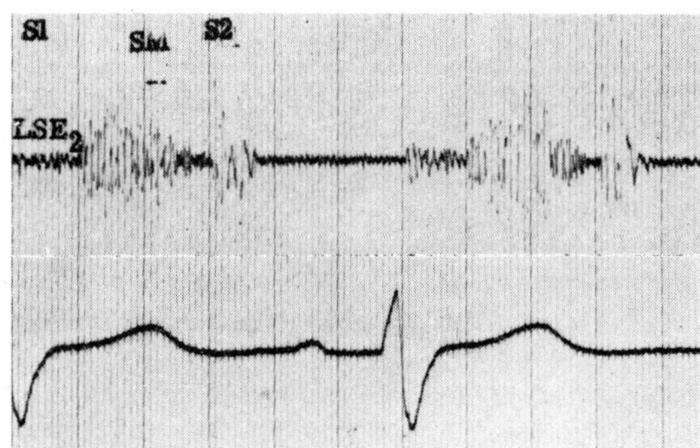

Figure 11–42. Phonocardiogram of a 5-year-old patient with coarctation of the aorta. Note the delay before the crescendo-decrescendo systolic murmur begins at the left sternal edge (LSE_2). (Reproduced, with permission, from Auerback ML, Sokolow M: Phonocardiography in acyanotic congenital heart disease. Pediatrics 24:1026, 1959.)

Collateral vessels are often present on the back. They are best seen and felt by feeling the intercostal arteries under the ribs and the enlarged arteries around the scapula as the patient bends forward.

B. Cardiac Signs: The heart is often enlarged, with a prominent left ventricular heave. Two varieties of murmur in coarctation of the aorta can usually be distinguished. One arises from the aortic obstruction and is late systolic in timing and ejection in type (Fig 11–42). The other is longer and more continuous and arises from the collateral vessels. Both are heard best in the back. The aortic valve closure sound is loud, and a third heart sound and a short delayed diastolic murmur arising from the mitral valve are occasionally heard.

C. Hemodynamic Findings: In coarctation of the aorta, the left ventricle pumps into a restricted arterial bed. This accounts for the high arterial pressure and pulse pressure seen in the upper extremities. However, the hemodynamics of coarctation are not as simple as they seem, and mechanical factors cannot account for all the findings. There may be disproportionate left ventricular hypertrophy and unexplained high resting cardiac output. The hypertension cannot be entirely explained on mechanical grounds, and a renal component has been suggested.

D. Electrocardiographic Findings: Some degree of left ventricular hypertrophy is present in all but the mildest cases. The ECG changes may be out of proportion to the level of arterial pressure. This suggests that aortic stenosis or left ventricular disease may also be present. Left bundle branch block is sometimes seen in older patients, and atrial fibrillation may occur.

E. X-Ray Findings: The characteristic radiologic sign is the so-called "3" sign in the region of the aortic knob. It is shown in Fig 11–41. The upper half of the 3 is formed by the left subclavian artery and the lower half by the poststenotic dilatation of the aorta below the coarctation. Rib notching is another radiologic sign closely associated with coarctation. It is caused by the large collateral intercostal arteries that erode the inferior surfaces of the ribs. The sign, which may be absent in childhood, is not invariably present in adults and is more significant in the outer portions of the ribs, 10 cm or more from the costovertebral junction. Left ventricular enlargement with prominence of the ascending aorta is seen in most cases.

F. Special Investigations: Patients with coarctation of the aorta present such a clear clinical picture that many are referred for surgical treatment without the need for special investigation. However, it is becoming more common to recommend measurement of the pressure difference across the obstruction (Fig 11–43), together with systemic cardiac output. The resistance offered by the involved segment cannot be measured because the volume of blood flowing across the obstruction is unknown. Aortography is often performed, but the outline of the lesion is often seen just as well on a plain x-ray.

Differential Diagnosis

Coarctation of the aorta enters into the differential diagnosis of systemic hypertension (see Chapter 9). It is more likely to be overlooked entirely than incorrectly diagnosed. Minor forms of the lesion without systemic hypertension cause more problems in diagno-

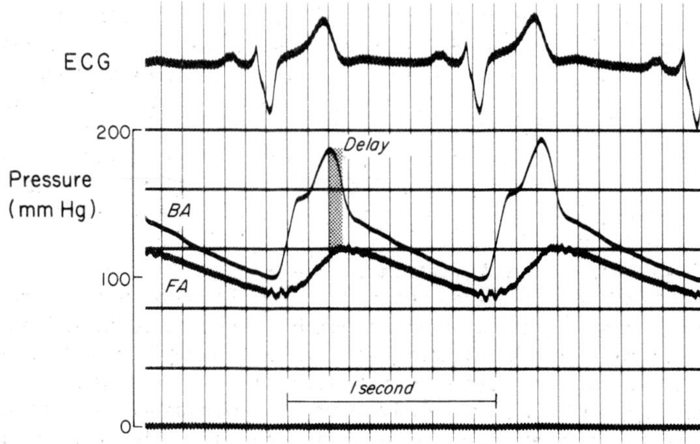

Figure 11–43. Pressure tracings above (BA) and below (FA) the site of obstruction in a patient with coarctation of the aorta. The delay of the peak systolic wave is indicated.

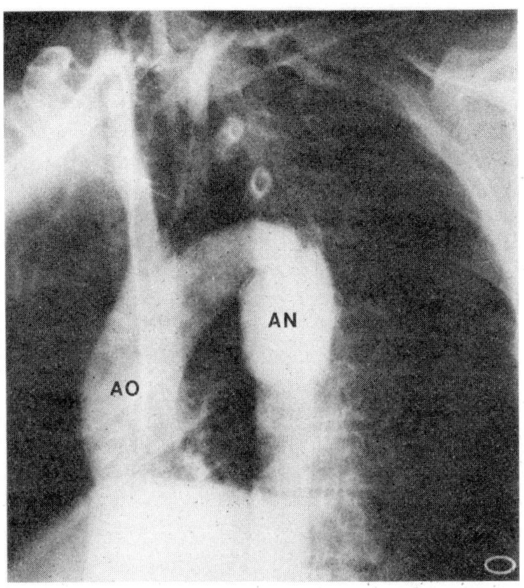

Figure 11–44. Angiogram showing a left anterior oblique view of the aorta. A traumatic false aneurysm (AN) is shown at the isthmus of the aorta (AO). The lesion resulted from an automobile accident and caused acquired coarctation.

sis, and when aortic stenosis or marked dilatation of the ascending aorta coexists, coarctation may be difficult to detect. Acquired forms of coarctation may occasionally cause problems in diagnosis. The aorta may rupture as a result of trauma, usually in road accidents. The site of rupture is almost always the isthmus of the aorta. Hematoma formation may narrow the lumen and cause acute coarctation with surprisingly little leakage of blood into the mediastinum or pleural space. Renal failure, acute systemic hypertension, and death may occur, and an aneurysm may form at the site of rupture, as shown in Fig 11–44.

Complications

Subarachnoid hemorrhage due to rupture of a congenital aneurysm in the circle of Willis, aortic rupture, and left ventricular failure were the common causes of death before surgical treatment became available. Infective endarteritis may occur at the site of coarctation. In this case, emboli are confined to the lower parts of the body.

Treatment

If the lesion is hemodynamically significant, surgical resection of the coarcted area should always be recommended. In most cases, the ends of the cut aorta can be sutured without the insertion of a graft. Although the operation is relatively easy in childhood, it can be extremely difficult in older patients with larger collateral vessels and friable aortic tissue. Reoperation to deal with an inadequate previous repair presents serious problems. The mortality rate is higher in older patients, being approximately 10% in patients over age 30. Fortunately, few patients now present in that age group.

A peculiar form of arteritis may occur after surgical relief of coarctation of the aorta. In patients with severe lesions, the sudden increase in perfusion pressure, especially of the gut and other abdominal organs, gives rise to an acute postoperative rise in blood pressure and an arterial lesion that histologically resembles the arteritis of malignant hypertension or polyarteritis nodosa. Abdominal pain may be severe enough to warrant exploratory laparotomy. Antihypertensive medication and expectant treatment are all that is required, and the lesions are short-lived. Paraplegia is another rare complication of surgery. Interference with the blood supply to the spinal cord at operation is responsible.

Prognosis

The prognosis in coarctation of the aorta is good when surgical treatment is performed in childhood. Blood pressure does not always return to normal, especially if the lesion is not corrected until adult life, and left ventricular hypertrophy may persist. The later development of aortic stenosis (which occurs when the bicuspid aortic valve, so commonly associated with coarctation, calcifies in middle life) tends to worsen the prognosis.

EBSTEIN'S MALFORMATION

This rare congenital malformation is illustrated in Fig 11–45 and represents about 1% of cases of adult congenital heart disease. It presents a sufficiently characteristic clinical picture to warrant separate description.

The basic abnormality is downward displacement of the tricuspid valve, with atrialization of a large part of the right ventricle. The principal variable is the presence or absence of an associated ostium secundum atrial septal defect. The atrialized portion of the ventricle hinders rather than helps the forward flow of blood, and the tricuspid valve is congenitally incompetent. The lesion is remarkably well tolerated and was first recognized clinically in a cyanotic form in patients who also had an atrial septal defect. More acyanotic cases without atrial defects have come to be recognized, and it now appears that the lesion probably occurs more commonly *without* an atrial defect. Pulmonary blood flow is reduced, especially when right-to-left shunting through an atrial defect is present.

Clinical Findings

A. Symptoms and Signs: Dyspnea and fatigue are the commonest presenting symptoms. Atrial arrhythmias commonly cause palpitations, and right heart failure occurs with increasing age. The pulse is of small amplitude, and the venous pressure is usually raised in adult patients. Atrial fibrillation is usually present after

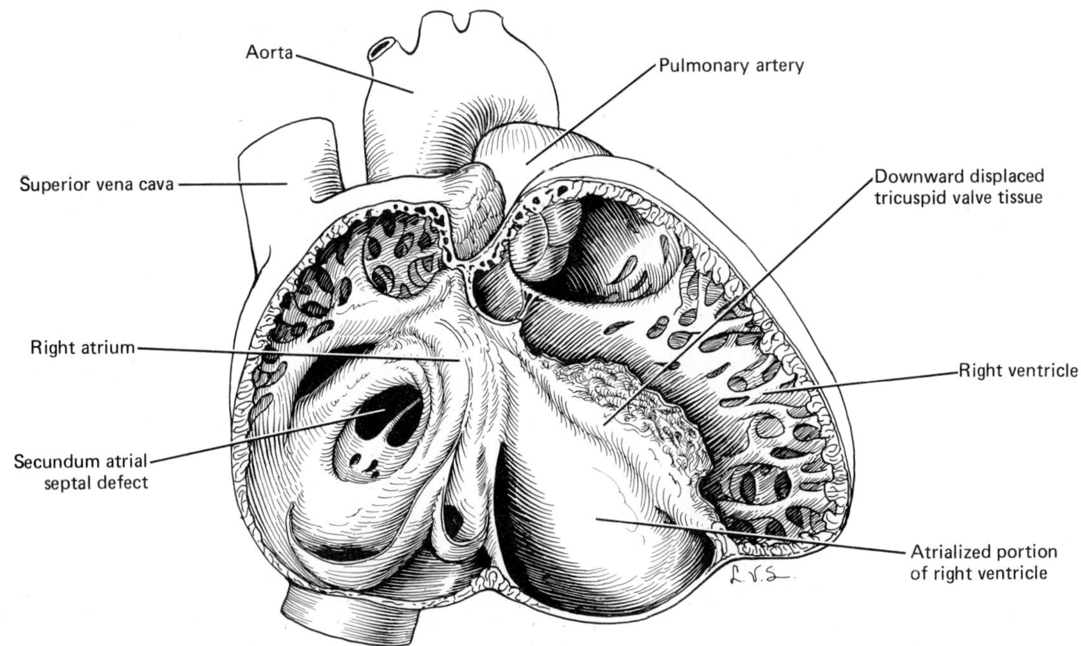

Figure 11–45. Anatomic features of Ebstein's malformation.

age 20. The heart is quiet, with distant heart sounds. There is usually a systolic murmur of tricuspid origin and wide splitting of the second heart sound. A short scratchy diastolic murmur or third heart sound arising from the tricuspid valve is usually heard at the left sternal edge. The murmurs tend to increase in intensity during inspiration.

B. Electrocardiographic Findings: The ECG usually shows incomplete or complete right bundle branch block and a low voltage.

C. X-Ray Findings: The heart is large, with a well defined border because its excursions are small. The lungs are oligemic, and the pulmonary artery is not enlarged (Fig 11–46). The cardiac enlargement is all right-sided.

D. Special Investigations:

1. **Noninvasive technics**–Echocardiography reveals delayed closure of the tricuspid valve coinciding with an early systolic click. There is rightward rotation of the heart, large excursions of the tricuspid valve, and downward displacement of the entire valve mechanism.

2. **Invasive technics**–Cardiac catheterization is generally performed to confirm the diagnosis. Right-sided pressures are all about the same level, and it is difficult to tell from the pressure tracings whether the catheter is in the pulmonary artery, the distal right ventricle, the proximal right ventricle, the right atrium, or the superior vena cava.

Intracardiac electrocardiography has been advocated as the definitive diagnostic test (Fig 11–47). The finding of right atrial pressure tracings at a level in the right heart at which the intracardiac ECG shows a right ventricular electrogram is said to be diagnostic, but there is some disagreement about the specificity of the finding. It has been said that it is dangerous to perform cardiac catheterization in patients with Ebstein's malformation, but in fact the procedure is well tolerated and is not contraindicated.

Differential Diagnosis

Massive cardiac enlargement due to pericardial disease can usually be distinguished on the basis of the

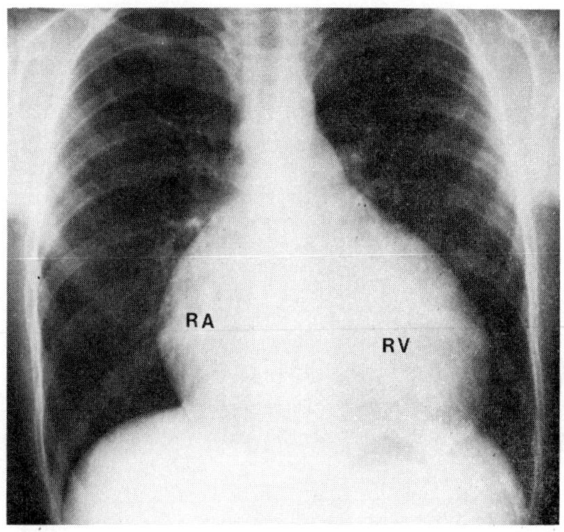

Figure 11–46. Chest x-ray showing cardiac enlargement in a patient with Ebstein's malformation.

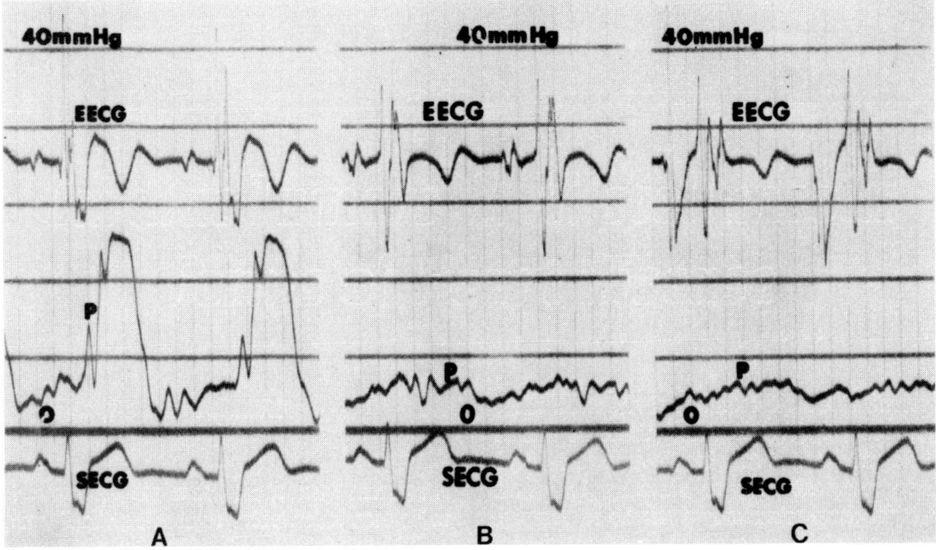

Figure 11–47. Simultaneous endocardial ECG (EECG), pressure tracing (P), and surface ECG (SECG) in a patient with Ebstein's malformation. In *A,* the catheter is in the right ventricle. In *B,* the catheter has been withdrawn to a position in which the EECG shows a ventricular complex but the pressure is atrial (atrialized ventricle). In *C,* the catheter is in the true atrium (atrial EECG and atrial pressure). (Courtesy of EH Botvinick.)

history. The cardiac enlargement will have developed recently, whereas in Ebstein's malformation there is a long history of heart disease. Severe right heart failure in patients with congenital pulmonary stenosis may produce a somewhat similar picture, and advanced rheumatic tricuspid valve disease can be recognized and ruled out because there will almost certainly be some associated mitral valve disease.

Complications

Atrial arrhythmias and right heart failure are sufficiently common to be considered as part of the disease rather than as complications.

Treatment

Plication of the right atrium, eliminating the atrialized portion of the ventricle, has been advocated. The operation is palliative rather than curative and is certainly not indicated in mild forms of the condition. The indications for surgery are not clear, and there has been little experience with the operation.

Prognosis

Patients with Ebstein's malformation have a reduced life expectancy and seldom reach age 50. Persons with milder forms of the disease can have an almost normal life span.

MORE COMPLEX & COMBINED CONGENITAL HEART LESIONS

The possible combinations of congenital heart lesions are too numerous to describe in detail in this book. There are, however, a number of complicated congenital heart lesions seen in infancy and childhood that are seldom seen in adult cardiology clinics.

1. TRANSPOSITION OF THE GREAT ARTERIES

In transposition of the great arteries, the aorta rises from the right ventricle and the pulmonary artery from the left ventricle. If the infant is to survive, there must be some form of septal defect to permit circulation of the blood. The pulmonary blood flow is usually increased in infants with this lesion, and only those who have large septal defects and who develop a raised pulmonary vascular resistance survive without surgery (Fig 11–48). This lesion can now be treated surgically by Mustard's operation, in which a baffle is inserted in the atrium after the atrial septal defect has been resected, and the systemic and pulmonary venous returns are redirected to the appropriate ventricles. In early infancy the patient's condition may deteriorate when the ductus arteriosus closes. In such cases, an atrial septal defect may be created or enlarged by a "noninvasive" palliative operation. A balloon catheter is passed into the left atrium and, after inflation, is

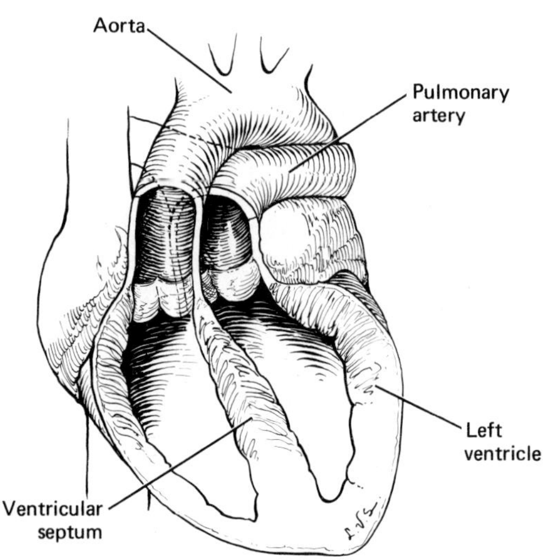

Figure 11–48. Typical transposition of the great arteries. The aorta arises from the morphologic right ventricle and is anterior to and slightly to the right of the pulmonary artery, which originates from the morphologic left ventricle. (Reproduced, with permission, from Dunphy JE, Way LW [editors]: *Current Surgical Diagnosis & Treatment,* 3rd ed. Lange, 1977.)

pulled forcefully back into the right atrium, tearing the septum. The procedure is surprisingly well tolerated.

2. CORRECTED TRANSPOSITION

In corrected transposition, the aorta arises from the embryonic right ventricle, whereas the pulmonary artery arises from the embryonic left ventricle. The term "corrected" indicates that unlike the situation in transposition of the great arteries, the systemic venous return goes to the lungs and the pulmonary venous blood passes out the aorta. The atrioventricular valves are transposed so that the venous "tricuspid" valve is mitral in shape, and the systemic "mitral" valve has 3 cusps (Fig 11–49). T'.e abnormality can be associated with almost any form of congenital heart disease, but ventricular septal defect and complete heart block are the lesions most commonly seen. The exact positions of the great vessels in relation to one another can vary, but the aorta is commonly on the left and in front of the pulmonary artery. The lesion can be seen in adult life and is presumably compatible with a normal life span if it is the sole abnormality. Problems may occur

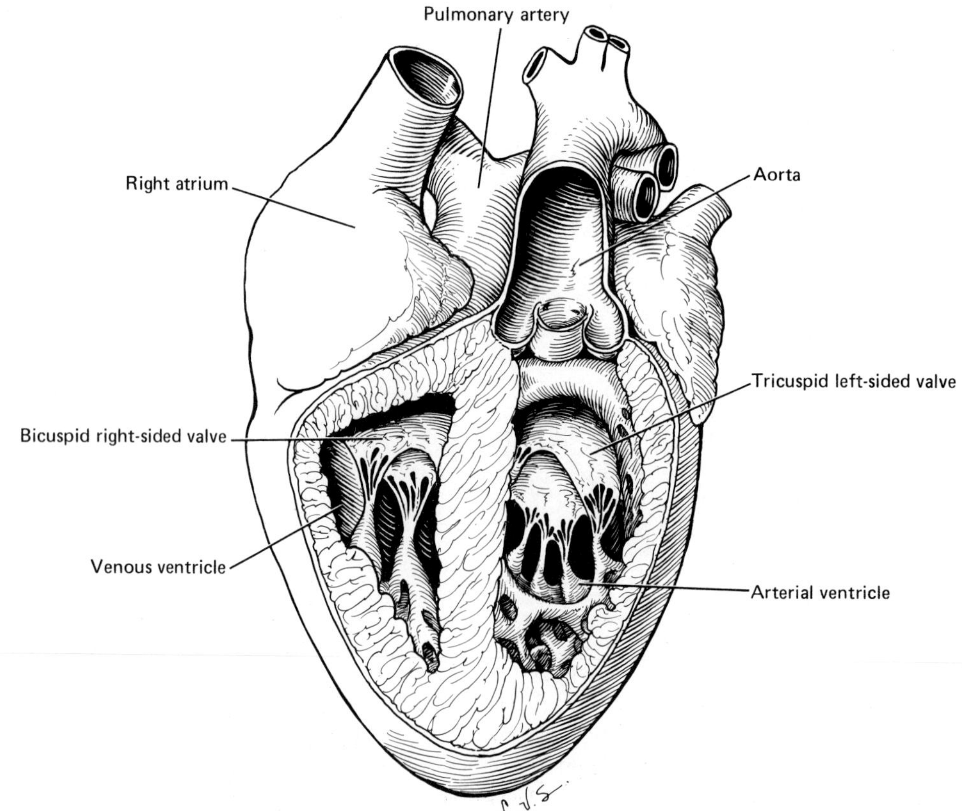

Figure 11–49. Drawing showing anatomic features of corrected transposition. The aorta arises in front and to the left of the pulmonary artery, but the great vessels are corrected to the appropriate ventricles (aorta to arterial ventricle; pulmonary to venous ventricle). The right-sided atrioventricular valve is bicuspid (mitral); the left-sided atrioventricular valve has 3 cusps.

during cardiac catheterization because it is difficult to enter the pulmonary artery. In such cases a Swan-Ganz balloon catheter will often float through the right ventricle and enter the pulmonary artery, making it possible to record the pulmonary arterial pressure, which is of clinical importance. Surgical treatment of other defects in patients with this lesion was for many years made difficult and dangerous by the fact that the right coronary artery often runs across the outflow tract of the right ventricle, over the usual site of ventriculotomy. Now that septal defects can be closed by a transatrial approach, operations on patients with corrected transposition have become less dangerous.

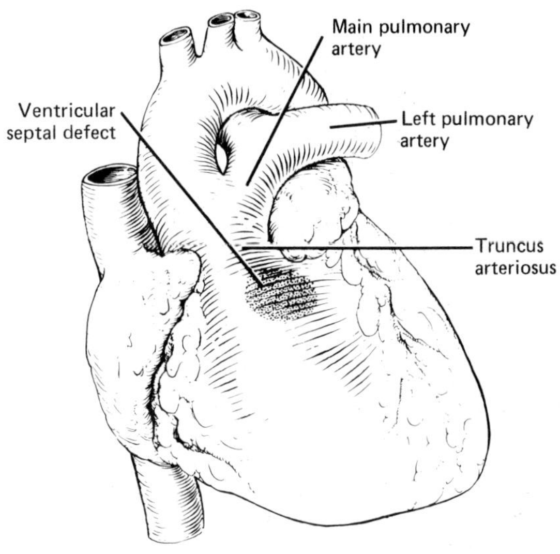

Figure 11–50. Truncus arteriosus. The main pulmonary artery arises from the truncus arteriosus downstream to the truncal semilunar valve. A ventricular septal defect is always present. (Modified and reproduced, with permission, from Dunphy JE, Way LW [editors]: *Current Surgical Diagnosis & Treatment,* 3rd ed. Lange, 1977.)

3. TRUNCUS ARTERIOSUS

In truncus arteriosus the blood vessels supplying blood to the lungs arise from the aorta (Fig 11–50). A ventricular septal defect is obligatory in this lesion. The level of pulmonary flow and pulmonary vascular resistance varies. Almost all patients who survive infancy have a raised pulmonary vascular resistance. The exact origin of the vessels supplying the lungs varies and does not greatly influence the clinical picture. When pulmonary blood supply is derived solely from bronchial collateral vessels, the lesion is indistinguishable from pulmonary atresia. In many cases, there is a

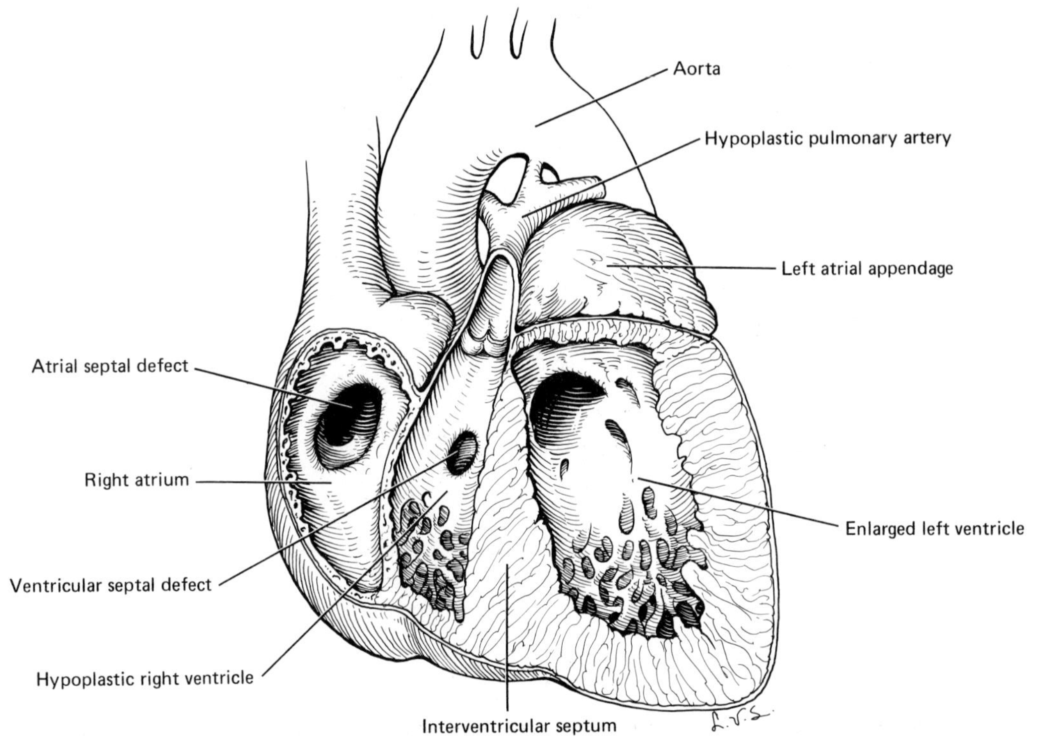

Figure 11–51. Tricuspid atresia, right-sided view.

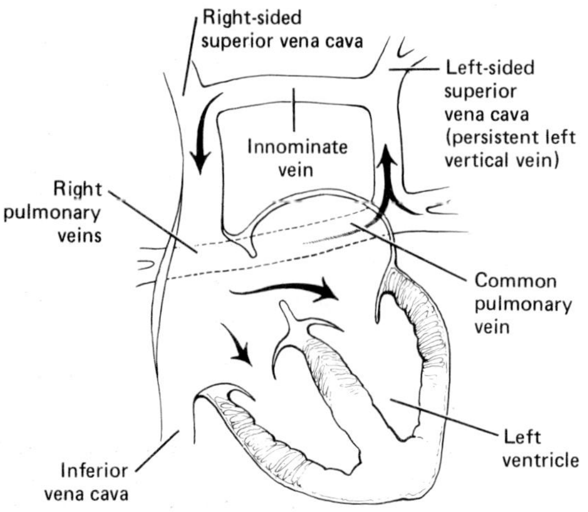

Figure 11–52. Common type of total anomalous pulmonary venous connection. The pulmonary veins connect to a persistent left-sided superior vena cava (left vertical vein), the innominate vein, and the right superior vena cava. (Reproduced, with permission, from Dunphy JE, Way LW [editors] : *Current Surgical Diagnosis & Treatment,* 3rd ed. Lange, 1977.)

common outflow valve with more than 3 cusps. This valve tends to be incompetent and causes a loud immediate diastolic murmur. The lesion can now be treated surgically provided that pulmonary vascular resistance is not too high. A plastic right ventricular prosthesis is interposed between the right atrium and the pulmonary arteries, which are removed from the aorta and sutured to the prosthesis. The ventricular defect is closed, and although the result is not a normal heart, the outcome is more favorable than was formerly the case.

4. TRICUSPID ATRESIA

In cases of atresia of the tricuspid valve, there must be an atrial defect through which all the systemic venous return reaches the left heart (Fig 11–51). As a result, there is left ventricular hypertrophy that shows up clearly on ECG as left ventricular dominance because the right ventricle is absent or not functional. Various associated lesions, especially transposition of the great arteries, may be present, and the origin of blood flow to the lungs is the principal variable. There may be associated pulmonary atresia with reduced pulmonary blood flow, or there may be a ventricular septal defect through which an increased pulmonary blood flow reaches the lungs. In rare cases, the tricuspid atresia is not complete, and there is a small underdeveloped right ventricle. In such patients the characteristic finding of the lesion (left ventricular hypertrophy on ECG) is still present. A right ventricular prosthesis interposed between the right atrium and the pulmonary artery (if one exists) is now the treatment of choice. Previously, an anastomosis was made between the superior vena cava and the right pulmonary artery (Glenn's operation).

5. TOTAL ANOMALOUS PULMONARY VENOUS DRAINAGE

In this lesion all the blood returning from the lungs enters the right heart (Fig 11–52). There must of necessity be an atrial septal defect. The principal variable is the route taken by the pulmonary venous return, which is most commonly via a left-sided superior vena cava to the innominate vein and thence to the right atrium via the superior vena cava. The other common pattern seen in infancy is via the inferior vena cava below the diaphragm. More rarely, other patterns of venous return are seen. The pulmonary blood flow and blood pressure vary, and the pulmonary venous return may be obstructed, leading to pulmonary venous congestion and edema. The variety of the lesion most commonly seen in older children is the pattern involving the innominate vein. The venous return is free, and there is usually raised pulmonary vascular resistance. In this lesion there is a characteristic chest x-ray picture called "snowman heart." The upper circular shadow is the anomalous venous pathway which lies above the lower circular shadow formed by the rest of the heart (Fig 11–53).

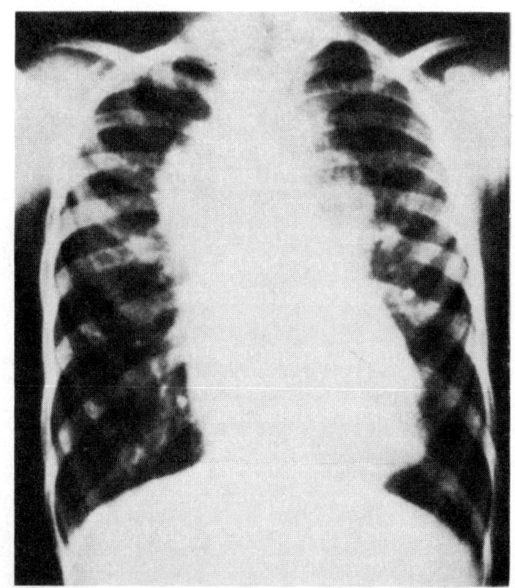

Figure 11–53. Chest x-ray showing typical "snowman" appearance due to total anomalous pulmonary venous drainage into left innominate vein. (Reproduced, with permission, from Wood P: *Diseases of the Heart and Circulation.* Lippincott, 1968.)

OTHER LESIONS

Dextrocardia with a mirror image heart in the right side of the chest can occur, with or without any other lesion, although situs inversus of the abdominal viscera is usually present. Dextroversion of the heart with abnormal rotation that leaves the heart mainly in the right chest can also occur. In this case the cardiac chambers are not in a mirror image position. Complete heart block may occur as an isolated congenital lesion or in association with other congenital heart lesions. Complete heart block is also a not infrequent complication of cardiac surgery performed to relieve congenital heart lesions.

Anomalies of the coronary circulation are also seen, either alone or in association with other lesions. The origin of the left coronary artery from the pulmonary artery is perhaps the most important (Fig 11–54). In this lesion, the blood flow through the anomalous vessel is into the pulmonary artery and a left-to-right shunt is seen. There is usually an ECG pattern of severe myocardial ischemia or infarction. Ligation of the abnormal vessel at the pulmonary artery level benefits the patient but does not cure the condition. Reanastomosis of the vessel to the aorta may eventually be the treatment of choice.

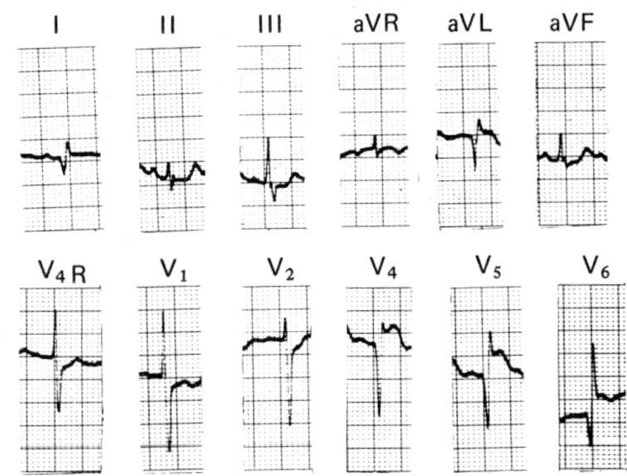

Figure 11–54. Representative ECG leads from a patient with anomalous left coronary artery originating from the aorta showing a current of injury pattern in the anterolateral left ventricular wall. (Reproduced, with permission, from Askenazi J, Nadas AS: Anomalous left coronary artery originating from the aorta. Circulation 51:976, 1976.)

In some cases the coronary arteries arise from abnormal sites, often from the wrong sinus of Valsalva. In some cases the coronary vessel may appear to become kinked as it follows its abnormal course. The lesion is occasionally found at autopsy in young persons who die suddenly; ventricular arrhythmia is believed to be the immediate cause of death.

• • •

References

Abrahams DG, Wood P: Pulmonary stenosis with normal aortic root. Br Heart J 13:519, 1951.

Ashby DW & others: The Holt-Oram syndrome: Associated skeletal and cardiac abnormalities. Q J Med 38:267, 1969.

Auerback ML, Sokolow M: Phonocardiography in acyanotic congenital heart disease. Pediatrics 24:1026, 1959.

Bacon APC, Matthews MB: Congenital bicuspid aortic valves and the aetiology of isolated aortic valvular stenosis. Q J Med 28:545, 1959.

Barber J & others: Atrial septal defect. Br Heart J 12:277, 1950.

Baron MG & others: Endocardial cushion defects: Specific diagnosis by angiocardiography. Am J Cardiol 13:162, 1964.

Bedford DE, Papp C, Parkinson J: Atrial septal defect. Br Heart J 3:37, 1941.

Bedford DE & others: Atrial septal defect and its surgical treatment. Lancet 1:1255, 1957.

Besterman EMM: Atrial septal defect with pulmonary hypertension. Br Heart J 23:587, 1961.

Blalock A, Taussig HB: The surgical treatment of malformations of the heart in which there is pulmonary stenosis or pulmonary atresia. JAMA 128:189, 1945.

Braunwald NS, Morrow AG: Incomplete persistent atrioventricular canal. J Thorac Cardiovasc Surg 51:71, 1966.

Brewer LA III & others: Spinal cord complications following surgery for coarctation of the aorta. J Thorac Cardiovasc Surg 64:368, 1972.

Brock RC: Pulmonary valvulotomy for the relief of congenital pulmonary stenosis. Br Med J 1:1121, 1948.

Campbell M: Congenital complete heart block. Br Heart J 5:15, 1943.

Campbell M: Natural history of persistent ductus arteriosus. Br Heart J 30:4, 1968.

Cartmill TB & others: Results of repair of ventricular septal defects. J Thorac Cardiovasc Surg 52:46, 1966.

Case RB & others: Anomalous origin of the left coronary artery: The physiologic defect and suggested surgical treatment. Circulation 17:1062, 1958.

Ceballos R, Kirklin JW: Long term anatomical results of intracardiac repair of tetralogy of Fallot. Ann Thorac Surg 15:371, 1973.

Chiariello L & others: Intracardiac repair of tetralogy of Fallot: 5 year review of 403 patients. J Thorac Cardiovasc Surg 70:529, 1975.

Corone P & others: Natural history of ventricular septal defect: A study involving 790 cases. Circulation 55:908, 1977.

Crafoord C, Nylin G: Congenital coarctation of the aorta and its surgical treatment. J Thorac Surg 14:347, 1945.

Crawford DW, Simpson E, McIlroy MB: Cardio-pulmonary function in Fallot's tetralogy after palliative shunting operations. Am Heart J 74:463, 1967.

Crews TL & others: Auscultatory and phonocardiographic findings in Ebstein's anomaly: Correlation of first heart sound with ultrasonic records of tricuspid valve movement. Br Heart J 34:681, 1972.

Damman JF, Ferenz C: The significance of the pulmonary vascular bed in congenital heart disease. Am Heart J 52:210, 1956.

Dexter L: Atrial septal defect. Br Heart J 18:209, 1956.

Dock W: Erosion of ribs in coarctation of the aorta: A note on the history of a pathognomonic sign. Br Heart J 10:148, 1948.

Dock W: Erosion of ribs in coarctation of the aorta: A note on the history of a pathognomonic sign. Br Heart J 10:148, 1948.

Ebstein W: Ueber einen sehr seltenen Fall von Insufficienz der Valvula tricuspidalis bedingt durch eine angeborene boch-gradige Missbildung derselben. Arch Anat Physiol 238, 1866.

Edie RN & others: Surgical repair of single ventricle. J Thorac Cardiovasc Surg 66:350, 1973.

Edwards JE: Functional pathology of the pulmonary vascular tree in congenital heart disease. Circulation 15:164, 1957.

Edwards WS, Bargeron LM Jr: The superiority of the Glenn operation for tricuspid atresia in infancy and childhood. J Thorac Cardiovasc Surg 55:60, 1968.

Eisenmenger V: Die angeborenen Defecte der Kammerscheid-wand des Herzens. Klin Med 32 (Suppl 1), 1897.

Ellis FH & others: Patent ductus arteriosus with pulmonary hypertension: An analysis of cases treated surgically. J Thorac Cardiovasc Surg 31:268, 1956.

Emanuel RW, Pattinson JN: Absence of the left pulmonary artery in Fallot's tetralogy. Br Heart J 18:289, 1956.

Fallot A: Contribution a l'anatomie pathologique de la maladie bleue (cyanose cardiaque). Marseille Med 25:77, 1888.

Fontan F & others: Repair of tricuspid atresia: Surgical considerations and results. Circulation 50 (Suppl 3):72, 1974.

Gault JH & others: Atrial septal defect in patients over the age of forty years: Clinical and hemodynamic studies and the effects of operation. Circulation 37:261, 1968.

Gerbode F & others: Endocardial cushion defects. Ann Surg 166:486, 1967.

Gomes MMR & others: Total anomalous pulmonary venous connection. J Thorac Cardiovasc Surg 60:116, 1970.

Greene DG & others: Pure congenital pulmonary stenosis and idiopathic congenital dilatation of the pulmonary artery. Am J Med 6:24, 1949.

Gross RE: Complete division for the patent ductus arteriosus. J Thorac Cardiovasc Surg 16:314, 1947.

Hoffman JIE: Natural history of congenital heart disease: Problems of its assessment with special reference to ventricular septal defects. Circulation 37:97, 1968.

Holt M, Oram S: Familial heart disease with skeletal malformations. Br Heart J 22:236, 1960.

Hultgren HN & others: The ejection click of valvular pulmonic stenosis. Circulation 40:631, 1969.

Jones JC: Twenty-five years' experience with the surgery of patent ductus arteriosus. J Thorac Cardiovasc Surg 50:149, 1965.

Keck EWO: Ventricular septal defect with aortic insufficiency. Circulation 27:203, 1963.

Keith JD, Rowe RD, Vlad P: *Heart Disease in Infancy and Childhood,* 2nd ed. Macmillan, 1967.

Kidd BSL, Keith JD (editors): *The Natural History and Progress in Treatment of Congenital Heart Defects.* Thomas, 1971.

Kimball KG, McIlroy MB: Pulmonary hypertension in patients with congenital heart disease. Am J Med 41:883, 1966.

Kirklin JW, Karp RB: *The Tetralogy of Fallot from a Surgical Viewpoint.* Saunders, 1970.

Leatham A: *Auscultation of the Heart and Phonocardiography,* 2nd ed. Churchill-Livingstone, 1975.

Leatham A, Gray I: Auscultatory and phonocardiographic signs of atrial septal defect. Br Heart J 18:193, 1956.

Leatham A, Segal B: Auscultatory and phonocardiographic signs of ventricular septal defect with left-to-right shunt. Circulation 25:318, 1962.

Lev M & others: Single (primitive) ventricle. Circulation 39:577, 1969.

Marfan AB: Un cas de déformation congenitale des quatre membres, plus prononceé aux extrémités, caractérisée par l'allongement des os avec un certain degré d'amincissement. Bull Soc Med Paris 13:220, 1896.

Møller I, Wennevold A, Lyngborg KE: The natural history of pulmonary stenosis: Long-term follow-up with serial heart catheterizations. Cardiology 58:193, 1973.

Morrow AG & others: Successful surgical repair of a ruptured aneurysm of the sinus of Valsalva. Circulation 16:533, 1957.

Mustard WT & others: The surgical management of transposition of the great vessels. J Thorac Cardiovasc Surg 48:953, 1964.

Nadas AS: Pulmonic stenosis: Indications for surgery in children and adults. N Engl J Med 287:1196, 1972.

Neill C, Mounsey P: Auscultation in patent ductus arteriosus. Br Heart J 20:61, 1958.

Parry LW, Scott LP: Anomalous left coronary artery from pulmonary artery. Circulation 41:1043, 1970.

Perloff JK: *The Clinical Recognition of Congenital Heart Disease.* Saunders, 1970.

Perloff JK: Pediatric congenital cardiac becomes a postoperative adult: The changing population of congenital heart disease. Circulation 47:606, 1973.

Potts WJ, Smith S, Gibson S: Anastomosis of the aorta to a pulmonary artery. JAMA 132:627, 1946.

Rudolph AM: *Congenital Diseases of the Heart.* Year Book, 1974.

Rudolph AM (editor): *Pediatrics,* 16th ed. Appleton-Century-Crofts, 1977.

Rytand DA: The renal factor in arterial hypertension with coarctation of the aorta. J Clin Invest 17:391, 1938.

Schuster SR, Gross RE: Surgery for coarctation of the aorta: A review of 500 cases. J Thorac Cardiovasc Surg 43:54, 1962.

Sellers RD & others: Secundum type atrial septal defects: Results with 275 patients. Surgery 59:155, 1966.

Starr A, Bonchek LI, Sunderland CO: Total correction of tetralogy of Fallot in infancy. J Thorac Cardiovasc Surg 65:45, 1973.

Steell G: The murmur of high pressure in the pulmonary artery. Med Chron 9:182, 1888.

Sutton G, Harris A, Leatham A: Second heart sound in pulmonary hypertension. Br Heart J 30:743, 1968.

Tofler OB: The pulmonary component of the second heart sound in Fallot's tetralogy. Br Heart J 25:509, 1963.

Trusler GA, Mustard WT: Palliative and reparative procedures for transposition of the great arteries: Current review. Ann Thorac Surg 17:410, 1974.

Verska JJ, DeQuattro V, Wooley MM: Coarctation of the aorta: The abdominal pain syndrome and paradoxical hypertension. J Thorac Cardiovasc Surg 58:746, 1969.

Whitaker W & others: Patent ductus arteriosus with pulmonary hypertension. Br Heart J 17:121, 1955.

Wood P: The Eisenmenger syndrome. (2 parts.) Br Med J 2:701, 755, 1958.

Wood P: Pulmonary hypertension. Br Med Bull 8:348, 1952.

12 . . .
Valvular Heart Disease; Mitral Valve Disease

Valvular heart disease presents some of the most important diagnostic problems in adult cardiology. Because of the vast range in types of lesions, valvular involvement, causes, and associated conditions, certain broad generalizations about valvular heart disease are inevitable.

Classification of Valvular Disease

Valvular disease can be classified according to the following factors:

A. Lesion: Valvular disease can be divided into 3 categories on the basis of the type of lesion: stenosis, incompetence, and mixed stenosis and incompetence (regurgitation, insufficiency).

B. Valvular Involvement: Lesions involving the mitral and aortic valves are more common than tricuspid and pulmonary valve lesions in adult valvular disease.

C. Cause: Rheumatic endocarditis is the most important cause of valvular heart disease; degenerative disorders and congenital disease are other prominent causes.

Associated lesions such as past or present myocardial damage due to rheumatic carditis, or degenerative changes due to hypertension, atherosclerosis, cardiomyopathy, or abnormal wear and tear secondary to the valvular lesion will affect the classification.

Hemodynamic Effects of Valvular Lesions

Mechanical lesions such as valvular stenosis or incompetence cause abnormal stresses on the heart.

A. Stenosis: In stenosis, the chamber behind the stenotic valve—the left ventricle in aortic stenosis and the left atrium in mitral stenosis—must work harder to maintain a normal cardiac output if a valvular lesion is present. Thus, left ventricular and left atrial hypertrophy are the first manifestations of significant obstruction at the aortic and mitral valves, respectively. Normal heart valves can handle flows that are 5–7 times the resting values; consequently, valvular stenosis must be severe before it causes life-threatening problems. Symptoms generally appear first during exercise.

B. Incompetence: If a valve is incompetent, both the chamber behind the valve and the chamber in front must bear an extra load. Thus, in mitral incompetence both the left atrium and the left ventricle are subject to increased stress; in aortic incompetence, the left ventricle and the aorta are affected. The stress in valvular incompetence is different from that in stenosis and more closely resembles the physiologic stress of muscular exercise. The heart must deal with an extra volume of blood with each heartbeat. The blood that flows backward across an incompetent valve in one phase of the cardiac cycle must flow forward during the other phase. This is in addition to the normal forward flow. In mitral and tricuspid disease, the incompetence is systolic, and diastolic flow is increased; conversely, in aortic and pulmonary incompetence, diastolic backflow occurs, and it is the systolic flow that is increased.

C. Mixed Stenosis and Incompetence: Valvular lesions are never entirely anatomically "pure," and both stenosis and incompetence occur almost invariably. For the purposes of clinical classification, however, it is convenient to think of lesions in terms of the predominant mechanical load they impose on the heart. This leads to the classification of valvular lesions into predominant stenosis, predominant incompetence, and mixed stenosis and incompetence.

Natural History

A. Chronic Valvular Lesions: Chronic valvular lesions tend to have a long course. Impairment of cardiac function may be detected even when the patient is asymptomatic. There is not necessarily a direct relationship between the severity of symptoms and the degree of functional impairment of cardiac performance, and the varying responses to disease make it virtually impossible to correlate a given degree of disability with a certain severity of valvular abnormality. The age, sex, race, occupation, and activity level of the patient and the presence and cause of other lesions are important variables influencing the clinical picture.

1. Effects of myocardial disease—Emphasis on the importance of the severity of the valvular lesion in valvular disease has varied. Before the advent of cardiac surgery for the relief of valvular disease, cardiologists felt that the state of the myocardium was the most significant factor. After cardiac surgery became widely available, myocardial function was considered to be of secondary importance. In actuality, both the severity of the lesion and the degree of myocardial dysfunction are important, and these factors are synergistic in their relation to each other. Thus, myocardial disease causes cardiac dilatation, thereby exaggerating the effects of valvular disease by increasing the severity of the effects of incompetence on the heart. Similarly, valvular disease augments the effects of myocardial disease by increasing the load on diseased heart muscle.

2. Causes of progression—The natural history and course of chronic valvular disease are long and difficult to follow. It is not easy to predict the course, nor is it clear how much of the progression is due to actual worsening of the anatomic lesion caused by the original valvular damage. A valve that is the site of an anatomic lesion is subject to abnormal mechanical stress and premature degenerative changes. Such changes as sclerosis, fibrosis, and calcification influence the progress of valvular lesions regardless of the original cause of the lesion.

3. Variation in clinical features—Because the course of chronic valvular disease often lasts for 20–30 years, it is much easier to gain experience based on several patients seen at different stages of the disease than it is to follow a single patient progressively through the different stages. Although it is relatively easy to see that disease has progressed in a given patient, the nature, timing, and rate of progress are difficult to determine. The natural progress of disease is also modified by treatment, and it is in valvular heart disease that the iatrogenic modification of cardiac disease is seen most clearly.

B. Acute Valvular Lesions: The clinical picture in patients with acute valvular lesions is different from that seen in classic chronic lesions associated with rheumatic fever. Pure valvular incompetence rather than stenosis is an example of the classic acute lesion. It has become increasingly important to distinguish the clinical features of an acute lesion—which develops over a period of minutes, days, or weeks—from the more readily recognized effects of chronic valvular lesions. Acute lesions are relatively rare (10%), and their importance depends on their severity. If the patient survives the onset of an acute lesion, compensatory responses to increased cardiac load occur, leading to hypertrophy or dilatation of the appropriate chambers. Such a lesion becomes chronic in about 1 year. In acute severe valvular lesions the heart tolerates the extra load poorly. In acute aortic and mitral incompetence, pulmonary congestion and edema tend to so dominate the clinical picture that separate clinical features must be distinguished. The lungs carry the brunt of the disease, and some of the cardiac manifestations associated with chronic valvular lesions may not appear for several weeks.

MITRAL VALVE DISEASE

Mitral valve disease is the commonest form of valvular heart disease and accounts for more than half of cases with significant valvular lesions. Rheumatic heart disease is the commonest cause of mitral valve disease in particular and all valve disease in general. Acute clinical manifestations of rheumatic fever are detected in only about half of patients who subsequently develop mitral valve disease. The presence or absence of a history of rheumatic fever makes no difference in the course of the disease or in its clinical, hemodynamic, or pathologic findings. In patients who have no history of rheumatic fever, it is generally assumed that a subclinical attack without overt signs of cardiac or joint involvement was responsible for the valvular lesion.

Classification of Mitral Valve Disease

Mitral valve disease has been classified somewhat arbitrarily into 3 types: mitral stenosis, mixed mitral stenosis and incompetence, and mitral incompetence.

It is difficult to distinguish between the different lesions in some cases, and in some patients the disease can on occasion shift from one category to another. The classification depends primarily on the physical findings rather than the history, although the history and course of the disease vary in the different lesions.

In mitral stenosis, the predominant lesion is obstruction to the diastolic flow of blood through the mitral valve. The hallmark of the lesion is the presence of a presystolic (atrial systolic) murmur indicating that mitral flow is still continuing when atrial contraction occurs and that the patient is still in sinus rhythm. Atrial fibrillation commonly accompanies mitral valve disease and occurs in all types of lesions. In mitral stenosis, however, it is seldom present when the patient first presents with symptoms. Predominant obstruction to mitral valve flow during diastole is such a potent cause of symptoms that patients with this lesion develop dyspnea early in adult life in all but the mildest cases.

In mixed mitral stenosis and incomptence, there is both obstruction to forward flow and leakage of blood from the left ventricle into the left atrium during systole. Mitral stenosis and incompetence have traditionally been thought to be mutually exclusive lesions that cannot coexist except in a mild form. The rationale for this category of mixed stenosis and incompetence may therefore warrant explanation. Mitral valvotomy may alter the natural history of mitral valve disease. In relieving mitral stenosis, the surgeon not infrequently renders the valve incompetent. Long-term follow-up of patients who have had mitral valvotomy shows that the operation is usually only palliative and that symptoms recur. Although some patients show evidence of restenosis, the majority present a clinical picture of mixed stenosis and incompetence, often with a fixed, calcified valve that neither opens nor shuts completely. The hallmark of the lesion is the absence of a presystolic murmur, which indicates that the obstruction is not severe enough to hinder forward flow at the end of diastole. It also implies that the patient is in atrial fibillation. Patients with mixed mitral stenosis and incompetence characteristically develop symptoms for the first time when their cardiac rhythm changes from sinus to atrial fibrillation. This usually takes place at about age 40. This course also occurs in some patients who have not had a previous mitral valvotomy.

Mitral incompetence differs from other kinds of mitral valve disease in that it has several forms and has a variety of causes. It is here divided into the following categories: (1) acute mitral incompetence and (2) chronic mitral incompetence (hemodynamically insignificant and significant).

The hallmark of mitral incompetence is the presence of a systolic murmur without any significant diastolic murmur to indicate the presence of obstruction to the diastolic forward flow across the valve. In acute lesions the onset is abrupt and caused by acute disruption of the mitral valve due to rupture or stretching of the chordae tendineae, weakening of the papillary muscles, or perforation of a valve cusp. In hemodynamically insignificant chronic lesions the characteristic feature is a late systolic murmur with or without a midsystolic ejection click. The murmur is associated with a specific clinical picture and a course that may lead in time to either a significant chronic lesion or an acute exacerbation. In chronic hemodynamically significant mitral incompetence there is a pansystolic murmur with a third heart sound and no diastolic murmur. The lesion is well tolerated, and even the onset of atrial fibrillation does not cause serious symptoms. Left ventricular stroke volume is increased in mitral incompetence, and the way the ventricle responds to the extra "flow" work determines the course of the disease.

Development of Rheumatic Mitral Lesions

A past history of rheumatic fever is present in about half of patients with mitral valve disease. It is least common in patients with acute mitral incompetence (15%), more common in chronic mitral incompetence (20%) and mitral stenosis (50%), and commonest in mixed mitral stenosis and incompetence (70%). The physical signs of rheumatic mitral valve lesions develop at different times after an acute attack of rheumatic fever. In the case of mitral incompetence or mixed mitral stenosis and incompetence, murmurs are usually audible during or shortly after the acute attack. In mitral stenosis, signs of rheumatic mitral valve lesions develop after several years. In all but the most severe cases, physical signs precede symptoms by many years. A murmur is usually present by age 20, and, since the majority of patients are women, pregnancy constitutes an important form of stress in the course of a disease which may last for 20–30 years. More severe cases of mitral stenosis cannot withstand the stress of pregnancy, but it is remarkable that many women who present in their 40s and 50s with mitral stenosis and pulmonary hypertension have had several pregnancies without difficulty.

Cause of Mitral Valve Disease

Rheumatic heart disease is, in effect, the sole cause of all mitral valve disease except mitral incompetence. Even in cases of mitral incompetence, however, rheumatic fever probably accounts for half of chronic lesions. Rheumatic heart disease is much more common in women than in men; the female:male ratio of 9:1 in mitral stenosis falls to 3:1 in mixed mitral stenosis and incompetence and 1:1 in mitral incompetence. The only nonrheumatic causes of mitral stenosis or mixed stenosis and incompetence are congenital heart disease and hypertrophic cardiomyopathy. Congenital heart disease is rare, being encountered in less than 1% of adult cases, and it is debatable whether hypertrophic cardiomyopathy should be considered as a form of mitral disease or as part of the differential diagnosis.

MITRAL STENOSIS

The cardinal features of mitral stenosis are shown in Fig 12–1. In mitral stenosis, rheumatic endocarditis scars the mitral valve and commonly causes fusion of the commissures and matting of the chordae tendineae, which interfere with the opening of the valve. The left atrium bears the brunt of the load, and the extent to which it dilates depends on its internal pressure and the state of the atrial myocardium. With time, calcification of the mitral valve renders it less mobile. In some patients with tight mitral stenosis, pulmonary vascular resistance rises because the pulmonary arteriolar smooth muscle responds to the increase in pulmonary venous pressure by vasoconstriction. The reasons for this response are not clear. The increase in resistance appears to be related to the rise in pulmonary venous pressure and does not occur when the rise is small. At first the changes are functional and reversible by drugs such as acetylcholine and tolazoline. Later, however, anatomic changes appear, with medial hypertrophy and intimal thickening of pulmonary arterioles occurring first at the base of the lungs, where venous pressure is higher because of the effects of gravity, and later throughout the lungs. Severe pulmonary vascular lesions with markedly raised pulmonary vascular resistance (> 7.5 mm Hg/l/min) are virtually limited to patients with severe mitral stenosis, whereas lesser increases in pulmonary vascular resistance are seen in other forms of mitral disease. When pulmonary vascular resistance rises, the course of mitral stenosis is strikingly altered; the brunt of the load is transferred from the left atrium to the right ventricle, and right ventricular failure eventually occurs if the stenosis is not relieved.

Passive pulmonary hypertension. The pulmonary arterial pressure must rise to maintain pulmonary blood flow in any patient whose left atrial pressure rises. Thus, when left atrial pressure rises to 25–30 mm Hg in mitral stenosis, the pulmonary arterial mean pressure inevitably increases to a mean level of 30–40 mm Hg. This "passive" pulmonary hypertension results in redistribution of the blood flow to the lungs, with more perfusion of the apexes. The load is not severe

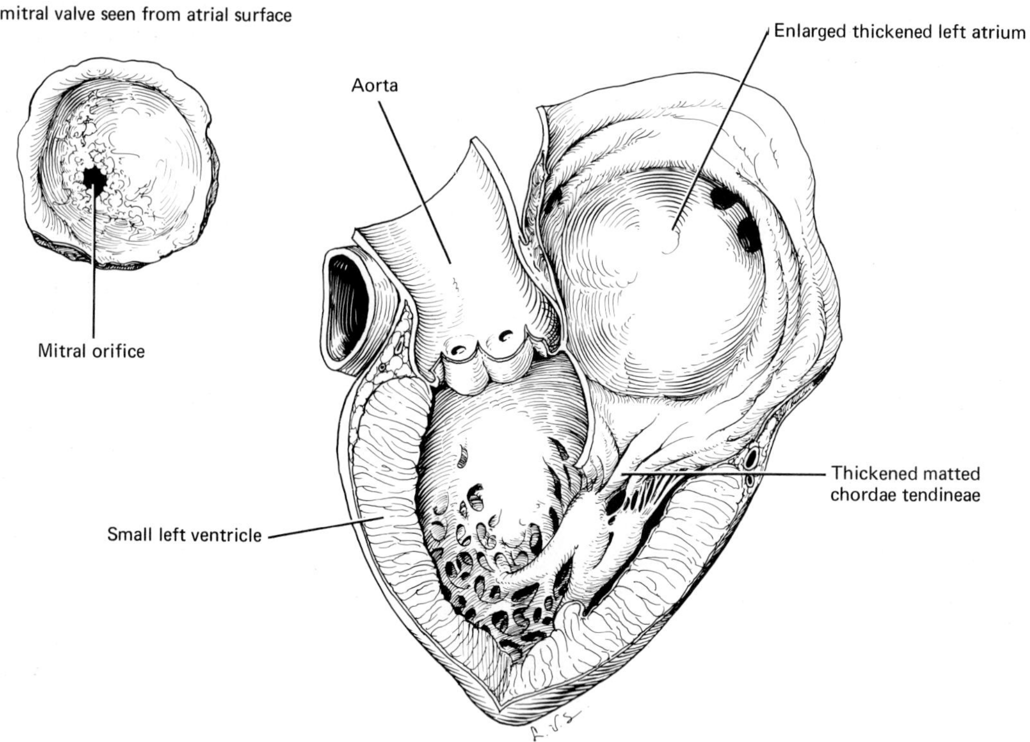

Drawing of left heart in left anterior oblique view showing anatomic features of mitral stenosis.

Cardinal features: *Thickening and fusion of mitral valve cusps; raised left atrial pressure; left atrial enlargement.*

Variable factors: *Severity of obstruction; severity of rheumatic myocarditis; level of pulmonary vascular resistance.*

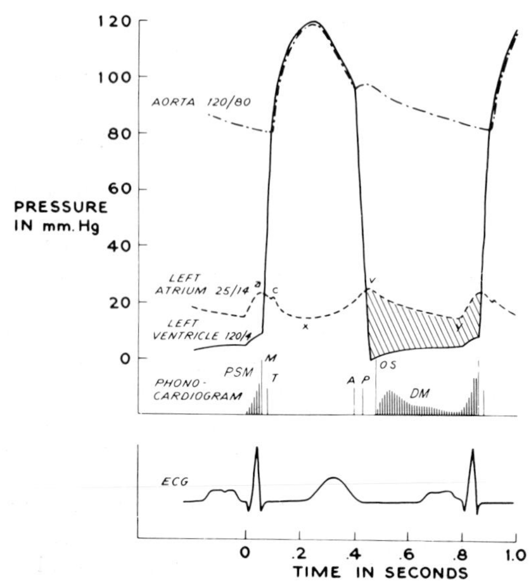

Diagram showing auscultatory and hemodynamic features of mitral stenosis.

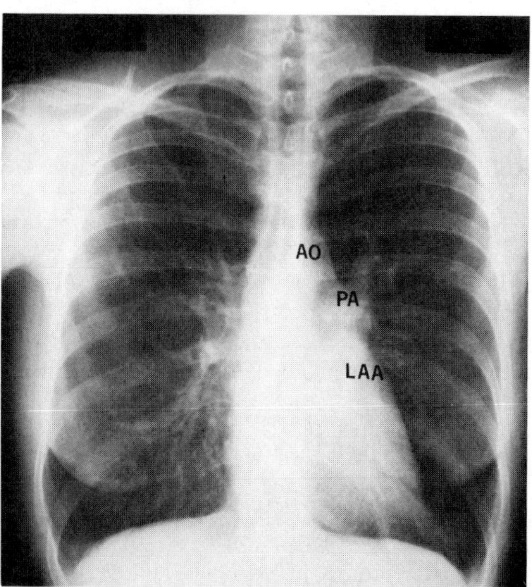

Chest x-ray of a patient with mitral stenosis showing left atrial appendage (LAA) enlargement. PA, pulmonary artery; AO, aorta.

Figure 12–1. Mitral stenosis. Structures enlarged: Left atrium; small left ventricle.

enough to cause right heart failure, and pulmonary congestion with orthopnea and paroxysmal dyspnea dominates the clinical picture. Before mitral valvotomy was available, some patients died of acute pulmonary edema. The right ventricle continued to pump blood into the congested lung, and leakage of fluid into the alveoli flooded the lungs and produced a fatal disturbance of gas exchange.

Onset of Atrial Fibrillation

In patients without pulmonary hypertension, atrial fibrillation almost always develops with the passage of time. Even if pulmonary hypertension is present, 30% of patients develop atrial fibrillation early in the course of the disease. Atrial fibrillation is most closely correlated with age, but it also depends on left atrial pressure and the severity of involvement of the left atrium in the rheumatic process.

Clinical Findings

A. Symptoms:

1. **Dyspnea**—The commonest presenting symptom (80%) in patients with mitral stenosis is shortness of breath on exertion. In women with severe lesions this is usually noticed in early adult life (age 20–30), while the patient is still in sinus rhythm, perhaps during pregnancy. The dyspnea is due to pulmonary congestion that results from a rise in left atrial pressure associated with an increase in heart rate and a decrease in left atrial emptying time. The increased stiffness of the lungs increases the work of breathing, and the fall in cardiac output which results from mitral valve obstruction leads to an increase in heart rate that further aggravates the congestion. Any factor that increases the heart rate is likely to aggravate dyspnea in mitral stenosis; anxiety, anemia, exposure to high altitude, pregnancy, thyrotoxicosis, and atrial arrhythmia are poorly tolerated. The onset of atrial fibrillation in a patient with significant mitral stenosis virtually always provokes dyspnea. In milder cases there may have been no dyspnea prior to the onset of arrhythmia, but in most instances the onset of atrial fibrillation exacerbates dyspnea rather than provoking it for the first time. Conversely, when a patient believed to have significant mitral stenosis develops atrial fibrillation without experiencing dyspnea, the diagnosis is in doubt and the lesion is at most mild.

2. **Paroxysmal nocturnal dyspnea**—The dyspnea in patients with mitral stenosis may be severe enough to progress to episodes of acute pulmonary edema, especially in the presence of some additional stress. Increased heart rate due to anxiety, atrial arrhythmia, fever due to intercurrent infection, excessive salt intake, or unaccustomed exertion should be sought. An acute episode of dyspnea often occurs at night, and the patient wakes from sleep with a choking sensation accompanied by cough. Relief is obtained by sitting or standing up. One episode of paroxysmal nocturnal dyspnea may cause the patient to sleep on several pillows indefinitely, and the association between recumbency and dyspnea is readily apparent to the patient. However, orthopnea is not necessarily present just because the patient uses several pillows. It is important to count the pulse and respirations and observe how well a change in posture is tolerated when the patient lies flat. Orthopnea should be treated as a sign rather than a symptom.

3. **Hemoptysis**—Hemoptysis is the second most common presenting symptom in mitral stenosis. There may be frank pulmonary hemorrhage from rupture of a pulmonary vein; frothy pink, blood-tinged sputum in pulmonary edema; or hemoptysis resulting from pulmonary infarction. Hemoptysis is seen in patients with raised pulmonary vascular resistance and in those with pulmonary congestion.

4. **Systemic embolism**—Presenting symptoms due to systemic embolism are infrequent in patients with mitral stenosis. Embolism is more common after atrial fibrillation has occurred and tends to occur later in the disease.

5. **Palpitations**—Palpitations are rarely the chief presenting complaint. Any arrhythmia is likely to provoke dyspnea, and the patient will usually complain of dyspnea rather than palpitations.

6. **Symptoms in patients with raised pulmonary vascular resistance**—Fatigue, coldness of the extremities, abdominal discomfort, and swelling of the abdomen and ankles are symptoms of right heart involvement. They suggest the presence of severe pulmonary hypertension and raised pulmonary vascular resistance with a low cardiac output and are thus indicative of severe mitral stenosis. Symptoms of right heart involvement can also occur in patients with associated organic involvement of the tricuspid valve. Chest pain that is indistinguishable from angina pectoris is occasionally noted in the presence of raised pulmonary vascular resistance or pulmonary embolism.

7. **Episodic symptoms**—Confusion in diagnosis sometimes occurs when the patient's symptoms are episodic. In this case arrhythmia should be suspected, and the physician should try to see the patient during an attack in order to record an ECG.

B. **Signs**: The physical signs in patients with mitral stenosis vary with the severity of the valvular lesion and also with the amount of increase in pulmonary vascular resistance. The classic signs of mitral stenosis shown in Fig 12–2 develop early in the natural course of the condition and can usually be noted before symptoms develop. However, the patient may have to engage in exercise in order to elicit the signs. In classic mitral stenosis the pulse is normal or small in amplitude, and the blood pressure and systemic venous pressure are normal.

1. **Loud first heart sound**—The heart is not enlarged, and on palpation there is an obvious localized tapping cardiac impulse. This represents the vibrations from the loud first heart sound that result from closure of the mitral valve (closing snap). There may also be a diastolic thrill with presystolic accentuation felt at the apex and a palpable opening snap felt at the base of the heart.

2. **Opening snap**—On auscultation the first sound

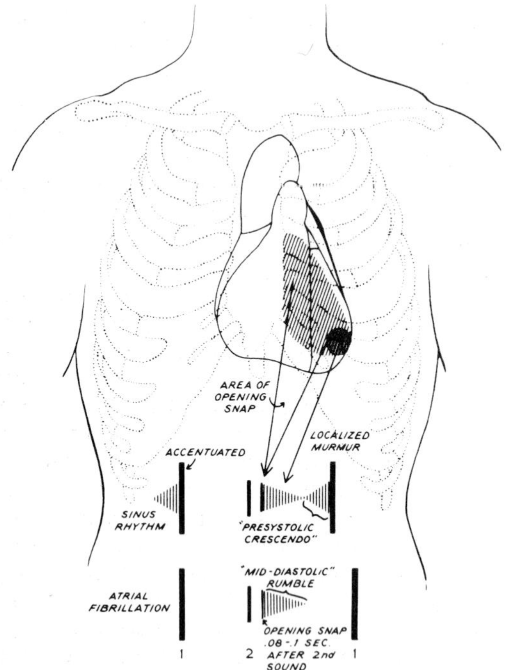

Figure 12–2. Diagram showing auscultatory signs of mitral stenosis. (Reproduced, with permission, from Krupp MA, Chatton MC [editors]: *Current Medical Diagnosis & Treatment 1977.* Lange, 1977.)

is loud, and the second sound is followed by a loud opening snap that is high-pitched and widely transmitted but heard best to the left of the sternum, near the base of the heart.

3. **Diastolic murmur with presystolic accentuation**—The characteristic finding in predominant mitral stenosis is a long, loud, rumbling mitral diastolic murmur with presystolic accentuation due to atrial systole (Fig 12–3). The murmur is often best heard in a localized area about 2.5 cm in diameter located at the apex of the heart. The patient should be on the left side after exercise, and the physician should use the bell of the stethoscope and light pressure on the chest. The murmur may be absent in mid diastole in mild cases but still show presystolic accentuation (Fig 12–4).

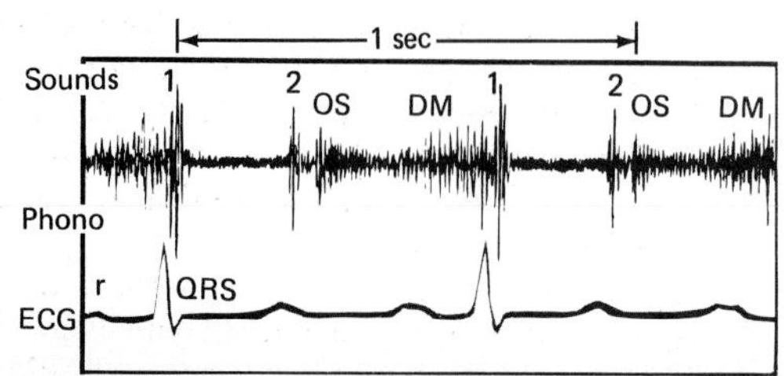

Figure 12–3. Typical phonocardiogram in mitral stenosis showing loud first sound and opening snap (SO), followed by long diastolic rumbling murmur (DM) with presystolic accentuation. (Courtesy of Roche Laboratories Division of Hoffman-La Roche Inc.)

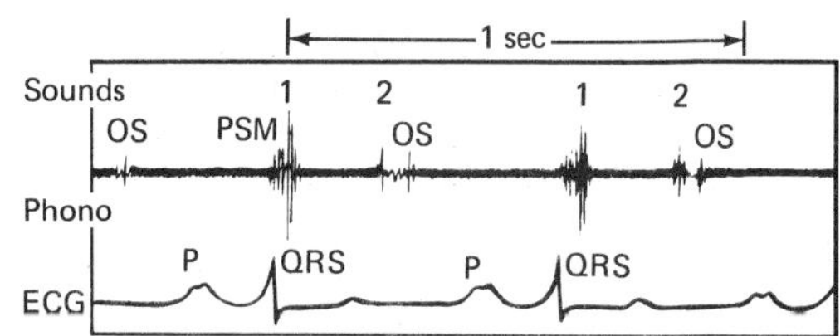

Figure 12–4. Phonocardiogram of loud first sound in mitral stenosis. Note presystolic murmur (PSM) and opening snap (OS) with no diastolic murmur following the snap. (Courtesy of Roche Laboratories Division of Hoffman-La Roche Inc.)

4. **S_2–OS interval**—The time elapsing between the aortic valve closure sound and the opening snap is roughly related to left atrial pressure. If left atrial pressure is high, the valve will open early because left atrial pressure soon comes to exceed left ventricular pressure. Conversely, if left atrial pressure is low, a longer time will elapse before left atrial pressure exceeds left ventricular pressure and filling starts. Thus, an early opening snap (0.05–0.07 sec after A_2) suggests more severe stenosis than a later (0.10–0.12 sec after A_2) opening snap. The presence of loud opening and closing snaps indicates that the mitral valve is flexible and suggests that mitral valvotomy rather than valve replacement will be appropriate treatment.

There is not infrequently a mitral systolic murmur in pure mitral stenosis. A long, rumbling diastolic murmur with presystolic accentuation during atrial contraction is the definitive auscultatory sign of mitral stenosis, and the presence of a presystolic (atrial systolic) murmur excludes a diagnosis of significant mitral incompetence. Thus, even though mild, hemodynamically insignificant mitral incompetence may cause a loud systolic murmur, this should not be construed as evidence of significant mitral incompetence when a patient has none of the other signs of mitral incompetence but some of the signs of mitral stenosis. The murmur may be due to tricuspid incompetence.

5. **Signs in the presence of atrial fibrillation**—When the patient develops atrial fibrillation, the presystolic murmur disappears. The heart rate becomes irregular, and after the heart rate has been slowed by digitalis therapy it becomes important to listen for the length of the diastolic murmur during the longest diastolic pauses. In patients with predominant mitral stenosis, the murmur should persist until the end of diastole even in cardiac cycles lasting 1 sec (Fig 12–2). A shorter murmur suggests either mixed mitral stenosis and incompetence or raised pulmonary vascular resistance. It is the length of the diastolic murmur and not the fact that it lasts until the next first heart sound that is important in the determination of the severity of mitral stenosis.

6. **Pulmonary signs**—Rales at the bases of the lungs are commonly found in mitral stenosis, but their absence does not exclude the possibility of pulmonary congestion or even edema. The patient is often orthopneic because the lungs become more congested when the patient is in a supine position, the respiratory rate

increases as the lungs become stiffer, and the patient becomes breathless. It is more reliable to have the patient lie flat and look for evidence of orthopnea than to ask whether shortness of breath occurs on recumbency.

7. **Signs in the presence of pulmonary hypertension**—When pulmonary vascular resistance is markedly raised (> 7.5 mm Hg/l/min), the physical signs of mitral stenosis tend to be different. The patient usually has a low cardiac output and is often thin, with peripheral cyanosis, cool extremities, and a pulse of small volume. Dilated veins on the cheeks combined with peripheral cyanosis give rise to a "mitral facies" that is also seen in other patients with a chronically low cardiac output. Systemic venous pressure is likely to be raised, with a prominent *a* wave visible in the jugular pulse if sinus rhythm is present. The heart may be enlarged, with a right ventricular substernal impulse. The auscultatory signs of mitral stenosis tend to be less florid than those in patients with low pulmonary vascular resistance because the cardiac output is lower. Less often, there is a diastolic thrill, but pulmonary valve closure is usually palpable. In about one-third of cases, either reduction in the cardiac output or valvular calcification modifies the classic physical signs, making the diagnosis difficult. Calcification of the valve may eliminate the opening snap but should not affect the murmur. Low output may eliminate the murmur but should not affect the snap. Calcification of the mitral valve does not always affect the physical signs, and more than half of patients with valvular calcification have an opening snap. There is often a pulmonary systolic ejection click and a short pulmonary systolic murmur in addition to a loud pulmonary valve closure sound.

a. **Pulmonary incompetence**—Pulmonary incompetence secondary to pulmonary hypertension may cause an immediate diastolic murmur at the base of the heart (Graham Steell murmur). In practice, associated hemodynamically insignificant aortic incompetence is a much more common cause of such a basal murmur.

b. **Tricuspid incompetence**—Pansystolic murmurs are common in patients with pulmonary hypertension and are usually due to secondary tricuspid incompetence, as shown by increased systemic venous pressure, a prominent *v* wave in the neck, and increased intensity of the murmur during inspiration. When right ventricular failure occurs, the right side of the heart may become so large that it occupies the whole front of the chest.

8. **Signs in the presence of low output**—In severely ill patients, the mitral diastolic murmur may vary in intensity because of changes in cardiac output or heart rate. The fact that one observer has heard the murmur and another has not should not be discounted, and repeated examinations may be helpful. A mitral diastolic murmur that is ordinarily inaudible may be heard by listening in the axilla, with the patient lying on the left side.

9. **Assessment of severity from physical signs**—Assessment of the severity of mitral stenosis based on physical signs is not of sufficient accuracy to be clinically valid. Patients with varying degrees of stenosis can all show fully developed classic physical signs. The timing of the opening snap confirmed by phonocardiography may be a guide to the severity of the disease, but this measurement must be assessed in relation to the rest of the clinical picture. The degree of pulmonary congestion shown on the chest x-ray and the findings at cardiac catheterization provide a more reliable index of severity.

C. **Electrocardiographic Findings**: The ECG is of little help in diagnosing or assessing the severity of predominant mitral stenosis with low pulmonary vascular resistance. A broad, notched, posteriorly oriented P wave (P mitrale) is usually all that is present. If right ventricular hypertrophy is present, pulmonary vascular resistance is almost certainly raised. ECG evidence of right ventricular hypertrophy is seen in 75% of patients whose pulmonary vascular resistance is over 7.5 mm Hg/l/min. In patients in sinus rhythm, right ventricular hypertrophy is manifested by right axis deviation, with an S wave and a tall R or R′ wave in V_1 and T wave inversion in V_{1-3}, and P mitrale. The absence of right ventricular hypertrophy on ECG does not rule out severe pulmonary hypertension, but some signs are usually present, and the progressive development of ECG changes (Fig 12–5) is an important clue to the diagnosis of raised pulmonary vascular resistance. ECG evidence of left ventricular hypertrophy suggests a diagnosis of systemic hypertension, aortic valve disease, or rheumatic myocardial disease rather than mitral incompetence.

D. **X-Ray Findings**: In predominant mitral stenosis with normal pulmonary vascular resistance, the overall heart size may be normal, as shown in Fig 12–6. The left atrium is enlarged, and the left atrial appendage is usually visible on the left cardiac border. The pulmonary artery is not greatly enlarged unless pulmonary arterial pressure is over 45 mm Hg. Minor enlargement of the pulmonary artery contributes to straightening of the left cardiac border when the pulmonary artery pressure is lower. The size of the left atrium is better discerned on the lateral and oblique views (Figs 12–6B, C, D) with barium in the esophagus. The left main bronchus may be elevated and lie more horizontally than normally in the left anterior oblique view (Fig 12–6D) if the left atrium enlarges upward. Posterior displacement of the barium-filled esophagus by the left atrium is seen on the lateral (Fig 12–6B) and right anterior oblique (Fig 12–6D) views. With moderate left atrial enlargement, the right border of the left atrium produces a double density on the right (posteroanterior view).

1. **Pulmonary changes**—The chest x-ray is useful in assessing the degree of pulmonary congestion. The most characteristic finding is the presence of Kerley's B lines, as shown in Fig 12–7. These are thickened interlobular septums that are usually seen at the outer edges of the lungs at the bases. They are evidence of chronic pulmonary congestion and are almost invariably associated with significantly increased pulmonary

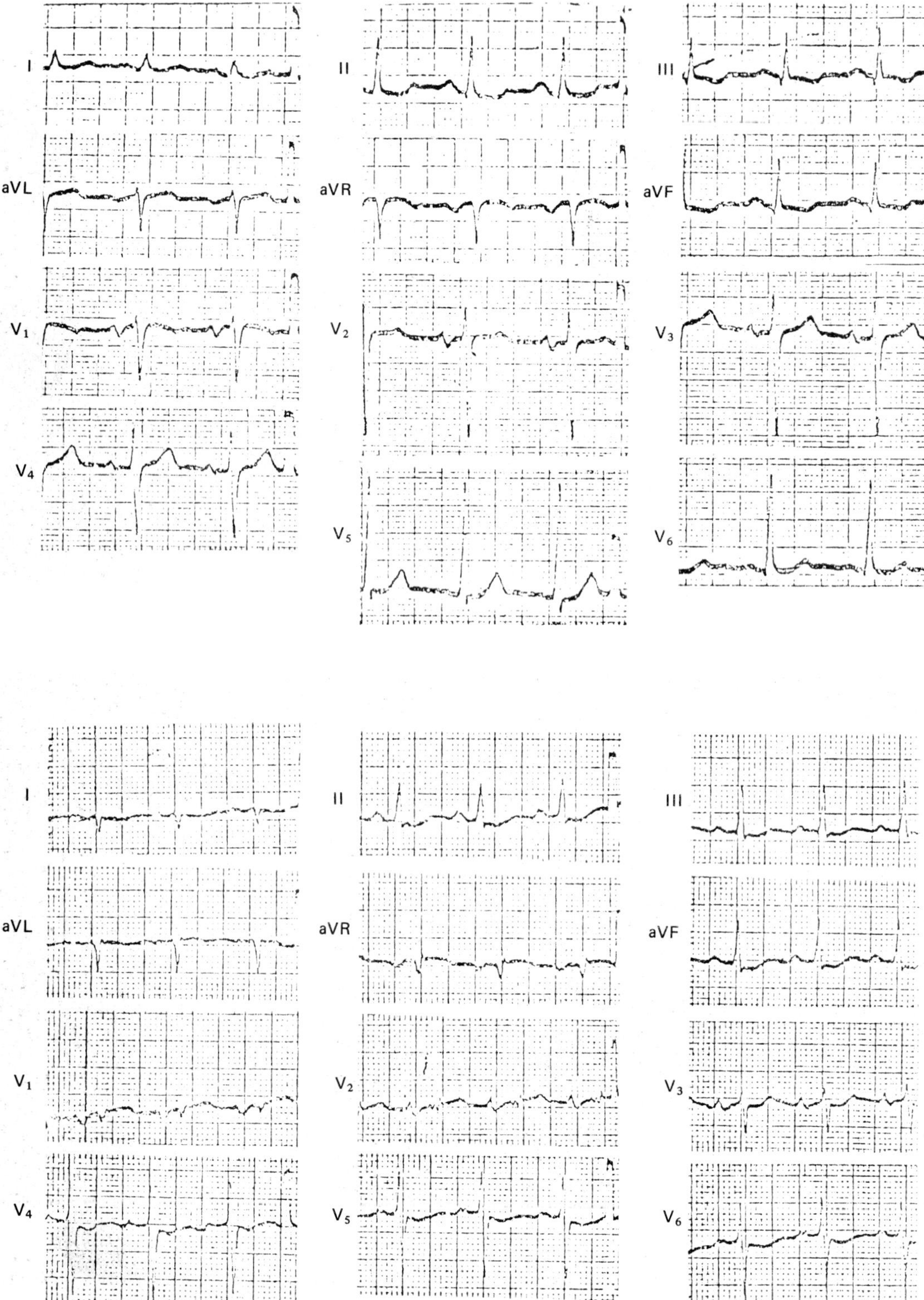

Figure 12–5. Two ECGs taken 3 years apart showing the development of right ventricular hypertrophy due to increasing pulmonary vascular resistance in a 48-year-old woman with mitral stenosis.

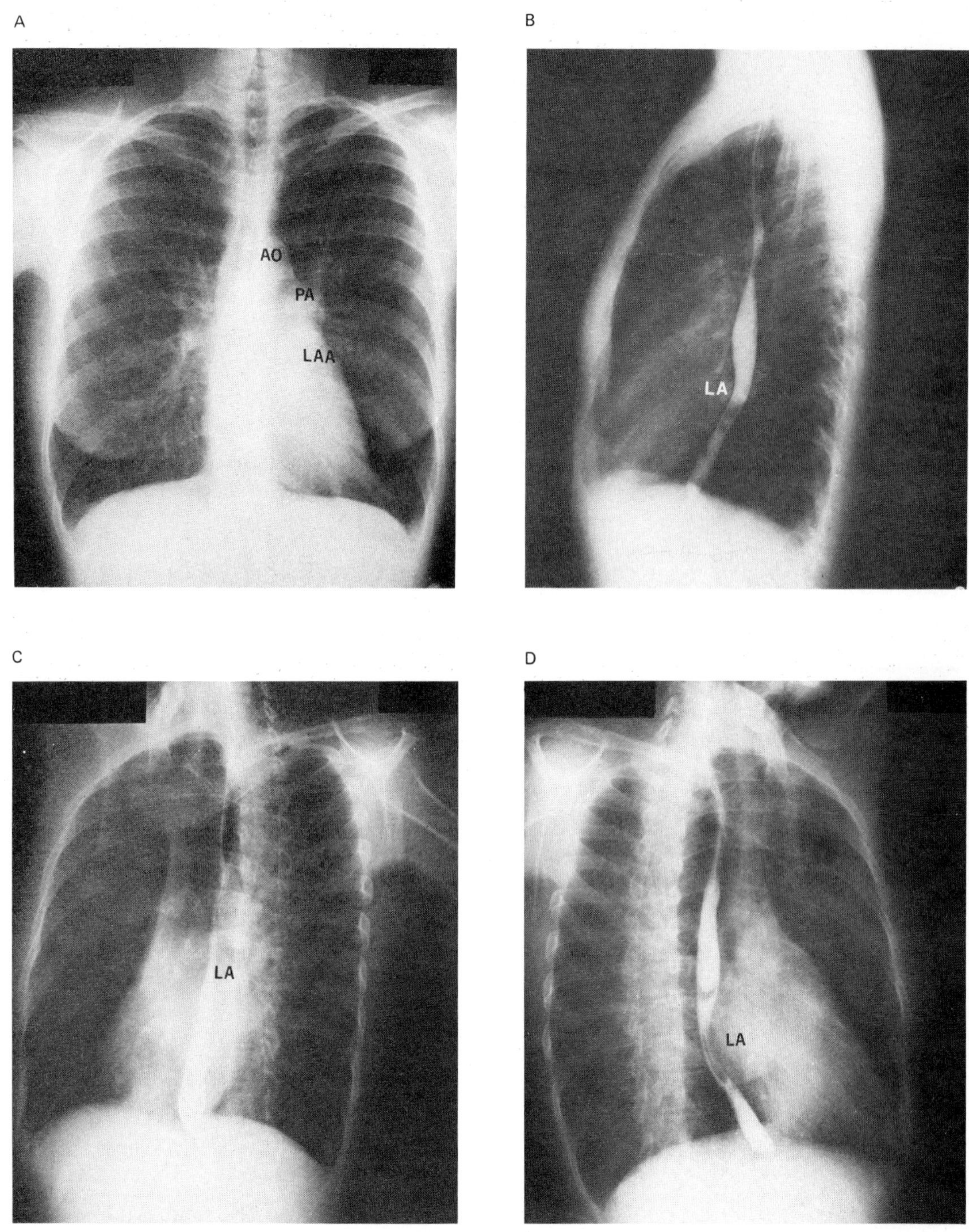

Figure 12–6. Cardiac series of chest x-rays of a 34-year-old woman with moderate mitral stenosis. Left atrial enlargement (LA) is seen on all views. The overall heart size is normal. *A,* posteroanterior view; *B,* lateral view; *C,* left anterior oblique view; *D,* right anterior oblique view.

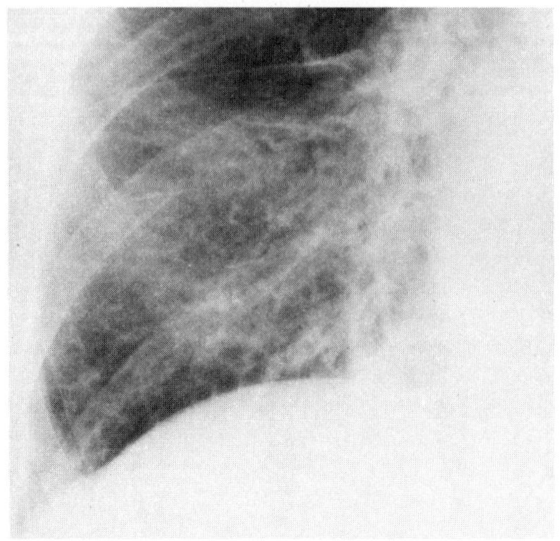

Figure 12–7. Close-up of chest x-ray of base of right lung of patient with mitral stenosis showing Kerley's B lines.

venous pressure. Diffuse pulmonary fibrosis in patients without evidence of heart disease occasionally causes Kerley's B lines. The pattern of pulmonary congestion in mitral valve disease is influenced by the effects of gravity. The bases of the lungs occupy the lowest position in the chest whether the patient is standing or in the supine position. The level of the pulmonary venous and arterial pressures is therefore highest at the base of the lungs.

2. Pulmonary hypertension–The response of pulmonary blood vessels to increased pressure is hypertrophy of their walls; consequently, pulmonary vascular disease is most marked at the base of the lungs. As the pulmonary arterioles thicken and develop an increased resistance to blood flow, redistribution of pulmonary blood flow occurs. As a result, the veins of the upper lobe of the lung become more prominent, and the lower lobes receive a smaller proportion of pulmonary blood flow. "Pruning" of the pulmonary arterial tree appears first at the base and later spreads to involve the entire lung. Occasionally, passive pulmonary venous congestion with intra-alveolar hemorrhage causes hemosiderosis, giving rise to a diffuse mottled pattern on the chest x-ray.

3. Assessment of severity–The accuracy of radiologic assessment of the level of pulmonary arterial and venous pressures is disappointing, and the correlation between hemodynamic and radiologic data is poor, although Kerley's B lines are always associated with significant disease. Calcification of the mitral valve is seldom seen in young persons with predominant mitral stenosis and is present in less than 10% of patients who present before their first valvotomy. Ventricular enlargement is not seen in patients with predominant mitral stenosis and low pulmonary vascular resistance.

4. Ventricular enlargement–When the heart is enlarged, it is not always easy to decide on purely radiologic grounds whether the right ventricle (Fig 12–8) or the left ventricle (Fig 12–9) is enlarged.

E. Special Investigations:

1. Noninvasive technics–The mitral valve is one

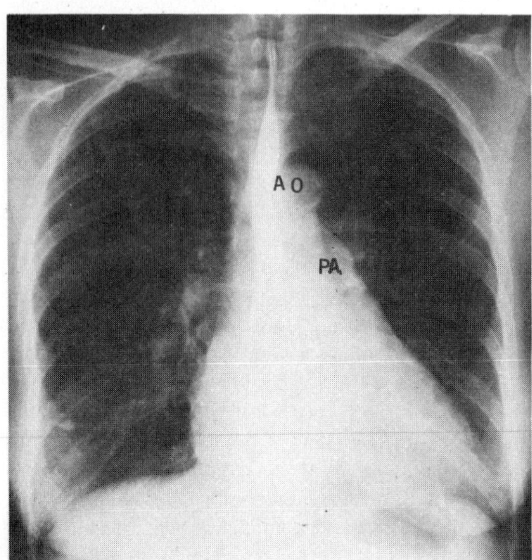

Figure 12–8. Chest x-ray of a 60-year-old woman with cardiac enlargement due to mitral stenosis with pulmonary hypertension. Ventricular enlargement is right-sided. AO, aorta; PA, pulmonary artery.

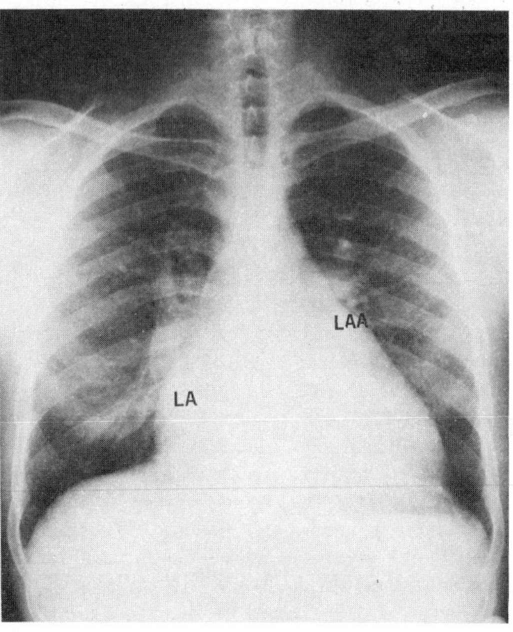

Figure 12–9. Chest x-ray of a 28-year-old man with mitral stenosis and incompetence. The ventricular enlargement is all left-sided. LA, left atrium; LAA, left atrial appendage.

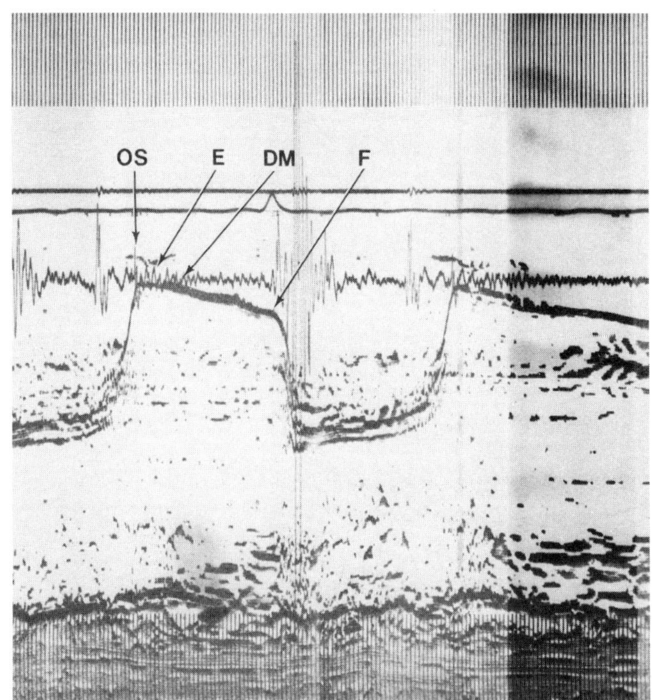

Figure 12–10. Echocardiogram showing slow diastolic posterior motion of stenotic mitral valve. Atrial fibrillation is present. OS, opening snap; E, point on mitral valve echo; F, F point on mitral valve echo; DM, diastolic murmur. (Courtesy of NB Schiller.)

of the structures that registers most clearly and consistently on echocardiography. The movements of the valve during systole and diastole and the effects of atrial contraction can usually be clearly discerned. Echocardiography is thus especially helpful in the diagnosis and clinical assessment of patients with mitral stenosis. The valve is thickened and less mobile than normally in patients with mitral stenosis, as shown in Fig 12–10. The thickened adherent mitral valve leaflets move together; and, while anterior valve motion may be less than normal, the posterior leaflet may in some cases move more than normally. Measurement of the mitral valve slope gives some indication of the severity of stenosis. The valve slope is the rate of change in the position of the fused mitral valve cusps that occurs as the valve closes during diastole. It is measured by drawing a straight line through the echo tracing and calculating the E → F slope in mm/sec. The normal E → F slope of 80 mm/sec or more falls to about 20 mm/sec in mitral stenosis, and the values obtained in different patients correlate significantly with the mitral valve area calculated from data obtained during cardiac catheterization. The measurement is not completely specific, since slow posterior valve motion is also seen in patients with extremely low cardiac output, and the way in which the line is drawn on the echo tracing is somewhat subjective. It therefore seems doubtful that echocardiography will prove to be a reliable substitute for cardiac catheterization in the preoperative assessment of patients. However, it may be valuable in following the course of the disease, since the effect of operation on the mitral valve slope can be clearly demonstrated (Fig 12–11).

2. Invasive technics–

a. Right heart catheterization is the definitive study for assessing the hemodynamic severity of mitral stenosis. It is almost always indicated before surgery, and studies should be repeated before a second operation is performed. It is rarely needed for diagnosis because the classification of patients into the categories of mitral stenosis, mixed mitral stenosis and incompetence, and mitral incompetence is not based on cardiac catheterization findings. The left atrial ("wedge") pressure, the left ventricular pressure, and the cardiac output are needed for full assessment of the severity of mitral stenosis. Measurements of pulmonary arterial pressure, the left atrial ("wedge") pressure, and the cardiac output are necessary to calculate pulmonary vascular resistance, which is an important feature in mitral stenosis. In most laboratories, the wedge pressure is considered to be an acceptable substitute for left atrial pressure. In some centers, however, direct left atrial pressure measurement by transseptal catheterization is preferred. In patients with distorted cardiac anatomy due to marked left atrial enlargement, kyphoscoliosis, unsuspected left atrial thrombus, or left atrial tumor, transseptal catheterization is less successful and more dangerous because of the likelihood of cardiac perforation and systemic embolization. It is not always possible to pass a catheter across the mitral valve in patients with mitral stenosis, even though the left atrium can be entered. On the other hand, left ventricular retrograde catheterization from the aorta is normally easy in such patients. For these reasons and because left ventricular angiography is now almost routinely performed, simultaneous measurements of wedge pressure and left ven-

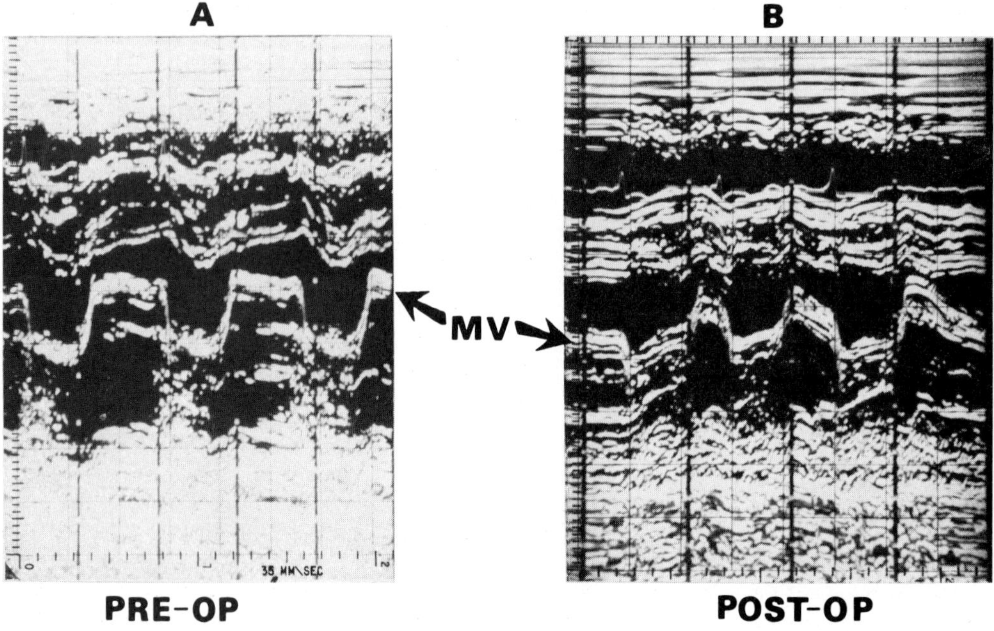

Figure 12–11. Preoperative *(A)* and postoperative *(B)* echocardiograms showing mitral valve (MV) motion in a patient with mitral stenosis. The diastolic slope of valve motion is steeper in *B.* (Reproduced, with permission, from Kleid J, Schiller NB: *Echocardiography Case Studies.* Med Exam Pub, 1974.)

tricular pressure are widely used in the study of patients with mitral stenosis.

(1) Hemodynamic measurement of severity—There is unfortunately no entirely satisfactory method for measuring the hemodynamic severity of mitral stenosis, even during cardiac catheterization. The calculation of mitral valve area by means of the hydraulic formula introduced by Gorlin and Gorlin is the best available method (see p 71). The 3 variables cardiac output, length of diastole, and pressure difference across the valve are included in the calculation. Mitral diastolic blood flow is only equal to cardiac output when there is no mitral incompetence, and the presence of significant mitral incompetence is the principal cause of error in applying the formula. When mitral incompetence is not taken into account, mitral diastolic flow is underestimated, giving a falsely low value in the measurement of valve area. Simpler alternative measurements of "gradient," ie, pressure difference across the valve, have been suggested. End-diastolic gradient, mean gradient, and the difference between mean wedge pressure and end-diastolic pressure have been advocated. Although these may give rough indications of the degree of stenosis in patients whose heart rates are in the normal range, they can never be as accurate as calculations that include the length of diastole. The patient's symptoms are best assessed by the level of the wedge pressure. In general, mild symptoms occur with resting wedge pressures below 20 mm Hg, moderate symptoms with wedge pressures between 20–30 mm Hg, and severe symptoms with resting wedge pressures over 30 mm Hg. Previously, patients with mitral stenosis underwent only right heart catheterization, and only the wedge pressure and cardiac output (not the left ventricular pressure) were measured. In practice, the omission of this measurement is not crucial because most patients with mitral stenosis have normal left ventricular diastolic pressures, and the association of left ventricular failure with mitral stenosis is rare.

(2) Technic for patients with pulmonary hypertension—In patients who have marked increases in pulmonary vascular resistance, wedge pressure measurement is critical and may occasionally prove difficult because the high pulmonary arterial pressure is associated with rapid tapering of the vessels. If a satisfactory wedge pressure tracing cannot be recorded using a conventional cardiac catheter, a Swan-Ganz balloon-tipped catheter should be passed into a peripheral branch of the pulmonary artery and the balloon inflated to obtain an indirect measure of left atrial pressure. Such a procedure is more likely to be necessary in patients whose pulmonary hypertension is due to causes other than mitral stenosis, eg, Eisenmenger's syndrome or primary pulmonary hypertension.

(3) Risks in severely ill patients—Patients with mitral stenosis and markedly raised pulmonary vascular resistance are often severely ill when they undergo cardiac catheterization. Although measurement of simultaneous wedge and left ventricular pressures and cardiac output is important, the patient may be so ill that a limited study is all that is warranted. Such patients tolerate angiography poorly, particularly when large volumes of contrast material are injected rapidly into the pulmonary arteries. Attempts to obtain information not absolutely essential for diagnosis should not be permitted to lead to complications in the basic procedure.

(4) Relationship between clinical and hemodynamic findings—The results of cardiac catheterization in patients with mitral stenosis are often surprising because the hemodynamic severity differs from what might be expected based on the clinical features of the case. In some patients with severe symptoms, the hemodynamic data are unimpressive; in other patients, the wedge pressure is markedly raised even when symptoms are relatively mild. Discrepancies between hemodynamic data and symptoms are even more common after surgical treatment, and heart rate and rhythm must always be considered in interpreting the results of cardiac catheterization in patients with mitral stenosis. Errors in calibrating strain gauges, collecting expired gas for the determination of oxygen consumption, and collecting and analyzing blood samples may provide false information. An unduly anxious or excited patient, failure to achieve a steady state, or even simple computational errors may give a false impression of the severity of the lesion.

(5) Indications for cardiac catheterization—In past years, many patients with mitral stenosis underwent mitral valvotomy without prior cardiac catheterization. Since it is now clear that valvotomy is usually only a first step in treatment and that a second valvotomy or mitral valve replacement will be needed in the future, it has become almost routine to obtain baseline hemodynamic data before performing any surgery. Since mitral valve replacement is a more serious operation than valvotomy, most cardiologists believe that complete left and right heart catheterization should always be done before the patient undergoes mitral valve replacement.

(6) Exercise during cardiac catheterization—Patients with mitral stenosis must sometimes exercise during cardiac catheterization because if the wedge pressure is only slightly raised, the pressure difference across the mitral valve may be too small to be measured accurately, and the calculation of mitral valve area may be unduly influenced by small pressure differences, especially when the heart rate is slow. When the patient exercises and increases the heart rate and cardiac output, it is possible to accentuate the hemodynamic findings and confirm or disprove resting values. As a rule, only mild exercise or such simple maneuvers as raising the legs will cause a significant increase in wedge pressure in patients with mitral stenosis. Accurate pressure measurements and cardiac output determinations during steady-state exercise at significant work loads are difficult to obtain. In routine studies, semiquantitative measurements are usually all that can be readily obtained. It should be remembered that the result of exercise is not to influence the hemodynamic severity of mitral stenosis but rather to increase the pulmonary capillary (wedge) pressure. Exercise testing thus provides evidence pertinent to the interpretation of the patient's symptoms rather than to the degree of mitral stenosis.

(7) Overall results—The results of cardiac catheterization in patients with mitral stenosis show considerable variation from case to case. However, the average values give some indication of the levels of pressure and flow. The data in Table 12–1 show the fall in cardiac output and the rise in pulmonary arterial systolic and diastolic pressures associated with raised pulmonary vascular resistance. Mean right atrial pressure is also raised in patients with high resistance.

b. Left ventricular angiography is now an important component of the overall study of patients with mitral stenosis. It is primarily used to evaluate left ventricular function and to determine the presence or absence of mitral incompetence. The multiple ectopic beats which so frequently follow the left ventricular injection of contrast material often cause mitral incompetence, even in patients with normal mitral valves. In patients with mitral stenosis, the small rigid orifice of the mitral valve may permit a small localized jet of contrast material to flow back into the left atrium. This finding does not invalidate the diagnosis of predominant mitral stenosis, however. It is important to assess the size of the left ventricle, measure its systolic and diastolic dimensions, and compare the measurements with the equivalent dimensions of the left atrium and the systemic cardiac output before concluding that significant mitral incompetence is present. Spurious mitral incompetence occurring after left ventricular injections of contrast material is useful in the diagnosis of left atrial myxoma because the contrast material which enters the atrium may outline the

Table 12–1. Cardiac catheterization data in patients with mitral stenosis.

	Pulmonary Vascular Resistance (mm Hg/l/min)	Indirect Left Atrial (Wedge) Pressure (mm Hg)	Cardiac Output (l/min)	Pulmonary Arterial Pressure (mm Hg)		Mean Right Atrial Pressure (mm Hg)
				Systolic	Diastolic	
Low resistance (< 4.0)	1.9 ± 1.0	26 ± 4	4.5 ± 1.1	47 ± 12	23 ± 6	7 ± 4
Intermediate resistance (4.0–7.5)	5.3 ± 1.0	29 ± 7	3.6 ± 1.1	71 ± 20	32 ± 8	8 ± 4
High resistance (> 7.5)	12.2 ± 5.0	31 ± 5	2.8 ± 0.7	94 ± 19	43 ± 8	13 ± 5

tumor and confirm the diagnosis. Injection of contrast material into the pulmonary artery can also be used for this purpose, but it is less often successful.

F. Assessment of Severity: The assessment of the severity of mitral stenosis presents important problems. The patient and the physician have different views of severity. To the patient, it is the severity of symptoms that matters most. Symptoms are closely related to activity in mitral stenosis because heart rate determines left atrial pressure, which in turn determines the degree of pulmonary congestion and dyspnea. For example, by restricting activity, a patient with severe mitral stenosis can often avoid dyspnea, whereas a person with a milder lesion and an occupation involving heavy labor may develop dyspnea at a relatively early stage.

To the cardiac surgeon, it is the hemodynamic severity of the basic mechanical lesion that is important because it can be relieved by operation. The severity of the lesion may not correspond to the severity of symptoms. For example, a patient with mild mitral stenosis who develops rapid, uncontrolled atrial fibrillation may have pulmonary edema when the heart rate is 180/min and yet have a hemodynamically mild lesion that is not severe enough to warrant operation. Conversely, a patient with hemodynamically severe mitral stenosis may lead such a restricted life that mitral valvotomy is necessary in spite of the absence of symptoms. Unfortunately, there is no completely satisfactory means of measuring the severity of mitral stenosis. Any measurement that fails to consider the heart rate is unsatisfactory in patients whose heart rates are outside the normal range. The patient's main symptom—dyspnea—is the one most closely correlated with the degree of pulmonary congestion, which in turn depends on the level of left atrial pressure.

In mitral stenosis, the mitral valve area—calculated by the Gorlin formula from the diastolic blood flow and pressure difference across the valve—provides the best assessment of severity. The inadequacies of this measurement have already been described (p 71), but it is still superior to "gradient" measurements, which although designed to express hemodynamic severity in terms of pressure differences, do not take into account either blood flow or the length of diastole. The advantage of accurate valve area calculations is that they provide information that is not dependent on the conditions prevailing during examination of the patient. Thus, they should give the same results at rest and during exercise, and at both slow and fast heart rates. Significant mitral incompetence is the most important factor causing inaccurate valve area calculations. Consequently, the physician cannot reduce the assessment of severity to a single number or set of figures.

Differential Diagnosis

Left atrial myxoma is the most important disorder in the differential diagnosis of mitral stenosis with or without raised pulmonary vascular resistance. The radiologic picture shown in Fig 12–12 closely resembles that of mitral stenosis, and left atrial appendage enlargement is seen. Episodic symptoms, variable heart murmurs, fever, systemic embolism, a raised sedimentation rate, and hyperglobulinemia suggest the possibility of myxoma. The lesion is 100 times less common than mitral stenosis and 100 times more common than the rare congenital lesion cor triatriatum, in which the left atrium is divided into an upper and a lower chamber by an incomplete transverse septum. Cor triatriatum may also simulate mitral stenosis. Echocardiography and angiocardiography with injection of contrast material into the left ventricle or the pulmonary artery are helpful in diagnosis.

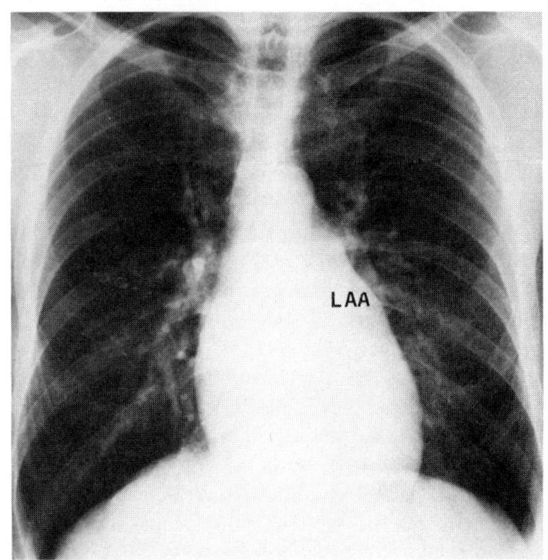

Figure 12–12. Chest x-ray in a 40-year-old man with left atrial myxoma. The left atrial appendage (LAA) is prominent.

In patients with raised pulmonary vascular resistance, pulmonary hypertension due to any other cause such as Eisenmenger's syndrome, idiopathic or thromboembolic pulmonary hypertension, or atrial septal defect with acquired pulmonary hypertension must be ruled out. Because mitral stenosis with pulmonary hypertension can be cured by surgery and patients with pulmonary hypertension due to other causes do not withstand exploratory thoracotomy well, it is essential to make the correct diagnosis.

Course & Complications

The course of mitral stenosis is long by nature and lasts 20 years or more in many instances. The natural history of the lesion can be altered by surgical treatment, and an almost normal life expectancy may be possible with optimal treatment. If the stenosis is moderate or severe, mitral valvotomy will almost certainly be required before age 40 for the relief of dyspnea unless the level of activity is seriously curtailed by the patient. Restenosis of the valve may necessitate a second valvotomy, and mitral valve replacement is likely to be required. Co-existent left ventricular myocardial disease plays a smaller part in the course of mitral stenosis than in any other valvular lesion. Patients with moderately severe mitral stenosis seldom have important associated rheumatic myocarditis.

A. Atrial Fibrillation: Atrial fibrillation occurs so frequently in the course of mitral stenosis that it hardly qualifies as a complication. The importance of both the effect of atrial fibrillation on the natural history of the lesion and its time of onset cannot be stressed too strongly. The circumstances precipitating atrial fibrillation and its clinical effects provide important diagnostic and prognostic information about the lesion. It is important to determine whether the onset of atrial fibrillation aggravated existing symptoms or heralded their appearance. If the onset of atrial fibrillation escapes notice in a patient with mitral stenosis, either the lesion is extremely mild, or increased pulmonary vascular resistance is present. In the latter situation, the patient has presumably been so disabled that the additional stress of the arrhythmia goes unnoticed. The earlier atrial fibrillation occurs, the worse the prognosis because of the implication that rheumatic carditis must have damaged the atrial muscle. Conversely, if atrial fibrillation has not developed by age 50 in a patient with mitral stenosis, the stenosis is almost invariably mild. It is therefore imperative to determine the circumstances surrounding the onset of atrial fibrillation and to assess the patient's tolerance of the arrhythmia.

B. Bronchitis: The congested lungs of patients with mitral disease are prone to bronchitis. This is seen more frequently in patients with mitral stenosis because pulmonary congestion is generally more severe than in other types of mitral valve disease.

C. Pulmonary Infarction: Pulmonary embolism and pulmonary infarction are common, especially in mitral stenosis with raised pulmonary vascular resistance. The lungs with their double arterial blood supply normally are not subject to infarction unless they are congested, and mitral stenosis is one of the commonest conditions in which pulmonary embolism is followed by pulmonary infarction. It is not always possible to determine the origin of the thrombus, and although emboli from the veins of the pelvis and legs are common, the possibility of thrombosis in situ should not be ruled out.

Treatment

A. Medical Treatment:

1. Penicillin prophylaxis to prevent recurrence of rheumatic fever—Prophylactic penicillin therapy to prevent recurrence of rheumatic carditis should be considered in all young patients with mitral stenosis. The younger the patient, the stronger the indication for treatment. The upper age limit for the initiation and cessation of prophylactic penicillin therapy is not clearly defined. Most physicians do not start prophylactic therapy if the patient is older than age 30 or if there has been no evidence of activity in the previous 5 years; treatment is seldom continued past age 40.

2. Prevention of infection endocarditis—Treatment to prevent infective endocarditis should always be recommended, especially if the valvular lesion is mild. The dangers of mechanical damage to the valve are greatest in patients with the most nearly normal valves. This subject is discussed in greater detail in Chapter 16.

3. Restoration of sinus rhythm by DC countershock—Restoration of sinus rhythm in patients with atrial arrhythmia is rarely indicated before surgery in mitral stenosis. A patient with atrial fibrillation and symptoms severe enough to warrant restoration of sinus rhythm would almost certainly benefit from surgery.

B. Surgical Treatment:

1. Mitral valvotomy—Surgery in mitral valve disease is seldom if ever curative. However, it is the treatment of choice. Mitral valvotomy is indicated in any patient with mitral stenosis who has significant symptoms and a mitral valve area of about 1 cm^2 or less. The operation, which is now usually performed under direct vision during cardiopulmonary bypass, is palliative; its benefits do not last indefinitely. Many surgeons feel that closed mitral valvotomy in which the surgeon's finger is introduced through the left atrial appendage to split open the valve requires so much skill and judgment that the results of the first 50–100 closed operations performed by any one surgeon are likely to be less satisfactory than they would be under direct vision. Now that the mortality rate of cardiopulmonary bypass is 1% or less, the indications for open mitral valvotomy are even stronger. Open mitral valvotomy improves the surgeon's ability to treat left atrial thrombus, and mitral incompetence is less likely to result. This operation also enhances the possibility of mobilizing subvalvular structures such as fused papillary muscles and matted chordae tendineae. The decision whether to proceed with mitral valvotomy or to replace the mitral valve ultimately rests with the surgeon and is often made during the operation. In some cases, during the actual valvotomy, the surgeon encounters problems which make valve replacement essential and lead to a change in plans. Mitral valvotomy is not dangerous in patients with mitral stenosis and low pulmonary vascular resistance. The mortality rate is less than 2%, and in most centers patients with class II symptoms are readily selected for operation. The principal cause of morbidity and mortality is embolism. Occasionally, massive cerebral embolism occurs with disastrous results. Mitral stenosis often occurs with little or no rheumatic myocardial involvement, and in such cases the mechanical effects of obstruction to mitral flow predominate so that the results of surgery are good. In patients with more evidence of myocardial disease, in older patients, in those with atrial fibrillation, and in those with enlarged hearts, the benefits of valvotomy are less dramatic. However, there is almost always some temporary benefit from surgery. There is often a discrepancy between improvement in the patient's symptoms, which is striking, and the objective evidence of benefit, which is often lacking.

2. Mitral valve replacement—Mitral valve replacement is seldom indicated as an initial operation in patients with mitral stenosis. If the patient is a woman, she is usually of childbearing age, and the use of long-term anticoagulation therapy, which is usually necessary after mitral valve replacement, is a distinct disadvantage. In patients with raised pulmonary vascular resistance, valve replacement may occasionally be indicated as an initial operation, especially in older patients with calcified valves. Valve replacement is generally performed only when mitral valvotomy has failed to control the patient's symptoms.

A second or even a third mitral valvotomy is not infrequently performed when stenosis recurs or when the first operation has not relieved the obstruction. Raised pulmonary vascular resistance does not contraindicate mitral valvotomy, and satisfactory reversal of pulmonary vascular disease following mitral valvotomy can be achieved. Since valve replacement became possible, however, the number of patients who have experienced a reversal in pulmonary hypertension following surgery has increased, implying that earlier valvotomy procedures were probably inadequate in some patients.

3. **Mortality rate in patients with pulmonary hypertension**—The mortality rate of surgery in patients with raised pulmonary vascular resistance is roughly related to the level of resistance. In patients with severe right heart failure, the mortality rate is 10–15%. Late deaths in heart failure (10%) and survivors with persistent irreversible pulmonary vascular disease as shown in Fig 12–13A and B bring the percentage of cases with unsatisfactory results to about 50%. This figure reflects the fact that many patients seek treatment at a late stage of the disease. Results in earlier stages and in younger patients are better.

Prognosis

The prognosis for patients with mitral stenosis is good now that mitral valve surgery is readily available. Although the lesion cannot be cured and any myocardial involvement due to rheumatic carditis is not affected by surgery, relief of dyspnea and prevention of attacks of pulmonary edema are assured. The long-term results of surgery are not yet fully known, but it is clear that most patients with mitral stenosis who have had mitral valvotomy will develop symptoms again some time later, probably with the onset of atrial fibrillation in early middle age. The benefits of mitral valvotomy in patients with mitral stenosis vary and tend to be best in those who develop severe stenosis at an early age and who have no evidence of myocardial disease. Patients with the severest stenosis and the least myocardial disease will derive the greatest benefit. Age is an important factor; if the indications for mitral valvotomy are strong and if the operation is on a young adult, the relief may last for 10–15 years, but if operation is not indicated in early adult life and is not performed until the patient is 50, the relief is likely to be short-lived. Results are better in patients who are in sinus rhythm, which probably reflects the influence of age on prognosis. It is clear that age-related degenerative changes both in the valve itself and in the atrial and ventricular myocardium play an important role and that coexisting rheumatic and degenerative heart disease are seen more frequently now that surgical treatment is more widely available.

Raised pulmonary vascular resistance worsens the prognosis of mitral stenosis. If developing pulmonary hypertension is diagnosed early and treatment is not delayed, the prognosis is better. In older patients, how-

A

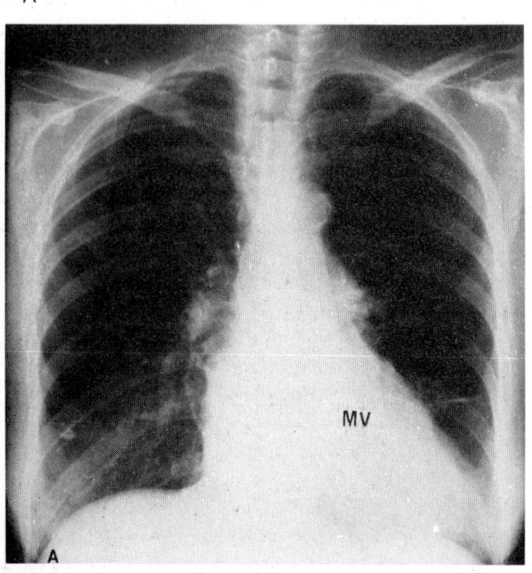

B

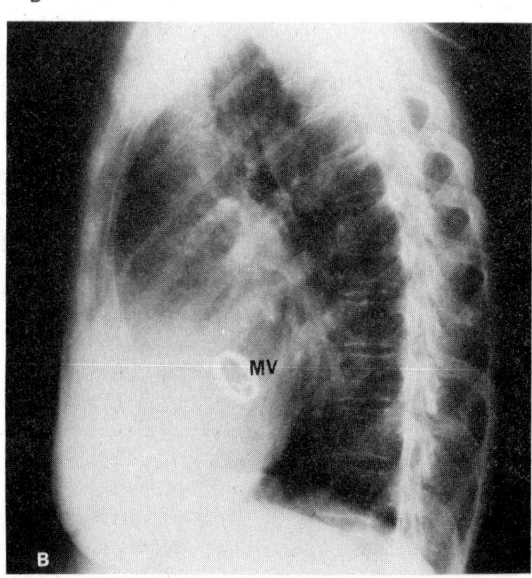

Figure 12–13. Postoperative chest x-rays of the 60-year-old woman whose preoperative x-ray is shown in Fig 12–8. Cardiac enlargement persisted after operation. The Björk-Shilley prosthetic valve (MV) is seen more clearly on the lateral view. *A*, postero-anterior view. *B*, lateral view.

ever, and in patients who do not receive early treatment, the prognosis is significantly worse. Relief of mitral stenosis reverses the course of pulmonary vascular disease; the speed of reversal depends on 2 factors: (1) how thoroughly the mitral stenosis has been eliminated and (2) how long the original pulmonary changes have been present. Improvement may continue for up to 2 years after operation.

MIXED MITRAL STENOSIS & INCOMPETENCE

In some cases the rheumatic involvement of the mitral valve leads to dilatation and stretching of the valve tissue and subsequent scarring and retraction in addition to narrowing. In this case, stenosis is present in addition to significant leakage through the valve. After severe mitral stenosis has been treated surgically, the stenosis is less severe, but the valve is still abnormal. With time, degenerative changes, fibrosis, and calcification stiffen and immobilize the valve and produce a mixture of stenosis and incompetence. The cardinal features of this lesion (Fig 12–14) include obstruction and leakage at the mitral valve, left atrial enlargement, and left ventricular enlargement (not hypertrophy). Variable features which may alter these findings are the severity of obstruction, the amount of regurgitation, and the severity of rheumatic myocardial damage.

Patients with mixed mitral stenosis and incompetence run a more constant clinical course than might be expected in view of the numerous possible combinations of severity of the components. Fig 12–15 illustrates the hemodynamic reasons for the constant clinical course. The blood that leaks back across the mitral valve during systole must flow forward during diastole, augmenting the normal forward stroke volume. Mitral incompetence thus increases mitral diastolic blood flow. The clinical severity of mitral valve disease is determined by left atrial pressure, which in turn depends on the length of ventricular diastole, the size and function of the left atrium, and mitral diastolic blood flow. The extra blood flow resulting from systolic mitral incompetence raises left atrial pressure and makes any mitral stenosis appear more severe. For these reasons, the clinical severity of mixed mitral stenosis and incompetence depends on the sum of the incompetence and the stenosis and tends to remain constant. If there is more stenosis than incompetence, there is a smaller amount of systolic backflow and a smaller diastolic forward flow across the valve. If there is more incompetence than stenosis, there is a larger systolic backflow and a larger diastolic forward flow. Thus, the symptoms in patients with mixed mitral lesions tend to vary less than might be expected. In contrast, the physical signs—which depend mainly on the volume of blood passing through the mitral valve during both systole and diastole—tend to depend on the severity of incompetence, and there is wide variation in the lengths and intensities of the systolic and diastolic mitral murmurs and in the degree of left ventricular volume overload.

Clinical Findings

A. Symptoms:

1. Dyspnea—Dyspnea is the commonest presenting symptom in patients with mixed mitral stenosis and incompetence. It seldom occurs while the patient is in sinus rhythm. The patient often presents with an acute episode of dyspnea associated with the development of atrial fibrillation. This onset commonly heralds the approach of other symptoms, and the patient, who may have been living a relatively normal life, becomes acutely ill with severe dyspnea and perhaps pulmonary edema. Atrial fibrillation is sometimes triggered by an intercurrent infection such as influenza or pneumonia, and a systemic or pulmonary embolism may occur simultaneously. This clinical picture is so common that it is important to consider the possibility of mitral stenosis and incompetence in any patient who suddenly becomes short of breath, especially if the heart rate is rapid and atrial fibrillation is present. The physical signs can be difficult to interpret in the acute stage when the heart rate is rapid. Episodic dyspnea may be present when there is paroxysmal atrial arrhythmia. In such circumstances it is important to see the patient during an attack.

2. Palpitations—Palpitations are common in patients with mixed mitral stenosis and incompetence. Palpitations are generally due to atrial arrhythmia; if the heart rate is rapid, dyspnea is likely to occur.

3. Systemic embolism—The first symptom of mixed mitral stenosis and incompetence may be due to acute systemic embolism. Sudden pain and coldness in the leg, sudden paralysis, acute loin pain due to renal infarction, flank pain due to infarction of the spleen, and infarction of the bowel due to mesenteric artery emboli sometimes occur. Embolism usually occurs in patients with atrial fibrillation, particularly when the rhythm changes, but it may happen when the patient is in sinus rhythm.

4. Pressure from a large left atrium—Symptoms due to pressure from a greatly enlarged left atrium on surrounding structures are occasionally seen. Thus, cough, hoarseness, and recurrent chest infection involving the left lower lobe may occur.

B. Signs: The physical signs in patients with mixed mitral stenosis and incompetence depend on the degree of mitral incompetence. When incompetence is the predominant lesion, the left ventricular systolic ejection rate is more rapid than normal, and the peripheral pulse resembles a miniature "water-hammer" pulse. In patients with mixed mitral stenosis and incompetence it is not always easy to assess the relative importance of the stenosis, the incompetence, or the overall severity of the lesion. Many of the patients with this lesion had mitral stenosis, and the mitral incompetence has resulted either from valvotomy or calcification and fixation of the deformed valve; degenerative, age-related changes; and increased wear and tear.

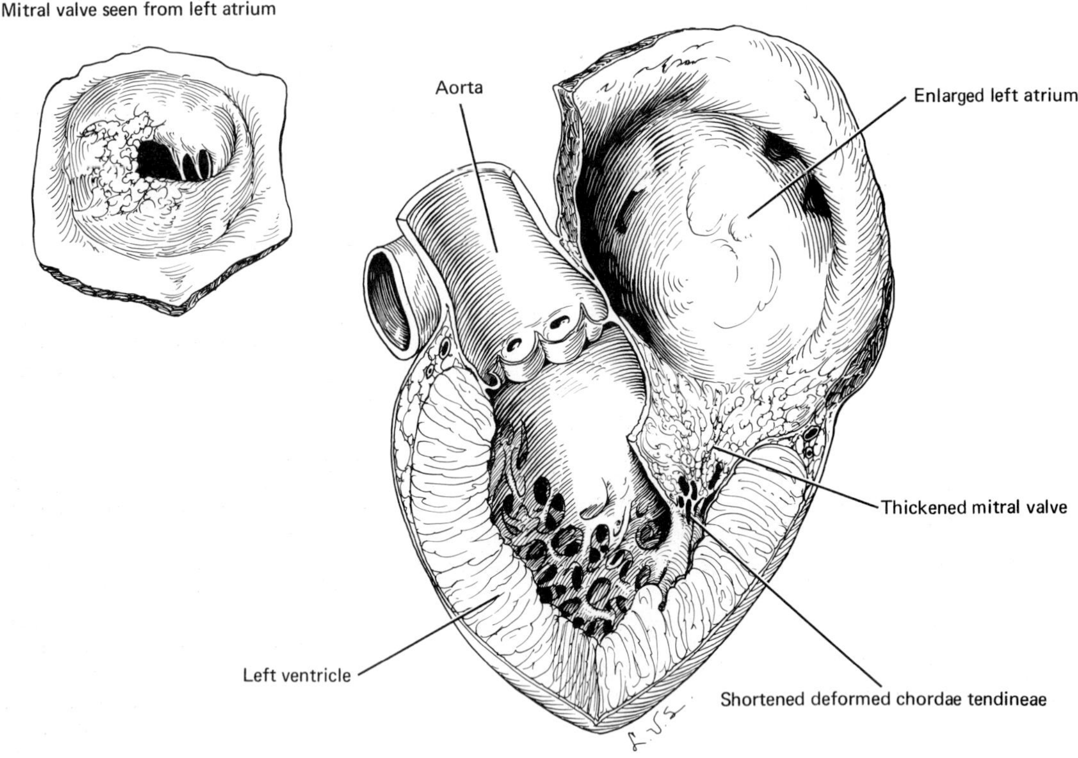

Drawing of left heart in left anterior oblique view showing anatomic features of mixed mitral stenosis and incompetence.

Cardinal features: *Obstruction and leakage at the mitral valve; left atrial enlargement; left ventricular enlargement (not hypertrophy).*

Variable factors: *Severity of obstruction; amount of leakage; severity of rheumatic myocardial damage.*

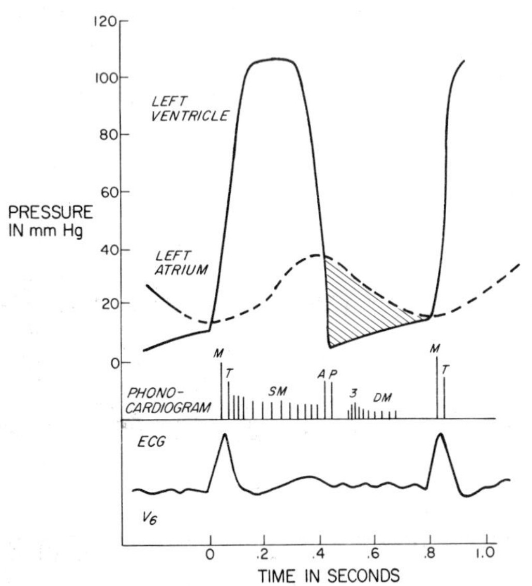

Diagram showing auscultatory and hemodynamic features of mixed mitral stenosis and incompetence.

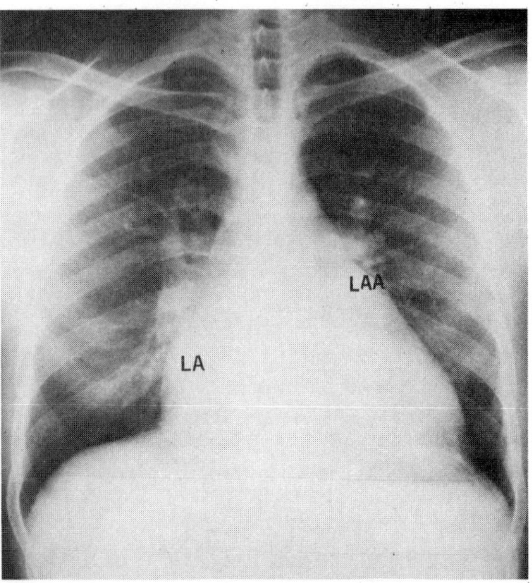

Chest x-ray showing left atrial (LA), left atrial appendage (LAA), and left ventricular (LV) enlargement in mixed mitral stenosis and incompetence.

Figure 12–14. Mitral stenosis and incompetence. Structures enlarged: Left atrium, left ventricle.

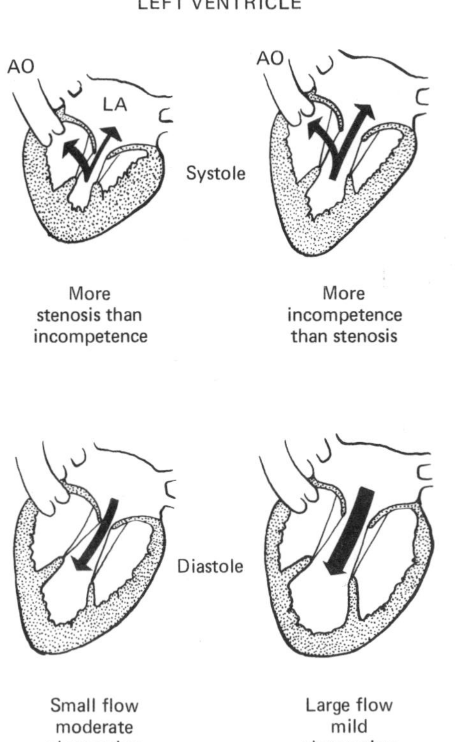

Figure 12–15. Diagram showing hemodynamic interaction between stenosis and incompetence in mixed mitral valve lesions.

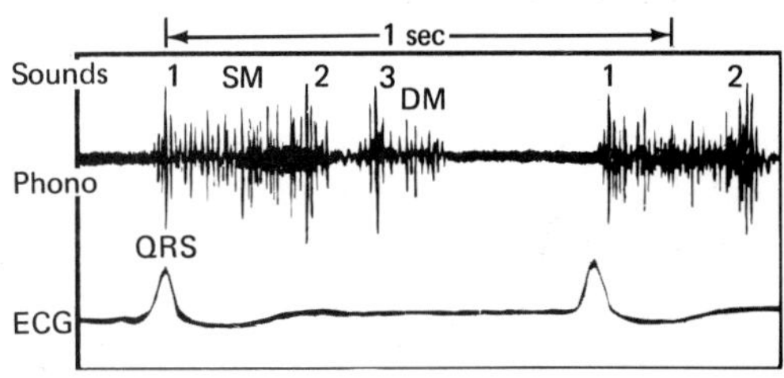

Figure 12–16. Phonocardiogram from a patient with mixed mitral stenosis and incompetence in atrial fibrillation. A pansystolic murmur (SM) and third heart sound (3) are followed by a short diastolic murmur (DM) at a slow heart rate. (Courtesy of Roche Laboratories Division of Hoffman-La Roche, Inc.)

The systemic venous pressure is not often raised unless there is associated tricuspid valve disease. Because pulmonary hypertension is seldom severe, the pulse is usually normal and the rhythm irregular in patients with atrial fibrillation. The heart is usually enlarged, with a hyperdynamic left ventricular impulse. The first sound may be loud and there may be an opening snap, especially if the patient has had a previous valvotomy for mitral stenosis. A third heart sound may also be heard, sometimes replacing the snap rather than accompanying it. Depending on the volume of mitral diastolic blood flow, there is a pansystolic mitral murmur transmitted to the axilla and a diastolic mitral murmur of variable length (Fig 12–16). In patients with moderate mitral incompetence, the murmur may last until the end of diastole at rapid heart rates (more than 100/min). The murmur is never accentuated during atrial systole because even if the patient is in sinus rhythm, the mitral stenosis is not sufficient to limit atrial emptying, and the force of contraction of the distended left atrium is reduced. In patients with atrial fibrillation, the length of the mitral diastolic murmur depends on the R–R interval of the preceding beat, as shown in Fig 12–17. A long diastolic pause allows time for equilibration between left atrial and left ventricular pressures. With long pauses, the murmur disappears toward the end of diastole. It is thus important to ascertain the length of the diastolic murmur during the longest pauses. In mixed mitral stenosis and incompetence, the murmur is less than full length at a normal heart rate of 70/min.

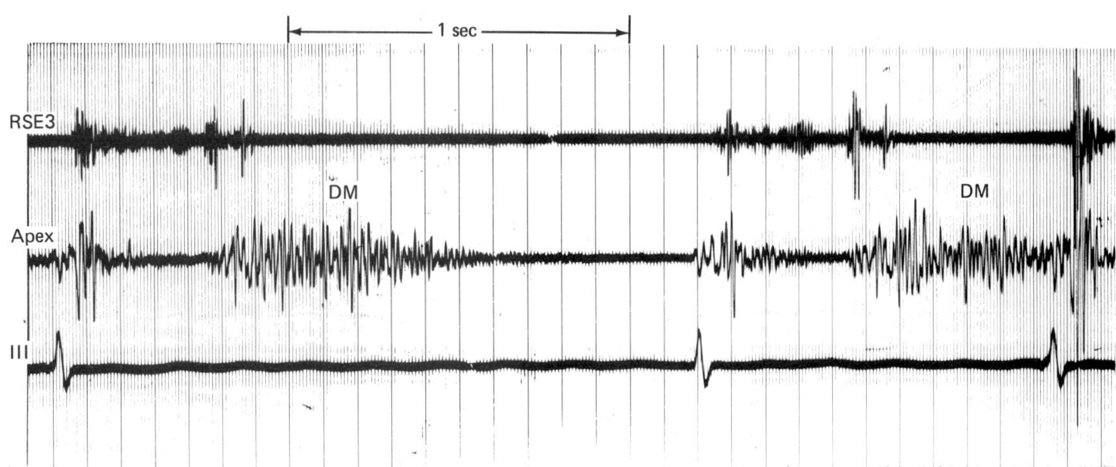

Figure 12–17. Rheumatic heart disease with mitral stenosis and insufficiency. Note relation of length of diastolic murmur (DM) to length of diastole. RSE3, right sternal edge third space.

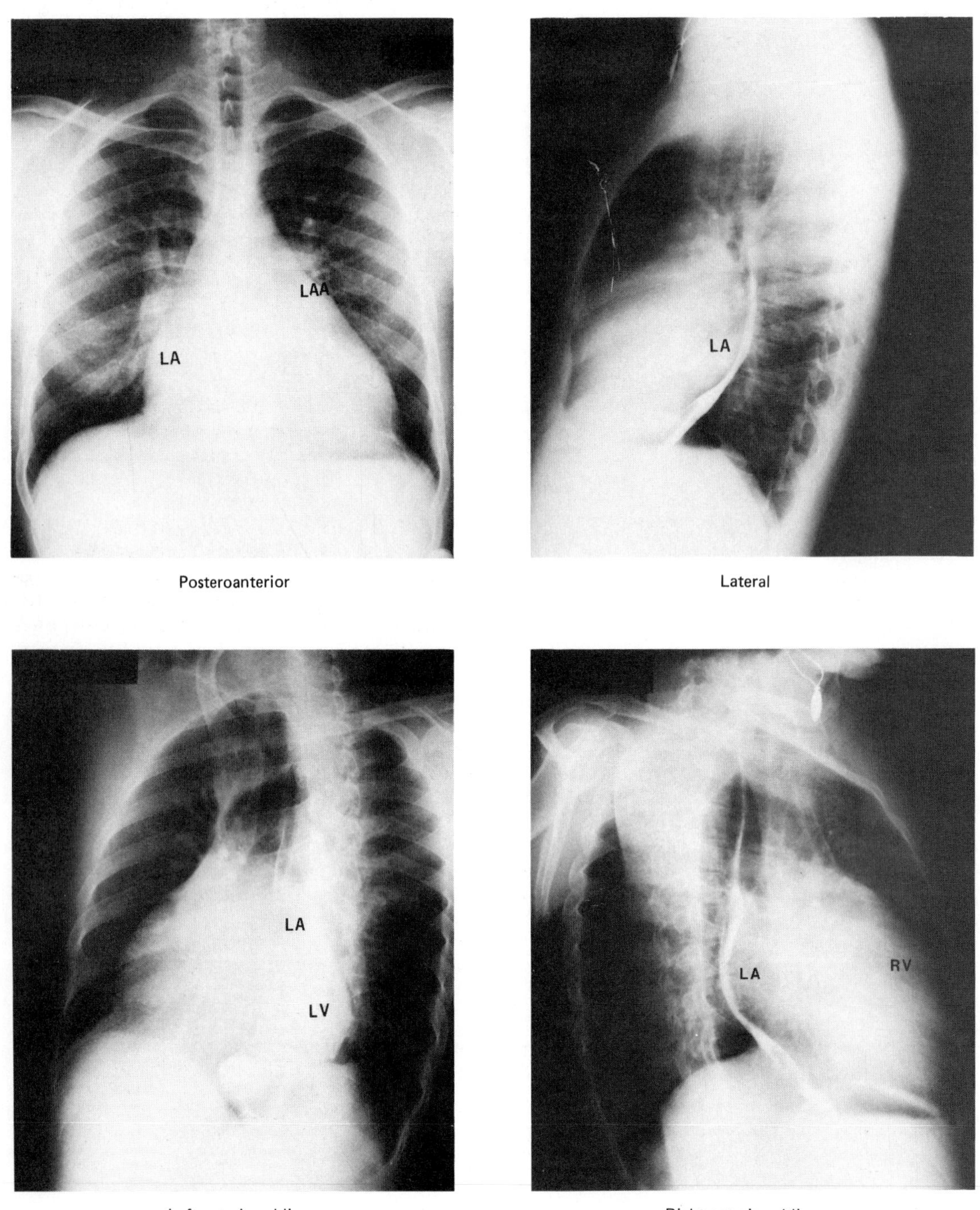

Figure 12–18. Cardiac series of chest x-rays of a 28-year-old man with mitral stenosis and incompetence. Left atrial (LA) and left ventricular enlargement (LV) are seen on several views, and the left atrial appendage (LAA) is prominent in the posteroanterior view.

Pulmonary congestion in mixed mitral valve disease is less marked than in mitral stenosis. Although pulmonary edema may occur at the onset of atrial fibrillation, control of the heart rate by digitalis usually leads to rapid improvement, and the symptom seldom recurs. Similarly, an increase in pulmonary vascular resistance seldom occurs and is not often severe in mixed mitral valve disease, presumably because left atrial pressure is lower than in pure stenosis. The most important factors to consider in mixed mitral valve disease are heart rate and heart rhythm. The whole clinical picture is greatly dependent on these factors, and the effects of changes in heart rate on the patient's condition offer the best means of assessing the severity of the lesion.

C. Electrocardiographic Findings: The ECG findings in patients with mixed mitral stenosis and incompetence are not of diagnostic value. A broad, notched, posteriorly oriented P wave (P mitrale) is seen if the patient is in sinus rhythm. Atrial fibrillation is usually present, whereas right ventricular hypertrophy is rarely seen. The increase in left atrial pressure is seldom great enough to provoke an increase in pulmonary vascular resistance.

Left ventricular hypertrophy on ECG is common but not invariable, even when mitral incompetence is more prominent than stenosis. The hypertrophy is more commonly due to systemic hypertension, aortic valve disease, or rheumatic myocardial disease than to the valve lesion.

D. X-Ray Findings: Left ventricular enlargement is seen in patients with mixed mitral stenosis and incompetence (Fig 12–18), and it is roughly proportionate to the severity of the lesion. Left atrial enlargement is seen as a double density on the right border of the heart (Fig 12–9). Posterior and upward displacement of the barium-filled esophagus is best appreciated on the oblique and lateral views. The downward sweep of the enlarged left ventricle, overlying the dorsal spine, is best seen in the left anterior oblique view.

Left atrial enlargement tends to be greatest in patients with mixed mitral stenosis and incompetence. In patients with giant left atrium, shown in Fig 12–19, in which the chamber assumes enormous proportions with a volume of one liter or more, mixed mitral lesions are almost always present. The left atrium forms both the right and left borders of the heart and the picture can be mistaken for that of pericardial effusion (see Chapter 18).

Enlargement of the left atrial appendage, seen on the left border of the heart, is almost invariably present.

E. Special Investigations:

1. Noninvasive technics—Because the mitral valve shows up so well on echocardiography, this form of investigation is particularly helpful in assessing the lesion. Echocardiography can determine the degree of stenosis, effects of incompetence, and the sizes of the left atrium and ventricle. The adequacy of left ventricular function can also be estimated from the motion of the left ventricular wall.

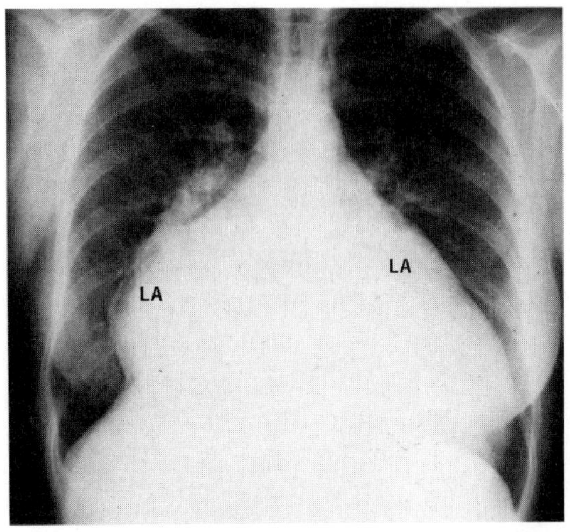

Figure 12–19. Chest x-ray of a 42-year-old woman with giant left atrium. The left atrium (LA) forms the left and right heart borders on the posteroanterior view.

2. Invasive technics—

a. Cardiac catheterization—Right and left heart catheterization are required before surgery in all patients with mixed mitral stenosis and incompetence. Simultaneous measurements of wedge pressure, left ventricular pressure, and cardiac output are essential. The patient is frequently in atrial fibrillation, and the effects of variation in the length of diastole from beat to beat can be clearly seen in Fig 12–20. The height and configuration of wedge pressure tracings depend on the severity of the lesion, the heart rate, and the compliance of the left atrium. Equalization of the pressures in the left atrium and left ventricle usually occurs by mid diastole at slow heart rates (less than 60/min). With faster heart rates (shorter diastolic intervals), wedge pressure rises, and an end-diastolic pressure difference usually occurs. The time course of the fall in left atrial pressure following the *v* wave is roughly exponential, and its time constant depends on the product of the resistance to flow across the mitral valve and the compliance of the left atrium. Thus, either mitral stenosis or a capacious left atrium may slow the rate of left atrial emptying and ventricular filling. It is unfortunate that the amount of left ventricular blood leaking back into the atrium cannot be accurately measured in mixed mitral lesions, with the result that mitral valve area cannot be accurately calculated. However, it is possible to calculate a lower limit, arbitrarily assume there is no incompetence, and estimate that the valve area is greater than a certain value. The left ventricular end-diastolic pressure is ordinarily normal in patients with mixed mitral valve disease, and pulmonary congestion results from relative mitral stenosis rather than left ventricular failure. A raised end-diastolic left ventricular pressure in a patient with mixed mitral valve disease suggests that independent left ventricular myocardial disease is present and requires further investiga-

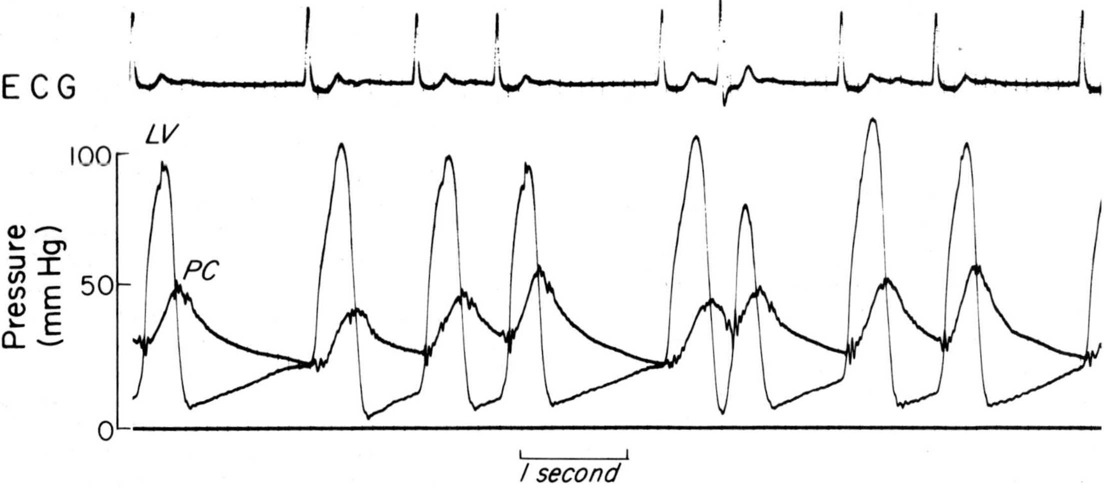

Figure 12–20. Wedge (PC) and left ventricular (LV) tracings from a patient with mixed mitral stenosis and incompetence in atrial fibrillation. The wedge pressure rises and the end-diastolic gradient increases when the heart rate increases. Lower wedge pressures are seen after a longer pause occurs between beats, and the end-diastolic gradient disappears.

tion. Unrecognized rheumatic myocardial damage, systemic hypertension, uncontrolled atrial fibrillation, aortic valve disease, and coronary disease should be considered as possible causes.

Cardiac catheterization is indicated to assess the relative severity of stenosis and incompetence rather than to confirm a diagnosis that has basically been established on physical examination.

b. Left ventricular angiography—Left ventricular angiography is needed in all patients. It provides the only means of measuring the amount of mitral incompetence. If the left ventricular stroke volume is subtracted from the forward stroke volume (calculated by means of the Fick principle), the difference is the volume of blood flowing back across the mitral valve per beat. This somewhat indirect measurement is not always accurate, but it is the best available. Left ventricular angiography also gives an indication of left ventricular function, which may be impaired because of either rheumatic myocardial damage or coronary artery disease.

Differential Diagnosis

A. Atrial Septal Defect: Atrial septal defect with normal pulmonary vascular resistance and hypertrophic obstructive cardiomyopathy enter into the differential diagnosis of patients with mixed mitral stenosis and incompetence. In atrial septal defect, atrial fibrillation, cardiac enlargement, and systolic and diastolic murmurs occur, and in the middle-aged patient an erroneous history of rheumatic fever in childhood is sometimes present. With these findings, the incorrect diagnosis of rheumatic heart disease is easily made. Radiologic examination is most useful because in atrial septal defect the chest x-ray shows a large pulmonary artery, a small aorta, a big heart, a big right atrium, and a left atrium that is usually unimpressive. ECG almost invariably shows an incomplete or complete right bundle branch block with an rsR′ pattern in lead V_1. This finding should always raise the suspicion that an atrial defect exists. Cardiac catheterization is ordinarily required to establish the diagnosis with certainty. The 2 lesions—mitral valve disease and atrial septal defect—may rarely coexist in Lutembacher's syndrome. In this condition, raised venous pressure, hepatomegaly, and peripheral edema are common, and the presence of right heart failure in a patient with mixed mitral stenosis and incompetence should always suggest the possibility of an associated atrial septal defect.

B. Hypertrophic Cardiomyopathy: Patients with hypertrophic cardiomyopathy (who tend to be confused with those with mixed mitral valve disease) have lesions of the left ventricular inflow tract, with or without outflow obstruction. This lesion is rare, but when it is present mitral systolic and diastolic murmurs and mitral incompetence are seen. Significant left ventricular hypertrophy is always seen on the ECG. Echocardiography shows narrowing of the left ventricular outflow tract and systolic anterior motion of the aortic cusp of the mitral valve. Left ventricular catheterization and angiography are needed to confirm the diagnosis.

Course & Complications

A. Atrial Fibrillation: As in pure mitral stenosis, atrial fibrillation is such a frequent occurrence that it hardly qualifies as a complication. The age at which it occurs depends to some extent on the severity of the lesion and on the rheumatic myocardial damage. In patients with severe, recurrent attacks of rheumatic carditis, atrial fibrillation may occur even in adolescence. In the Western world, the onset is usually delayed until about age 40. The onset of atrial fibrillation often heralds the onset of dyspnea, and the combination of an increased heart rate, irregular heartbeat, and loss of coordinated atrial contraction aggravates the condition.

B. Rheumatic Myocarditis: Acute rheumatic myocarditis is an important complication of valve disease. It is common in patients with mixed mitral stenosis and incompetence and is so difficult to diagnose that it is usually only in retrospect that it can be identified. The standard major and minor criteria for rheumatic fever activity are seldom present. The early onset of atrial fibrillation, disproportionate cardiac enlargement, disproportionate tachycardia, and left ventricular hypertrophy or left bundle branch block on ECG all point to rheumatic myocardial damage. On cardiac catheterization, low cardiac output, high left ventricular end-diastolic pressure, and diminished left ventricular ejection fraction indicate an important myocardial factor, which is generally assumed to be active rheumatic carditis in patients under age 40. Since histologic evidence of rheumatic activity in the form of Aschoff's nodes can be found in the left atrial appendage in virtually all patients undergoing operation, even the usual histologic criteria for the diagnosis of active rheumatic carditis are of doubtful value in identifying patients with clinically important rheumatic myocarditis. Patients with severe myocardial damage have a worse prognosis following surgery than patients with pure mechanical lesions, but management of the patient is not altered significantly by the finding.

C. Coronary Artery Disease: In older patients, atherosclerotic coronary arterial disease may influence the clinical picture with a myocardial factor that alters prognosis.

D. Systemic Embolism: Systemic embolization is a frequent and important complication. Embolism is detected in about 20% of cases, but the true incidence is almost certainly higher when asymptomatic cases are included. Cerebral, femoral, renal, intestinal, and coronary emboli comprise most of the clinically recognized cases. Left atrial thrombi form because of stasis and account for most emboli in mixed valvular disease. The emboli resulting from left atrial thrombus clear more readily than those associated with endocarditis. Embolism is more common in patients with atrial fibrillation and is more likely to occur when heart rhythm changes, either at the onset of atrial fibrillation or at the restoration of sinus rhythm.

E. Infective Endocarditis: Endocarditis is a serious complication in patients with mixed mitral stenosis and incompetence. It occurs more frequently than in mitral stenosis, but not as often as in mitral incompetence. The patient is almost invariably in sinus rhythm at the time of onset (see Chapter 16).

Treatment

A. Medical Treatment:

1. Prophylactic penicillin—Since rheumatic myocarditis is so commonly associated with mixed mitral stenosis and incompetence, prophylactic penicillin treatment to prevent recurrence of rheumatic fever is essential in all cases. The younger the patient, the more important the treatment. Penicillin prophylaxis should be continued up to about age 40 and is seldom started in patients over age 30.

2. Prevention of endocarditis—Antibiotic therapy to prevent infective endocarditis should always be recommended, especially if the lesion is mild. It should be administered before the patient undergoes major dental work or minor surgical procedures.

3. Restoration of sinus rhythm by DC conversion—Restoration of sinus rhythm before surgery is sometimes indicated. If the patient develops atrial fibrillation with a rapid heart rate during an intercurrent infection or in relation to some other special stress, the mitral valve lesion may be too mild to warrant surgical treatment. In this case, restoration of sinus rhythm by DC countershock (as described in Chapter 7) may be effective in maintaining sinus rhythm for several years. In general, however, the results of cardioversion are poor, not because the patient fails to obtain relief but because atrial fibrillation soon recurs. Propranolol for the control of heart rate may be useful in some patients. The deleterious effects of the drug on myocardial function may be outweighed by the benefits of a reduced heart rate, but, in general, medical treatment provides only temporary relief.

4. Anticoagulant therapy—Anticoagulant therapy is often advised in patients with atrial fibrillation who are not treated surgically. Unfortunately, it does not always prevent embolism, and if embolism occurs in a patient who has been given anticoagulants in full doses, hemorrhage into the area of infarction may be disastrous. Thus, the decision to start anticoagulation is controversial.

B. Surgical Treatment: Mitral valve replacement is the only operation indicated for the treatment of mixed mitral stenosis and incompetence. Starr-Edwards valves have generally proved to be the most satisfactory. Annuloplasty, valvuloplasty, and other conservative reconstructive operations on the mitral valve have not proved successful. Mitral valvotomy is contraindicated because significant mitral stenosis is not present by definition. Since mixed mitral stenosis and incompetence is a mechanically less severe lesion than mitral stenosis, the results of surgery are less dramatic. By the time the question of surgery arises, patients are older, there is a greater likelihood of associated myocardial disease, and atrial fibrillation has almost inevitably occurred. Since mitral valve replacement is a more serious operation than valvotomy, surgery is generally undertaken with much greater caution than in mitral stenosis. It is important to observe the response to medical treatment in patients presenting with dyspnea at the onset of atrial fibrillation. It may be possible to postpone mitral valve replacement for several years if the arrhythmia has been precipitated by some intercurrent illness; if the heart rate was extremely rapid at the onset but has slowed significantly with digitalis therapy; and if the patient can lead a quiet life. The decision to replace the mitral valve in patients with mixed mitral stenosis and incompetence is always a serious one because the mortality rate of the operation is about 10% and improvement is seldom dramatic. On the other hand, if the operation will ultimately be necessary, it may be advantageous to do it before increasing age, degenerative changes, and coronary artery disease increase the mortality rate. There is no doubt that the increased load of the valvular lesion increases wear and tear on the heart, and it is difficult to strike a balance between the different factors and select the right time for valve replacement.

1. **Influence of myocardial disease on surgery**—A frequent problem confronting the physician who treats patients with mixed mitral stenosis and incompetence is to determine the relative severity of the mechanical and the myocardial elements of the lesion. Many patients who have had previous mitral valvotomy are left with either mild mitral stenosis or mixed stenosis and incompetence. The patient may have symptoms, but on cardiac catheterization the lesion does not seem to be significant enough to warrant the drastic step of mitral valve replacement. The dilemma is one of choosing between temporizing measures such as cardioversion on the one hand and valve replacement on the other. It is generally helpful to compare the original catheterization data with the more recent studies to try to decide whether the patient's status is the same as that which prompted the original surgery. It is always important to remember that the most mitral valve replacement can offer is palliation of dyspnea of effort, ie, dyspnea will come on less readily than before, but the patient will not have normal exercise tolerance. Whether valve replacement affects longevity in patients with mixed mitral stenosis and incompetence is not yet known, since the operation has been in wide use for only a relatively short time. Although there is absolutely no doubt about the life-saving potential of even closed mitral valvotomy in young patients who have severe mitral stenosis with or without pulmonary hypertension, mixed lesions are less severe and the benefits are consequently less dramatic.

2. **Restoration of sinus rhythm after surgery**—Restoration of sinus rhythm by DC countershock should always be considered after surgery in patients who are not in sinus rhythm. It is probably not indicated in patients with giant left atrium or other lesions with marked cardiac enlargement, however. Quinidine should always be used in an attempt to prevent recurrence of atrial fibrillation. The results of cardioversion are not encouraging, but it is not possible at this time to predict which patients will benefit. If sinus rhythm can be maintained for a year or two, most patients will benefit.

3. **Digitalization and heart rate**—The immediate treatment of a patient with mixed mitral stenosis and incompetence and atrial fibrillation often consists of controlling the heart rate with digitalis because patients so commonly present with this arrhythmia. The diagnosis by ascultation of mixed mitral stenosis and incompetence can be difficult at this stage since murmurs are more difficult to hear when the heart rate is rapid and cardiac output is low. The physician must assume that any patient presenting with rapid atrial fibrillation, dyspnea, and pulmonary congestion has mitral disease until it is proved otherwise, and full digitalization is indicated. Prophylactic digitalis may be indicated for patients in sinus rhythm in whom atrial fibrillation is expected. There is some evidence that the heart rate may be slower when atrial fibrillation occurs, but lack of certain knowledge of the blood level of digitalis complicates the emergency management of an acutely ill patient. The control of heart rate is often a serious problem, and the easier it is to achieve such control, the easier it is to manage the patient. Mitral valve replacement seldom makes the heart rate easier to control, and the anticipation that surgery will help in difficult cases should not be used as an indication for operation. Propranolol has proved valuable in some cases. A search for precipitating factors such as intercurrent chest infection, a febrile illness, anemia, or thyrotoxicosis is always indicated.

Prognosis

The prognosis in mixed mitral stenosis and incompetence is not greatly influenced by surgery because there is usually an important myocardial factor influencing the overall clinical picture. Rheumatic myocardial disease is more likely to be present in mixed valvular disease, and the severe mechanical lesions seen in pure mitral stenosis do not occur. If a patient with mixed mitral stenosis and incompetence experiences significant dyspnea before age 30, the prognosis is poor because rheumatic myocarditis is almost certainly present. If myocardial function is good and the heart is not overly large, the patient can usually live a relatively normal sedentary life, and the heart rate can be controlled by digitalis. Systemic embolization is always a hazard but usually causes morbidity rather than mortality. Patients with extreme cardiac enlargement can nonetheless live strikingly long lives and are relatively uninfluenced by surgical treatment. Such patients develop a chronic low output state and, although seriously incapacitated by fatigue and dyspnea, manage to live a sedentary existence for 10–15 years after the lesion has become too far advanced for surgery. If embolic complications are not considered, it is the state of the myocardium that dominates the prognosis. The effect of anticoagulation on the prognosis is difficult to determine, and it is important to remember the possibility that hemorrhage into a cerebral infarct can be disastrous.

MITRAL INCOMPETENCE

Mitral incompetence differs from other forms of mitral valve disease in that it occurs as both an acute and a chronic lesion. The chronic lesions are further subdivided into hemodynamically insignificant and significant lesions. The hemodynamically insignificant form is present in those patients with the "click-murmur" syndrome described by Barlow, sometimes referred to as the floppy valve syndrome or mitral valve prolapse, but these terms are unsatisfactory because prolapse and "floppy valves" may cause acute mitral incompetence and imply a pathologic process that cannot be determined at the bedside.

The cardinal features of mitral incompetence (Fig 12–21) include left ventricular enlargement (hypertrophy in acute lesions), systolic backflow into the left atrium, and left atrial enlargement. The variable features that influence atrial and ventricular enlargement are the severity of the leak and the acuteness or chronicity of the process. The causes of mitral incompetence are variable, as is the severity of associated left ventricular disease.

Causes of Mitral Incompetence

The causes of mitral incompetence are diverse and are different for acute and chronic lesions.

A. Rheumatic Fever: Rheumatic carditis is responsible for about half of cases of mitral incompetence seen in the Western world. A history of rheumatic fever is present in about 25% of cases; taking into account that rheumatic fever is subclinical in about 50% of cases, this figure suggests that a rheumatic cause is present in about 50% of patients with mitral incompetence. The lesion may be of any degree of hemodynamic severity.

B. Degenerative Changes: Degenerative changes in the mitral valve figure prominently in the development of mitral incompetence, and the effects of abnormal wear and tear on a slightly abnormal valve may be important in the aggravation of mitral incompetence. Stretching, tearing of the chordae tendineae, atrophy of valve tissue, and myxomatous degeneration are commonly found at operation in both acute and chronic cases. It is not clear whether the degenerative changes are superimposed on congenital or mild rheumatic lesions, or whether they occur in previously normal valves. However, it is striking that a history of a previous murmur is present in half of patients with acute mitral incompetence. This suggests that degenerative changes occur more readily in abnormal valves and that patients with the click-murmur syndrome may develop acute mitral incompetence.

C. Infective Endocarditis: Infective endocarditis plays a particularly important role in the clinical course of mitral incompetence. It is both a causative factor and a complication. A valve that is the site of a minor, hemodynamically insignificant lesion seems to be especially prone to endocarditis, with the subsequent exacerbation of mitral incompetence in patients with click-murmur syndrome. Endocarditis is also a direct cause of mitral incompetence when highly invasive organisms become established in the bloodstream and lodge on a normal mitral valve. The resulting mitral incompetence is of varying degrees of severity; rarely, repeated attacks of infective endocarditis may be the sole cause of chronic mitral incompetence.

D. Ischemic Heart Disease: Ischemic heart disease may be important in the development of mitral incompetence. Posteroinferior myocardial infarctions may cause ischemia or even rupture of the papillary muscle supporting the valve. Acute rupture is usually fatal, but less severe degrees of ischemia may lead to ruptured chordae tendineae or produce acute mitral incompetence in the course of myocardial infarction. After myocardial infarction, temporary interference with the function of the mitral valve sufficient to cause a murmur of mitral incompetence commonly occurs. It is difficult to decide whether such lesions are hemodynamically significant.

E. Congenital Heart Disease: Congenital mitral incompetence may be more important in the development of mitral incompetence than was once thought. Clefts in the mitral and tricuspid valves are part of atrioventricular canal lesions. They are also part of the lesion in endocardial cushion defects, which are seen in association with ostium primum atrial septal defects. Isolated mitral incompetence seen in association with Marfan's syndrome or osteogenesis imperfecta is congenital in origin, and it may be that the click-murmur syndrome seen in young women is often congenital in origin. There seems to be an association between abnormalities of the coronary circulation and mitral incompetence, and some cases of click-murmur syndrome have been found to have abnormalities of the coronary circulation which may be responsible for the tendency toward ventricular arrhythmia in this condition. Another rare cause of mitral incompetence is coronary arteriovenous fistula. The mechanism underlying this association is not known.

F. Mitral Valve Ring Calcification: Complete calcification of the mitral valve ring is a rare cause of mitral incompetence. It occurs in elderly women and produces a pathognomonic radiologic picture (see p 381). The calcified mitral valve is shaped like an onion ring and moves up and down with each heartbeat.

G. Traumatic Heart Disease: Trauma is another rare but important cause of mitral incompetence and is usually acute. Steering wheel chest injuries in automobile accidents and other forms of direct trauma to the thorax, or even the effort of attempting to lift a heavy object, may apparently cause acute disruption of the mitral valve, usually by rupture of the chordae tendineae. The patient may have forgotten the episode of trauma and must be questioned directly about accidents while the history is being taken.

Classification of Mitral Incompetence

A. Acute Lesions: In acute mitral incompetence, the degree of pulmonary congestion is much greater than in chronic lesions. A large proportion of the force of left ventricular contraction is expended in pumping blood back across the incompetent valve into a noncompliant atrium of normal size. The volume of blood flowing forward through the aortic valve falls, reducing arterial pressure and causing reflex tachycardia and peripheral vasoconstriction, which aggravate the lesion. Pulmonary venous pressure rises, and pulmonary congestion and edema occur acutely. If the acute mitral incompetence is severe, the patient cannot survive

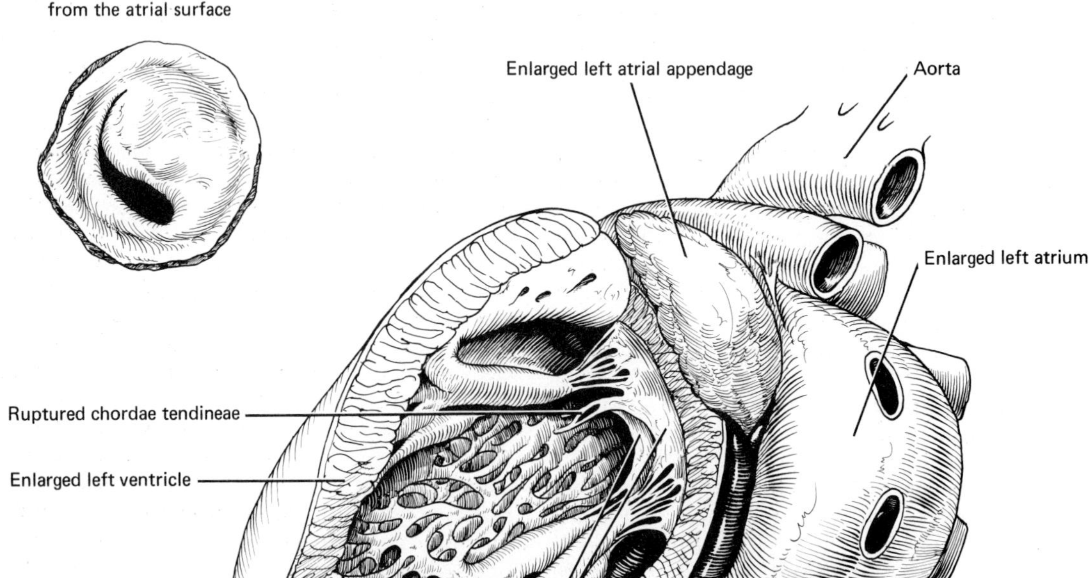

Drawing of left heart in left lateral view showing anatomic features of mitral incompetence.

Cardinal features: *Systolic backflow into left atrium; left atrial enlargement; left ventricular enlargement (hypertrophy in acute lesions).*

Variable factors: *Severity of leak; acuteness or chronicity; etiology; severity of associated left ventricular disease.*

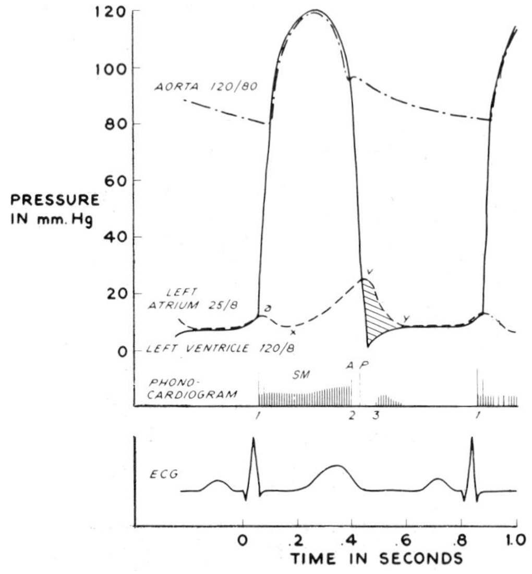

Diagram showing auscultatory and hemodynamic features of mitral incompetence.

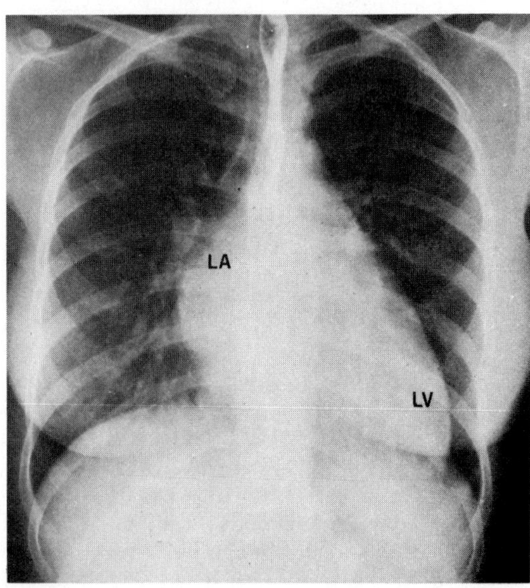

Chest x-ray of a patient with mitral incompetence showing left atrial (LA) and left ventricular (LV) enlargement.

Figure 12–21. Mitral incompetence. Structures enlarged: Left atrium and left ventricle.

without surgical treatment. With time, pulmonary vascular resistance rises, and right heart failure ultimately develops if the patient does not die in pulmonary edema. In less severe cases, the hemodynamic picture gradually changes, and the left atrium dilates and becomes more compliant. The left ventricle enlarges, and as left atrial pressure falls, the resistance against which the left ventricle pumps decreases. In this way the left ventricular pressure load of acute mitral incompetence gradually changes to the volume load of chronic mitral incompetence. In the acute, severe stage of mitral incompetence, left ventricular hypertrophy occurs, and it is possible that part of the left ventricular hypertrophy sometimes seen on the ECG in chronic mitral incompetence may be due to a previous acute lesion.

1. **Hemodynamic effects**–The hemodynamic picture in acute mitral incompetence is shown in Fig 12–22. The findings are unique because there is pulmonary congestion with raised left atrial pressure but no left ventricular failure and no mitral stenosis. The systolic left atrial pressure is markedly raised owing to the late *v* wave, but the wedge pressure falls to normal levels by the end of diastole, and there is no appreciable end-diastolic pressure difference across the mitral valve. However, the average left atrial pressure is high enough to cause pulmonary edema, especially when diastole is shortened by tachycardia. Thus, the patient with acute mitral incompetence suffers from "relative" mitral stenosis and not from left ventricular failure in the initial stages.

2. **Associated left ventricular disease**–The hemodynamic changes mentioned above are seen in pure mechanical lesions, but the clinical picture is different in patients whose mitral incompetence is due to left ventricular disease. Hemodynamic studies are the only sure means of making the distinction between patients with relative mitral stenosis and those with left ventricular failure.

The unique hemodynamic state of the patient with acute mitral incompetence is particularly susceptible to changes in systemic arterial resistance. The left ventricle pumps against 2 impedances in parallel during systole–aortic impedance and the impedance of the left atrium seen through the mitral valve. The magnitude of each impedance determines the overall load. If aortic impedance is reduced by vasodilator therapy, aortic flow will increase and mitral incompetence will decrease, lowering left atrial pressure and relieving any tendency toward pulmonary edema. This principle forms the basis for the successful use of nitroprusside and nitroglycerin in the treatment of acute mitral incompetence. If the patient survives, the acute lesions come to look more and more like those of chronic mitral incompetence, and, after about a year, mitral incompetence that had an acute onset is usually indistinguishable from the chronic form of the lesion.

B. Chronic Lesions: Chronic mitral incompetence is the best tolerated of all the major valvular lesions. The commonest form of chronic mitral incompetence is a hemodynamically insignificant lesion with only a heart murmur. Hemodynamically important chronic lesions of varying degrees of severity account for about one-third of cases of chronic mitral incompetence.

1. **Hemodynamically insignificant mitral incompetence**–Hemodynamically insignificant mitral incompetence is a common coincidental finding in patients with many types of cardiac disease. The click-murmur syndrome, which is synonymous with hemodynamically insignificant mitral incompetence, is being diagnosed with increasing frequency in young women, although the lesion is seen in patients of all ages and occurs in men also. When echocardiographic criteria are used for the diagnosis, it has been seen in as many as 6% of the general female population in the age range from 20–30 years. Some patients have clicks without murmurs, and some have only murmurs. It is not clear

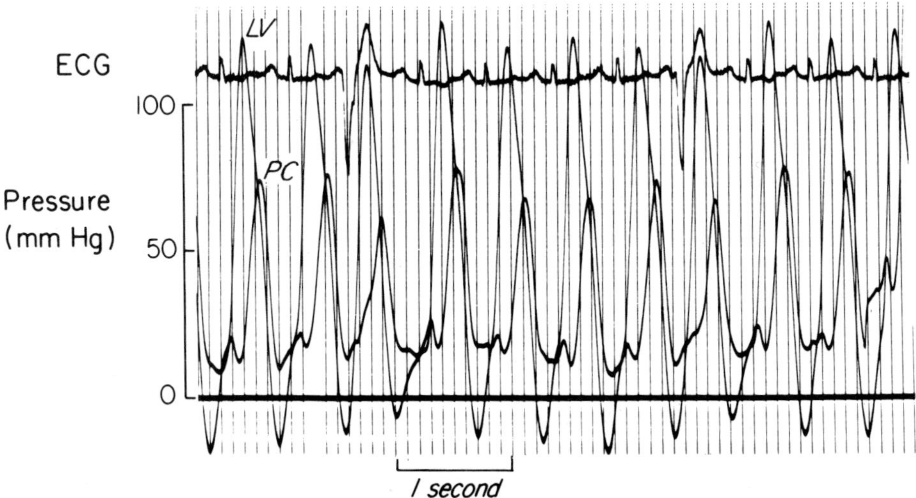

Figure 12–22. Pressure tracings in a patient with acute severe mitral incompetence showing large (70 mm Hg) *v* wave in wedge (PC) tracing and nearly normal left ventricular (LV) diastolic pressure.

how important hemodynamically insignificant mitral incompetence is in the natural history of mitral incompetence. It certainly predisposes to the development of infective endocarditis, which in turn leads to the development of acute mitral incompetence. A history of a heart murmur is such a common finding in patients with acute disruption of the mitral valve that it seems likely that patients with hemodynamically insignificant lesions are also especially prone to rupture of the chordae tendineae, leading to acute episodes of mitral incompetence in later life. In an older patient, the long course of mitral incompetence makes it difficult to ascertain whether a chronic lesion has developed slowly over the years or whether it has suddenly become worse and then stabilized.

2. **Hemodynamically significant mitral incompetence**–Chronic mitral incompetence causes less hemodynamic stress than any other left-sided lesion. The left atrium bears the brunt of the load and in chronic cases dilates and become more compliant than normal. The mean left atrial pressure in chronic cases is thus usually less than 20 mm Hg, and left ventricular ejection against the low atrial pressure results in a pure volume overload on the left ventricle. Left ventricular stroke volume is increased, but left ventricular hypertrophy does not necessarily follow. Associated left ventricular disease due to hypertension, coronary artery disease, or even possibly normal aging processes plays an important part in aggravating the hemodynamic effects of mitral incompetence. A raised systemic vascular resistance increases the leak through the mitral valve and compromises the left ventricular output. A low output causes tachycardia and peripheral vasoconstriction, which further aggravate the lesion. Thus, age-related degenerative changes in left ventricular function may be the precipitating cause of symptoms. Left atrial dilatation secondary to mitral incompetence usually leads to atrial fibrillation in middle age, but, since there is no obstruction to mitral diastolic flow, patients with mitral incompetence withstand this arrhythmia better than do patients with any degree of mitral stenosis. The commonly held view is that chronic mitral incompetence of moderate or severe degree results in left ventricular hypertrophy on the ECG and leads to left ventricular failure. In our experience, this is incorrect. Undoubtedly, some patients with mitral incompetence have both of these features. It is equally clear, however, that some patients with severe lesions do not, and if the hemodynamic load were responsible for these findings, left ventricular hypertrophy and left heart failure would be the almost inevitable result in severe cases, as seen in patients with aortic valve disease (either incompetence or stenosis).

C. **Mitral Incompetence Secondary to Left Ventricular Failure:** Mitral incompetence also occurs as a secondary lesion in patients with left ventricular dilatation due to hypertensive heart disease or cardiomyopathy. It is also seen temporarily during the course of myocardial infarction. If these "functional" forms are included in the category of mitral incompetence, it becomes the commonest of all valvular lesions. It seems reasonable, however, to discount these temporary lesions and concentrate instead on those cases in which actual valve disease is present.

Clinical Findings

A. **Symptoms:**

1. **Acute lesions**–Dyspnea is the principal presenting symptom in patients with acute mitral incompetence. The onset may be acute, (eg, when a cusp perforates or tears), or subacute (eg, when the mitral valve gradually shrinks and retracts after treatment of endocarditis). Dyspnea may progress to acute pulmonary edema with acute circulatory collapse, shock, and frothy pink, blood-tinged sputum. The patient may be ill at the time of onset, with a high fever and septicemia. Episodic attacks of dyspnea may occur and are associated with minor increases in cardiac output in response to the exertion of meals, washing, bowel movements, or even the excitement of visitors. Left atrial pressure is markedly dependent on the peripheral resistance in this lesion, and any increase in arterial pressure may provoke an attack of dyspnea.

2. **Chronic lesions**–In hemodynamically insignificant lesions, the patient has no significant dyspnea. There are usually no symptoms other than perhaps some palpitations, unless the patient knows about the murmur and becomes nervous. In hemodynamically significant lesions, dyspnea is the principal presenting symptom. It is not usually as severe as in mitral stenosis, and the effects of an increase in heart rate are less prominent. The onset of atrial fibrillation is generally well tolerated and does not provoke the acute symptoms seen in patients who have mitral stenosis. Palpitations are more common than in other forms of mitral disease; atrial fibrillation is the commonest cause. Patients do not usually present with symptoms due to systemic embolism, but such symptoms can occur, especially in the presence of endocarditis.

B. **Signs:** The physical signs are depicted in Fig 12–23. The first heart sound is usually buried in the pansystolic murmur, but there is never an opening snap. The presence of an opening snap indicates that significant rheumatic mitral stenosis is present. There is almost invariably a loud third heart sound associated with the rapid phase of left ventricular filling. It is a dull, low-pitched, thudding sound occurring about 0.10–0.18 sec after the second sound (Fig 12–24). Some observers may consider it long enough to be called a diastolic murmur. Differences of opinion may arise about whether any degree of mitral stenosis is present. The characteristic murmur is a loud, high-pitched, pansystolic apical murmur transmitted to the axilla. It is louder on expiration and decreases when systemic vascular resistance decreases acutely, as occurs with amyl nitrite inhalation.

Signs of right heart failure and raised pulmonary vascular resistance are rare except in patients with severe acute mitral incompetence resulting from acute disruption of the valve. The presence of right-sided failure with increased venous pressure in a patient with mitral incompetence should suggest the possibility of

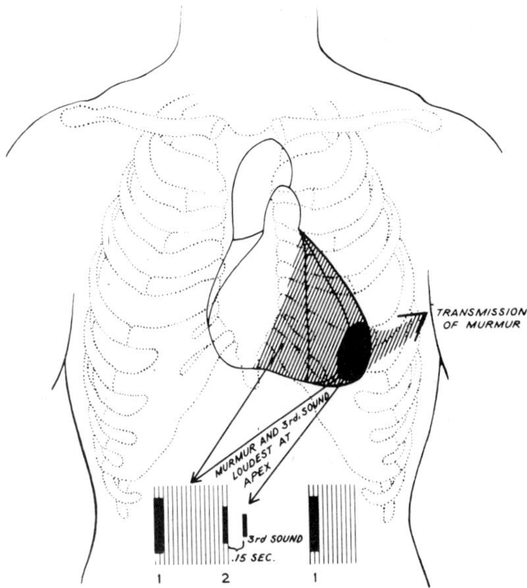

Figure 12–23. Diagram showing auscultatory signs of mitral incompetence. (Reproduced, with permission, from Krupp MA, Chatton MJ [editors]: *Current Medical Diagnosis & Treatment 1977.* Lange, 1977.)

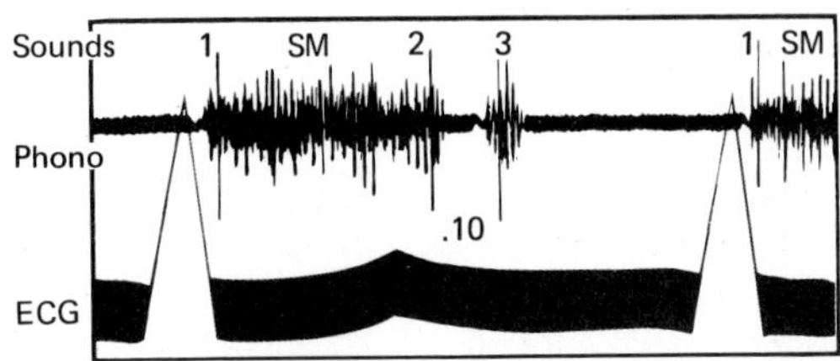

Figure 12–24. Phonocardiogram in a patient with hemodynamically significant mitral incompetence. The pansystolic murmur (SM) lasts until the second heart sound (2). The third heart sound (3) occurs 0.10 sec after S_2 and lasts for about 0.05 sec. Atrial fibrillation is present. (Courtesy of Roche Laboratories Division of Hoffman-La Roche, Inc.)

associated organic tricuspid valve disease.

1. Hemodynamically insignificant lesions—In hemodynamically insignificant lesions, the only abnormalities are usually auscultatory in nature. The characteristic sign is a late systolic murmur, as shown in Fig 12–25. It is often preceded by one or more midsystolic clicks. This condition is being seen more frequently and is referred to as the click-murmur syndrome. The murmur increases in intensity up to the second heart sound, making it difficult to time and often leading to an incorrect diagnosis of diastolic murmur. It may become pansystolic with exercise and may even be heard without a stethoscope. It often has a honking quality and may vary with posture, often being louder on standing. It is not uncommonly the only abnormal finding on examination, and its timing is its most consistent feature.

2. Hemodynamically significant lesions—In patients with more severe mitral incompetence, the cardiac impulse is hyperdynamic. The pulse is jerky and has been called a "small water-hammer pulse" because it resembles the pulse of aortic incompetence and has a rapid upstroke. The size of the heart varies with the severity and acuteness of the lesion. Chronic severe lesions show large overactive hearts because of increased systolic and diastolic flows across the incompetent valve. A prominent substernal impulse is sometimes seen as a result of the wide amplitude of the left atrial pressure pulse, and this impulse is often confused with right ventricular overactivity. In acute or less severe lesions, the heart is small, but it is still hyperdynamic, especially in acute disruption of the valve.

C. Electrocardiographic Findings: ECG evidence of left ventricular hypertrophy is more likely to occur in patients with acute rather than chronic lesions. The ventricle pumps into a small noncompliant left atrium and generates systolic pressures of up to 80 mm Hg in the atrium. This is a greater load than occurs in chronic mitral incompetence, and some evidence of left ventricular hypertrophy may be found. The ECG changes are not usually severe, and in most cases only high

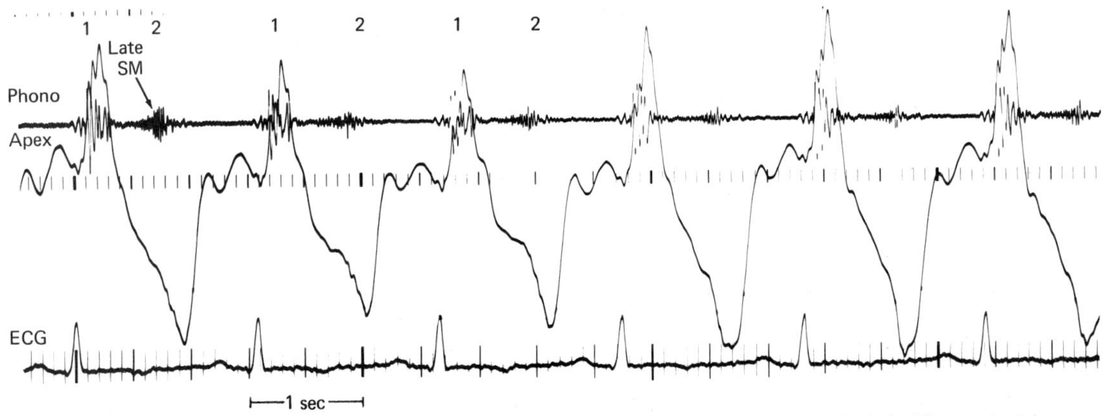

Figure 12–25. Phonocardiogram, apexcardiogram, and ECG from a patient with hemodynamically insignificant mitral incompetence. The late systolic accentuation of the murmur (late SM) can be seen.

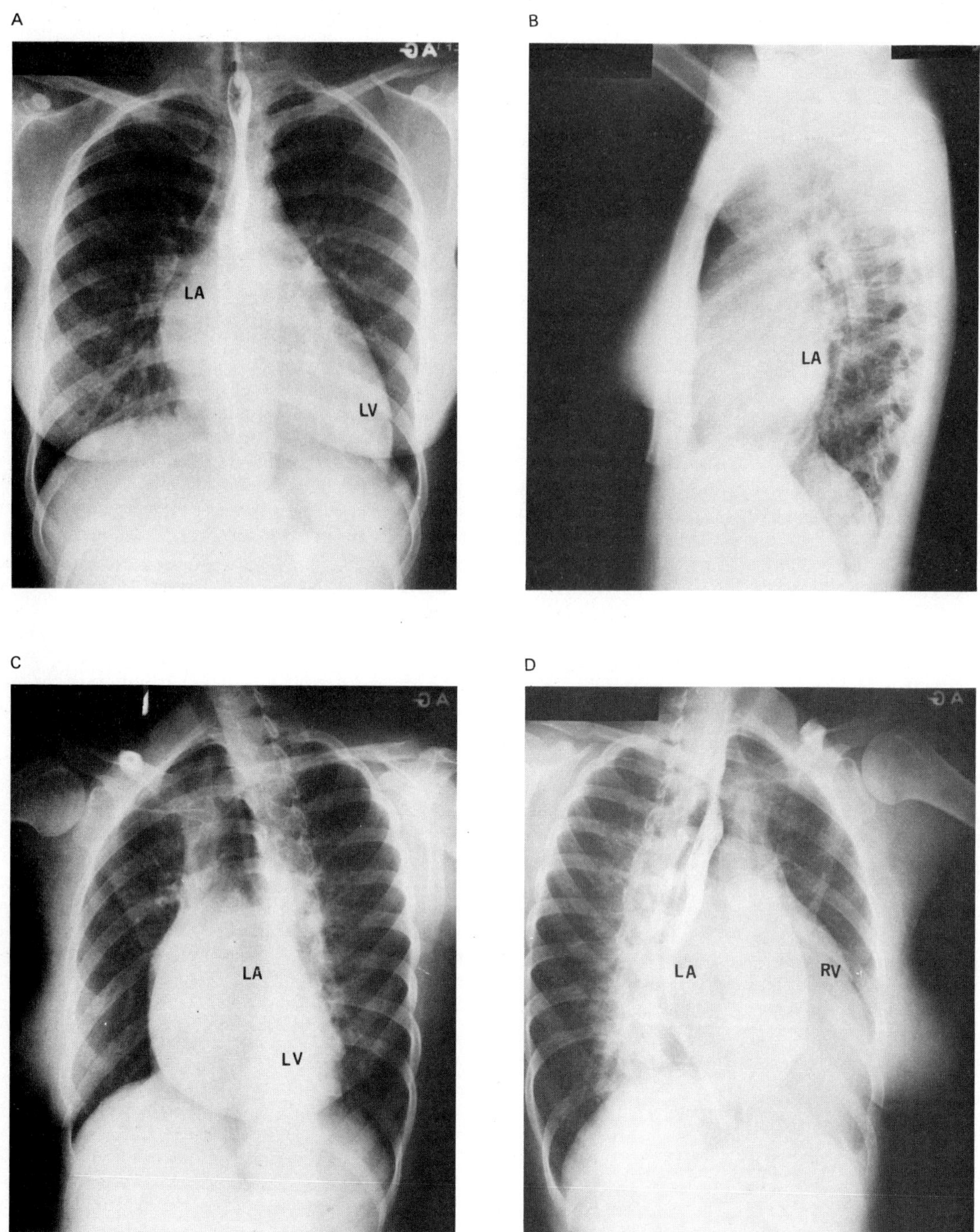

Figure 12–26. Cardiac series of chest x-rays of a 25-year-old asymptomatic woman with mitral incompetence. Left atrial (LA) and left ventricular (LV) enlargement are seen on several views. *A,* posteroanterior view; *B,* lateral view; *C,* left anterior oblique view; *D,* right anterior oblique view.

voltage is found. An incomplete right bundle branch block pattern (rsR′ in lead V_1) is seen in about 5% of patients with incompetence. Left bundle branch block is less common and is evidence of left ventricular disease. In patients in whom acute mitral incompetence is not treated in the early stages, right ventricular hypertrophy may ultimately develop owing to raised pulmonary vascular resistance. Atrial arrhythmias almost inevitably develop with time in patients with mitral incompetence. Although atrial premature beats, atrial tachycardia, and atrial flutter are occasionally seen, atrial fibrillation is much more common. Atrial arrhythmia may be paroxysmal at first and become chronic later. The onset of atrial fibrillation is more closely related to the patient's age than to any other variable in mitral incompetence. It is least common in acute mitral incompetence. The absence of atrial fibrillation in a symptomatic patient is also important. Significant symptoms in the presence of sinus rhythm suggest acute mitral incompetence. In patients with click-murmur syndrome, there may be a P mitrale. Atrial and ventricular premature beats are often present, and atrial and ventricular arrhythmias can be important.

D. X-Ray Findings: In patients with acute mitral incompetence, the heart is often of normal size at the outset, and marked pulmonary congestion and edema may be the only visible signs. Starting within a week or two, however, the left atrium and ventricle enlarge and reach the proportions seen in chronic cases by the end of a year if the patient survives.

In hemodynamically insignificant lesions, the heart is normal in size, and even the slight left atrial enlargement seen in mild cases may be absent. In hemodynamically significant chronic lesions, the left ventricle and left atrium are enlarged in proportion to the severity of the lesion. In the example shown in Fig 12–26A, B, C, and D, the lesion is severe and the left atrium and left ventricle can be seen on several views.

The principal form of mitral incompetence in which cardiac fluoroscopy is valuable is mitral ring calcification. In this lesion, which is virtually confined to elderly women, the radiologic picture is striking (Fig 12–27). The entire calcified mitral ring can be seen moving up and down with the heart beat, and the lesion can be distinguished from calcification of other sites in the chest.

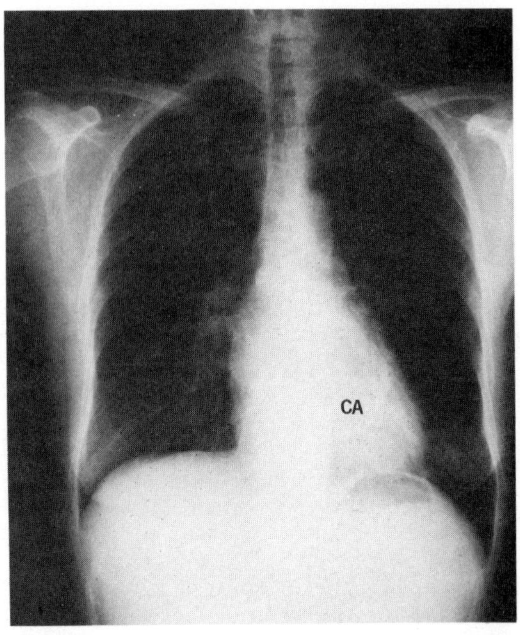

Figure 12–27. Chest x-ray of a 69-year-old woman with progressive mitral incompetence showing calcification (CA) of the mitral valve ring.

E. Special Investigations:

1. Noninvasive technics–Mitral incompetence can be diagnosed echographically (Fig 12–28), especially in acute disruption of the mitral valve. The late systolic posterior movements of the prolapsing valvular tissue can be seen in Fig 12–28A, and even in hemodynamically insignificant lesions, echocardiographic tracings are abnormal. Echocardiography appears to be a particularly sensitive means of detecting minor degrees of mitral valve prolapse, and abnormalities are seen in patients who have no heart murmur and in whom a mid- or late systolic click is the only finding. In addition to the valve itself, the size of the relevant heart chambers (left atrium and left ventricle) can be measured in the planes that are accessible to echographic investigation. Enlargement in one plane generally correlates with enlargement in other planes, and by concentrating on echographic views that show the mitral valve in a consistent manner, the physician can obtain reproducible tracings that can be used to follow changes in chamber size.

2. Invasive technics–

a. Acute mitral incompetence–Right and left heart catheterization are required in virtually all patients with acute disruption of the mitral valve in order to differentiate the mechanical effects of the lesion from those of associated myocardial disease. The hallmark of acute severe mitral incompetence is a wide pulse pressure in the wedge or left atrial tracing. The giant *v* wave, averaging over 50 mm Hg with values as high as 80 mm Hg in some cases, is quite characteristic. The *v* wave can usually also be seen in the pulmonary arterial pressure tracing as a second systolic peak which may equal that due to right ventricular contraction (Fig 12–29). The level of the diastolic left atrial pressure is also important as a clue to the state of the myocardium. In lesions that are mainly mechanical, the left ventricular and left atrial diastolic pressures are both about 15 mm Hg, indicating that there is no left ventricular failure. The mean left atrial pressure in a group of 20 patients with this lesion was 28 mm Hg, indicating that pulmonary congestion was moderately severe. Considerable emphasis should be placed on the measurement of left atrial pulse pressure in such cases, since it provides a simple means of assessing left ventricular function. A wide atrial pulse pressure with a

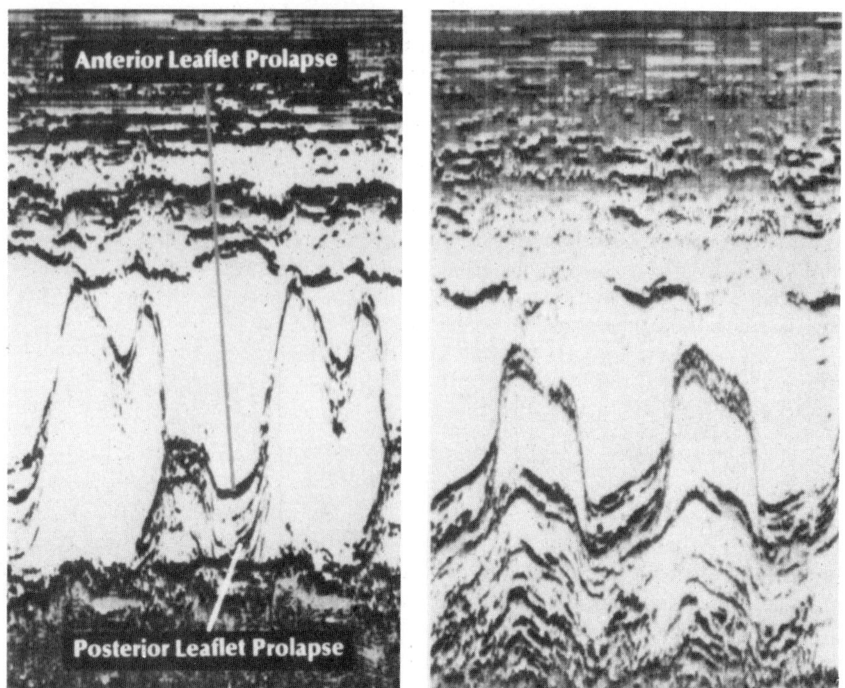

Figure 12–28. Two types of mitral regurgitation are shown. In *A,* from a patient with mild mitral prolapse, both anterior and posterior leaflets abruptly move posteriorly in late systole. In *B,* in another patient with severe mitral regurgitation secondary to rheumatic heart disease, there is no abnormal systolic motion, but, because the leaflets are thickened, they are moving (abnormally) parallel to each other in diastole. (Reproduced, with permission, from Fortuin NJ: Echocardiography. Hosp Pract 10:78, Nov 1975.)

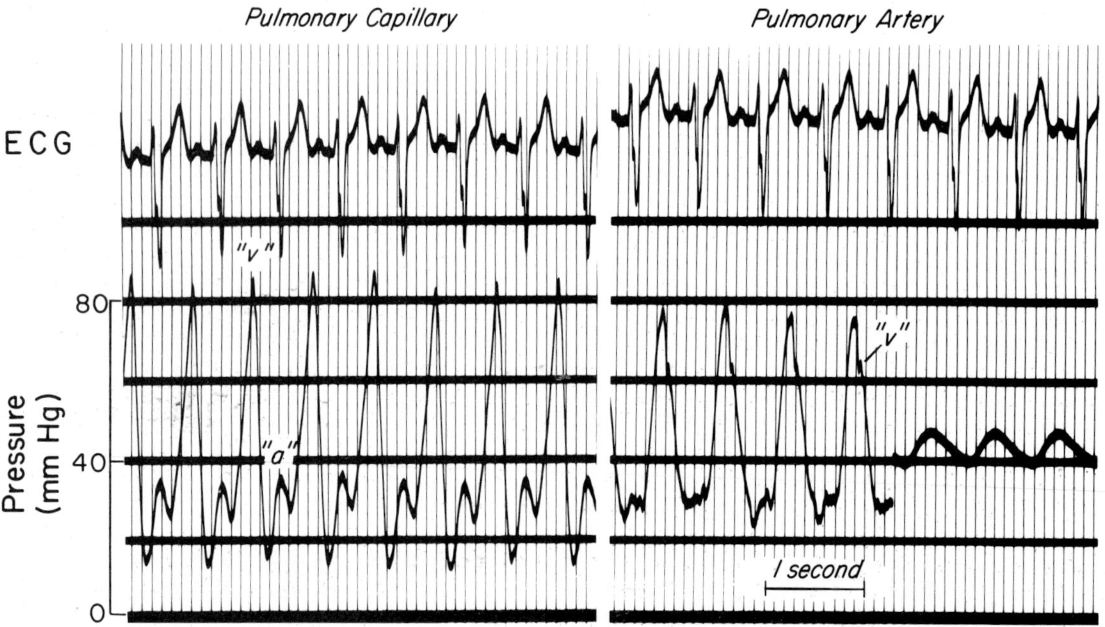

Figure 12–29. Pulmonary capillary (wedge) and pulmonary artery pressure tracings in a patient with acute mitral incompetence. The giant *v* wave seen in the wedge tracing is also visible in the pulmonary arterial pressure tracing.

high systolic and a low diastolic pressure indicates a powerfully contracting left ventricle with a low filling pressure. Conversely, a low systolic pressure with a high diastolic pressure indicates a poorly contracting left ventricle with a high filling pressure. Left ventricular angiography is an essential part of the study because it shows the magnitude of mitral incompetence and demonstrates the hyperdynamic state found in pure mechanical lesions, as opposed to the sluggish ventricular contraction with less forceful mitral incompetence occurring in lesions that have poor left ventricular function. In patients who have cardiac pain and any suggestion of prior infarction, coronary angiography is indicated. In about 15% of cases, especially in younger patients, the raised left atrial pressure resulting from acute disruption of the mitral valve may cause a marked increase in pulmonary vascular resistance. If the patient survives the acute stage of the lesion or if the acute incompetence is less severe, circulatory adaptations occur. The left atrium and ventricle become more compliant, and left atrial pressure falls. The hemodynamic picture then comes to resemble that of chronic mitral incompetence, and raised pulmonary vascular resistance may persist.

b. Chronic hemodynamically insignificant mitral incompetence–Since the diagnosis of chronic hemodynamically insignificant mitral incompetence is based on the clinical and ECG findings and because the patient, by definition, has no significant symptoms, cardiac catheterization is not indicated to establish the diagnosis. However, if cardiac catheterization is performed, the findings are not striking. The right-sided pressures, including the wedge pressure, are normal, and although mitral incompetence can be demonstrated by left ventricular angiography, cardiac chambers arc normal in size. The incompetence may appear more severe than it actually is upon measurement of left ventricular stroke volume and forward stroke volume.

c. Chronic hemodynamically significant mitral incompetence–In symptomatic patients with hemodynamically significant mitral incompetence, cardiac catheterization is indicated to determine the severity of the lesion before considering surgery. Left atrial pressure is usually only moderately raised, with a *v* wave of up to 30 mm Hg. The size of the left atrium is an important determinant of the hemodynamic findings, and in patients with a large atrium, the pressures are not usually impressive. The end-diastolic left ventricular pressure is of considerable importance. If it is raised, hypertension, active or inactive rheumatic myocarditis, or coronary disease should be suspected. The cardiac output may be abnormally low in patients with chronic mitral incompetence, especially in older persons, and the hemodynamic findings in patients with severe lesions may be unimpressive if this is the case. It is important to remember these factors when assessing the need for surgery, since valve replacement in patients with wedge pressures of less than 20 mm Hg may have surprisingly good results. Assessment of left ventricular function by left ventricular angiography is essential in any patient with mitral incompetence. Measurements of left ventricular ejection fraction and left ventricular wall motion should be obtained. The more obvious the mechanical lesion is on angiography, the higher the chances the patient will benefit from surgery. Selective coronary angiography is becoming a routine procedure, but this investigation increases morbidity and mortality and is of doubtful value in patients with no cardiac pain or other evidence (eg, ECG) of coronary disease.

It is difficult to determine the severity of mitral incompetence. Combined angiographic and physiologic measurements of left ventricular systolic and diastolic volumes and forward stroke volume provide the best information, but the 2 measurements are seldom made simultaneously, and they are both subject to error. The physician must depend on an overall, integrated assessment based on the entire clinical picture in order to determine severity. Since other variables such as left ventricular function and the nature of the lesion (acute or chronic) influence the clinical picture, the process is far from satisfactory.

Differential Diagnosis

Mitral incompetence must be distinguished from hypertrophic cardiomyopathy. There is a long pansystolic murmur in both conditions, and although the murmur in mitral incompetence is usually higher-pitched, has a timing that is not of the ejection type, and is transmitted to the axilla rather than centrally, the 2 lesions can be confused on diagnosis. Both show a third heart sound and a prominent left ventricle.

Ventricular septal defect is another condition that can be confused with mitral incompetence. Again, the auscultatory findings are similar, with an overactive left ventricle, a pansystolic murmur, and third heart sound. Chest x-ray may be helpful if the ventricular septal defect is large enough to cause increased lung markings resulting from increased pulmonary blood flow, but even these markings can be confused with those due to pulmonary congestion. Endocardial cushion defects with an associated ostium primum atrial defect and mitral incompetence are also difficult to differentiate from pure mitral incompetence, and cardiac catheterization is almost invariably needed to confirm the diagnosis. In the case of acute lesions, especially in patients who have suffered a recent myocardial infarction, the distinction between acquired ventricular septal defect due to rupture of the ventricular septum and acute mitral incompetence due to papillary muscle involvement can be extremely difficult. Here, too, as in all significant lesions, cardiac catheterization and angiography are necessary to confirm the diagnosis before surgery.

Complications

A. Systemic Embolism: Systemic embolization is an important complication. It is more common in mixed mitral stenosis and incompetence, but it also occurs in pure mitral incompetence, where it is more frequently due to infective endocarditis. Embolism is detected in about 20% of cases and almost certainly occurs more frequently without causing symptoms. Cerebral, femoral, renal, intestinal, and coronary emboli comprise most of the clinically recognized cases. Left atrial thrombi do not occur as frequently in mitral incompetence as in mitral stenosis because there is less stasis. The emboli resulting from left atrial thrombus clear more readily than those associated with endocarditis. Embolism is more common in patients with atrial fibrillation and is more likely to occur when the rhythm changes, either when atrial fibrillation begins or when sinus rhythm is restored.

B. Infective Endocarditis: Infective endocarditis is an important complication of mitral valvular disease in general and occurs most frequently in patients with mitral incompetence (20%). The patient is almost invariably in sinus rhythm at the onset of this complication (see also Chapter 16).

C. Rheumatic Myocarditis: See above under Mixed Stenosis and Incompetence for discussion of rheumatic myocarditis as a complication.

D. Coronary Artery Disease: In older patients, atherosclerotic coronary arterial disease may influence the clinical picture with a myocardial factor that alters prognosis. This is especially true of those patients with mitral incompetence, whose lesions are frequently degenerative in origin. Coronary arterial disease, hypertension, and atherosclerosis are almost invariably present in elderly patients with mitral incompetence, and distinguishing between the mechanical and myocardial components of the lesion in a given patient often presents an insoluble problem. The decision to advocate surgical treatment is extremely difficult even if complete studies have been performed preoperatively.

E. Ventricular Arrhythmias and Sudden Death: Patients with click-murmur syndrome are likely to develop ventricular arrhythmias, and there is undoubtedly an increased incidence of sudden death in persons with this lesion. An echocardiogram demonstrating mitral valve prolapse in a 26-year-old woman with palpitations is shown in Fig 12–30. This patient subsequently died suddenly, and, since no obvious cause was found at autopsy, arrhythmia was felt to be responsible. The incidence of sudden death is not known, but even 0.1% per year would be important because click-murmur syndrome is so common.

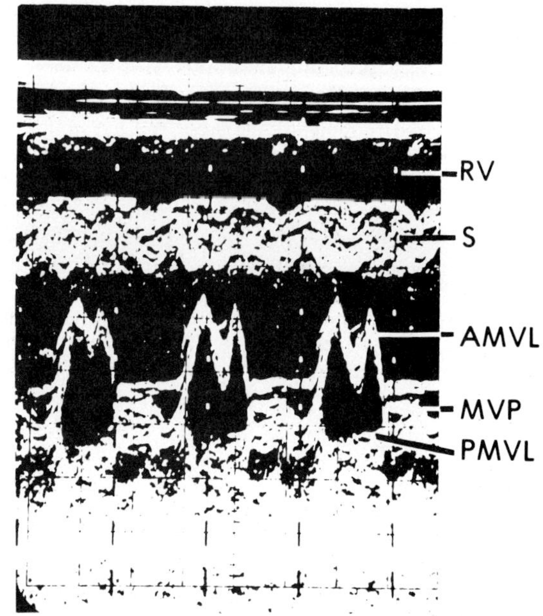

Figure 12–30. Echocardiogram showing mitral "click-murmur" syndrome in a patient who subsequently died suddenly. RV, right ventricle; S, septum; AMVL, anterior, and PMVL, posterior mitral valve leaflets; MVP, mitral valve prolapse. (Courtesy of NB Schiller.)

Treatment

A. Medical Treatment: See above under Mitral Stenosis for a discussion of medical measures used in the treatment of mitral incompetence.

B. Surgical Treatment:

1. Valvuloplasty in acute mitral incompetence–Acute mitral incompetence is the major disorder that can be treated satisfactorily with mitral valvuloplasty. In cases in which the chordae tendineae supporting the posterior (mural) cusp of the mitral valve are torn, wedge resection of the affected part of the cusp gives excellent results. This operation has the advantage of not requiring long-term anticoagulant therapy. The only comparable palliative operation for mitral incompetence is the suturing of the cleft in the mitral valve in a patient with an endocardial cushion defect. This procedure is undertaken in young persons, for whom a lifetime of anticoagulation is the only other alternative until the long-term effectiveness of heterograft porcine valves is established.

2. Mitral valve replacement in mitral incompetence–Mitral valve replacement is the treatment of choice in almost all cases of mitral incompetence. In acute lesions it may be difficult to decide when to operate. In patients with infective endocarditis or acute myocardial infarction, surgery should be delayed, if possible, until the acute lesion is completely healed. The hemodynamic load of acute mitral incompetence is generally not as severe as that of acute aortic incompetence, and it is usually possible to delay, particularly if systemic vasodilator therapy (afterload reduction) is employed. In most acute cases, surgery will be needed eventually, and there is some justification for operating before left atrial dilatation and atrial fibrillation have occurred. These changes ordinarily take from several months to a year to develop following an acute episode, and the optimal time for operation is 6 weeks to 3 months after the episode. The timing of surgery is most critical in patients suffering from endocarditis following intravenous drug abuse or endocarditis caused by drug-resistant organisms. No satisfactory regimen has yet been established for the management of such cases, and the long-term results are dismal whether valve replacement is performed early or late in the course of the disease. Patients with known associated left ventricular disease also present problems in management. In patients with a narrow left atrial pulse pressure, left ventricular diastolic pressure over 25 mm Hg, and a reduced left ventricular ejection fraction (less than 40%), surgery is not indicated, but in borderline cases, especially those with previous myocardial infarction, the decision to withhold surgery can be extremely difficult. Studies during cardiac catheterization in which afterload reduction is carried out, ie, in which systemic arterial resistance is acutely lowered by vasodilator drugs such as intravenous nitroprusside, may be helpful. If cardiac output rises by 1 liter or more per minute and the left atrial pressure falls by 5–10 mm Hg, the outlook for surgery may be more encouraging.

3. Timing of surgery—In acute mitral incompetence the problem facing the cardiologist is no longer one of diagnosis because the clinical features distinguishing acute lesions are becoming widely recognized. Instead, the problem now is to decide when to operate on patients with endocarditis and how to determine the relative proportions of mechanical load and myocardial damage in patients with ischemic heart disease. Cardiac surgery generally has significant acute but reversible damaging effects on myocardial function, and if sufficient relief of the mechanical lesion is not afforded by operation, the surgical mortality rate will be high. However, in patients who have both a mechanical and a myocardial lesion, the mechanical lesion seriously burdens an already damaged myocardium, and the extra load should be relieved surgically whenever possible. It is difficult to predict the outcome of surgery in such mixed lesions, and the decision to operate depends to a large extent on local facilities, experience, and philosophy. Cardiac surgery is expensive in terms of time, energy, money, and personal psychic trauma for all concerned. It seems clear that there are levels of mortality that are intolerable for the surgical team. The level of mortality that is unacceptable is not clearly defined, but it is difficult to maintain morale when the mortality rate is greater than 25%.

In hemodynamically insignificant mitral incompetence, the principal problem is one of management. Patients are now being seen at earlier stages. In hemodynamically insignificant mitral incompetence, sudden death from arrhythmia is a possibility in a small percentage of patients. No form of treatment has yet been shown to affect this complication, but quinidine or propranolol should be given if premature beats are shown to be frequent (see Chapter 15). Patients with this lesion do not in general lead happier lives when they are aware of the possibility of this complication. The physician must exercise extreme care to ensure that patients with hemodynamically insignificant mitral incompetence do not become cardiac invalids. The physician should make a clear mental distinction between the patient who presents with no complaint and whose lesion is therefore discovered on routine or incidental examination and the patient who has consulted a physician because of some specific symptom thought to be related to cardiac disease.

Prognosis

A. Acute Mitral Incompetence: In patients with mitral incompetence the prognosis depends more on the cause of the valvular lesion than on its severity and acuteness. The prognosis in acute mitral incompetence is good with surgery provided that myocardial infarction or uncontrollable infective endocarditis is not the basic cause. Early diagnosis and operation performed as soon as any associated lesions have healed improve the prognosis by preventing the changes of chronic mitral incompetence.

B. Hemodynamically Insignificant Lesions: The prognosis of hemodynamically insignificant mitral incompetence is not yet clear. The results of 20-year follow-up studies of patients with a late systolic murmur as the only finding are just now appearing. They indicate that infective endocarditis and acute disruption of the mitral valve due to rupture of the chordae tendineae are not infrequent sequelae. This finding correlates well with the information obtained from the history of patients with significant mitral incompetence. A long history of a heart murmur is found in 3 types of patients with mitral incompetence: those with infective endocarditis, those with acute mitral valve disruption, and those with chronic hemodynamically significant mitral incompetence. It seems likely that many of these have had hemodynamically insignificant lesions that subsequently become more severe. As in rheumatic mitral valve disease, it is clear to physicians who are now treating more patients in older age groups that age-related degenerative changes figure more prominently in the development of sequelae than was first thought. The mitral valve is a common site for degenerative changes of a calcific, myxomatous, or mechanical nature. Mechanical degenerative changes are due to stretching of tissues weakened by age.

• • •

References

Allen H, Harris A, Leatham A: Significance and prognosis of an isolated late systolic murmur: A 9 to 22-year follow-up. Br Heart J 36:525, 1974.

Austen WG & others: Ruptured papillary muscle. Circulation 32:597, 1965.

Barlow JB & others: Late systolic murmur and non-ejection ("mid-late") systolic clicks. Br Heart J 30:203, 1968.

Barnes CG, Finlay HVL: Cor triatriatum. Br Heart J 14:283, 1952.

Besterman EMM: The use of phenylephrine to aid auscultation of early rheumatic diastolic murmurs. Br Med J 2:205, 1951.

Bower BD & others: Two cases of congenital mitral stenosis treated by valvotomy. Arch Dis Child 28:91, 1953.

Braunwald E: Mitral regurgitation: Physiologic, clinical, and surgical considerations. N Engl J Med 281:425, 1969.

Braunwald E & others: Effects of mitral valve replacement on the pulmonary vascular dynamics of patients with pulmonary hypertension. N Engl J Med 273:509, 1965.

Brickman RD & others: Cor triatriatum. J Thorac Cardiovasc Surg 60:523, 1970.

Brigden W, Leatham A: Mitral incompetence. Br Heart J 15:55, 1953.

Brown OR & others: Aortic root dilatation and mitral valve prolapse in Marfan's syndrome: An echocardiographic study. Circulation 52:651, 1975.

Chatterjee K & others: Beneficial effects of vasodilator agents in severe mitral regurgitation due to dysfunction of subvalvular apparatus. Circulation 48:684, 1973.

Criley JM & others: Prolapse of the mitral valve: Clinical and cine-angiocardiographic findings. Br Heart J 28:488, 1966.

Davis RH & others: Myxomatous degeneration of the mitral valve. Am J Cardiol 28:449, 1971.

Ellis LB, Ramirez A: The clinical course of patients with severe "rheumatic" mitral insufficiency. Am Heart J 78:406, 1969.

Goodman DJ & others: Effect of nitroprusside on left ventricular dynamics in mitral regurgitation. Circulation 50:1025, 1974.

Goodwin JF: Diagnosis of left atrial myxoma. Lancet 1:464, 1963.

Hancock EW, Cohn K: The syndrome associated with midsystolic click and late systolic murmur. Am J Med 41:183, 1966.

Jeresaty RM: Mitral valve prolapse-click syndrome. Prog Cardiovasc Dis 15:623, 1973.

Kirklin JW: Replacement of the mitral valve for mitral incompetence. Surgery 72:827, 1972.

Kirklin JW, Pacifico AD: Surgery for acquired valvular heart disease. N Engl J Med 288:133, 1973.

Littler WA, Epstein EJ, Coulshed N: Acute mitral regurgitation resulting from ruptured or elongated chordae tendineae. Q J Med 42:87, 1973.

Lundstrom NR: Echocardiography in the diagnosis of congenital mitral stenosis and in evaluation of the results of mitral valvotomy. Circulation 46:44, 1972.

Markiewicz W & others: Mitral valve prolapse in one hundred presumably healthy young females. Circulation 53:464, 1976.

Marshall R, McIlroy MB, Christie RV: The work of breathing in mitral stenosis. Clin Sci 13:137, 1954.

McCall BW, Price JL: Movement of mitral valve cusps in relation to first heart sound and opening snap in patients with mitral stenosis. Br Heart J 29:417, 1967.

McIntosh CL, Michaelis LL, Morrow AG: Atrio-ventricular valve replacement with the Hancock porcine xenograft: A five-year clinical experience. Surgery 78:768, 1975.

Mills P & others: Long-term prognosis of mitral-valve prolapse. N Engl J Med 297:13, 1977.

Pocock WA, Barlow JB: Etiology and electrocardiographic features of the billowing posterior mitral leaflet syndrome. Am J Med 51:731, 1971.

Popp RL & others: Echocardiographic abnormalities in the mitral valve prolapse syndrome. Circulation 49:428, 1974.

Rapaport E & others: Natural history of aortic and mitral valve disease. Am J Cardiol 35:221, 1975.

Reichek N, Shelburne JC, Perloff JK: Clinical aspects of rheumatic valvular disease. Prog Cardiovasc Dis 15:491, 1973.

Reid JVO: Mid-systolic clicks. S Afr Med J 35:353, 1961.

Rizzon P & others: Familial syndrome of midsystolic click and late systolic murmur. Br Heart J 35:245, 1973.

Roberts WC, Perloff JK: Mitral valvular disease: A clinicopathologic survey of the conditions causing the mitral valve to function abnormally. Ann Intern Med 77:939, 1972.

Rowe JC & others: The course of mitral stenosis without surgery: Ten- and twenty-year perspectives. Ann Intern Med 52:741, 1960.

Sanders CA & others: Etiology and differential diagnosis of acute mitral regurgitation. Prog Cardiovasc Dis 14:129 1971.

Selzer A, Cohn KE: Natural history of mitral stenosis: A review. Circulation 45:878, 1972.

Shappell SD & others: Sudden death and the familial occurrence of mid-systolic click, late systolic murmur syndrome. Circulation 48:1128, 1973.

Smith ER & others: Angiographic diagnosis of mitral valve prolapse: Correlation with echocardiography. Am J Cardiol 40:165, 1977.

Wells BG: Prediction of mitral pressure gradient from heart sounds. Br Med J 1:551, 1957.

Wigle ED, Auger P: Sudden, severe mitral insufficiency. Can Med Assoc J 96:1493, 1967.

Winkle RA & others: Life-threatening arrhythmias in the mitral valve prolapse syndrome. Am J Med 60:961, 1976.

Wood P: An appreciation of mitral stenosis. (2 parts.) Br Med J 16:1051, 1113, 1954.

Wood P & others: The effect of acetylcholine on pulmonary vascular resistance and left atrial pressure in mitral stenosis. Br Heart J 19:279, 1957.

Wynn A: Gross calcification of the mitral valve. Br Heart J 15:214, 1953.

13 . . .
Aortic Valve Disease; Combined Valve Disease

Aortic valve disease is the next most common form of valvular heart disease after mitral disease and accounts for about 35% of patients with significant valvular lesions. Classification is difficult because of the varied causes, hemodynamic severity, acuteness or chronicity, anatomic site, and nature of the lesion.

Classification

Aortic valve disease has been classified in this text into 3 main categories: (1) hemodynamically insignificant aortic valve disease, (2) hemodynamically significant predominant aortic stenosis, and (3) hemodynamically significant predominant aortic incompetence.

In hemodynamically insignificant aortic valve disease, it is impossible to determine whether stenosis or incompetence is predominant because the lesion is so mild. There is no evidence of cardiac enlargement or hypertrophy and no limitation of exercise tolerance. It is not possible to predict whether the lesion will progress, or if it does, whether aortic stenosis or aortic incompetence will predominate. Hemodynamically insignificant aortic valve disease accompanying other forms of heart disease such as hypertension, atherosclerosis, or disease of other valves complicates the classification. In such cases, complete investigation is often needed to confirm the diagnosis; the existence of predominant aortic stenosis is often suspected before left heart catheterization is performed, and the correct diagnosis is not established until the investigations have been completed.

Hemodynamically significant aortic valve lesions range from pure stenosis through mixed stenosis and incompetence to pure incompetence. It is thus difficult to know how to separate patients into groups for the purposes of classification. Because aortic stenosis is a more serious lesion than aortic incompetence, the lesions of all patients with any element of stenosis are classified as predominantly stenotic rather than incompetent.

An indirectly recorded brachial arterial diastolic blood pressure of 70 mm Hg or more is used as an arbitrary measurement below which hemodynamically significant aortic incompetence is present. This cutoff point is naturally not entirely satisfactory, but it represents the best single figure on which to base a classification. In practice, the level of the systolic arterial pressure, the rate of rise of the carotid pulse, the pulse pressure, the quality of the left ventricular impulse, the degree of left ventricular hypertrophy, and the presence or absence of left ventricular failure all assist the cardiologist in determining whether the lesion is predominantly stenotic or incompetent and whether it is hemodynamically significant or not.

Interaction of Stenosis & Incompetence

Patients with hemodynamically insignificant lesions probably represent an earlier stage of disease, and they may subsequently develop either predominant stenosis or incompetence. Predominant aortic stenosis is almost always calcific in adults, and the presence or development of calcification plays an important role in the stiffening and immobilization of the valve. On the other hand, aortic incompetence is virtually never calcific, and it is shrinkage, retraction, atrophy, or perforation of valve tissue or dilatation of the root of the aorta that is responsible for valvular incompetence. Aortic stenosis and aortic incompetence load the left ventricle in different ways. In the purest forms of stenosis, the extra left ventricular work is performed almost entirely against increased pressure, with no increase in flow. In pure incompetence there is an almost pure flow load with an increase in stroke volume, because the ventricle must eject both its normal stroke volume and the blood which returns as backflow through the valve during diastole. Falling between these 2 extremes is a spectrum of lesions in which the ventricular load consists partly of increased volume and partly of increased flow. Severe stenosis and severe incompetence cannot coexist; therefore, in mixed lesions neither component is severe. As is true also in mitral valvular disease, the incompetence and stenosis interact in such a way that the clinical picture in mixed lesions is relatively independent of the mix of stenosis and incompetence. If incompetence is greater than stenosis, the stroke volume is larger, and the pressure difference between the left ventricle and the aorta is exaggerated because of the large flow. If stenosis is more severe than incompetence, the narrower orifice permits less backflow during diastole, but the pressure difference during systole is large because the stenosis is relatively severe. Since the left ventricle tolerates pressure loads less easily than volume loads, stenotic lesions are more important than incompetent ones. Therefore, all cases with significant stenosis are in-

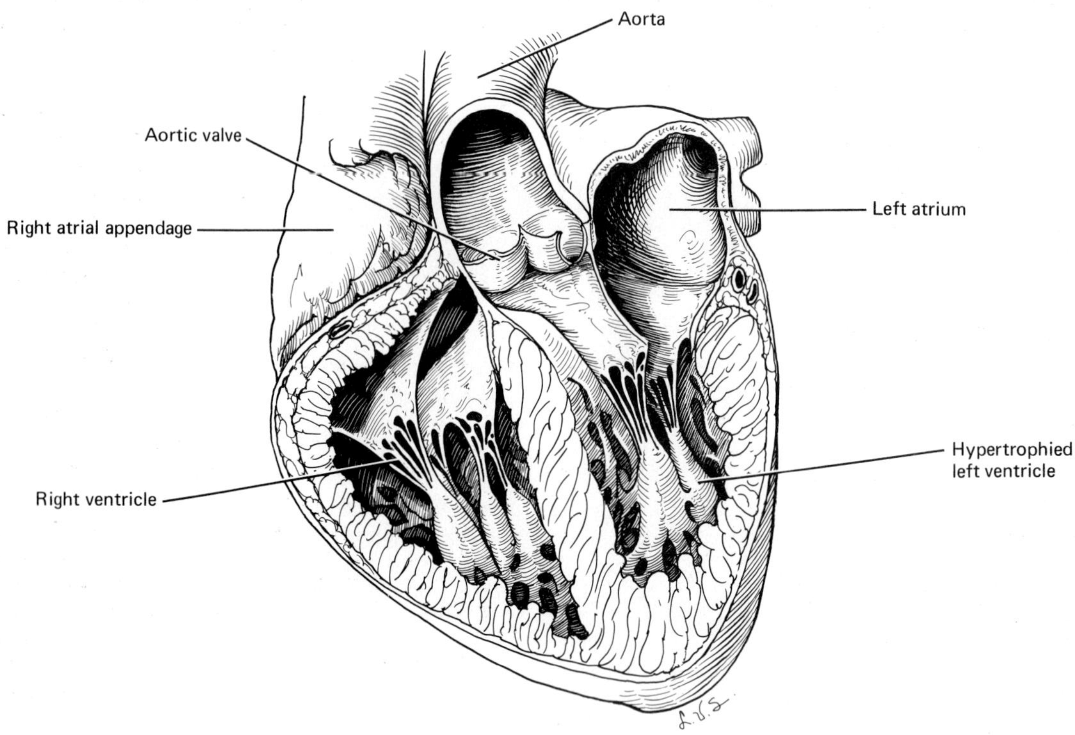

Drawing of left heart in left anterior oblique view showing anatomic features of hemodynamically insignificant aortic valve disease.

Cardinal features: *Normal heart size and hemodynamics; systolic ejection murmur.*

Variable factors: *Systolic ejection click; short aortic diastolic murmur.*

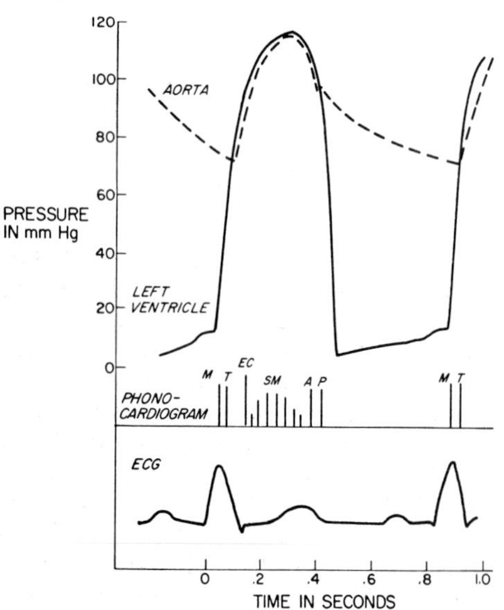

Diagram showing auscultatory and hemodynamic features of hemodynamically insignificant aortic valve disease. Note the absence of a gradient across the aortic valve. M, mitral; T, tricuspid; A, aortic, P, pulmonary valve; EC, ejection click; SM, systolic ejection murmur.

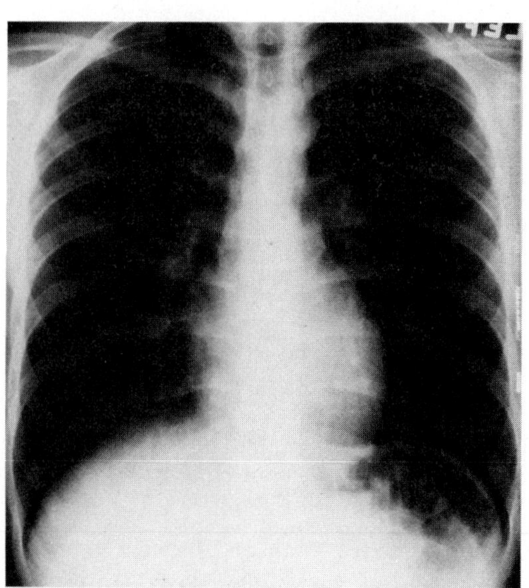

Chest x-ray showing normal heart size and shape.

Figure 13–1. Hemodynamically insignificant aortic valve disease. Structures enlarged: None.

cluded in one group (predominant aortic stenosis), and predominantly incompetent lesions form another.

Subvalvular & Supravalvular Aortic Stenosis

Among patients with predominant aortic stenosis is a small group (1% of cases) who do not have disease affecting the valves but rather congenital supravalvular or subvalvular lesions. Supravalvular aortic stenosis usually results from congenital hypoplasia of the ascending aorta, whereas subvalvular stenosis is due to the presence of a fibrous ring or shelf of tissue immediately below the valve. Supravalvular stenosis occurs in a familial form in physically underdeveloped children with characteristic elfin facies and prominent ears. Surgical relief of the aortic obstruction is often difficult because of the diffuse hypoplasia of the aorta.

Subvalvular stenosis is also congenital and is due to ring lesions which are especially amenable to surgical relief, in contrast to those of supravalvular stenosis. The clinical picture resembles that of predominant aortic stenosis, and the valve often leaks, perhaps because the subvalvular ring interferes with normal valve closure. The condition is diagnosed by supravalvular angiography. The ring is often so close to the aortic valve that withdrawal pressure tracings may fail to detect the lesion. In hypertrophic obstructive cardiomyopathy, the obstruction lies lower in the ventricle, and the clinical picture is different (see Chapter 17, p 522).

Acute & Chronic Aortic Incompetence

Aortic incompetence, like mitral incompetence, occurs in both the acute and the chronic forms. Acute lesions are almost always due to the effects of infective endocarditis but may rarely occur when acute aortic dissection involves the aortic root. The acute load on the left ventricle causes a clinical picture that is different from that seen in chronic lesions. Acute left ventricular failure with severe pulmonary congestion and edema can occur within a few hours or days, and the lesion is often fatal if valve replacement is not performed. The degree of acuteness varies from case to case. Some of the most severe lesions are seen when an aortic cusp is torn or perforated. In acute aortic incompetence, the patient's condition seldom stabilizes without valve replacement, but in a few cases in which the onset is less acute, the changes associated with chronic aortic incompetence—left ventricular hypertrophy and dilatation—develop over several weeks, and after a year the clinical picture is indistinguishable from that seen in chronic aortic incompetence.

Causes of Aortic Valve Lesions

To detect both the cause and severity of aortic valve lesions is difficult by ordinary clinical means. There is often a discrepancy between the patient's symptoms and the hemodynamic severity of the lesions, and the cause often remains in doubt, even after autopsy. Both aortic stenosis and aortic incompetence may run long clinical courses lasting 20–30 years, and the physician is often confronted with patients who have hemodynamically significant lesions and yet no symptoms. Just as frequently, the patient has symptoms that are out of proportion to the hemodynamic findings. Because aortic valve lesions can run such a long clinical course, it is difficult to determine what factors are responsible for the progressive deterioration of the patient's clinical state that often occurs over a short period of a few weeks or months. Long-term changes may be due to valvular calcification or myocardial fibrosis, but an acute exacerbation often cannot be explained. The lesions themselves do not seem to change clinically, but the patient nonetheless suddenly develops left ventricular failure, and the disease runs a rapid downhill course that is not always reversed by surgical treatment.

As in mitral valve disease, rheumatic fever is an important cause of aortic valvular lesions. A history of previous rheumatic fever is present in 20% of patients with predominant stenosis and in 25% of those with predominant incompetence. Since congenital aortic valve lesions are relatively common, some patients who have been diagnosed as having had rheumatic fever in childhood actually have congenital aortic valve lesions. Seventy-five percent of patients with predominant aortic stenosis who have a past history of rheumatic fever are women, whereas 75% of those with pure incompetence who have a past history of rheumatic fever are men. This agrees with the finding in mitral valve disease that stenosis occurs more commonly in females and incompetence in males. Aortic valve disease is more prevalent in males by a factor of 3:1 in predominant stenosis and 3:2 in predominant incompetence. These proportions vary in different series for the reason that causes vary in different geographic areas.

HEMODYNAMICALLY INSIGNIFICANT LESIONS

The cardinal features of hemodynamically insignificant aortic lesions (Fig 13–1) include normal heart size and hemodynamics and a systolic ejection murmur. The variable features are a systolic ejection click and a short aortic diastolic murmur. Auscultatory physical signs arising from the aortic valve are usually the sole abnormality. These lesions constitute 10% of cases seen in university hospital practice but make up a much larger percentage in private practice. These cases probably represent a presymptomatic phase of aortic valve disease that if followed long enough would be seen to develop into either aortic stenosis or aortic incompetence. The most important complication in such cases is the development of infective endocarditis, with associated development or exacerbation of aortic incompetence. These lesions are seen in patients of all ages. Congenital, rheumatic, and atherosclerotic causes account for two-thirds of cases; no causative factor is identified in the others.

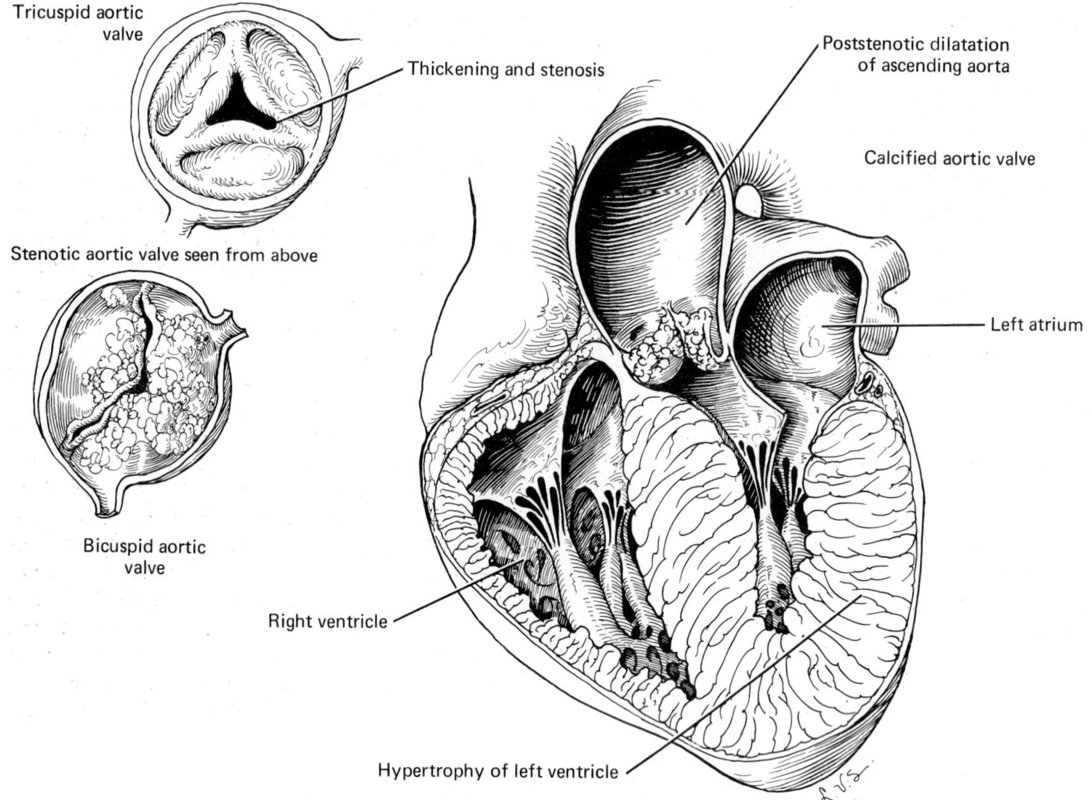

Drawing of left heart in left anterior oblique view showing anatomic features of aortic stenosis.

Cardinal features: *Left ventricular hypertrophy; systolic ejection murmur.*

Variable factors: *Severity; site of obstruction; cause; valvular calcification.*

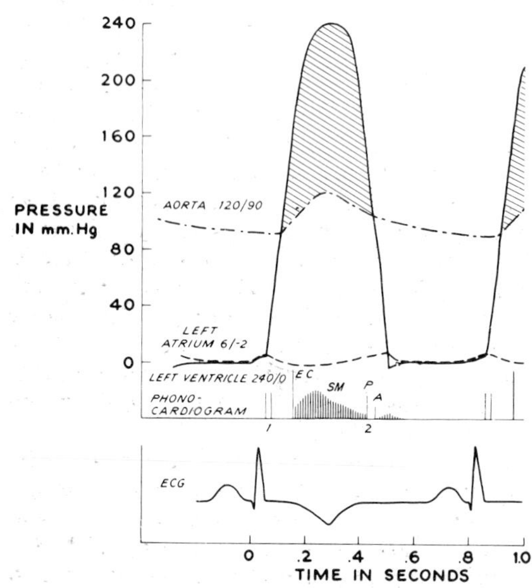

Diagram showing auscultatory and hemodynamic features of predominant aortic stenosis.

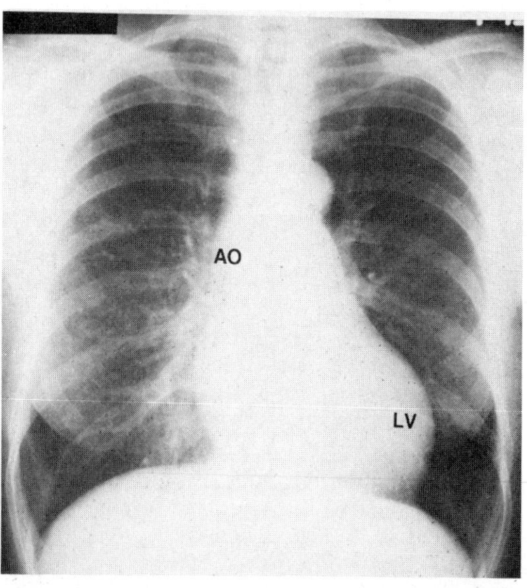

Chest x-ray of a patient with aortic stenosis showing left ventricular (LV) and aortic (AO) enlargement.

Figure 13–2. Aortic stenosis. Structures enlarged: Left ventricle (thickened); poststenotic dilatation of the aorta.

Clinical Features

More than half of cases are entirely asymptomatic. In the others, palpitations, fatigue, dizziness, and noncardiac dyspnea occur but without evidence of heart failure. Symptoms are more common in patients who are aware that they have a heart murmur. The pulse and blood pressure are normal; a collapsing pulse or a slow-rising pulse is, by definition, absent. The heart is not enlarged on clinical or x-ray examination, and no evidence of ventricular hypertrophy is detectable. (If any of these signs are present, the lesion is no longer hemodynamically insignificant.) There is always a systolic murmur at the base of the heart, preceded by an ejection click in one-third of cases and followed by a faint aortic diastolic murmur in one-third. Slight aortic dilatation is occasionally seen, but valvular calcification is not necessarily present.

Cardiac catheterization is not indicated for diagnosis, but if it is performed, intracardiac pressures are normal, and there is no significant pressure difference between the left ventricle and the aorta. Such patients can subsequently develop predominant aortic stenosis, but the course in individual cases is difficult to predict. Long-term follow-up of 20 years or more is often necessary.

The role of the deposition of calcium in these slightly abnormal valves is difficult to determine, but it seems likely that valvular calcification immobilizes and narrows the valve, causing stenosis that gradually progresses but does not significantly load the left ventricle until the valve is narrowed to about one-fourth its normal area (5.0 $cm^2 \rightarrow 1.25\ cm^2$).

The other important development in such cases is infective endocarditis. Patients with hemodynamically insignificant aortic lesions are particularly prone to this complication, and the valve is likely to become acutely and severely incompetent as a result. Thus, the prevention and early recognition of endocarditis are important aspects of the management of patients with this lesion. Antibiotic prophylactic therapy preceding major dental work or minor surgery and early blood culture during febrile illnesses are mandatory. Intravenous drug abuse is particularly likely to result in infective endocarditis because contaminated needles and syringes are often used, and the drugs are seldom sterile. When a rheumatic origin for the lesion is suspected, prophylactic penicillin treatment is warranted to prevent recurrences of rheumatic fever (see p 533).

PREDOMINANT AORTIC STENOSIS

The cardinal features of predominant aortic stenosis (Fig 13–2) are left ventricular hypertrophy and a systolic ejection murmur. The variable factors are the severity, which affects the hypertrophy; the site of the obstruction; the cause; and the presence or absence of valvular calcification.

Importance of Aortic Stenosis

Predominant aortic stenosis has an importance in clinical cardiology that is out of proportion to its frequency. The reason for this is that both the diagnosis and the assessment of severity of the lesion are often extremely difficult. Aortic stenosis is easily missed on clinical examination, especially if the patient is in severe left ventricular failure and the cardiac output is so low that the aortic systolic murmur that might point toward a diagnosis of aortic stenosis is virtually inaudible. Aortic stenosis is often suspected in patients in whom there is no significant obstruction to aortic flow. In these cases, it is the presence of an aortic systolic murmur, often associated with calcification of the aortic valve on fluoroscopy, that indicates possible aortic stenosis. Although echocardiography may be valuable in ruling out a diagnosis of aortic stenosis, left heart catheterization is always indicated to confirm that obstruction is severe. Approximately 10% of patients undergoing cardiac catheterization in a university hospital subsequently prove to have hemodynamically unimportant lesions despite a diagnosis of aortic stenosis before the procedure, but the risks of missing the correct diagnosis so far outweigh the dangers of cardiac catheterization that the study should be performed if there is the slightest doubt about the diagnosis.

Cause of Aortic Stenosis

The cause of aortic stenosis has been the subject of controversy for many years. In most cases (70%), there is no clinical clue to the cause. At autopsy the valve is usually so disorganized by calcification that it is difficult to count the number of cusps. Now that aortic valve replacement has become routine, the valve is available for study at an earlier stage of the disease, and it is easier to see if there are 2 or 3 cusps. Even so, separate cusps cannot be identified in some patients (15%). Since the normal aortic valve has 3 cusps, the finding of a bicuspid valve in 50% of patients indicates that the basic lesion is congenital in patients with predominant aortic stenosis who undergo surgery or die of the disease. Patients with bicuspid valves often have other congenital lesions, most commonly coarctation of the aorta. Some are known to have had a murmur since early infancy, but the majority (two-thirds) have had a murmur first heard only after age 20. This latter group generally does not have congenital aortic stenosis but rather a minor congenital valvular lesion that apparently makes the valve more than normally susceptible to wear and tear.

Congenital aortic stenosis is rarely seen in adults and constitutes about 5% of cases. In such cases, a murmur has almost always been heard in infancy, and symptoms usually have developed in early adult life. All patients with predominant aortic stenosis tend to develop valvular calcification with increasing age, and, after age 40, valvular calcification is present in virtually all cases, irrespective of the cause of the lesion. Age-related degenerative changes in the valve thus seem to be important in the progression of the lesion.

In a small but increasing number of patients, atherosclerotic, age-related degenerative changes in a normal valve appear to be the sole cause of aortic stenosis. In this group, the valve is tricuspid, the patient is over age 60, and a murmur has not been present for more than 5 years. This group of patients constitutes about 10% of cases. There is some suggestion that aortic stenosis may develop rapidly in such patients and run a shorter course.

Progression of Aortic Stenosis

The role played by the deposition of calcium in the cusps and the consequent progression of the disease seems unpredictable. Physicians must learn to recognize the signs of increasing severity of stenosis: progressive cardiac enlargement, decreasing peripheral pulse pressure, slowing of carotid upstroke, and increasing left ventricular hypertrophy on the ECG and echocardiograms. Aortic valve replacement is so much more successful in patients who have not yet developed left ventricular failure that early diagnosis and recognition of increasing severity are of the utmost importance. A special problem is the increased incidence of acquired aortic stenosis due to atherosclerosis in elderly persons. The disease can be extremely insidious and difficult to diagnose.

Clinical Findings

In all forms of aortic stenosis a fixed, disorganized, calcified, thickened, radiopaque mass of tissue replaces the normal flexible, thin, filmy valve structure. In congenital aortic stenosis the valve is often dome-shaped, and no cusps can be distinguished. Calcification is most closely related to age and occurs at the earliest in the late teens and 20s. The development of calcification is commonly associated with the development of an aortic systolic ejection murmur.

Aortic stenosis increases the work of the left ventricle. In cases of pure stenosis, hypertrophy first occurs at the expense of the left ventricular cavity, causing a decrease in ventricular compliance. The ventricle becomes more rounded, but overall heart size is not increased. If there is associated aortic incompetence, the left ventricle is larger, and in most cases heart size is increased by the time symptoms appear. The narrowing of the aortic valve produces turbulence and often causes a jet stream of blood to impinge on the anterior and right walls of the aorta, resulting in a localized, poststenotic dilatation of the aorta. The calcification of the aortic valve may spread to the valve ring and thence to the anterior (aortic) cusp of the mitral valve and the membranous part of the interventricular septum, where it may involve the atrioventricular conduction system and cause heart block. The coronary vessels are usually large and not atherosclerotic in younger patients with bicuspid valves, but calcific emboli may occur and cause coronary occlusion or other serious systemic embolism. Aortic stenosis developing de novo in elderly persons is more likely to be associated with coronary artery disease, and the combination of the 2 conditions carries a poor prognosis.

Blood is subject to extremely severe mechanical stress as it passes through the turbulent areas associated with a stenotic aortic valve. Damage to red cells in the form of excessive hemolysis may occur in patients with aortic stenosis, especially if the cells are abnormally fragile. This rare form of hemolytic anemia is also seen after aortic valve replacement.

A. Symptoms: Symptoms appear late in the course of aortic stenosis, and many patients with hemodynamically significant lesions have no complaints. The disease is not recognized in its earlier stages, usually because the patient does not seek medical advice. In some cases, the murmur has been present without any symptoms for so many years that the physician overlooks the possibility of aortic stenosis until it becomes severe.

The stage at which symptoms develop depends to some extent on the patient's activity level. In sedentary people the disease may be far advanced before the patient complains of symptoms. Half of patients with surgically significant aortic stenosis have had at least one episode of left ventricular failure before they undergo surgery for stenosis. In active persons, dyspnea on exertion occurs before overt left ventricular failure develops, but especially in sedentary people, an episode of paroxysmal nocturnal dyspnea may be the first symptom of disease.

That aortic stenosis runs a long presymptomatic course is evident from the finding that significant stenosis—as judged by the presence of a systolic murmur and left ventricular hypertrophy on the ECG—may be present for 20 years without causing any symptoms. The course of the disease after symptoms develop is rapid. Progressive left ventricular failure leads to death in 2–8 years if surgery is not performed. The symptoms in the later stages of aortic stenosis are some of the most difficult to manage in the entire spectrum of cardiac disease. Nightly attacks of paroxysmal dyspnea, with sweating, collapse, extreme restlessness, and intractable shortness of breath, cause severe distress. Morphine and potent diuretics are the drugs of choice in the medical management of such patients, but physicians who have had to treat patients at this stage of the disease tend to favor surgical treatment for all patients with significant aortic stenosis, regardless of age.

Dyspnea on exertion is the commonest presenting symptom (75% of cases) in predominant aortic stenosis. As in other forms of left ventricular overload, shortness of breath is quantitatively related to exertion and is often accompanied by a heavy, tight feeling in the chest that is discomfort rather than pain and is only perceived in association with dyspnea. This sensation may occasionally radiate to the arms and is often interpreted as angina pectoris. Dyspnea on effort ordinarily precedes the episodes of paroxysmal nocturnal dyspnea which herald the onset of left ventricular failure. Dizziness (10% of patients) and cardiac pain (10%) are the next most common presenting symptoms of aortic stenosis; syncope on unaccustomed effort is the other principal symptom. It occurs in about 5% of cases, usually early in the disease before the left ventricle has failed. In many patients it only occurs once, because the patient associates the syncope with overexertion and subsequently avoids lifting heavy objects, shoveling snow, running upstairs, or performing whatever activity precipitated the first attack. Loss of consciousness is usually preceded by dyspnea, which the patient disregards, perhaps because of the circumstances surrounding the overexertion. Recovery from the syncopal attack is rapid, and sudden death, which is common in aortic stenosis, seldom occurs. It is of great importance to obtain a clear history of the circumstances surrounding a syncopal episode in a patient suspected of having aortic stenosis. If syncope is provoked only by severe effort, stenosis is already severe. Syncope unrelated to excessive effort is more common than effort syncope in aortic stenosis (10%) but is not necessarily an indication that severe stenosis is present. Such syncope is often due to arrhythmia rather than an inadequate increase in cardiac output during stress. It is often confused with transient cerebral ischemic attacks due to atherosclerosis of the cerebral vessels in patients who have aortic systolic murmurs but no aortic stenosis.

Cardiac pain in patients with aortic stenosis is attributed either to failure of coronary blood flow to meet the increased demands of the hypertrophied left ventricular myocardium or to associated coronary disease in older patients. It is important to distinguish 2 types of cardiac pain in aortic stenosis. The commonest form is a heavy substernal discomfort, described as a bursting, choking, constricting feeling that only comes when the patient is dyspneic. It may occur more readily after meals and radiate to the arms, but it never occurs without dyspnea. It differs from true angina of effort, in which the pain or discomfort is clearly the primary event and occurs before dyspnea. If both of these forms of cardiac distress are termed angina, then the commonest symptom of aortic stenosis is indeed angina. However, if the term angina is reserved for pain that is not associated with or preceded by dyspnea, then angina is the presenting symptom of only 10% of patients with aortic stenosis.

B. Signs: The arterial pulse in patients with predominant aortic stenosis is of small amplitude and is slow-rising because left ventricular ejection time through the narrowed aortic valve is prolonged. Such an arterial pulse is termed an anacrotic pulse, plateau pulse, or pulsus tardus, because the wave takes longer than normal to pass beneath the examiner's fingers. The examiner should also feel the radial, brachial, femoral, and carotid pulses. The carotid pulse, being closest to the aortic valve, gives the most accurate information. The rise time is slowed and the time taken to reach peak pressure is increased in the central pulse in aortic stenosis. Pressure tracings may show an anacrotic notch on the upstroke; the lower on the upstroke it occurs, the more severe the lesion. In patients with mixed lesions in whom there is also aortic incompetence, the upstroke of the pulse is more rapid, and a double-peaked pulse (pulsus bisferiens) may be found (Fig 13–3). Pulsus bisferiens is more likely to be present in a more peripheral artery (eg, radial or brachial) and is not usually seen in the central aortic pulse. The presence of pulsus bisferiens is not of diagnostic significance. Before aortic valve replacement was available, pulsus bisferiens was taken as evidence that aortic incompetence was too severe to warrant aortic valvotomy. This operation, like mitral valvotomy, tended to convert pure stenosis to mixed stenosis and incompetence.

Blood pressure is ordinarily low, with a narrow pulse pressure, and reflects the small stroke volume in aortic stenosis. However, it may be normal, especially in patients with mixed lesions. Systemic hypertension, although uncommon, does not rule out surgically significant aortic stenosis. An *a* wave may be seen in the jugular venous pulse if the ventricular septum bulges to the right and impairs right ventricular filling, or if se-

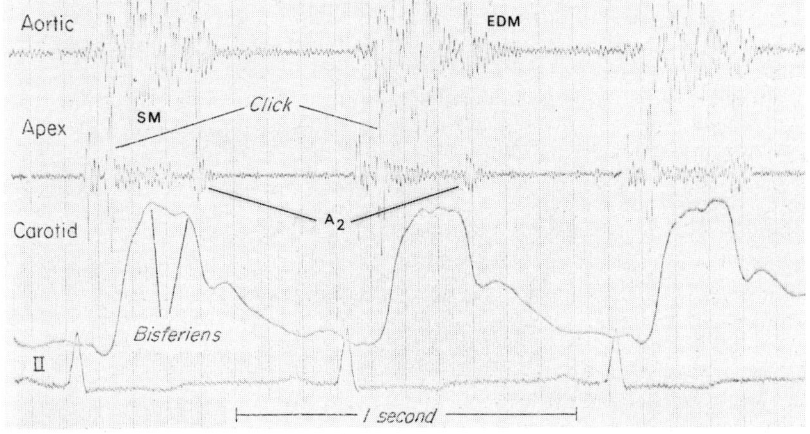

Figure 13–3. Phonocardiogram of a 36-year-old man with aortic stenosis and insufficiency. Note systolic ejection click, crescendo-decrescendo systolic murmur (SM), and short early aortic diastolic murmur (EDM). First sound faint at aortic area. Clinically, thought to be triple rhythm with presystolic gallop. The carotid pulse shows 2 peaks (bisferiens) whose relative heights vary.

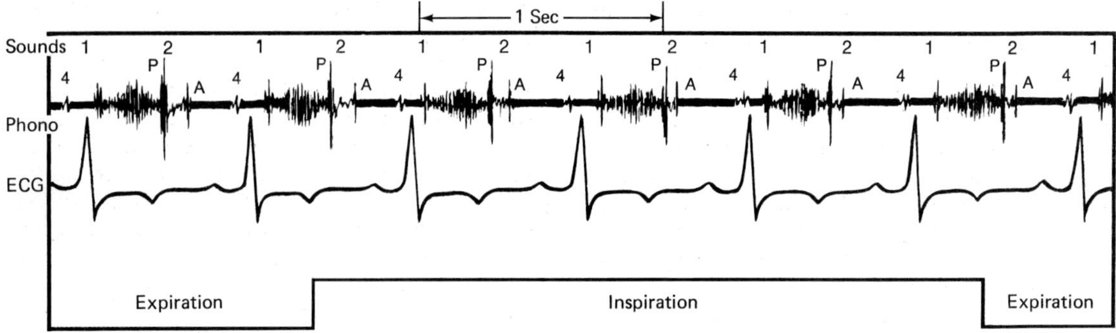

Figure 13–4. Phonocardiogram and ECG in aortic stenosis. The phonocardiogram shows ejection murmur, presystolic gallop (4), soft late A_2, and paradoxic splitting of the second heart sound (2). (Courtesy of Roche Laboratories Division of Hoffman-La Roche, Inc.)

vere pulmonary hypertension develops. The heart rate is usually regular, but about 10% of patients are in atrial fibrillation at the time of surgery. The incidence of atrial fibrillation in cases with a past history of rheumatic fever is no greater than in those with congenitally bicuspid aortic valves, but atrial fibrillation should always alert the physician to the possibility of coexisting associated mitral valve disease. The degree of left ventricular hypertrophy on physical examination—as shown by the prominence of the left ventricular heave—depends on the severity and purity of the stenosis. If the chest wall is thin, a left ventricular heave is readily seen and felt, but in many patients it is necessary to rely on the ECG for evidence of left ventricular hypertrophy. The degree of left ventricular enlargement on physical examination depends largely on the degree of aortic incompetence accompanying the aortic stenosis. The examining hand readily perceives the dynamic quality of the ventricular impulse, which primarily reflects left ventricular stroke volume. The degree of left ventricular enlargement is better detected on the chest x-ray than on physical examination, especially when left ventricular failure has reduced the stroke volume.

Since in most cases the aortic valve is thickened, immobilized by calcification, and stenotic, it does not close properly, and some degree of aortic incompetence is usually present. The greater the incompetence, the larger the heart. Predominant aortic stenosis varies from cases with no incompetence to those with an aortic leak sufficient to give a normal or slightly widened pulse pressure and a slightly hyperdynamic left ventricular impulse.

Depending on the anatomy of the valve, an aortic valve closure sound may or may not be present. If A_2 is audible, paradoxic (reversed) splitting of the second heart sound may be heard if severe stenosis or left bundle branch block is present (Fig 13–4). Third and fourth heart sounds are commonly heard. The characteristic murmur of aortic stenosis is harsh and chugging, and its timing is ejection in nature, starting after isometric contraction has occurred, ie, 0.06 sec or more after the first heart sound (Fig 13–5). It is usually associated with a systolic thrill at the base. It is preceded by an ejection click (Fig 13–3) only in mild cases, when the aortic valve is more flexible and ventricular ejection more rapid. The murmur may be heard at the base or the apex of the heart. It is often heard well in the neck, but this does not mean it is aortic in origin, since pulmonary systolic murmurs and bruits of carotid artery stenosis are also well heard there. The murmur starts after the first heart sound and stops before the second heart sound. It is louder after a long pause following an ectopic beat, and it varies with cardiac filling in atrial fibrillation. It may be audible only at the apex of the heart and can be

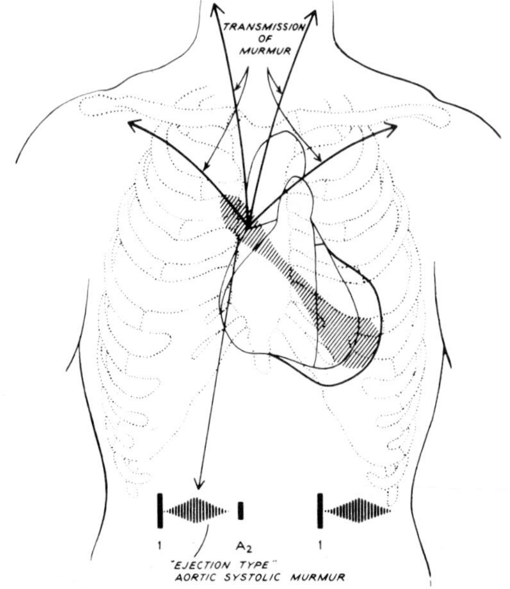

Figure 13–5. Diagram showing auscultatory signs of aortic stenosis. (Reproduced, with permission, from Krupp MA, Chatton MJ [editors]: *Current Medical Diagnosis & Treatment 1977.* Lange, 1977.)

easily missed if the patient is in severe left ventricular failure. A faint aortic diastolic murmur along the left sternal edge is usually present, but its loudness does not necessarily correspond to the severity of associated aortic incompetence, which is judged instead by the character of the pulse, the size of the heart, and the dynamic qualities of the left ventricular impulse.

Rales at the base of the lungs are heard in patients with left ventricular failure, and signs of right ventricular failure with raised jugular venous pressure, hepatomegaly, and peripheral edema are late manifestations of the disease. They are generally due to the development of a raised pulmonary vascular resistance (> 3.5 mm Hg/min), which occurs in a small proportion (about 10%) of cases.

C. Electrocardiographic Findings: ECG evidence of left ventricular hypertrophy is characteristically severe in predominant aortic stenosis. In about 10% of cases, left—or equally commonly—right bundle branch block or even complete block is found. Left bundle branch block interferes with the electrocardiographic recognition of left ventricular hypertrophy, but right bundle branch block does not. Significant aortic stenosis may be present in patients in whom the ECG shows little or no evidence of left ventricular hypertrophy (Fig 13–6). Moderately severe or gross evidence of left ventricular hypertrophy on the ECG is seen in about 75% of cases. Relatively slight ECG changes occur in patients whose stenosis has developed more rapidly and in persons (most often women) who have refrained from physical exertion. Changes due to associated myocardial ischemia or myocardial infarction may be present and make electrocardiographic interpretation difficult.

D. X-Ray Findings: The chest x-ray shows a rounded shadow forming the left border of the heart; this represents the hypertrophied left ventricle. The overall heart shadow is enlarged in patients with left ventricular failure and in those with significant aortic incompetence, but not necessarily in those with early stenotic lesions in whom the left ventricle hypertrophies at the expense of the left ventricular cavity. The progression of the lesion over 10 years is shown in Fig 13–7A and B. Poststenotic dilatation confined to the origin of the ascending aorta is the rule and is produced by the jet of blood from the narrowed aortic valve orifice impinging on the aortic wall. It is best seen on the left anterior oblique view (Fig 13–8). If the jet is not directed to the right, the characteristic poststenotic dilatation is absent. Calcification of the aortic valve, although often visible on the x-ray, should be sought at fluoroscopy. The characteristic dense shadow of the calcified aortic valve lies surprisingly low in the cardiac silhouette, moves up and down with the heartbeat, and lies more medially and less posteriorly than a calcified mitral valve. Cinefluoroscopy should be employed and permanent records of the study maintained. The presence of calcium in the aortic valve can readily be detected during cardiac catheterization when the catheter comes up against the aortic valve, or during angiocardiography. Signs of pulmonary congestion and slight left atrial enlargement are common, but prominence of the pulmonary artery is only seen in a few patients (5%) presenting late in the course of the disease.

E. Special Investigations:

1. Noninvasive technics—Systolic time intervals, indirect carotid pulse tracings, apexcardiography, echo-

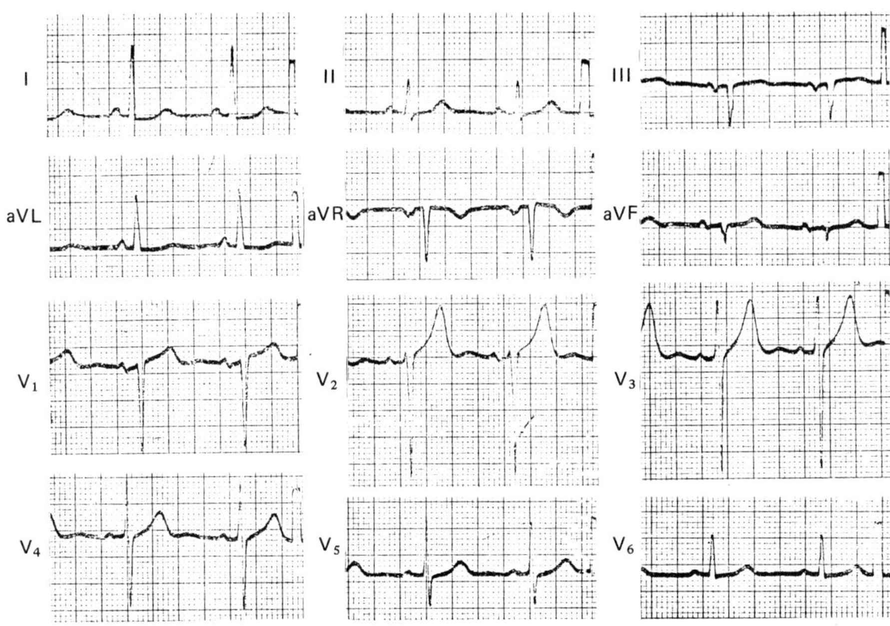

Figure 13–6. ECG of a 77-year-old woman with severe aortic stenosis. Left ventricular pressure 260/5 mm Hg; aortic pressure 130/67 mm Hg. There is little ECG evidence of left ventricular hypertrophy.

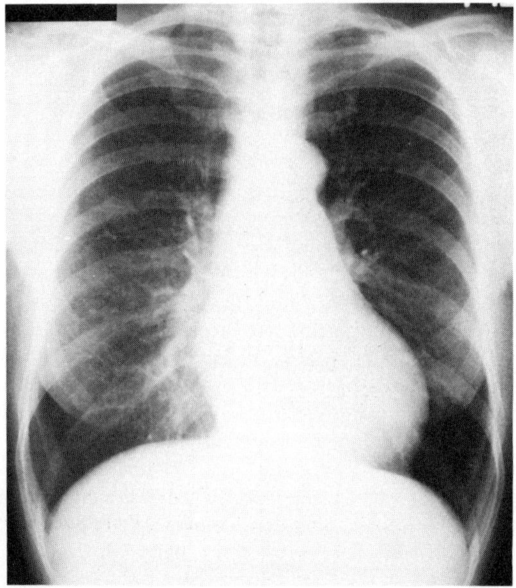

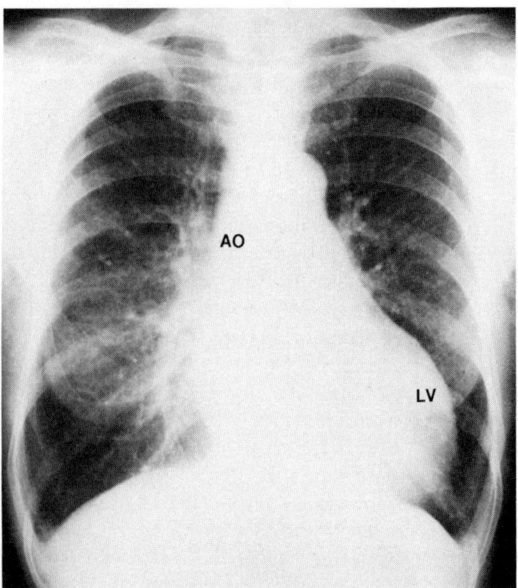

Figure 13-7. Serial chest x-rays of a patient with aortic stenosis taken 10 years apart. The left ventricle (LV) and aorta (AO) are prominent in both x-rays. The heart is larger and the right hilar vessels more prominent in the film shown at right, which was taken after the development of symptoms. Pressure tracings from this patient are shown in Fig 13–10.

cardiography, and exercise testing are all helpful in assessing the severity of aortic stenosis. Echocardiography is most helpful in excluding aortic stenosis by demonstrating that the aortic valve echo is normal. Unfortunately, this form of noninvasive investigation cannot determine the severity of aortic stenosis because it can only detect the thickening and lack of motion of the valve, as shown in Fig 13–9. Abnormalities of the aortic valve with calcification occurring in patients in whom there is no significant obstruction to left ventricular outflow can give echocardiographic findings similar to those in patients with severe stenosis.

Figure 13–8. Chest x-ray showing poststenotic dilatation (PSD) of the aorta on left anterior oblique view in a patient with aortic stenosis.

It is essential to assess the hemodynamic severity of predominant aortic stenosis in all patients suspected of having this lesion, and the fact that one particular noninvasive study can lead to the correct diagnosis in most cases is not sufficient evidence on which to base any crucial therapeutic decision, such as valve replacement.

2. **Invasive technics**–

a. **Right and left heart catheterization**–The definitive study for the assessment of severity is always the measurement of the pressure difference between the left ventricle and the aorta, together with the systolic blood flow across the aortic valve; therefore, left heart catheterization is always indicated. Right heart catheterization may show a large right atrial *a* wave, raised pulmonary arterial pressure, and even moderately raised pulmonary vascular resistance in patients with severe lesions who are seen late in the course of the disease. In most cases, the right-sided pressures are normal, and the left atrial (wedge) pressure shows a large left atrial *a* wave due to increased force of left atrial contraction against a poorly compliant left ventricle. Left heart catheterization is most commonly performed using the retrograde aortic route following cutdown on the right brachial artery.

Retrograde percutaneous femoral arterial catheterization is less often successful. Transseptal catheterization passing a catheter across the mitral valve into

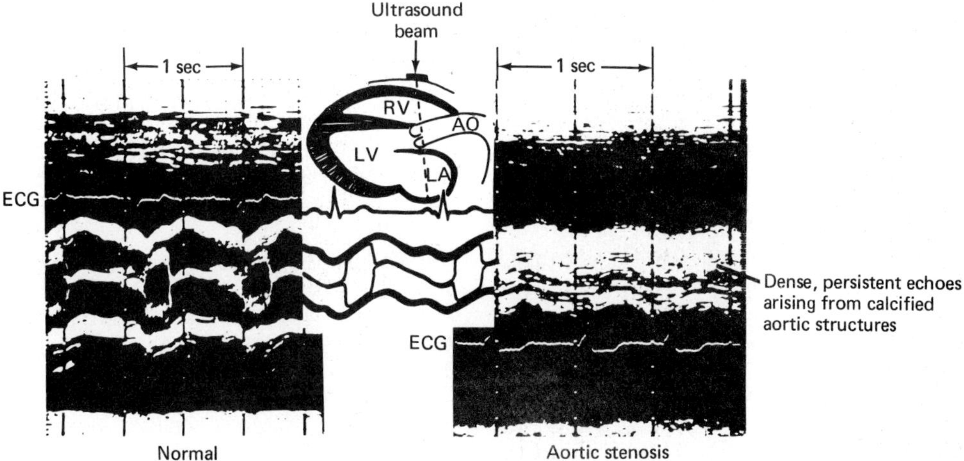

Figure 13–9. Comparison of echocardiograms of normal and stenotic aortic valves. RV, right ventricle; AO, aorta; LV, left ventricle; LA, left atrium. (Reproduced, with permission, from Kleid J, Schiller NB: *Echocardiography Case Studies.* Medical Examination Publishing Company, 1974.)

the left ventricle and simultaneous retrograde aortic catheterization are preferred in some centers, and this approach succeeds in about 85% of cases. It is important to measure left ventricular pressure, aortic pressure, and cardiac output simultaneously. An example of left ventricular and aortic pressure tracings in a patient with severe aortic stenosis is shown in Fig 13–10. Calculation of the valve area by the Gorlin formula is the most valuable index of severity. As in mitral disease, the presence of incompetence invalidates the measurement of valve area, but the Gorlin formula can provide a minimal value for valve area if it is assumed that incompetence is absent.

If it proves difficult to pass a catheter across the aortic valve, supravalvular angiography may be helpful in indicating the position of the aortic valve orifice, but the angiographic findings cannot be used as an indication of the severity of stenosis. In retrograde

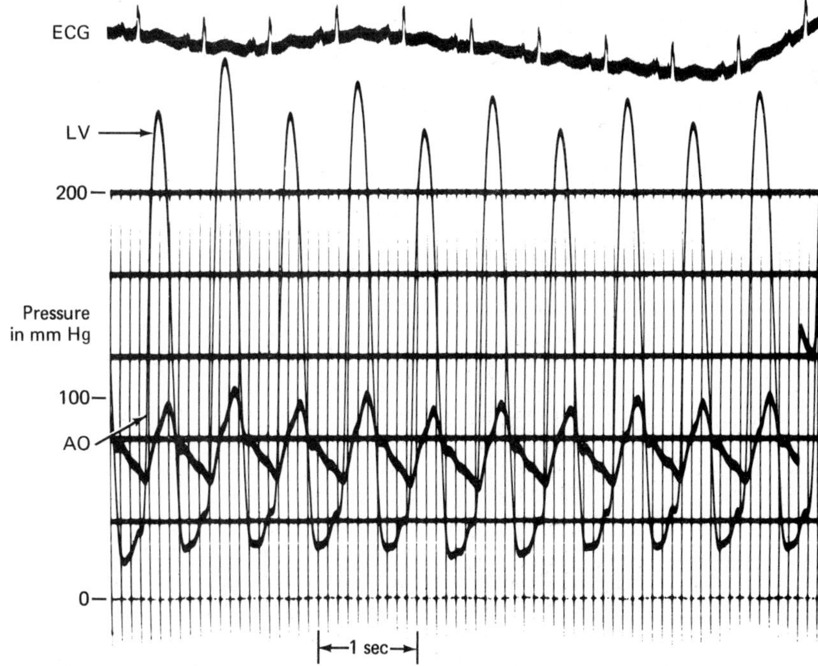

Figure 13–10. Simultaneous left ventricular (LV 270–240/40) and aortic (AO 100/60) pressure tracings in the patient whose chest x-rays are shown in Fig 13–7A and B. Pulsus alternans is present and is more prominent on the left ventricular tracing.

studies, the severity of aortic stenosis does not correlate directly with the ease with which a catheter can be passed across a stenotic valve. The degree of aortic dilatation and the position of the valve are more important factors in determining success of the procedure. Passing a catheter across the aortic valve in a patient with aortic stenosis constitutes the most frequent and difficult problem in cardiac catheterization in acquired heart disease.

b. **Left ventricular puncture**—When retrograde aortic catheterization fails, direct left ventricular puncture via the apex of the heart is indicated. In some centers, transseptal catheterization may be tried before resorting to this procedure, but in most hospitals the last resort is left ventricular puncture. The procedure is performed with a 20 gauge lumbar puncture needle under fluoroscopic control, using 50–100 mg of intravenous meperidine as an analgesic. It is surprisingly well tolerated and usually painless. Satisfactory tracings are obtained in about 85% of cases, and since the left ventricle is almost invariably hypertrophied, the dangers of hemorrhage and tamponade are minimal. A small pneumothorax is the most frequent complication and occurs in about 10% of cases. The patient must be monitored for several hours after the procedure in order to detect any early evidence of complications.

c. **Selective coronary angiography**—Some cardiologists advocate coronary arteriography in all patients with aortic stenosis. If the surgeon plans to perfuse the coronary arteries, the investigation may indeed be indicated in order to confirm that the anatomy of the main branches of the coronary vessels is normal. In general, however, the state of the coronary vessels alters the prognosis of aortic stenosis but not the treatment or the decision to operate, which depend on the severity of the obstruction. Because coronary arteriography increases the morbidity and mortality rate of an already difficult investigation, it is not advised in patients with severe or moderately severe aortic stenosis. In cases in which the hemodynamic severity of the stenosis does not definitely warrant surgery, coronary angiography can help the cardiologist decide whether or not to operate. Coronary angiography is definitely indicated in those patients with prominent angina pectoris or in those who have suffered myocardial infarction. Coronary angiography is sometimes advocated as a routine measure because patients may prove to need an aortocoronary bypass when adequate systemic circulation cannot be restored following valve replacement. However, since the mortality rate of aortic valve replacement in aortic stenosis is less than 5%, the possible morbidity and mortality imposed by coronary angiography outweigh the possible benefits. In our opinion, only a specific reason such as angina pectoris or previous myocardial infarction warrants coronary angiography in a patient with predominant aortic stenosis. However, this view may have to be modified in the light of increasing experience with older patients (over age 70).

F. Hemodynamic Values: The means and standard deviations of measurements obtained during cardiac catheterization in patients with predominant aortic stenosis are shown in Table 13–1. In addition to the values in the entire group of patients, the results have been broken down in 2 subgroups: those with clear evidence of left ventricular failure and those without. This difference is not reflected in the length of history, the cardiac output, or the hemodynamic severity of the stenosis, but only in the level of the wedge pressure.

Diagnosis

The most pressing problems in the diagnosis of aortic stenosis are (1) to detect when left ventricular failure will occur in the course of the disease, (2) to accurately assess the severity of stenosis, and (3) to decide whether to recommend surgery for asymptomatic and mildly symptomatic patients. The presence of left ventricular hypertrophy on the ECG or physical examination may raise the possibility of surgery but is not an absolute indication for further clinical investigation, since a patient with the disease can be asymptomatic for up to 20 years with moderate left ventricular hypertrophy.

On the other hand, the possibility that dyspnea, syncope, dizziness, or cardiac pain is due to aortic stenosis is a strong indication for left heart catheterization. Echocardiography can reduce the number of patients in whom cardiac catheterization is performed by showing that the aortic valve is thin and mobile, but it cannot be used to establish a diagnosis of aortic stenosis. The physician must maintain a strong index of suspicion and a sense of urgency in dealing with patients whose symptoms may be due to aortic stenosis, because delay is more dangerous in aortic stenosis than in any other cardiac lesion in adults. There is no substitute for left heart catheterization as a means of determining the severity of obstruction; physical signs, an ECG, presence of aortic valve calcification, aortic angiography, and the shape or movement of the valve on

Table 13–1. Cardiac catheterization data, including length of history, in patients with predominant aortic stenosis.

	Mean Wedge Pressure (mm Hg)	Left Ventricular Systolic Pressure (mm Hg)	Aortic Systolic Pressure (mm Hg)	Aortic Diastolic Pressure (mm Hg)	Cardiac Output (l/min)	Length of History (Years)
Predominant aortic stenosis	20 ± 10	208 ± 40	132 ± 28	69 ± 13	4.7 ± 1.5	2.4 ± 2.0
Without left ventricular failure	13 ± 6	215 ± 40	138 ± 26	73 ± 14	4.8 ± 1.5	2.2 ± 1.8
With left ventricular failure	28 ± 9	202 ± 41	126 ± 29	85 ± 13	4.6 ± 1.5	2.6 ± 2.2

echocardiography are all incapable of providing consistently correct assessments of severity, although they may lead to a correct diagnosis in 85% of cases.

Differential Diagnosis

A. Left Ventricular Failure: Aortic stenosis enters into the differential diagnosis of all patients with left ventricular failure, especially when there is a basal systolic murmur and a history of syncope, dizziness, or heart block. The possibility of aortic stenosis must be considered in hypertension, cardiomyopathy, and even in coronary artery disease, especially when heart failure is severe. It is important to recognize the systolic murmur and rule out the possibility of aortic stenosis by all available means, including cardiac catheterization. In many centers, all patients with cardiomyopathy undergo cardiac catheterization in order to rule out aortic stenosis.

B. Hypertrophic Obstructive Cardiomyopathy: Aortic stenosis should not be confused with hypertrophic obstructive cardiomyopathy. In the latter condition (see Chapter 17, p 522), the pulse is jerky and the upstroke rapid and often bifid, in contrast to the slow-rising pulse of aortic stenosis. If there is associated aortic incompetence modifying the upstroke of the pulse in a patient with predominant aortic stenosis, there will almost certainly be an aortic diastolic murmur, which virtually rules out a diagnosis of obstructive cardiomyopathy. The murmur of hypertrophic cardiomyopathy is longer and harsher and usually heard best to the left of the sternum. The variation occurring in the murmur when diagnostic measures are used to influence the extent of outflow tract narrowing is helpful in establishing the diagnosis of obstructive cardiomyopathy. Echocardiography is particularly helpful in differential diagnosis because it shows systolic anterior motion of the mitral valve in hypertrophic cardiomyopathy and aortic valve thickening in aortic stenosis. Left heart catheterization and left ventricular angiography are generally used to confirm the diagnosis.

C. Other Lesions: The physical signs in mitral incompetence and ventricular septal defect are seldom confused with those of predominant aortic stenosis. In these disorders, the murmur is pansystolic, and the carotid upstroke is rapid. When the patient has both aortic stenosis and mitral incompetence, it is difficult to distinguish between them, and clinical assessment of the relative severity of the 2 lesions is usually impossible. In some cases there is a characteristic high-pitched "seagull cry" murmur (see p 413).

Coarctation of the aorta is another lesion which may occasionally coexist with aortic stenosis and be confused with it. The murmur of coarctation occurs later in systole and reaches its peak about the time of the second heart sound. There is characteristically a prominent carotid arterial pulsation as well as delay between the peaks of the brachial and femoral pulses, with hypertension in the arms (see Chapter 11). Although coarctation of the aorta is commonly associated with bicuspid aortic valve, the coarctation is likely to cause problems long before the abnormal valve gives rise to difficulties that are associated with the development of aortic stenosis resulting from calcification of the abnormal valve.

Complications

A. Sudden Death: Patients with predominant aortic stenosis are likely to die suddenly. The incidence of sudden death is unknown and is likely to be underestimated. As in other forms of sudden death, the mechanisms involved are difficult to investigate. Sudden death is clearly not confined to patients with severe stenosis, since it is one of the common causes of late death following aortic valve replacement. This finding suggests that residual myocardial damage may cause arrhythmias or that valve malfunction may occur acutely. The general consensus is that arrhythmia is responsible for most cases of sudden death in aortic stenosis. In aortic stenosis, the effects of a sudden fall in arterial pressure resulting from arrhythmia are probably greater than normal for both mechanical and reflex reasons. In terms of mechanics, cardiac output takes longer to return to normal after an arrhythmia has developed. In terms of reflexes, the central nervous system tends to receive contradictory information from the carotid and aortic baroreceptors on the one hand and the left ventricular stretch receptors (von Bezold receptors) on the other because left ventricular pressure is high and aortic pressure is relatively low.

B. Left Ventricular Failure: Left ventricular failure is an almost inevitable consequence of aortic stenosis and occurs relatively late. It is the strongest possible indication for surgical treatment because it is consistently relieved by surgery. Medical measures for its control should be regarded as part of the preoperative preparation and not as a substitute for surgery.

C. Heart Block: Complete atrioventricular block occasionally complicates aortic stenosis, and its association with slow heart rates and large stroke volumes makes clinical assessment of the lesion difficult. The hemodynamic signs of aortic stenosis seem more severe when the heart rate is slow. The heart is larger, the systolic murmur and thrill are more impressive, and the pressure difference between the left ventricle and the aorta is greater. These factors may require that cardiac pacing be performed to study the effects of changes in heart rate on hemodynamic findings. Usually, however, all that is necessary is a calculation of the aortic valve area by means of the Gorlin formula, since the heart rate does not influence the calculation of valve area.

D. Infective Endocarditis: Infective endocarditis is an important but rare complication of aortic stenosis. It occurs in about 2% of cases and is less common than in mitral or aortic incompetence. It is more important in the presymptomatic stage of the disease, when the valve is more readily damaged by the infective process.

Treatment

A. Medical Treatment: It is important that the treatment for left ventricular failure in aortic stenosis not be restricted to medical means. Surgery is the first and not the last resort. Digitalis, diuretics, and salt restriction are effective in left ventricular failure caused by aortic stenosis, and they should be used preoperatively. However, the marked benefit that follows their use should not prompt the physician to delay surgery, as this merely increases the mortality rate of any subsequent operation. Surgical treatment in severe aortic stenosis is a matter of some urgency. Patients not infrequently die while waiting for the completion of a clinical investigation or for surgery.

B. Surgical Treatment:

1. Aortic valve replacement—Replacement of the aortic valve is required in all patients with moderate or severe stenosis (pressure difference 50 mm Hg or more or aortic valve area 0.8 cm^2 or less). Age is no bar to surgery, and the discomfort of intractable left ventricular failure should be avoided if at all possible. In young patients (under age 30), palliative open aortic valvotomy may be justified because the long-term hazards of valve replacement are not yet known. The physician should remember that after valvotomy a second operation to replace the aortic valve will almost certainly be necessary in a decade or two.

The choice of artificial valve rests with the surgeon. Homograft, heterograft, ball, flap, and disk valves have been used (Fig 13–11). The Starr-Edwards ball and cage valve has been used most frequently and has proved most successful. It is generally thought that homograft and heterograft tissue valves do not require postoperative anticoagulant therapy indefinitely, as opposed to all types of prosthetic valves, in which lifetime anticoagulation is needed. The mortality rate of aortic valve replacement depends on the stage of the disease at the time of surgery; the average is 5–10%. The mortality rate is greatest in patients with marked left ventricular hypertrophy or severe heart failure.

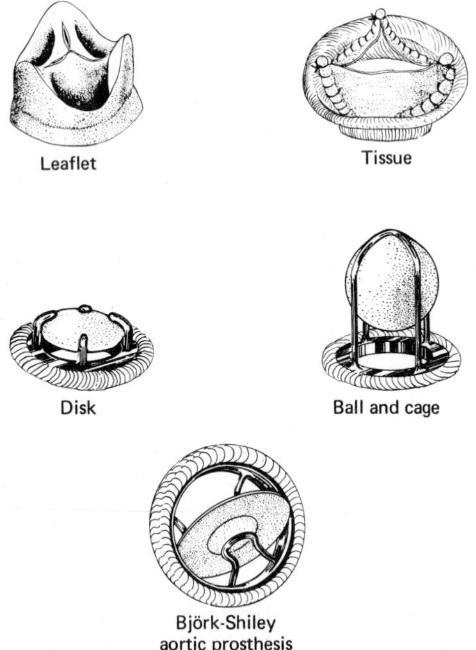

Figure 13–11. Examples of artificial heart valves. (Reproduced, with permission, from Dunphy JE, Way LW [editors]: *Current Surgical Diagnosis & Treatment,* 3rd ed. Lange, 1977.)

2. Surgical treatment of nonvalvular lesions—Supravalvular aortic stenosis is more difficult to treat than valvular stenosis because the ascending aorta is often hypoplastic. Congenital subvalvular ring stenosis can be excised, bringing dramatic relief. Valve replacement is not needed.

3. Results of surgery—Like the mortality rate, the results of surgical treatment vary depending on when operation is performed and whether coronary artery disease or other valve lesions are present. If the left ventricle is markedly dilated as a result of longstanding left ventricular failure, results will be worse than in early cases with hearts of normal size. Ideally, patients should be closely followed and operation recommended at the first sign of significant symptoms. In practice, however, diagnosis is made late in the course of the disease in about half of cases, usually because the patient does not seek help, and sometimes because the correct diagnosis is missed.

Prognosis

The prognosis in aortic stenosis after the development of signs and symptoms of heart failure is poor. With modern treatment of heart failure, the patient may live for up to 8 years, but distressing episodes of recurrent left ventricular failure with pulmonary edema make the average survival time shorter. The long-term (20-year) results of aortic valve replacement are not yet known, but a reasonable number of patients have lived for 10 years or more with Starr-Edwards valves. The long-term results of homograft valves are less satisfactory because the cusps of the valves tend to stiffen with time, and the valves leak after several years. Fresh homograft aortic valves are difficult to obtain and store. Consequently, enthusiasm for this form of valve replacement has been highest in the small number of centers that have had more experience with its use. The more recently introduced porcine heterograft valves do not yet have an established position in the hierarchy of surgical treatments.

When the long-term results of valve replacement are better known, it may become reasonable to recommend surgery in earlier cases, but at present definite symptoms must be noted before surgery can be advised. In order to elicit the degree of disability and show that the lesion is severe, it may be necessary to perform studies while the patient is exercising. In some stoic patients the physician must exert pressure to persuade the patient to submit to study and operation. Aortic valve replacement for predominant stenosis is the most satisfactory of all valve replacement operations and will probably become a prophylactic measure within the next few years.

PREDOMINANT AORTIC INCOMPETENCE

The cardinal features of hemodynamically significant predominant aortic incompetence (Fig 13–12) include a large hypertrophied left ventricle, a large aorta, increased stroke volume, and wide pulse pressure. Variable factors include the severity of the process, the nature of the lesion (acute or chronic), and the cause.

Hemodynamically significant aortic incompetence creates an important extra load on the left ventricle. The blood that flows back aross the aortic valve during diastole must be ejected during systole, and the consequent large stroke volume increases the work of the heart. The extra work is mainly "flow" work rather than "pressure" work, but peak systolic pressure tends to be raised and aortic diastolic pressure lowered because of rapid runoff of aortic blood into the peripheral arterial bed and back into the left ventricle. The arbitrary basis on which aortic incompetence is classified as hemodynamically significant here is the level of diastolic pressure. As stated on p 387, a value of less than 70 mm Hg constitutes the dividing line, and patients with aortic incompetence and arterial diastolic pressures higher than that are generally considered to have hemodynamically insignificant aortic incompetence. Exceptions do exist, especially in patients in severe heart failure, in whom peripheral vasoconstriction has occurred and caused an increase in diastolic pressure.

Acute Lesions

Aortic incompetence occurs both as an acute lesion (20% of cases) and as a single chronic lesion (80% of cases). Acute aortic incompetence occurs when valve lesions develop either instantaneously–when a cusp perforates or tears–or over a few days or weeks–when valve tissue is gradually eroded by infection, or when fibrosis, associated with healing of an infection, scars and contracts the valve. Acute aortic incompetence throws a more serious load on the left ventricle than acute mitral incompetence, and the chances that the patient's hemodynamic status will stabilize without surgical treatment are small. If the damage is less severe or less acute, the possibility for survival is better; and if the patient survives, the clinical picture in acute aortic incompetence by the end of about one year resembles that in chronic lesions. The hemodynamic load in acute lesions tends to fall mainly on the lungs, and acute left ventricular failure usually develops before left ventricular hypertrophy or dilatation has had time to occur. If the patient has marked pulmonary edema, the peripheral signs of aortic incompetence, with wide pulse pressure and low diastolic pressure, may be masked because arteriolar vasoconstriction has occurred in response to impaired perfusion, but there should still be an obvious aortic diastolic murmur.

Chronic Lesions

Chronic aortic incompetence results in marked peripheral vasodilatation, which is attributable in part to reflex baroreceptor effects. The wide aortic and carotid pulse pressures cause reflex vasodilatation and relative bradycardia. With exercise, the cardiac output increases, there is peripheral vasodilatation of the muscular capillaries, and a further fall in systemic vascular resistance occurs. As a result, the proportion of the left ventricular stroke volume returning to the left ventricle during diastole falls, and the hemodynamic status becomes closer to that seen in normal subjects. In contrast, anything that increases the systemic vascular resistance, such as isometric exercise, exposure to cold, sympathetic nervous system stimulation, mental stress, or cardiac failure, tends to increase the volume of blood returning to the ventricle during diastole and makes the load on the heart more a "pressure" load and less a "flow" load.

Left Ventricular Hypertrophy & Dilatation

Aortic incompetence leads to left ventricular dilatation, which constitutes an important stimulus to hypertrophy of the left ventricular muscle. Hypertrophy involves an increase in the size of muscle cells and an increase in the connective tissue elements of the heart. In time, long-standing hypertrophy almost inevitably leads to myocardial fibrosis and becomes irreversible, so that heart muscle cells do not return to normal when the stimulus causing the hypertrophy is removed. With time, the left ventricle fails, probably as a result of myocardial fibrosis and age-related changes in ventricular muscle. This occurs relatively late in the course of chronic lesions. The development of ventricular failure is influenced by the severity of the incompetence and the state of myocardium, which in turn depend on the degree of atherosclerosis or the extent of rheumatic myocardial damage. It is also possible that the patient's activity level may play a part; earlier failure may develop in patients with more strenuous occupations. When it occurs, left ventricular failure is often acute and severe because reflex vasoconstriction takes the place of the normal vasodilatation seen in chronic lesions, and it further aggravates ventricular failure by increasing systemic vascular resistance and hence the amount of incompetence. The most striking clinical manifestations of left ventricular failure are an increase in arterial diastolic pressure and the change from vasodilatation to vasoconstriction that often accompanies failure and tends to obscure peripheral signs of aortic incompetence.

Causes of Aortic Incompetence

A. Acute Lesions: The most important cause of acute aortic incompetence is infective endocarditis. Patients with initially normal aortic valves may contract infective endocarditis when the organism is highly invasive or when the patient is debilitated because of immunosuppressive therapy, chronic illness, or intravenous drug abuse; in these cases, organisms of minimal pathogenicity may be the infective agent. Infective endocarditis also affects valves that are already diseased as a result of rheumatic or congenital involvement. The milder the original valve disease, the greater the potential for acute hemodynamic deterioration.

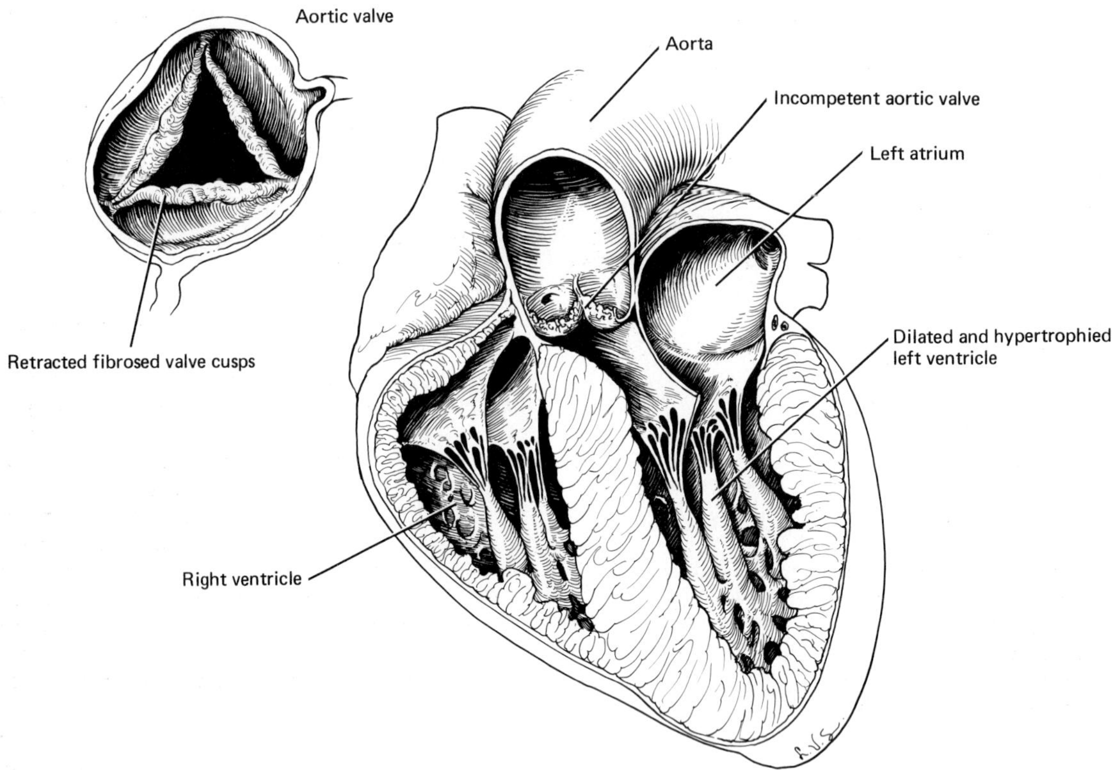

Drawing of left heart in left anterior oblique view showing anatomic features of aortic incompetence.

Cardinal features: *Large hypertrophied left ventricle; large aorta; increased stroke volume; wide pulse pressure.*

Variable factors: *Severity; acuteness or chronicity; cause.*

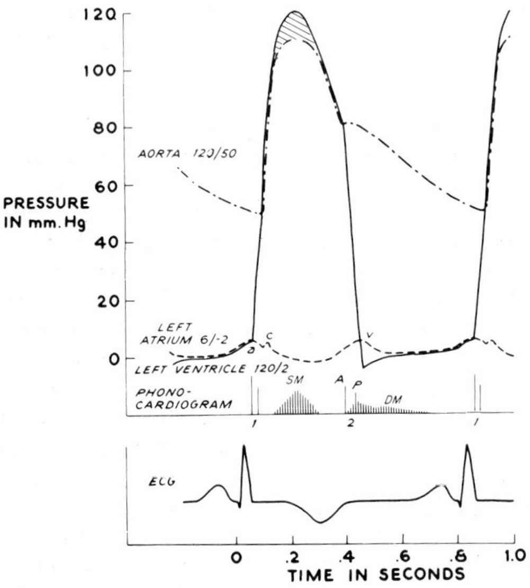

Diagram showing auscultatory and hemodynamic features of predominant aortic incompetence.

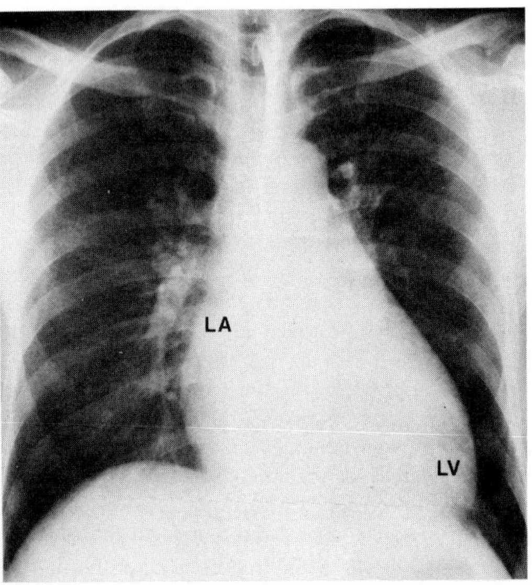

Chest x-ray of a patient with aortic incompetence and no signs of left heart failure. The long shadow of the enlarged left ventricle (LV) and slight left atrial (LA) enlargement can be seen.

Figure 13–12. Aortic incompetence. Structures enlarged: Left ventricle, aorta.

Thus, patients with severe chronic aortic incompetence are at less risk than those with mild lesions, not from the point of view of infection or its control but from the dangers of acute exacerbation of aortic incompetence.

The only other major cause of acute aortic incompetence is aortic dissection. In this condition, a tear in the aortic intima extends to the neighborhood of the noncoronary cusp of the aortic valve and causes the valve lesion. The cystic medial necrosis of Marfan's syndrome, aortic atherosclerosis with hypertension, and arteritis are the main causes of aortic dissection.

B. Chronic Lesions: Chronic aortic incompetence has several causes and occurs at all ages. It is more common in males by a factor of 3:2 and appears in our experience to be the commonest valvular lesion in black males. Rheumatic fever probably still accounts for the majority of cases. If it is assumed that rheumatic fever is subclinical in 50% of cases, a confirmed history of previous rheumatic fever in 25% of cases of chronic aortic incompetence indicates that about half of cases are rheumatic in origin.

Syphilis is a decreasingly common cause of aortic incompetence, but it is still found in 10% of cases. The average age of these patients is over 60 years, and associated atherosclerosis is almost always present.

Cases in which a congenital cause is confirmed account for about 10%, but this may be an underestimate; a congenital cause should be suspected when associated lesions such as ventricular septal defect, patent ductus arteriosus, or coarctation of the aorta are seen, when noncardiac congenital lesions such as Marfan's syndrome are present, or when the murmur is heard in infancy.

Ankylosing spondylitis and Reiter's syndrome are rare causes of aortic incompetence (5% of cases) in which the atrioventricular conduction system may be involved. The characteristic hip or sacroiliac joint involvement of ankylosing spondylitis may precede or follow the valve lesion and is sometimes only detected on x-ray examination.

Hypertension and atherosclerosis are rarely (3% of cases) the cause of hemodynamically significant aortic incompetence. More commonly these conditions produce an aortic diastolic murmur, with only slight widening of the aortic pulse pressure and no lowering of the aortic diastolic pressure.

Clinical Findings

In rheumatic lesions, fibrosis and retraction of the valve cusps start early in the course of rheumatic infection and progress slowly over several years. Syphilis attacks the aortic valve secondarily, by extension of disease from the aorta. Endarteritis obliterans of the vasa vasorum of the aorta is the basic pathologic lesion of syphilitic aortitis, and aortic dilatation with swelling and thickening of the intima involves the root of the aorta and perhaps also the coronary ostia, leading to myocardial ischemia. In congenital lesions, the valve lesion is often secondary to aortic dilatation, as in Marfan's syndrome, or to prolapse of unsupported valvular tissue, as in association with ventricular septal defects involving the membranous part of the interventricular septum. There is no associated myocarditis in congenital cases; as a result, muscle damage is less prominent. In ankylosing spondylitis and Reiter's syndrome, the pathologic lesion is again primarily in the aorta and in the connective tissues supporting the valve. In atherosclerotic lesions, too, it is aortic involvement that secondarily affects the valve, principally by means of dilatation.

A. Symptoms:

1. Acute lesions—Dyspnea is the commonest presenting cardiac symptom in acute lesions (50% of cases). Since infective endocarditis is by far the commonest cause, the patient usually is febrile and may be acutely ill with septicemia at the time that the aortic valve lesion develops. In other cases, the onset is slower and subacute: the aortic lesion appears or worsens as endocarditis heals, and the valve shrinks as it fibroses weeks or months after the endocarditis has responded to antibiotic therapy. In other patients, systemic embolism may be the presenting symptom, with a cerebrovascular accident, an acute coronary occlusion, or a cold, painful leg as the first sign of acute aortic incompetence. Acute aortic incompetence occurring in a person who is not ill with infective endocarditis suggests the possibility of acute aortic dissection involving the noncoronary cusp of the aortic valve. This uncommon lesion is not always painful. If either the left or right coronary artery is involved, the patient almost inevitably dies.

The dyspnea of acute aortic incompetence is often paroxysmal and associated with orthopnea and cough, with frothy pink sputum due to acute pulmonary edema. Chest pain may occur because of acute myocardial ischemia and peripheral circulatory collapse. Symptoms of shock, with anxiety, confusion, and mental obtundation are occasionally seen.

2. Chronic lesions—

a. Symptoms unrelated to severity—There are 2 varieties of symptoms in chronic aortic incompetence, those due to the patient's awareness of increased force of the heartbeat and those due to left ventricular disease and heart failure. One-third of patients with hemodynamically significant aortic incompetence not infrequently complain of palpitations, which on questioning turn out to be associated with sensations arising from forceful left ventricular contraction. The patient often notices the symptoms when lying in bed at night. These sensations sometimes provoke the symptoms of anxiety seen in cardiac neurosis, with stabbing inframammary pain, fatigue, and dyspnea with sighing respirations. The patient may have ventricular premature beats that further accentuate the symptoms. These symptoms usually occur in early adult life and can be present for 20 years or more without significant progression of the valvular lesion. More frequently (two-thirds of cases), the patient has no symptoms and is able to lead a surprisingly normal, active life in spite of a hemodynamically serious lesion. It is important to recognize certain symptoms as "functional" in patients with aortic incompetence and not interpret them as a necessary indication for surgery. Ventricular arrhythmia is probably the most important cause of symptoms at this stage since it is thought that it may precede ventricular tachycardia or fibrillation, and these developments may account for the sudden death that is rarer in aortic incompetence than in stenosis but which nevertheless occurs. The presence of symptoms in a patient with aortic incompetence is always an indication for thorough investigation; but if the valvular lesion is well tolerated, the patient (especially if young) should usually simply be closely followed, and the physician should watch for the development of more serious symptoms.

b. **Symptoms of left ventricular failure**–When aortic incompetence is the sole lesion, serious symptoms due to left ventricular failure occur late in the course of the disease. Dyspnea is by far the commonest symptom (75% of cases) and may be associated with a feeling of heaviness in the chest and substernal discomfort. If significant dyspnea occurs before age 30 and left ventricular failure is found, it is most likely that past or present rheumatic myocardial involvement is influencing the clinical picture. Left ventricular failure due solely to chronic aortic incompetence usually occurs after age 40, and patients who lead sedentary lives may not be aware of the insidious progression of pulmonary congestion because they have never exerted themselves sufficiently. In these patients, an acute episode of paroxysmal nocturnal dyspnea or frank pulmonary edema may be the presenting event. Chest pain is the next most common symptom in aortic incompetence. It is particularly common in patients with syphilitic lesions and in older persons with associated coronary arterial disease. Anginal pain may be present at rest or during exercise; in general, it is due to increased metabolic demands of the hypertrophied myocardium rather than to decreased supply resulting from obstructive atherosclerotic lesions in major coronary vessels. Syncope and dizziness are less common than in patients with predominantly stenotic lesions, and syncope during unaccustomed effort (the type seen in aortic stenosis) does not occur.

c. **Development of left ventricular failure**–The late symptoms in aortic incompetence carry a poor prognosis. This is in part due to reflex factors that cause a vicious cycle. When cardiac output falls as the left ventricle fails, the normal peripheral vasodilatation seen in aortic incompetence is replaced by vasoconstriction because the carotid and aortic baroreceptors no longer transmit inhibitory sensory information via the glossopharyngeal nerve. This peripheral vasoconstriction increases the work of the left ventricle, increases aortic incompetence, and aggravates left ventricular failure. The relatively high arterial diastolic pressure that results may mislead the physician into thinking that significant aortic incompetence is not present. Left ventricular failure is thus especially sudden in aortic incompetence and is often provoked by factors involving autonomic nervous system control of blood pressure and blood volume, such as excitement, excessive sodium intake, recumbency, overexertion, excessive mental stress, and violent dreams, all of which cause a rise in systemic arterial pressure. The patient's occupation may also influence the occurrence of left ventricular failure. Patients with strenuous jobs involving heavy manual labor may develop larger hearts corresponding to a given level of severity in the lesion and hence develop left ventricular failure earlier than patients who avoid excessive exertion. The role of mental stress may also be important in patients with this lesion, because it is increased systemic arterial pressure and increased peripheral resistance that tend to aggravate incompetence more than any increase in cardiac output.

d. **Sweating**–Patients with predominant aortic incompetence have a tendency to sweat more, a finding that is unexplained. The mechanism is thought to involve the cholinergic sympathetic vasodilator fibers and be in some way related to the wide pulse pressure, since a similar tendency is seen in other high output states such as thyrotoxicosis and Paget's disease.

B. Signs: The rapid runoff of blood from the aorta during diastole dominates the physical signs of hemodynamically significant aortic incompetence. Prominent carotid pulsations in the neck, throbbing peripheral arteries, and a prominent left ventricular impulse that moves the whole left side of the chest produce easily visible evidence of the large left ventricular stroke volume and increased rate of systolic ejection seen in this lesion. These peripheral circulatory signs are seen in both acute and chronic lesions and are present in all patients except those in severe left ventricular failure. The rapid aortic runoff is due to increased blood flow back into the left ventricle and into the dilated peripheral arterial bed. It is important to remember that rapid runoff from the aorta into cardiac chambers or blood vessels other than the left ventricle is an equally potent cause of the peripheral signs ordinarily associated with aortic incompetence. Large patent ductus arteriosus, aortopulmonary window, rupture of an aneurysm of the aortic sinus (sinus of Valsalva) with consequent left-to-right shunt, or a major systemic arteriovenous fistula may produce similar physical signs.

Systemic arterial pressure is the most readily measured indication of the severity of the peripheral signs of rapid aortic runoff. There is a wide pulse pressure, with high systolic and low diastolic pressure. Arterial pressure measured indirectly with a blood pressure cuff is not always accurate, and a diastolic pressure reading of zero, indicating that there is an audible sound over the artery with no cuff in position, is never an accurate physical finding although it is often seen in patients with aortic incompetence. The wide pulse pressure gives rise to the typical collapsing pulse in which the pulse wave rises rapidly to a peak and falls away quickly. Secondary physical signs due to rapid aortic runoff are numerous and usually have eponymic designations. Head movement in time with the heartbeat is called Musset's sign after the French poet Alfred de Musset, in whom it was noticed by his brother, who was a physician. Quincke's pulse denotes capillary pulsation in the extremities; Duroziez's sign refers to systolic and diastolic murmurs over the femoral artery; and Hill's sign denotes increased blood pressure in the legs above that measured in the arms. Corrigan's pulse refers to the collapsing pulse, which is also called a "water-hammer" pulse after a 19th century child's toy of that name. Pulsations in the digital and ulnar arteries are readily felt, and the hands and feet are warm and sweaty.

It is important to remember that rapid aortic runoff is a nonspecific clinical finding. Pulsation can also be seen in the second and third intercostal spaces to the right of the sternum when the aorta is dilated, especially in syphilitic lesions with or without associated aortic dissections. It is seen best from the side of the bed, with the examiner's eye at chest level.

In chronic aortic incompetence, the left ventricular impulse is heaving and hyperdynamic, and the apex beat is displaced downward and to the left. These physical signs depend largely on the size of the heart and are less obvious in acute aortic incompetence in which left ventricular hypertrophy has not yet developed. The characteristic physical sign on auscultation is a high-pitched, blowing diastolic murmur beginning immediately after the second sound at the start of diastole (Fig 13–13). It is called an "immediate" diastolic murmur to distinguish it from the "delayed" diastolic murmur of mitral stenosis, which does not start until left ventricular pressure has fallen below the level of left atrial pressure, ie, about 0.1 sec after the start of diastole. The diastolic murmur of aortic incompetence lasts until backflow through the valve stops;

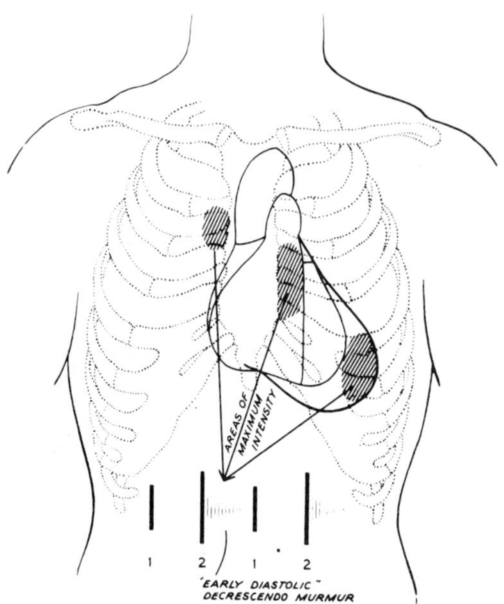

Figure 13–13. Diagram showing auscultatory signs of aortic incompetence. (Reproduced, with permission, from Krupp MA, Chatton MJ [editors]: *Current Medical Diagnosis & Treatment 1977.* Lange, 1977.)

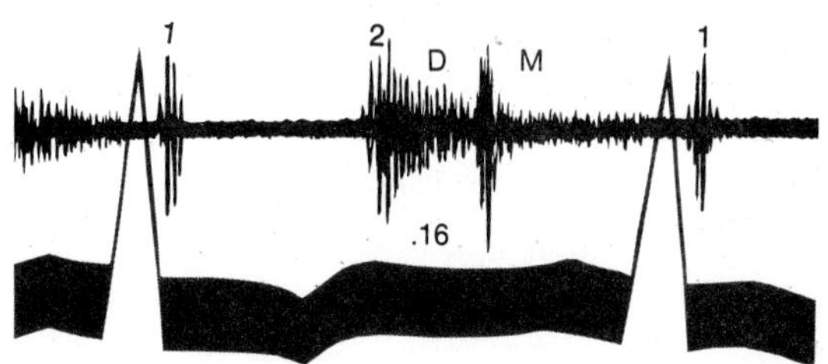

Figure 13–14. Phonocardiogram of a patient with aortic incompetence. A third sound is buried in the murmur (DM) which follows immediately after the second sound (2). (Courtesy of Roche Laboratories Division of Hoffman-La Roche, Inc.)

the length of the murmur thus depends on the severity of the lesion and the compliance of the left ventricle. In severe cases, the murmur lasts throughout diastole and may be associated with gallop rhythm (Fig 13–14).

The inevitable increase in left ventricular stroke volume ordinarily causes a systolic murmur that is of no value in diagnosis or in the differentiation of aortic incompetence from predominant aortic stenosis. The site at which the immediate diastolic murmur of aortic incompetence is heard best depends on the degree of aortic dilatation. If the aorta is large, as in syphilitic lesions, the murmur is heard best to the right of the sternum. If the aorta is small, as in rheumatic lesions, the murmur is heard best to the left of the sternum. The murmur of aortic incompetence is sometimes only heard in the lower intercostal spaces (fourth or fifth) beside the sternum and is usually not heard well at the apex. When aortic incompetence is severe, an additional, separate apical diastolic murmur is heard. This murmur, which is called an Austin Flint murmur (Fig 13–15), is middiastolic or presystolic and is thought to be due to fluttering of the anterior, aortic cusp of the mitral valve as it is caught between the 2 streams of blood flowing into the ventricle during diastole, one from the aorta and the other from the left atrium. Atrial contraction can influence the pattern of flow in this region and cause presystolic accentuation of the murmur, which is only heard in patients with severe aortic incompetence. Thus, the differential diagnosis is not between mitral stenosis and aortic incompetence, but between aortic incompetence and aortic incompetence plus mitral stenosis.

Although murmurs of aortic incompetence are similar in both the acute and the chronic form, the physical signs due to the hemodynamic effects of aortic incompetence may be strikingly different in the 2 lesions. For example, left ventricular dilatation and hypertrophy and aortic dilatation are not seen at the onset of acute aortic incompetence, whereas peripheral circulatory collapse, sweating, marked tachycardia, and signs of shock with tachypnea, basal rales, and other signs of acute severe incompetence are not seen in patients with chronic lesions, except in severe left ven-

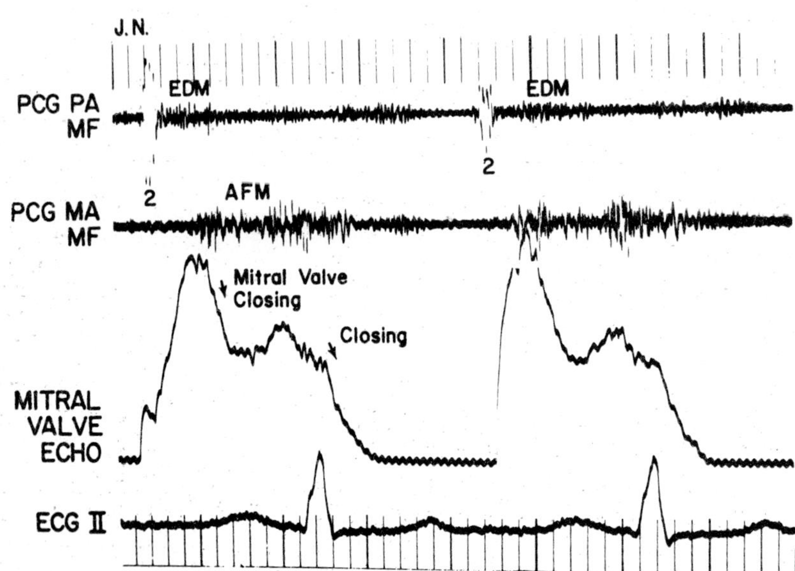

Figure 13–15. Phonocardiogram, echocardiogram, and ECG of a patient with a 2-component Austin Flint murmur (AFM). The murmur has its onset in mid diastole as the early diastolic aortic murmur (EDM) is diminishing, and it occurs while the mitral valve is closing. The second component of the murmur occurs coincidentally with atrial systole. At the time of this murmur, the mitral valve opens incompletely. The mitral valve echocardiogram shows the position of the anterior cusp. The rapid backward motion associated with mitral valve closure is interrupted by atrial systole. (Reproduced, with permission of the American Heart Association, Inc., from Fortuin NJ, Craige E: On the mechanism of Austin Flint murmur. Circulation 45:558, 1972.)

tricular failure. The aortic diastolic murmur and the pulse pressure are the 2 signs that should be monitored continuously in patients with infective endocarditis who are at risk of developing aortic incompetence.

C. Electrocardiographic Findings: ECG evidence of left ventricular hypertrophy is always present in patients with chronic hemodynamically significant aortic incompetence unless left bundle branch block or complete heart block obscures the changes. The degree of left ventricular hypertrophy—as judged by the height of the R wave in the left-sided chest leads, the depth of the S wave in the right-sided leads, and the associated ST–T changes—is moderate or considerable in more than half of patients. In about 10% of patients, right or, more commonly, left bundle branch block or even complete atrioventricular block is present. Atrial fibrillation is less common than in any other isolated left-sided lesion (5% of patients), perhaps because left ventricular failure is seldom chronic, and unrecognized mitral valve disease occurs less frequently. In acute aortic incompetence, left ventricular hypertrophy may be absent when the patient is first seen and may develop over a period of 3 weeks to 6 months, as shown in Fig 13–16. In other patients in whom aortic incompetence is present before infective endocarditis develops, left ventricular hypertrophy may become progressively more severe. Age does not prevent the development of left ventricular hypertrophy, as shown by the full-blown changes that have appeared in a 6-month period after infective endocarditis in a 78-year-old man with aortic incompetence.

D. X-Ray Findings: The cardiac silhouette in severe aortic incompetence shows evidence of both dilatation and hypertrophy of the left ventricle, as shown in Fig 13–12. The long wide curve of the left lateral wall of the heart on the posteroanterior view extends below the diaphragm; on the left anterior oblique view, the posterior sweep of the left ventricle overlies the dorsal spine and extends posterior to the inferior vena caval shadow. The physician must exercise care in interpreting x-ray evidence of left ventricular enlargement since the left and right ventricles can on occasion be confused with one another. Electrocardiographic confirmation is always helpful and is required before the physician concludes that x-ray findings are due to the enlargement of a particular ventricle. Aortic dilatation, as shown in Fig 13–17, is an important finding in patients with nonrheumatic aortic incompetence. Although calcification of the aortic valve is rare (less than 10% of cases), linear "eggshell" calcification of the ascending aorta (Fig 20–2) is diagnostic of aortitis and almost pathognomonic of a syphilitic lesion. Calcification of the arch and descending portions of the aorta is not as important as a diagnostic sign and is commonly seen in older, atherosclerotic patients.

In acute aortic incompetence, left ventricular enlargement on the chest x-ray may be absent when the patient is first seen. If the patient survives, the left ventricle enlarges at about the same rate as the electrocardiographic changes of hypertrophy develop (3 weeks–6 months). X-ray evidence of pulmonary con-

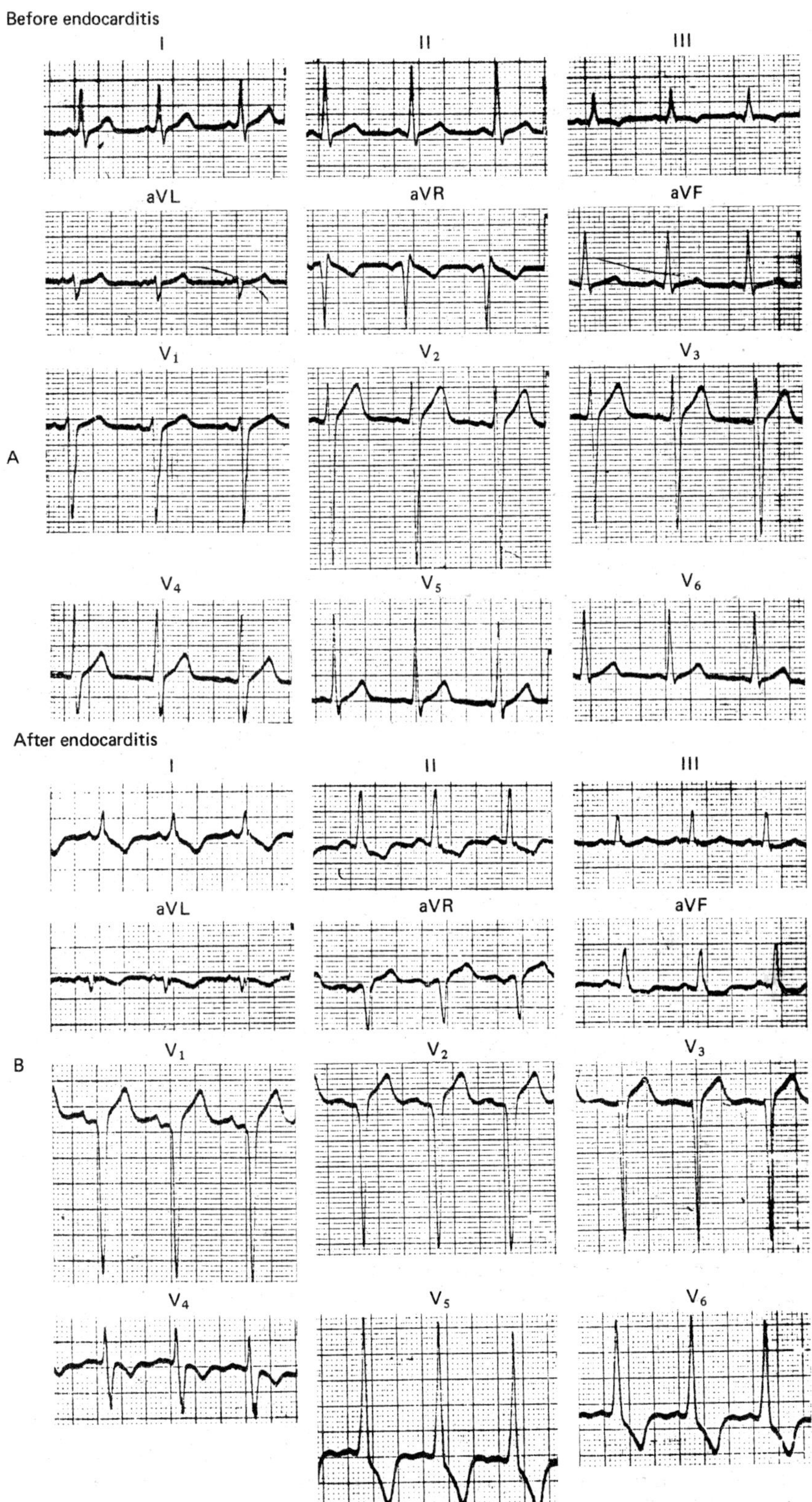

Figure 13–16. Serial ECGs taken 11 months apart in a 30-year-old man with hemodynamically insignificant aortic valve disease who developed acute severe aortic incompetence after infective endocarditis. The ECG changes of severe left ventricular hypertrophy seen in *B* developed over the months following treatment of infective endocarditis.

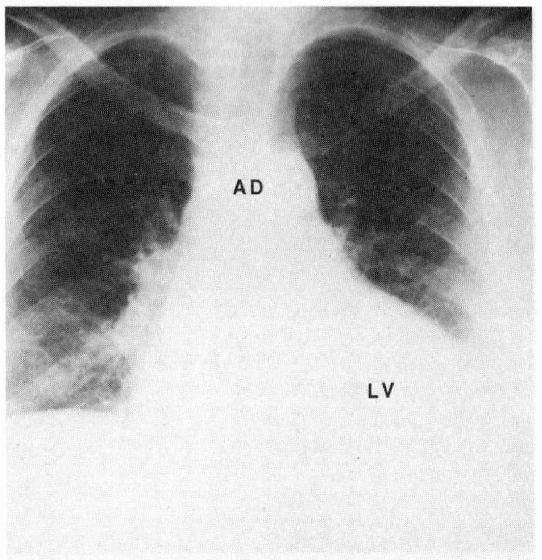

Figure 13–17. Chest x-ray of a patient with severe aortic incompetence and left heart failure. The large left ventricle (LV) and aortic dilatation (AD) are clearly seen.

gestion with acute or subacute pulmonary edema is commonly seen in acute lesions. It is important to distinguish these changes from those seen in pulmonary infarction or pneumonia. The lesions are almost always bilateral but not always symmetric, and the characteristic "bat's wing" distribution of subacute pulmonary edema with shadows extending out from the roots of the lungs is often seen.

E. Special Investigations:

1. Noninvasive technics–Noninvasive methods of investigation are valuable in recording the clinical manifestations of aortic incompetence. Prolongation of the ejection time following a rapid upstroke of the indirect carotid pulse, increased amplitude of the tracing obtained from the apexcardiogram, and diastolic fluttering of the aortic leaflet of the mitral valve during diastole on echocardiography are usually noted (Fig 13–18), but in general such findings are confirmatory rather than diagnostic. In severe, acute cases of aortic incompetence, the mitral valve closes early in diastole as the diastolic rush of blood from the aorta enters the ventricle. Although this echocardiographic sign has been used as an indication of severity, it is probably not always valid, because in patients with a slow heart rate and large stroke volume due to any cause, the mitral valve may drift into a closed position relatively early in diastole. The sign is useful, however, in following patients with endocarditis in whom aortic incompetence may be developing.

2. Invasive technics–

a. Cardiac catheterization–Cardiac catheterization and angiocardiography are mandatory in any patient in whom surgical treatment is contemplated. It is essential to demonstrate that the aortic valve is the site of the lesion and that it is the cause of the peripheral signs of rapid aortic runoff. In rare cases, especially in acute lesions, paravalvular lesions or rupture of an aortic sinus (sinus of Valsalva) aneurysm may not be suspected until the time of study. Although difficulties in diagnosis occur more commonly in acute cases of aortic incompetence that are due to infective endocarditis, even chronic cases of incompetence may be incorrectly diagnosed as *valvular* aortic incompetence when in fact the valve is intact and a paravalvular leak or ruptured aortic sinus is responsible for the lesion. The danger of an incorrect diagnosis lies in the increased mortality rate at surgery.

Since left ventricular failure occurs so late in the

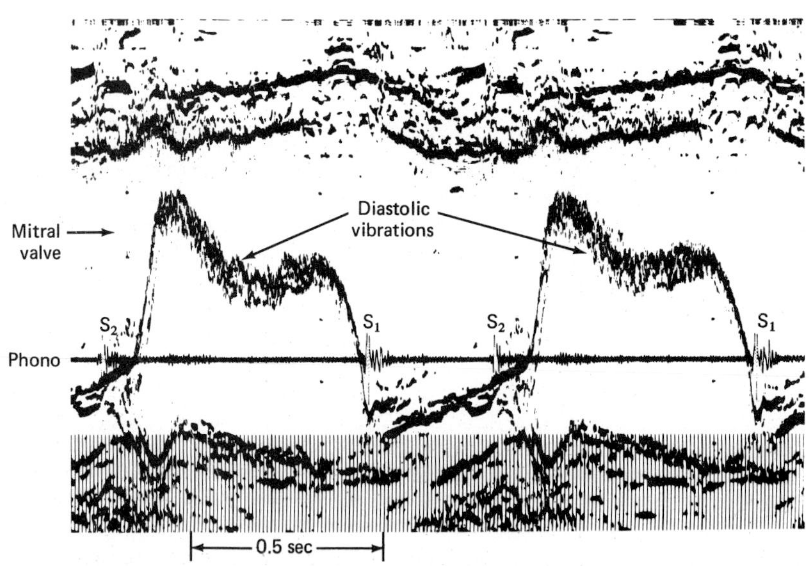

Figure 13–18. Echocardiogram showing diastolic vibration of mitral valve leaflet in a patient with aortic incompetence.

Table 13–2. Cardiac catheterization data in patients with hemodynamically significant predominant aortic incompetence.

	Mean Wedge Pressure (mm Hg)	Left Ventricular Systolic Pressure (mm Hg)	Aortic Systolic Pressure (mm Hg)	Aortic Diastolic Pressure (mm Hg)	Cardiac Output (l/min)
Pure aortic incompetence					
Chronic	18 ± 9	158 ± 31	157 ± 31	56 ± 12	5.1 ± 1.4
Acute	32 ± 10	134 ± 24	135 ± 24	54 ± 12	5.1 ± 1.7

course of aortic incompetence, most patients with chronic lesions show normal right heart pressures when they are first studied. In older patients with clinical evidence of left heart failure, raised wedge and left ventricular diastolic pressures are found, although the cardiac output is usually normal or even slightly raised. The pressure levels are usually lower than expected, and pulmonary vascular resistance is rarely increased (less than 10% of cases); the increase is at most moderate (3.5–7.5 mg Hg/l/min). In acute lesions, the hemodynamic findings are much more impressive, as shown in Table 13–2, and the wedge pressure and left ventricular diastolic pressures are often at a level at which pulmonary edema is likely to occur (more than 35 mm Hg). The pressure in the left ventricle may rise rapidly during diastole to high levels, and a reversed gradient across the mitral valve may be seen in severe cases (Fig 13–19). This finding correlates reasonably well with the echocardiographic evidence of early mitral valve closure. The characteristic finding of a wide aortic pulse pressure is present in all cases except those in severe left ventricular failure. The aortic pulse pressure is usually less than that in a peripheral artery, and that in turn is less than the indirectly recorded pulse pressure. As left ventricular failure develops, left ventricular diastolic pressure rises, establishing a lower limit to the aortic pressure of about 40 mm Hg. The level of left ventricular diastolic pressure varies with the compliance of the left ventricle. This is greater in large dilated ventricles in chronic lesions. The highest ventricular diastolic pressures are seen in patients with acute lesions and small hearts. In such patients, values of 60 mm Hg can occur, as seen in Fig 13–20.

b. **Angiography**—Supravalvular angiocardiography is important in assessing aortic incompetence. The speed at which the left ventricle opacifies is roughly proportionate to the severity of the leak. Angiocardiography establishes the valvular nature of the lesion and provides opacification of the left ventricle sufficient to assess left ventricular function without having to pass a catheter into the chamber. Angiography also makes it possible to detect or rule out associated mitral incompetence with greater certainty because ectopic beats (which often produce spurious mitral incompetence) occur less frequently, and positioning of the catheter to avoid interfering with the action of the mitral valve apparatus is not a problem. The end-diastolic volume of the left ventricle is increased in aortic incompetence, often with a normal end-diastolic pressure, indicating increased compliance of the ventricle. The total stroke volume is always greater than normal, and the ejection fraction is reasonably well maintained until left ventricular failure occurs. If the forward stroke volume is measured independently from the systemic cardiac output, it is possible to calculate the volume of blood flowing back across the aortic valve during diastole. This is usually expressed as a proportion of the total stroke volume. A value of 50% or more is found in patients with severe lesions and indicates that half the stroke volume returns to the ventricle during diastole. Unfortunately, the measurements obtained by angiographic and physiologic means cannot readily be made simultaneously, and they are thus not really comparable, since the heart rate during angiography is usually more rapid. Coronary arteriography is now more frequently performed as a routine procedure in patients with aortic incompetence, but as in aortic stenosis, the state of the coronary arteries should not influence the decision to operate, which depends instead on the hemodynamic severity of the aortic valve lesion. As in aortic stenosis, it seems more logical to reserve coronary arteriography for those patients in whom angina pectoris is suggested by the history.

F. **Hemodynamic Values**: Hemodynamic data obtained at cardiac catheterization in a group of patients with aortic incompetence are shown in Table 13–2. Cardiac output is well maintained in both acute and chronic lesions. The pulse pressure is larger in chronic cases, although aortic diastolic pressure is reduced in both groups.

Differential Diagnosis

A. **Pulmonary Incompetence**: The murmur of aortic incompetence can be readily confused with the murmur of pulmonary incompetence in patients with severe pulmonary hypertension. Pulmonary incompetence rarely occurs in patients who do not have moderate or severe pulmonary hypertension. In patients with pulmonary hypertension, the hypertrophied right ventricle relaxes at about the same time as the left ventricle, causing the characteristic immediate, high-pitched diastolic murmur that is indistinguishable from that of aortic incompetence. On the basis of statistics, aortic incompetence is always the more likely lesion when an immediate diastolic murmur is present. However, full study is usually needed to confirm the cause of the murmur, and the associated signs of pulmonary hypertension and right ventricular hypertrophy are ultimately always more important in diagnosis than the characteristics of the murmur.

In patients with low pulmonary arterial pressure,

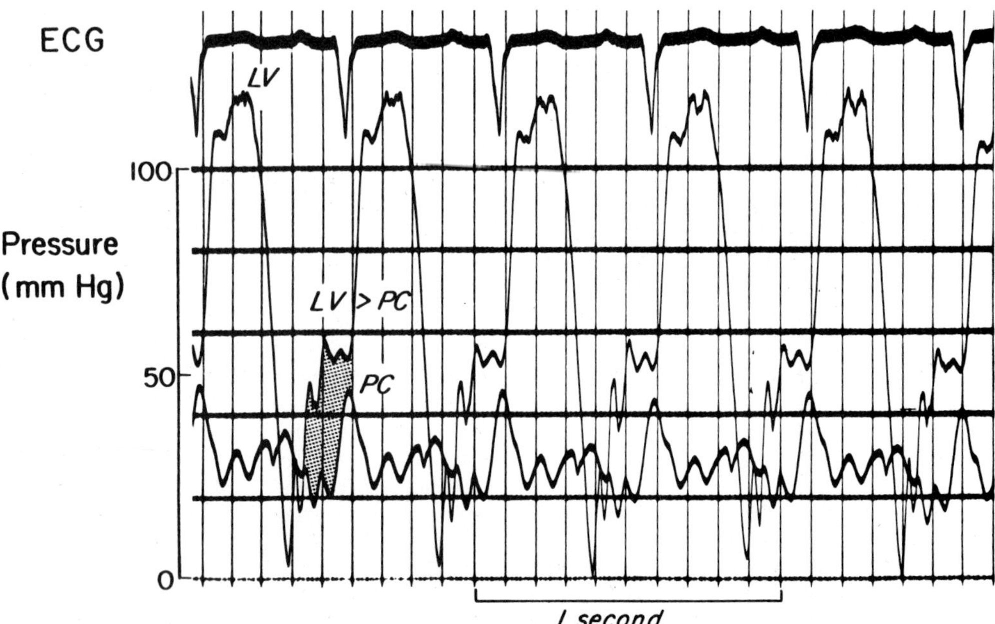

Figure 13–19. Left ventricular (LV) and wedge (PC, pulmonary capillary) pressure tracings in a patient with acute severe aortic incompetence. During the crosshatched period of diastole, the left ventricular pressure exceeds the pulmonary capillary pressure; this constitutes the reverse mitral gradient.

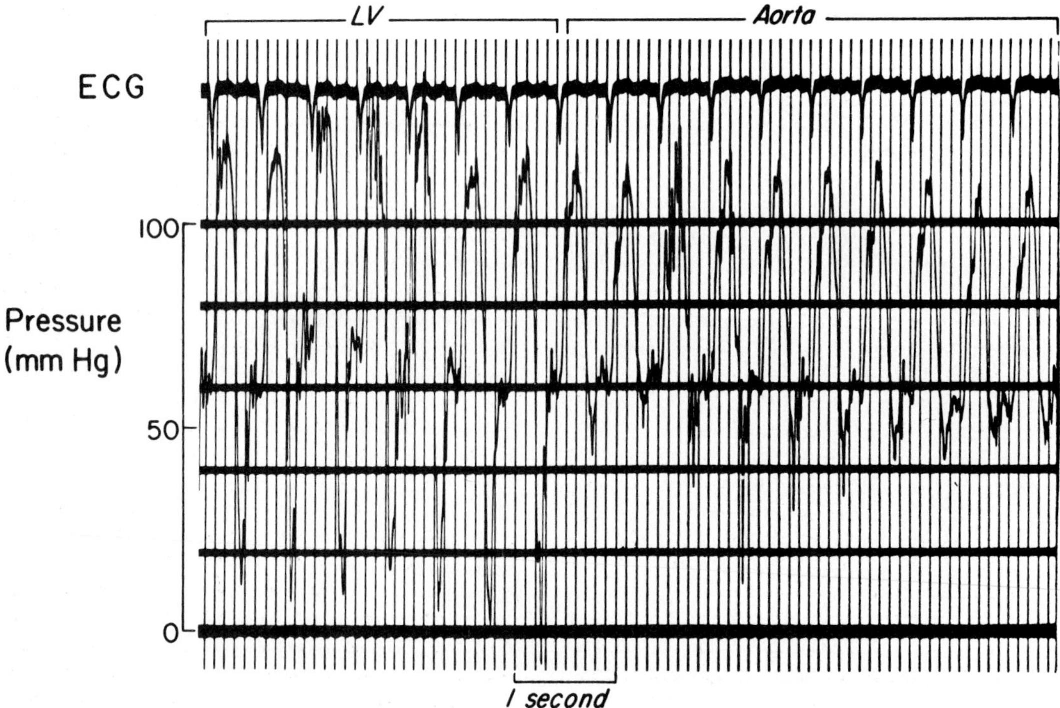

Figure 13–20. Withdrawal pressure tracing from left ventricle (LV) to aorta in a patient with acute severe aortic incompetence showing equalization of end-diastolic pressure at 60 mm Hg.

the murmur of pulmonary incompetence is different and is therefore not likely to be confused with an aortic murmur. When pulmonary arterial pressure is low, the right ventricle relaxes more slowly and the murmur starts later and is not as high-pitched.

B. Rapid Aortic Runoff in Other Conditions: Disorders other than aortic incompetence can cause the characteristic physical signs of rapid runoff of blood from the aorta into some low pressure area or into other areas in the circulation. These disorders include patent ductus arteriosus, aortopulmonary window, aortic-to-right-ventricular or atrial fistula, systemic arteriovenous fistula, truncus arteriosus, and associated ventricular septal defect. Anemia without organic valvular disease occasionally causes aortic incompetence.

Course & Complications

A. Left Ventricular Failure: Left ventricular failure occurs late in the course of uncomplicated chronic aortic incompetence and should be thought of as part of the disease rather than a complication. The part played by myocardial fibrosis in causing left heart failure is difficult to determine. Myocardial hypertrophy results in an increase in connective tissue elements of the heart as well as an increase in the size of the individual muscle cells. The relationship among the increase in cell size, cell nutrition, and oxygen and substrate requirements is not well understood, but it seems likely that over the long course of the lesion, progressive myocardial fibrosis occurs. The role of absolute or relative myocardial ischemia is similarly not certain, but it appears likely that the compensatory mechanisms of left ventricular hypertrophy are limited and that ultimately myocardial fibrosis occurs. The progress of myocardial fibrosis is probably also influenced by inflammatory changes due to current or previous rheumatic myocarditis, which lead to left ventricular failure in younger patients. The diagnosis of active rheumatic myocardial disease is usually impossible except by retrospective analysis of the history.

Severe coronary arterial disease is not usually present in patients with hemodynamically significant aortic incompetence who present in a hospital, presumably because the 2 lesions together are not compatible with life and are mutually exclusive. In syphilitic aortic incompetence, coronary ostial stenosis is an important associated finding that may cause transient edema of the aortic intima, resulting in acute ostial obstruction and acute myocardial ischemia.

Left ventricular failure is difficult to predict in aortic incompetence, and the premonitory symptoms of increasing dyspnea with decreasing effort over several months or years are not always seen. The onset of left ventricular failure is more abrupt in aortic incompetence than in any other form of chronic left ventricular disease, probably because the change from marked peripheral vasodilatation to severe vasoconstriction associated with a falling cardiac output is so abrupt. There are no reliable guidelines to indicate impending left ventricular failure.

B. Infective Endocarditis: Infective endocarditis is the most important complication of aortic incompetence. It is both a cause and a complication of the lesion. In the preantibiotic era, *Streptococcus viridans* was the commonest causative organism. Therapeutic advances, increased use of intravenous medication by physicians and patients, and the use of immunosuppressive drugs have since increased both the variety of organisms and the range of pathogenicity. Infective endocarditis is a greater hazard at the aortic valve than at any other site and is most dangerous when aortic incompetence is mild. Patients with mild lesions and those with no aortic valve disease at all are likely to suffer the most severe hemodynamic insults. Patients who have already developed significant aortic incompetence and whose cardiovascular systems have already adapted to the lesion are not exposed to comparable hemodynamic risks. The reason that endocarditis involving the aortic valve carries such a poor prognosis is that the valve is of crucial hemodynamic importance and is situated very close to the main coronary vessels and conduction system. Ulcerative lesions of the cusps and the aortic root can cause acute, subacute, or chronic exacerbation of aortic incompetence, with or without perforation into adjacent cardiac chambers. (See Chapter 16 for details of treatment of infective endocarditis.)

C. Heart Block: Heart block is an occasional complication, especially in patients with ankylosing spondylitis or Reiter's syndrome. In patients with marked left ventricular hypertrophy and dilatation, left bundle branch block may occur, and all varieties of heart block up to and including complete block are seen.

Treatment

Aortic valve replacement is the only effective treatment for aortic incompetence. However, this lesion is the one with the most problematic indications for surgery. Both the timing of surgery and the choice of prosthetic valve are still controversial. Since aortic valve replacement has become widely available, surgical treatment of chronic aortic incompetence has been instituted at progressively earlier stages of the disease. The principal difficulty is that if surgery is delayed until obvious heart failure has developed, the results of operation are poor because the large, hypertrophied, dilated, and often fibrotic heart does not recover normal function because irreversible myocardial fibrosis has irrevocably compromised left ventricular function.

The dilemma is that heart failure develops late in the course of the disease, and its onset cannot be predicted with sufficient accuracy to enable the surgeon to make a rational decision about surgical treatment. If the long-term durability of prosthetic valves were good and the surgical mortality rate were negligible, earlier valve replacement could be recommended. However, since the long-term (20-year) durability of prosthetic valves is not yet known and because as yet neither the mortality and morbidity rates of aortic valve replacement nor the long-term lack of complications associated with artificial valves or homografts is sufficiently low, prophylactic valve replacement is not warranted.

Since physicians cannot predict when serious problems may arise, most of them are reluctant to recommend aortic valve replacement until they are certain that the patient actually needs this major life-threatening step, particularly in view of the fact that continuous anticoagulant therapy may be required after operation and a second valve replacement operation may be needed when the initial artificial valve wears out.

If surgery is performed, an additional difficulty lies in anchoring the valve securely. In aortic stenosis there is almost always a firm fibrous or calcific ring of tissue around the valve that holds surgical sutures securely, but in aortic incompetence, this ring is not present. Furthermore, there is often associated disease of the aortic wall that makes sutures more likely to tear out and necessitate a second open heart operation. Severe morbidity or even death may then result.

A 20-year-old asymptomatic patient with uncomplicated hemodynamically significant aortic incompetence can probably expect an average of about 20 years of life free from symptoms. Some more precise indications for surgery, such as massive cardiac enlargement, an arbitrary age (eg, 40 years), or the hemodynamic response to some stress such as salt loading or angiotensin infusion, might be more logical than the present situation in which some "excuse" is generally required before surgery is recommended in an asymptomatic patient. When significant dyspnea and left heart failure develop, surgery is mandatory. Medical treatment of left ventricular failure should only be a prelude to operation. Long-term digitalis therapy is not indicated because a patient in need of digitalis is in need of valve replacement. Unfortunately, there is no satisfactory index of left ventricular function that can be used as a guide to the need for operation.

Exercise testing is less helpful than might be expected because the patient with aortic incompetence generally tolerates exercise well. Signs of increasing left ventricular hypertrophy on the ECG and chest x-ray are not too helpful, since both have been documented 20–30 years before left ventricular failure occurred. Our recommendation is that patients with isolated hemodynamically significant aortic incompetence be followed at yearly intervals and observed for signs of left ventricular failure. If a patient shows an increasing heart size and progression of ECG changes indicative of left ventricular hypertrophy between ages 35–40, valve replacement is advisable, and this operation should be given serious consideration in any patient reaching age 40. The development of left ventricular failure in a patient under age 30 who has chronic aortic incompetence suggests the presence of associated myocardial damage—usually rheumatic carditis or unrecognized mitral valve disease. Although the results of surgery in such patients are not good, operation is still indicated in order to relieve the load on the left ventricle.

In patients with acute or acutely exacerbated lesions, surgery is almost always needed, and acute and progressive hemodynamic deterioration may force operation. Patients with infective endocarditis, especially those with acute fulminant lesions, should be treated at a center where emergency cardiac surgery is available, because the need for operation may arise at any time in the course of the disease. When endocarditis is present, surgery should be delayed if possible until the infection involving the valve has been controlled and sufficient healing has occurred to ensure that there is adequate tissue to hold the sutures securing the valve. Achieving such a result in actual practice is difficult. The course of infective endocarditis is so unpredictable and varies so widely with the type of causative organism, the prior state of the valve, and the general health of the patient that it is impossible to set up any rational guidelines for the management of patients with this lesion. Medical treatment alone is unlikely to stabilize the hemodynamic status of patients with aortic incompetence occurring de novo. In these patients, aortic valve replacement is almost inevitable, and the principal question is the timing of surgery.

Serious problems arise in patients who are addicted to heroin and in whom saprophytic organisms and fungi are often present. The reinfection rate is extremely high, and the prognosis is dismal. In our opinion, the most logical course to follow in the management of acute aortic incompetence with infective endocarditis is to wait and follow the patient as closely as possible and to use digitalis and diuretic therapy where indicated but withhold vasodilator therapy with nitroprusside infusion except for emergency use, just to maintain the patient for the few hours needed to prepare for open heart surgery. There is little doubt that satisfactory results can be obtained in no more than 50% of patients. The patient must be closely followed for over one year because hemodynamic deterioration following infective endocarditis may occur late in the disease when healing causes retraction and fibrosis of the damaged valvular tissue. Another complicating feature is toxic myocarditis accompanying endocarditis, but there is some disagreement about the existence and significance of this complication.

As it does in aortic stenosis, the choice of artificial valve rests with the surgeon. Homograft aortic valves have the advantage of not requiring long-term anticoagulation, but this factor must be balanced against their tendency to stiffen, calcify, and leak with time. The mortality rate of surgery depends on the clinical status of the patient and the experience of the surgeon and averages 2–5% in chronic cases. The mortality rate is always higher in second operations and in patients with acute lesions who undergo surgery when infection is still present.

Prognosis

Aortic incompetence has a better prognosis than aortic stenosis since the load on the ventricle is better tolerated, primarily because it is an increased flow load. The lesion is not as well tolerated as mitral incompetence, in which the systolic pressure against which the left ventricle does its extra work is always lower. In acute lesions, aortic incompetence carries a worse prognosis than mitral incompetence because there is an increased possibility of coronary arterial involvement; because a severe systemic infection is often present when the lesion develops; and because fistula formation and heart block are more likely to occur.

The prognosis of left ventricular failure in aortic incompetence is poor because it occurs at such a late stage in the disease. In milder lesions, the threat of endocarditis is the most important and least predictable factor in prognosis.

MULTIPLE VALVE INVOLVEMENT

Combined Mitral & Aortic Valve Disease

Involvement of both aortic and mitral valves is almost pathognomonic of rheumatic heart disease, and patients with lesions of both valves have a higher incidence of infection in childhood (70%) than any other group of patients with valve disease. When both aortic and mitral valves are involved, the variability of the clinical picture greatly increases. The importance of the lesion at each valve can vary; the nature of each lesion (stenosis, incompetence, or mixture of the 2) is diverse; and rheumatic myocardial involvement tends to play a more important part in the clinical course because the rheumatic infection is more severe and more often recurrent in these cases. It can be seen from the classification of mitral and aortic disease in this text that 20 or more subclassifications of different mixed valvular diseases can be described. It is beyond the scope of this text to do more than point out some of the more obvious relationships between aortic and mitral disease and to make a few general comments about the clinical picture. Combined mitral and aortic valve disease constitutes about 10% of cases of valvular disease. Such patients have hemodynamically significant disease of each valve. Predominant aortic and predominant mitral disease are about equal in frequency in combined lesions. Mitral stenosis decreases the apparent severity of aortic disease, particularly in aortic incompetence, and the combination of mitral stenosis and aortic incompetence is surprisingly well tolerated. After mitral stenosis has been relieved by valvotomy, aortic incompetence often appears to be more severe, and the presence on ECG of left ventricular hypertrophy due to aortic incompetence in a patient with predominant mitral stenosis is sufficient warning to warrant serious consideration of aortic valve replacement at the time of mitral valve surgery.

Mitral stenosis and aortic stenosis tend to mask one another, so that one or the other appears to be the dominant lesion clinically. The significance of the less dominant lesion is often underestimated.

When aortic valve disease is the major lesion, significant mitral incompetence is more serious than mitral stenosis. In either aortic stenosis or aortic incompetence, mitral incompetence is aggravated, and extreme cardiac enlargement and early heart failure are common.

Among the characteristic clinical pictures of combined valvular disease which should be mentioned is the combination of aortic stenosis with insignificant or mild mitral incompetence. This lesion gives rise to a characteristic high-pitched "seagull cry" murmur. In some cases, extension of aortic calcification into the aortic cusp of the mitral valve can be demonstrated, and this is one of the few combined aortic and mitral valve lesions that does not always have a rheumatic origin.

Clinical Course of Combined Lesions

Patients with combined mitral and aortic valve lesions tend to be symptomatic at an earlier age than patients with single valve lesions. The heart is usually larger, and atrial fibrillation tends to develop at an earlier age. The disease of each valve is less advanced in combined lesions because the valvular lesions are additive and because myocardial disease is so often present. Physical signs are more difficult to interpret in mixed lesions, and it is not always easy to distinguish the delayed diastolic or presystolic murmur of severe aortic incompetence (Austin Flint murmur) from the murmur of associated mitral stenosis. Similarly, an immediate basal diastolic murmur of pulmonary incompetence (Graham Steell murmur) in mitral stenosis with a raised pulmonary vascular resistance can be confused with the murmur of associated aortic incompetence. In patients with predominant aortic valve disease, the distinction between functional and organic mitral incompetence is often difficult. In the presence of left heart failure, a systolic murmur of mitral incompetence is often found, but it may be difficult to distinguish from the aortic systolic murmur; in mixed mitral stenosis and incompetence, the organic nature of the systolic murmur can be more readily recognized. In combined aortic and mitral valve disease, either valve lesion may become acutely worse in the course of infective endocarditis. The presence of a chronic lesion of one valve exaggerates the effects of an acute lesion of the other valve. Infective endocarditis and systemic embolism are as common in combined aortic and mitral valve disease as they are in aortic or mitral incompetence alone.

Double Valve Replacement

Surgical replacement of both valves, or aortic valve replacement with mitral valvotomy, generally leads to less satisfactory results than single valve replacement. This is probably because more extensive myocardial disease is present in patients with combined lesions. Simultaneous valve replacement is preferable to serial valve replacement, since the second cardiotomy is always more difficult than the first. The surgeon should have as much information as possible on which to base the decision whether to replace one valve or two, and full preoperative hemodynamic studies are mandatory. Long-term survival after double valve replacement is not significantly shorter than after single valve replacement. This may be because valve lesions are additive, and double valve replacement is therefore usually undertaken at an earlier stage of development of each individual valve lesion.

The management of patients with combined aortic and mitral valve lesions always presents problems because the cases are naturally more complex and different, and sufficient experience of treatment regimens is generally lacking. Fortunately, the number of patients with combined mitral and aortic disease is decreasing in the Western world.

Combined Mitral & Tricuspid Valve Disease

Functional tricuspid incompetence has already been mentioned as a common complication of mitral stenosis with raised pulmonary vascular resistance (see Chapter 12). In about 2% of patients with mitral valve disease, organic tricuspid valve disease is present and causes right heart failure. The mitral valve lesion is almost always mixed mitral stenosis and incompetence, and pulmonary vascular resistance is not greatly raised (average 2 mm Hg/l/min). Markedly raised systemic venous pressure (average 24 mm Hg) is the most striking clinical feature, and cardiac enlargement is usually massive, but not as great as in giant left atrium. Low cardiac output and atrial fibrillation are almost inevitable, and the lesions tend to run a chronic course in which valve replacement provides less benefit than in disease of the mitral valve alone. Isolated tricuspid valve disease without mitral valve involvement can theoretically occur, but for practical purposes it is rare enough to be of negligible importance.

Triple Valve Disease

The remarks that have been made about double valve disease are even more applicable to triple valve disease, in which aortic, mitral, and tricuspid valves are involved. Since the lesions are additive and rheumatic myocarditis is almost inevitably present, the results of surgery are never as satisfactory as in disease affecting a single valve. All artificial valves currently available are functionally inferior to a normal valve. The presence of 3 such valves in series in the heart is likely to cause a significant load on the myocardium and tends to make the prognosis worse and decrease the degree of functional improvement that the patient experiences after surgery. In spite of these disadvantages, the necessity for inserting 3 valves still occurs in a few cases, and there is usually no alternative to operation because of the severe effects of the combined valve lesions.

CARCINOID VALVULAR HEART DISEASE

Carcinoid tumors that arise from the chromaffin tissue in the gastrointestinal tract–usually in the ileum–produce vasoactive substances such as serotonin, bradykinin, and tryptophan. These vasoactive substances cause endothelial damage to the right side of the heart, resulting in fibrosis and thickening of the heart valves. Tricuspid incompetence and, less frequently, pulmonary stenosis are the end results of the damage, which also affects the endocardium of the right atrium and ventricle. The primary tumors can be small, and hepatic metastases are usually present in patients with cardiac involvement. The pathologic features of the condition (Fig 13–21) include massive dilatation of the right heart with fibrosis and thickening of the right atrium and ventricle involving the tricuspid valve.

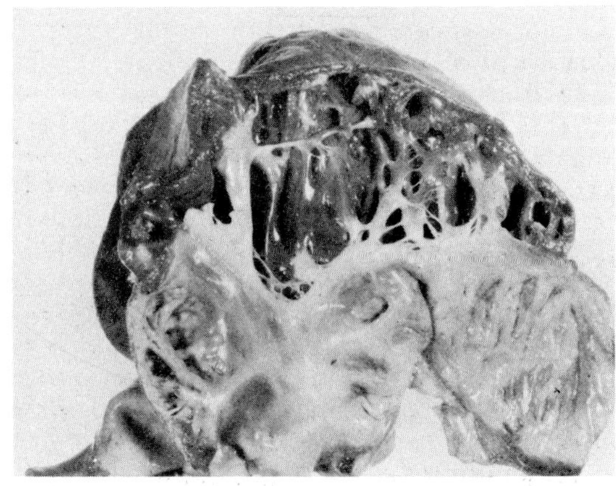

Figure 13–21. The heart in carcinoid syndrome. Note dilatation of the right atrium and fibrosis and insufficiency of the tricuspid valve. (Courtesy of O Rambo.)

Clinical Findings

A. Symptoms: Patients with carcinoid syndrome complain of episodes of facial and upper trunk flushing in response to alcohol ingestion, eating, and emotional reactions. The release of vasoactive substances into the bloodstream is thought to be responsible. Abdominal pain, diarrhea, and renal and hepatic failure are also seen. Dyspnea is uncommon.

B. Signs: Hepatic enlargement and a peculiar violaceous color of the face and neck are often seen, and abdominal distention and ascites occur. The cardiac signs are not present in all cases, but the physician should search for them by looking at the venous pressure and pulse in the neck and listening for heart murmurs. A systolic murmur of tricuspid incompetence is the commonest finding. It is louder on inspiration and often associated with *a* and *v* waves in the jugular venous pulse. A systolic ejection murmur due to pulmonary stenosis is less common, and diastolic murmurs are a late manifestation. Frank right heart failure with edema appears late in the disease and may be difficult to assess in the presence of severe hepatic involvement.

C. Electrocardiographic Findings: P wave abnormalities are usually all that are seen, and right ventricular hypertrophy is rare.

D. X-Ray Findings: Dilatation of the right heart occurs late in the disease.

E. Special Investigations: The diagnosis of carcinoid tumor is established by finding 5-hydroxyindoleacetic acid in the urine. It is a metabolic product of serotonin. A value of more than 25 ng/24 hours is considered diagnostic and usually implies hepatic metastases. An amount exceeding 200 ng/24 hours is usually found in patients with cardiac involvement. A variety of foods (bananas, apples) or drugs (phenothiazines) may cause false-positive reactions. Liver scans may reveal defects from metastases, and biopsy of the liver or the primary tumor shows the characteristic histologic findings.

Echocardiography may show dilatation of the right heart and abnormal motion of the ventricular septum. Cardiac catheterization is seldom indicated because the cardiac involvement is usually not severe.

Differential Diagnosis

Isolated tricuspid incompetence is rare in rheumatic heart disease and infective endocarditis involving the tricuspid valve, and tumor involving the right atrium is the most important differential diagnostic problem.

Course & Complications

The tumor grows slowly in most cases, although it metastasizes early. The cardiac manifestations rarely cause serious problems but can progress to the stage at which valve replacement must be considered. Atrial fibrillation may occur in severe cases. In some patients the vasoactive substances are not inactivated in the lungs, and left-sided lesions have been reported.

Treatment

Resection of the primary tumor is the most helpful procedure. Chemotherapy with cytotoxic drugs (eg, cyclophosphamide) is used to treat hepatic metastases. Various serotonin antagonists (eg, methysergide) have been used to treat the flushing attacks, with generally disappointing results. Phenothiazines have been useful in some cases. Digitalis and diuretics are used for the treatment of right heart failure, and tricuspid or pulmonary valve replacement is seldom needed.

Prognosis

The disease is more slowly progressive than might be expected, and survival for 5–10 years after the initial symptoms develop is not uncommon. The cardiac involvement seldom influences the prognosis, which depends on the hepatic metastases.

IATROGENICALLY MODIFIED VALVULAR HEART DISEASE

Mitral Valvotomy

Mitral commissurotomy is the most important iatrogenic factor modifying the course of valvular heart disease. Tight mitral stenosis and mitral stenosis with raised pulmonary vascular resistance were usually fatal in early middle life before the advent of mitral valve surgery. Even relatively ineffective closed mitral valvulotomy was—and still is—capable of influencing the clinical course of mitral stenosis. The operation is palliative rather than curative, and in 2–15 years after valvotomy the patient is likely to experience a recurrence of dyspnea. In some cases (about 20%), a second valvotomy is performed, but in most cases mitral valve replacement is necessary at the second operation. The clinical features of these patients with iatrogenically modified mitral stenosis warrant description.

Clinical Findings

A. Symptoms: In patients who have had a previous mitral valvotomy, symptoms are difficult to assess. Dyspnea is the commonest symptom, and, as in all patients with mitral valve disease, the relation between the onset of atrial fibrillation and the onset of dyspnea is of prime importance. A clinical picture resembling that of mixed mitral valve disease is common. Patients who have gained relief through mitral valvotomy are likely to experience a significant increase in dyspnea when atrial fibrillation occurs at about age 40. There is often a relationship between the length of the asymptomatic interval following valvotomy and the age of the patient. A woman who has had a mitral valvotomy in her 20s is likely to have 15 symptom-free years before atrial fibrillation develops, whereas a 35-year-old woman is likely to develop atrial fibrillation within about 5 years of operation. It seems that mitral valvotomy is a means of shifting the patient from the category of pure tight mitral stenosis to that of mixed mitral stenosis and incompetence.

B. Signs: The physical signs in iatrogenically modified cases usually reflect the preoperative findings. A loud opening snap and loud first heart sound are often present, and the timing of the opening snap reflects the preoperative and not the postoperative status of the patient. In such cases, the length of the diastolic murmur measured at the bedside becomes the best indicator of the severity of stenosis. A systolic murmur may appear after surgery, but, as is the case in patients who have not undergone operation, its significance is open to question, and other clinical evidence of mitral incompetence must always be sought.

C. Electrocardiographic Findings: In a few cases, regression of the changes of right ventricular hypertrophy is seen, as shown in Fig 13–22, but in most patients the ECG shows little change from the preoperative tracing. Sooner or later, atrial fibrillation will almost certainly develop.

D. X-Ray Findings: The absence of the left atrial appendage as a bulge on the left heart border is a characteristic finding in patients who have undergone operation (Fig 13–23). If the pulmonary artery was enlarged before operation, it seldom returns to normal size, and the same is true of the left atrium. Changes in the degree of pulmonary congestion are perhaps the best indicators of the success of surgical treatment.

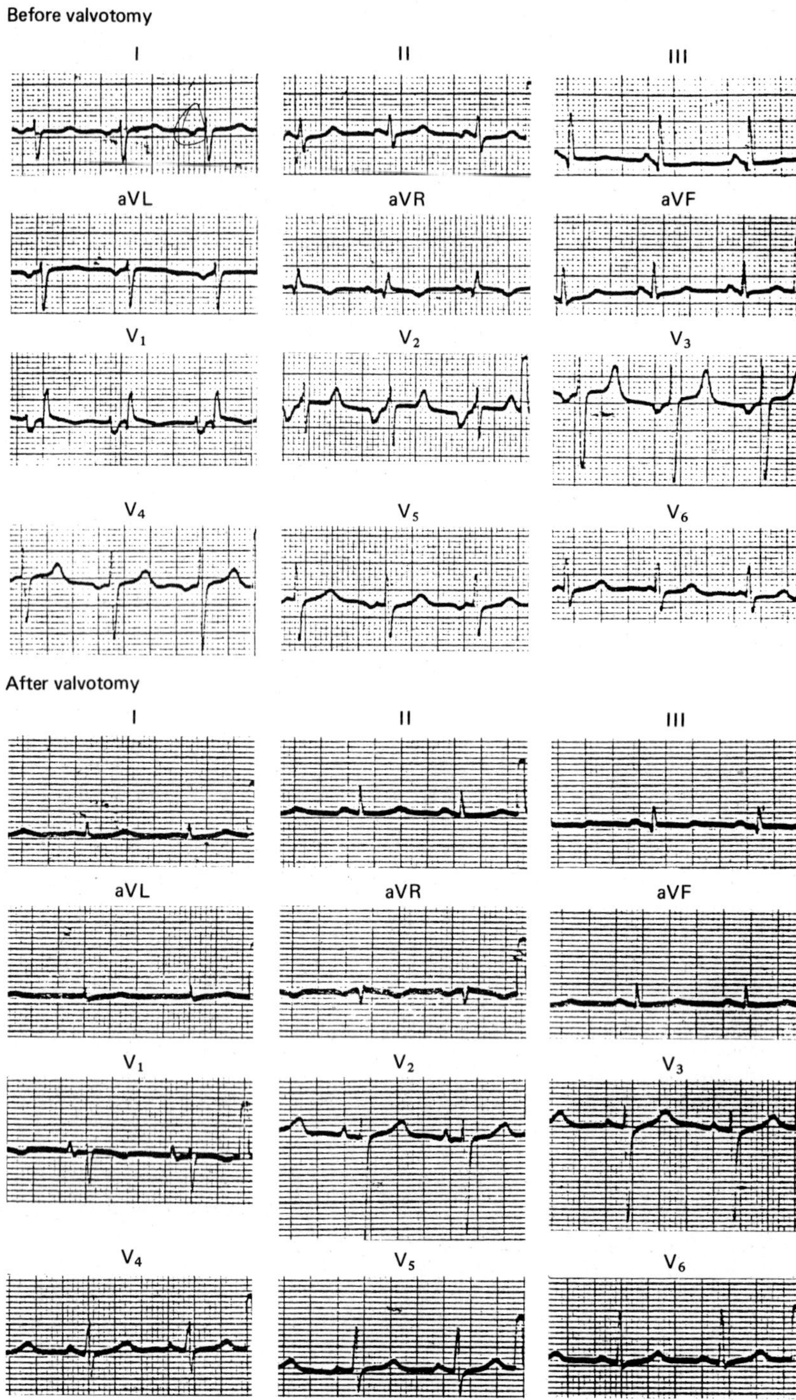

Figure 13–22. Serial ECGs taken before and 1 year after mitral valvotomy in a 25-year-old woman with mitral stenosis and raised pulmonary vascular resistance (12 mm Hg/l/min). ECG evidence of right ventricular hypertrophy and left atrial enlargement is not present after operation. The inverted P wave in lead I before valvotomy is unexplained. The upright T wave in lead I is against reversal of right and left arm leads in the presence of right ventricular hypertrophy. Two possible explanations for the inverted P in lead I are (1) a left atrial rhythm and (2) marked rightward deviation (as well as posterior deviation resulting from the left atrial hypertrophy) of the P vector from right atrial enlargement secondary to the marked pulmonary hypertension. The precordial leads are the important ones for diagnosing the condition and for demonstrating the change after surgery.

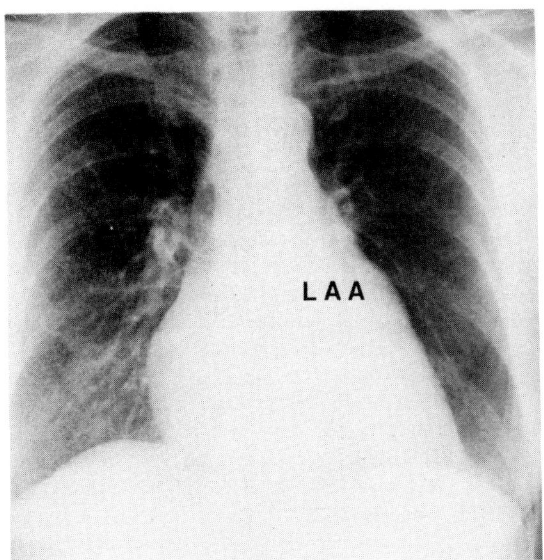

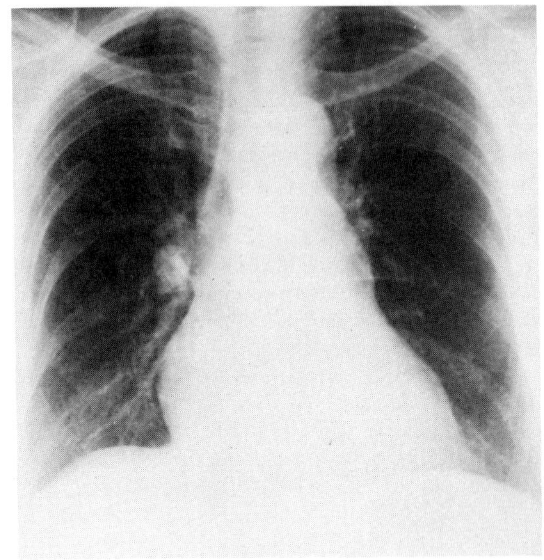

Figure 13–23. Preoperative and postoperative chest x-rays of a patient with mitral stenosis. The left atrial appendage (LAA) has been resected.

E. Special Investigations: Exercise testing and echocardiography are helpful noninvasive technics used in screening patients to decide whether they should undergo catheterization again. However, echocardiographic findings tend to be influenced by the preoperative status of the valve. Cardiac catheterization, with measurement of the wedge pressure, left ventricular pressure, and cardiac output, constitutes the only acceptable objective evidence of the patient's postoperative status. It is thus highly advantageous to have a preoperative study available for comparison. The decision to perform a second operation is important since the chances are high (80%) that valve replacement will be needed at that time.

Treatment

Almost all patients who have had mitral valvotomy ultimately require valve replacement. Temporizing with a second valvotomy is generally attempted when the valve is flexible and shows little or no calcification. It is unusual for a second valvotomy to be performed after the menopause in female patients, but the clinical picture in patients who have undergone surgical treatment is quite variable.

The principal problem posed by patients who have had a previous valvotomy is for the physician to decide when the patient's condition has deteriorated sufficiently to require further surgery. The subjective improvement after mitral valve surgery is so much more impressive than the objective evidence of improvement that the decision to operate again is often somewhat arbitrary.

A later form of iatrogenically modified mitral valve disease occurs after mitral valve replacement. Pulmonary vascular disease is sometimes irreversible, and when its development is arrested, cardiac function often continues to deteriorate as degenerative age-related changes occur. Patients with raised pulmonary vascular resistance often develop chronic severe right heart failure that responds poorly to treatment. In such cases, left ventricular failure may also be present, as shown by a rise in end-diastolic left ventricular pressure. This finding may be due to the mechanical effects of extreme right-sided enlargement and resembles that seen in patients with atrial septal defect who are in heart failure or patients with primary pulmonary hypertension. There is often an extreme posterior displacement of the left ventricle. Patients with such lesions are usually subjected to repeated investigation in the hope of finding some surgically treatable lesion, but in practice they are usually exhibiting the long-term effects of rheumatic carditis.

PATIENTS WITH ARTIFICIAL VALVES

Patients who have had mitral or aortic valve replacement are becoming more common in everyday medical practice. By far the largest number of such patients have Starr-Edwards ball and cage prostheses. Other forms of plastic and metal valves, such as the Björk-Shiley disk valve, and homograft or heterograft (Hancock) tissue valves are also used.

The clinical picture in patients who have had valve replacement varies greatly and depends on the type of valve used, the nature of the original lesion, the stage at which operation was performed, and the success of the operation. Few patients are free of symptoms; the problems encountered are most commonly related to thrombosis, embolism, leakage or obstruction of the valve, and hemorrhage from excessive anticoagulant therapy.

Clinical Findings

A. Symptoms: Many patients with artificial valves have residual shortness of breath on exertion. Most have at least a small pressure gradient across the valve at rest that becomes larger when the cardiac output and heart rate increase during exercise. The patient may also complain of the loud noise made by the artificial valve as it opens and closes with each heartbeat, but most patients become accustomed to the sensation within a few weeks after operation.

B. Signs: The physical signs arising from an artificial valve depend on the nature and type of valve used. Tissue valves do not give rise to the loud opening and closing clicks heard with metal and plastic prostheses. However, they do tend to leak with the passage of time as the tissue stiffens and calcifies. Thus, mitral systolic and aortic diastolic murmurs are not uncommon. The opening and closing clicks of plastic and metal valves are characteristic for each individual brand of valve. In general, there is a loud opening click at the start of systole and a loud closing click at the end of systole. The clicks are usually louder than the normal heart sounds and interfere with auscultation of natural valves. Systolic and diastolic murmurs are difficult to interpret in patients with artificial valves, and more importance should be given to changes in the auscultatory findings than to the findings themselves.

Signs of pulmonary congestion and right heart failure with edema and a raised venous pressure are found when surgical results are poor.

C. Electrocardiographic Findings: There are no characteristic ECG changes in patients with artificial heart valves. Postoperative ECG changes reflect surgical results.

D. X-Ray Findings: Artificial heart valves composed of metal are clearly seen on chest x-rays. Even the plastic ball can usually be seen moving up and down with the heartbeat on cinefluoroscopy. The position of the artificial valve varies considerably from case to case, and a change in the position of the valve or in its movement during the cardiac cycle is important evidence of valvular dysfunction. Tissue valves may calcify with time and become visible on chest x-ray.

E. Special Investigations:

1. **Noninvasive technics**–Because plastic and metal valves reflect ultrasound well, they are readily detected by echocardiography. However, it is difficult to determine valve function by this means of study.

2. **Invasive technics**–Cardiac catheterization and angiography are usually needed to decide whether prosthetic valve malfunction is severe enough to warrant reoperation. Most physicians carefully avoid passing a catheter through a prosthetic valve for fear of causing damage. When catheters have been inadvertently passed through artificial valves, little ill effect has been noticed. The most important information sought in studies of patients with artificial valves is the pressure difference across the valve and the flow through it. Angiography is commonly used to test for valvular incompetence.

Differential Diagnosis

The principal problem in differential diagnosis is distinguishing artificial valve malfunction from disease of another valve. Full study of the patient is needed in such cases, and the findings vary greatly in individual patients.

Complications

Thrombosis around the artificial valve, with consequent stenosis and systemic embolism, is the commonest complication of artificial valves. Anticoagulant therapy is needed in all types of valves except tissue valves, and hemorrhage due to excessive anticoagulation is also encountered. When thrombus forms around a prosthetic valve, it may disturb valve function and interfere with both the opening and the closing of the valve. Thus, both stenosis and incompetence can result from thrombus formation around an artificial valve. In some cases, especially early after operation, valve displacement due to tearing out of the sutures anchoring the valve leads to paravalvular leak. In other cases the valve mechanism itself may fail and cause leakage. Sudden death is still an important complication of valve replacement. The mechanism is not always clear, but escape of a worn ball from the cage mechanism has been reported. In other cases, the valve mechanism sticks shut. Hemolysis may occur after valve replacement. Mechanical trauma to the red cells resulting from contact with the artificial valve is thought to be responsible. Infective endocarditis can also occur when the endothelialized surface of the prosthetic valve becomes infected. Infection at this site is particularly difficult to eradicate, and removal of the infected prosthesis and replacement are often necessary.

Treatment

A second valve replacement is the only effective therapy for artificial valve malfunction. Both the patient and the physician are naturally reluctant to take this major step, and clear evidence of malfunction is required before a second artificial valve is inserted. In some cases, one of the natural valves proves to be the cause of the problem and needs replacement.

Prognosis

The long-term prognosis of patients with artificial valves is not yet established. Current data show that most of the problems occur in the first year after surgery and that once this period has passed, fewer complications arise.

• • •

References

Aroesty JM & others: Carcinoid heart disease. Circulation 34:105, 1966.

Bacon APC, Matthews MB: Congenital bicuspid aortic valves and the aetiology of isolated aortic valvular stenosis. Q J Med 28:545, 1959.

Barratt-Boyes BG: Homograft aortic valve replacement in aortic incompetence and stenosis. Thorax 19:131, 1964.

Bean WB & others: The syndrome of carcinoid and acquired valve lesions of the right side of the heart. Circulation 12:1, 1955.

Bernhard WF & others: Progress and problems in the surgical management of congenital aortic stenosis. J Thorac Cardiovasc Surg 66:404, 1973.

Biörck G, Axen O, Thorson A: Unusual cyanosis in a boy with congenital pulmonary stenosis and tricuspid insufficiency: Fatal outcome after angiography. Am Heart J 44:143, 1952.

Botvinick EH & others: Echocardiographic demonstration of early mitral valve closure in severe aortic insufficiency: Its clinical implications. Circulation 51:836, 1975.

Braunwald E & others: Congenital aortic stenosis: Clinical and hemodynamic findings in 100 patients. Circulation 27:426, 1963.

Bristow JD, Kremkau DL: Hemodynamic changes after valve replacement with Starr-Edwards prostheses. Am J Cardiol 35:716, 1975.

Bulkley B, Roberts WC: Ankylosing spondylitis and aortic regurgitation: Description of the characteristic cardiovascular lesion from study of eight necropsy patients. Circulation 48:1014, 1973.

Campbell M: Calcific aortic stenosis and congenital bicuspid aortic valve. Br Heart J 30:606, 1968.

Cohen LS, Friedman WF, Braunwald E: Natural history of mild congenital aortic stenosis elucidated by serial hemodynamic studies. Am J Cardiol 30:1, 1972.

Davies CE, Steiner RE: Calcified aortic valve: Clinical and radiological features. Br Heart J 8:733, 1949.

Denie J, Verheugt SP: Supravalvular aortic stenosis. Circulation 18:902, 1958.

Eddleman EE Jr & others: Critical analysis of clinical factors in estimating severity of aortic valve disease. Am J Cardiol 31:687, 1973.

Eyster E, Mayer K, McKenzie S: Traumatic hemolysis with iron deficiency anemia in patients with aortic valve lesions. Ann Intern Med 68:995, 1968.

Fenoglio JJ Jr others: Congenital bicuspid aortic valve after age 20. Am J Cardiol 39:164, 1977.

Fleming PR: The mechanism of the pulsus bisferiens. Br Heart J 19:519, 1957.

Fortuin NJ, Craige E: On the mechanism of the Austin Flint murmur. Circulation 45:558, 1972.

Frank S, Johnson A, Ross J Jr: Natural history of valvular aortic stenosis. Br Heart J 35:41, 1973.

Gault JH & others: Left ventricular performance following correction of free aortic regurgitation. Circulation 42:773, 1970.

Goldschlager N & others: The natural history of aortic regurgitation. Am J Med 54:577, 1973.

Grahame-Smith DG: The carcinoid syndrome. Am J Cardiol 21:376, 1968.

Griffin FM Jr, Jones G, Cobbs CG: Aortic insufficiency in bacterial endocarditis. Ann Intern Med 76:23, 1972.

Hirshfeld JW & others: Indices predicting long-term survival after valve replacement in patients with aortic regurgitation and patients with aortic stenosis. Circulation 50:1190, 1974.

Hunt D & others: Quantitative evaluation of cineaortography in the assessment of aortic regurgitation. Am J Cardiol 31:696, 1973.

Kerzacky AK & others: Combined mitral and aortic valve disease. Am J Cardiol 25:588, 1970.

Kirklin JW, Pacifico AD: Surgery for acquired valvular heart disease. (2 parts.) N Engl J Med 288:133, 194, 1973.

Kloster FE: Diagnosis and management of complications of prosthetic heart valves. Am J Cardiol 35:872, 1975.

Lee SJK & others: Circulatory changes in severe aortic regurgitation before and after surgical correction. Am J Cardiol 28:442, 1971.

Lee SJK & others: Hemodynamic changes following correction of severe aortic stenosis using the Cutter-Smeloff prosthesis. Circulation 42:719, 1970.

Mengel CE: Carcinoid and the heart. Mod Concepts Cardiovasc Dis 35:75, 1966.

Mundth ED, Austen WG: Postoperative intensive care in the cardiac surgical patient. Prog Cardiovasc Dis 11:229, 1968.

Najafi H: Aortic insufficiency: Clinical manifestations and surgical treatment. Am Heart J 82:120, 1971.

Najafi H & others: Acute aortic regurgitation secondary to aortic dissection: Surgical management without valve replacement. Ann Thorac Surg 14:474, 1972.

Pacifico AD, Karp RB, Kirklin JW: Homografts for replacement of the aortic valve. Circulation 45 (Suppl 1):1, 1972.

Pansegrau DG & others: Supravalvular aortic stenosis in adults. Am J Cardiol 31:535, 1973.

Paton BC & others: Ruptured sinus of Valsalva. Arch Surg 90:209, 1965.

Paulus HE, Pearson CM, Pitts W Jr: Aortic insufficiency in five patients with Reiter's syndrome: A detailed clinical and pathologic study. Am J Med 53:464, 1972.

Perloff JK: Clinical recognition of aortic stenosis: The physical signs and differential diagnosis of the various forms of obstruction to left ventricular outflow. Prog Cardiovasc Dis 10:323, 1968.

Pernow B, Waldenstrom J: Paroxysmal flushing and other symptoms caused by 5-hydroxytryptamine and histamine in patients with malignant tumors. Lancet 2:951, 1954.

Pluth JR, McGoon DC: Current status of heart valve replacement. Mod Concepts Cardiovasc Dis 43:65, 1974.

Reis RL & others: Congenital fixed subvalvular aortic stenosis. Circulation 43 (Suppl 1):11, 1971.

Reis RL & others: The flexible stent: A new concept in the fabrication of tissue heart valve prostheses. J Thorac Cardiovasc Surg 62:683, 1971.

Rotman M & others: Aortic valvular disease: Comparison of types and their medical and surgical management. Am J Med 51:241, 1971.

Shine KI & others: Combined aortic and mitral incompetence: Clinical features and surgical management. Am Heart J 76:728, 1968.

Spagnuolo M & others: Natural history of rheumatic aortic regurgitation: Criteria predictive of death, congestive heart failure, and angina in young patients. Circulation 44:368, 1971.

Ureles AL: Diagnosis and treatment of malignant carcinoid syndrome. JAMA 229:1346, 1974.

Weinstein L: Infected prosthetic valves: A diagnostic and therapeutic dilemma. N Engl J Med 286:1108, 1972.

Wigle ED, Labrosse CJ: Sudden, severe aortic insufficiency. Circulation 32:708, 1965.

Wise JR & others: Urgent aortic-valve replacement for acute aortic regurgitation due to infective endocarditis. Lancet 2:115, 1971.

Wood P: Aortic stenosis. Am J Cardiol 1:553, 1958.

Yacoub MH, Keeling DH: Chronic haemolysis following insertion of Ball valve prosthesis. Br Heart J 30:676, 1968.

14 . . .
Conduction Defects

NORMAL ELECTROPHYSIOLOGY & CONDUCTION*

Disorders of the formation (initiation) and conduction (transmission) of the cardiac impulse are among the most common and important problems in cardiology. Disturbances of cardiac rhythm have intrigued cardiologists for many years because the mechanisms involved are so complex, because the clinical situations in which arrhythmias occur are so variable, and because their proper management requires expert clinical judgment. Our understanding of the electrophysiology of the heart has been greatly expanded by the development of the Graham-Girard glass microelectrode, which permits measurement of intracellular electrical activity and has provided the background for an understanding of the action potential. Much of what we know about clinical arrhythmias is based on electrophysiologic studies of the properties of single cardiac cells and correlation of those studies with clinical data on ECG abnormalities, the clinical course of arrhythmias, and patients' responses to treatment. The limitations of these extrapolations will of course be obvious.

Advances have resulted also from technical developments such as continuous ambulatory monitoring of the ECG; bedside monitoring with memory loops, permitting study of events in the 30–60 sec prior to the start of an arrhythmia or conduction defect; His bundle recordings, which distinguish supraventricular and ventricular origins of disturbances of rhythm; timed intracardiac stimulation and recording; rapid atrial pacing; and precise determination of refractory periods and antegrade and retrograde conduction. Continuous monitoring has shown the great frequency of ventricular arrhythmias in patients with acute myocardial infarction, ventricular aneurysm, and chronic coronary heart disease. The newer electrophysiologic studies combined with intracardiac stimulation and recording have incriminated reentry rather than increased automaticity as the usual mechanism for paroxysmal atrial tachycardia. At the same time, they have demonstrated that many of the junctional rhythms that occur in acute myocardial infarction and digitalis toxicity result from increased automaticity of the junctional tissues rather than reentry.

*The discussion here is pertinent also to the subject matter of Chapter 15, Cardiac Arrhythmias.

ELECTROPHYSIOLOGY OF THE HEART

Transmission of Cardiac Impulse

Excitation of the heart is due to propagation of an impulse which starts in the sinoatrial node and is transmitted by the specialized conduction system sequentially through intranodal atrial tracts, the atrioventricular node, the bundle of His, the bundle branches, the Purkinje fibers, and finally, by arborization, the ordinary ventricular muscle (Fig 14–1). The sequential firing is highly organized in normal subjects, and the timing allows orderly contraction of the vari-

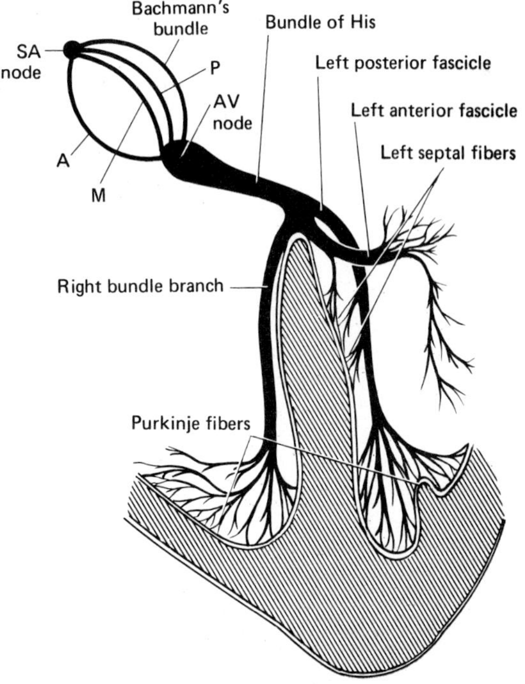

Figure 14–1. The conduction system. A, M, P, anterior, medial, and posterior interatrial tracts. (Adapted and reproduced, with permission, from Goldman MJ: *Principles of Clinical Electrocardiography*, 9th ed. Lange, 1976.)

ous cardiac chambers and thus efficient cardiac contraction. The cardiac cells are all interconnected and can transmit excitatory stimulation one to the other, but the velocity of conduction through the specialized conduction system and the differences in refractory period act to couple excitation with contraction to generate an effective cardiac output. The action potential (see below), conduction velocity, and recovery of excitability (refractory period) vary in different portions of the heart as well as in different cells of the specialized conduction system. This provides a mechanism by which the cardiac impulse is transmitted to different parts of the heart, permitting a proper sequence of contraction and preventing tetanic contraction such as can occur in skeletal muscle. The refractory period of skeletal muscle is short. The muscle responds to an impulse in a single direction from a single nerve supplying the muscle. In contrast, the refractory period in cardiac muscle is longer, the impulse can be spread in all directions, and direct nervous stimulation does not occur.

A. Conduction to Atrioventricular Node: There are at least 3 interatrial tracks as well as the Bachmann bundle* whereby the excitation wave spreads from the sinoatrial node to the atrioventricular node, whose conduction and refractory characteristics slow the spread of the impulse and thus prevent inordinately rapid ventricular rates. The long effective refractory period of the atrioventricular node prevents it from responding rapidly to impulses received from the sinus node or from the atria.

One may think of the atrioventricular node as a protective mechanism to prevent the ventricles from responding regularly to rapid atrial stimuli, whereas the specialized cells below the sinus node and in particular below the atrioventricular node may be considered protective in that secondary and tertiary pacemakers initiate the heartbeat if the primary pacemakers should fail. They may be considered as junior officers who take over command of the ship when the captain collapses. This is in contrast to ectopic pacemakers, which are active and not passive originators of an impulse beginning in one of the specialized cells anywhere along the specialized conduction pathway below the normal sinoatrial node and which "take command" with a rate of pacing faster than the inherent pacemaker activity of the sinoatrial node. The conduction system both initiates and conducts impulses; conduction abnormalities and cardiac arrhythmias often have similar mechanisms and coexist.

B. Bundle of His and Bundle Branches: When the excitation wave leaves the atrioventricular node, it arrives at the bundle of His and travels down its 2 branches, the left and right bundles. The right bundle does not branch until its distal portion. The left bundle is usually described as dividing into 2 major subdivisions (fascicles)—the left anterior superior and the left posterior inferior branches—although the anatomy of the left bundle is really much more complex and variable, ie, in addition to the 2 main subdivisions there may be many distal interconnections between the bundles and the fascicles (Massing, 1976). The 2 main branches of the left bundle plus the right bundle can be thought of as 3 fascicles of the bundle of His. The terms unifascicular, bifascicular, and trifascicular block have come into use because electrophysiologic studies, including His bundle recordings, have demonstrated that one can distinguish dominant conduction delay in one or more of these 3 fascicles.

C. Purkinje System and Myocardium: The conduction velocity of the depolarization wave (see below) varies, so that the impulse travels rapidly via the peripheral Purkinje cells in the endocardium to activate both ventricles and then, more slowly, to activate the ventricular muscle.

Action Potential

The initiating event in the propagation of the cardiac impulse is the development of an action potential in the sinoatrial nodal cells. The electrical events leading to the contraction of the heart involve a sequential process whereby the resting cell membrane is first depolarized and then repolarized. The resting cell membrane potential (−90 mV) is a manifestation of the asymmetric distribution of sodium and potassium ions across the cell membrane, with the interior of the cell high in potassium and low in sodium. This electrochemical gradient for sodium and potassium is produced by the continued action of the ionic sodium pump. The sequential depolarization and repolarization of the cell has conventionally been divided into 5 phases (see p 424). The ability of cardiac tissue to be depolarized by a stimulus from a neighboring cell or by spontaneous depolarization is called excitability, which is maximal just before depolarization.

The depolarization of the cell (phase 0, Fig 14–2), which initiates the action potential, results from the change in the electrical properties of the cell brought about initially by a rapid change in the permeability of the cell membrane to sodium ions. The mechanism by which the cell membrane becomes permeable to sodium ions is not completely known. There is a channel or pore in the cell membrane controlled by "gates" which open, allowing a rapid inward current of sodium into the cell. Repolarization follows in what has been called phase 2, owing to cessation of increased permeability to sodium ions followed by a slow inward current of calcium ions through a different channel. Increased permeability of the cell membrane to potassium causes repolarization. The calcium influx through the "slow" calcium channel apparently results in increased availability of calcium ions from intracellular stores, which affect the actin-myosin interaction and result in contraction of the cell fibers. The sequence is known as excitation-contraction coupling.

Fig 14–2 illustrates the action potential of a Purkinje fiber combined with ionic fluxes during var-

*See Fig 14–1. Bachmann's bundle is a bypass bundle that forms a direct connection with the sinoatrial and atrioventricular nodes.

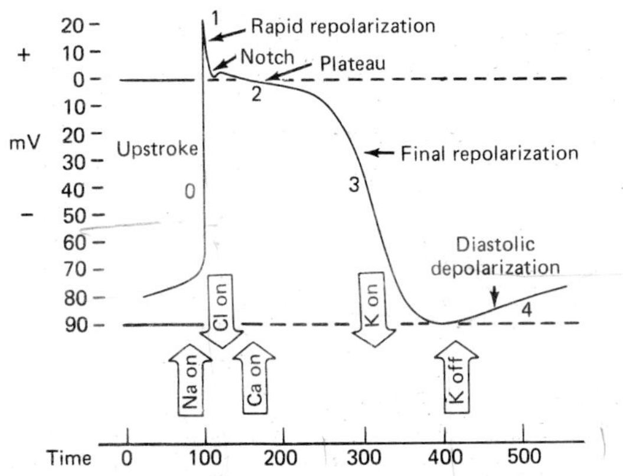

Figure 14–2. Diagrammatic representation of a cardiac action potential, emphasizing characteristics of the Purkinje fiber (false tendon) action potential. Each distinctive phase is labeled where the ionic events related to it are discussed. The arrows below the diagram refer to the approximate time when the indicated ion is influencing membrane potential. They point in the direction of the effect on the membrane potential, upward for depolarization and downward for repolarization. (Reproduced, with permission, from Fozzard HA, Gibbons WR: Action potential and contraction of heart muscle. Am J Cardiol 31:182, 1973.)

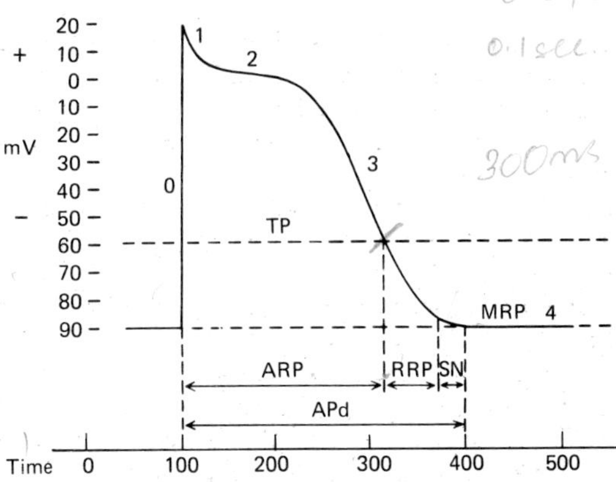

Figure 14–3. Diagram of the action potential of a ventricular muscle cell. MRP, membrane resting potential; 0, depolarization; 1, 2, 3, phases of repolarization; 4, diastolic phase, MRP; APd, duration of action potential; TP, threshold potential; ARP, absolute refractory period; RRP, relative refractory period; SN, supernormal period. (Reproduced, with permission, from Goldman MJ: *Principles of Clinical Electrocardiography,* 9th ed. Lange, 1976.)

ious phases of the action potential. Phase 0 is the rapid upstroke which carries the maximum resting membrane potential from about –90 mV to +25 mV. It lasts only a few milliseconds and, as stated above, results from the rapid inward flow of sodium, which accelerates as the membrane potential reaches threshold value at about –55 or –60 mV.

The maximum negative resting potential (normally about –90 mV) decreases (becomes less negative) with ischemia, fibrosis, hypoxia, acidosis, and increased extracellular potassium concentration and as a result of the action of various antiarrhythmia agents such as quinidine. As will be seen later under the discussion of conduction, the maximum rate of depolarization (phase 0 of the action potential) is a function of the magnitude of the maximum resting potential when depolarization begins. As the maximum negative resting membrane potential decreases (becomes less negative), the rate of rise of phase 0 slows from the normal rate of 500 V/sec to 300 V/sec when the membrane potential decreases to –70 mV (Watanabe, 1975).

Fig 14–3 shows an action potential from a ventricular muscle cell. Phase 4 is flat in atrial and ventricular muscle but has an upward slope in the sinoatrial node, as in the Purkinje fibers and in any portion of the specialized conduction system capable of spontaneous depolarization. The steeper upward slope of phase 4 ultimately reaches threshold potential and so initiates depolarization.

Five Phases of the Action Potential

The 5 phases of the action potential are phases 0, 1, 2, 3, and 4:

Phase 0: Rapid depolarization from –90 to about +25 mV.

Phase 1: This is short and represents early repolarization when the electrical potential falls to about 0.

Phase 2: The plateau phase of repolarization, corresponding to the ST segment of the ECG and lasting about 150 msec.

Phase 3: This is short, lasting about 50 msec. It corresponds to the T wave and ends with the membrane potential returning to resting potential. During most of phase 3 the cell is unable to respond to any stimulus, no matter how strong (absolute refractory period*). In the last part of phase 3, as the membrane potential approaches the threshold value, the cardiac cell is now only relatively inexcitable (the relative refractory period) and will respond to a strong stimulus either by propagation from a neighboring cell or from early spontaneous depolarization of the succeeding phase.

Phase 4: The action potential gradually returns to a resting value of –90 mV in all but the specialized automatic cells, in which the voltage rises to or toward a threshold of –75 mV (see below).

A. Slope of Phase 4: The slope of phase 4 is normally zero in nonspecialized cells, whereas in the specialized conduction cells (automatic cells), phase 4 gradually becomes less negative and depolarizes until it reaches threshold potential (about –75 mV), when it may spontaneously generate a new action potential which may then propagate in all directions. Because

*See discussion of refractory period under Properties of the Heart on p 9 as well as Fig 14–3, which illustrates the absolute refractory period.

the upward slope of phase 4 in the sinoatrial node is normally steeper than in any other part of the specialized conduction system, threshold potential is reached first at this site, making the sinoatrial node the pacemaker of the heart and the initiator of the sequence of events leading to cardiac contraction.

This function of all of the specialized conduction cells of the heart is known as automaticity (see below); such cells are also known as automatic or latent pacemaker cells. Automaticity is a fundamental property of specialized cells and is influenced not only by the maximum resting membrane potential but also by sympathetic impulses, which enhance it; by factors (fever, sympathetic stimuli, drugs, etc) that increase the slope of phase 4; or by pathologic states such as hypoxia, hypercapnia, ischemia, and cardiac dilatation that likewise increase the slope of phase 4. Parasympathetic impulses flatten the slope of phase 4 and thus slow the heart rate by increasing the time taken to reach the threshold potential. The mechanisms by which pacemaker cells can be provoked to initiate impulses are related to changes in membrane permeability to ions such as sodium, potassium, and calcium. Fig 14–2 shows ionic changes during the Purkinje action potential. The permeability of the cell membrane that initiates the ionic fluxes is related to disease processes and varies in different parts of the heart.

B. Varied Configuration of Action Potential in Disease States: The configuration of the action potential described above, characteristic of Purkinje cells, differs in different parts of the heart, so that the duration of the action potential, both depolarization and repolarization, varies in such a way as to ensure orderly sequential cardiac contraction. Disease states, electrolyte concentrations, and drug effects alter the configuration of the action potential by changing the maximum resting potential, the slope of phase 0, and the duration of the action potential and its various components, thus influencing the velocity of conduction and excitation-contraction coupling.

C. Calcium Influx: Calcium influx is significant, especially when the maximum resting membrane potential decreases and the fast inward current of sodium is decreased. An example is the new drug verapamil (not approved by the FDA in the USA but used extensively in Europe), which, by blocking the inward calcium current, slows conduction through the atrioventricular node and so is useful in treating and preventing reentry paroxysmal atrial tachycardia and other arrhythmias. Calcium influx is increased by catecholamines and therefore speeds conduction.

Properties of Specialized Cells

Knowledge of the inherent characteristics of specialized cells is basic to the understanding of cardiac arrhythmias. These include automaticity, excitability, conductivity, refractoriness, and capacity for reentry.

A. Automaticity: Certain cells of the specialized conduction system are able to spontaneously initiate an action potential which sequentially activates the entire heart. Maximum automaticity is characteristic of the sinoatrial nodal cells that initiate the cardiac impulse, because their spontaneous slow depolarization during phase 4 has the steepest slope of any of the specialized cells in the heart. These cells thus serve as the pacemaker of the heart. The inherent slope of phase 4 is more gradual as one descends from the sinoatrial node to the atrioventricular junction and finally to the Purkinje fibers. With failure of any of the more proximal pacemakers, a more distal latent pacemaker cell may become the pacemaker of the heart, preventing cardiac standstill and producing "escape" pacemaker rhythms. The rate of automatic discharge slows as the escape pacemaker becomes more distal, and it is common to have the "escape" rhythms originating in the junctional tissues near the atrioventricular node, in the bundle of His, or in the Purkinje system when the primary pacemakers in the sinoatrial node fail for any reason. This is in contrast to actively increased automaticity (by disease, drugs, or overactivity of the sympathetic nervous system) of subsidiary pacemaker cells which may allow the cells to assume the role of cardiac pacemaker at more rapid rates. When secondary pacemakers take command of the heart by default, it is because of failure of the primary pacemakers. When the subsidiary pacemakers take command because of increased automaticity, it is akin to mutiny because the competing impulse opposes the primary pacemakers, which are still functioning. Under ordinary circumstances, the heart rate is determined by the slope of diastolic depolarization of the sinus node cells. The sinoatrial node is under the influence of the autonomic nervous system; stimulation of the vagus nerve, either spontaneously, by reflex, or by drugs, decreases the slope of phase 4 and therefore slows the heart rate. Sympathetic cardiac stimulation by drugs or via the central nervous system directly or reflexly increases the heart rate by increasing the slope of phase 4. Latent or subsidiary pacemakers, although capable of becoming enhanced and taking command of the heart, are basically protective and provide a backup mechanism in the event that the more proximal automatic cells fail to "fire."

B. Excitability: The ability of a cell to respond to a stimulus and initiate an action potential is called excitability. The term also denotes the ability of a cell to respond to a propagated impulse from a neighboring cell. The action potential itself serves as a stimulus to excite neighboring cells, and in this way, in a sequential and orderly manner, the heart is depolarized.

C. Conductivity: Conduction of an electrical impulse from one cell to another is a fundamental property of cardiac tissue and results from the spread of electrical activity from one specialized cell to another and finally to myocardial cells. The velocity of conduction varies in different tissues of the heart and is 100 times more rapid in the Purkinje system than in the atrioventricular node. It is about 20–30 mm/sec in the atrioventricular node, 3000–5000 mm/sec in the Purkinje system, and about 500–600 mm/sec in the ventricle. Slow conduction through the atrioventricular node prolongs the absolute refractory period in nodal cells and prevents rapid atrial impulses from activating the ventricles at the same rapid rate as the atria. In normal adults, this prevents them from beating so rapidly that they cannot maintain a normal cardiac output. Infants do not have the same conduction delay in the atrioventricular node and can have atrial arrhythmias with ventricular rates as high as 300/min.

Velocity of conduction. The velocity of conduction is related to the magnitude of the resting membrane potential when the action potential begins. The velocity is slower and there is a decreased rate of rise of phase 0 when the resting membrane potential is less negative. The velocity of the conduction is also related to the heart rate. Decrease in the slope and amplitude of phase 4 depolarization increases the time between successive action potentials and the velocity of conduction in the subsequent beat. When the velocity of conduction is slowed sufficiently as a result of decreased maximum resting membrane potential, conduction may be sufficiently impaired so that it decreases as the depolarization wave spreads distally, with the result that the impulse may not be propagated throughout the entire conduction system. The ability of the excitation wave to propagate may progressively deteriorate. The term decremental conduction refers to the progressive decrease in conduction that results from alterations in the characteristics of the action potential owing to cellular abnormalities in the conduction pathway until ultimately a propagated impulse cannot be sustained. Decremental conduction may leave in its wake cells which have been incompletely repolarized and therefore have become refractory to an oncoming antegrade stimulus. It may not be obvious on the ECG and is one form of concealed conduction, which may also result when premature beats partially penetrate but do not pass through the atrioventricular node to the remainder of the conduction system. Such failure to conduct completely is called concealed conduction regardless of whether the spread is antegrade from the atria or retrograde from the ventricles. Decreased conduction may cause conduction delay or block anywhere along the normal pathway. Failure or delay in conduction may not be uniform, ie, it may be more manifest in one fiber than in a neighboring one and may be important in setting up a reentry circuit, causing premature beats or tachycardia (see below). Failure of conduction is usually due to disease such as fibrosis, ischemia, hypoxia, acidosis, or drugs or hyperkalemia, any of which decreases the maximum resting membrane potential or shortens repolarization, allowing the resting membrane potential during diastole to be closer to the threshold potential. This decreases the velocity of the upstroke of phase 0 of depolarization, which determines the velocity of conduction.

D. Refractoriness: Refractoriness is the property by which cardiac cells fail to respond to an oncoming stimulus because repolarization is incomplete and the voltage of the interior of the cell has not become sufficiently negative to initiate or propagate an action potential. It is related to excitability in that the cell is totally unexcitable when the voltage is less negative than threshold and no stimulus, no matter how strong, can evoke a propagated response. This is the absolute refractory period (Fig 14–3). As the voltage of the cell becomes more negative at the end of phase 3, the resting membrane potential may not have reached its normal value of −90 mV but may be sufficiently negative that a powerful stimulus can evoke a response even though it may not be sufficiently strong to be fully propagated and may depolarize a few neighboring cells. Shortly after this relative refractory period and before the normal resting maximum diastolic pressure potential has been reached, there is a short "supernormal" phase corresponding to the downstroke of the T wave, during which time a smaller than usual current can induce a propagated response. This brief period of increased excitability follows the relative refractory period and has been termed the supernormal phase of excitability (Fig 14–3). The supernormal or vulnerable phase is responsible for the so-called R on T phenomenon, in which a ventricular premature beat falling on the descending limb of the T wave may induce repetitive ventricular ectopic discharges, including ventricular fibrillation.

The refractory period varies in different parts of the heart, being shortest in the atrium and longest in the Purkinje system and in the atrioventricular node. This variability of recovery of excitability or refractoriness is exaggerated in portions of the ventricle or conduction system in diseases such as ischemic heart disease. Altered, uneven recovery of excitability in ischemic cells may be responsible for the frequency of ventricular arrhythmias in coronary heart disease. Recovery of refractoriness, excitability, and conduction velocity varies from one cell to another and from one tissue region to another. This variability affects repolarization, heart rate, and duration of the action potential and can thus initiate reentry arrhythmias (Han, 1966). Drugs rather than disease may exaggerate these changes; digitalis, for example, shortens the action potential, whereas quinidine prolongs it. Hypokalemia lengthens and hyperkalemia shortens the action potential.

E. Capacity for Reentry:

1. Mechanism of arrhythmias—Reentry is not a property of cardiac cells per se but is thought to be the mechanism by which arrhythmias can develop in any portion of the heart through disturbances in the fundamental properties noted above. An automatic cell, by increasing the slope of phase 4 depolarization and increasing its automaticity, can become the pacemaker of the heart, producing either a premature beat or tachycardia. Similarly, through operation of a reentry mechanism, a premature beat can be propagated by a circuitous route through an area of the heart and permit continuous repetitive depolarization and tachycardia.

Fig 14–4 shows in schematic fashion a reentrant pathway and how it can be modified.

2. Requirements for reentry—Normally, the cardiac impulse propagates evenly through the distal conducting system to the ventricles, with equal velocity in

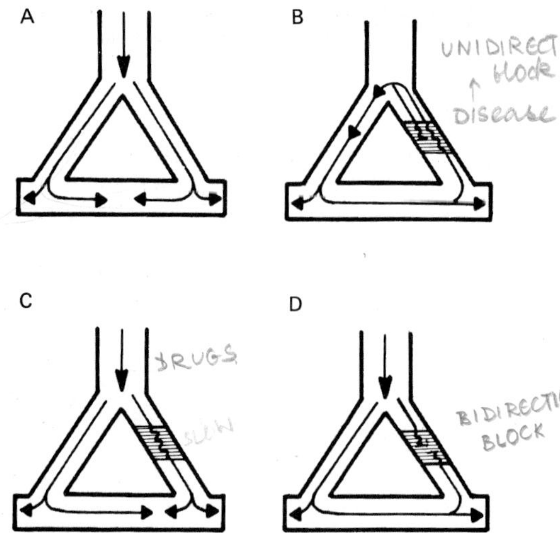

Figure 14–4. Schematic diagram of reentrant pathway and means for its modification. *A:* Normal propagation through the distal conducting system to the ventricle. Conduction proceeds with equal velocity through both limbs of a terminal Purkinje fiber bundle and then activates the myocardium. *B:* Shaded area indicates diseased tissue, including partially depolarized Purkinje fibers. Antegrade activation through the site is blocked. Activation proceeds normally through the other limb to the myocardium and then activates the depressed segment in a retrograde direction. This impulse succeeds in propagating slowly through the depressed segment and reenters the proximal conducting system. *C:* If physiologic changes occur or appropriate pharmacologic agents are administered (see text), conduction may improve through the depressed segment and result in reestablishment of antegrade activation and abolition of reentry. *D:* If changes occur (or are induced) which result in block of retrograde activation as well as antegrade activation, then bidirectional conduction block occurs. This condition, too, would suppress a reentrant arrhythmia. (Reproduced, with permission, from Rosen MR & others: Electrophysiology and pharmacology of cardiac arrhythmias. 5. Cardiac antiarrhythmic effects of lidocaine. Am Heart J 89:526, 1975.)

each of the closely related cardiac fibers (for purposes of illustration called "limbs" of a terminal Purkinje fiber bundle, as illustrated in Fig 14–4). Use of the term limb is not meant to imply that every area of the Purkinje system has only 2 fibers. Reentry requires that one portion of the myocardial fiber in a bundle of fibers be blocked in one direction (usually antegrade) because that "limb" is partially depolarized and cannot conduct properly (unidirectional block). Reentry also requires that antegrade activation through the other limb of the distal Purkinje fiber be slowed but spread in the normal direction to the ventricle. It then returns to the point of origin in a retrograde manner and activates the initially blocked limb or fiber. The impulse proceeds slowly in retrograde fashion through the segment that had antegrade block until it reaches the proximal conducting fiber, which by this time has recovered its excitability and is no longer refractory as a result of excitation; this allows a retrograde impulse from the originally blocked segment to reenter the normal segment or limb, setting up a reentry circuit which may then become repetitive.

Reentry requires, then, both impaired conduction (in one limb) and unidirectional block (in the other). Decremental conduction (as discussed above) may slow conduction in one fiber or produce antegrade unidirectional block in another fiber and so foster reentry. Parts C and D of Fig 14–4 show how the reentry rhythm can be terminated, either by improving conduction in the depressed segment and thus allowing the initial impulse to spread equally through both limbs of the fibers, or by increasing the retrograde block in the blocked segment so that the original impulse cannot be conducted to the proximal site.

A new stimulus, either from an atrial premature beat or from retrograde excitation of the atria by ventricular premature beats, is the usual mechanism for initiating paroxysmal atrial tachycardia, with the reentry circuit involving the atrioventricular node. A repetitive reentry circuit can be interrupted by drugs such as digitalis or verapamil if the reentry circuit involves the atrioventricular node. These drugs increase atrioventricular block, prolonging conduction in the atrioventricular node and making it refractory to any new impulse that reaches the atrioventricular node as part of the reentry circuit. Return or echo beats find the atrioventricular node unexcitable so that it cannot continue to propagate the reentry circuit impulse.

Occurrence and causes of reentry. A reentry circuit can occur anywhere in the heart. In paroxysmal atrial tachycardia it usually includes the atrioventricular node. Atrial flutter is thought to result from a reentry pathway in the atria. In the ventricle it may occur in a diseased portion of the tissue. If there is an "excitable gap" between the head and tail of the reentry pathway (circus movement), there may be a continuous excitation wave that sets up a paroxysm of arrhythmia. Unidirectional block in one segment may be induced by ischemia, hypoxia, acidosis, potassium leak from necrotic cells, or (experimentally) by cooling. As a result of the relative automaticity of one group of cells, currents may be set up that stimulate neighboring cells and may lead to a propagated paroxysmal arrhythmia either via the reentry mechanism or via a direct ectopic rhythm (automaticity). Pathologic states such as ischemia do not affect all fibers uniformly, and irregular distribution of ischemia with resulting irregular return of cells to their maximum resting diastolic potential, with varying conduction velocity, may lead to cardiac arrhythmias. Ventricular arrhythmias may be due to propagation from an ectopic site which has assumed greater automaticity because of early recovery of excitability; in other instances, reentry may be the mechanism. Recovery of excitability and altered refractory periods are common, especially in the border zone between necrotic and surviving cells that behave as chronically ischemic cells. This may explain the high incidence of arrhythmias after myocardial infarction has healed and why unexpected ventricular fibrillation and sudden death may occur.

CAUSES OF CONDUCTION DEFECTS

Causes of Chronic Defects

Chronic sinoatrial and atrioventricular conduction defects are most commonly due to degenerative disease of the specialized conduction system. This is the mechanism responsible for over half of cases of chronic heart block. Coronary disease and cardiomyopathy are the 2 other major causes, and chronic congenital atrioventricular block is rare. The degenerative changes are mostly sclerofibrotic and may be quite extensive, involving any area of the conduction system from the atrioventricular node to the Purkinje fibers. The degenerative process usually begins after age 60, and many patients with fibrosis of the conduction system are in their seventh and eighth decades, but it may be present in younger persons. The cause of the fibrosis is not known. The usual presenting symptoms are those due to Stokes-Adams attacks.

Congestive Cardiomyopathy

Although persistent chronic conduction defects—atrial, ventricular, or bundle branch block—are commonly associated with ischemic heart disease, conduction defects that develop during the course of acute myocardial infarction do not commonly persist after the infarction heals. Whether coronary disease is a cause of or merely a concurrent disease in chronic conduction defects is the subject of debate at present. Idiopathic cardiomyopathy is a frequent cause.

Unknown Cause

Right or left bundle branch block or partial atrioventricular block is a common finding on routine ECGs in patients who have no clear history of disease to account for it. There was a time when it was thought that diphtheria, rheumatic fever, and other inflammatory myocarditides were responsible, but persistence of conduction defects in patients who develop them during these acute inflammatory disorders is uncommon. Partial atrioventricular block, for example, which is the most common ECG sign of acute rheumatic fever, was found to be persistent in only 4% of a large group of patients. Even meticulous pathologic studies of the conduction system are often insufficient to explain conduction defects during life in many patients. Serial sections of the conduction system correlate reasonably well with electrophysiologic studies in bundle branch block, but there are great variations in the anatomy of the conduction system even in normal hearts.

Causes of Acute Defects

Acute reversible conduction defects are usually due to drugs such as digitalis which produce atrioventricular block, acute myocardial infarction, acute myocarditis including rheumatic fever, and metabolic disorders such as hyperkalemia or hypokalemia. These account for most of the acute atrioventricular conduction defects. In some instances the cause is unknown, although subsequent observation sometimes reveals subtle manifestations of connective tissue disorders, scleroderma, cardiomyopathy, or sarcoidosis.

PATHOLOGY OF CONDUCTION SYSTEM ABNORMALITIES

As indicated above in the section on etiology, the commonest pathologic finding in cardiac conduction defects is sclerofibrosis involving the specialized conduction system anywhere from the sinoatrial node to the ventricles. An exception is congenital atrioventricular block, in which the pathologic process is not fibrosis but a degenerative process relatively well localized to the atrioventricular node. Most patients with chronic conduction defects have widespread lesions throughout the system, although the distribution may be spotty. On microscopic examination the lesions are often incomplete, although the ECG may appear complete. The term conduction delay or conduction defect is better than block because the pathologic process rarely produces complete block in chronic disease. It may occur in acute occlusion of the anterior descending coronary artery with resultant necrosis of an area of the septum which includes a portion of the conduction system. Although on the basis of the ECG or His bundle recordings one may speak of block or defect in one area of the impulse pathway, lesions can often be found in other parts of the conduction system as well. The ECG abnormality underestimates the extent of the disease process.

Control of Sinoatrial Node in Bradycardia

James (1970) has shown that the sinus node is controlled by both cholinergic and adrenergic nerves. Efferent impulses from the hypothalamus and cerebral cortex or from any part of the body may be transmitted to the sinus node via the autonomic nervous system. Noncardiac causes of sinus bradycardia involving this system must always be considered and evaluated in the light of the function of the sinus node as the common end pathway for many efferent impulses from the central nervous system.

Influence of Myocardial Infarction on Bradycardia

The artery to the sinus node arises in most people from the right coronary artery, but in about one-third of individuals it arises from a branch of the left circumflex artery; sinus bradycardia, therefore, is usually found in patients with acute inferior myocardial infarction resulting from occlusion of the right coronary artery. These slow heart rates are often transient or reversible, owing to ischemia of the sinus node and increased vagal tone, and can be reversed with time or with atropine. The slow heart rate is significant for 2 reasons: (1) By decreasing cardiac output, bradycardia may interfere with coronary perfusion and thus extend the infarction; and (2) a slow ventricular rate with variable conduction delay and repolarization may allow ectopic impulses to take over the rhythm of the heart in the ischemic or damaged ventricular muscle supplied by the right coronary artery. The role of drugs—especially beta-adrenergic blocking agents, opiates, tranquilizers, and phenothiazines—must always be considered in sinus bradycardia. The decreased phase 4 depolarization slope that occurs in hypothyroidism and other metabolic disturbances should also be considered in the analysis of sinus bradycardia.

Definition of Bradycardia; Relationship to Age

The assessment of sinus bradycardia is difficult since the definition itself is by no means uniform. Many authorities state that any regular sinus rate less than 60/min constitutes sinus bradycardia. Others use lower figures, such as 55 or 50/min. The age of the patient plays a role because slower heart rates (< 55/min) are more prevalent in healthy young individuals, especially athletes, are usually attributed to high vagal tone, are rarely associated with symptoms, and require no special investigative studies or treatment. Equivalent slow rates or more marked bradycardia (< 45/min) may produce symptoms in older individuals because, with the development of coronary artery disease and impaired left ventricular function, stroke volume may not be able to increase to compensate for the slow heart rate and there may be a fall in cardiac output. Sinus bradycardia at any age is fairly common unless one defines it as a rate less than 40/min.

Table 14–1. Holter monitoring findings in 95 patients with dizziness or syncope.*†

Clinical Findings	Number of Patients
No abnormalities detected	22
Findings definitely correlating with symptoms	46
Paroxysmal atrial fibrillation	6
Paroxysmal atrial flutter	1
Paroxysmal atrial tachycardia	11
Ventricular tachycardia	10
Sinus bradycardia	3
Sinoatrial block or standstill	5
Atrioventricular block, second degree	4
Atrioventricular block, third degree	3
Defective pacemaker	5
Findings possibly related to symptoms	42
Frequent premature atrial contractions	11‡
Frequent premature ventricular contractions	31§
Findings not related to symptoms	17
Sinus tachycardia (⩾ 120 beats/min)	8
Sinus bradycardia (⩽ 50 beats/min)	1
Intermittent bundle branch block	3
Atrioventricular block, first degree	5

*Reproduced, with permission, from Van Durme JP: Tachyarrhythmias and transient cerebral ischemic attacks. Am Heart J 89:538, 1975.

†Whenever a patient presented different types of arrhythmia or conduction defect, he was always listed under each separate item.

‡Five patients developed paroxysmal atrial tachycardia; 2 patients developed atrial fibrillation.

§Ten patients developed ventricular tachycardia.

DIFFERENTIAL DIAGNOSIS OF BRADYCARDIA

Because there is evidence that sinus bradycardia may not be as benign as once thought and because varying degrees of sinus node and atrial dysfunction as well as atrioventricular conduction defects may develop over a period of years, a 12- to 24-hour Holter monitor ECG recording should be obtained on older patients (over age 50) with otherwise unexplained rates less than 50/min at rest to rule out transient unrecognized atrial arrhythmias or conduction defects. Ambulatory monitoring is more strongly indicated if the rate is slower, if there is concomitant evidence of intraventricular conduction defects such as right or left bundle branch block or bifascicular block (usually right bundle branch block and left anterior hemiblock), or if the patient complains of dizziness. (See section on atrioventricular conduction defects, below.) If the patient is young, with no symptoms and only modest bradycardia (eg, < 50/min), and has normal exercise tolerance, further investigation is not indicated, but the patient should be seen once a year and told to report any unusual symptoms such as near syncope or dizziness or awareness of cardiac arrhythmias. If dizziness, palpitations, or syncope occurs, a 24-hour ECG monitor should be employed to determine the presence or absence of tachy- or bradyarrhythmias (Table 14–1).

SINOATRIAL-HIS BUNDLE CONDUCTION

Normal Conduction

The sinoatrial node is a small group of cells situated at the junction of the superior vena cava and the right atrium that initiates the cardiac impulse and results in normal sinus rhythm. Spread of the impulse throughout the heart can be recognized on the ECG by the well-known P wave, QRS complex, ST segment, and T wave, which are the "surface" representation of sequential spread of the excitatory electrical impulse as it passes through the heart. His bundle recordings (see below and Fig 14–5) have shown that the P–R interval includes the spread of the impulse from the sinoatrial node through the atria and the bundle of His as well as the first part of its 2 main branches. The current from the His bundle is of sufficiently small magnitude so that the surface ECG does not pick up its individual potentials. It can be recorded by an electrode catheter placed across the tricuspid valve near the His bundle and can be seen to occur during the P–R interval of the surface ECG. The activity and timing of the conduction system between the sinoatrial node and the ventricles can then be determined. His bundle recordings have enhanced our understanding of the pathophysiology of atrioventricular conduction defects, especially the diagnostic, prognostic, and ther-

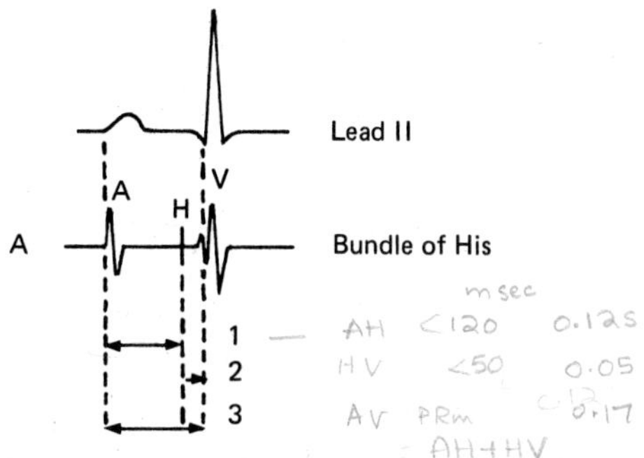

Figure 14–5. Diagrammatic illustration of His bundle recordings with normal AV conduction. (1), A–H interval, approximately 120 msec, which is the time from beginning of atrial depolarization to the beginning of the bundle of His spike. (2), H–V interval, approximately 50 msec (upper limits of normal are 55–60 msec), which represents the time from the bundle of His spike to the beginning of ventricular depolarization. (3), A–V time, which is the P–R interval. (Reproduced, with permission, from Goldman MJ: *Principles of Clinical Electrocardiography,* 9th ed. Lange, 1976.)

apeutic significance of pacemaker activity above, in, and below the atrioventricular node.

Mechanism of Sinoatrial Dysfunction

The mechanism of sinoatrial dysfunction varies. Some patients have sinoatrial block, with adequate atrial transmission function, and some have adequate sinus node function but disturbance of conduction through the atria. The clinical significance of sinus bradycardia or sinus node or atrial dysfunction depends on whether atrioventricular junctional escape pacemakers or His bundle escape pacemakers take over the rhythm of the heart at rates that are only slightly slower than the normal sinus rate. If there is concomitant involvement of both sinoatrial and atrioventricular nodal areas, so that bundle branch or ventricular pacemakers are required, the prognosis for life is worse because these lower pacemakers are slower and less reliable, and artificial pacemakers are often indicated.

The fibrotic process responsible for sick sinus syndrome (see below) or atrioventricular conduction defect must be sufficiently extensive to interfere with function and produce symptoms. Localized fibrosis may be insufficient to produce conduction delays and symptoms.

Sinus Tachycardia

Sinus tachycardia (more than 100 beats/min) can occur in any condition that increases the slope of phase 4 depolarization of the sinus node cells, which therefore reach "threshold" sooner and thus result in rapid heart rates. This occurs in exercise, anemia, fever, emotional stress, thyrotoxicosis, or following administration of adrenergic drugs such as epinephrine. When it occurs in acute myocardial infarction it increases the work of the heart and may extend the size of the myocardial infarction. If the patient has an obstructive lesion such as mitral stenosis, tachycardia decreases the duration of ventricular filling and causes an increase in the pulmonary artery wedge pressure that induces pulmonary venous congestion and dyspnea.

BRADYCARDIA-TACHYCARDIA SYNDROME
(Sick Sinus Syndrome)

The bradycardia-tachycardia syndrome, consisting of alternating bradycardia due to sinus arrest, sinus bradycardia, or sinoatrial exit block combined with tachycardia from paroxysmal atrial or junctional arrhythmias, may produce symptoms referable to either the slow or the fast heart rates (Short, 1954). It is being reported with increasing frequency as its importance becomes recognized. The term sick sinus syndrome is offered by Ferrer (1974) because the symptoms due to the slow rate result from failure of impulse formation in the sinoatrial node or its conduction to the atrioventricular node, causing dizziness, syncope, and bradycardia. The term bradycardia-tachycardia syndrome is preferred by others because patients characteristically have paroxysmal atrial or junctional tachyarrhythmias in addition to the slow heart rates; this is because the pathologic process, usually fibrosis, is not confined to the sinoatrial node but may involve parts of the atrium, the atrioventricular node, and the bundle of His. Recent pathologic investigations have shown that the process is much more common than was once thought. The mechanism of bradycardia-tachycardia syndrome can therefore be sinus bradycardia, sinus node arrest, sinoatrial conduction defect, or disease of the atrioventricular node.

Clinical Findings

A. Symptoms and Signs: Characteristic findings are intermittent symptoms referable to a slow heart rate or to rapid supraventricular arrhythmia (paroxysmal atrial or junctional tachycardia, atrial flutter, or atrial fibrillation).

In some patients, the fast and slow rates may alternate. On one occasion the patient may have paroxysmal arrhythmia with palpitations and impaired cerebral, coronary, and extremity flow from rapid ventricular rates, and, on another occasion, bradycardia and similar symptoms, including syncope due to a slow rather than a rapid ventricular rate.

The slow heart rate caused by dysfunction of the sinus node or transmission from the sinoatrial to the atrioventricular node may result in inadequate perfusion of the brain, with dizziness, impaired cerebral function, and either presyncope or syncope. Impairment of coronary flow may result in angina pectoris or symptoms of cardiac failure or general weakness. In patients who present with paroxysmal atrial arrhythmias, the disorder of the sinus node or sinoatrial conduction dysfunction may only be recognized by the presence of sinus bradycardia between attacks or by noting that when the tachycardia is terminated (either with drugs or with cardioversion) the sinoatrial node shows a period of standstill and slow return to normal function. Five to 10% of cases of cardiovascular syncope were found by Easley and Goldstein (1971) to occur in this manner. A history of syncope which immediately follows the cessation of tachycardia suggests the diagnosis.

In a prospective study (Rokseth, 1974), sinoatrial or sinus node disease occurred in about one-third of all clinical conduction defects, the other two-thirds being atrioventricular block. Many patients were seen by a neurologist because the symptoms were vague and misinterpreted. Sixty percent of patients had atrial arrhythmias, and the incidence was higher if long-term ambulatory ECG monitoring was used. It is estimated that over a 5- to 10-year period about half of patients with sinoatrial dysfunction will have symptoms suggesting Stokes-Adams attacks (Ferrer, 1974).

Sinus bradycardia, especially in older individuals, should be looked on with suspicion and not dismissed as a sensitive carotid sinus or "vagotonia." Patients with marked sinus bradycardia or with symptoms that could be related to a slow heart rate should have ambulatory ECG monitoring for 12–24 hours or more (Table 14–2); episodes may be found of short or long paroxysmal atrial arrhythmias (paroxysmal atrial tachycardia, atrial fibrillation, or atrial flutter), many of which were not suspected on the basis of the clinical history. His bundle recordings of atrial and His bundle depolarizations may show a variety of conduction disturbances between the sinoatrial node and other parts of the specialized conduction system (not solely the atrioventricular node) in a reentry circuit, as is usual in paroxysmal atrial tachycardia.

Although most patients with bradycardia-tachycardia syndrome are older (usually at least in the seventh decade), the disease may occur in young people, and the possibility of degenerative disease of the sinoatrial node and the atria should not be dismissed on the basis of age. Patients who develop angina pectoris should be investigated for possible episodic bradycardia or tachycardia.

Table 14–2. Incidence of sinus abnormalities and atrioventricular block in patient population.*

	Number of Cases†	Percentage of Total Cases
Sinus		
Bradycardia	129	7.7
Tachycardia	429	25.6
Pause, arrest, or sinoatrial block	63	3.8
Atrioventricular block		
First degree	32	1.9
Second degree	39	2.3
Third degree (complete)	10	0.6

*Reproduced, with permission, from Bleifer SB & others: Diagnosis of occult arrhythmias by Holter electrocardiography. Prog Cardiovasc Dis 16:569, 1974.

†These are not mutually exclusive, since a patient may demonstrate more than one abnormality.

B. Special Studies: In addition to continuous ECG monitoring over a period of hours, either while the patient is ambulatory or in the coronary care unit, other studies may be helpful in making the diagnosis. His bundle recordings, atrial pacing, atrial extrastimulus testing, and overdrive suppression of the sinus node may reveal dysfunction of the sinoatrial node or its connections to the atrioventricular node. Examples of such dysfunction are delayed recovery of the sinus node following rapid atrial pacing (sinoatrial node recovery time) and delayed sinoatrial conduction time after atrial extrastimulus testing with progressively increasing prematurity. These studies are still investigational, and their role in diagnosis is uncertain. The atrial arrhythmias are often due to chance reexcitation of already repolarized fibers; differences in the rate of repolarization result from variable refractory periods which are prevalent when the heart rate is slow. Han (1966) has shown that vagal stimulation decreases the refractory period unevenly in different parts of the atrium, which might lead to reentry atrial arrhythmias.

If the patient with sinus bradycardia is asymptomatic and yet has both bifascicular block and a prolonged P–R interval on the ECG, suggesting trifascicular block, the hazard of complete heart block is sufficient to make one follow the patient closely and proceed with His bundle and other specialized studies if symptoms appear.

Precautions Before Undertaking Special Investigations in Chronic Sinoatrial Disease

Before resorting to invasive technics such as atrial pacing and His bundle recordings, one should (as indicated earlier) rule out paroxysmal arrhythmias, drug effects, hypothyroidism, anemia due to blood loss or hematologic disorders, postural hypotension, transient ischemic attacks, what in early days was called swooning (vasovagal attacks), and the vague dizziness and confusion of cerebral vascular disease without focal neurologic signs. Nonspecific dizziness and weakness in elderly people are complex symptoms, and the differential diagnosis includes many noncardiac conditions. This problem is discussed in more detail in Chapter 2. Twenty-four hour ECG monitoring is indicated in all such patients to exclude a tachy- or bradyarrhythmia that is amenable to treatment, as illustrated in Table 14–1. Myocardial ischemia induced by effort may be associated with hypotension and cerebral symptoms. ECG monitoring may identify these patients. The specialized studies discussed below require equipment which is available only in larger centers. Simple noninvasive tests (eg, exercise tests or 24-hour ECG monitoring) (see pp 89 and 91) should be performed in symptomatic patients before referral to a major center for invasive studies.

Differential Diagnosis

Differential diagnosis includes all conditions causing bradycardia and atrial tachyarrhythmias. In addition, because the symptoms are often vague and nonspecific, one must consider psychophysiologic reactions, transient ischemic attacks due to cerebrovascular disease, vasovagal fainting, and all conditions in which elderly individuals may have transient cerebral symptoms other than sinus, sinoatrial, or atrioventricular conduction disturbances. Cerebral symptoms are nonspecific when due to conduction defects and may result from abnormalities anywhere in the transmission system from the sinus node to the Purkinje system. Special studies are needed to identify the site of delay in conduction.

If vague symptoms suggesting cerebral or cardiac ischemia appear with exercise and the sinus rate is slow (usually < 45/min), one should exercise the patient to determine if the atrial rate can be increased appropriately. If the cardiac rate does not increase following moderate exercise to more than 110/min or if symptoms suggest decreased perfusion of the brain or heart, one can conclude that bradycardia is responsible for the symptoms and proceed to evaluate the effect of atropine.

Atropine Test

Atropine sulfate, 0.5 mg intravenously, usually increases the heart rate in normal individuals to over 100/min. In a group of patients with bradycardia-tachycardia syndrome, Rosen (Rosen & others, 1971) found that no patient developed a heart rate greater than 90/min after administration of 1 mg of atropine intravenously.

Sinoatrial & Atrial Conduction Defects

One must differentiate atrioventricular from sinoatrial conduction defects when patients complain of syncope because, as stated previously, the degenerative fibrosis may be widespread along the entire conduction system and disease of the sinoatrial node, atrioventricular node, or bundle of His may dominate the clinical picture. Electrocardiographic study, including His bundle recordings if necessary, may reveal that the conduction defect responsible for the symptoms is in the atrioventricular node or distal to the bundle of His and not in the sinoatrial node or sinoatrial conduction system. Approximately one-third of patients with bradycardia-tachycardia syndrome have associated atrioventricular conduction defects, and sinus bradycardia may be the initial manifestation.

Caution with atropine treatment. Although atropine can be used as a test of the ability of the sinoatrial node to increase its rate of discharge, there are occasions when atropine produces tachycardia and may induce angina pectoris or an arrhythmia, especially in the presence of coronary heart disease. Small doses (eg, 0.25 or 0.5 mg intravenously) should be given first, therefore, and the effect on heart rate noted before larger doses are used. An initial effort should be made to increase the sinus rate because slow heart rates with varying rates of recovery of excitability in different parts of the atrium lead to reentry atrial premature beats and perhaps atrial tachycardia or fibrillation. If the patient is asymptomatic but the atrial rate fails to increase with exercise, and the rate is nonetheless still not slow enough to warrant a ventricular pacemaker, one may try to increase the atrial rate with atropine or ephedrine combined with a mild sedative. If, in addition to a slow heart rate that fails to respond adequately to exercise and to atropine, the patient has symptoms of cerebral insufficiency suggesting sinoatrial syncope, a demand right ventricular pacemaker should be considered.

Treatment

A. Change in Attitude Toward Treatment: Prior to 1954 (Short), it was commonly believed that sinus node dysfunction was of no clinical importance and did not require treatment. Recent experience indicates that many patients with bradycardia-tachycardia syndrome do require treatment. Treatment is often difficult because cardiac depressant drugs given to suppress an atrial tachyarrhythmia also depress the rate of sinus discharge and may induce more severe sinus bradycardia or sinoatrial block, with resulting symptoms from the slow heart rate. Drugs that increase the rate of sinus discharge, such as atropine, sublingual isoproterenol, or ephedrine, are rarely effective in relieving the bradycardia and may enhance atrial irritability. The most effective method of therapy in symptomatic patients is insertion of an artificial demand transvenous pacemaker in the right ventricle to maintain an adequate heart rate and prevent syncopal attacks. The physician can then use antiarrhythmia drugs to prevent atrial tachyarrhythmias without being concerned about their cardiac depressant effects. With the improvement in cardiac function that follows restoration of a normal heart rate by the introduction of a demand pacemaker, the atrial arrhythmias may not recur. Sinus node dysfunction with bradycardia-tachycardia syndrome is the indication for implantation of about one-third of all demand pacemakers for cardiac syncope.

B. Rule Out Bradycardia Caused by Drugs: Before considering the use of potent drugs or artificial right ventricular pacemakers in the treatment of bradycardia-tachycardia syndrome, the physician should make certain that the symptoms and slow heart rate are not due to phenothiazines, or to quinidine or propranolol given to prevent atrial arrhythmias. Digitalis given in large doses to prevent or treat paroxysmal atrial fibrillation may cause or prolong the period of sinus arrest. Withdrawal of medication is an important first step before use of a pacemaker.

C. Need for Pacemaker Therapy in Syncope Due to Chronic Sinoatrial Disease: Although patients with sinoatrial disease average about 10 years younger than those with atrioventricular conduction disease and generally have a more benign prognosis than those with atrioventricular block, major Stokes-Adams attacks may occur with sinoatrial disease. A pacemaker should be inserted when it is apparent that presyncope or syncope is due to sinoatrial disease.

1. Noninvasive methods of estimating need for pacemaker therapy—Before an artificial pacemaker is inserted, atrial pacemaker function should be evaluated by noting the heart rate when the patient is in the upright posture after exercise, after Valsalva's maneuver, after squatting and leg raising, and by means of Holter monitoring.

2. The decision to start pacemaker therapy—The slow progression of bradycardia-tachycardia syndrome to complete atrioventricular block makes it difficult sometimes to decide whether to be conservative or aggressive in treatment. In general, as long as the patient is asymptomatic or has not developed bi- or trifascicular block, nothing is necessary except to carefully note the response to noninvasive procedures such as exercise, posture, Valsalva's maneuver, squatting, or atropine. If the cause has been identified as coronary heart disease, if the progress of the disease seems rapid, or if the patient develops symptoms due to both bradycardia and tachycardia, then definitive pacemaker therapy should be initiated. Before a permanent transvenous pacemaker is introduced—especially if there is doubt about the relationship between the cerebral symptoms and bradycardia—a temporary pacemaker should be tried, and the effect of increased heart rate on the cerebral symptoms should be noted.

The physician should be alert to the development of manifestations that warrant more vigorous treatment—especially evidence of impaired perfusion of vital organs, blunting of the response of the sinus node to simple maneuvers that ordinarily increase the heart rate, and the development of atrial arrhythmias that are difficult to control with drugs. When management with drugs is difficult or when involvement of the atrioventricular node or an area of the specialized conduction system distal to the bundle of His occurs, the physician must anticipate that the patient may alternate between Stokes-Adams attacks (or their equivalent) and cardiac arrhythmias, producing an unstable clinical picture. Further prospective studies are necessary before definitive statements can be made about the effect of pacemaker therapy on the ultimate prognosis, but it is now sufficiently clear that demand transvenous pacing should be started when symptoms interfere with ordinary life activities. Because the rate of progress is slow, there is usually time to study the patient thoroughly and initiate demand transvenous pacemaker therapy when it is obvious that medical treatment has failed. Sinus bradycardia, which is the earliest manifestation of the syndrome, is 5–10 times more frequent than bifascicular block, which presents the physician with similar problems in deciding when to actively intervene with transvenous pacing. Pacemakers are not innocuous (see Chapter 7, p 118) and should be used only on adequate indications, but it is just as wrong not to use pacemakers when they are clearly indicated as to recommend their introduction unnecessarily. The results of transvenous pacing in patients with bradycardia-tachycardia syndrome have been uniformly good with respect to relief of symptoms from slow heart rates, but additional drugs are often necessary to control the paroxysmal arrhythmia.

Prognosis

Because the most common pathologic process is fibrosis of the conduction system, which is usually slowly progressive, the physician should follow the patient even if there are no apparent symptoms in order to note the development of any symptoms or atrioventricular conduction defects that may presage the development of Stokes-Adams attacks. Atypical symptoms may not be interpreted correctly, and sinoatrial disease may be found only if special studies such as 24-hour ECG monitoring are periodically undertaken. Unexplained cerebral symptoms are most important to note in patients with bradycardia. Unexplained atrial fibrillation, especially when associated with bradycardia occurring between paroxysmal attacks, should also alert the physician to the possibility of the condition and its long-term guarded prognosis. The time required for progression from sinus bradycardia to sinus arrest, sinoatrial block, and atrioventricular conduction defects is not known. However, once clinical symptoms develop, their importance should not be discounted.

ATRIOVENTRICULAR CONDUCTION DEFECTS

As stated previously, symptoms of syncope and Stokes-Adams attacks may result from lesions anywhere in the transmission system from the sinoatrial node to the peripheral conduction system, and efforts should be made to identify the site of the conduction delay. Atrioventricular conduction defects are considerably more common than sinoatrial conduction defects. They may be acute and transient or chronic and permanent, and they may require insertion of an electronic ventricular pacemaker to prevent sudden death.

1. ACUTE ATRIOVENTRICULAR CONDUCTION DEFECTS

Acute Myocardial Infarction & Conduction Defects*

Continuous ECG monitoring of patients in coronary care units has shown that atrioventricular conduction defects are much more common in acute myocardial infarction than formerly thought. Overall, complete atrioventricular block occurs in 6–10% of cases, depending on the sample of patients, and is associated with a high mortality rate not necessarily as a result of the heart block itself. Heart block, especially in the presence of anterior myocardial infarction, implies a large infarct with considerable myocardial damage in the area of the septum and consequent cardiac failure or cardiogenic shock.

*See also Chapter 8.

Differentiation of Atrioventricular Conduction Defects in Anterior & Inferior Infarcts

A. Inferior Infarcts: When atrioventricular conduction defects occur in inferior infarction, the damage to the conduction tissue is usually reversible and transient. It is due to temporary ischemia or edema of the atrioventricular node caused by occlusion of the atrioventricular nodal artery–a branch of the right coronary artery–and is characterized by progression through all degrees of atrioventricular block to complete atrioventricular block, though Stokes-Adams attacks are uncommon. The QRS complex is almost always normal in width. With complete atrioventricular block, there is a functional pacemaker, resulting in a heart rate greater than 50/min. His bundle recordings indicate that the atrioventricular block is usually in the atrioventricular node and rarely involves the bundle of His or its branches, and the prognosis is correspondingly better than when the block is infranodal. Artificial cardiac pacemakers are less often required than in anterior infarction and in many centers are not used at all unless the patient has episodes of syncope. The conduction defect usually lasts for a few days–rarely as long as a week–and the prognosis is good for the acute episode. The frequency of transient complete atrioventricular block in inferior infarctions is at least twice what it is in anterior infarctions.

B. Anterior Infarcts: In anterior myocardial infarction with conduction defects, there is usually widespread necrosis of the septum involving the bundle of His and its branches, usually preceded by the sudden onset of unifascicular or bifascicular block–most often right bundle branch block or left anterior hemiblock (see p 444). The sequential change to and from bundle branch block to left anterior hemiblock and complete atrioventricular block as well as various arrhythmias may be rapid and take place over minutes to an hour. His bundle recordings show that the conduction defect is below the atrioventricular node, the QRS duration is usually widened, the interval between the bundle of His spike and the beginning of the QRS complex (the H–V interval) is prolonged, the heart rate is usually less than 40 beats/min, and the escape pacemaker is in the bundle branches or lower in the Purkinje system. Stokes-Adams attacks and sudden death are an ever-present danger. For this reason, the development of conduction defect in a patient with anterior myocardial infarction usually indicates severe stenosis of the left anterior descending artery or the left main coronary artery and is much more serious than is the case in inferior infarctions. Insertion of a prophylactic demand ventricular pacemaker is indicated when certain manifestations of ventricular conduction defect such as bilateral bundle branch block or type II second degree (Mobitz type II) atrioventricular block develop during the course of acute anterior infarction because complete atrioventricular block and Stokes-Adams attacks may appear rapidly. The mortality rate is high when atrioventricular conduction defects develop for the first time in anterior infarction because the necrosis is extensive and left ventricular function is severely impaired, with decreased cardiac output, raised left ventricular filling pressure, decreased ejection fraction, and a low stroke work index. There may be ventricular hypokinesia and even an abrupt development of ventricular aneurysm, septal perforation, or mitral insufficiency. The mortality rate is high even if a pacemaker is introduced, because cardiac function is sufficiently impaired by the widespread necrosis so that even if Stokes-Adams attacks are prevented the patient may die of "pump failure," cardiogenic shock, or ventricular fibrillation. If the patient survives the episode of complete atrioventricular block with Stokes-Adams attacks in anterior infarction, it may be wise to replace the temporary ventricular pacemaker with a permanent one because there are some (though few) data that these patients have a high incidence of sudden death within the next 1–2 years if they are not paced. The incidence of complete heart block and sudden death is said to be higher in unpaced than in permanently paced patients who demonstrate complete atrioventricular block with an acute anterior infarction. This is still a controversial subject.

The mortality rate is doubled or tripled when complete atrioventricular block or ventricular conduction defects appear in the presence of acute myocardial infarction (Mullins, 1976).

2. CHRONIC ATRIOVENTRICULAR CONDUCTION DEFECTS

General Considerations & ECG Features

Discussion of atrioventricular conduction defects requires detailed description of the ECG findings, both conventional and in association with intracardiac recordings, including His bundle recordings and observation after programmed stimulation. The patient may have no symptoms, and evaluation and treatment may depend on specialized ECG studies. Recent studies with His bundle recordings have increased our understanding and insight into the mechanism and perhaps the prognosis of conduction defects, but one of the physician's major concerns is to determine when pacing is necessary. ECGs and His bundle recordings illustrating various types of atrioventricular conduction defects are shown in Figs 14–6 to 14–10.

A. Partial (First Degree) Atrioventricular Block: Partial atrioventricular block consists of prolongation of the P–R interval to 0.21 sec or more at normal heart rates, usually in the absence of symptoms, and represents a delay in conduction of the cardiac impulse from the sinoatrial node to the ventricles recognized only on the ECG. The ECG alone does not enable the physician to determine the location of the conduction delay, and His bundle recordings have been helpful in clarifying the site of the block.

Exercise in atrioventricular block. In partial atrioventricular block, exercise may provide a clue to whether the block is in the atrioventricular node or

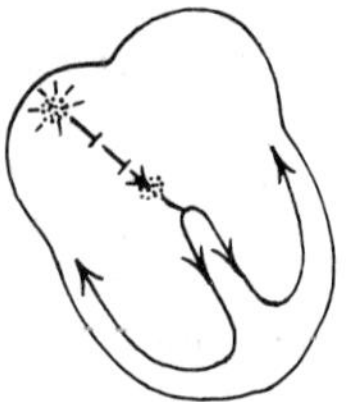

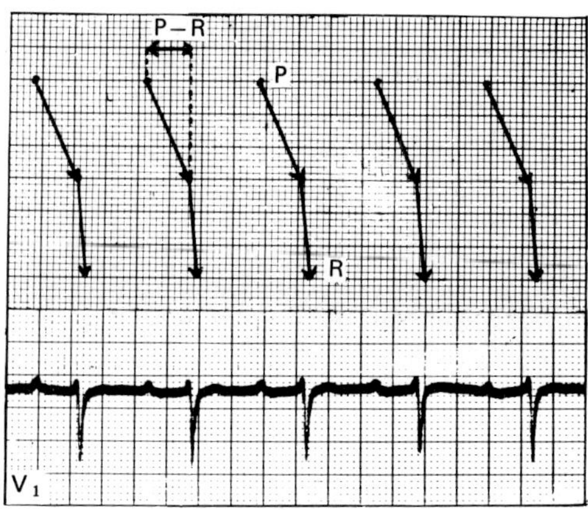

Figure 14–6. First degree atrioventricular block. The P–R interval is prolonged to 0.28 sec. (Reproduced, with permission, from Goldman MJ: *Principles of Clinical Electrocardiography,* 9th ed. Lange, 1976.)

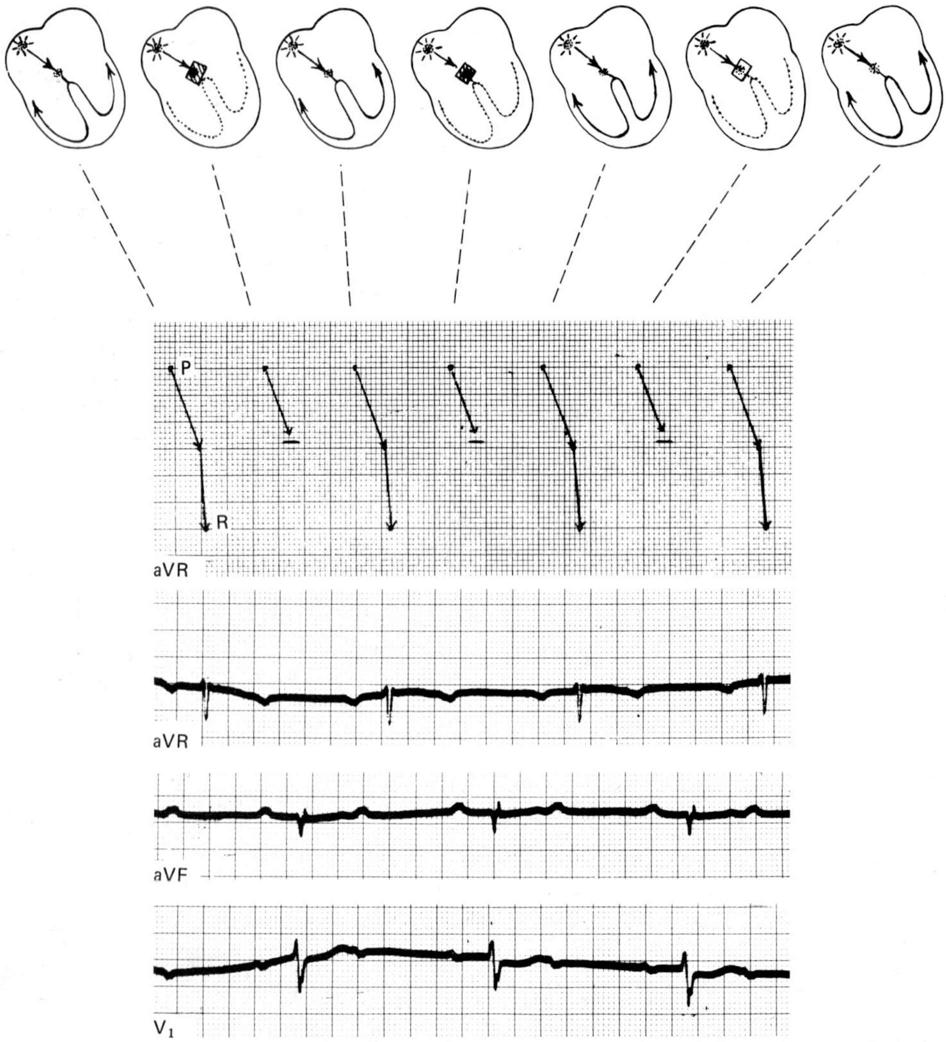

Figure 14–7. 2:1 atrioventricular block. The atrial rhythm is regular at a rate of 82/min. Every other atrial beat produces ventricular stimulation. (Reproduced, with permission, from Goldman MJ: *Principles of Clinical Electrocardiography,* 9th ed. Lange, 1976.)

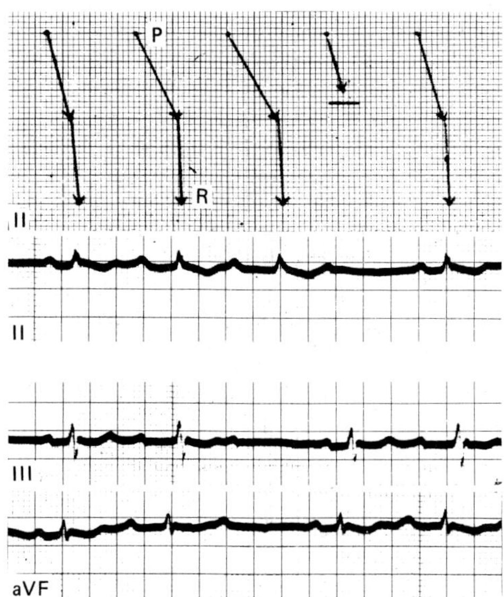

Figure 14–8. Second degree atrioventricular block of Wenckebach type. The atrial rhythm is regular. In lead II, the first P–R interval = 0.18 sec, the second = 0.28 sec, and the third = 0.36 sec. The fourth atrial beat fails to activate the ventricle. In leads III and aVF, the cycle consists of only 2 sinus conducted beats followed by the dropped ventricular beat. (Reproduced, with permission, from Goldman MJ: *Principles of Clinical Electrocardiography*, 9th ed. Lange, 1976.)

distal to it. When exercise shortens the P–R interval, His bundle recordings have shown the reduction to be due to shortening of the A–H interval without effect on the H–V interval, indicating that the block is in the atrioventricular node. When the block is distal to the bundle of His, exercise may not affect the P–R interval but may prolong the H–V interval and shorten the A–H interval (so as to keep the P–R interval unchanged).

1. His bundle recordings–The P–R interval has been shown by His bundle recordings to divide into the A–H interval (65–145 msec), representing the spread of the impulse from the low atrial region to the bundle of His, and the H–V interval (35–55 msec), representing the spread of the impulse from the bundle of His to the beginning of the QRS complex. Electrophysiologic studies have shown that when the prolongation of the P–R interval is due to prolongation of the A–H interval, the disease process is in the atrioventricular node; when the H–V interval is prolonged, the pathologic processes are distal to the His bundle. The A–H interval is prolonged by drugs such as digitalis and by acute myocarditis, thyrotoxicosis, acute inferior infarction, and rapid atrial pacing. In general, a long A–H interval is of less prognostic significance because Stokes-Adams attacks are rare even if the block progresses to third degree (complete). When the A–H interval is normal but the H–V interval is prolonged (especially to more than 70 msec) in partial atrioventricular block, it indicates that the conduction delay is distal to the His bundle or its branches. This infranodal delay is more serious because it indicates disease of the ventricular conduction system, with more chronic myocardial disease, so that Stokes-Adams attacks, sudden death, and cardiac failure are more likely to occur (Scheinman, 1977). Exactly what constitutes an abnormal H–V

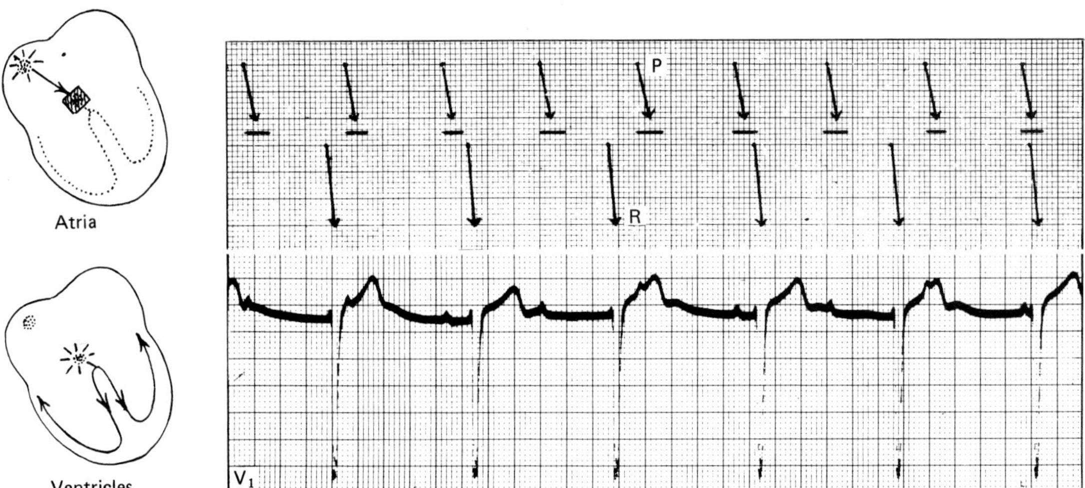

Figure 14–9. Diagram of complete heart block. The atria are activated by impulses arising normally in the sinoatrial node. In this example, the atrial rate = 72/min. The atrial impulses do not activate the ventricles. A second cardiac pacemaker is located near the atrioventricular node and stimulates the ventricles. The ventricular rate = 54/min. The atrial and ventricular rhythms are independent of each other. (Reproduced, with permission, from Goldman MJ: *Principles of Clinical Electrocardiography*, 9th ed. Lange, 1976.)

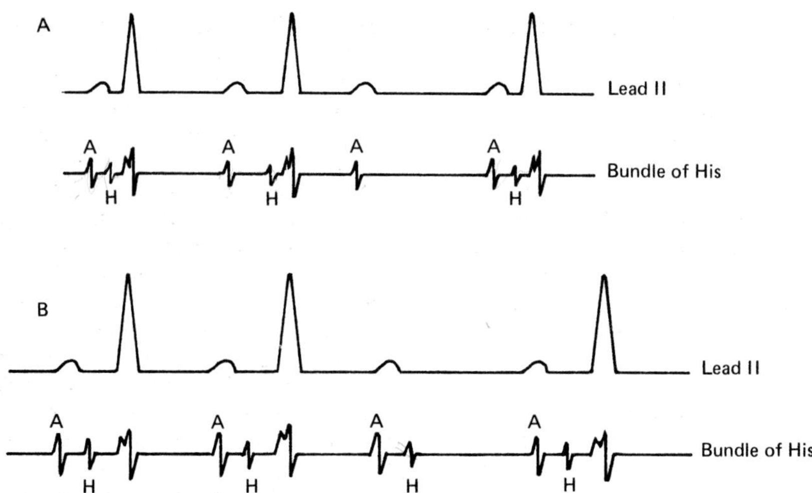

Figure 14–10. Diagrammatic illustrations of bundle of His recordings in second degree atrioventricular block. *A:* Mobitz type I (Wenckebach) block: The first complex has a normal P–R interval with normal A–H and H–V intervals. The second complex has a prolonged P–R interval owing to lengthening of the A–H interval. The third P wave is not conducted and is not followed by a bundle of His spike. This indicates that the site of the block is proximal to the His bundle, in the atrioventricular node. *B:* Mobitz type II block: The first 2 beats are sinus conducted with a prolonged P–R interval owing to lengthening of the H–V interval. The third P wave is not conducted and is followed by a His spike. This indicates that the block is distal to the His bundle. The P–R interval is constant for the conducted beats, and the QRS interval is prolonged. (Reproduced, with permission, from Goldman MJ: *Principles of Clinical Electrocardiography,* 9th ed. Lange, 1976.)

interval has been the subject of some dispute; 55 msec is usually called the upper limit of normal, although some authorities use 60 msec. In general, the longer the H–V interval, the more severe the disease in the distal conduction system and the greater the likelihood of Stokes-Adams attacks or sudden death.

2. Trifascicular block with prolonged P–R and H–V intervals and bundle branch block–This consists of an H–V interval greater than 70 msec in the presence of left or right bundle branch block. If symptoms related to atrioventricular block develop, a permanent prophylactic pacemaker should be inserted to prevent Stokes-Adams attacks due to complete atrioventricular block. Not everyone agrees with Scheinman (1977) with respect to prophylactic pacemakers (Denes, 1977), and further prospective data are required before any definitive opinion can be offered. Patients with prolonged H–V intervals are more apt to have a greater degree of cardiac failure, and deaths may be due to this cause. There are insufficient data describing the course of patients with prolonged H–V intervals and cardiac failure treated with artificial pacemakers. If the atrioventricular block is associated with a prolonged A–H interval only, one can conclude that although heart disease is present, the risk of complete atrioventricular block is minimal.

3. Clinical diagnosis of partial atrioventricular block–Clinically, patients with partial atrioventricular block alone are usually asymptomatic, and the diagnosis is made on routine electrocardiography. It may be suspected clinically if there is a very soft first heart sound, as noted 30 years ago by Levine, who showed the inverse relationship between the P–R interval and the loudness of the first sound. With long P–R intervals, the mitral valve leaflets have become nearly apposed prior to ventricular systole; when they finally close completely with ventricular systole, closure of the valve is associated with minimal sound. Conversely, a loud first heart sound indicates that the mitral valve leaflets were wide apart just before ventricular systole, making first degree atrioventricular block unlikely. This is correlated with a normal or short P–R interval.

Although there is conduction delay between the atria and the ventricles in partial atrioventricular block, each atrial impulse is transmitted regularly to the ventricles. Conduction is delayed following an early premature beat, and partial atrioventricular block may be seen only in one or 2 beats following the long pause after an early premature beat. The refractory period of the atrioventricular node and of the ventricular myocardium is inversely proportionate to the preceding cycle length (Han, 1971). Partial atrioventricular block that occurs unexpectedly in one or 2 beats should suggest an atrial premature beat (often nonconducted) or a His bundle premature beat that may not be easily visible on the ECG; this has been termed concealed conduction by Langendorf (1948) and refers to incomplete penetration of the atrioventricular node by the atrial premature beats that are not discernible on the routine ECG but which can be seen in His bundle recordings. The next sinus beat finds the atrioventricular node partially refractory, which results in prolongation of the P–R interval. An abrupt, transient prolonged P–R interval may thus justify the inference that conduction has been delayed by an event such as an atrial premature beat that is not visible by conventional means. The finding has no more significance than the atrial premature beat itself.

B. Second Degree Atrioventricular Block: In second degree atrioventricular conduction delay, not every sinus impulse reaches the ventricles, with the result that failure of ventricular contraction occurs and is apparent on auscultation at the bedside by the absence (dropping) of the beat, which is subsequently confirmed by ECG. The failure of conduction on the part of the ventricles allows the conduction system to recover so that a subsequent beat is transmitted to the ventricles.

Classification & Definition of Second Degree Atrioventricular Block

The basic definitions and classification of second degree atrioventricular block are those proposed by Mobitz (Mobitz type I and Mobitz type II; see below). These definitions have been in common usage for many years but currently are in a state of flux, clarified in part by His bundle recordings and electrical stimulation of the heart.

The division of the P–R interval into the A–H interval and the H–V interval (see p 435) by His bundle recordings has led to an attempt to classify second degree atrioventricular block by the duration of the H–V interval (nodal if the H–V interval is normal; infranodal if it is prolonged). But measurement of the H–V interval is imprecise, and the interval may be either normal or abnormal with either a normal or abnormal P–R interval or with evidence of infranodal ventricular conduction defect such as left or right bundle branch block or hemiblock (see below). In the discussion that follows, the standard definitions are used, but particular note is taken of exceptions to the conventional generalizations (see ¶ 2, below) and when controversy exists.

1. Two types of second degree atrioventricular block–Second degree atrioventricular block may be of 2 forms: partial progressive atrioventricular block, in which the P–R interval progressively increases, culminating in a dropped beat (Wenckebach or Mobitz type I); or 2:1 block, in which every other beat is not conducted but the P–R interval is not progressively prolonged in the beat prior to the dropped beat (usually Mobitz type II as commonly defined) (Fig 14–11). The classification of Mobitz type I and Mobitz type II is only partially helpful because some patients demonstrate both type I and type II in the same lead and because the site of the block in 2:1 block cannot be predicted with complete reliability. Although in most patients with 2:1 block the block is distal to the bundle of His, it may be in the atrioventricular node. The width of the QRS complex in the conducted beats is helpful in locating the block–narrow if the block is in the atrioventricular node and wide if below it. Multiple blocks may also be present.

Clinical correlation has shown that Mobitz type I or partial progressive atrioventricular block is usually due to conduction delay in the atrioventricular node and associated with a QRS complex of normal width and a heart rate of more than 50 beats/min; it rarely produces Stokes-Adams attacks. This is in contrast to Mobitz type II, which has been shown by His bundle recordings to be due in most cases to conduction delay within or distal to the bundle of His but definitely distal to the atrioventricular node; this form is usually associated with a wide QRS complex, is more apt to progress to complete atrioventricular block with Stokes-Adams attacks, and is associated with a prolonged H–V interval in about half of cases. It seems paradoxic that 2:1 atrioventricular block may be associated with a normal H–V interval in the conducted beat, but this occurs because of variable conduction delay in different parts of the system. A similar situation obtains in complete atrioventricular block without a phase of partial or complete atrioventricular block.

2. Exception to generalizations about Mobitz type I and II block–There are exceptions to the basic rule that Mobitz block type I is due to delay in the

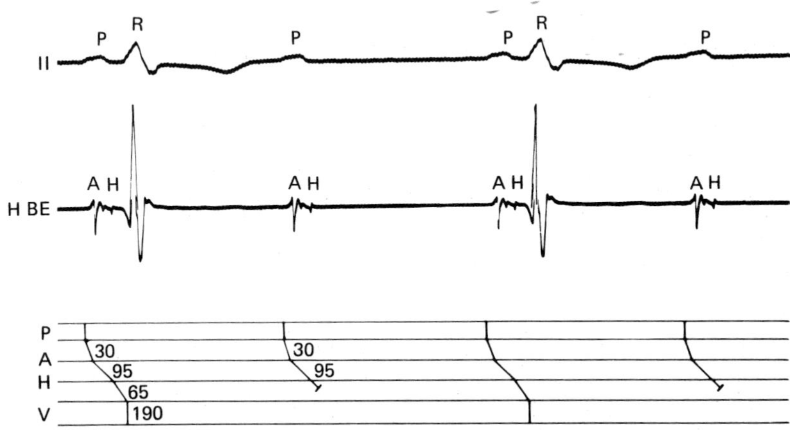

Figure 14–11. Second degree atrioventricular block (Mobitz type II). Every other atrial impulse is blocked. The QRS is wide (0.12 sec). The block occurs below the His bundle owing to a sudden decrement in conduction below the His bundle. (Reproduced, with permission, from Dreifus LS & others: Atrioventricular block. Am J Cardiol 28:371, 1971.)

atrioventricular node and is benign whereas Mobitz type II is distal to the atrioventricular node and is more apt to be clinically significant. Type I second degree block may be distal to the atrioventricular node and type II may be due to a delay in the atrioventricular node; one cannot tell for certain from the routine ECG. In some patients, Mobitz type I and Mobitz type II may be present within a short interval or in the same lead of the ECG, indicating conduction delay both in the atrioventricular node and in the ventricular conduction system distal to it. In acute infarction, type I is usually associated with acute inferior infarction and type II with acute anterior septal myocardial infarction with septal myocardial necrosis.

3. **Wenckebach pauses**–In partial progressive atrioventricular block (Wenckebach type), the increment in P–R interval between the first and second conducted beats is usually greater than in subsequent conducted beats, with the P–R intervals becoming longer and the R–R shorter with each beat. The pauses may vary, so that the rhythm can be 2:1, 4:3, 5:4, etc. Although in Mobitz type II the second degree block is usually associated with a 2:1 rhythm, there may be other intervals such as 3:1 or 4:1. As implied above, His bundle recordings are required in 2:1 block to determine whether the H–V interval is prolonged and whether the block is proximal or distal to the His bundle.

4. **Dropped beats**–Dropped beats must be differentiated from premature beats by noting that there is no heart sound at the apex. Premature beats, even when quite premature, can usually be heard (unless they are blocked supraventricular premature beats) faintly at the apex although not necessarily felt at the wrist. Patients are usually unaware of the dropped beat, and the diagnosis is often made incidentally from a routine ECG or during continuous ECG monitoring.

C. **Complete (Third Degree) Atrioventricular Block**: This form of atrioventricular conduction defect may be due to a lesion in the atrioventricular node or to one distal to the His bundle. It is often part of a more generalized pathologic process (Table 14–3) and associated with bilateral bundle branch block, but it may occur without any conduction defect in either the right or the left bundle branches. Block usually progresses from first to second to third degree (Fig 14–12), but complete block may occur without preceding partial block, or the P–R interval may be normal immediately after a period of complete block. Runs of ventricular tachycardia or fibrillation may interrupt complete atrioventricular block and may be the mechanism for a Stokes-Adams attack (Fig 14–13). The site of the complete atrioventricular block is often suggested by the width of the QRS complex and the ventricular rate. The former is usually normal, and the escape pacemaker has a rate of more than 50/min in atrioventricular nodal complete block (Narula & others, 1971). The QRS complex is usually widened and the heart rate slower when the block is distal to the His bundle. Because of the block, there is dissociation between the atrial and ventricular contractions, but atrioventricular dissociation is not synonymous with atrioventricular block. Atrioventricular dissociation is always present in complete atrioventric-

Table 14–3. Causes of complete atrioventricular block.

1. Congenital.
2. Valvular heart disease (especially aortic stenosis and aortic insufficiency associated with spondylitis).
3. Connective tissue disorders (sarcoidosis, scleroderma, amyloidosis, systemic lupus erythematosus, etc).
4. Myocardial infarction or ischemia without infarction.
5. Metabolic disease (hemochromatosis, thyroid disease, etc).
6. Surgical heart block.
7. Hyperkalemia and following antiarrhythmia drugs.
8. Cardiac tumors (usually secondary but sometimes primary).
9. Chagas' disease of the heart (and, rarely, syphilitic gumma).
10. Drug toxicity: digitalis, quinidine, phenothiazines, tricyclic antidepressants.

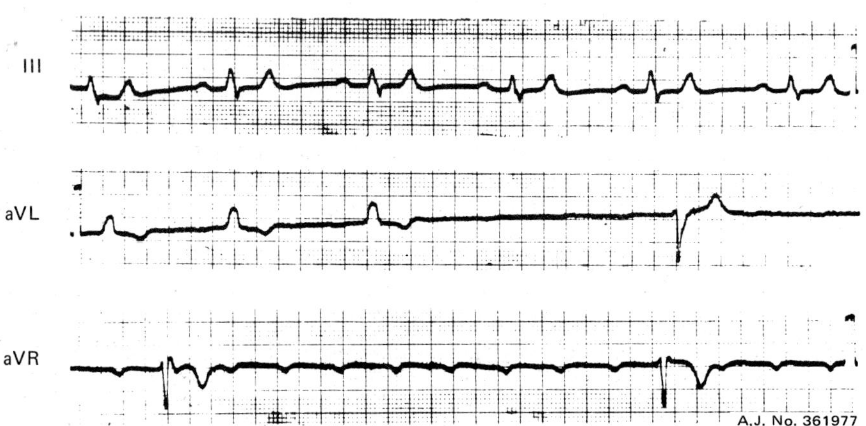

Figure 14–12. Transition from 2:1 atrioventricular block to complete block with ventricular escape following a period of ventricular standstill in a man age 53.

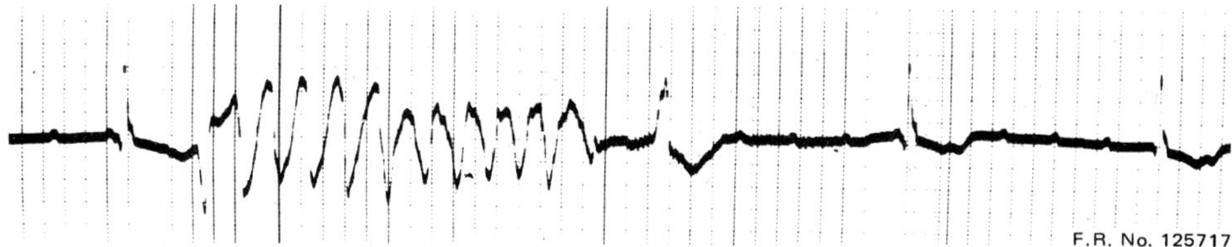

Figure 14–13. Complete atrioventricular block with run of ventricular tachycardia in a woman age 55 with atrial flutter.

ular block but may also be present in its absence, as in nonparoxysmal junctional tachycardia or ventricular tachycardia. In these situations, the junctional or ventricular pacemaker rate is faster than the sinus rate and does not permit the latter to activate the ventricles.

1. **"Escape" pacemakers**–In complete atrioventricular block, survival of the patient depends upon activation of pacemakers distal to the block which are called "escape" pacemakers. When the block is in the atrioventricular node, the pacemaker may be in the bundle of His, which has an inherently faster rate of spontaneous phase 4 depolarization than do pacemakers lower in the Purkinje system. When the atrioventricular block is distal to the bundle of His, the "escape" pacemaker may be in one of the bundle branches or in the ventricles. These are less reliable and may fail temporarily, leading to cessation of ventricular activity, with Stokes-Adams attacks.

2. **Stokes-Adams attacks**–Stokes-Adams attacks, manifested by cerebral symptoms due to cerebral ischemia from ventricular asystole in complete heart block or ventricular conduction defects. Ventricular asystole may follow a period of ventricular fibrillation; therefore, a patient seen late may be thought to have primary ventricular asystole when in fact it was preceded by ventricular fibrillation. In almost all cases of cardiac arrest observed at onset, the mechanism is ventricular fibrillation followed by asystole. The latter obviously can occur de novo. The cerebral symptoms reflect a continuum from momentary transient giddiness to loss of consciousness, convulsions, and sudden death depending upon the duration of interruption of the cardiac output. The momentary lapse of consciousness resembles a petit mal episode and may last only a few seconds. The attacks are abrupt and unpredictable, can occur without warning many times a day or at intervals of days to years, are variable in severity (duration of syncope), and occur in recumbency as well as in the erect position. The patient falls to the ground without warning and becomes pale and pulseless but rapidly recovers when the ventricles resume beating. There is usually a postischemic flush, and the reactive hyperemia is often so obvious that both the patient and witnesses can describe it. As soon as the ventricles resume beating, the patient feels well and can resume activity. This is in sharp contrast to epilepsy or vasovagal fainting, in which the patient has premonitory symptoms and feels weak and nauseated both before and after. Absence of premonitory symptoms, pallor during and hyperemia after the attack, and rapid recovery are characteristic of Stokes-Adams attacks.

3. **Signs of complete atrioventricular block**–The physical signs of complete atrioventricular block are due to the slow ventricular rate, the long period of variable diastolic ventricular filling, the large stroke volume resulting from the slow heart rate, and the presence of independent atrial and ventricular contractions. The slow ventricular rate increases only slightly (approximately 5 beats/min) with exercise or following a sympathomimetic drug and is associated with a wide pulse pressure and raised systolic pressure. The large stroke volume produces a variable pulmonary ejection systolic murmur and third heart sound. The most important signs are those related to independent atrial and ventricular contractions with evidence of atrioventricular dissociation. Depending upon the timing of the contractions of the atrium and ventricles, the first sound varies in intensity, so that there may be intermittent loud first sounds as well as atrial sounds. There may be intermittent "cannon" *a* waves when the right atrium contracts against a closed tricuspid valve.

4. **Symptoms other than syncope**–Depending upon the heart rate and the underlying condition of the ventricle, the patient may be totally asymptomatic despite the presence of complete atrioventricular block or may complain of fatigue and weakness because a normal cardiac output cannot be maintained at the slow rate, especially with physical activity. Any manifestations of cardiac failure or cerebral symptoms due to impaired cerebral perfusion may then develop. A ventricular rate of more than 40/min is usually necessary for the patient to be free of symptoms. When the ventricular rate is less than 30/min, the patient is often weak, dyspneic, and somewhat confused, especially on exercise. There may be episodes of transient dizziness rather than typical Stokes-Adams attacks if the duration of ventricular standstill is short. If ventricular fibrillation occurs, defibrillation is necessary. Asystole lasting 2–3 minutes is usually fatal if not treated.

5. **Special investigations**–Patients with slow ventricular rates and symptoms should have continuous (Holter) ECG monitoring to determine if the episodes of near syncope or syncope are associated with the development of complete atrioventricular block. Dizziness is a common symptom in older people, and it must be definitely established that the symptom is due to complete block before inserting a pacemaker. Even with other evidence of conduction delay in the bundle

branches with bilateral bundle branch block or a prolonged H–V interval by His bundle recording, dizziness and weakness may be due to other arrhythmias, postural hypotension, anemia, diffuse cerebral arteriosclerosis, or general debility and not to complete block. This is especially important in patients with bilateral bundle branch block with or without a prolonged P–R interval, who have syncope or near syncope. His bundle recordings have shown that whether or not the P–R interval or H–V interval is prolonged, one cannot automatically assume that episodes of syncope or near syncope are due to intermittent complete atrioventricular block. The longer the H–V interval, the more likely that episodic syncope is due to the development of complete atrioventricular block, but this is not invariable.

Bilateral Bundle Branch Block & Pacemakers

In bilateral bundle branch block (right bundle branch block and left anterior hemiblock, right bundle branch block and left posterior hemiblock, or right or left bundle branch block with prolonged P–R interval) or alternating right and left bundle branch block, the heart presumably depends on the remaining fascicle for conduction of the atrial impulse to the ventricle. At one time it was estimated that about 1% of adults have bifascicular block and that about 0.1% develop complete atrioventricular block after a few years. Recent prospective studies, however, have indicated that these data must have come from a select population. The true incidence of complete atrioventricular block is probably considerably less than 10% in unselected asymptomatic patients found or known to have bifascicular block, but it does occur, as shown by Lenegre (Fig 14–14). Temporary pacemakers are not indicated in asymptomatic patients with bifascicular block even if they have a prolonged P–R or H–V interval. Individuals with bilateral bundle branch block who have cerebral symptoms with documented bradyarrhythmias (Dhingra, Circulation, 1976) and whose H–V intervals exceed 70 msec may be an exception (Scheinman, 1977), but the decision regarding implantation of a right ventricular pacemaker is a controversial one. Only 20% of patients with bifascicular block and syncope had documented bradyarrhythmias requiring electronic pacing. Furthermore, there were no significant differences in the incidence of sudden death in patients with bifascicular block with and without syncope (Dhingra, Circulation, 1976). His bundle recordings of H–V intervals could not predict sudden death (Denes, 1977).

The presence of an atrioventricular conduction defect, whether it be a prolonged H–V interval or second degree block, does not necessarily mean that Stokes-Adams attacks are likely or that a pacemaker is necessary. *Further prospective studies and clinical judgment are required before pacemaker implantation can be justified solely on the basis of the ECG or His bundle findings in the absence of symptoms shown to be due to bradyarrhythmias.*

Patients with right bundle branch block and left anterior hemiblock do not need temporary ventricular pacing for noncardiac surgery. They rarely develop

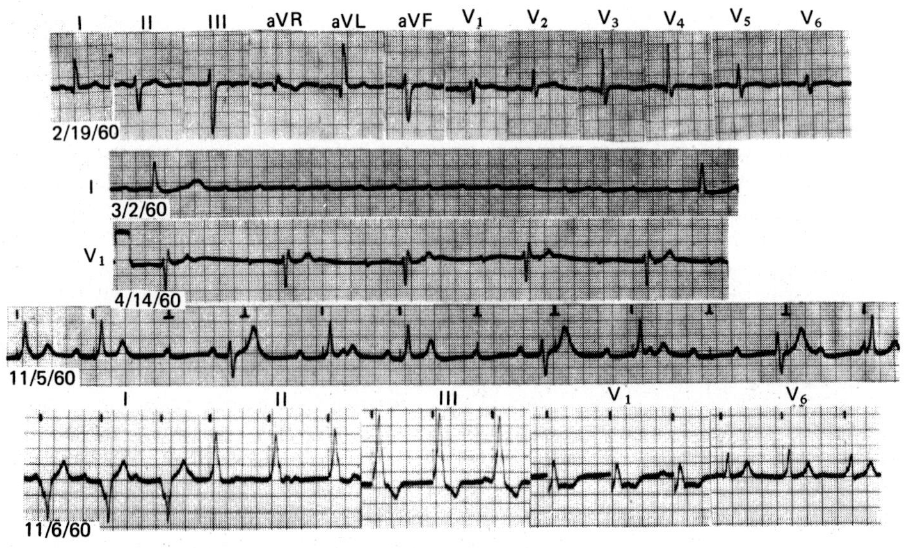

Figure 14–14. Five successive ECGs of a man age 58 suffering from Stokes-Adams attacks. First tracing, February 12, 1960. Regular sinus rhythm 66/min, practically normal P–R interval measuring 0.20 sec, atypical right bundle branch block with QRS axis −60 degrees and left anterior hemiblock (bifascicular block), T axis +20 degrees, QRS duration = 0.12 sec, rSr′ pattern in V_1 (r′ delay = 0.08 sec), qr or QR pattern in aVR and aVL; measured in aVL, the left ventricular activation time would be delayed to 0.09 sec. The second and third tracings, recorded on March 2 and April 14, 1960, showed a complete atrioventricular block (76/36) with a right ventricular delay (identical in pattern as when in sinus rhythm) and a ventricular pause of 7 sec. The last 2 tracings, recorded after electrical stimulation, showed one an intermittent and the other a regular response. (Reproduced, with permission, from Lenegre J: Etiology and pathology of bilateral bundle branch block in relation to complete heart block. Prog Cardiovasc Dis 6:409, 1964.)

complete atrioventricular block under these circumstances. The usual procedure is for the patient to be monitored with an oscilloscope during the surgical procedure with a standby pacemaker should atrioventricular block develop. If the patient is symptomatic and it can be shown by Holter monitoring that the symptoms are related to transient complete atrioventricular or sinoatrial block, it is wise to insert a permanent ventricular demand pacemaker so that the patient is not dependent on a distal "escape" pacemaker in the event of ventricular standstill. Pacemakers should not be used unless there is a clear indication (see Chapter 7).

3. TREATMENT OF ATRIOVENTRICULAR CONDUCTION DEFECTS

Partial (First Degree) Atrioventricular Block

Treatment usually involves careful serial observation with frequent ECGs if the conduction defect is chronic in an attempt to discern any progression to more advanced block. Attempts should also be made to eliminate the cause if the block is due to digitalis, other antiarrhythmia agents, propranolol, quinidine, procainamide, hyperkalemia, or myocarditis. A decrease in the P–R interval following exercise is a helpful sign, indicating that the conduction defect is apt to be benign and in the atrioventricular node, because exercise increases the adrenergic impulses to the atrioventricular node. If the patient is symptomatic, with episodic dizziness or syncope suggesting intermittent Stokes-Adams attacks, 24-hour continuous Holter ECG monitoring is indicated to see if the symptoms are due to complete atrioventricular block or to something else not related to bradyarrhythmia. His bundle recordings should be reserved for symptomatic patients with atrioventricular block in order to determine if the block is distal to the His bundle.

The question when to insert an artificial pacemaker in patients with partial (first degree) atrioventricular block is controversial. If the patient has *cerebral symptoms proved to be due to bradyarrhythmia,* insertion of a pacemaker is generally advisable. If the patient is *asymptomatic,* and the H–V interval is 70 msec or more, opinion is divided. Narula (1975) and Scheinman (1977) believe the risk of sudden death from complete atrioventricular block is sufficiently great that a pacemaker should be inserted, especially if the patient also has bifascicular block (see below). Dhingra (Circulation, 1976) and Denes (1977) find the H–V interval in asymptomatic patient an inadequate reason for permanent pacing. If the atrioventricular block is due to a prolonged A–H interval and a normal H–V interval, the conduction defect is atrioventricular nodal or supranodal, and the risk of development of complete atrioventricular block is minimal even in the presence of known heart disease. It is clear that further prospective observation in patients studied both clinically and by His bundle recording is necessary to reconcile the differing opinions.

Second Degree Atrioventricular Block

As indicated above, if second degree block is in the atrioventricular node (Mobitz type I), even with inferior myocardial infarction, clinical observation is usually sufficient because progression to complete atrioventricular block and Stokes-Adams attacks is much less common than when the second degree block is Mobitz type II and in or distal to the His bundle. There are still differences of opinion about whether a temporary demand pacemaker should be introduced in patients with inferior myocardial infarction with complete atrioventricular block. Although the likelihood of Stokes-Adams attacks is less than in complete atrioventricular block distal to the atrioventricular node, it is still significant, and we believe it is wise in inferior infarction to insert a pacemaker when the patient develops complete atrioventricular block, especially if he develops symptoms suggesting Stokes-Adams attacks. In chronic Mobitz type II atrioventricular block, careful observation with serial ECGs is usually sufficient unless the patient has symptoms suggesting episodic syncope or its equivalent or unless the block develops acutely in the setting of acute anterior infarction with the acute development of bifascicular block, in which case a temporary demand pacemaker is immediately indicated. The decision on what course of action to take will depend upon the age of the patient and the degree of associated atherosclerosis. It is important to determine whether the bifascicular block preceded the acute infarction because in this instance the prognosis is better and a pacemaker need not be inserted, as would be the case if the bifascicular block developed after the acute infarction.

Complete Atrioventricular Block

The treatment of asymptomatic complete atrioventricular block discovered accidentally is a matter of some dispute. The prognosis is worse without a pacemaker than with one because patients with complete block, especially if over age 60, may develop Stokes-Adams attacks, ventricular arrhythmias, or cardiac or cerebral perfusion abnormalities. Young patients (15–35 years) with asymptomatic congenital complete block whose ventricular rate increases with exercise do not need a pacemaker and can be observed at yearly intervals. If the patient has had a single unequivocal Stokes-Adams attack, a demand pacemaker should be introduced because recurrent attacks are the rule, and any individual episode may be fatal. When atrioventricular block is varying from 2:1 to complete, a demand pacemaker should be inserted because during the transition there may be ventricular asystole with Stokes-Adams attacks and the patient is at greater risk of ventricular fibrillation. Dramatic improvement in cardiac failure, relief of cerebral symptoms and of syncope or near syncope, and improved survival result from the use of pacemakers in patients with permanent or intermittent complete atrioventricular block. The artificial pacemaker should be set at 70–80/min. It is always well to determine the effect of a temporary pacemaker before placing it permanently. Even though it may not be established that dizziness or near syncope is due to complete atrioventricular block, this diagnosis is strongly suspected if a patient has partial or 2:1 atrioventricular block. If the symptoms are thought to be due to complete atrioventricular block which has not been documented, a temporary ventricular pacemaker should relieve the symptoms and clarify the diagnosis. If the patient has documented complete atrioventricular block with Stokes-Adams attacks, a temporary pacemaker is not required and a permanent pacemaker should be inserted promptly.

A. Use of Drugs in Complete Atrioventricular Block: Drugs are rarely used today in complete atrioventricular block because of the almost universal availability of pacemakers. During the interval between recognition of a Stokes-Adams attack and introduction of a temporary or permanent pacemaker, it is wise for the patient to be in the hospital with continuous ECG monitoring and an intravenous infusion of isoproterenol available.

B. Proper Functioning of Pacemakers: (See Chapter 7.) After being provided with a demand pacemaker, the patient should be closely observed to confirm its proper functioning, especially during the first month. Recurrence of symptoms suggests that positioning of the electrode catheter has been faulty or that the catheter has moved, and Holter ECG monitoring should be employed to correlate symptoms with the possibility of such faulty pacing. The patient should be instructed to report to the physician so that the rate of the pacemaker and its functioning can be checked periodically—weekly for the first month, monthly for 1–2 years, and then more frequently as battery failure is anticipated. The patient or a family member should be taught to count the pulse rate, learn the significance of changes in rate, and immediately report such changes to the physician.

Atrioventricular conduction defects represent the most common indication for cardiac pacing. Sinoatrial defects account for about one-third of cases.

BUNDLE BRANCH BLOCK

Bundle branch block is an ECG finding, usually an unexpected one. As with other conduction defects, pathologic lesions may also be found elsewhere in the system although they may be expressed electrocardiographically as isolated bundle branch block, either right or left. Bundle branch block is diagnosed when the QRS complex exceeds 0.11 sec, with late delay in the right precordial leads in right bundle branch block and in the left ventricular leads in left bundle branch block, combined with depressed ST and asymmetrically inverted T waves opposite to the direction of the QRS delay in the leads with late delay in the QRS complex (rsR′ complexes). The block may be intermittent or develop over a period of years (Fig 14–15).

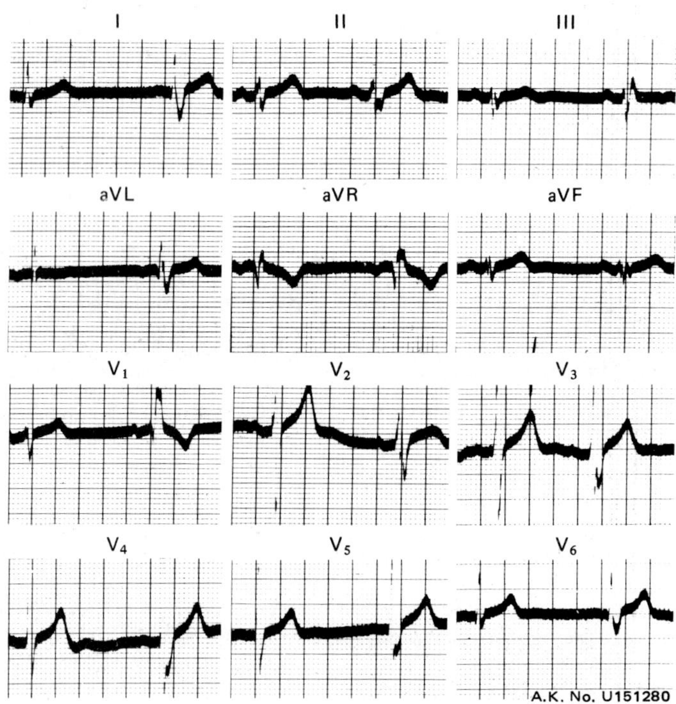

Figure 14–15. Intermittent right bundle branch block in a man age 61 with no clinical evidence of heart disease. Right bundle branch block complexes occur with every other beat.

Branches of the bundle of His are part of the normal conduction pathway system from the atria to the ventricles. Delay in one or both parts of the bundle branches is a common phenomenon in clinical medicine, often in asymptomatic individuals. In such persons, when conduction delay in either bundle branch occurs as an isolated finding without symptoms or other evidence of cardiac disease, the prognosis is usually good. The concept of bundle branch block, whether right or left, implies that the branch is in fact blocked, whereas anatomically and functionally there is merely a delay in conduction in the bundle branches. The term conduction delay rather than block is therefore preferable, and the degree of the delay can be expressed as minor, incomplete, or complete. Even the last term is a misnomer. In some patients with bundle branch block with a QRS duration of 0.12–0.14 sec, the duration may be extended to 0.16–0.18 sec in certain circumstances such as potassium excess or quinidine therapy. One cannot say, however, that the block is then "more complete." For this reason, the terms "complete left" and "complete right" bundle branch block are rarely used, though the term incomplete is used when the QRS duration is borderline and the R′ wave in either the left or the right ventricular leads is only modestly abnormal and delayed.

Left Bundle Branch Block

Left bundle branch block is most frequently found in individuals with clinical evidence of heart disease. In the absence of other evidence of heart disease, it can be associated with many years of normal life. Despite complete study, including coronary angiography and exercise stress ECGs, cardiac disease cannot be found in many such patients. Insurance data have confirmed this finding.

The left bundle is not a discrete entity, as is the right bundle, and the division into left anterior and right posterior divisions is purely arbitrary. When left bundle branch block occurs in the presence of anterior myocardial infarction, the prognosis is better and the incidence of complete atrioventricular block lower than when right bundle branch block is present in association with acute myocardial infarction. The mortality rate of left bundle branch block varies from 22–65% in different series but was 65–67% in right bundle branch block (Norris, 1972; Lie, Circulation, 1974). Complete atrioventricular block developed in about 12% of cases of left bundle branch block (Bigger, 1977) but in about 30% of cases of right bundle branch block (Norris, 1972). The worse prognosis in the latter group may be because right bundle branch block, when it appears in acute myocardial infarction, is due to septal necrosis, usually associated with left anterior hemiblock and followed rapidly by complete atrioventricular block. Left bundle branch block obscures the ECG diagnosis of acute myocardial infarction; radioisotopic methods (see Chapter 8) may be useful in diagnosis under these circumstances.

Right & Left Bundle Branch Block

Right bundle branch block, especially incomplete block, occurs in many normal individuals. If one includes as right ventricular conduction defects those ECGs with an r′ in the right precordial leads, the percentage in the general population may be as high as 10%. When a right or left bundle branch block occurs in the presence of associated cardiac disease, its significance depends on the nature of the cardiac disease, associated defects in the fascicles of the left bundle, a prolonged P–R interval, and symptoms suggesting intermittent, more advanced heart block. Bundle branch block may be intermittent (Fig 14–15) or may progress over a period of years (Fig 14–16). Transient

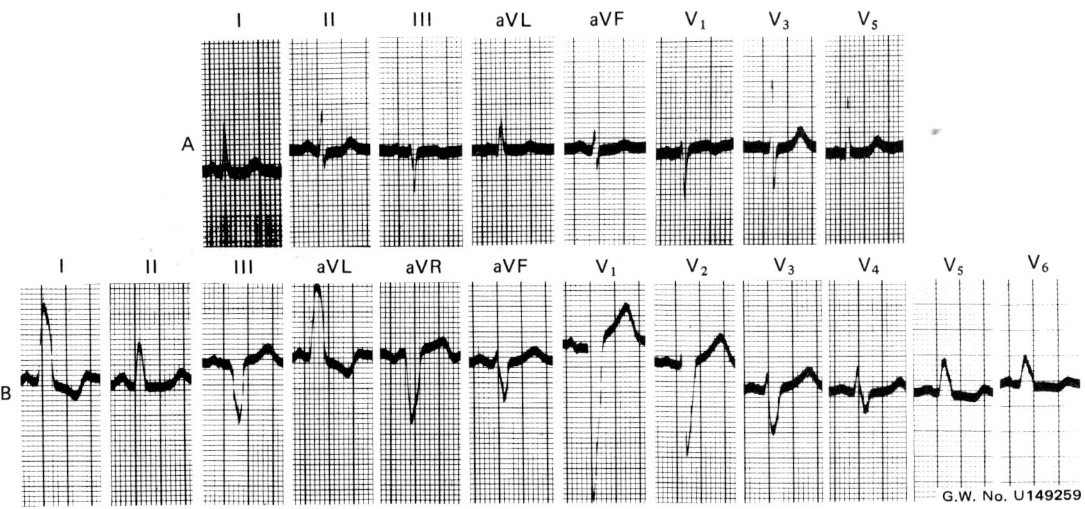

Figure 14–16. Left bundle branch block developing in a 53-year-old woman. Note wide slurred R waves in leads V_5, V_6, I, and aVL in *B* as compared to normal conduction in *A*.

right bundle branch block (complete or incomplete) may follow the development of acute right ventricular dilatation in acute pulmonary embolism. Pulmonary hypertension develops transiently, causing right ventricular dilatation and an ECG pattern of right ventricular conduction defect. Depending upon the site of the pulmonary embolus (proximal or distal pulmonary entry), the conduction defect may be slight, incomplete, or complete.

As indicated earlier, right bundle branch block is more common in acute myocardial infarction than is left bundle branch block and may be rapidly followed by complete atrioventricular block, especially if the patient has associated left anterior hemiblock. The right bundle is supplied anatomically by the first septal perforator branch of the left anterior descending artery. Right bundle branch block, therefore, is common when necrosis of the proximal portion of the septum occurs as a result of occlusion of the proximal left anterior descending artery. In chronic right just as in chronic left bundle branch block, His bundle recordings have shown that H–V prolongation, indicating extension of the conduction defect to the more distal branches of the right and left bundles, is present in many instances of left bundle branch block (less so in right bundle branch block) whether the P–R interval is normal or prolonged. The likelihood of the prolonged H–V interval is greater if there is first degree atrioventricular block in conjunction with either left or right bundle branch block, but the H–V interval may be prolonged even if the P–R interval is normal. A normal H–V interval may occur in either left or right bundle branch block with both normal and abnormal P–R intervals. Therefore, one cannot predict whether or not the H–V interval will be prolonged without a His bundle study in patients with bundle branch block (Levites, 1974). This is of importance because the incidence of cardiac failure and cardiac enlargement is higher in patients with prolonged H–V intervals, in contrast to those with normal H–V intervals in partial atrioventricular block. The combination of bundle branch block and partial atrioventricular block implies bilateral bundle branch block, as will be explained in the next section on bifascicular block.

Examination over a period of months or years or ECG monitoring for 24 hours in patients with either right or left bundle branch block will often reveal paroxysmal atrioventricular block, indicating that the ventricular conduction defects precede and may be the earliest precursors of complete atrioventricular block. Review of old records of patients who develop atrioventricular block often discloses asymptomatic bundle branch block with a normal P–R interval. Further studies, therefore, such as 24-hour ECG monitoring and careful clinical observation, are indicated in patients with isolated bundle branch block who have symptoms suggesting bradyarrhythmia.

Unifascicular & Bifascicular Block

The main left bundle branch of the bundle of His usually divides into 2 main branches, the left anterior superior and the left posterior fascicles. Anatomically, the division is often much more complex, but for clinical purposes it is sufficient to assume only the 2 divisions. Left anterior hemiblock is diagnosed when the frontal plane QRS axis is to the left and superior, between −45 and −90 degrees in association with right bundle branch block. There is an r wave and a prominent S wave in leads II and III. There are also q waves in leads I and aVL. The differentiation from an old inferior myocardial infarction is not always easy. Left posterior hemiblock is diagnosed when there is right axis deviation greater than 120 degrees, provided that right ventricular hypertrophy or old lateral myocardial infarction (both of which may cause right axis deviation) can be excluded.

Left anterior hemiblock is much more common than left posterior hemiblock. When complete atrioventricular block develops in anterior myocardial infarction, the usual sequence is that of right bundle branch block, left anterior hemiblock, and then complete atrioventricular block.

The causes of bifascicular block are chiefly those of ventricular conduction defects anywhere: hypertensive or coronary heart disease, fibrosis of the conduction system, and primary myocardial disease. Bifascicular block is more common in men. The average age of patients when first seen is about 60 years. Dyspnea, cardiac enlargement, and congestive heart failure are more common when the H–V interval is prolonged (Dhingra, Circulation, 1974; Am J Cardiol, 1976).

In bifascicular block with right bundle branch block and left anterior or left posterior hemiblock, it is assumed that 2 of the 3 fascicles which are extensions from the bundle of His are involved, and survival depends on adequate functioning of the remaining third fascicle. It must be reemphasized that the concept of the 3 fascicles is a considerable oversimplification of the anatomic complexity of the main bundle. Furthermore, the disease in the atrioventricular conduction system is usually more extensive than would be inferred from the ECG; considerable portions of the conduction system are usually involved. Left axis deviation—a frontal plane QRS axis to the left of 0 degrees (some would say −30 degrees)—appearing after a previously documented normal axis represents an intraventricular conduction defect, with or without left anterior hemiblock (an arbitrary criterion). Many of these individuals are asymptomatic, and the incidence of complete heart block and Stokes-Adams attacks in these patients over a period of years is not precisely known, although in patients who present to physicians with symptoms of syncope, dizziness, or neurologic symptoms it is estimated to be about 3% per year (Denes, 1977). More follow-up time is required before a definitive statement can be made, but recent prospective data over relatively few years of observation indicate that bifascicular block is more benign than formerly thought. Careful follow-up is sufficient in asymptomatic bifascicular block unless the patient develops cerebral symptoms thought (or found by Holter monitoring) to be due to atrioventricular block. If the symptoms strongly suggest Stokes-Adams attacks and the diagnosis is supported by continuous ECG monitoring, if the patient has partial atrioventricular block, or if the H–V interval on His bundle recording exceeds 70 msec, a prophylactic right ventricular pacemaker should probably be implanted (Scheinman, 1977), although this is a matter of some dispute (see section above on first degree atrioventricular block). Because of the hazard of abrupt onset of complete atrioventricular block and syncope, a conservative course of action is *not* advised in acute anterior myocardial infarction, in which a pacemaker should be promptly introduced when left anterior hemiblock with right bundle branch block (bifascicular block) develops.

Bifascicular block with right bundle branch block and left posterior hemiblock is often overdiagnosed because right axis deviation exceeding 110 degrees can be found in normal thin individuals or those with right ventricular hypertrophy. A marked superior axis, even to the right, can occur with some varieties of anterolateral myocardial infarction. Left posterior hemiblock is an uncommon condition.

Intermittent or Rate-Dependent Conduction Defects

Conduction defects are not static, and ECG abnormalities may be present on one occasion and absent at other times (Figs 14–15 and 14–16). Atrioventricular block, bundle branch block, and bifascicular block may vary with the heart rate and be either bradycardia- or tachycardia-dependent. Perfusion of the conduction pathways may be influenced by small changes in heart rate or in cardiac output. Intermittent conduction defects are common, and, while they indicate the presence of disease, they do not usually require treatment. Of course, one should be alert for the development of complete atrioventricular block regardless of where the conduction defect manifests itself in the ECG. It must be reemphasized that pathologically the disease occurs in multiple sites both proximal and distal to the bundle of His.

VENTRICULAR PREEXCITATION
(Accelerated Conduction Syndrome; Wolff-Parkinson-White Syndrome)

Preexcitation may occur by a number of accessory pathways (Fig 14–17). In addition to the normal spread of activation from the atria to the ventricles via the atrioventricular node, early activation of the ventricle occurs along a complex system of accessory pathways, as shown by epicardial mapping and surgical interruption of the pathways (Gallagher, 1977). The lateral accessory pathway (bundle of Kent) enters a portion of the ventricular myocardium from the atrium. Mahaim fibers may pass from the bundle of His to the ventricular myocardium, and pathways may spread from the internodal atrial tracks to the ventricular myocardium, bypassing the upper part of the atrioventricular node via the James fibers. The precise anatomy of the bypass track is not known until epicardial mapping is performed. Determination of the orientation of the delta wave gives a clue to the location of the accessory pathways, which may be anterior, posterior, septal, lateral, or a combination of these sites (Gallagher, 1977).

Wolff-Parkinson-White syndrome may be constant or intermittent, the latter often brought on by a change in atrial rate. Because the ventricle is activated both via the accessory pathway and through the normal atrioventricular nodal pathway, fusion ventricular beats may occur. The syndrome occurs in 0.5–2% of the population, and paroxysmal atrial arrhythmias occur in half of affected individuals.

Types of Preexcitation

A. Lown-Ganong-Levine Syndrome: The forme fruste of Wolff-Parkinson-White syndrome is the Lown-Ganong-Levine syndrome (Lown, 1952), characterized on the ECG by a short P–R interval and normal QRS interval without a delta wave. It is thought to represent a variety of short-circuiting of the upper part of the atrioventricular node (via James fibers) and is also associated with increased frequency of paroxysmal atrial arrhythmias. The arrhythmias observed in Lown-Ganong-Levine syndrome include mostly atrial and ventricular premature beats; however, one-fifth of patients have paroxysmal atrial tachycardia, and smaller numbers of other arrhythmias occur during 24-hour ECG monitoring (Monahan, 1975). Aberrancy occurs because the ventricular complex resulting from the atrial premature beat occurs during the relative refractory period of the preceding depolarization before repolarization is complete. Ventricular depolarization following the atrial premature beat begins, therefore, at a less negative maximum resting potential and alters phase 0 of the action potential.

We know of no attempts at surgical correction. This may be because a dual pathway in the atrioventricular node rather than an accessory bypass track may be responsible for the preexcitation.

B. Wolff-Parkinson-White Syndrome: Preexcitation due to Wolff-Parkinson-White syndrome (Wolff, 1930) has been classified according to the location of the accessory bypass, but the classification is incomplete because a variety of subtypes have recently been discovered by electrophysiologic study. Conventionally, type A preexcitation is from the left accessory bypass, producing an ECG pattern in V_1 resembling right ventricular hypertrophy or right bundle branch block. Type B preexcitation results from early activation via the right lateral accessory pathway, producing an ECG change similar to that of left bundle branch block (Figs 14–18 and 14–19). Subgroups can be identified by special invasive technics which allow the physician to identify candidates for epicardial mapping and perhaps surgery. The ECG classification originally proposed by Rosenbaum (1945), has been extended by the work of Gallagher, Wallace, and associates (1976, 1977 [in press]) with special reference to the polarity

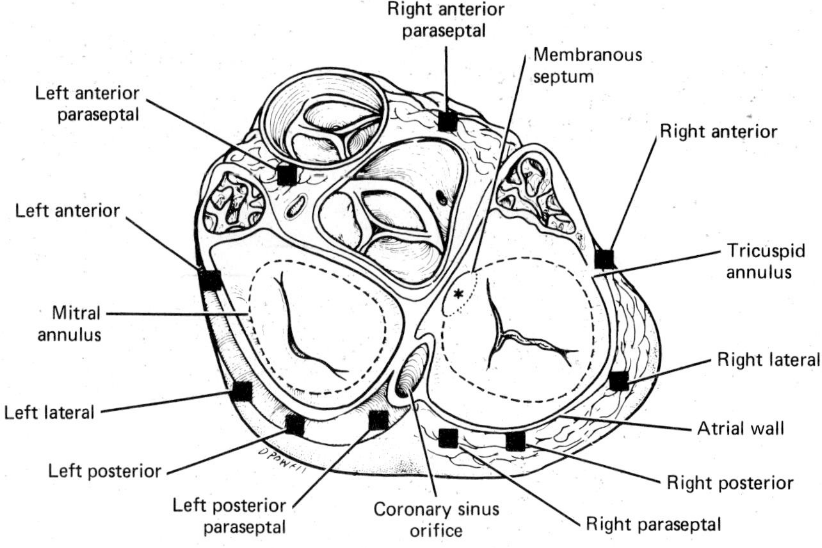

	I	II	III	aVR	aVL	aVF	V_1	V_2	V_3	V_4	V_5	V_6
1	+	+	+(±)	-	±(+)	+	±	±	+(±)	+	+	+
2	+	+	-(±)	-	+(±)	±(-)	±	+(±)	+(±)	+	+	+
3	+	±(-)	-	-	+	-(±)	±	±	±	+	+	+
4	+	-	-	-	+	-	±(+)	±	+	+	+	+
5	+	-	-	-(+)	+	-	±	+	+	+	+	+
6	+	-	-	-	+	-	+	+	+	+	+	+
7	+	-	-	±(+)	+	-	+	+	+	+	+	-(±)
8	-(±)	±	±	±(+)	-(±)	±	+	+	+	+	-(±)	-(±)
9	-(±)	+	+	-	-(±)	+	+	+	+	+	+	+
10	+	+	+(±)	-	±	+	±(+)	+	+	+	+	+

DELTA WAVE POLARITY

± = Initial 40 msec delta wave isoelectric
+ = Initial 40 msec delta wave positive
− = Initial 40 msec delta wave negative

Figure 14–17. Epicardial preexcitation. (Reproduced, with permission, from Gallagher JJ & others: The preexcitation syndromes. Prog Cardiovasc Dis [in press].)

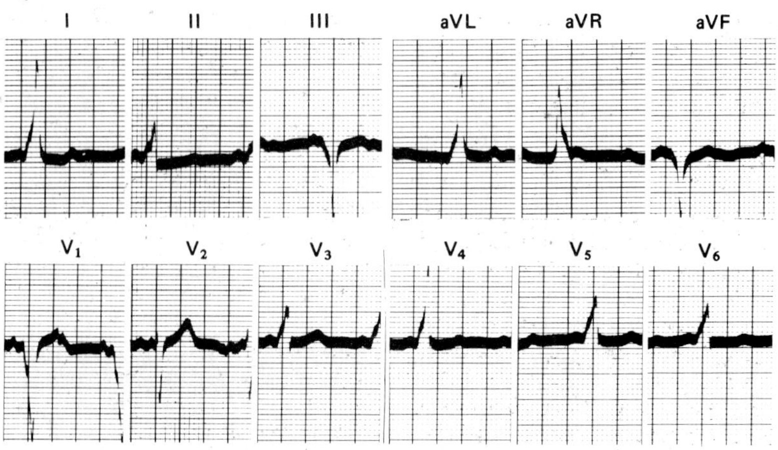

Figure 14–18. Wolff-Parkinson-White syndrome in a woman age 26. The superior orientation of the delta vector type B produces QS complexes in aVF which simulate inferior infarction.

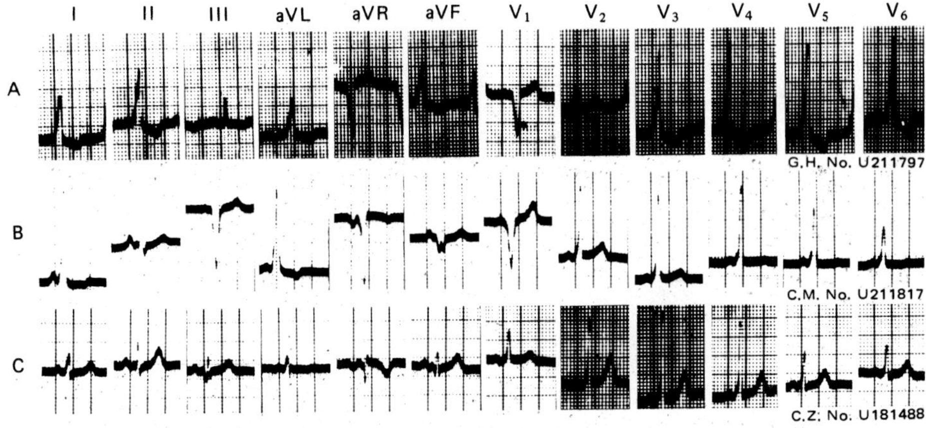

Figure 14–19. Three examples of Wolff-Parkinson-White syndrome. *A:* Woman age 17. *B:* Man age 39. *C:* Woman age 57.

of the delta wave, resulting in probable identification of 10 different anatomic locations of accessory pathways.

The spatial orientation of the delta vector in patients with Wolff-Parkinson-White syndrome gives some indication of the location of the accessory pathway, but electrophysiologic studies are required for precise localization. Some pathways are difficult to identify, but some can be inferred. The polarity of the delta wave in various types of epicardial preexcitation is illustrated in Fig 14–17. Epicardial mapping to determine the site of the accessory pathways should be performed only if the patient has disabling atrial arrhythmias and cardiac surgery is contemplated. On the other hand, His bundle recordings with programmed electrical stimulation are desirable in almost all cases of Wolff-Parkinson-White syndrome to determine the refractory period of the accessory pathway. If the refractory period is short, drugs such as digitalis, which shorten it further, are hazardous, especially if the patient has atrial fibrillation.

Fig 14–17 justifies the inference that there are many intermediate types between type A and type B because of the highly variable position of the accessory tracks; the delta wave orientation allows inferences about the site of the anomalous pathway causing the preexcitation. Multiple muscular connections between the atrium and ventricle may result in both type A and type B at different times.

The effective refractory period of the accessory pathway ranges from 200 msec to as long as 900 msec, with most of the periods between 200–400 msec (Gallagher, 1976). This wide range must be appreciated, as must the significance of the short refractory periods, which may result in rapid ventricular responses to atrial fibrillation.

In addition to the characteristic ECG changes, Wolff-Parkinson-White syndrome is frequently associated with paroxysmal atrial arrhythmias, usually atrial tachycardia.

Approximately one-third of patients with Wolff-Parkinson-White syndrome develop atrial fibrillation at some time. Knowing the duration of the refractory period of the accessory pathway is of considerable therapeutic importance. The physician should determine the effective refractory period at different heart rates, because with rapid rates the refractory period might shorten as it does normally. Gallagher believes that in patients who are shown to have a short effective refractory period of the accessory pathway, atrial fibrillation should be induced experimentally by rapid atrial stimulation to determine the ventricular rate under these circumstances.

The mechanism of the atrial arrhythmia is that of reentry, in which impulses from the atria usually pass through the normal atrioventricular conduction system to the ventricle and then return in retrograde fashion to the atria via the anomalous pathway (Fig 14–20). When the atria, the atrioventricular junction, and the atrioventricular node are no longer refractory, the retrograde impulse may reexcite portions of the specialized normal atrioventricular pathway which conduct to the ventricles and so set up a self-perpetuating circuit and normalize the QRS. Recent electrophysiologic studies have shown that the circuit is antegrade through the normal atrioventricular pathway and retrograde through the anomalous bypass pathway because the refractory period of the latter is usually (not always) shorter. Rarely, the reverse pathway may be the mechanism of the reentry tachycardia. The impulse is retrograde via the atrioventricular node and antegrade through the accessory pathway (Fig 14–20), and the pattern thus simulates ventricular tachycardia because of the aberrant QRS complexes.

His Bundle & Intracardiac Recording in Wolff-Parkinson-White Syndrome

His bundle recordings and epicardial mapping have further delineated the mechanisms of Wolff-Parkinson-White syndrome.

The relationship of the His bundle spike to the delta wave is a function of the A–H interval. When

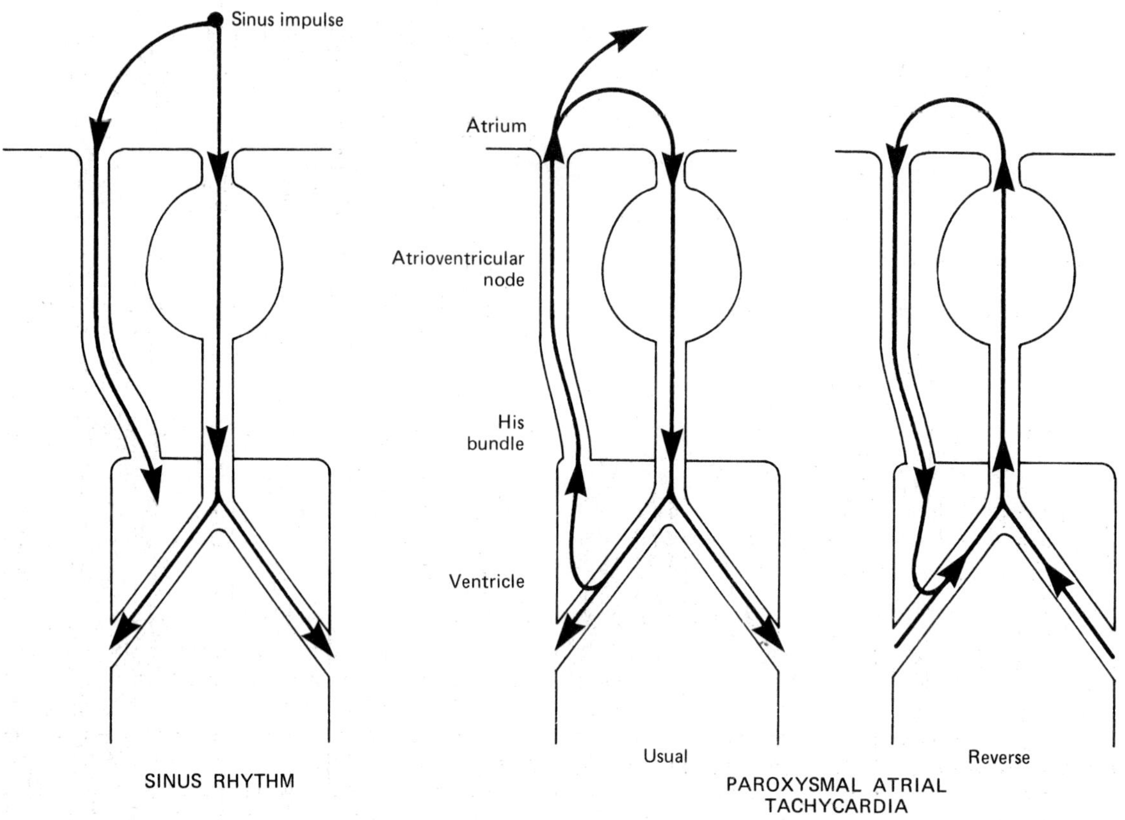

Figure 14–20. Diagram of the normal conduction system and the accessory atrioventricular connection showing the conduction sequence during sinus rhythm in the left hand panel and during tachycardia in the 2 right hand panels. (Arrows show the direction of the reverse of the conduction sequence during tachycardia if the impulse spreads from the atrium via the bypass accessory pathway and returns through the atrioventricular node in retrograde fashion.) (Reproduced, with permission, from Spurrell RAJ, Krikler DM, Sowton E: Problems concerning assessment of anatomical site of accessory pathway in Wolff-Parkinson-White syndrome. Br Heart J 37:127, 1975.)

conduction from the atrioventricular node is prolonged, the H spike may either follow the delta wave or be "lost" in the QRS complex because excitation of the ventricles precedes that of the His bundle presumably by bypass tracks.

Wellens (1974) found an almost linear relationship between the shortest R–R interval (the most rapid ventricular response) during atrial fibrillation and the effective refractory period of the accessory pathway. When the effective refractory period was 200 msec, the R–R interval was 200 msec. When the effective refractory period was 300 msec, the shortest R–R interval during atrial fibrillation was 300 msec. This was true not only in a series of 16 patients but also in the same patients when consecutive R–R intervals were measured. The duration of the refractory period following administration of various antiarrhythmia agents was determined by Wellens (1975). All of the common antiarrhythmia agents either increased the refractory period of the accessory pathway or had no effect–with the exception of digitalis, which decreased it. Procainamide and quinidine increased the H–V interval, but digitalis, phenytoin, atropine, propranolol, lidocaine, and verapamil had no effect. The drugs had contrasting effects on the refractory period of the atrioventricular node. Digitalis, propranolol, and verapamil prolonged it; quinidine had a variable effect, decreasing it in some and increasing it in others; and atropine decreased the refractory period of the atrioventricular node, as did lidocaine (Wellens: Effect of..., 1975). Procainamide may increase the refractory period of the accessory pathways from 275 to 400 msec and is therefore a safe drug to use in Wolff-Parkinson-White syndrome. Epicardial mapping reveals the basis of the ECG in Wolff-Parkinson-White syndrome and identifies the accessory pathways by noting the activation of the ventricles that coincides with the delta wave. Fig 14–21 shows this graphically. At 2 the delta wave coincides with the antegrade activation of the right ventricle at the time of the delta wave. The latter part of the QRS is a fusion wave which results from activation of the ventricle from both the accessory

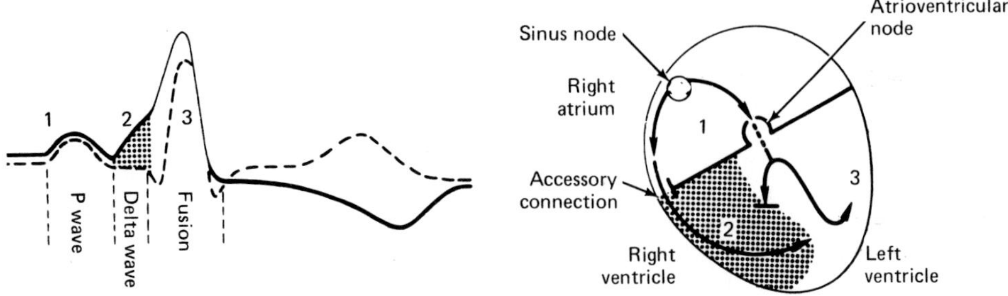

Left: Electrocardiogram

Right: Epicardial mapping

1. Normal P waves with shortened P–R interval. — Antegrade conduction from the sinus node to the atrioventricular node.
2. Premature activation of the ventricle from the accessory pathway, which forms the delta wave.
3. Late fusion of both ventricular depolarizations.

Figure 14–21. Basis of the ECG in Wolff-Parkinson-White syndrome. (Reproduced, with permission, from Boineau JP & others: Epicardial mapping in Wolff-Parkinson-White syndrome. Arch Intern Med 135:422, 1975.)

pathway and the normal pathway. When the ventricle is activated early but the QRS complex is normal in duration, the connection between the atria and the His bundle is by way of the James fibers, bypassing the upper part of the atrioventricular node. This is probably the mechanism of the Lown-Ganong-Levine syndrome.

The technic of epicardial mapping is described in detail by Boineau and associates (1975). The timing of the arrival of the excitation wave in various parts of the ventricle defines the site of the accessory pathway and is best predicted by the delta vectors as in Fig 14–17.

Clinical Findings in Wolff-Parkinson-White Syndrome

The diagnosis is made electrocardiographically, even in patients who do not have a history of paroxysmal arrhythmia. During the arrhythmia it may be difficult to see the characteristic pattern, especially if there is a rapid atrial rate. The typical findings include a short P–R interval, a wide QRS complex, and a slurred delta wave at the onset of the QRS, representing ventricular preexcitation via the bypass through the accessory pathway. The total P–R interval plus the QRS interval is essentially normal (Fig 14–19). The delta wave is usually short—about 0.05 sec—and the P–R interval in rare cases may be essentially normal. About half of patients have no symptoms; the remainder have episodes of paroxysmal atrial arrhythmia which in some cases may only be noted by 12- to 24-hour Holter monitoring. Palpitations due to arrhythmia are the presenting symptom in many patients; they may last a few seconds and produce trivial or no concern or may last hours and be disabling. It was once thought that death was rare during an attack of arrhythmia. This opinion has been modified, possibly because of the very rapid ventricular rates that may occur if the patient has atrial fibrillation and because of the adverse effect of digitalis in such circumstances, with occasional deterioration to ventricular fibrillation and death. Digitalis increases conduction through the accessory pathway and does not slow the ventricular rate.

Determination of the refractory periods of the accessory pathway and of the atrioventricular nodal–Purkinje system and their responses to antiarrhythmia agents is essential, especially in patients with atrial fibrillation, in order to anticipate and avoid shortening of the refractory period of the accessory pathway and so risk the rapid atrial beats activating the ventricle. These determinations require His bundle recordings and extensive atrial and ventricular pacing at different sites and at different rates.

Treatment

Asymptomatic patients in whom the condition is discovered by chance during a routine ECG should be informed of the nature and significance of the syndrome for future reference. Electrophysiologic investigation of paroxysmal arrhythmias is indicated in patients whose attacks of tachycardia are severe and not readily prevented or treated or if the arrhythmia is paroxysmal atrial fibrillation. The most important feature of these special investigations is to determine the effective refractory period of the accessory pathway and the effect of pharmacologic agents on it, not only to be certain that the drug selected does not decrease the refractory period of the accessory pathway but also to determine which of several drugs effectively terminates the reentry circuit. The effects of various drugs on the refractory period of the accessory pathway, the atrioventricular node, and the H–V interval of atrioventricular conduction have already been discussed. Three drugs not approved in the USA but used extensively in Europe—ajmaline, verapamil, and amiodarone—are of clinical interest. Amiodarone prolongs the effective refractory period of both the atrium and the ventricle, preventing the initiation of reentry tachycardia as well as prolonging the refractory period of the accessory pathway.

Procainamide, clonidine, and ajmaline have been given intra-atrially to demonstrate prolongation of the refractory period of the accessory pathway (Wellens, 1974).

As already noted, the effective refractory period of the accessory pathway in different patients with Wolff-Parkinson-White syndrome is not uniform but can be estimated by noting the shortest R–R interval occurring during atrial fibrillation. The faster the ventricular rate (the shorter the R–R interval), the shorter the effective refractory period.

A. Hazard of Digitalis When Atrial Fibrillation Occurs in Wolff-Parkinson-White Syndrome: If the atrial arrhythmia is fibrillation, digitalis should *not* be used because it increases the block in the atrioventricular node while decreasing the refractory period of the anomalous pathway, permitting favored passage of the cardiac impulse via the accessory pathway. The rapid atrial impulses may then be transmitted without the protective blocking action of the atrioventricular node directly to the ventricle, and rapid ventricular rates of atrial fibrillation, ventricular tachycardia, or even ventricular fibrillation may ensue. Drugs that prolong the refractory period of the accessory pathway (procainamide, quinidine) are preferable and safer.

B. Management of Paroxysmal Atrial Arrhythmia in Wolff-Parkinson-White Syndrome: Patients who have episodes of paroxysmal atrial arrhythmia require a different approach; some authorities believe it wise in all patients to determine the refractory period of both the normal and the anomalous pathways to the ventricle so as to avoid drugs that decrease the refractory period of the anomalous pathway. Most cases of paroxysmal atrial tachycardia can be treated in the usual fashion, ie, with interruption of the reentry circuit. This can be achieved by increasing the block in the atrioventricular node by maneuvers such as carotid sinus massage or with drugs that stimulate the vagus nerve—or with digitalis if the rhythm is paroxysmal atrial tachycardia and not atrial fibrillation. Drugs that *increase* the block in the anomalous pathway—procainamide and quinidine—are the most effective. Propranolol and verapamil (the latter not yet approved by FDA) have little effect on the anomalous pathway but a selective blocking effect on the atrioventricular node.

1. Atrial pacing—Atrial pacing has been used therapeutically with the hope that a random beat might by chance excite a portion of the reentry pathway, making it refractory to the oncoming circuit wave. There is a risk that atrial pacing may increase the impulses to the ventricles via the anomalous pathway and so raise the ventricular rate.

2. Emergency treatment—DC shock (cardioversion) or intravenous procainamide should be considered in emergency situations. It may be unwise to use propranolol and verapamil because, although they do not decrease the refractory period of the accessory pathway per se, they decrease it *relative* to that of the atrioventricular node. The refractory period of the atrioventricular node is prolonged by propranolol and verapamil. Further experience is necessary before the precise role of these 2 drugs in Wolff-Parkinson-White syndrome is clarified. If the attacks of atrial arrhythmia are frequent and difficult to control, major efforts to prevent the arrhythmia are indicated (drugs, atrial pacing, and surgery).

3. Prevention of atrial arrhythmias in the preexcitation syndromes—Drugs that prevent the reentry phenomena by slowing conduction in the atrioventricular node or increasing the refractory period of the atrioventricular node may be helpful, as in paroxysmal atrial tachycardia in the absence of Wolff-Parkinson-White syndrome. Quinidine and procainamide are valuable, and, *if one is certain that the arrhythmia is not atrial fibrillation,* digitalis may prevent the attacks. Drugs used in combination rather than one alone may sometimes be more effective in preventing atrial arrhythmias. Side-effects may prevent one drug from being used to maximum effect, eg, bradycardia complicating propranolol therapy. A ventricular pacemaker may be inserted and may be activated externally by a magnet or by a radiofrequency signal in the hope that a chance premature beat may interrupt the reentry cycle.

4. Operative treatment—Surgical interruption of the anomalous pathway is being performed with increasing frequency in selected centers, preceded by careful electrophysiologic studies and epicardial mapping at the time of surgery to determine the area of earliest ventricular excitation. When the anomalous pathway is clearly mapped, resection may interrupt the pathway and prevent both the delta wave and the subsequent arrhythmias. The procedure is difficult and should not be undertaken lightly, because the sequence of ventricular activation varies in different patients.

Cryosurgical ablation of the accessory atrioventricular connections is a new technic now being used in some centers, which if found to be consistently beneficial is a considerable addition to surgical treatment, because thoracotomy alone rather than cardiopulmonary bypass is sufficient, decreasing operating time by several hours. The site of preexcitation can be abolished by local application of the cryoprobe at −60 °C. Evidence of preexcitation and arrhythmias disappeared in these patients, as described by Gallagher and associates (1977).

Type B Wolff-Parkinson-White syndrome has been treated surgically with more success because of its more accessible location, but type A has also been successfully treated. New understanding of the accessory pathways is still being acquired, and it is now clear that such pathways are not uniform in Wolff-Parkinson-White syndrome. A patient may have multiple accessory pathways, and highly technical study in selected centers is mandatory before surgical treatment is undertaken.

• • •

References

Abbott JA & others: Graded exercise testing in patients with sinus node dysfunction. Am J Med 62:330, 1977.

Akhtar M, Damato AN: Clinical uses of His bundle electrocardiography. (Part 1.) Am Heart J 91:520, 1976.

Akhtar M & others: Electrophysiologic effects of atropine on atrioventricular conduction studied by His bundle electrogram. Am J Cardiol 33:333, 1974.

Aranda JM, Befeler B, Castellanos A Jr: His bundle recordings, bundle branch block, and myocardial infarction. Ann Intern Med 86:106, 1977.

Bahl OP, Walsh TJ, Massie E: Left axis deviation: An electrocardiographic study with postmortem correlation. Br Heart J 31:451, 1969.

Barold SS, Coumel P: Mechanisms of atrioventricular junctional tachycardia: Role of reentry and concealed accessory bypass tracts. Am J Cardiol 39:97, 1977.

Barold SS, Friedberg HD: Second degree atrioventricular block: A matter of definition. Am J Cardiol 33:311, 1974.

Bigger JT Jr & others: Ventricular arrhythmias in ischemic heart disease: Mechanism, prevalence, significance, and management. Prog Cardiovasc Dis 19:255, 1977.

Bleifer SB & others: Diagnosis of occult arrhythmias by Holter electrocardiography. Prog Cardiovasc Dis 16:569, 1974.

Boineau JP & others: Epicardial mapping in Wolff-Parkinson-White syndrome. Arch Intern Med 135:422, 1975.

Breithardt G, Seipel L, Loogen F: Sinus node recovery time and calculated sinoatrial conduction time in normal subjects and patients with sinus node dysfunction. Circulation 56:43, 1977.

Briant RH & others: Assessment of selective beta-adrenoceptor blockade in man. Br J Pharmacol 49:106, 1973.

Campbell M, Suzman SS: Congenital complete heart-block. Am Heart J 9:304, 1934.

Cannom DS, Goldreyer BN, Damato AN: Atrioventricular conduction system in left bundle-branch block with normal QRS axis. Circulation 46:129, 1972.

Caracta AR & others: Electrophysiologic studies in the syndrome of short P–R interval, normal QRS complex. Am J Cardiol 31:245, 1973.

Castellanos A, Castillo CA, Agha AS: Contribution of His bundle recordings to the understanding of clinical arrhythmias. Am J Cardiol 28:499, 1971.

Castellanos A Jr, Lemberg L: Diagnosis of isolated and combined block in the bundle branches and the divisions of the left branch. Circulation 43:971, 1971.

Castellanos A Jr & others: Factors regulating ventricular rates during atrial flutter and fibrillation in preexcitation (Wolff-Parkinson-White) syndrome. Br Heart J 35:811, 1973.

Childers R: Concealed conduction. Med Clin North Am 60:149, 1976.

Cohen HC & others: Tachycardia and bradycardia-dependent bundle branch block alternans: Clinical observations. Circulation 55:242, 1977.

Cohen SI & others: Atrioventricular conduction in patients with clinical indications for transvenous cardiac pacing. Br Heart J 37:583, 1975.

Conde CA & others: Effectiveness of pacemaker treatment in the bradycardia-tachycardia syndrome. Am J Cardiol 32:209, 1973.

Coumel P & others: "Incessant" tachycardias in Wolff-Parkinson-White syndrome. 2. Role of atypical cycle length dependency and nodal-His escape beats in initiating reciprocating tachycardias. Br Heart J 38:897, 1976.

Davies MJ: *Pathology of Conducting Tissue of the Heart.* Appleton-Century-Crofts, 1971.

Denes P & others: The effects of cycle length on cardiac refractory periods in man. Circulation 49:32, 1974.

Denes P & others: Sudden death in patients with chronic bifascicular block. Arch Intern Med 137:1005, 1977.

DePasquale NP, Bruno MS: Natural history of combined right bundle branch block and left anterior hemiblock (bilateral bundle branch block). Am J Med 54:297, 1973.

DeSanctis RW: Diagnostic and therapeutic uses of atrial pacing. Circulation 43:748, 1971.

Dhingra RC & others: Prospective observations in patients with chronic bundle branch block and marked H–V prolongation. Circulation 53:600, 1976.

Dhingra RC & others: Significance of A–H interval in patients with chronic bundle branch block: Clinical, electrophysiologic and follow-up observations. Am J Cardiol 37:231, 1976.

Dhingra RC & others: The significance of second degree atrioventricular block and bundle branch block: Observations regarding site and type of block. Circulation 49:638, 1974.

Dhingra RC & others: Syncope in patients with chronic bifascicular block: Significance, causative mechanisms, and clinical implications. Ann Intern Med 81:302, 1974.

Dighton DH: Sinoatrial block: Autonomic influences and clinical assessment. Br Heart J 37:321, 1975.

Dollery CT, Paterson JW, Conolly ME: Clinical pharmacology of beta-receptor blocking drugs. Clin Pharmacol 10:765, 1969.

Dreifus LS: Atrioventricular block. Am J Cardiol 28:371, 1971.

Dreifus LS & others: Sinus bradycardia and atrial fibrillation associated with the Wolff-Parkinson-White syndrome. Am J Cardiol 38:149, 1976.

Durrer D, Wellens HJJ: The Wolff-Parkinson-White syndrome anno 1973. Eur J Cardiol 1:367, 1974.

Durrer D & others: The role of premature beats in the initiation and the termination of supraventricular tachycardia in the Wolff-Parkinson-White syndrome. Circulation 36:644, 1967.

Easley RM Jr, Goldstein S: Sino-atrial syncope. Am J Med 50:166, 1971.

Eraut D, Shaw DB: Sinus bradycardia. Br Heart J 33:742, 1971.

Erlanger J: On the physiology of heart block in mammals, with especial reference to the causation of Stokes-Adams disease. J Exp Med 8:8, 1906.

Escher DJW: Follow-up of the patient with an implanted cardiac pacemaker. Mod Concepts Cardiovasc Dis 63:77, 1974.

Escher DJW: Historical aspects of pacing. Pages 1–15 in: *Cardiac Pacing.* Samet P (editor). Grune & Stratton, 1973.

Ferrer MI: Preexcitation. Am J Med 62:715, 1977.

Ferrer MI: *The Sick Sinus Syndrome.* Futura, 1974.

Fisch C & others: Potassium and the monophasic action potential, electrocardiogram, conduction and arrhythmias. Prog Cardiovasc Dis 8:387, 1966.

Flensted-Jensen E: Wolff-Parkinson-White syndrome: A long term follow-up of 47 cases. Acta Med Scand 186:65, 1969.

Fozzard HA: Cardiac muscle: Excitability and passive electrical properties. Prog Cardiovasc Dis 19:343, 1977.

Fozzard HA, DasGupta DS: Electrophysiology and the electrocardiogram. Mod Concepts Cardiovasc Dis 44:29, 1975.

Fraser GR, Froggatt P, James TN: Congenital deafness associated with electrocardiographic abnormalities, fainting attacks and sudden death: A recessive syndrome. Q J Med 33:361, 1964.

Gallagher JJ & others: The preexcitation syndromes. Prog Cardiovasc Dis. [In press.]

Gallagher JJ & others: The Wolff-Parkinson-White syndrome and the preexcitation dysrhythmias: Medical and surgical management. Med Clin North Am 60:101, 1976.

Gallagher JJ & others: Wolff-Parkinson-White syndrome: The problem, evaluation, and surgical correction. Circulation 51:767, 1975.

Gilchrist AR: Clinical aspects of high grade heart block. Scott Med J 3:53, 1958.

Godman MJ, Lassers BW, Julian DG: Complete bundle branch block complicating acute myocardial infarction. N Engl J Med 282:237, 1970.

Goldman MJ: *Principles of Clinical Electrocardiography*, 9th ed. Lange, 1976.

Goldreyer BN, Damato AN: Sino-atrial node entrance block. Circulation 44:789, 1971.

Grant RP: Left axis deviation: An electrocardiographio-pathologic correlation study. Circulation 14:233, 1956.

Haber E, Leatham A: Splitting of heart sounds from ventricular asynchrony in bundle-branch block, ventricular ectopic beats, and artificial pacing. Br Heart J 27:691, 1965.

Haft JI: Clinical indications for the His bundle electrogram. Cardiovasc Med 2:449, 1977.

Haft JI, Herman MV, Gorlin R: Left bundle branch block: Etiologic, hemodynamic, and ventriculographic considerations. Circulation 43:279, 1971.

Han J: The concepts of re-entrant activity responsible for ectopic rhythm. Am J Cardiol 28:253, 1971.

Han J & others: Temporal dispersion of recovery of excitability in atrium and ventricle as a function of heart rate. Am Heart J 71:481, 1966.

Harris A & others: Management of heart block. Br Heart J 27:469, 1965.

Helfant RH, Scherlag BJ: *His Bundle Electrocardiography*. Medcom Press, 1974.

Hinkle LE Jr, Carver ST, Stevens M: The frequency of asymptomatic disturbances of cardiac rhythm and conduction in middle-aged men. Am J Cardiol 24:629, 1969.

Hoffman BF, Cranefield PF: *The Electrophysiology of the Heart*. McGraw-Hill, 1960.

Hudson REB: Surgical pathology of the conducting system of the heart. Br Heart J 29:646, 1967.

Ikkos D, Hanson JS: Response to exercise in congenital complete atrioventricular block. Circulation 22:583, 1960.

James TN: The connecting pathways between the sinus node and the A–V node and between the right and left atrium in the human heart. Am Heart J 66:498, 1963.

James TN & others: Adrenergic mechanisms in the sinus node. Arch Intern Med 125:512, 1970.

Jensen G, Sigurd B, Sandoe E: Adams-Stokes seizures due to ventricular tachyarrhythmias in patients with heart block: Prevalence and problems of management. Chest 67:43, 1975.

Johansson BW: Longevity in complete heart block. Ann NY Acad Sci 167:1031, 1969.

Jordan JL, Yamaguchi I, Mandel WJ: The sick sinus syndrome. JAMA 237:682, 1977.

Kaplan BM: Tachycardia-bradycardia syndrome. Med Clin North Am 60:81, 1976.

Kastor JA: Atrioventricular block. (2 parts.) N Engl J Med 292:462, 572, 1975.

Kirk JE, Kvorning SA: Sinus bradycardia: A clinical study of 515 consecutive cases. Acta Med Scand 266 (Suppl):625, 1952.

Kunkel F, Rowland M, Scheinman MM: The electrophysiologic effects of lidocaine in patients with intraventricular conduction defects. Circulation 49:894, 1974.

Lagergren H & others: Three hundred and five cases of permanent intravenous pacemaker treatment for Adams-Stokes syndrome. Surgery 59:494, 1966.

Lancaster MC, Schechter E, Massing GK: Acquired complete right bundle branch block without overt cardiac disease. Am J Cardiol 30:32, 1972.

Landegren J, Biörck G: The clinical assessment and treatment of complete heart block and Adams-Stokes attacks. Medicine 42:171, 1963.

Langendorf R: Concealed A–V conduction: The effect of blocked impulses on the formation and conduction of subsequent impulses. Am Heart J 35:542, 1948.

Langendorf R, Cohen H, Gozo EG Jr: Observations on second degree atrioventricular block, including new criteria for the differential diagnosis between type I and type II block. Am J Cardiol 29:111, 1972.

Lenegre J: Bilateral bundle branch block. Cardiologia 48:134, 1966.

Lenegre J: Etiology and pathology of bilateral bundle branch block in relation to complete heart block. Prog Cardiovasc Dis 6:409, 1964.

Lev M: The normal anatomy of the conduction system in man and its pathology in atrioventricular block. Ann NY Acad Sci 111:819, 1964.

Lev M: The pathology of atrioventricular block. Cardiovasc Clin 4:159, 1972.

Levites R, Haft JI: Significance of first degree heart block (prolonged P–R interval) in bifascicular block. Am J Cardiol 34:256, 1974.

Lewis CH & others: Coronary arteriographic appearances in patients with left bundle branch block. Circulation 41:299, 1970.

Lewis JK: Stokes-Adams disease: An account of important historical discoveries. Arch Intern Med 101:130, 1958.

Lewis T: *The Mechanism and Graphic Registration of the Heart Beat*, 3rd ed. Shaw & Sons, 1925.

Lie KI & others: Factors influencing prognosis of bundle branch block complicating acute antero-septal infarction: The value of His bundle recordings. Circulation 50:935, 1974.

Lie KI & others: Mechanism and significance of widened QRS complexes during complete atrioventricular block in acute inferior myocardial infarction. Am J Cardiol 33:833, 1974.

Lister JW, Kline RS, Lesser ME: Chronic bilateral bundle-branch block: Long-term observations in ambulatory patients. Br Heart J 39:203, 1977.

Lloyd-Mostyn RH, Kidner PH, Oram S: Sinu-atrial disorder including the brady-tachycardia syndrome. Q J Med 42:41, 1973.

Lown B, Ganong WF, Levine SA: The syndrome of short P–R interval, normal QRS complex, and paroxysmal rapid heart action. Circulation 5:693, 1952.

Lown B, Kosowsky BD: Artificial cardiac pacemakers. (3 parts.) N Engl J Med 283:907, 971, 1023, 1970.

Luy G, Bahl OP, Massie E: Intermittent left bundle branch block. Am Heart J 85:332, 1973.

Mackenzie J: *Diseases of the Heart*. Oxford, 1908.

Mandel WJ, Danzig R, Hayakawa H: Lown-Ganong-Levine syndrome: A study using His bundle electrograms. Circulation 44:696, 1971.

Mandel WJ, Laks MM, Obayshi K: Sinus node function: Evaluation in patients with and without sinus node disease. Arch Intern Med 135:388, 1975.

Margolis JR & others: Digitalis and the sick sinus syndrome. Circulation 52:162, 1975.

Marriott HJL, Menendez MM: A-V dissociation revisited. Prog Cardiovasc Dis 8:522, 1966.

Massing GK, James TN: Anatomical configuration of the His bundle and bundle branches in the human heart. Circulation 53:609, 1976.

McGuire LB, O'Brien WM, Nolan SP: Patient survival and instrument performance with permanent cardiac pacing. JAMA 237:558, 1977.

Mendez C, Gauhzit CC, Moe GK: Influence of cycle length upon refractory periods of auricles, ventricles and A–V node in the dog. Am J Physiol 184:287, 1956.

Merideth J, Pruitt RD: Disturbances in cardiac conduction and their management. Circulation 47:1098, 1973.

Moe GK, Mendez C: The physiologic basis of reciprocal rhythm. Prog Cardiovasc Dis 8:461, 1966.

Monahan JP, Denes P, Rosen KM: Portable electrocardiographic monitoring: Performance in patients with short P–R intervals without delta waves. Arch Intern Med 135:1188, 1975.

Moore EN, Knoebel SB, Spear JF: Concealed conduction. Am J Cardiol 28:406, 1971.

Moss AJ, Davis RJ: Brady-tachy syndrome. Prog Cardiovasc Dis 16:439, 1974.

Mullins CB, Atkins JM: Prognoses and management of ventricular conduction blocks in acute myocardial infarction. Mod Concepts Cardiovasc Dis 45:129, 1976.

Nakamura FF, Nadas AS: Complete heart block in infants and children. N Engl J Med 270:1261, 1964.

Narula OS (editor): *His Bundle Electrocardiography and Clinical Electrophysiology.* Davis, 1975.

Narula OS, Gann D, Samet P: Prognostic value of H–V intervals. Pages 437–449 in: *His Bundle Electrocardiography and Clinical Electrophysiology.* Narula OS (editor). Davis, 1975.

Narula OS, Samet P: Right bundle branch block with normal, left or right axis deviation: Analysis by His bundle recordings. Am J Med 51:432, 1971.

Narula OS & others: Atrioventricular block: Localization and classification by His bundle recordings. Am J Med 50:146, 1971.

Norris RM, Mercer CJ, Croxson MS: Conduction disturbances due to anteroseptal myocardial infarction and their treatment by endocardial pacing. Am Heart J 84:560, 1972.

O'Rourke RA: The Stokes-Adams syndrome: 1. Definition and etiology. West J Med 117:96, 1972.

Parsonnet V, Manhardt M: Permanent pacing of the heart: 1952 to 1976. Am J Cardiol 39:250, 1977.

Penton GB, Miller H, Levine SA: Some clinical features of complete heart block. Circulation 13:801, 1956.

Puech P: Atrioventricular block: The value of intracardiac recordings. Page 81 in: *Cardiac Arrhythmias. The Modern Electrophysiological Approach.* Krikler DM, Goodwin JF (editors). Saunders, 1975.

Radford DJ, Julian DG: Sick sinus syndrome: Experience of a cardiac pacemaker clinic. Br Med J 3:504, 1974.

Reuter H: Dependence of slow inward current in Purkinje fibres on the extracellular calcium concentration. J Physiol (Lond) 192:479, 1967.

Rodstein M & others: Mortality study in bundle branch block. Arch Intern Med 87:663, 1951.

Rokseth R, Hatle L: Prospective study on the occurrence and management of chronic sinoatrial disease, with follow-up. Br Heart J 36:582, 1974.

Rosen KM: The contribution of His bundle recording to the understanding of cardiac conduction in man. Circulation 43:961, 1971.

Rosen KM & others: Cardiac conduction in patients with symptomatic sinus node disease. Circulation 43:836, 1971.

Rosen KM & others: Chronic heart block in adults. Arch Intern Med 131:663, 1973.

Rosen MR & others: Electrophysiology and pharmacology of cardiac arrhythmias: 5. Cardiac antiarrhythmic effects of lidocaine. Am Heart J 89:526, 1975.

Rosenbaum FF & others: The potential variations of the thorax and the esophagus in anomalous atrioventricular excitation (Wolff-Parkinson-White syndrome). Am Heart J 29:281, 1945.

Rosenbaum MB & others: The differential electrocardiographic manifestations of hemiblocks, bilateral bundle branch block and trifascicular blocks. Pages 145–182 in: *Advances in Electrocardiography.* Schlant RC, Hurst JW (editors). Grune & Stratton, 1972.

Rossi L: Histopathology of conducting system in left anterior hemiblock. Br Heart J 38:1304, 1976.

Rotman M, Triebwasser JH: A clinical and follow-up study of right and left bundle branch block. Circulation 51:477, 1975.

Rowe JC, White PD: Complete heart block: A follow-up study. Ann Intern Med 49:260, 1958.

Rubenstein JJ & others: Clinical spectrum of the sick sinus syndrome. Circulation 46:5, 1972.

Samet P: *Cardiac Pacing.* Grune & Stratton, 1973.

Scarpelli FM, Rudolph AM: The hemodynamics of congenital complete heart block. Prog Cardiovasc Dis 6:327, 1964.

Schamroth L, Ziady F, de Kock J: Acute inferior wall myocardial infarction associated with complete atrioventricular block and left posterior hemiblock. Br Heart J 37:471, 1975.

Scheinman MM, Brenman B: Clinical and anatomic implications of intraventricular conduction blocks in acute myocardial infarction. Circulation 46:753, 1972.

Scheinman MM & others: Atrial pacing in patients with sinus node dysfunction. Am J Med 61:641, 1976.

Scheinman MM & others: Electrophysiologic effects of procainamide in patients with intraventricular conduction delay. Circulation 49:522, 1974.

Scheinman MM & others: Prognostic value of infranodal conduction time in patients with chronic bundle branch block. Circulation 56:240, 1977.

Scherlag BJ & others: Catheter technique for recording His bundle activity in man. Circulation 39:13, 1969.

Schuilenburg RM, Durrer D: Observations on atrioventricular conduction in patients with bilateral bundle-branch block. Circulation 41:967, 1970.

Sellers TD, Bashore TM, Gallagher JJ: Digitalis in the preexcitation syndrome: Analysis during atrial fibrillation. Circulation 56:260, 1977.

Sellers TD Jr & others: Effects of procainamide and quinidine sulfate in the Wolff-Parkinson-White syndrome. Circulation 55:15, 1977.

Short DS: The syndrome of alternating bradycardia and tachycardia. Br Heart J 16:208, 1954.

Siddons H, Nowak K: Surgical complications of implanting pacemakers. Br J Surg 62:929, 1975.

Siddons H, Sowton E: *Cardiac Pacemakers.* Thomas, 1967.

Singer DM, Lazzara R, Hoffman B: Interrelationships between automaticity and conduction in Purkinje fibers. Circ Res

21:537, 1967.

Spurrell RAJ, Kerkler DM, Sowton E: Problems concerning assessment of anatomical site of accessory pathway in Wolff-Parkinson-White syndrome. Br Heart J 37:127, 1975.

Strauss HC & others: Electrophysiologic evaluation of sinus node function in patients with sinus node dysfunction. Circulation 53:763, 1976.

Svenson RH & others: Electrophysiological evaluation of the Wolff-Parkinson-White syndrome: Problems in assessing antegrade and retrograde conduction over the accessory pathway. Circulation 52:552, 1975.

Thilenius OG & others: Hemodynamic studies in children with congenital atrioventricular block. Am J Cardiol 30:13, 1972.

Titus JL: Cardiac arrhythmias. 1. Anatomy of the conduction system. Circulation 47:170, 1973.

Tonkin AM, Gallagher JJ, Wallace AG: Tachyarrhythmias in Wolff-Parkinson-White syndrome: Treatment and prevention. JAMA 235:947, 1976.

Tonkin AM & others: Refractory periods of the accessory pathway in the Wolff-Parkinson-White syndrome. Circulation 52:563, 1975.

Trevino AS, Beller BM: Conduction disturbances of the left bundle branch system and their relationship to complete heart block. 2. A review of differential diagnosis, pathology and clinical significance. Am J Med 51:374, 1971.

Van Durme JP: Tachyarrhythmias and transient cerebral ischemic attacks. Am Heart J 89:538, 1975.

Vera Z & others: Prolonged His–Q interval in chronic bifascicular block: Relation to impending complete heart block. Circulation 53:46, 1976.

Vohra J & others: The effect of toxic and therapeutic doses of tricyclic antidepressant drugs on intracardiac conduction. Eur J Cardiol 3/3:219, 1975.

Watanabe Y, Dreifus LS: Factors controlling impulse transmission with special reference to A-V conduction. Am Heart J 89:790, 1975.

Watt TB, Pruitt RD: Character, cause and consequence of combined left axis deviation and right bundle branch block in human electrocardiograms. Am Heart J 77:460, 1969.

Wellens HJJ: Contribution of cardiac pacing to our understanding of the Wolff-Parkinson-White syndrome. Br Heart J 37:231, 1975.

Wellens HJJ: Effect of drugs on Wolff-Parkinson-White syndrome. Page 367 in: *His Bundle Electrocardiography and Clinical Electrocardiography.* Narula O (editor). Davis, 1975.

Wellens HJJ, Durrer D: Effect of digitalis on A–V conduction and circus movement tachycardias in patients with the Wolff-Parkinson-White syndrome. Circulation 47:1229, 1973.

Wellens HJJ, Durrer D: Wolff-Parkinson-White syndrome and atrial fibrillation: Relation between refractory period of accessory pathway and ventricular rate during atrial fibrillation. Am J Cardiol 34:777, 1974.

Wenckebach KF: Zur analyse des unregelmässigen pulses. Z Klin Med 36:181, 1899.

Williams EM: Classification of anti-arrhythmic drugs. Page 449 in: *Symposium on Cardiac Arrhythmias.* Sandor E, Flensted-Jensen E, Olesen KH (editors). Elsinore, 1970.

Wohl AJ & others: Prognosis of patients permanently paced for sick sinus syndrome. Arch Intern Med 136:406, 1976.

Wolff L, Parkinson J, White PD: Bundle branch block with short P–R interval in healthy young people prone to paroxysmal tachycardia. Am Heart J 5:685, 1930.

Wright KE Jr, McIntosh HD: Artificial pacemakers. Circulation 47:1108, 1973.

15...
Cardiac Arrhythmias

The electrophysiologic principles applicable to the study of cardiac arrhythmias are included with the discussion of that subject in Chapter 14.

Causes of Cardiac Arrhythmias

A. Diseases and Drug Effects: Cardiac arrhythmias can occur in any condition, such as coronary heart disease or hypoxia, in which impulse formation is enhanced, or in which impulse conduction is impaired, or in which a combination of these factors is present. Enhancement of automaticity of latent pacemaker cells by increased sympathetic discharge is a common cause of arrhythmias, and this may explain the relatively high frequency of all types of supraventricular arrhythmias in patients with no known heart disease. Ventricular arrhythmias are also due to this cause. Disturbances in rhythm are common in healthy persons during emotional crises; in patients with any cardiac condition involving the left ventricle such as coronary heart disease, hypertension, acute myocarditis, or cardiomyopathy; in patients with connective tissue disorders such as lupus erythematosus, scleroderma, and polyarteritis nodosa; and in patients with mitral valve prolapse, sick sinus syndrome, and preexcitation with Wolff-Parkinson-White syndrome. Atrial fibrillation occurs commonly in mitral stenosis and insufficiency, in which an enlarged left atrium facilitates ectopic atrial rhythms. Atrial fibrillation is rare in pure aortic valve lesions, in cor pulmonale, and in infective endocarditis. Ingestion of large quantities of alcohol during a short period may precipitate transient atrial fibrillation. Coffee, tea, and tobacco may occasionally cause disturbances in cardiac rhythm, especially ventricular premature beats, but in the authors' opinion their importance has been overestimated. Cigarette smoking is undoubtedly an important cause of arrhythmias in patients with coronary heart disease who have ventricular premature beats, and smoking may in fact be responsible for the onset of ventricular fibrillation and sudden death.

In many cases the cause of a cardiac arrhythmia, regardless of its type, cannot be determined. One then assumes that the cause is that of any associated cardiac disease. Common causes of arrhythmias that are sometimes overlooked are extracardiac disorders (eg, thyrotoxicosis); electrolyte (hyperkalemia or hypokalemia) and acid-base disorders; hypotension, hypoxia, and hypercapnia due to poor ventilation in chronic lung disease or after pulmonary surgery; and adverse effects of drugs such as digitalis, quinidine, propranolol, aminophylline, and beta-adrenergic agonists.

Although each of the factors mentioned above may precipitate a cardiac arrhythmia, the physiologic disturbances resulting from the arrhythmia may be a combination of both the arrhythmia itself and the underlying cardiac state. Potent cardiac drugs have the paradoxic effect of both reversing and producing arrhythmias, as in the case of quinidine.

B. Prevalence of Arrhythmias in Relation to Age: Paroxysmal atrial tachycardia is common in younger people, often in the absence of evidence of heart disease, whereas it is uncommon in older individuals although it may complicate acute myocardial infarction. The most common cause of ventricular arrhythmias in older people is coronary heart disease, but ECG monitoring for 12–24 hours has shown that there is a high incidence of ventricular premature beats in asymptomatic ambulatory men without known cardiac disease who have normal coronary arteriograms and a good prognosis. This is in contrast to ventricular premature beats that complicate acute or chronic coronary heart disease. The likelihood of sudden death is enhanced in patients with ventricular premature beats secondary to coronary heart disease, especially if the premature beats occur in multifocal pattern or are frequent, early, in pairs, or associated with short or long runs of ventricular tachycardia.

Impact on the Heart; Pathogenesis & Pathophysiology

The consequences of a cardiac arrhythmia depend upon its effect on cardiac hemodynamics; on cerebral, coronary, and renal perfusion; on blood pressure, left ventricular function, and cardiac rate (rapid or slow); on the duration of the arrhythmia; and on the presence or absence of underlying heart disease. If the arrhythmia occurs in a young person with no underlying heart disease and the increase in ventricular rate is only modest (< 160/min), hemodynamic function is rarely impaired, and perfusion of vital organs (brain, heart, and kidneys) and extremities is adequate. Cardiac output and left ventricular filling pressure do not worsen. The patient may complain of palpitations (awareness of a rapid heartbeat) or may have no symptoms.

If the arrhythmia occurs in an older patient with coronary heart disease, severe symptoms of near syncope, chest pain, palpitations, dyspnea, and disturbed left ventricular function with low cardiac output may develop.

Whether the disturbance in rhythm is regular or irregular has an important influence on the patient's ability to tolerate it; an irregular rhythm such as atrial fibrillation is less well tolerated than paroxysmal atrial tachycardia at an identical rate. Incomplete ventricular filling from the absence of atrial systole can significantly influence cardiac output in a cardiac arrhythmia in such conditions as atrial septal defect, mitral valve prolapse, mitral stenosis, or cardiomyopathy with decreased ventricular compliance. A rapid ventricular rate is catastrophic in patients with severe mitral stenosis, who require adequate diastolic time to fill the left ventricle and empty the left atrium. Atrial fibrillation is relatively unimportant in aortic valvular disease or mitral regurgitation, because there is no obstruction to left ventricular filling and diastolic filling time is thus less important. However, the lack of effective atrial contraction with decrease in late ventricular filling can reduce the cardiac output.

Clinical Features of Tachyarrhythmias in General

A. Initial Assessment of the Nature of the Arrhythmia and Its Impact on the Patient: The approach to the patient with a cardiac arrhythmia requires first an assessment of the precise diagnosis of the arrhythmia and an estimate of its severity (ie, the impact of the arrhythmia on left ventricular function, blood pressure, cerebral and coronary perfusion, and renal function). The importance of the heart rate, the duration of the arrhythmia, and the presence of underlying heart disease must be reemphasized. As stated in the general introduction, the arrhythmia may be trivial or urgent depending upon the age of the patient, the cause of the arrhythmia, and the effect of the arrhythmia on the circulation. The disturbance in rhythm may be intermittent, and its presence must be documented by continuous ambulatory ECG monitoring in doubtful cases because palpitations, which are subjective sensations of the patient, may be due to increased forcefulness of the heartbeat and not to arrhythmia.

B. Variable Difficulty of Diagnosis: The diagnosis may be simple—at the bedside or after routine ECG—or it may be very complex, requiring extensive studies with carotid sinus massage, Valsalva's maneuver, rapid atrial pacing, His bundle studies with intracardiac recording and stimulation, and, in selected cases, coronary arteriography and left ventricular cineangiograms to rule out cardiac aneurysm. It may be necessary to determine the relationship of the QRS complex and the P wave to the His bundle deflection, the effect of posture and drugs, and the adequacy of the baroreceptor reflexes in order to identify the type of arrhythmia and determine whether it is ventricular or supraventricular. The arrhythmia may be intermittent or short-lived. The relationship of the P waves to the QRS complexes requires careful study. A long ECG strip with each P wave and QRS complex identified is essential in the study of antegrade and retrograde conduction. Conduction delays or blocks may occur in limitless combinations and in both directions. New depolarizations in various parts of the heart, intermittent conduction with entrance and exit block to an ectopic focus (as in parasystole), and multiple arrhythmias may follow each other in rapid sequence. This is particularly true in acute myocardial infarction, in which, over a period of an hour, the patient may have multiple arrhythmias combined with conduction defects anywhere in the specialized conduction system. In most instances, however, careful consideration of the ECG evidence will allow the diagnosis to be made without the need for invasive procedures.

C. Previous Attacks: In assessing the importance of any given episode of arrhythmia, the examiner should obtain a history of previous episodes, an indication of the patient's tolerance for them, their frequency and duration, the extent of circulatory impairment, and the response to treatment if any. Some arrhythmias last seconds or minutes, while others, such as atrial fibrillation, last hours or days or indefinitely. The examiner should keep separate the clinical features and treatment of an acute episode from measures taken to prevent a recurrent attack.

D. Symptoms:

1. Identification of arrhythmia—The patient may have no symptoms at all, and the arrhythmia may be discovered on routine examination in which the patient is found to have premature beats, atrial fibrillation or flutter, or even ventricular tachycardia or transient brief episodes of ventricular fibrillation. Many patients with mitral stenosis have short bouts of atrial fibrillation without being aware of it. On the other hand, the onset of atrial fibrillation may be devastating, producing acute dyspnea, pulmonary edema, and an abrupt worsening of the clinical and hemodynamic state because of the inability to empty the left atrium and fill the left ventricle during the short diastolic pauses that are due to the rapid ventricular rate and the loss of atrial systole and dilatation of the left atrium. The usual history is of a sudden onset of palpitations which the patient may describe as regular or irregular, although it may not always be possible to characterize them one way or the other. It may help if the physician taps out various rhythms and rates and asks, "Is it like this? Or like this?" etc. The patient may not complain of palpitations but rather of the consequences of the arrhythmia, such as weakness, chest pain, dizziness, dyspnea, and confusion. In paroxysmal atrial tachycardia the patient may pass a large quantity of urine within a few minutes of onset, a phenomenon which is thought to be due to inhibition of vasopressin secretion by the posterior pituitary, although the hypothesis has not been proved. The mechanism by which this occurs is not known. Hemodynamic studies in paroxysmal atrial tachycardia may in some cases show not only a marked increase in heart rate but also prolongation of the P–R interval, fall in arterial pressure, decrease in the cardiac index, and

increase in the pulmonary artery diastolic pressure and right atrial pressure (Goldreyer, 1976).

2. Progressive deterioration of cardiac function—The symptoms of an arrhythmia may not be apparent at the onset. In arrhythmias of longer duration, there may be progressive deterioration of cardiac function, with impaired perfusion of vital organs from decreased cardiac output. The patient may then develop symptoms resulting from inadequate perfusion of the brain, heart, kidneys, skin, and extremities. The fact that the patient tolerates the arrhythmia at the outset does not guarantee that circulatory embarrassment will not develop with time. This is especially true in patients in the coronary care unit, in whom cardiac failure may develop gradually.

SUPRAVENTRICULAR OR ATRIAL ARRHYTHMIAS

PREMATURE BEATS

Supraventricular premature beats originate, as does supraventricular tachycardia, anywhere above the bundle of His. They can be atrial, atrionodal, or junctional or may arise in the bundle of His itself. They may be single, rare or frequent, and similar in configuration to the sinus (or basic) beat, or they may have multiple sites of origin (multifocal) and, depending upon the time in diastole when they occur (their degree of prematurity), may induce aberrant conduction, producing wide QRS complexes simulating ventricular ectopic beats. The QRS configuration in aberrant conduction varies depending in part upon how early in diastole they occur and in part upon the duration of refractoriness and recovery of excitability in different parts of the conduction system. The most common pattern, because the refractory period of the right bundle is longer than that of the left, is that of right bundle branch block (rsR′ pattern in V_1) with or without left anterior hemiblock. Atrial premature beats may occur in runs or pairs and may induce atrial fibrillation or atrial tachycardia. When they occur early in diastole—ie, when the ventricles are still partially refractory, not having recovered fully from the preceding beat—they may be nonconducted and recognized only on the ECG as an extra-atrial depolarization not disturbing the fundamental pattern of ventricular beats or by a prolonged P–R interval in the succeeding beat.

Importance of Premature Beats

As explained in the section on electrophysiology in Chapter 14, premature beats are important only if they interfere with the hemodynamic function of the left ventricle, impair cardiac output, decrease perfusion to vital organs, or if they are precursors of more serious arrhythmias. Supraventricular premature beats are rarely important in this sense and, when single or infrequent, do not interfere with left ventricular function, do not decrease the blood flow to any of the vital organs, and rarely produce symptoms other than the feeling of a skipped beat or the sensation of the more powerful beat that follows the pause. In community prospective studies, supraventricular beats are not related to sudden death, as are ventricular premature beats in coronary disease. Atrial premature beats are conducted in antegrade or retrograde manner; they commonly depolarize the sinus node, and therefore there may be a pause following the premature beat which is longer than the pause between 2 normally conducted sinus beats. With the exception of hypertrophic cardiomyopathy, in which the stroke output following a pause is usually weaker than normal, the ventricular beat following the pause is usually stronger, and the patient may have a variety of symptoms referable to awareness of the strength of this beat. As is typical of tachycardia in general, systemic symptoms may occur depending on the state of the heart and the frequency of the premature beats. When supraventricular beats are frequent or occur in runs, such beats may decrease the cardiac output and impair perfusion to the essential organs, causing mental confusion, dyspnea, angina, palpitations, or weakness. Usually, however, unless the underlying state of the heart is precarious or unless the premature beats induce tachycardia with a rapid irregular rate, patients with supraventricular premature beats have few or no symptoms.

Relation to Atrial Fibrillation

Supraventricular premature beats are more apt to occur if there is atrial or conduction system disease such as left atrial enlargement in mitral stenosis. When the beats occur under these circumstances, they may presage the development of atrial fibrillation. When atrial fibrillation is converted to sinus rhythm by cardioversion or quinidine, reappearance of atrial premature beats often indicates that atrial fibrillation will soon recur.

Clinical Findings

Supraventricular premature beats, like ventricular premature beats, may be recognized at the bedside when an extra beat is heard that disturbs the dominant rhythm. The origin of the extra beat, whether supraventricular or ventricular, is difficult to distinguish on auscultation. If the premature beat retrogradely penetrates the sinus node and discharges it, the next normal sinus beat is delayed, but the pause is not "compensatory" and the basic rhythm is altered since the sinus node has been prematurely depolarized. Unless the premature beats occur near the junction of the atria and the atrioventricular node (junctional premature beats), cannon waves do not occur. They may occur if the atria contract when the tricuspid valve is closed, since both atria and ventricles contract within a short interval. In the usual atrial premature beat, atrial and ventricular contractions are normally sequential and

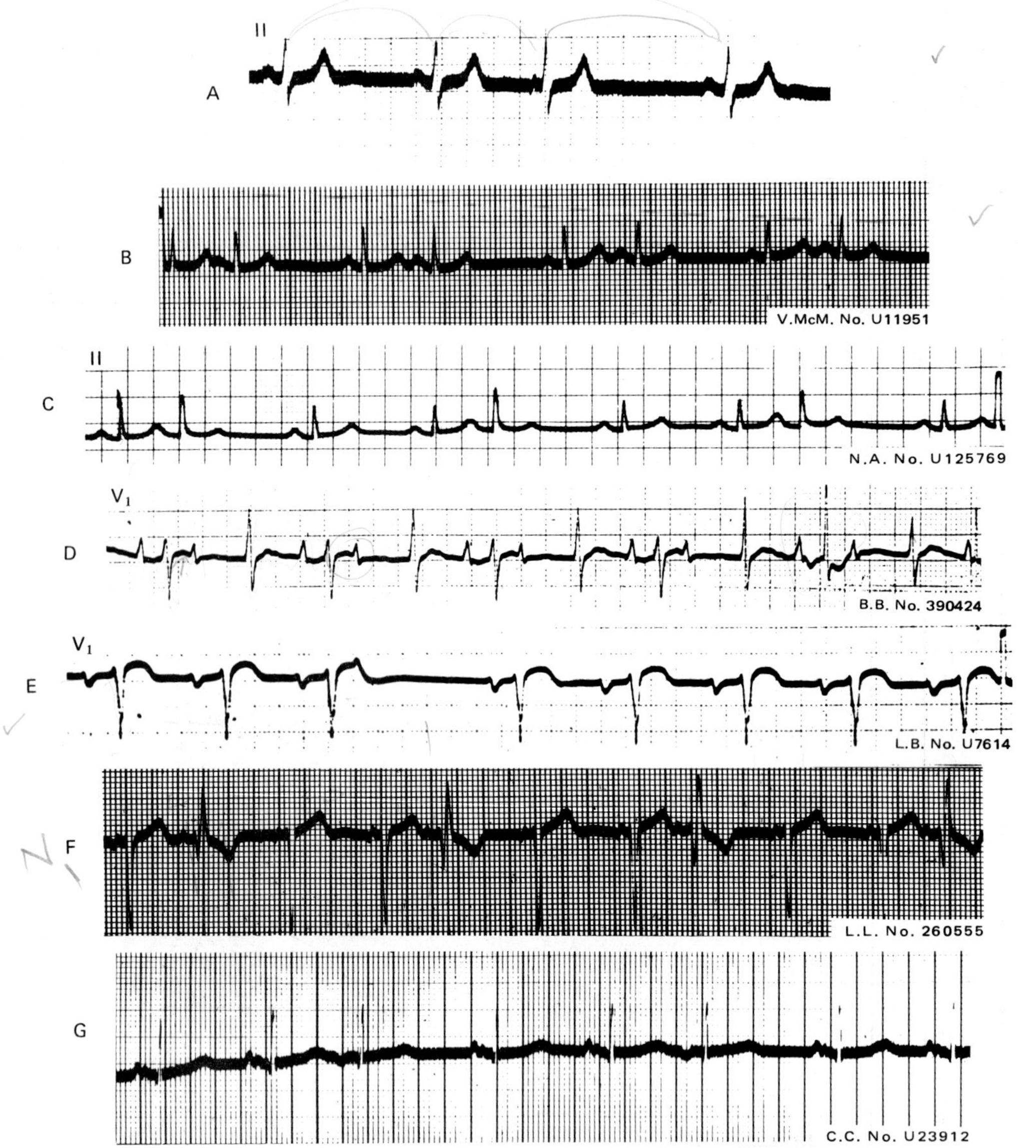

Figure 15–1. Atrial premature beats. *A:* Atrial premature beats, lead II. *B:* Atrial bigeminal rhythm, lead II, in a woman age 62. *C:* Atrial premature beats with slight aberrant conduction and subtle changes when P is superimposed on T waves, lead II; man age 61. *D:* Normal sinus rhythm with atrial bigeminy which represents either nonconducted premature beats followed by junctional escape beats with aberrant intraventricular conduction or atrial premature beats with prolonged P–R interval, lead V_1. *E:* Nonconducted atrial premature beat after third QRS complex, lead V_1. *F:* Atrial premature beats with aberrant conduction of right bundle branch block pattern, lead V_1; man age 51. *G:* Atrial or junctional premature beats, lead II; man age 53.

cannon waves do not occur, as may happen if there is atrioventricular dissociation or in the case of some ventricular premature beats.

A. ECG Recognition of Premature Beats: Supraventricular premature beats are best recognized on the ECG, especially after careful inspection of a long strip (Fig 15–1). The usual pattern is that of P waves having a contour different from that of regular sinus P waves. These P waves are premature and may be associated with an aberrant QRS complex that usually has a right bundle branch block configuration. They may be nonconducted if they occur early and may be missed unless careful inspection of the T wave preceding a pause shows that it is slurred or notched or otherwise different from other T waves in the lead, thus indicating that a premature P wave is buried in the T wave complex.

The ectopic (premature) P wave has been called P′ and should be carefully sought if the R–R interval or the dominant rhythm is disturbed or if the P–R interval in the succeeding beat is prolonged because of concealed conduction in the atrioventricular node.

Search for P′ complexes may often explain unsuspected bradycardia. When atrial premature beats occur in bigeminy, ie, in every other beat, the patient may be thought to have 2:1 block or sinus bradycardia when in fact the rhythm is that of atrial premature beats, which are clinically less significant.

B. Concealed Atrial Premature Beats: Occasionally, the premature beat or P′ beat may be isoelectric to the lead examined and thus not obvious and only suspected or recognized by its effects on the subsequent P–R interval or by the pause that follows the so-called "concealed" premature beat. Atrial premature beats may be "concealed" when they partially penetrate the atrioventricular node and do not spread onto the ventricles, but they nonetheless influence the refractory period of the atrioventricular node and so alter the succeeding P–R interval. Supraventricular beats may not be recognized despite careful inspection but may be found and proved by His bundle recording which reveals a premature atrial or His bundle spike. If the presence of a premature beat that is not obvious on the ordinary ECG is strongly suspected, the ECG can be recorded at double standardization, or different leads that tend to exaggerate the size of the P′ wave may be employed.

Other means of amplifying the size of the supra-

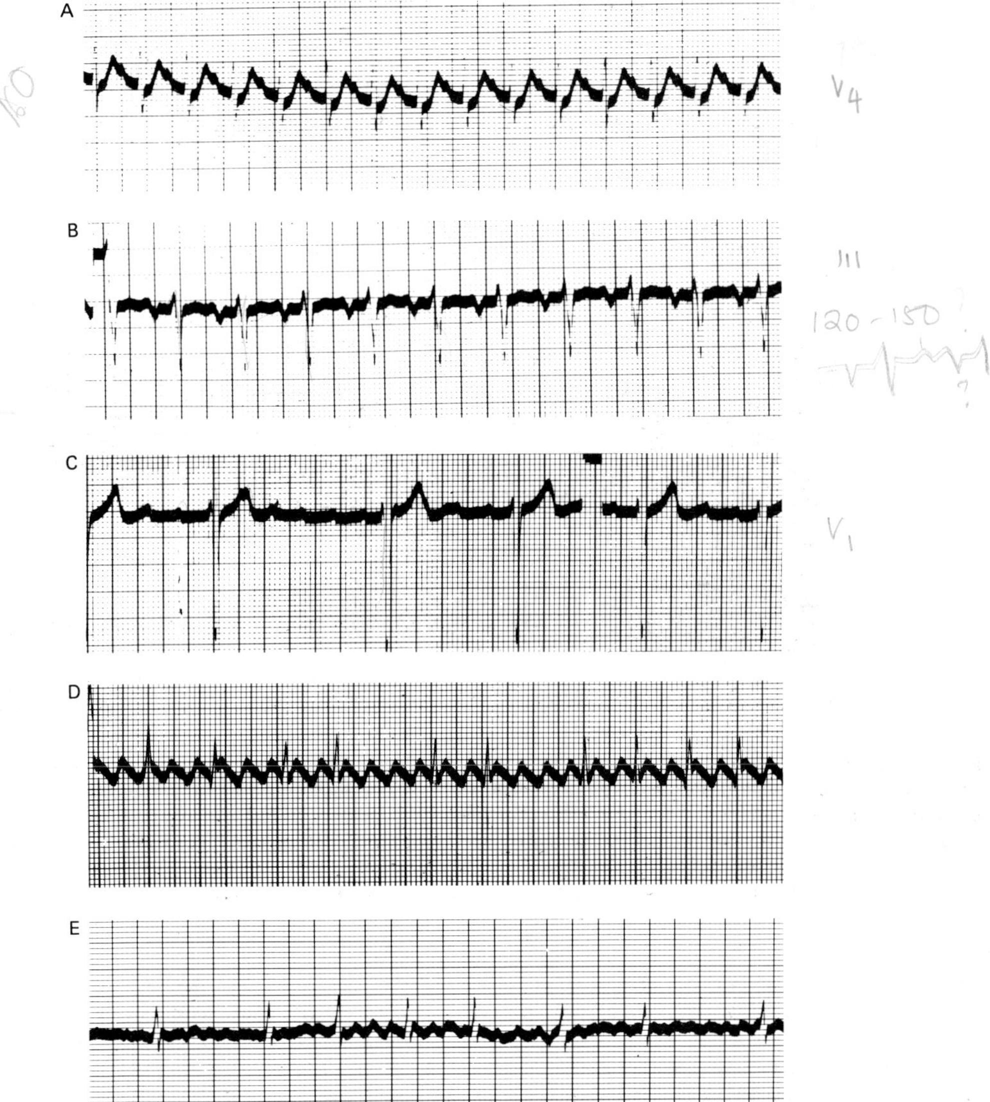

Figure 15–2. Supraventricular tachycardia. *A:* Atrial tachycardia, lead V_4. *B:* Junctional or atrial tachycardia, lead III. *C:* Atrial flutter, lead V_1. Atrial rate approximately 300/min. *D:* Atrial flutter, lead III. Atrial rate approximately 300/min. *E:* Atrial fibrillation, lead aVF. (See Figs 15–3, 15–4, and 15–5 for ladder diagrams.) There is variable atrioventricular conduction in *C* and *D*, so the ventricular rate is irregular.

ventricular depolarizations include the bipolar Lewis lead (see also p 487) (right arm electrode in the second intercostal space to the right of the sternum 2 interspaces above lead V_1 and left arm electrode in the fourth intercostal space to the right of the sternum, the normal position for lead V_1, and both recorded on lead I), esophageal leads (electrode directly posterior to the left atrium), and right atrial electrode catheters which display large P′ as well as P waves. The P′ or ectopic atrial depolarization usually has a polarity different from the normal sinus P wave and may be inverted in leads II, III, and aVF and upright in aVR. These are low atrial or junctional.

Features of Special Importance

The pause that follows the premature beat may allow the physician to diagnose the underlying cardiac condition, and it is useful to listen carefully to the postpause beat. In aortic stenosis, for example, the murmur may be louder as a result of the more forceful ventricular contraction following the pause. However, this is not the case in mitral regurgitation. The long pause with increased left ventricular volume may produce or increase left ventricular outflow obstruction in hypertrophic cardiomyopathy (see Chapter 17), and the first sound may be diminished in the postpause beat. When long pauses are felt at the wrist or at the carotid arteries, the possibility of a "dropped" beat due to atrioventricular block must be considered. Even early premature beats can be heard with the stethoscope (unless they are nonconducted atrial premature beats), whereas during "dropped" beats there is no ventricular sound.

Initiation of Paroxysmal Tachycardia

If the atrial premature beats occur at a critical time after the previous QRS complex (so-called critical coupling interval) and if conduction delay through a portion of the conduction system, usually the atrioventricular node, is present, a reentry circuit may be established and the premature atrial beat may initiate supraventricular tachycardia. Programmed electric stimulation, inducing atrial premature beats with a progressively shorter coupling interval combined with delay in conduction through the atrioventricular node, has been shown to be the causal mechanism in most cases of supraventricular tachycardia, although such tachycardias may be due to increased automaticity such as occurs in coronary disease or following digitalis. (Examples of atrial arrhythmias are shown in Fig 15–2.)

SUPRAVENTRICULAR TACHYCARDIA

When there is a rapid, regular rhythm varying from 150–250/min in which the QRS complex is normal in appearance and similar to that seen in sinus rhythm, the term supraventricular tachycardia is used. If ectopic P waves or P′ waves are seen distorting the T waves or occurring prior to the QRS complexes with a 1:1 conduction and a normal P–R interval, then atrial tachycardia is present. If the P′ wave immediately (Figs 15–3, 15–4, and 15–5) precedes or is coincident with the QRS complex, then a junctional or His bundle rhythm can be diagnosed and proved by His bundle recordings. Often, however, no P′ can be seen, and the site of origin of the ectopic focus cannot be identified other than to say that it is above the ventricles. If the QRS complex is distorted and wide, the rapid regular rhythm may be confused with ventricular tachycardia, and a number of clinical features have been described to help in the differentiation (see below under diagnosis). A bizarre, aberrant QRS complex in a rapid ventricular rhythm does not establish the site of origin as ventricular; a narrow QRS complex does not automatically mean that the site of origin is in the atria because it may be in the bundle of His. When the origin of the P′ is inferior, indicating a low origin spreading superiorly, it favors atrial flutter; the reverse is true of atrial tachycardia.

Significance of Supraventricular Tachycardia

Supraventricular tachycardia is due to the same causes as premature beats. It often occurs in individuals with no evident heart disease, in which case it is thought to result from central nervous system-mediated sympathetic influences. It may result from disease of the atria or bundle of His, as in atrial septal defect, mitral stenosis, or coronary disease involving the artery to the sinoatrial or atrioventricular node. The latter is usually confined to acute myocardial infarction, and paroxysmal supraventricular tachycardia is infrequent in patients with chronic coronary heart disease. Tobacco, coffee, stimulant drugs, and, most importantly, alcohol have been invoked as causal factors. Most often, however, the individual has no history of abnormal consumption of alcohol, tobacco, or coffee—just as the appearance of a single premature beat may have no readily discernible cause.

Diagnosis (Fig 15–6)

Supraventricular tachycardia is recognized by a sudden increase in heart rate to 150–250/min, although rates of 300/min have been observed in infants, probably because atrioventricular conduction is accelerated in infants and the refractory period of the atrioventricular node is shorter. This is speculative because very limited electrophysiologic studies have been done in infants. Young adults may have ventricular rates of 300/min for short periods at the onset that may result in syncope. Many normal individuals have rapid heart rates with paroxysmal atrial tachycardia but do not develop "ischemic" ST segments during the attack or after it, or, if they do, the ST changes may last only minutes to hours. Since patients rarely die during an attack, pathologic confirmation is not available. Some patients who develop "ischemic" ST segments during paroxysmal atrial tachycardia but who do not have angina on effort when they are in sinus rhythm may over a period of a few years develop angina pectoris, suggesting that subclinical coronary disease was unmasked by the rapid rate of the paroxysmal atrial tachycardia. The amount of ischemia or cellular damage that results from rapid rates with paroxysmal atrial tachycardia must be small because few of these patients develop serum enzyme abnormalities or clinical manifestations suggesting subendocardial infarction. Nevertheless, it is common to find ischemic ST segment changes during paroxysmal atrial tachycardia in patients who have no symptoms and who do not have angina pectoris between attacks.

Palpitations may be the only symptom, but if there is underlying heart disease the patient may complain of weakness, dizziness, anginal pain, or dyspnea. Central nervous system disturbances, when they occur, are usually diffuse in nature and not focal, as they are apt to be in cerebral ischemic attacks due to internal carotid artery disease. Angina pectoris may appear with the onset of the tachycardia even if the patient has had no history of angina. The patient may be unaware of the rapid heart rate and complain only of angina, and it is important to consider the onset of arrhythmia as a cause of the angina pectoris that appears at rest or during the night and which is unrelated to exercise. The presence of underlying coronary dis-

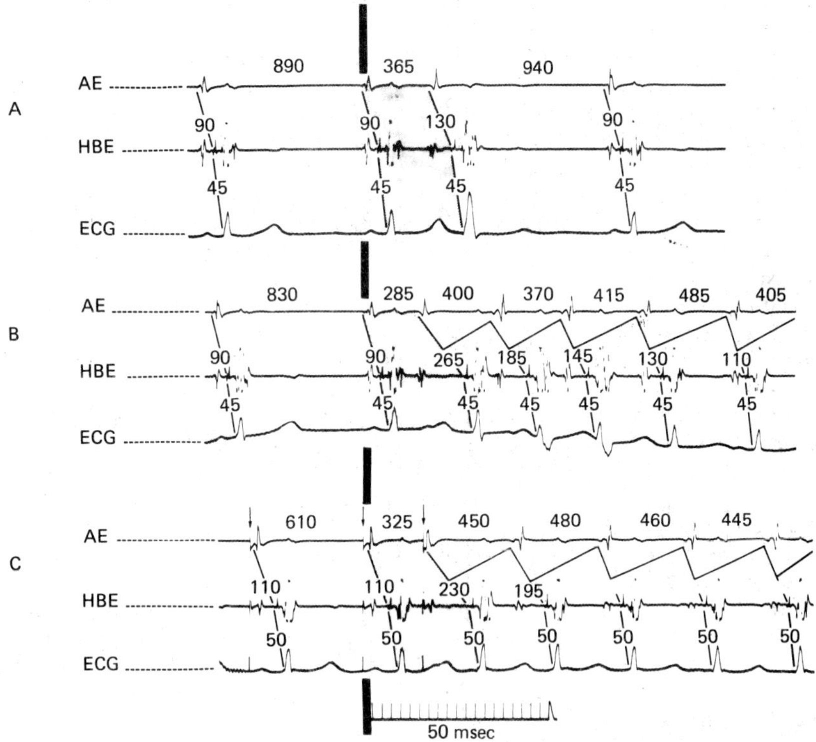

Figure 15–3. His bundle activity during the spontaneous and stimulated onset of supraventricular tachycardia. Atrial electrogram (AE), His bundle electrogram (HBE), and surface electrocardiogram (ECG) are recorded. Intervals in milliseconds between successive atrial depolarizations are given above each atrial electrogram. Atrioventricular conduction times in milliseconds are given on each diagonal line. The heavy vertical bar aligns the last atrial depolarization prior to an atrial premature depolarization; one atrial cycle appears to the left of the bar. Time markers at 50-msec intervals are shown at the bottom. *A:* During sinus rhythm, cycle length is 890 msec, A–H interval is 90 msec, H–V interval is 45 msec. A spontaneous atrial premature depolarization occurs 365 msec after the sinoatrial beat and shows a prolonged A–H interval (130 msec), indicating that the atrial premature depolarization occurred during the atrioventricular nodal relative refractory period. The H–V interval is unchanged. Atrial reentry does not occur, and sinus rhythm resumes after a 940-msec interval. *B:* A spontaneous atrial premature depolarization at a 285-msec interval exhibits prolonged atrioventricular conduction (A–H interval, 265 msec); the H–V interval remains constant. Atrial reentry occurs 400 msec after the atrial premature depolarization, and supraventricular tachycardia is initiated. During subsequent beats of supraventricular tachycardia, the A–H interval progressively shortens to 110 msec but remains longer than during sinus rhythm. The first 3 beats of supraventricular tachycardia have a right bundle branch block configuration-rate-related aberration. *C:* During atrial pacing at a cycle length of 610 msec, the A–H interval is 110 msec and the H–V interval 50 msec. Stimuli are indicated by arrows. An atrial premature depolarization at a 325-msec interval shows a markedly prolonged A–H interval (230 msec), whereas the H–V interval again remains constant. The prolonged atrioventricular nodal conduction time allows atrial reentry to occur 450 msec after the atrial premature depolarization, and a sustained episode of supraventricular tachycardia is initiated. (Reproduced, with permission of the American Heart Association, Inc., from Goldreyer BN, Bigger JT Jr: Site of reentry in paroxysmal supraventricular tachycardia in man. Circulation 43:15, 1971.)

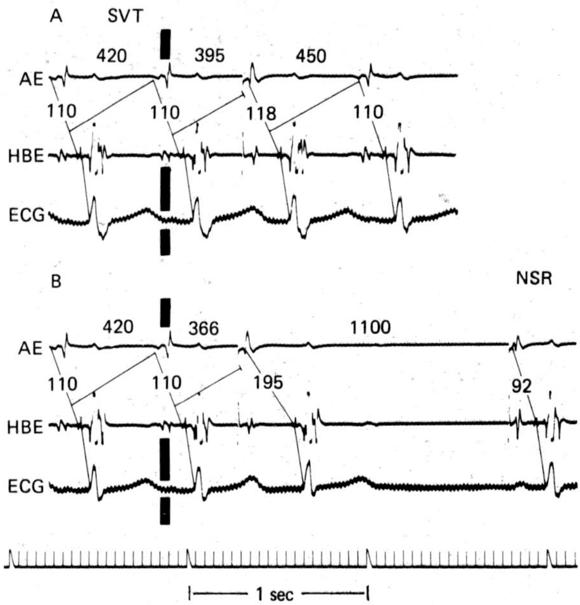

Figure 15–4. His bundle activity during the termination of supraventricular tachycardia by single stimulated atrial premature depolarization. The heavy vertical bar aligns the last atrial depolarization of supraventricular tachycardia before the introduction of a stimulated atrial premature depolarization. *A:* During supraventricular tachycardia at a cycle length of 420 msec, the A–H interval is 110 msec. A stimulated atrial premature depolarization with a coupling interval of 395 msec results in prolongation of the A–H interval (118 msec), but reentry is sustained and supraventricular tachycardia continues. *B:* During the same episode of supraventricular tachycardia at cycle length 420 msec and A–H interval 110 msec, a stimulated atrial premature depolarization is introduced 366 msec after the atrial depolarization indicated by the vertical bar. The A–H interval of the atrial premature depolarization is markedly prolonged (195 msec), and the episode of supraventricular tachycardia is terminated. After 1100 msec, the stimulator initiates another atrial beat with normal A–H interval (92 msec); when the stimulator is turned off, sinus rhythm (NSR) is resumed. (Reproduced, with permission of the American Heart Association, Inc., from Goldreyer BN, Bigger JT Jr: Site of reentry in paroxysmal supraventricular tachycardia in man. Circulation 43:15, 1971.)

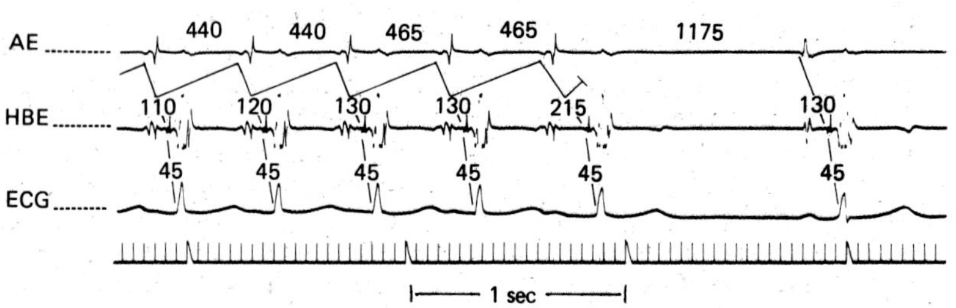

Figure 15–5. Termination of sustained supraventricular tachycardia by carotid sinus massage. AE, HBE, and ECG are recorded along with time markers at 1-sec and 50-msec intervals. Intervals in msec between successive atrial depolarizations are shown above AE. Here, during stable supraventricular tachycardia with a cycle length of 440 msec, carotid sinus massage is begun. During massage, conduction time across the atrioventricular node (A–H interval) progressively lengthens (110, 120, 130, 130, 215 msec). The interval between atrial depolarizations lengthens only slightly (440 to 465 msec). During the terminal cycle of supraventricular tachycardia, the A–H interval is markedly prolonged (215 msec), and retrograde conduction fails. Sinus rhythm resumes 1175 msec later. The A–H interval of the first sinus cycle is 130 msec, showing the effect of carotid sinus massage. Over the next few sinus cycles the A–H interval returns to the control value of 90 msec. (Reproduced, with permission of the American Heart Association, Inc., from Goldreyer BN, Bigger JT Jr: Site of reentry in paroxysmal supraventricular tachycardia in man. Circulation 43:15, 1971.)

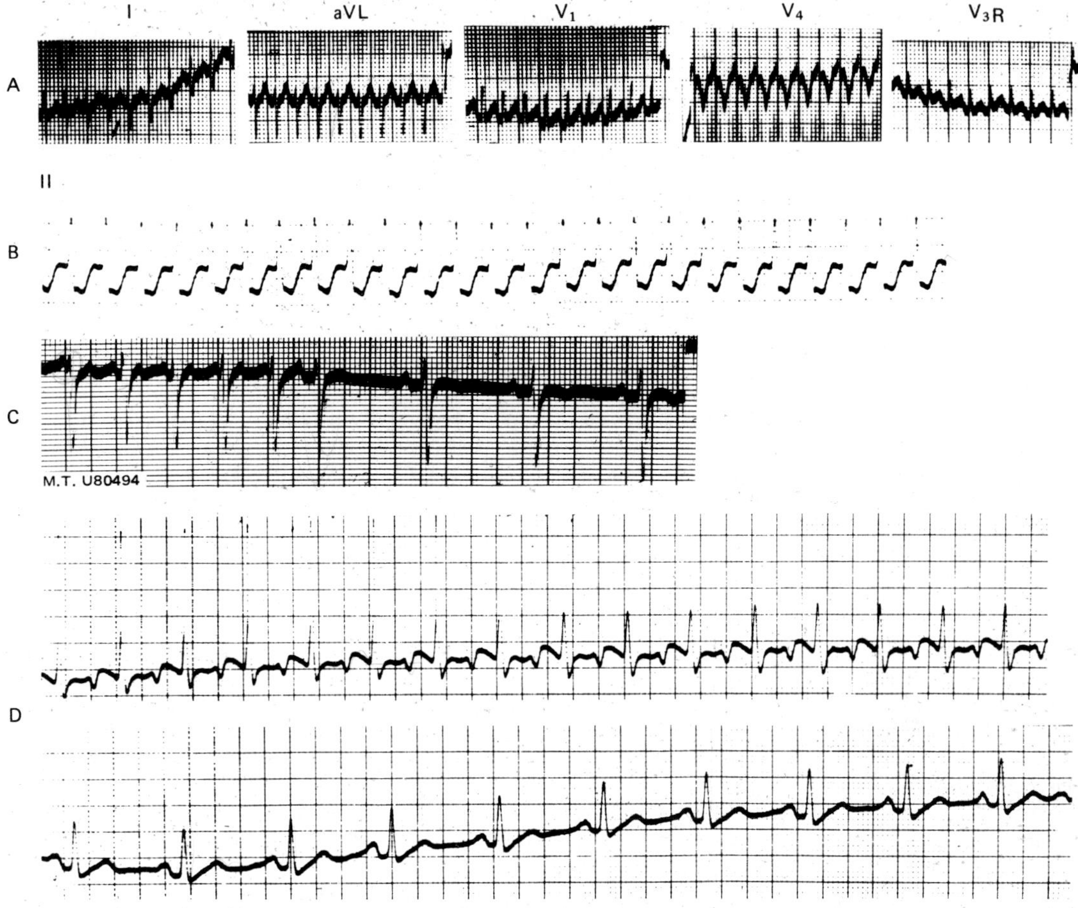

Figure 15–6. Supraventricular tachycardia. *A:* Supraventricular tachycardia in 3-week-old girl with a heart rate of 300/min. *B:* Probable myocardial ischemia during supraventricular tachycardia at a rate of 220/min. *C:* Supraventricular tachycardia with spontaneous subsidence in a 57-year-old woman. *D:* Paroxysmal atrial tachycardia with 1:1 conduction. Change in height of R waves indicates altered ventricular conduction converted by cardioversion in a 36-year-old woman to 2:1 conduction.

ease is suggested not only by the appearance of angina during the tachycardia but also by the appearance of typical ischemic ST segments on the ECG during the attack of rapid heart action and their persistence for 1–2 weeks after the tachycardia has stopped. Infants, especially if the heart rate exceeds 300/min, may develop heart failure that often is the presenting manifestation of supraventricular tachycardia.

Diagnostic Features of Paroxysmal Atrial Tachycardia

A. Degree of Atrioventricular Conduction: Conduction is almost always 1:1, and there is no clinical evidence of atrial and ventricular asynchrony, so that there is nothing abnormal to be heard at the bedside other than the rapid heart rate. The first sound does not vary in intensity, and no cannon waves can be seen in the jugular venous pulse. The major exception occurs when the atrial tachycardia is due to digitalis toxicity, in which instance, because digitalis also decreases conduction through the atrioventricular node, 2:1 block is frequent and may be overlooked when the atrial rate is about 150/min and the ventricular rate about 75/min. As the ventricular rate is normal, the patient has no palpitations or other symptoms, and, were it not for the ECG evidence of rapid atrial rates with 2:1 ventricular response, digitalis toxicity could be overlooked. Fig 15–7 shows ECGs in coronary heart disease before and after treatment. Although digitalis is the usual cause of atrial tachycardia with 2:1 conduction, there are well-documented instances in which the patient has not received digitalis; the physician is thus not warranted in diagnosing digitalis toxicity by the arrhythmia alone.

Digitalis toxicity is less commonly manifested by atrial tachycardia with 1:1 conduction or complete atrioventricular block with or without atrial tachycardia or atrial fibrillation. Not only may digitalis cause atrial tachycardia with 2:1 conduction; it may also produce partial progressive atrioventricular block with Wenckebach phenomenon, as shown in Fig 15–7C.

B. Jugular Venous Pulse: It is helpful to study the

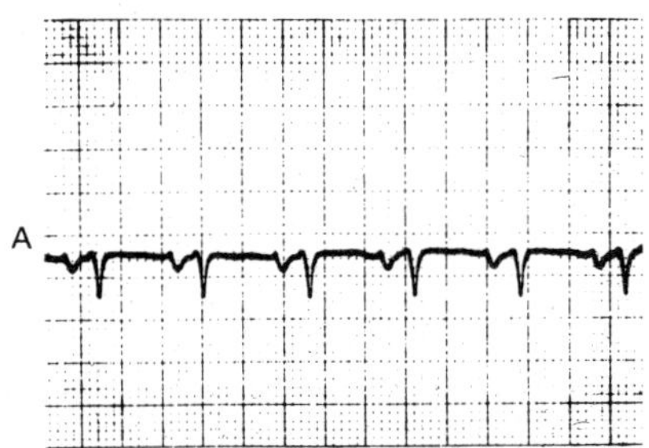

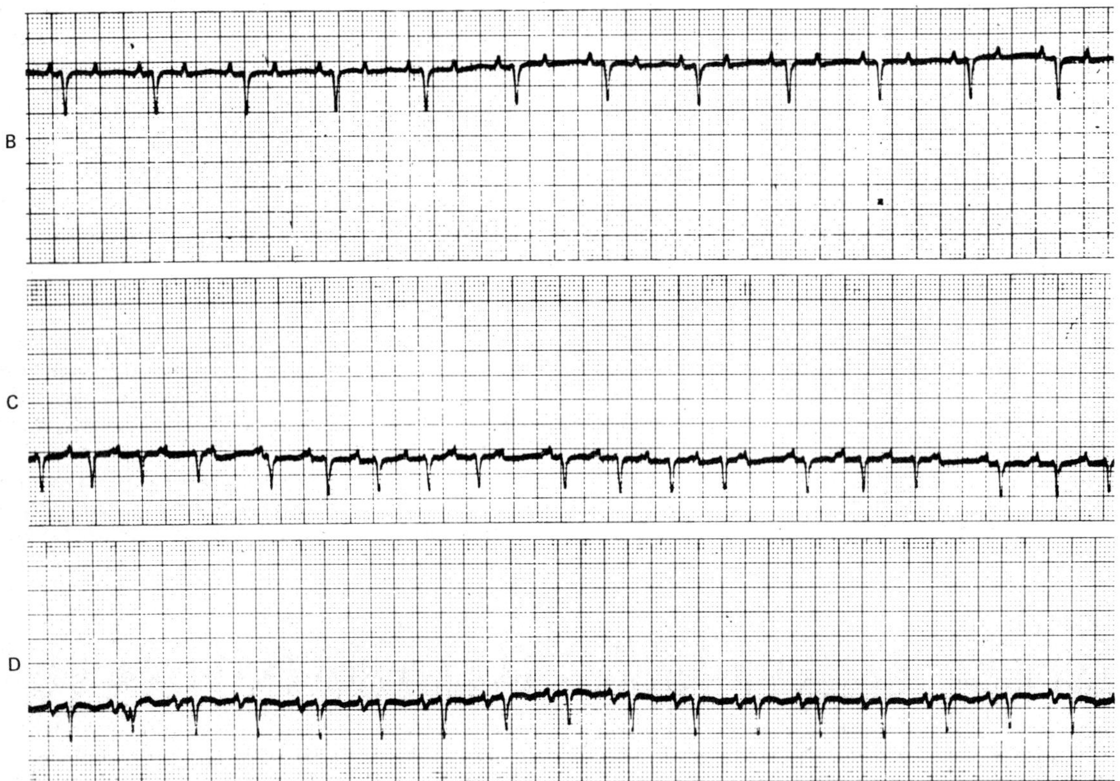

Figure 15–7. Atrial tachycardia before, during, and after treatment in a man age 52 weighing 60 kg, with coronary heart disease. *A*: 5:00 pm 7/22/55. Coronary heart disease before treatment with digoxin and a mercurial diuretic (Mercuhydrin, 2 ml IM). Note sinus rhythm. *B:* Atrial tachycardia with an atrial rate of 150/min and a ventricular rate of 75/min with 2:1 block after digoxin, 2.5 mg, and Mercuhydrin, 1 ml IM in 24 hours, with weight loss of 3.6 kg not recognized. On second day, a further dose of 1 mg digoxin and 1 ml Mercuhydrin was given, with weight loss of 5.9 kg in 48 hours. *C:* 9:00 pm 7/25/55, four hours after administration of 11 mEq potassium orally. Atrial tachycardia (rate 125/min) with Wenckebach phenomenon is now present. *D:* 11:45 pm 7/25/55, one hour and 45 minutes after a second dose of 11 mEq potassium. Sinus tachycardia is now present.

jugular venous pulse carefully in these instances; rapid *a* waves at twice the rate of the ventricular response may lead to the correct diagnosis. The same is true in atrial flutter (see below), when the conduction from the atria to the ventricles is 4:1 and the ventricular rate at 75/min does not make one suspect that the atria are beating at a more rapid rate. At times the rapid atrial rate can be discerned during cardiac fluoroscopy and confirmed by inspection of the jugular pulse. The ECG can usually define the atrial rate unless the atrial waves are isoelectric.

C. Differentiation From Atrial Flutter: Atrial flutter is an atrial arrhythmia, thought to be due to a circus movement, arising low in the atria, with atrial rates varying from 150–350/min; at the lower range, it may be difficult to distinguish from atrial tachycardia, just as atrial tachycardia with a rapid atrial rate may be difficult to distinguish from atrial flutter. One must then rely upon probabilities. In the usual case of supraventricular tachycardia the atrial rate is less than 200/min, and in most cases of atrial flutter the atrial rates are approximately 300/min. Therefore, the rate of the tachycardia, as well as the age of the patient, immediately weights the diagnosis in one direction or another. Furthermore, atrial or supraventricular tachycardia usually occurs in younger individuals, often those with no heart disease or with heart disease that obviously involves the atria; it can then be inferred that the rapid supraventricular rhythm is more likely to be supraventricular tachycardia than atrial flutter. In contrast, atrial flutter, like atrial fibrillation, is more apt to occur in older individuals with obvious heart disease such as coronary heart disease or mitral stenosis. The age and underlying heart condition may make atrial flutter a more likely diagnosis than supraventricular tachycardia. A conduction delay from atria to ventricles of 4:1–or variable conduction such as alternating 2:1, 3:1, 4:1–occurs in atrial flutter but is uncommon in supraventricular tachycardia.

NONPAROXYSMAL JUNCTIONAL TACHYCARDIA

When sinoatrial nodal function is depressed, as is the case with digitalis therapy, in acute myocardial infarction, or often after open heart surgery, supraventricular tachycardia with a rate usually less than 130/min may occur, either because the secondary junctional pacemakers "escape" as a result of depressed sinus node function or because the automaticity of the junctional tissues is enhanced by metabolic abnormalities secondary to hypoxia, ischemia, and associated digitalis therapy.

This condition is called nonparoxysmal junctional tachycardia and is usually associated with a narrow QRS complex. The junctional pacemaker may activate the atria retrogradely or may beat independently of the atria and result in atrioventricular dissociation. Knoebel (1974) believes that most of these tachycardias are due to increase in automaticity of the junctional tissues and are not passive escape rhythms, because the ventricular rate is often faster than in passive rhythms (usually less than 60/min) and because atrioventricular dissociation occurs, indicating that both sinus and junctional pacemakers are intact.

When the mechanism is not "escape" but enhanced automaticity, it is postulated that the released metabolites or potassium from the ischemic and hypoxic myocardial cells may increase the slope of phase 4 diastolic depolarization of the action potential of the involved cells, leading to increased automaticity of the junctional tissues.

Atrioventricular Dissociation

In some instances, both the sinus node and the junctional area "fire" independently, and atrioventricular dissociation occurs. This can be recognized on the ECG by noting intermittent capture of the ventricles by a sinus impulse which fortuitously reaches the ventricle when it has recovered excitability following depolarization from the junctional beat. Pick (1957) described nonparoxysmal junctional tachycardia and noted that the ventricular rate was slower than with ordinary supraventricular tachycardia. In contrast to the sudden onset and sudden offset that characterize supraventricular tachycardia, nonparoxysmal junctional tachycardia has a gradual onset and offset and is often seen transiently in the first few days after acute myocardial infarction. Although the QRS interval is often normal, it may be wide and slurred if there is aberrant conduction to the ventricles.

Differential Diagnosis

Nonjunctional paroxysmal tachycardia with aberrancy must be differentiated from slow accelerated idioventricular rhythm during acute myocardial infarction, but this is often not possible with conventional ECGs. This latter condition usually has more abnormal ventricular complexes, but His bundle recordings may be necessary if a clear diagnosis is felt to be clinically required. The ventricular origin is also more obvious when the clinical situation abruptly worsens or when the signs of ventricular tachycardia (see Clinical Differentiation, below) can be elicited. If fusion beats or gradual onset and offset occur, the rhythm is probably ventricular in origin.

In sinus tachycardia, the rate is rapid, essentially regular at short intervals, and almost always less than 180/min. It may be slightly irregular and vary with simple maneuvers such as posture, mild exercise, respiration, breath-holding, or carotid sinus pressure. The regularity of the heart rate in paroxysmal atrial tachycardia may differentiate this rhythm from sinus tachycardia, in which the heart rate may be rapid and apparently regular but can be altered by position, respiration, or slight exercise. If the heart rate is counted for a full minute, especially after changes in position and other maneuvers mentioned in the preceding sentence, it will be shown to be slightly irregular and variable in sinus tachycardia. In paroxysmal atrial tachycardia, however, the heart rate is not influenced by these procedures unless the attack is terminated abruptly. In ventricular tachycardia, careful inspection of the ECG or careful counting of the heart rate for 1 minute will show that the ventricular rate is often slightly irregular.

It is wise to count the heart rate for a full minute at intervals after these procedures because in sinus tachycardia the rate will change, whereas in paroxysmal atrial or junctional tachycardia it is usually regular and uninfluenced unless the attack is terminated abruptly.

Sinus tachycardia also has a background of one of a number of causative factors, eg, fever, infection, anemia, anxiety, leukemia, thyrotoxicosis, or connective tissue disorders.

A. Differentiation of Ventricular and Supraventricular Rhythms on ECG: The differentiation between ventricular tachycardia and supraventricular tachycardia with aberrant conduction is often difficult (Fig 15–8). It is easy if the QRS complex is narrow and preceded by P waves; the difficulty arises when one cannot see P waves and the QRS complexes are wide. The key to the differentiation is identification of the P waves and their relationship to the ventricular complex. In ventricular tachycardia, atrioventricular disso-

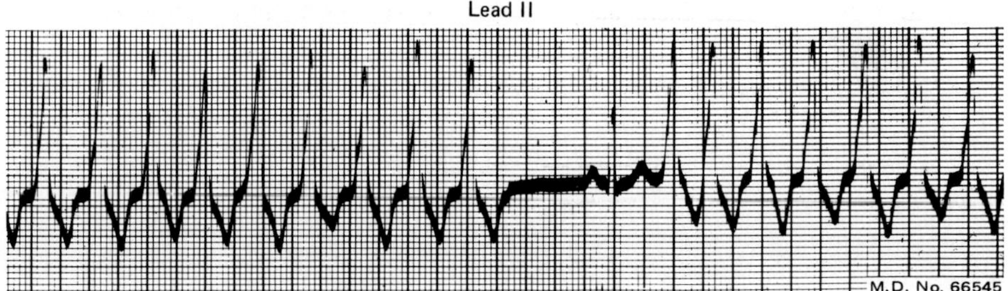

Figure 15–8. Tachycardia (ventricular or junctional) interrupted by single normal beat in a 43-year-old man.

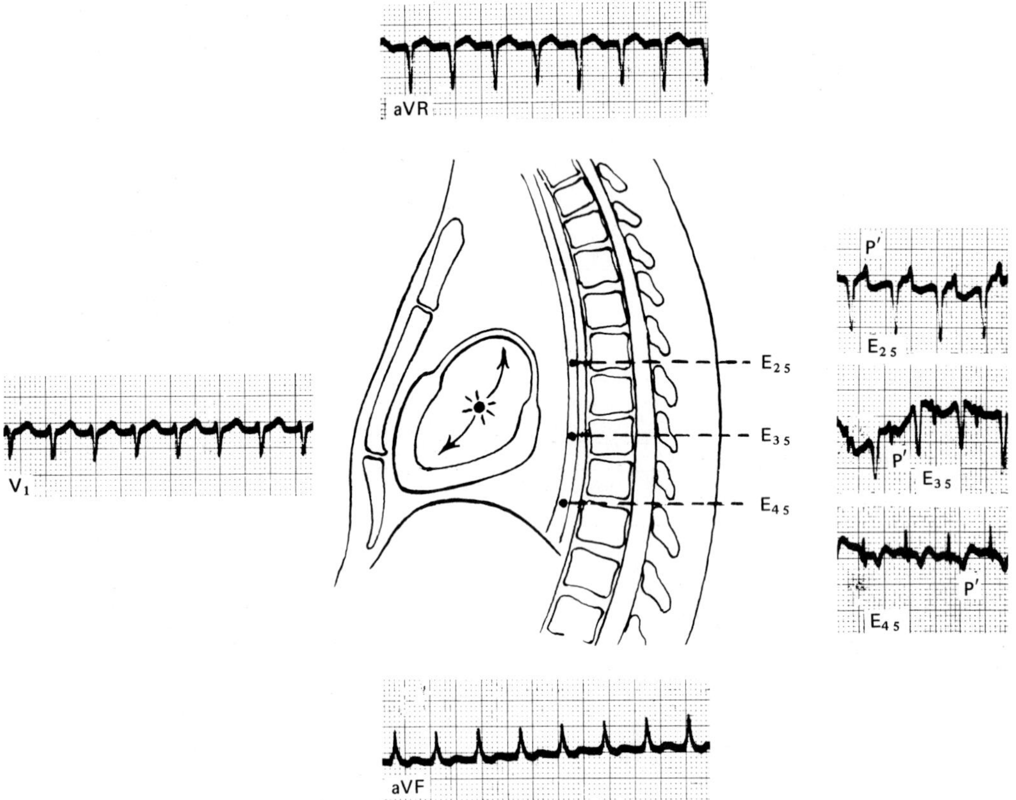

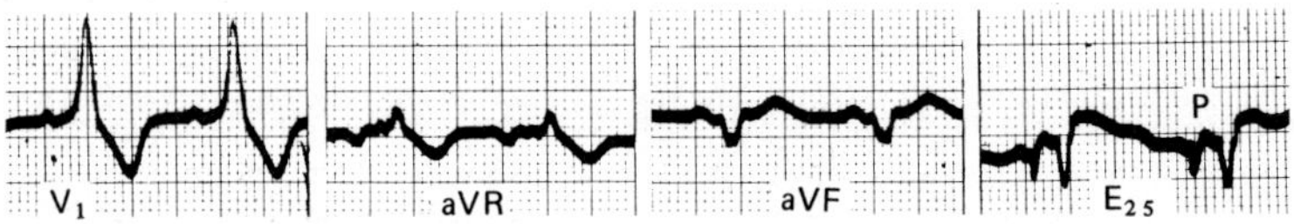

Figure 15–9. Supraventricular paroxysmal atrial or junctional tachycardia, diagnosed with the aid of esophageal leads which amplify the P waves. (Reproduced, with permission, from Goldman MJ: *Principles of Clinical Electrocardiography,* 9th ed. Lange, 1976.)

ciation occurs, although in rare cases there may be retrograde conduction to the atria, with retrograde 1:1 conduction and one P wave for every QRS complex. Usually, however, the ventricles are beating at a faster rate than the atria in ventricular tachycardia, whereas they are both the same in paroxysmal atrial tachycardia. Careful inspection of the T waves and QRS complexes for the possible presence of "buried" P waves is important in determining the atrial rate and in deciding if there are 2 independent pacemakers. Multiple conventional or Lewis leads, esophageal leads, right atrial electrode catheter electrograms, or His bundle recordings may be required to amplify the P waves or to relate them to the QRS complexes (Figs 15–9 and 15–10).

When the QRS complex is wide and irregular, the differentiation between ventricular tachycardia and supraventricular tachycardia with aberrant conduction is more difficult. Supraventricular tachycardia is inferred when the pattern in lead V_1 is that of right bundle branch block with an rSr′ or rsR′ pattern because of a prolonged refractory period in the right bundle or when the QRS configuration in the first few beats of tachycardia is similar to the pattern of premature beats that may have been present previously. These criteria are only probable and not absolute indications of supraventricular tachycardia. Although the odds favor supraventricular tachycardia on the basis of what has been said, the rSR′ pattern in lead V_1 could still represent junctional tachycardia with

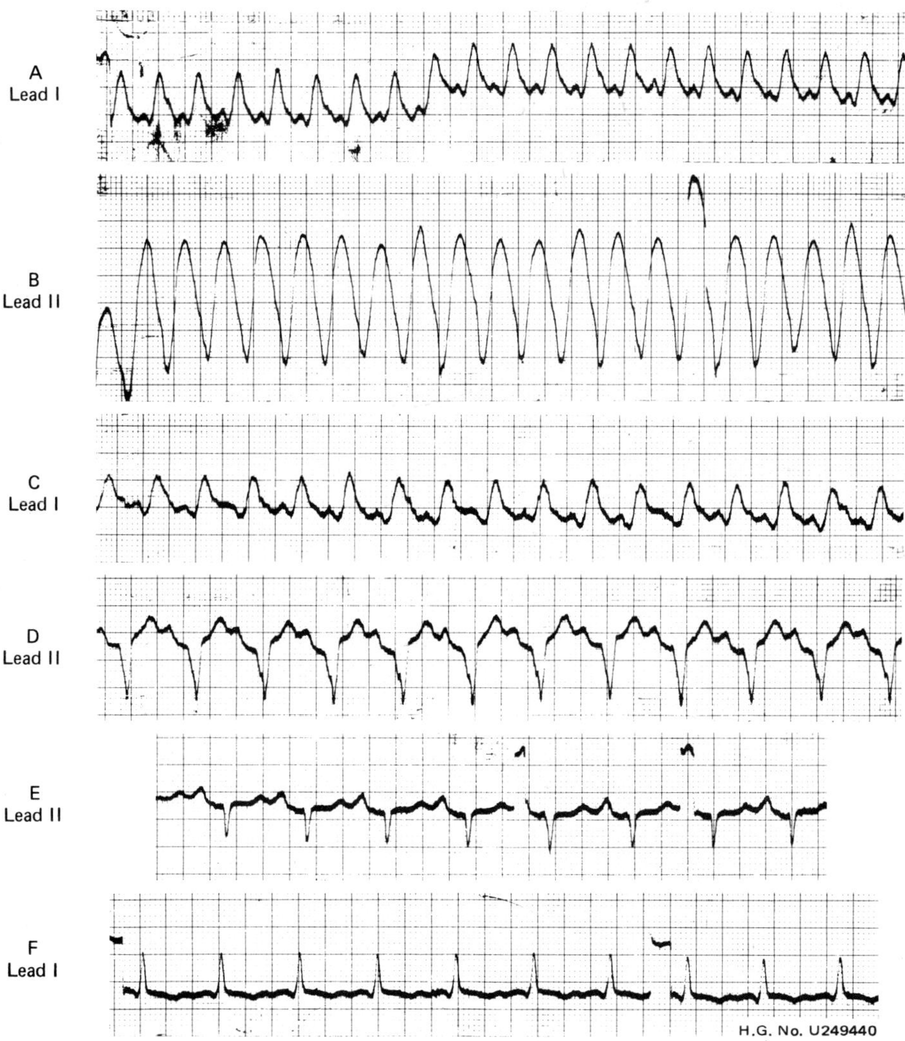

Figure 15–10. Paroxysmal supraventricular tachycardia 7 days after aortoiliac thromboendarterectomy. Sudden tachycardia after bowel movement. *A* and *B:* Before treatment. The pattern resembles ventricular tachycardia because of the wide QRS complexes, but a P wave is seen before each QRS complex in *A,* indicating that the rhythm is atrial tachycardia with aberrant conduction. *C:* Ventricular slowing following administration of 400 mg of procainamide intravenously (2 hours after 1 g quinidine gluconate intramuscularly in 4 hours with a quinidine blood level of 3.1 mg/ml). *D:* Sinus rhythm with intraventricular block at time of conversion. *E* and *F:* 10 minutes later, showing normal intraventricular conduction.

aberrancy and not paroxysmal atrial tachycardia. Ventricular tachycardia is the more likely diagnosis if the QRS pattern is of the left bundle branch type or has a QR pattern in lead V_1. If the patient has had ventricular premature beats on a previous ECG which are similar in configuration to the QRS complexes of the current tachycardia, ventricular tachycardia is the more probable diagnosis.

B. Clinical Differentiation: Clinical bedside evaluation may be valuable to provide evidence of atrial and ventricular asynchrony, eg, varying intensity of the first heart sound and cannon waves in the jugular venous pulse. The signs of atrioventricular asynchrony may occur in His bundle or junctional tachycardia with atrioventricular dissociation, but this is uncommon. Cannon waves are large abrupt *a* waves in the jugular venous pulse ("venous Corrigan waves") occurring as the atria contract when the tricuspid valve is closed (see Chapter 3). They are often seen best when the patient is sitting and can be important clinical evidence, suggesting ventricular tachycardia when the ECG is doubtful.

C. Value of Underlying Condition in Differentiation: The age of the patient and the setting in which the tachycardia occurs are helpful in diagnosis. Ventricular tachycardia is more likely if the patient has acute myocardial infarction, coronary heart disease, or other disease of the left ventricle, such as hypertrophic cardiomyopathy, aortic stenosis, or hypertensive disease. As noted previously, if the patient is young and free of heart disease and the precipitating factor was an acute emotional event, supraventricular tachycardia is the more likely diagnosis. It must be emphasized again, however, that none of these criteria are absolute and all indicate only the probable site of origin of the tachycardia. About 5–10% of patients with ventricular tachycardia have no known or obvious heart disease, whereas supraventricular tachycardia may occur in patients with known heart disease even if the patient is young, so that one cannot rely exclusively on the age and underlying cardiac disease criteria. If it is essential to make the differentiation in order to determine therapy, His bundle recordings are helpful by demonstrating the presence of a His bundle spike preceding the QRS complex, in which case the tachycardia is supraventricular. His bundle recordings with intracardiac stimulation by programmed, critically timed supraventricular premature beats may establish the supraventricular origin of a tachycardia of unknown cause, but such procedures are indicated only if therapy is ineffective and the prognosis doubtful. In troublesome cases, treatment should be directed toward the more serious condition, ventricular tachycardia; lidocaine with or without DC electric shock is helpful in both supraventricular and ventricular tachycardia.

Treatment

In the treatment of supraventricular tachycardia, drugs should be given orally unless serious cardiovascular deterioration indicates the need for rapid reversion to sinus rhythm. It is most important for the physician to estimate the degree of urgency. This estimate is made in part by observing how the patient is handling the rapid rate and whether the tachycardia is producing dyspnea, angina, faintness, confusion, hypotension, or oliguria. The history of previous attacks is most helpful in determining not only their usual duration but also the degree of disability produced. The duration of the current attack when the patient is first seen is of importance because, if arrhythmia has been present for hours or days and the patient is still asymptomatic, the urgency is not great unless the patient's age and the presence of underlying heart disease such as mitral stenosis or coronary heart disease suggest that hemodynamic abnormalities can be expected if the attack continues. Therapeutic decisions are also influenced by ineffective treatment that the patient may already have received or by a history of therapeutic agents that have or have not succeeded in stopping previous attacks. If the patient is in a coronary care unit, a Swan-Ganz catheter may be inserted to allow bedside hemodynamic observations of pulmonary capillary wedge pressure, pulmonary artery pressure, cardiac output, and stroke work index, as in patients with acute myocardial infarction. If the patient is hypotensive, raising the arterial pressure with pressor agents may stop the attack or allow other therapeutic agents to become effective, and this form of treatment is often the most valuable immediate measure.

In general, if the situation is urgent, the physician should treat the patient urgently; otherwise, the patient should be treated conservatively, especially since paroxysmal supraventricular tachycardia is rarely fatal and large doses of potent drugs may do more harm than the underlying tachycardia.

A. Treat the Underlying Condition: Treatment of underlying metabolic abnormalities such as hypoxia, ischemia, alkalosis, acidosis, or anemia is of first importance. Treatment of ventilatory problems is more important than the use of cardiac drugs in postoperative patients or in patients with chronic lung disease.

B. Drug Treatment: If the ventricular rate is not too fast, ie, not over 150–180/min in a patient who has no or minimal heart disease with good left ventricular function and who is tolerating the tachycardia without symptoms other than palpitation—and especially if the attack was precipitated by an acute emotional event—sedation may be the initial and sole therapeutic agent for the first few hours. Seconal, 0.1–0.2 g orally, or diazepam (Valium), 5–10 mg orally, or flurazepam (Dalmane), 30 mg orally, may relax the patient and induce sleep, and the tachycardia may abruptly stop. If this fails or if the patient has dyspnea, severe palpitations, cerebral symptoms, polyuria, fall in blood pressure, or angina, one should immediately try maneuvers to increase atrioventricular block by stimulating the vagus nerve to increase the refractory period of the atrioventricular node and delay atrioventricular nodal transmission of the impulse. This interrupts the reentry circuit and closes the "gap" between the head and the tail of the reentry pathway.

C. Vagal Stimulation: Noninvasive methods of stimulating the vagus may be used first, eg, carotid sinus massage, Valsalva's maneuver, breath-holding, squatting, or placing the face in ice water for a few seconds. Placing the face in ice water induces a strong vagal stimulus which has been shown to rapidly stop paroxysmal atrial tachycardia, but it has not been used extensively. As is true of all methods of increasing vagal stimulation, patients may have a few ventricular premature beats or a short run of them at the time of conversion, and, rarely, ventricular fibrillation may develop. For this reason, when any of these therapeutic maneuvers are attempted, resuscitative equipment should be immediately available and the physician should be aware of the hazard of ventricular fibrillation. Gentle carotid sinus massage should be performed for 10–20 seconds with the patient's head comfortably supported by a pillow rather than carotid sinus pressure and should be first on one side and then the other but not both together. Eyeball pressure should be avoided because of the risk of retinal detachment. Inducing vomiting is an unpleasant measure but may be effective.

If noninvasive maneuvers fail, drugs can be used that directly increase atrioventricular conduction. Examples are edrophonium (Tensilon), 5–15 mg intravenously; verapamil (Isoptine), 10 mg intravenously or 15 mg by intravenous infusion over an 8-hour period (not yet approved by FDA); digitalis (digoxin), 0.75–1 mg intravenously; neostigmine, 0.5–2 mg subcutaneously or intramuscularly; or other cholinergic agents. Fig 15–11 shows the ECG picture of supraventricular tachycardia promptly abolished by means of intravenous lanatoside C therapy. As with vagal stimulation, intravenous digitalis may result in ventricular premature beats at the time of conversion of supraventricular tachycardia to sinus rhythm. These premature beats are similar to those that occur after carotid sinus massage or placing the face in ice water; therefore, it is doubtful that they are due to digitalis toxicity, but this is still a possibility. Furthermore, the ST segment is normal 5 minutes later, without premature beats, making digitalis toxicity unlikely.

If these drugs fail, one of the noninvasive methods of stimulating the vagus (such as carotid sinus massage) should be used during the time of drug action to produce additive vagal stimulation. If the tachycardia persists, therapeutic agents which reflexly increase vagal stimulation can be used, including such pressor drugs as phenylephrine, 2–4 mg subcutaneously or 0.1-0.2 mg intravenously, which raise blood pressure and stimulate the baroreceptor reflexes. Caution should be used; one should begin with small doses to avoid excess hypertension.

D. Drugs to Decrease Automaticity: (See Table 15–5.) Drugs that decrease excitability and automaticity may occasionally be helpful in an acute paroxysm of tachycardia. Give quinidine sulfate, 0.2–0.4 g orally every 4 hours; procainamide, 100 mg/5 min intravenously to a total of 1 g; or phenytoin or lidocaine, 50–100 mg of either drug intravenously followed by an infusion of 1–2 mg/min. (See Table 15–6 and p 481 for further details of treatment schedules.) Quinidine is most effective in atrial arrhythmias but may produce hypotension and ventricular arrhythmias when used intravenously. Propranolol, 20–40 mg 2–4 times daily orally or in small doses (0.1–2 mg) intravenously, may be used to increase atrioventricular block. Its mechanism of action is to block beta-adrenergic receptors, increase atrioventricular nodal transmission time, and block the reentry circuit. Begin with 0.1 mg every 1–5 minutes, until the desired effect is obtained or early toxic manifestations force one to abandon this therapy (Tables 15–5 and 15–6).

E. Cardioversion: If the above measures fail to stop the tachycardia, cardioversion can be used, especially in atrial flutter, unless the patient has been taking digitalis, in which case cardioversion should be

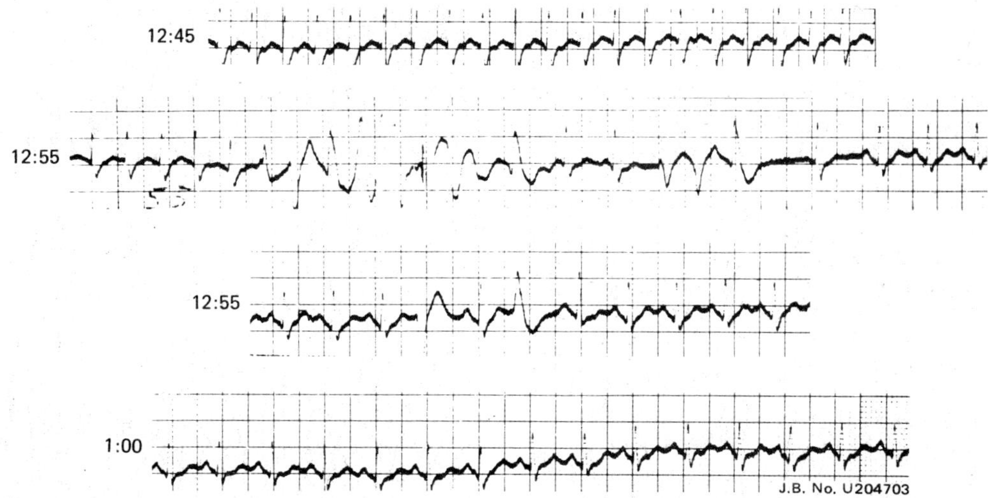

Figure 15–11. Supraventricular tachycardia promptly abolished with intravenous lanatoside C therapy in a 59-year-old man. Note the ventricular premature beats lasting 3 seconds at the time of reversion to sinus rhythm.

avoided or used in small increments of current beginning with 5–10 J, since it can produce serious ventricular arrhythmias.

F. Rapid Atrial Pacing: If there is digitalis toxicity, if supraventricular tachycardia occurs following cardiac surgery, or if the patient fails to convert to sinus rhythm with vigorous pharmacologic therapy, rapid atrial pacing to produce overdrive suppression of the ectopic focus may be the treatment of choice (Waldo, 1976; Haft, 1974). Pacing of the atrium at heart rates above that of the ectopic tachycardia may terminate the arrhythmia during pacing or immediately after pacing is stopped or may induce atrioventricular block, effectively slowing the ventricular rate. Discontinuing the atrial pacing causes transient depression of both the ectopic tachycardia and the sinus node; the latter recovers first, restoring sinus rhythm. Atrial pacing not only restores sinus rhythm by this "overdrive suppression," but it may interrupt the reentry circuit of the paroxysmal atrial tachycardia by depolarizing the atrium so that the reentry pathway is refractory to an oncoming pulse. Occasionally, atrial pacing may induce atrial fibrillation, which may then spontaneously revert to sinus rhythm.

G. Use of Pacemaker: As a last resort—especially if attacks are frequent and produce disabling symptoms—insertion of a permanent atrial pacemaker activated by an external magnet or controlled by an external radio frequency transmitter to convert the demand to a fixed mode pacemaker may allow random ectopic beats to interrupt the reentry wave because the tissue has just been depolarized. This method of treatment is effective only with the reentry mechanism of supraventricular tachycardia.

H. Paroxysmal Atrial Tachycardia With Block: As indicated previously, paroxysmal atrial tachycardia with block is usually (not always) due to digitalis toxicity. It is wise to stop digitalis and diuretics to minimize potassium loss and, if the situation is not urgent, allow tachycardia with block to gradually disappear over 1–3 days. If the serum potassium is less than 3 mEq/l, potassium chloride may be given in a dosage of 40–100 mEq orally; or, if the need is urgent or deemed possibly so, the potassium can be given intravenously in a dosage of 10–20 mEq/hour. Cardioversion should be avoided in the presence of digitalis toxicity because of the risk of inducing ventricular arrhythmias.

I. Treatment of Junctional Rhythms With Atrioventricular Dissociation: This rhythm is usually due to increased automaticity, most commonly from digitalis toxicity, and the treatment is the same as for paroxysmal atrial tachycardia with block. Digitalis and diuretics should be stopped, and, if the serum potassium is low, potassium may be given intravenously at a rate of 10–20 mEq/l/hour. If the abnormal rhythm is due to acute myocardial infarction, treatment should be directed at the acute infarction and should consist of rest, oxygen, and other therapy monitored by frequent determination of hemodynamic indices, noting the response of the patient (see Chapter 8).

ATRIAL FIBRILLATION & ATRIAL FLUTTER

(See Fig 15–12.)

Atrial fibrillation is the most common atrial arrhythmia in older people. It can be paroxysmal or established, as is true of atrial flutter (see p 472). Paroxysmal attacks usually last hours or days rather than seconds or minutes and almost never longer than 2 or 3 weeks. If the rhythm persists after this period, atrial

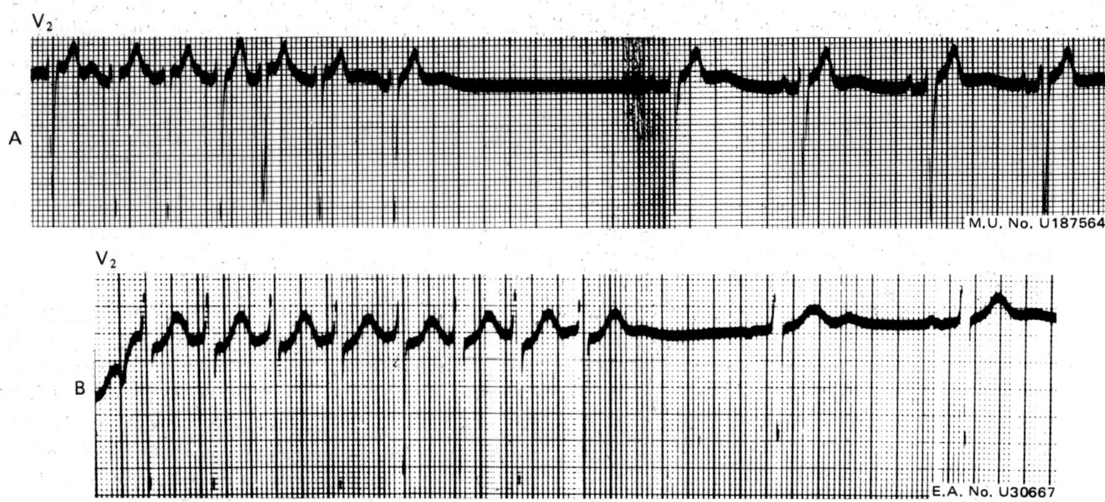

Figure 15–12. Spontaneous changes in atrial fibrillation. *A:* Spontaneous conversion of atrial fibrillation with rapid irregular ventricular response to sinus rhythm in a 71-year-old woman. *B:* Spontaneous subsidence of supraventricular tachycardia followed by junctional escape prior to sinus rhythm in a 62-year-old woman.

fibrillation is said to be established or chronic; this is in contrast to supraventricular tachycardia, which rarely lasts days or weeks and usually lasts minutes or hours. Paroxysmal atrial fibrillation may occur without known heart disease or other obvious reason but most commonly occurs after pulmonary or cardiac surgery or in older individuals with mitral stenosis, atrial septal defect, myocarditis, thyrotoxicosis, or constrictive pericarditis. It is most common in older people with left atrial enlargement due to any cause. It may be precipitated by an acute emotional event even if the patient has underlying cardiac disease such as mitral stenosis. It is not especially common in chronic coronary heart disease and is infrequent in acute myocardial infarction, although continuous monitoring has shown that it may occur. It is common when hypoxia and infection occur in chronic lung disease with cor pulmonale. Following pulmonary surgery—perhaps as a result of hypoxia from inadequate ventilation or pericardial injury—as many as one-third of patients may develop paroxysmal atrial fibrillation. Transient atrial fibrillation is also common following cardiac surgery, especially mitral valve surgery. Even if the rhythm reverts to sinus rhythm preoperatively, it often recurs after surgery. It is common during the course of untreated thyrotoxicosis and usually disappears spontaneously when the thyrotoxicosis is treated. It may be precipitated by cardiac catheterization in patients with mitral stenosis or atrial septal defect. For reasons that are not clear, atrial fibrillation is infrequent prior to infective endocarditis. It is common after the endocarditis is established in aortic or mitral valvular heart disease but uncommon in acute endocarditis in drug users with tricuspid and aortic valve lesions. Although it has been stated that coarse fibrillation (prominent fibrillation waves) is more common in atherosclerotic heart disease, we believe this differentiation is unreliable and too variable to depend on.

Atrial fibrillation is rare in pure aortic valve disease in the absence of failure, and its presence should prompt the physician to think of associated mitral valve disease even if the typical murmurs are not readily heard.

Clinical Course

The onset of atrial fibrillation may produce immediate symptoms of dyspnea in the patient with mitral stenosis and may also produce cardiac failure in the patient with atrial septal defect, when the rapid ventricular rate prevents atrial emptying and left ventricular filling. In mitral stenosis, left atrial pressure may rise quickly, producing pulmonary venous congestion, severe dyspnea, and acute pulmonary edema. The atrial transport function of atrial systole may be required to preserve adequate left ventricular filling in patients with low cardiac reserve; the onset of atrial fibrillation may produce severe left ventricular failure in these patients. Some individuals merely have palpitations; a few may have no symptoms whatever, and the atrial fibrillation in these cases is discovered accidentally.

Atrial Fibrillation in Mitral Stenosis

Even when the ventricular rate at rest is controlled with digitalis, the onset of atrial fibrillation may convert an asymptomatic patient with moderate or severe mitral stenosis to a cardiac invalid because of the disproportionate rise in ventricular rate that occurs as atrioventricular conduction improves with exercise. The increased ventricular rate with exercise decreases left ventricular filling, raises left atrial pressure, and produces pulmonary venous congestion. Individuals who are totally asymptomatic with normal pulmonary capillary wedge pressures during sinus rhythm may have marked symptoms and a considerable rise in pulmonary capillary wedge pressure when they develop atrial fibrillation. Patients with mitral stenosis who have similar ventricular rates at rest when they are in sinus rhythm or atrial fibrillation with a controlled ventricular rate may have a considerable rise in ventricular rate even with mild exercise when in atrial fibrillation. Mild exercise may produce a ventricular rate of 90/min when the patient is in sinus rhythm and 120–130/min when the rhythm is atrial fibrillation (Wetherbee, 1952). When the patient reverts to sinus rhythm spontaneously or after cardioversion or quinidine therapy, the cardiac output may increase up to 30% because atrial systole is restored, but the smaller rise in ventricular rate with exercise is more important in preventing pulmonary venous congestion when the patient is in sinus rhythm. Atrial fibrillation is tolerated better when the patient has dominant mitral regurgitation because there is no obstruction to left ventricular filling. The manner in which the patient with mitral stenosis handles atrial fibrillation is a clue to the severity of the lesion; if the patient merely has palpitations and a sense of irregularity of heart rate without significant dyspnea, it can be inferred that the mitral stenosis is trivial.

Chronic Atrial Fibrillation

In chronic atrial fibrillation—especially if the ventricular rate is controlled with digitalis—the patient may be asymptomatic and may be unaware of the atrial fibrillation or its irregularity except when exercising. Some patients describe what they think are paroxysmal episodes of atrial fibrillation when in fact they have chronic fibrillation but are aware of the rapid, irregular ventricular rate only with exercise or emotion.

Risk of Systemic Emboli

In addition to the possibility that pulmonary venous congestion and decreased cardiac output may occur when atrial fibrillation supervenes in mitral valve disease, patients with chronic atrial fibrillation have the added risk of systemic emboli, which are uncommon in patients with supraventricular tachycardia. Before mitral valve surgery became available, systemic emboli occurred in about one-third of patients with mitral stenosis and were the cause of death in about 20% of patients. Systemic embolism may be the initial clinical manifestation of mitral stenosis, eg, cerebral embolization with hemiplegia, and a major embolus to an extremity may require surgery. The likelihood of emboli is greatest in the year following onset of atrial fibrillation, but the course is unpredictable and patients may develop major emboli after they have had fibrillation for several years. Systemic emboli are much less common in nonrheumatic types of heart disease and are rare in thyrotoxicosis.

Atrial Rate & Ventricular Response

The atrial rate in atrial fibrillation is approximately 450–600/min, and the ventricular response is almost always irregular because of variable "concealed" conduction in the atrioventricular node. Without treatment, the ventricular rate usually varies between 130–160/min, but it may be less than 100/min. The so-called F (fibrillation) waves seen on the ECG reflecting the circus movements thought to be the cause of atrial fibrillation, with multiple wave fronts simultaneously exciting the atria, may be obvious on the ECG or may be fine and difficult to see. The differentiation of so-called coarse and fine atrial fibrillation is rarely of clinical importance. When the ventricular rate is rapid and only slightly irregular, the presence of obvious F waves is helpful in diagnosis. When the ventricular rate is rapid or when it is slow as a result of digitalis therapy, the irregularity may not be gross or obvious unless the ventricular rate is timed carefully. A helpful sign–both electrocardiographically and clinically–is the presence of pauses that follow previous pauses. Atrial premature beats, for example, occur early and are followed by a noncompensatory pause, and if one listens carefully or examines the ECG strip closely one will find that whenever there are pauses they are preceded by "quick" beats, ie, early beats with short cycle length from the beat before. In atrial fibrillation, however, one can detect pauses that are not preceded by quick beats but may be preceded by pauses of different lengths. These irregular pauses and irregular beats cause the "irregular irregularity" of atrial fibrillation.

If the ventricular rate is rapid, atrial fibrillation with aberrant conduction may be confused with ventricular tachycardia. The presence of a right bundle branch block pattern in lead V_1 is helpful, as noted previously in the differential diagnosis of tachycardia, and favors aberrancy of nodal conduction.

Pulse Deficit

Before treatment is given, there is a substantial difference in ventricular rate as determined at the apex of the heart and that which is felt at the radial pulse–the so-called pulse deficit. This occurs because the more rapid beats may not result in a sufficient stroke output to cause a pulse wave to reach the wrist. Following digitalis therapy, when the ventricular rate is slowed, each beat has a more forceful output and the pulse deficit diminishes. If the apical and radial rates are plotted before and during digitalis therapy, the disappearance or decrease of the pulse deficit is often a good index of adequate therapy.

Atrial Flutter

Atrial flutter is similar to atrial fibrillation in its age distribution and causative factors, but it is less common then atrial fibrillation in mitral valve disease and atrial septal defect. It may be paroxysmal or established, as in atrial fibrillation, but the atrial rate is slower, usually 260–350/min, and the ventricles usually respond to every other atrial excitation wave, so that the pattern is a 2:1 atrioventricular conduction with an atrial rate of about 300/min and a regular ventricular rate of 150/min. In some patients, atrioventricular conduction may be variable and show alternating 2:1, 3:1, or 4:1 conduction with an irregular ventricular rate, simulating atrial fibrillation. Atrioventricular conduction is less predictable than in atrial fibrillation, and patients may have abrupt changes from 4:1 to 2:1 with postural changes or excitement or while eating. They may have a ventricular rate of 75/min when recumbent and 150/min when sitting. They may then have an abrupt onset of palpitations and symptoms without a change in the basic atrial flutter due only to a change in the ventricular response to the flutter.

For these reasons, atrial flutter is a more unstable and troublesome rhythm than atrial fibrillation. The abrupt jumps in ventricular rate with minor activities such as sitting up may produce unpredictable pulmonary venous congestion if the patient has underlying cardiac disease such as severe mitral stenosis. This is in contrast to atrial fibrillation, in which there is a more gradual and smaller increase in ventricular response following trivial activity. Atrial flutter and atrial fibrillation may occur in the same patient on different occasions, as may atrial tachycardia. The fact that some patients have each of the 3 rhythms on different occasions led Prinzmetal (1952) to suggest that the basic mechanism of all 3 was an ectopic focus in the atria which varied in its rate of discharge. This is in contrast to the prevailing opinion that atrial arrhythmias usually are due to circus movements and reentry (see Supraventricular Tachycardia, p 460). In atrial flutter with variable atrioventricular conduction, the ventricular rate is irregular and may clinically or electrocardiographically simulate atrial fibrillation.

Quinidine in Treatment of Atrial Fibrillation

Almost all patients with atrial fibrillation who are treated with quinidine go through a transitional phase of atrial flutter prior to the development of sinus rhythm because quinidine slows the atrial rate. It has a vagolytic action which improves atrioventricular conduction, leading to a more rapid ventricular rate as the atrial rate slows. Digitalis is therefore given before quinidine to prevent a rapid ventricular rate. In these instances, the atrial rate varies from 150–300/min and may be irregular. Some physicians call this rhythm atrial flutter-fibrillation. Electrocardiographically, the atrial rate in the untreated patient is the best differential point because it is rare for atrial flutter to have an atrial rate greater than 350/min, whereas this is exceeded in almost all cases of atrial fibrillation, in which the atrial rate varies from 350–600/min. The atrial rate is variable in atrial fibrillation because the circus movement and reentry circuits vary from segment to segment in the atria, whereas atrial flutter is more apt to be due to a reentry circuit of a larger segment of atrium, with a more regular pattern. Atrial flutter is less apt to be chronic than atrial fibrillation, and it is usually paroxysmal. The clinical features of atrial flutter and atrial fibrillation have been discussed under the clinical features of arrhythmias in general. The irregularity of the ventricular response contributes to its deleterious effect independently of tachycardia.

Treatment of Atrial Fibrillation

The principal aim of therapy, whether the patient has acute or chronic atrial fibrillation, is to slow the ventricular rate by increasing atrioventricular block with digitalis. A secondary consideration is restoration of sinus rhythm, and a third very important therapeutic aim is to prevent recurrences.

A. Digitalis: When restoration of sinus rhythm is not urgent because severe symptoms of dyspnea, angina, palpitations, confusion, or hypotension are absent, digitalis* is the treatment of choice and can be used orally or parenterally, depending upon the urgency of the need to slow the ventricular rate by increasing the atrioventricular block. Once the ventricular rate is controlled, the decision to attempt restoration of sinus rhythm can be undertaken in nonurgent circumstances. Digitalis is often relatively ineffective in slowing the ventricular rate in acute atrial fibrillation or in chronic atrial fibrillation in the setting of severe cardiovascular disease. In these cases there is little relation between the "therapeutic" serum digoxin levels (0.8–2 ng/ml) and the ventricular rate (Goldman, 1975).

B. Cardioversion: Restoration of sinus rhythm is usually performed by electric shock "cardioversion." If an electric defibrillator is not available, quinidine can be used. Fig 15–13 shows the relationship between the daily dose of quinidine, peak serum quinidine concentrations, and myocardial toxicity. As the dose of quinidine in grams per day is increased, there is an average progressive increase in serum quinidine concentration, but there are many departures from the average. Serum levels of 8–10 μg/ml may be achieved with doses of 2–2.5 g/day in some patients, whereas serum concentrations below 7 μg/ml can be obtained in others with 3 g quinidine per day. Myocardial toxicity is more closely related to the serum concentration than to the dose and progressively increases as the serum concentration reaches approximately 11 μg/ml. If quinidine is used to restore sinus rhythm because countershock is not available, it can be started at a dose of 0.2 g every 2 hours for 5 doses on day 1 with serum levels obtained 2 hours after the last dose. Each day the individual dose can be increased by 0.1 g, but it is unwise to increase the dose beyond 3 g/day unless the physician is familiar with the use of quinidine, serum concentrations of the drug can be obtained, and the patient can be seen before each dose. It should be reemphasized that cardioversion is the treatment of choice in attempted conversion of chronic atrial fibrillation and that quinidine is used only if cardioversion is not possible.

*See Table 15–5 and Chapter 10 for details of dosage of digitalis preparations.

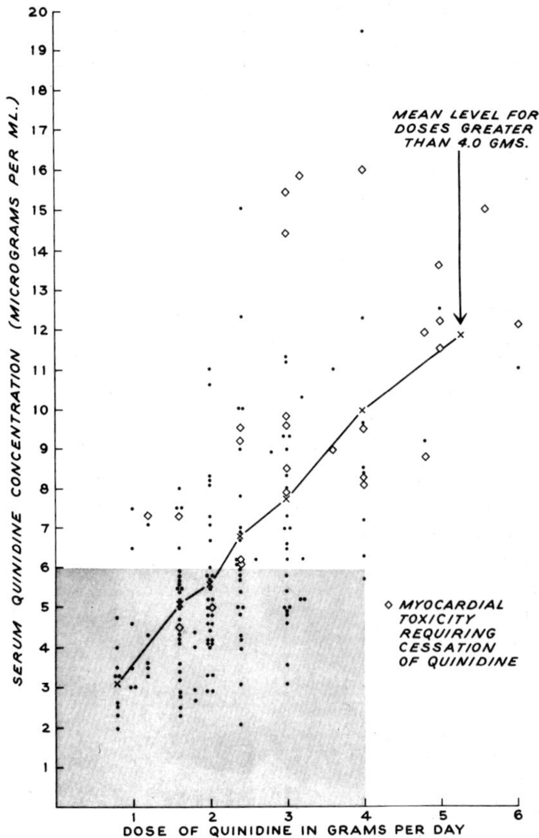

Figure 15–13. Relationship between daily dose, peak serum quinidine concentration, and myocardial toxicity. (Reproduced, with permission of the American Heart Association, Inc., from Sokolow M, Ball RE: Factors influencing conversion of chronic atrial fibrillation with special reference to serum quinidine concentration. Circulation 14:568, 1956.)

External countershock should be used with caution in the presence of digitalis toxicity. If large doses of digitalis have been required to slow the ventricular rate, it is wise to stop digitalis for one or more days and to attempt cardioversion with small stimuli such as 5 J, increasing as necessary. Because atrial fibrillation recurs so often, quinidine is usually begun 2 days before cardioversion to build up an adequate blood level of the drug in order to prevent recurrence of the arrhythmia. When quinidine (0.3 g 4 times daily) is given, about 20% of patients convert to sinus rhythm, and countershock cardioversion is not necessary. This dose of quinidine may produce a blood quinidine concentration of 2–4 μg/ml, which may be sufficient to convert the rhythm from atrial fibrillation to sinus

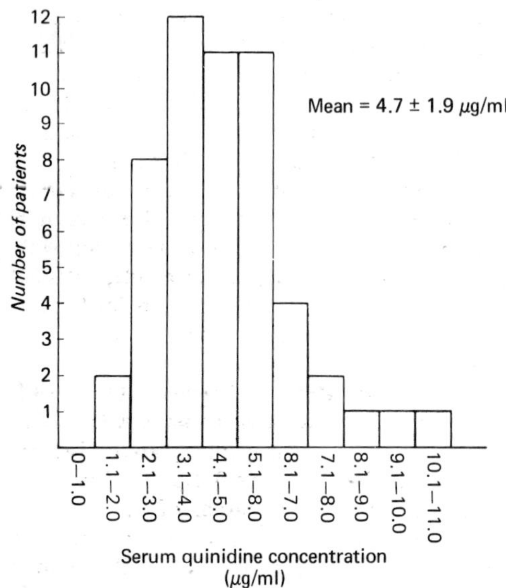

Figure 15–14. Distribution of 2:00 pm serum quinidine levels, dose of 0.4 g 4 times daily for at least 3 days (53 patients). (Reproduced, with permission of the American Heart Association, Inc., from Sokolow M, Ball RE: Factors influencing conversion of chronic atrial fibrillation with special reference to serum quinidine concentration. Circulation 14:568, 1956.)

rhythm. It is also a level which is usually adequate to prevent recurrences.

C. Anticoagulation Prior to Cardioversion: A controversial area with respect to cardioversion is the necessity for anticoagulation prior to conversion to sinus rhythm. The incidence of systemic emboli following restoration of sinus rhythm without anticoagulation is small—about 0.5%—although some authors have reported rates as high as 2–3%. If the patient has had recent systemic emboli or has a large left atrium, anticoagulant therapy with a coumarin drug for several weeks prior to countershock is desirable, although many physicians do not use anticoagulants prior to cardioversion. The argument is similar to that which prevailed when quinidine was the only method of restoration of sinus rhythm, ie, the risks of anticoagulation may be as great as the risk of systemic emboli.

D. Rapid Atrial Pacing: If atrial fibrillation or flutter with rapid ventricular rates cannot be controlled by conventional pharmacologic therapy, especially following open heart surgery, continuous rapid atrial pacing at rates of 450/min can be initiated. Pacing increases the atrioventricular block, slowing the ventricular rate. If atrial flutter is the arrhythmia, atrial pacing may induce atrial fibrillation with a slower ventricular rate; digitalis may then increase the atrioventricular block and further slow the ventricular rate (Waldo, 1976). The use of rapid atrial pacing for paroxysmal atrial tachycardia is discussed above (p 470). As with paroxysmal atrial tachycardia, atrial flutter may abruptly stop when rapid atrial pacing is discontinued.

E. Prevention of Recurrences: Because the recurrence rate following cardioversion is high, especially in patients who have long-standing atrial fibrillation or considerable enlargement of the heart or whose arrhythmias developed following cardiac surgery, it becomes a matter of judgment whether to control the ventricular rate with digitalis and leave the patient in chronic atrial fibrillation or to attempt to restore normal sinus rhythm with electric cardioversion. Quinidine is effective in preventing frequent recurrent attacks of paroxysmal atrial fibrillation of relatively short duration (usually hours to days), the dose and frequency of administration being gradually increased until the attacks no longer occur or are less frequent.

Fig 15–14 depicts the serum quinidine concentration measured at 2:00 pm in patients given 0.4 g 4 times a day. Although the mean value is 4.7 ± 1.9 μg/ml, the serum concentration ranges from 2–11 μg/ml, indicating differences in absorption, distribution, and metabolism of the drug. Myocardial toxicity may occur with increasing doses of quinidine, as in treating atrial fibrillation to restore sinus rhythm, and is manifested by the presence of ventricular arrhythmias—usually ventricular premature beats but occasionally ventricular tachycardia or even ventricular fibrillation. Ventricular fibrillation occurs infrequently when

Table 15–1. Effects of quinidine on 2 patients with coronary heart disease, paroxysmal atrial fibrillation, and paroxysmal atrial flutter.

	Dose of Quinidine	Average Midday Blood Level	Comment
Male, age 57 years Coronary heart disease. Paroxysmal atrial fibrillation 2–4 times per month for 12 years.	None	0	4 attacks in 6 weeks
	0.2 g 3 times daily	0.5 μg/ml	3 attacks in 6 weeks
	0.4 g 3 times daily	2.9 μg/ml	8 attacks in 24 weeks
	0.4 g 4 times daily	3.2 μg/ml	3 attacks in 6 weeks
	0.4 g 4 times daily (Enseals)	1.5 μg/ml	2 attacks in 1 week
	0.6 g 3 times daily	4.5 μg/ml	2 attacks in 6 weeks
	0.5 g 4 times daily	5.2 μg/ml	No attacks in 6 months
Male, age 54 years Coronary heart disease. Paroxysmal atrial flutter 2–4 times per week for 4 years.	0.2 g 5 times daily	1.3 μg/ml	No effect
	0.4 g 4 times daily	1.9 μg/ml	Slight decrease in attacks
	0.4 g 5 times daily	2.7 μg/ml	1 attack in 9 weeks
	0.4 g 5 times daily	3.7 μg/ml	1 attack in 6 weeks
	Quinidine stopped	0	Many attacks within 48–72 hours
	0.6 g 4 times daily	4.6 μg/ml	No attacks for 3 months

quinidine is given with the patient in a stable state with no other drug therapy, but the likelihood of fibrillation is enhanced when patients are receiving increasing doses of digitalis with or without diuretic therapy and resultant hypokalemia. Prolongation of the Q–T interval is common and represents the electrophysiologic action of quinidine delaying the velocity of conduction. Intraventricular block or bundle branch block which develops after quinidine is due to more marked conduction defect. When the QRS duration exceeds 50% of the control value, it is wise to stop quinidine.

If quinidine is given at regular intervals (eg, 4 times daily), a blood level plateau is reached in 48–72 hours. A larger dose or administration at shorter intervals is required to achieve higher, more effective blood levels.

Not only is the recurrence rate of atrial fibrillation high after cardioversion in patients with large hearts and a long history of atrial fibrillation, but the drug that is most effective in preventing recurrences is quinidine, which is unpleasant for some patients to take because of its side-effects: diarrhea, nausea, and tinnitus. The same symptoms occur when quinidine is used to convert atrial fibrillation to sinus rhythm, and various medications can be used to counteract the symptoms, but this is unwise in patients receiving chronic quinidine therapy. In patients whose atrial fibrillation has lasted less than 6 months and whose hearts and left atria are normal in size or only slightly enlarged, cardioversion is almost always desirable at least once, combined with an effort to prevent recurrences with oral quinidine therapy, 0.2–0.3 g 4 times daily, or long-acting quinidine preparations that require only twice-daily dosage. Under these circumstances, one-fourth to one-third of patients remain in sinus rhythm and are much more comfortable than when they were in atrial fibrillation, primarily because of relief of disproportionate tachycardia with mild exercise. Patients who have been repeatedly converted to sinus rhythm almost always indicate that their cardiac function is much better when they are in sinus rhythm. There are well-documented data that the use of quinidine decreases the recurrence rate of atrial fibrillation after restoration of sinus rhythm. In a multicenter study from Stockholm, approximately 50% of patients were still in sinus rhythm a year after treatment of atrial fibrillation or flutter when they received quinidine, whereas only 25% of the control group remained in sinus rhythm (Södermark, 1975).

Long-acting quinidine was superior to short-acting quinidine in maintaining sinus rhythm after DC cardioversion. After 18 months, 65% of patients remained in sinus rhythm on long-acting quinidine and 30% on short-acting quinidine of comparable dosage (Normand, 1976). In the whole series, sinus rhythm was maintained for 18 months in 50% of patients, which is consistent with the results of the Stockholm study.

F. Value of Addition of Propranolol: In chronic atrial fibrillation or in paroxysmal fibrillation when the ventricular rate cannot be controlled with digitalis (especially during exercise), propranolol (10–20 mg orally 4 times daily and increased as needed) can be added with benefit to slow the ventricular rate during exercise. It should be used with caution if the patient has a history of asthma or left ventricular failure, atrioventricular conduction defects, or bradycardia. Propranolol can be added to quinidine in an effort to prevent recurrences, and there are some data to suggest that the combination is more effective than quinidine alone. If quinidine alone or in combination with propranolol is not tolerated, procainamide, 250–500 mg orally 3 or 4 times a day alone or combined with quinidine, is sometimes effective but should be used cautiously.

G. Adverse Effects in Patients With Mitral Stenosis or Coronary Disease: In patients with minimal or moderate mitral valve or coronary artery disease, control of atrial fibrillation or flutter is often decisive in determining whether symptoms of dyspnea or angina are due to the arrhythmia or to the anatomic defect. If the former, drug therapy and not surgery is the treatment of choice to control the arrhythmia. Hemodynamic study with cardiac catheterization is often necessary to determine the magnitude of the structural defect. Cardiac catheterization should be delayed until the ventricular rate is controlled and the patient is in a steady state. The severity of mitral stenosis, for example, can be overestimated if cardiac catheterization is done when the ventricular rate is rapid, in which instance the pulmonary capillary wedge pressure may be high and evidence of pulmonary venous congestion present. The various formulas for determining the valve areas are theoretically not influenced by rapid ventricular rates, but this is often not the case.

Treatment of Atrial Flutter

Paroxysmal atrial flutter responds dramatically to cardioversion in about 95% of cases, and this is the treatment of choice in almost all cases. Patients should not be allowed to remain in chronic atrial flutter because of the instability of the rhythm, as noted above.

Before electric cardioversion became available, digitalis was used in large doses (1.5 mg orally followed by 0.25–0.5 mg orally every 4–6 hours until atrial fibrillation occurred) to convert atrial flutter to atrial fibrillation and thus allow the ventricular rate to be more easily controlled. In some patients, atrial fibrillation then reverted spontaneously to sinus rhythm, but this occurred in only a minority of cases and required large doses of digitalis. Quinidine by mouth is a relatively ineffective method of treatment of chronic atrial flutter and should be used only to prevent recurrences. If the patient has a history of paroxysms lasting hours which are not prevented by quinidine or quinidine plus propranolol, digitalis can be used to increase the atrioventricular block and slow the ventricular rate. Systemic emboli are much less frequent than in atrial fibrillation because atrial systole is made stronger by the slower atrial rate and more uniform atrial contractions, decreasing the likelihood of atrial thrombus formation. As in chronic atrial fibrillation, it is wise to begin

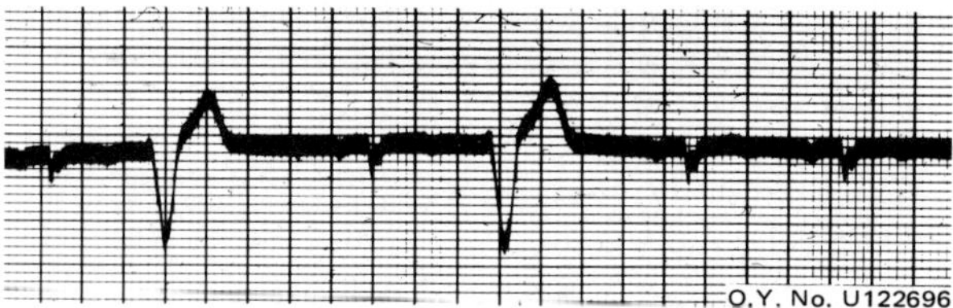

Figure 15–15. Ventricular premature beats with bigeminy in a 48-year-old man not receiving digitalis.

quinidine therapy 1–2 days prior to cardioversion if the patient has recurrent episodes of atrial flutter and to realize that an increased ventricular rate may result. The usefulness of digitalis to prevent recurrences should not be overlooked because it may increase the atrioventricular block. Digitalis is always worth a trial, because if it is successful, the patient can be maintained on a single daily dose, which is tolerated much better than multiple doses of quinidine.

See p 474 for discussion of rapid atrial pacing in the treatment of atrial flutter.

VENTRICULAR ARRHYTHMIAS

VENTRICULAR PREMATURE BEATS

Ventricular premature beats are the most common of all arrhythmias (Figs 15–15 and 15–16). In the absence of heart disease they are usually not of great clinical significance, but in patients with coro-

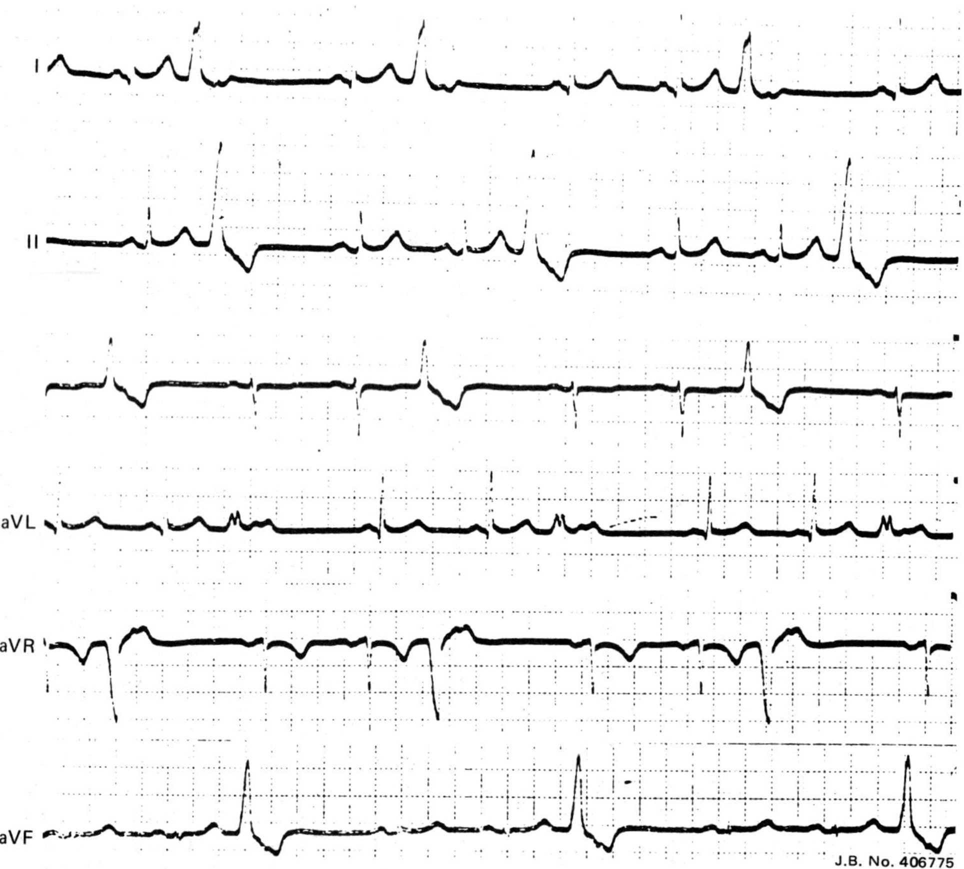

Figure 15–16. Sinus rhythm with frequent unifocal premature ventricular beats occurring in bigeminy (every other beat) and trigeminy (every third beat). The basic ventricular rate is 75/min. What appear to be retrograde P waves follow each ventricular complex, best seen in lead aVR. These could be nonconducted atrial premature beats, but the absence of any atrial premature beats elsewhere in the record except following the ventricular premature beats makes the assumption of retrograde P waves more likely.

nary heart disease they represent a constant danger of ventricular tachycardia or fibrillation and sudden death. Many epidemiologic studies of the incidence and prognostic significance of ventricular premature beats have been performed in recent years in the hope of identifying and perhaps treating a high-risk group liable to sudden death. Whereas in the past a single ECG was used to determine the presence of ventricular premature beats, more recent epidemiologic studies have used 6-, 12-, or 24-hour ambulatory ECG monitoring or continuous ECGs during graded exercise to evaluate the type and frequency of ventricular premature beats in population groups. It has been shown, for example, that multihour ambulatory monitoring reveals at least 10 times as many premature beats, as well as complex arrhythmias, as does a single routine ECG recording. Ventricular premature beats may cause concern in as many as one-third of patients convalescing from acute myocardial infarction. Lown (1977) has devised a grading system for ventricular premature beats that is shown in Table 15–2. Since sudden deaths are most apt to occur in people with known coronary disease–especially with ventricular premature beats–efforts have been made to identify those who have frequent or complex premature beats spontaneously or after exercise that might warrant long-term antiarrhythmia therapy, especially if the angiographically identified disease is severe. However, premature beats are capricious and variable in coronary disease, and, just as in normal subjects, they may be present on one occasion and absent on another. They are also common in asymptomatic patients with coronary disease (Table 15–3). Even in the coronary care unit, it has been shown that conventional ECG monitoring has limitations, and many arrhythmias are missed with ordinary monitoring technics. The number of diagnostic errors resulting from such unreliable estimates of the frequency of ventricular arrhythmias and their response to treatment has led to greater reliance on computer detection and analysis of ventricular arrhythmias in the coronary care unit. The frequency of ventricular arrhythmias, including multifocal and complex varieties as well as ventricular tachycardia, has been underestimated, and refinements of the computer method are under way to determine its clinical usefulness (Vetter, 1975; Knoebel, 1976).

In community epidemiologic studies, some middle-aged men with no history of angina or other evidence of coronary heart disease and no risk factors develop ventricular premature beats following graded exercise on a treadmill or bicycle ergometer. These men have an incidence of sudden death similar to those who do not develop premature beats with exercise. To further complicate the task of clinical assessment, antiarrhythmia therapy in patients with coronary heart disease during convalescence from acute myocardial infarction is of only limited benefit and does not eliminate the arrhythmia in many cases, and the side-effects of drug therapy may be significant. Further prospective studies are necessary to determine the prognostic significance of simple and complex ventricular premature beats that occur during ambulatory monitoring and following exercise and the benefits of various antiarrhythmia regimens, including newer drugs not yet approved by the FDA.

The prevention of ventricular fibrillation is an important goal in the treatment of ventricular premature beats, but there is no unanimity of opinion on how to distinguish the 50% of patients whose premature beats are unimportant prognostically from the other half in whom ventricular fibrillation or hemodynamic effects are produced. It seems established, however, that in coronary disease, frequent complex arrhythmias, those that occur in short runs, those that occur early on the T wave, or those that are associated

Table 15–2. A grading system for ventricular premature beats.*†

Grade	Characteristics of Beat
0	No ventricular beats
1A	Occasional, isolated ventricular premature beats (less than 30/hr): Less than 1/min
1B	Occasional, isolated ventricular premature beats (less than 30/hr): More than 1/min
2	Frequent ventricular premature beats (more than 30/hr)
3	Multiform ventricular premature beats
4A	Repetitive ventricular premature beats: Couplets
4B	Repetitive ventricular premature beats: Salvos
5	Early ventricular premature beats (ie, abutting or interrupting the T wave)

*Reproduced, with permission, from Lown B, Graboys TB: Sudden death: An ancient problem newly perceived. Cardiovasc Med 2:219, 1977.

†This grading system is applied to a 24-hour monitoring period and indicates the number of hours within that period that a patient has ventricular premature beats of a particular grade.

Table 15–3. Incidence of various ventricular arrhythmias in patient population.*

Arrhythmias	Number of Cases	Percent of Total Cases
Premature beats (unifocal)		
< 6/min†	523	31.3
6–12/min†	90	5.4
> 12/min†	70	4.2
Premature beats (multifocal)		
< 6/min†	206	12.3
6–12/min†	81	4.8
> 12/min†	69	4.1
Paired premature ventricular contractions	169	10.1
R wave encroaching on the T wave	72	4.3
Tachycardia	69	4.1
Fibrillation	0	0

*Reproduced, with permission, from Bleifer SB & others: Diagnosis of occult arrhythmias by Holter electrocardiography. Prog Cardiovasc Dis 16:569, 1974.

†In *any* 1-minute period.

with longer bursts of ventricular tachycardia, predispose to sudden death. Every effort should be made to suppress these premature beats with careful attention to precipitating factors, ventilation, iatrogenic factors such as cardiac catheters or pacemakers, attention to central nervous system autonomic influences, sedation, and antiarrhythmia drugs. Graded exercise and long-term monitoring should be used to count the various types of ventricular premature beats as an aid in deciding whether or not to give treatment. Monitoring should be continued during the recovery period after exercise because most premature beats occur during this period. Monitoring should be repeated months following recovery from a myocardial infarction because the incidence of subsequent sudden death is at least tripled when there are many ventricular premature beats as compared to when there are none.

Hazards of Ventricular Premature Beats

The greatest hazards of ventricular premature beats—in contrast to atrial premature beats—are ventricular tachycardia and ventricular fibrillation. Any tachycardia, atrial or ventricular, may have adverse hemodynamic effects if sufficiently rapid. Ventricular tachycardia, because it is more apt to occur in a setting of organic heart disease—particularly coronary heart disease or cardiomyopathy—is feared because of the likelihood of abrupt hemodynamic worsening or of ventricular fibrillation and sudden death.

Ventricular premature beats are common in older people with no heart disease. They increase in frequency with age, and the patients are often asymptomatic; but, as with atrial premature beats, the premature beat may produce symptoms referable to the postpause forceful beat that produces a thump, a sense of skipping or of emptiness in the chest, or a twinge of local pain. The premature beats may be the first sign of coronary heart disease, especially when they occur following exercise, but by themselves they are not a reliable sign of coronary disease. They are apt to occur in patients with slow heart rates because the long diastolic pause slows the subsequent velocity of conduction, increases the likelihood of variable refractory periods among cells, and favors the development of both reentry and automatic ectopic foci. In coronary disease, there may be scattered areas of ischemia or fibrosis, with different rates of recovery of excitability in neighboring fibers. This nonuniform recovery of excitability during the relative refractory period may induce chaotic propagation of the cardiac impulse and lead to ventricular fibrillation. This may occur with ventricular premature beats or with supraventricular premature beats with aberrant conduction. Aberrantly conducted beats also increase the likelihood of ventricular fibrillation, especially if the premature beats are closely coupled (Yoon, 1975). Prematurity and variable responsiveness are conditions within segments of the cardiac muscle of the ventricle that lead to reentry rhythms. If there is persistent ischemia, hypoxia, ventricular aneurysm, or left ventricular dilatation, phase 4 of the action potential may have an increased slope, with resultant increased automaticity. Ventricular premature beats may then be due to increased automatic ectopic firing rather than to reentry. Patients whose premature beats occur when the heart rate is slow are often benefited by increasing the rate, as with exercise, but when the rate slows following exercise, the premature beats may reappear. It is generally thought that premature beats are more significant when they occur only during or following exercise, but this requires further validation by prognostic studies. Premature beats occurring during acute myocardial infarction are discussed in Chapter 8.

Role of Central Nervous System

The role of the central nervous system in ventricular premature beats is particularly important because excitement, anxiety, or fear increases autonomic adrenergic stimuli to the heart and may induce increased automaticity in the Purkinje fibers, leading to premature beats. It is common to note ventricular premature beats in patients in the day or so preceding elective surgery only to have them disappear spontaneously in the postoperative period after successful surgery. Lown (Circulation 48, 1973) has shown that premature beats, while frequent during the day, may be less frequent or even absent during sleep. Alcohol is a notable offender with respect to ventricular premature beats, and tobacco and coffee may be important causes. Premature beats may come and go and are more apt to be present during periods of emotional stress even if the precise source of the stress is not clearly defined.

Identification of Simple & Complex Beats by Monitoring & Exercise

Various studies have shown that ambulatory monitoring and graded treadmill exercise may complement each other in identifying the presence of ventricular premature beats, neither procedure being clearly superior. At least 6 hours are required for ambulatory monitoring. In some patients, exercise is more effective in inducing ectopic beats than ambulatory monitoring; in others, the opposite is true. In prospective studies, therefore, both methods should be used. Ventricular premature beats should be counted and noted as being unifocal, multifocal, occurring in pairs or runs or appearing early on the T wave (during the "vulnerable" period), or occurring in short runs of ventricular tachycardia or ventricular fibrillation.

Clinical Findings

Patients may be asymptomatic or may complain of a forceful heartbeat that follows the extrasystolic pause. In contrast to atrial premature beats, when there is a normal sequence of conduction via the atrioventricular node through to the ventricles, ventricular premature beats by retrograde activation depolarize the atrioventricular node and interrupt the normal sequence.

A. Cannon Waves: Right atrial systole may find the tricuspid valve closed because of recent intermittent ectopic ventricular systoles and produce, irregular-

frequency of ventricular tachycardia, which is hemodynamically important, it does not minimize the potential of this arrhythmia to precipitate ventricular fibrillation. Short or longer paroxysms of ventricular tachycardia may occur in the same record with single premature beats.

Ventricular tachycardia is most common in the presence of acute myocardial infarction, usually in the first 1–3 hours, when by continuous monitoring it may be found in as many as 40% of cases depending on how early the monitoring is started. The incidence falls precipitously with the passage of hours, and in only 5% is the onset after the first day. Patients who have ventricular tachycardia early in the course of acute myocardial infarction do not necessarily have recurrences later in the disease or following convalescence, even after exercise. Ventricular tachycardia and ventricular fibrillation occurring very early (in the first few minutes or hours) in acute myocardial infarction are thought to be due to myocardial ischemia resulting in reentry or to automatic ectopic ventricular discharge. Patients with large infarcts and cardiac failure are more apt to have ventricular tachycardia and ventricular fibrillation. The former may occur in the setting of sinus bradycardia with inferior myocardial infarction and is less likely to occur when the ventricular rate is increased by administration of small doses of atropine. Large doses of atropine (1 mg or more intravenously) may induce ventricular arrhythmias because of the induced sinus tachycardia and the variable recovery of excitability in different portions of the infarcted heart. Ventricular tachycardia early in the course of acute myocardial infarction must be differentiated from nonparoxysmal junctional tachycardia with aberrant conduction. In the latter the rate is usually slower (70–120/min), and a careful search for P waves (see above) may indicate its supraventricular origin. Accelerated idioventricular rhythm (Fig 15–19) looks the same, but there is atrioventricular dissociation and perhaps capture or fusion beats.

Accelerated Idioventricular Rhythms

Accelerated idioventricular rhythms (Fig 15–19) may "escape" when there is suppression of higher pacemakers due to sinoatrial and atrioventricular block but may also represent "slow" ventricular tachycardia due to reentry or increased automaticity due to ischemia. Norris (1974), in his experience with 61 patients with accelerated idioventricular tachycardia in acute myocardial infarction, noted that the attacks of tachycardia consisted of paroxysms of relatively short duration which were relatively slow (less than 100/min),

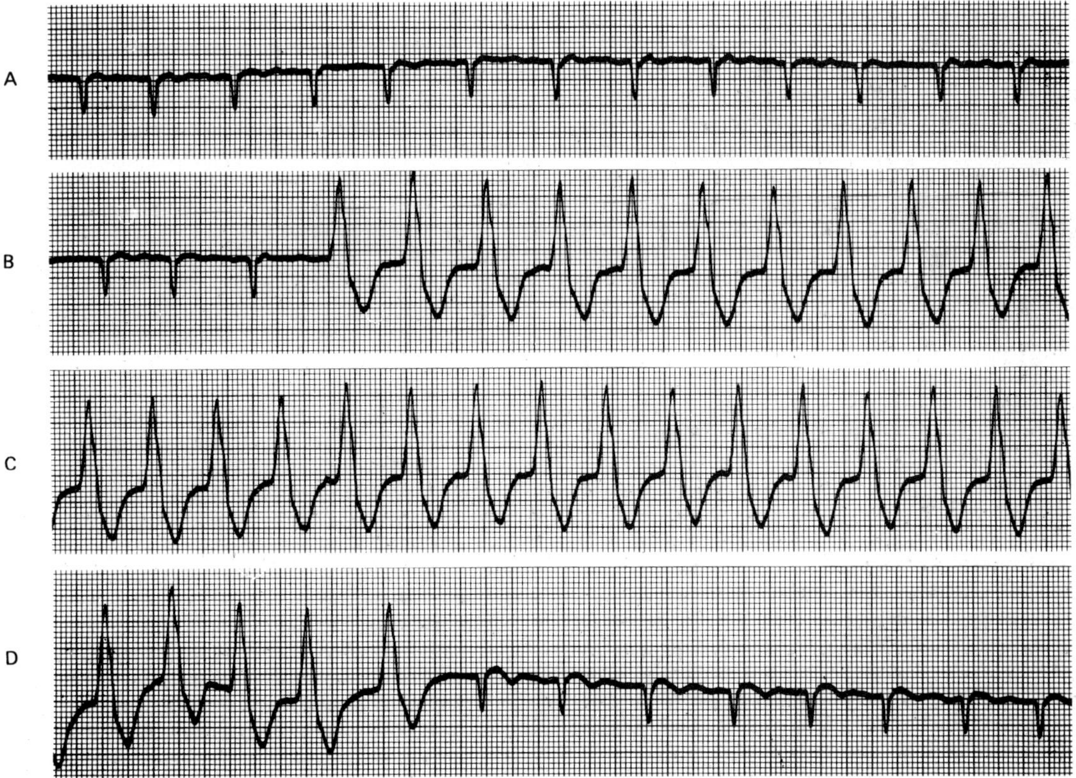

Figure 15–19. Accelerated idioventricular rhythm. Continuous recording of lead V_1 in a patient with acute myocardial infarction. *A:* Atrial fibrillation with irregular ventricular response, rate = 100. *B–C:* Appearance of idioventricular rhythm which initially has a rate of 100 and then increases to 120. *D:* Spontaneous reversion. (Reproduced, with permission, from Goldman MJ: *Principles of Clinical Electrocardiography*, 9th ed. Lange, 1976.)

often beginning with sinus bradycardia or sinoatrial block, and therefore were probably escape rhythms because the sinus node was depressed. The first beat occurs almost always after a long diastolic pause; the initial and final beats of a paroxysm may have a normal, nonpremature P wave and a QRS configuration combining sinus and ventricular origin (fusion beats). The incidence of ventricular fibrillation is only about one-fourth what it is in patients with ectopic (non-escape) ventricular tachycardia with a more rapid rate. Atrioventricular dissociation occurs in most patients with accelerated idioventricular rhythms because although the ventricular rhythm is usually "escape" in nature, the sinus node still discharges at a slower rate.

Accelerated idioventricular rhythms must be differentiated from idioventricular rhythm which occurs in complete atrioventricular block with ventricular rates less than 40/min. Not only is the ventricular rate slower, but evidence of complete atrioventricular block can be found on the ECG and by the clinical features noted above under complete atrioventricular block. In congenital atrioventricular block when the ventricular rate is faster (approximately 60–70/min), the differentiation may be more difficult, but it still depends upon the presence of complete atrioventricular block. Atrioventricular dissociation, such as occurs in accelerated idioventricular rhythm, also has independent atrial and ventricular pacemakers, but atrioventricular block is not present. Atrioventricular dissociation is always present in complete atrioventricular block but may occur in its absence when the atria and ventricles depolarize independently.

Clinical Findings in Ventricular Tachycardia
(Fig 15–20)

Ventricular tachycardia should be strongly suspected when an abrupt tachycardia occurs in an older patient with coronary heart disease, especially if the patient had ventricular premature beats before the tachycardia and the QRS complexes are wide and bizarre, with QR or QS complexes in lead V_1, or if the complexes are similar to those seen in the ventricular premature beats present on a prior occasion. The T wave is usually large and in the direction opposite to that of the QRS complex.

A. Asynchrony of Atrial and Ventricular Contractions: The most important clinical feature of ventricular tachycardia is asynchrony of atrial and ventricular contractions, with the atria beating at a slower rate. On auscultation, because of the wide QRS complexes and atrioventricular dissociation, there is wide splitting of the first and second heart sounds, beat-to-beat variation in arterial pressure and systolic murmurs, changing intensity of the first heart sound depending upon the relation of the P wave to the QRS complex, and intermittent, large cannon *a* waves in the jugular venous pulse. When the atria contract with the tricuspid valve closed, large cannon waves appear in the jugular venous pulse unless the patient has atrial fibrillation or flutter or 1:1 retrograde conduction to the atria. When the relationship between atrial and ventricular contraction is such that the mitral and tricuspid valves are wide open at the onset of ventricular systole, they close with a snap and the first heart sound is louder. When the atria and the ventricle contract close together, the mitral valve leaflets are relatively closed and the first sound is soft. The systolic blood pressure varies from beat to beat depending upon the sequence of the atrial and ventricular contraction and the contribution of atrial systole to ventricular filling. If ventricular excitation is transmitted backward to the atrium or sinus node, the result is 1:1 ventriculoatrial conduction with

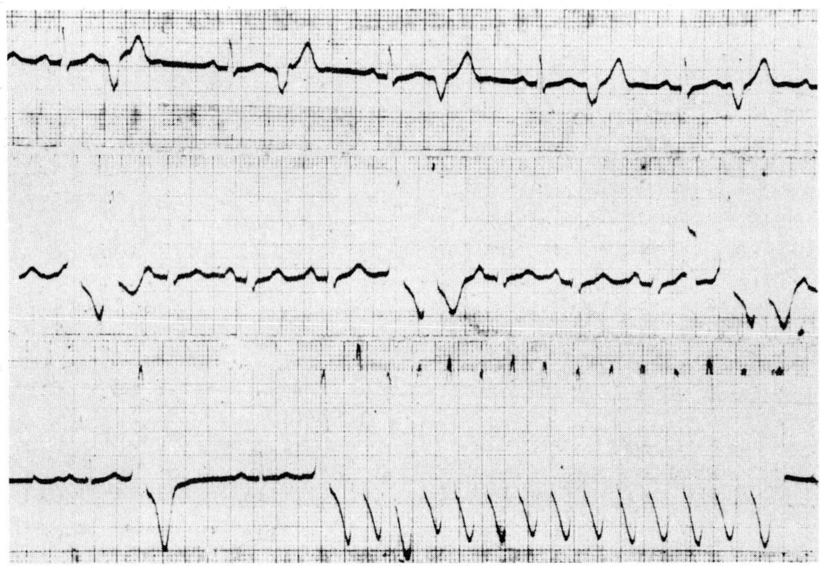

Figure 15–20. Ventricular tachycardia in a young woman with no obvious heart disease with single or paired premature beats of the same contour seen earlier in the continuous record.

no variation in the intensity of the first heart sound and no cannon waves in the jugular venous pulse.

B. Capture Beats and Supraventricular Tachycardia With Aberrant Conduction: The appearance of "capture" beats with normal QRS duration between the abnormal ventricular beats suggests ventricular tachycardia and indicates that a supraventricular impulse conducted across the atrioventricular node has "captured" the ventricles, a sign of the presence of atrioventricular dissociation rather than atrioventricular block.

Supraventricular tachycardia can only be diagnosed with confidence when P waves are found with the same frequency as the QRS complexes. They may precede or be buried in the QRS complex or may be retrograde when atrioventricular nodal junctional tachycardia is present. If the P waves cannot be definitely distinguished, one should explore the right precordial leads, obtain a Lewis lead (see p 460), and do esophageal or right atrial electrograms (Fig 15–9). Fusion beats (Dressler beats) are those in which an impulse from the sinus node fortuitously "captures" an independent ventricular beat to produce a QRS complex that resembles a ventricular premature beat but is a fusion of both atrial and ventricular depolarizations. Carotid sinus pressure or edrophonium may impair atrioventricular conduction and allow P waves to be seen in supraventricular tachycardia with aberration.

It bears reemphasis that rapid (> 250/min) tachycardia with wide, slightly irregular QRS complexes should suggest atrial fibrillation with Wolff-Parkinson-White conduction and lead to a search for slurred initial delta waves.

C. Search for P waves on the ECG: Review of long strips of the ECG in different leads with double sensitivity and a careful search for P waves may show independent atrial beats at a rate slower than the ventricular tachycardia. These are often not seen or may be buried in the QRS complex. The absence of P waves on a routine ECG does not exclude ventricular tachycardia. Furthermore, in junctional or ventricular tachycardia there may be retrograde activation of the atria that prevents independent atrial beats. Onset of tachycardia with an ectopic P wave is strong evidence of supraventricular tachycardia with aberrant conduction.

D. His Bundle Recordings: His bundle recordings may establish the diagnosis by noting the relationship of the His spike and the P wave to the QRS complexes. In supraventricular arrhythmia, the P wave and the His spike precede the QRS complex, whereas in ventricular tachycardia the QRS complex with retrograde conduction precedes the His potential.

E. Comparison of Previous Premature Beats and the Tachycardia: The diagnosis can be clarified in retrospect if, after cessation of the tachycardia, ventricular premature beats can be seen that have a configuration similar to that seen during the tachycardia. As mentioned in the discussion of supraventricular arrhythmias, if the initial or first few QRS complexes of a tachycardia are normal in configuration and later ones become bizarre, this favors a supraventricular over a ventricular origin. ECG monitoring during graded exercise may produce short bursts of ventricular tachycardia as well as ventricular premature beats and clarify the nature of the preceding tachycardia.

Treatment of Ventricular Tachycardia*

In the relatively asymptomatic patient with coronary disease whose premature beats are frequent or occur in short runs of tachycardia, treatment can be started with procainamide, 250–500 mg orally every 4–6 hours, or quinidine, 0.2–0.4 g orally 4 times daily, or lidocaine, 50–100 mg as an intravenous bolus. If the runs are prolonged or the patient is symptomatic, lidocaine, 50–100 mg intravenously, or procainamide, 100 mg/5 min intravenously up to a total of 1 g, can be given as an emergency measure while the patient is being prepared for external countershock. Fig 15–21 shows ECG changes resulting from treatment with intravenous procainamide. Fig 15–22 shows the effects of intramuscular quinidine gluconate. If 50–100 mg of intravenous lidocaine do not terminate the arrhythmia, a second injection can be given in 2–5 minutes with the hope of achieving blood levels of 1.5–4 μg/ml. If this is ineffective or if the patient has important clinical symptoms, cardioversion preceded by intravenous anesthesia, usually diazepam, 5–15 mg, should be accomplished promptly; almost all patients convert to sinus rhythm, often with low energy currents. A thump over the chest should be tried prior to electric external countershock; it may be successful in restoring sinus rhythm. Most instruments for defibrillation deliver 10 J as the minimum average. If this amount of energy is insufficient, repetitive and larger amounts of energy—up to 400 J—should be given as soon as possible to convert the arrhythmia to sinus rhythm. In patients with recurrent attacks, hypoxia and metabolic or electrolyte factors should all be corrected since they may be predisposing factors. Bedside hemodynamic monitoring with appropriate treatment may also help improve the function of the left ventricle and eliminate factors that predispose to ventricular tachycardia. Management of these hemodynamic abnormalities revealed by hemodynamic monitoring is discussed in detail in the chapter on coronary heart disease (see Chapter 8).

A. Role of Anxiety in the Coronary Care Unit: The role of anxiety in patients in the coronary care unit must be given considerable weight. Drugs such as diazepam, 5–10 mg orally as needed, or other tranquilizers should be given to decrease anxiety. Propranolol, 80–160 mg/day orally in divided doses, is occasionally effective early in the course of acute myocardial infarction to counteract the effects of autonomic discharge; later, this drug may be dangerous because it may increase the likelihood of left ventricular failure.

B. Emergency Cardioversion and Prevention of Recurrences: External direct current countershock

*The details of dosage and other information about antiarrhythmia drugs are presented in Tables 15–4 to 15–8.

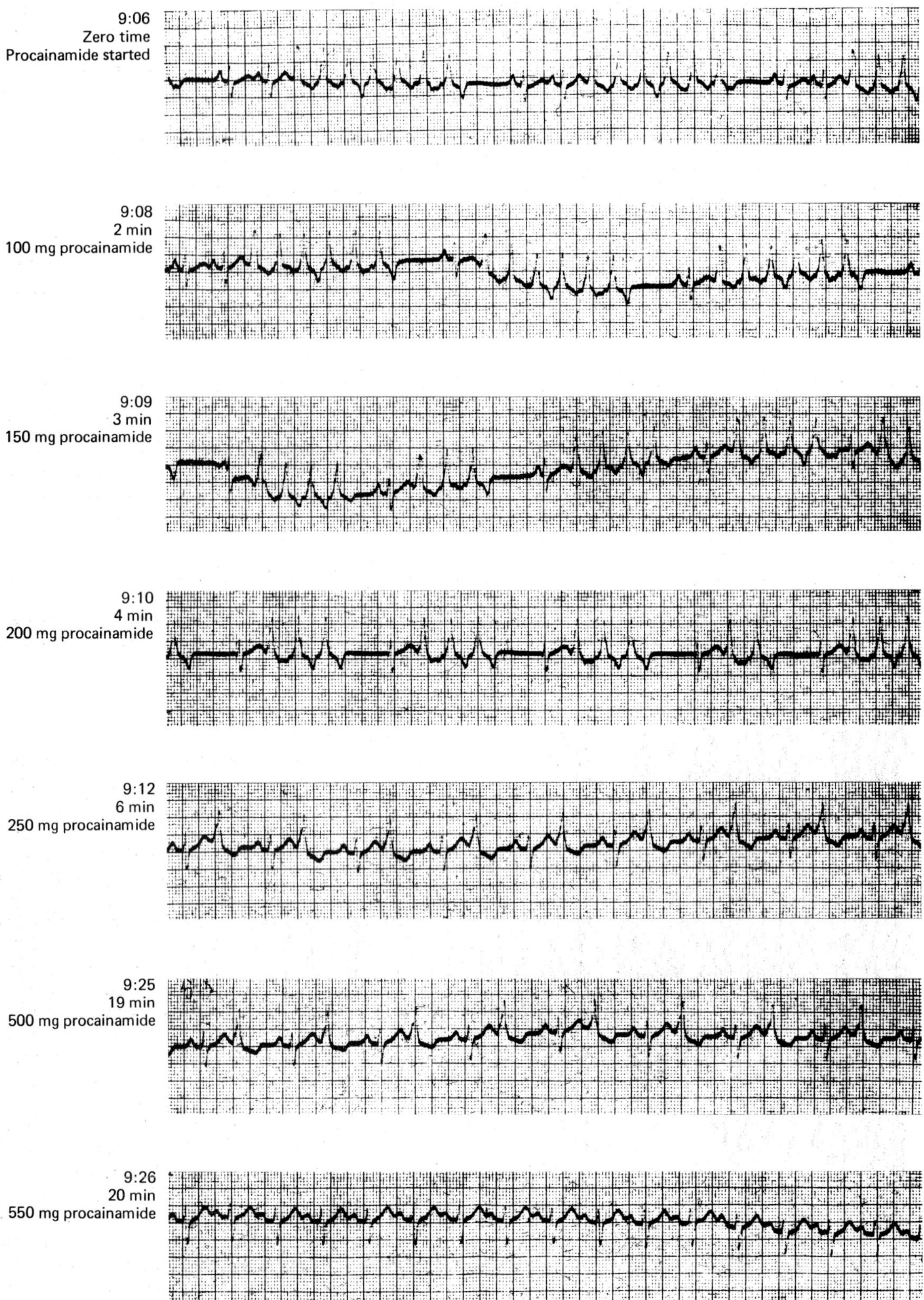

Figure 15–21. This continuous record of a 52-year-old man shows that as the dose of procainamide is increased, the bursts of ventricular tachycardia consist of progressively fewer beats, decreasing to runs of 6, 5, 4, 3, bigeminy, and finally sinus rhythm. Each run of ventricular tachycardia, as well as the ventricular bigeminy, begins on the downstroke of the T wave.

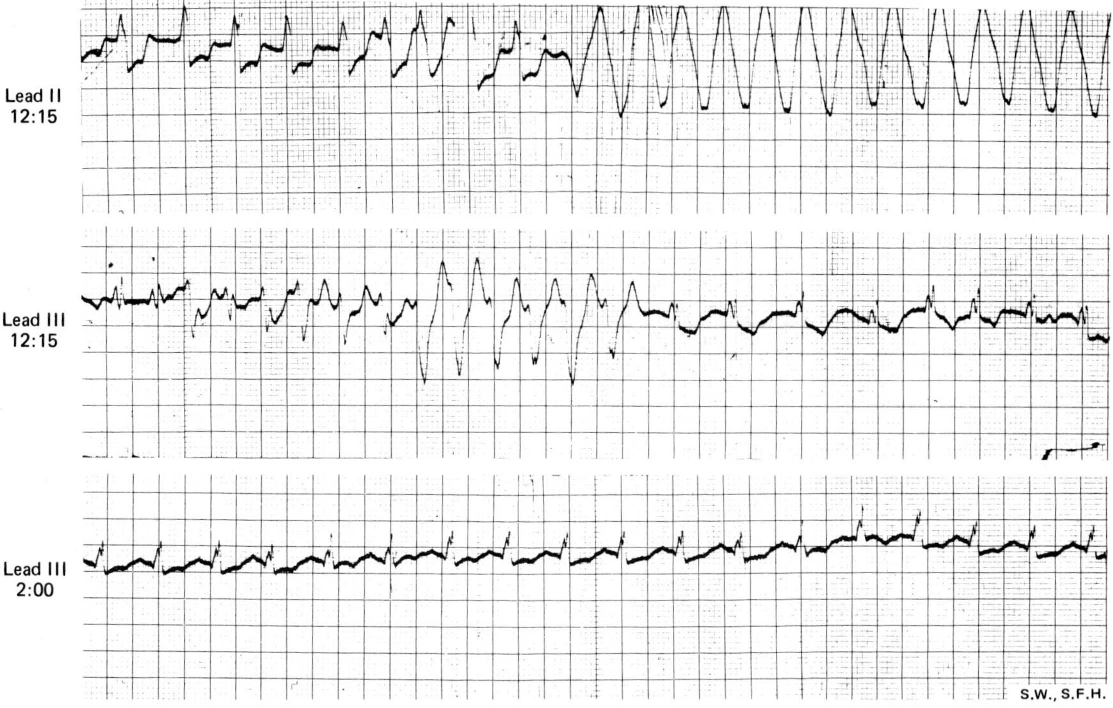

Figure 15–22. Woman age 30 years with myocarditis and runs of ventricular tachycardia at 12:15 pm. Quinidine gluconate (0.8 g) given intramuscularly at 12:30 pm. Sinus rhythm without premature beats noted at 2:00 pm. Blood quinidine level at this time was 4.8 μg/ml.

should be employed promptly if the ventricular tachycardia is life-threatening, after which pharmacologic therapy should be employed to prevent recurrence. Following electric cardioversion, the patient should be given prophylactic intravenous infusions of lidocaine, 1–4 mg/min, which, if ineffective, should be supplemented with quinidine, 0.2–0.6 g orally 3–4 times daily, or procainamide, 250–500 mg orally every 4 hours. One should avoid large doses of lidocaine over long periods because the patient may develop central nervous symptoms with dizziness, blurred vision, and excitement. Lidocaine blood levels are linearly dose-related and can be very helpful in avoiding toxicity. Lidocaine is metabolized in part by the liver, and smaller doses should be used in the presence of impaired liver function. If doses greater than 3–4 mg/min in an infusion must be exceeded or continued, one should consider combining lower doses of lidocaine with drugs such as quinidine and procainamide.

C. Overdrive Suppression by Rapid Pacing: If drugs and attention to precipitating factors are unsuccessful in preventing attacks of ventricular tachycardia, overdrive suppression of the ectopic focus by atrial or ventricular pacing may help prevent attacks. One should attempt to stop the initial attack and then use pacing at a rate somewhat faster than the ordinary sinus rate to prevent subsequent attacks. Overdrive suppression is ordinarily useful only as a temporary measure, although long-term pacing has been used with success in some centers.

D. Search for Ventricular Aneurysm: If episodes of ventricular tachycardia occur frequently (some patients have 75–100 attacks over a period of days or weeks), the possibility of ventricular aneurysm should be considered and cardiac catheterization with left ventricular angiography performed to establish the presence of a localized expansile pulsation of the left ventricle which might be treated surgically. Recurrent ventricular tachycardia unrelieved by other measures may be prevented in some cases by resection of the ventricular aneurysm, and cardiac failure may be reversed (see Chapter 8). ECG monitoring may continue to show ventricular premature beats following resection of the aneurysm, but the runs of ventricular tachycardia that are disabling are usually abolished.

E. Resection of Ischemic Zone of Increased Excitability: In a few patients with recurrent ventricular tachycardia producing severe hemodynamic abnormalities that cannot be prevented by the methods described above, epicardial mapping at thoracotomy may identify the earliest area of activation by which the excitation wave induces ventricular tachycardia and demonstrate that the abnormal ventricular beat arises from the ventricular aneurysm. Resection of this area has resulted in cessation of attacks of ventricular tachycardia. This procedure is highly experimental at present.

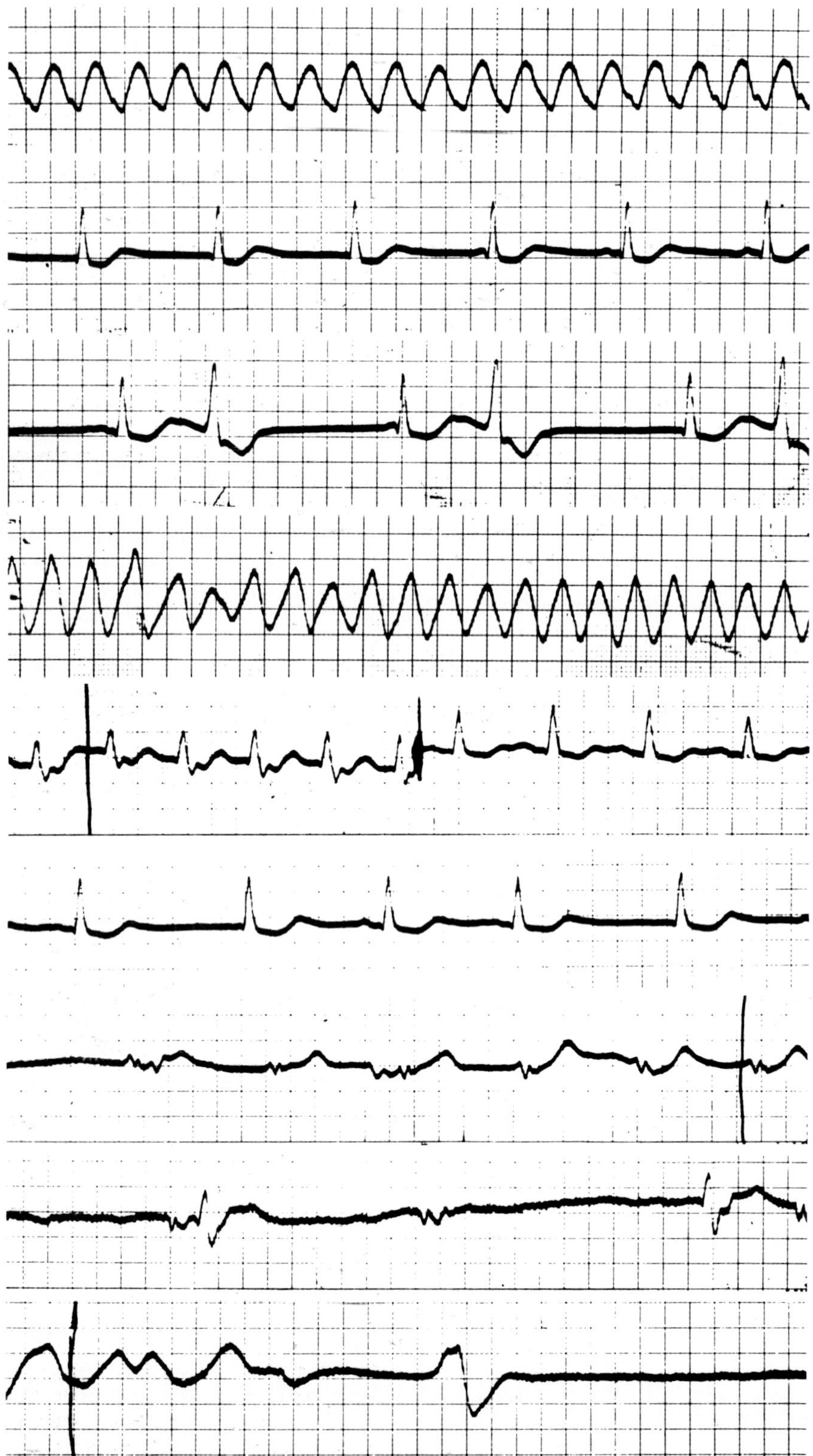

Figure 15–23. Progressive deterioration over a period of 2 hours from ventricular fibrillation to sinus bradycardia to asystole, lead II. The fourth strip is ventricular fibrillation; the eighth strip is idioventricular rhythm with bradycardia.

VENTRICULAR FIBRILLATION

Ventricular fibrillation (shown in Figs 15–23 and 15–24) is the most feared arrhythmia because of its relationship to sudden cardiac death.

Uncoordinated cardiac impulses spread rapidly across the ventricle from multiple areas of reentry and through pathways that vary in size and direction. As a result, there is a failure of the normal sequential contraction of the heart and only a rapid, irregular heartbeat. A heart in ventricular fibrillation is seen as a mass of multiple small twitches. The pressure within the ventricle does not rise, and the peripheral tissues are not perfused because there is no effective cardiac output. In effect, the heart is in a state equivalent to cardiac arrest. The random reentry pathways of the excitatory wave result in perpetuation of the dysrhythmia; although spontaneous episodes of ventricular fibrillation may terminate without therapy, the frequency of this happy event is not known. If the ventricular fibrillation persists for more than a few minutes, perfusion of the heart and brain essentially stops, and even if the patient is subsequently resuscitated irreversible brain damage may have occurred. As a result, efforts aimed at recognizing the high-risk patient susceptible to ventricular fibrillation have been employed to alert everyone concerned to the need for immediate treatment should the arrhythmia occur. As indicated in the sections on ventricular tachycardia and ventricular premature beats, most instances of ventricular fibrillation are preceded by less severe varieties of ventricular arrhythmia, but some patients, particularly those in the early minutes or hours of acute myocardial infarction, may have primary ventricular fibrillation without warning arrhythmias. Furthermore, in patients who have fortuitously developed an acute myocardial infarction while being monitored, the immediate phase of the infarction was not associated with ventricular arrhythmias which developed later, within minutes to an hour. The frequency of ventricular arrhythmias—especially ventricular fibrillation—while well established in coronary heart disease (see Chapter 8), is a matter of dispute in prolapsed mitral valve syndrome. Some authorities (Koch, 1976) believe that sudden death due to ventricular fibrillation is an important risk of mitral valve prolapse, whereas Mills (1977) found ventricular fibrillation in only one of 53 patients with mitral valve prolapse followed for a mean period of 13 years.

Prehospital Ventricular Fibrillation & Its Treatment

In selected communities, mobile teams have been trained so that an ambulance or fire department rescue vehicle with a trained crew can reach a stricken individual within 5 minutes. In Seattle, the average time between receiving the call in the emergency room and the appearance of the resuscitation crew at the scene was 3 minutes (Cobb, 1975). Pantridge's group in Belfast (Adgey, 1969) report on average time of 4 minutes. Experience with out-of-hospital onset of ventricular fibrillation has shown that only about one-fourth of patients will have unequivocal evidence of acute myocardial infarction by ECG criteria—perhaps half if one includes enzyme changes. Sixty to 70% of patients are resuscitated, and about 20% of resuscitated victims leave the hospital alive (Baum, 1974) (Table 15–9 and Fig

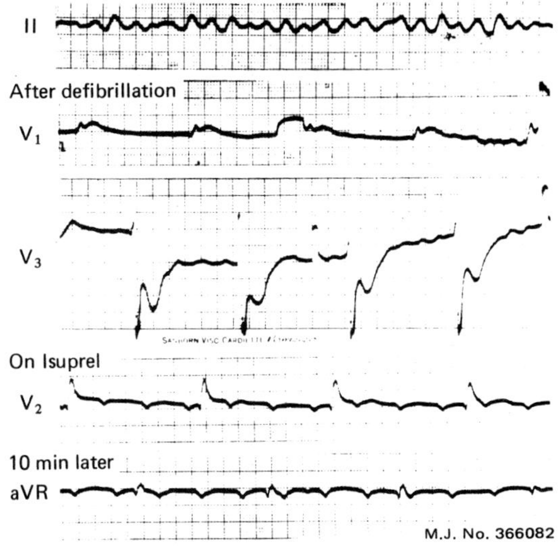

Figure 15–24. Ventricular fibrillation in a 67-year-old patient. Electric defibrillation was followed by atrial fibrillation with complete atrioventricular block and marked myocardial ischemia. After isoproterenol, sinus rhythm with rate of 112/min has appeared but atrioventricular block persists. Patient did well with implanted pacemaker.

Table 15–9. Hospital follow-up data on surviving patients who had defibrillation.*

	Hospital Deaths (Percent)	Discharged Survivors (Percent)	Totals (Percent)
Acute myocardial infarction	37	31	35
Ischemia without infarction	34	29	32
No acute electrocardiographic change	10	26	17
Complete left bundle branch block†	19	14	17
Complete right bundle branch block	24	7	17
Repeat ventricular fibrillation	50	24	40
Congestive heart failure	69	53	63
Cardiogenic shock	39	5	25
Severe pulmonary complications‡	41	44	42
Severe neurologic deficit	95	12	61
Partial neurologic deficit	5	28	15
No neurologic deficit	. . .	60	25

*Reproduced, with permission, from Liberthson RR & others: Prehospital ventricular defibrillation: Prognosis and follow-up course. N Engl J Med 291:317, 1974.

†Possibly masking an acute myocardial change.

‡Aspiration pneumonia or flail chest.

15–24). The resuscitation efforts are therefore clearly worthwhile.

Many patients who develop ventricular fibrillation have unwitnessed episodes that may be instantaneous or last only minutes and die before medical help can be obtained. In many communities, efforts are under way to train lay people to perform resuscitative measures with the hope that external cardiac massage and artificial respiration will be instituted pending the arrival of a trained ambulance or fire department rescue team.

Background of Patients Who Develop Ventricular Fibrillation

Most patients who develop ventricular fibrillation have known coronary heart disease or a history of hypertension, hypercholesterolemia, ventricular premature beats, or some other evidence of heart disease. Since approximately 60% of all coronary deaths are sudden and since most sudden deaths occur in patients with known coronary disease, identification of coronary patients at greatest risk of cardiac arrest and preventive treatment must take precedence over treatment of cardiac arrest itself if one hopes to decrease the mortality rate from sudden cardiac death.

Although many patients have seen their physician within the month preceding the ventricular fibrillation—and about one-fifth on the day of the arrest because of chest pain, dyspnea, or palpitations—most patients collapse instantaneously and therefore could not be saved by mobile teams but could only be saved if the episode was witnessed by a trained person who immediately instituted restorative measures. The American Heart Association makes available a film for the purpose of encouraging citizens, especially relatives or coworkers of patients who have once been defibrillated or have known coronary heart disease, to take special courses in resuscitation. Cobb (1975) has analyzed the types of activities immediately preceding ventricular fibrillation and notes that only about one-sixth have had unusual physical or mental stress. About one-third of cases occur during sleep, and the great majority of cases of ventricular fibrillation occur during ordinary activities at work or at home. Efforts should probably be concentrated on men under age 60 since these are the individuals most apt to develop ventricular fibrillation.

Course of the Disease: Sudden Cardiac Death
(Table 15–10)

Without treatment, the patient with acute myocardial infarction who develops ventricular fibrillation almost always dies within an hour, with a sequence of ventricular premature beats, complex premature beats, and ventricular tachycardia which then degenerates to ventricular fibrillation. Most cases of cardiac arrest have been found to be due to ventricular fibrillation, although a small percentage are due to cardiac standstill. Some patients have a slow idioventricular rhythm with acute myocardial infarction and then cardiac arrest. It is not known whether cardiac arrest, which is more common in unwitnessed attacks, is always preceded by ventricular fibrillation.

Table 15–10. Breakdown of the patient population showing the follow-up data on 301 subjects with prehospital ventricular fibrillation. (Reproduced, with permission, from Liberthson RR & others: Prehospital ventricular defibrillation: Prognosis and follow-up course. N Engl J Med 291:317, 1974.)

	Patients Alive	Deaths
Monitored prehospital ventricular fibrillation patients	301	102
Defibrillation attempted	199	98
Sent to hospital	101	59
Discharged from hospital	42	

In addition to the poor prognosis of untreated ventricular fibrillation, prospective follow-up of patients who have been resuscitated is unfavorable, with a 30% 1-year mortality rate and a 50% 3-year mortality rate. Most of the recurrences of "sudden cardiac death" occur within the first few months, and patients and their families should be instructed regarding resuscitation and the need to get professional help immediately if another attack occurs during this vulnerable period (Schaffer, 1975).

On physical examination, the patient with ventricular fibrillation is usually unconscious, pulseless, with obvious poor perfusion and cold skin, and apparently dead.

Treatment of Ventricular Fibrillation

Treatment consists of *immediate* emergency resuscitative measures (see Chapter 7) to restore the circulation by external cardiac massage combined with mouth-to-mouth breathing. External massage is given by means of a sharp downward thrust over the lower sternum at a rate of approximately 80/min, combined with 2 or 3 quick breaths with the nose closed and the neck extended (see Chapter 7), and continued at a rate of 18/min until help arrives. If 2 people are available, the inflations and the massage should be continued without interruption until help arrives. The patient must be intubated and defibrillated at the earliest possible moment. In the coronary care unit, with ECG monitoring, resuscitation should be accomplished within 30 seconds after the onset of ventricular fibrillation. Specially trained nurses in the coronary care unit should defibrillate the patient if a doctor is not available. Defibrillation is accomplished with 400 J, repeated if necessary. Lack of tissue perfusion causes anaerobic metabolic acidosis, and it is necessary to give sodium bicarbonate, 44 mEq intravenously every 5–10 minutes, for the duration of arrest. The accumulation of pyruvic and lactic acids and hypercapnia from absent ventilation lead to a low pH, which in turn may induce further arrhythmias and interfere with defibrillation by electric countershock. Arterial pH should be monitored when resuscitation is achieved so that excessive bicarbonate is not given to produce alkalosis.

In the coronary care unit, defibrillation is almost always successful, at least initially, but fibrillation may be recurrent, usually within the first day or so, and antiarrhythmia therapy such as with lidocaine infusion (1–4 mg/min) should be started promptly after the patient is resuscitated.

A. Subsequent Course Following Resuscitation Outside the Hospital: Although about one-half to two-thirds of patients with ventricular fibrillation outside the hospital are satisfactorily defibrillated by ambulance or fire department rescue squads, most of these patients die in the hospital. However, at least 20–25% are discharged alive, often with only mild evidences of cardiac failure or pulmonary complications. Subsequent coronary arteriography almost always shows extensive coronary disease, and approximately half have left ventricular wall motion abnormalities. Severe neurologic deficits are uncommon in patients who are promptly defibrillated. Impaired memory is described by Cobb (1975) as the most common late neurologic sequela. The high incidence of recurrence of fibrillation within the months following release from the hospital indicates that chronic myocardial ischemia is still present. The incidence of recurrence of ventricular fibrillation is greater among persons who show no evidence of myocardial infarction than in those who do.

1. Question of bypass coronary surgery–Because of the extensive coronary disease found on coronary arteriography in most patients recovered from ventricular fibrillation, bypass surgery has been recommended to prevent recurrence. The data are meager, but it is not established that bypass surgery can prevent recurrent attacks of ventricular fibrillation.

2. Prophylactic drugs to prevent recurrences–The same can be said for antiarrhythmia drugs such as quinidine, procainamide, and phenytoin (especially in digitalis toxicity). A number of studies have shown that these drugs may decrease the number of simple or complex ventricular premature beats seen on 24-hour monitoring, but the side-effects are significant and there is as yet only minimal evidence that they will in fact prevent sudden cardiac death even though the number of ventricular premature beats seems to be decreased (Jelinek, Circulation, 1974). New drugs to treat ventricular arrhythmias and prevent ventricular fibrillation are urgently needed. One such drug, mexiletene, available in England but not the USA, seems to have particular promise (Ross, 1974); the dosage is 200–500 mg intravenously given over 5 minutes, followed by an infusion at a rate of 60 mg/hour until its effects can be determined. Others used elsewhere but not yet approved are ajmaline and amiodarone. The unpredictability of the ventricular fibrillation is an especially devastating aspect of this fatal arrhythmia, and efforts are being made to preselect a high-risk group from the coronary heart disease population in which various forms of therapy can be prospectively tested.

3. Value of beta-adrenergic blockade–Various beta-adrenergic blocking agents that are more cardioselective than propranolol (timolol, atenolol, aprenolol) are the only drugs that have decreased the incidence of sudden death when used prophylactically in studies in Europe. The threshold for ventricular fibrillation in dogs exposed to a stressful environment is decreased 50% by a cardioselective beta-adrenergic blocker, tolamolol hydrochloride (not approved by FDA) (Amsterdam, 1976). Propranolol can be used for this purpose in patients who do not have left ventricular failure or bronchospasm. The value of beta-blocking drugs emphasizes the role of adrenergic central nervous system stimuli in causing ventricular arrhythmias. Decreasing these adrenergic stimuli with drugs such as tranquilizers, diazepam, and propranolol may prove to be more valuable than using purely antiarrhythmia drugs such as quinidine and procainamide.

4. Resection of ventricular aneurysms–One group of patients who might benefit from cardiac surgery are those who, following an acute myocardial infarction, develop a ventricular aneurysm with refractory ventricular arrhythmias that might degenerate into ventricular fibrillation, possibly because of persistence of a rim of viable but ischemic tissue on the edge of the aneurysm or the presence of cardiac failure. Resection of the aneurysm, when it is sharply localized with paradoxic motion, may be successful in eliminating the ventricular arrhythmia even if bypass surgery has not been performed. Large, flabby ventricles with dyskinesia or akinesia but without a well-marked or demarcated aneurysm should not be treated by resection of the poorly contracting segments.

B. Control of Risk Factors: Control of risk factors that increase the likelihood of clinical coronary events is a reasonable measure even though it has not been proved that control of hyperlipidemia and hypertension has a significant beneficial effect once coronary heart disease and ventricular fibrillation have occurred. Patients who have had ventricular fibrillation and have been resuscitated should be strongly advised to stop smoking. It is of considerable interest that overt diabetes is uncommon in this group of patients; however, diabetes should be treated if present.

Holter monitoring at monthly intervals following recovery from acute myocardial infarction or from an episode of ventricular fibrillation may identify some individuals in whom spontaneous cardiac pain occurs coincidentally with the development of complex ventricular arrhythmias. This group may benefit from intensive antiarrhythmia or propranolol therapy.

• • •

ANTIARRHYTHMIA DRUGS

The use, mechanisms, and effectiveness of various antiarrhythmia drugs are summarized in Tables 15–4 to 15–8. Further details of drug treatment are discussed throughout the chapter in the sections on treatment of the various arrhythmias.

• • •

References

Achuff SC & others: Mexiletine in the prevention of ventricular dysrhythmias in acute myocardial infarction. Circulation 52 (Suppl 2):147, 1975.

Adgey AAJ & others: Incidence, significance and management of early bradyarrhythmia complicating acute myocardial infarction. Lancet 2:1097, 1968.

Adgey AAJ & others: Management of ventricular fibrillation outside hospital. Lancet 1:1169, 1969.

Allen H, Harris A, Leatham A: Significance and prognosis of an isolated late systolic murmur: A 9- to 22-year follow-up. Br Heart J 36:525, 1974.

Amsterdam EA & others: Efficacy of cardioselective beta adrenergic blockade with intravenously administered tolamolol in the treatment of cardiac arrhythmias. Am J Cardiol 38:195, 1976.

Anderson R & others: Relation between metabolic acidosis and cardiac dysrhythmias in acute myocardial infarction. Br Heart J 30:493, 1968.

Armbrust CA Jr, Levine SA: Paroxysmal ventricular tachycardia: Study of 207 cases. Circulation 1:28, 1950.

Arnsdorf MF: Electrophysiologic properties of antidysrhythmic drugs as a rational basis for therapy. Med Clin North Am 60:213, 1976.

Arnsdorf MF: Membrane factors in arrhythmogenesis: Concepts and definitions. Prog Cardiovasc Dis 19:413, 1977.

Aviado DM, Salem H: Drug action, reaction and interaction. 1. Quinidine for cardiac arrhythmias. J Clin Pharmacol 15:477, 1975.

Ayres SM, Grace WJ: Inappropriate ventilation and hypoxemia as causes of cardiac arrhythmias. Am J Med 46:495, 1969.

Barold S: Therapeutic uses of cardiac pacing in tachyarrhythmias. Page 407 in: *His Bundle Electrocardiography and Clinical Electrophysiology.* Narula OS (editor). Davis, 1975.

Barold SS, Coumel P: Mechanisms of atrioventricular junctional tachycardia: Role of reentry and concealed accessory bypass tracts. Am J Cardiol 39:97, 1977.

Baum RS, Alvarez H III, Cobb LA: Survival after resuscitation from out-of-hospital ventricular fibrillation. Circulation 50:1231, 1974.

Befeler B & others: Electrophysiologic effects of the antiarrhythmic agent disopyramide phosphate. Am J Cardiol 35:282, 1975.

Bigger JT Jr & others: Ventricular arrhythmias in ischemic heart disease: Mechanism, prevalence, significance, and management. Prog Cardiovasc Dis 19:255, 1977.

Bleifer SB & others: Diagnosis of occult arrhythmias by Holter electrocardiography. Prog Cardiovasc Dis 16:569, 1974.

Bloomfield AL: A bibliography of internal medicine: Auricular fibrillation. Arch Intern Med 102:302, 1958.

Bloomfield SS & others: Quinidine for prophylaxis of arrhythmias in acute myocardial infarction. N Engl J Med 285:979, 1971.

Campbell RWF & others: Comparison of procainamide and mexiletine in prevention of ventricular arrhythmias after acute myocardial infarction. Lancet 1:1257, 1975.

Cantwell JD, Dawson JE, Fletcher GF: Supraventricular tachyarrhythmias: Treatment with edrophonium. Arch Intern Med 130:221, 1972.

Chapman JH, Schrank JP, Crampton RS: Idiopathic ventricular tachycardia: An intracardiac electrical, hemodynamic and angiographic assessment of six patients. Am J Med 59:470, 1975.

Chaudron JM & others: Attacks of ventricular fibrillation and unconsciousness in a patient with prolonged QT interval: A family study. Am Heart J 91:783, 1976.

Chung EK: *Principles of Cardiac Arrhythmias.* Williams & Wilkins, 1971.

Cobb LA & others: Resuscitation from out-of-hospital ventricular fibrillation: Four year follow-up. Circulation 52(Suppl 3):223, 1975.

Cohen H, Langendorf R, Pick A: Intermittent parasystole: Mechanism of protection. Circulation 48:761, 1973.

Collinsworth KA, Kalman SM, Harrison DC: The clinical pharmacology of lidocaine as an antiarrhythmic drug. Circulation 50:1217, 1974.

Conrad KA, Molk BL, Chidsey CA: Pharmacokinetic studies of quinidine in patients with arrhythmias. Circulation 55:1, 1977.

Corday E, Lang TW: Hemodynamic consequences of cardiac arrhythmias. Pages 498–502 in: *The Heart, Arteries and Veins,* 3rd ed. Hurst JW & others (editors). McGraw-Hill, 1974.

Cramer G: Early and late results of conversion of atrial fibrillation with quinidine: A clinical and hemodynamic study. Acta Med Scand, Suppl 490, 1968.

Cranefield PF, Wit AL, Hoffman BF: Genesis of cardiac arrhythmias. Circulation 47:190, 1973.

Crawford M & others: Comparative effectiveness of exercise testing and continuous monitoring for detecting arrhythmias in patients with previous myocardial infarction. Circulation 50:301, 1974.

Crouthamel WG: The effect of congestive heart failure on quinidine pharmacokinetics. Am Heart J 90:335, 1975.

Danilo P Jr, Rosen MR: Cardiac effects of disopyramide. Am Heart J 92:532, 1976.

De Leon AC Jr, Harvey WP: Pharmacological agents and auscultation. Mod Concepts Cardiovasc Dis 44:23, 1975.

Denes P & others: Electrophysiological studies in patients with chronic recurrent ventricular tachycardia. Circulation 54:229, 1976.

De Sanctis RW, Babb JW: The role of pacing in the management of cardiac tachyarrhythmias. Pages 223–240 in: *Cardiac Pacing.* Samet P (editor). Grune & Stratton, 1973.

DeSanctis RW, Block P, Hutter AM: Tachyarrhythmias in myocardial infarction. Circulation 45:681, 1972.

Easley RM Jr, Goldstein S: Differentiation of ventricular tachycardia from junctional tachycardia with aberrant conduction: The use of competitive atrial pacing. Circulation 37:1015, 1968.

Epstein SE, Braunwald E: Beta-adrenergic receptor blocking drugs: Mechanism of action and clinical applications. N Engl J Med 275:1106, 1966.

Evans GL, Charles MA, Thornsvard CT: Ventricular tachycardia with retrograde conduction: Simplified diagnostic approach. Br Heart J 38:772, 1976.

Faris JV & others: Incidence and reproducibility of ventricular arrhythmias during maximal exercise testing in normal men. Am J Cardiol 35:136, 1975.

Ferrer MI, Harvey RM: Some hemodynamic aspects of cardiac arrhythmias in man: A clinico-physiologic correlation. Am

Heart J 68:153, 1964.

Fisch C: Relation of electrolyte disturbances to cardiac arrhythmias. Circulation 47:408, 1973.

Fisch C (editor): Symposium on electrophysiological correlates of clinical arrhythmias, (3 parts.) Am J Cardiol 28:243, 371, 499, 1971.

Fisch C: Treatment of arrhythmias due to digitalis. J Indiana State Med Assoc 60:146, 1957.

Fisch C, Knoebel SB: Junctional rhythms. Prog Cardiovasc Dis 13:141, 1970.

Fisch C, Noble RJ: Ventricular tachycardia. Am Heart J 89:551, 1975.

Fowler NO & others: Electrocardiographic changes and cardiac arrhythmias in patients receiving psychotropic drugs. Am J Cardiol 37:223, 1976.

Friedlander RD, Levine SA: Auricular fibrillation and flutter without evidence of organic heart disease. N Engl J Med 211:624, 1934.

Froment R, Gallavardin L, Cohen P: Paroxysmal ventricular tachycardia: A clinical classification. Br Heart J 15:172, 1953.

Gallagher JJ, Damato AN, Lau SH: Electrophysiologic studies during accelerated idioventricular rhythms. Circulation 44:671, 1971.

Gaughan CE & others: Acute oral testing for determining antiarrhythmic drug efficacy. 1. Quinidine. Am J Cardiol 38:677, 1976.

Gettes LS, Surawicz B: Long-term prevention of paroxysmal arrhythmias with propranolol therapy. Am J Med Sci 254:257, 1967.

Gey GO & others: Quinidine plasma concentration and exertional arrhythmia. Am Heart J 90:19, 1975.

Gibson D, Sowton E: The use of beta-adrenergic receptor blocking drugs in dysrhythmias. Prog Cardiovasc Dis 12:16, 1969.

Gillette PC: The mechanisms of supraventricular tachycardia in children. Circulation 54:133, 1976.

Goel BG, Han J: Atrial ectopic activity associated with sinus bradycardia. Circulation 42:853, 1970.

Goldbarg AN: Exercise stress testing in the uncovering of dysrhythmias. Med Clin North Am 60:315, 1976.

Goldman S & others: Inefficacy of "therapeutic" serum levels of digoxin in controlling the ventricular rate in atrial fibrillation. Am J Cardiol 35:651, 1975.

Goldreyer BN: Intracardiac electrocardiography in the analysis and understanding of cardiac arrhythmias. Ann Intern Med 77:117, 1972.

Goldreyer BN: Mechanisms of supraventricular tachycardias. Annu Rev Med 26:219, 1975.

Goldreyer BN, Kastor JA, Kershbaum KL: The hemodynamic effects of induced supraventricular tachycardia in man. Circulation 54:783, 1976.

Goldschlager N, Cake D, Cohn K: Exercise-induced ventricular arrhythmias in patients with coronary artery disease: Their relation to angiographic findings. Am J Cardiol 31:434, 1973.

Gouaux JL, Ashman R: Auricular fibrillation with aberration simulating ventricular paroxysmal tachycardia. Am Heart J 34:366, 1947.

Gradman AH & others: Suppression of premature ventricular contractions by acebutolol. Circulation 55:785, 1977.

Greenblatt DJ, Koch-Weser J: Drug therapy: Clinical pharmacokinetics. (2 parts.) N Engl J Med 293:702, 964, 1975.

Grossman JJ, Cooper JA, Frieden J: Hemodynamic and antiarrhythmic effects of edrophonium chloride (Tensilon). Circulation 40 (Suppl 3):97, 1969.

Haft JI: Treatment of arrhythmias by intracardiac electrical stimulation. Prog Cardiovasc Dis 16:539, 1974.

Han J: Mechanisms of ventricular arrhythmias associated with myocardial infarction. Am J Cardiol 24:800, 1969.

Han J & others: Incidence of ectopic beats as a function of basic rate in the ventricle. Am Heart J 72:632, 1966.

Harvey WP, Ronan JA Jr: Bedside diagnosis of arrhythmias. Prog Cardiovasc Dis 8:419, 1966.

Helfant RH & others: The clinical use of DPH (Dilantin) in the treatment and prevention of cardiac arrhythmias. Am Heart J 77:315, 1969.

Heng MK & others: Effects of intravenous verapamil on cardiac arrhythmias and on the electrocardiogram. Am Heart J 90:487, 1975.

Henry WL & others: Relation between echocardiographically determined left atrial size and atrial fibrillation. Circulation 53:273, 1976.

Hillestad L & others: Quinidine in maintenance of sinus rhythm after electroconversion of chronic atrial fibrillation. Br Heart J 33:518, 1971.

Hinkle LE, Carver ST, Argyros DC: The prognostic significance of ventricular premature contractions in healthy people and in people with coronary heart disease. Acta Cardiol (Brux) Suppl 18:5, 1974.

Hinkle LE Jr, Carver ST, Stevens M: The frequency of asymptomatic disturbances of cardiac rhythm and conduction in middle-aged men. Am J Cardiol 24:629, 1969.

Hirschfeld DS & others: Clinical and electrophysiological effects of intravenous quinidine in man. Br Heart J 39:309, 1977.

Hoffman BF: The genesis of cardiac arrhythmias. Prog Cardiovasc Dis 8:319, 1966.

Hoffman BF, Bigger JT Jr: Antiarrhythmic drugs. Pages 824–852 in: *Drill's Pharmacology in Medicine,* 4th ed. DiPalma JR (editor). McGraw-Hill, 1971.

Hoffman BF, Rosen MR, Wit AL: Electrophysiology and pharmacology of cardiac arrhythmias. 3. The causes and treatment of cardiac arrhythmias. (Part A). Am Heart J 89:115, 1975.

Hoffman BF, Rosen MR, Wit AL: Electrophysiology and pharmacology of cardiac arrhythmias. 7. Cardiac effects of quinidine and procaine amide. (2 parts.) Am Heart J 89: 804; 90:117, 1975.

Holter NJ: New method for heart studies: Continuous electrocardiography of active subjects over long periods is not practical. Science 134:1214, 1961.

Hornbaker JH Jr, Humphries JO, Ross RS: Permanent pacing in the absence of heart block: An approach to the management of intractable arrhythmias. Circulation 39:189, 1969.

Hurst JW, Myerburg RJ: Cardiac arrhythmias: Evolving concepts (2 parts.) Mod Concepts Cardiovasc Dis 37:73, 79, 1968.

James TN: Congenital deafness and cardiac arrhythmias. Am J Cardiol 19:627, 1967.

James TN: Pathogenesis of arrhythmias in acute myocardial infarction. Am J Cardiol 24:791, 1969.

Jelinek MV, Lohrbauer L, Lown B: Antiarrhythmic drug therapy for sporadic ventricular ectopic arrhythmias. Circulation 49:659, 1974.

Jelinek MV, Lown B: Exercise stress testing for exposure of cardiac arrhythmia. Prog Cardiovasc Dis 16:497, 1974.

Jones DT, Kostuk WJ, Gunton RW: Prophylactic quinidine for the prevention of arrhythmias after acute myocardial infarction. Am J Cardiol 33:665, 1974.

Josephson ME & others: The effects of carotid sinus pressure in reentrant paroxysmal supraventricular tachycardia. Am Heart J 88:649, 1974.

Josephson ME & others: Electrophysiological evaluation of disopyramide in man. Am Heart J 86:771, 1973.

Julian DG: Toward preventing coronary death from ventricular fibrillation. Circulation 54:360, 1976.

Julian DG, Valentine PA, Miller CG: Disturbances of rate, rhythm, and conduction in acute myocardial infarction: A prospective study of 100 consecutive unselected patients with the aid of electrocardiographic monitoring. Am J Med 37:915, 1964.

Kahn A, Morris JJ, Citron P: Patient-initiated rapid atrial pacing to manage supraventricular tachycardia. Am J Cardiol 38:200, 1976.

Kastor JA: Digitalis intoxication in patients with atrial fibrillation. Circulation 47:888, 1973.

Kastor JA, DeSanctis RW: The electrical conversion of atrial fibrillation. Am J Med Sci 253:511, 1967.

Katz LN, Pick A: *Clinical Electrocardiography.* Part 1: *The Arrhythmias.* Lea & Febiger, 1956.

Killip T: Management of arrhythmias in acute myocardial infarction. Hosp Pract 7:131, April 1972.

Kimball JT, Killip T: Aggressive treatment of arrhythmias in acute myocardial infarction: Procedures and results. Prog Cardiovasc Dis 10:483, 1968.

Kistin AD: Problems in the differentiation of ventricular arrhythmia from supraventricular arrhythmia with abnormal QRS. Prog Cardiovasc Dis 9:1, 1966.

Kleiger R, Lown B: Cardioversion and digitalis. 2. Clinical studies. Circulation 33:878, 1966.

Knoebel SB, Fisch C: Accelerated junctional escape: A clinical and electrocardiographic study. Circulation 50:151, 1974.

Knoebel SB & others: Computer detection of premature ventricular complexes: A modified approach. Am J Cardiol 38: 440, 1976.

Koch FH, Hancock EW: Ten year follow-up of forty patients with middiastolic click/late systolic murmur syndrome. Am J Cardiol 37:149, 1976.

Koch-Weser J, Klein SW: Procainamide dosage schedules, plasma concentrations, and clinical effects. JAMA 215:145, 1971.

Konecke LL, Knoebel SB: Nonparoxysmal junctional tachycardia complicating acute myocardial infarction. Circulation 45:367, 1972.

Kosowsky BD & others: Occurrence of ventricular arrhythmias with exercise as compared to monitoring. Circulation 44:826, 1972.

Koster RW, Wellens HJJ: Quinidine-induced ventricular flutter and fibrillation without digitalis therapy. Am J Cardiol 38:519, 1976.

Kotler MN & others: Prognostic significance of ventricular ectopic beats with respect to sudden death in the late postinfarction period. Circulation 47:959, 1973.

Krikler D: Verapamil in cardiology. (Review article.) Eur J Cardiol 2:3, 1974.

Langendorf R, Pick A, Katz LN: Ventricular response in atrial fibrillation: Role of concealed conduction in the A–V junction. Circulation 32:69, 1965.

Langendorf R, Pick A, Winternitz M: Mechanisms of intermittent ventricular bigeminy: 1. Appearance of ectopic beats dependent upon length of the ventricular cycle, the "rule of bigeminy." Circulation 11:422, 1955.

Lefkowitz RJ: β-Adrenergic receptors: Recognition and regulation. N Engl J Med 295:323, 1976.

Levi GF, Proto C: Combined treatment of atrial fibrillation with quinidine and beta-blockers. Br Heart J 34:911, 1972.

Levitt B & others: Role of the nervous system in the genesis of cardiac rhythm disorders. Am J Cardiol 37:1111, 1976.

Levitt B & others: Ventricular rhythm disorders and sudden cardiac death. Am J Med 61:449, 1976.

Lewis T: Auricular fibrillation and its relationship to clinical irregularity of the heart. Heart 1:306, 1909–1910.

Lewis T: *Clinical Disorders of the Heartbeat.* Shaw & Sons, 1912.

Liberthson RR & others: Prehospital ventricular defibrillation: Prognosis and follow-up course. N Engl J Med 291:317, 1974.

Lie KI & others: Lidocaine in the prevention of primary ventricular fibrillation: A double-blind, randomized study of 212 consecutive patients. N Engl J Med 291:1324, 1974.

Lie KI & others: Observations on patients with primary ventricular fibrillation complicating acute myocardial infarction. Circulation 52:755, 1975.

Lown B: Electrical reversion of cardiac arrhythmias. Br Heart J 29:469, 1967.

Lown B, Levine SA: The carotid sinus: Clinical value of its stimulation. Circulation 23:766, 1961.

Lown B, Levine SA: Current concepts in digitalis therapy. N Engl J Med 250:866, 1954.

Lown B, Temte JV, Arter WJ: Ventricular tachyarrhythmias: Clinical aspects. Circulation 47:1364, 1973.

Lown B, Verrier RL: Neural activity and ventricular fibrillation. N Engl J Med 294:1165, 1976.

Lown B & others: Effect of a digitalis drug on ventricular premature beats. N Engl J Med 296:301, 1977.

Lown B & others: Monitoring for serious arrhythmias and high risk of sudden death. Circulation 51, 52 (Suppl 3):189, 1975.

Lown B & others: Sleep and ventricular premature beats. Circulation 48:691, 1973.

Lynch JJ & others: Psychological aspects of cardiac arrhythmia. Am Heart J 93:645, 1977.

Marriott HJL: Differential diagnosis of supraventricular and ventricular tachycardia. Geriatrics 25:91, 1970.

Matta RJ, Verrier RL, Lown B: The repetitive extrasystole as an index of vulnerability to ventricular fibrillation. Am J Physiol 230:1461, 1976.

McCord MD, Blount SG: Auricular flutter: A hemodynamic basis of clinical features. Am Heart J 50:731, 1955.

McHenry PL, Morris SN, Kavalier MD: Exercise-induced arrhythmias: Recognition, classification and clinical significance. Cardiovasc Clin 6:245, 1974.

Michaelson SP, Wolfson S: Treatment of supraventricular arrhythmias with propranolol. Cardiovasc Med 1:213, 1976.

Mills P & others: Long-term prognosis of mitral-valve prolapse. N Engl J Med 297:13, 1977.

Morris JJ Jr & others: The changes in cardiac output with reversion of atrial fibrillation to sinus rhythm. Circulation 31:670, 1965.

Moss AJ, Aledort LM: Use of edrophonium (Tensilon) in the evaluation of supraventricular tachycardias. Am J Cardiol 17:58, 1966.

Moss AJ & others: Prognostic grading and significance of ventricular premature beats after recovery from myocardial infarction. Circulation 51, 52 (Suppl 3):204, 1975.

Normand JP & others: Comparative efficacy of short-acting and long-acting quinidine for maintenance of sinus rhythm after electrical conversion of atrial fibrillation. Br Heart J 38:381, 1976.

Norris RM, Mercer CJ: Significance of idioventricular rhythms in acute myocardial infarction. Prog Cardiovasc Dis 16:455, 1974.

Parkinson J, Campbell M: Paroxysmal auricular fibrillation: A record of 200 patients. Q J Med 24:67, 1930.

Parkinson J, Papp C: Repetitive paroxysmal tachycardia. Br Heart J 9:241, 1947.

Paulk EA Jr, Hurst JW: Clinical problems of cardioversion. Am Heart J 70:248, 1965.

Perloff D, Sokolow M: Selected topics in cardiac arrhythmias. Geriatrics 22:190, 1967.

Pick A: Mechanisms of cardiac arrhythmias, from hypothesis to physiological fact. Am Heart J 86:249, 1973.

Pick A, Dominguez P: Nonparoxysmal A–V nodal tachycardia. Circulation 16:1022, 1957.

Pick A, Langendorf R: Differentiation of supraventricular and ventricular tachycardias. Prog Cardiovasc Dis 2:391, 1960.

Pick A, Langendorf R: Recent advances in the differential diagnosis of AV junctional arrhythmia. Am Heart J 76:553, 1968.

Prinzmetal M & others: *The Auricular Arrhythmias.* Thomas, 1952.

Puech P: Ectopic ventricular rhythms: Ventricular tachycardia and His bundle recordings. Page 243 in: *His Bundle Electrocardiography and Clinical Electrophysiology.* Narula O (editor). Davis, 1975.

Ricks WB & others: Surgical management of life-threatening ventricular arrhythmias in patients with coronary artery disease. Circulation 56:38, 1977.

Rodstein M, Wolloch L, Gubner RS: Mortality study of the significance of extra-systoles in an insured population. Circulation 44:617, 1971.

Romero CA Jr: Holter monitoring in the diagnosis and management of cardiac rhythm disturbances. Med Clin North Am 60:299, 1976.

Rosen KM: Junctional tachycardia: Mechanisms, diagnosis, differential diagnosis, and management. Circulation 47:654, 1973.

Rosen MR, Hoffman BF, Wit AL: Electrophysiology and pharmacology of cardiac arrhythmias. 5. Cardiac antiarrhythmic effects of lidocaine. Am Heart J 89:526, 1975.

Rosen MR, Wit AL, Hoffman BF: Electrophysiology and pharmacology of cardiac arrhythmias. 1. Cellular electrophysiology of the mammalian heart. Am Heart J 88:380, 1974.

Rosen MR, Wit AL, Hoffman BF: Electrophysiology and pharmacology of cardiac arrhythmias. 6. Cardiac effects of verapamil. Am Heart J 89:665, 1975.

Rosenbaum MB & others: Intraventricular trifascicular blocks: Review of the literature and classification. Am Heart J 78:450, 1969.

Ross JC, Paalman ACA, Dunning AJ: Electrophysiological effects of mexiletine in man. Br Heart J 38:1261, 1976.

Runge P & others: Variability of ambulatory arrhythmias during weekly ECG monitoring. Circulation 49, 50 (Suppl 3):111, 1974.

Rutkowski MM, Doyle EF, Cohen SN: Drug therapy of heart disease in pediatric patients. 3. The therapeutic challenge of supraventricular tachyarrhythmias in infants and children. Am Heart J 86:562, 1973.

Ryan M, Lown B, Horn H: Comparison of ventricular ectopic activity during 24-hour monitoring and exercise testing in patients with coronary heart disease. N Engl J Med 292:224, 1975.

Samet P: Hemodynamic sequelae of cardiac arrhythmias. Circulation 47:399, 1973.

Sandler IA, Marriott HJL: The differential morphology of anomalous ventricular complexes of RBBB-type in lead V_1: Ventricular ectopy versus aberration. Circulation 31:551, 1965.

Schaffer WA, Cobb LA: Recurrent ventricular fibrillation and modes of death in survivors of out-of-hospital ventricular fibrillation. N Engl J Med 293:259, 1975.

Schamroth L: The pathogenesis and mechanism of ventricular arrhythmias. Pages 75–111 in: *Progress in Cardiology.* Yu PN, Goodwin JR (editors). Lea & Febiger, 1974.

Scheinman MM, Hutchinson JC: Cavitary left atrial electrograms after open-heart surgery. J Thorac Cardiovasc Surg 57: 400, 1969.

Scherf D, Cohen J: Atrioventricular rhythms. Prog Cardiovasc Dis 8:499, 1966.

Scherf D, Schott A: Pages 381–441 in: *Extrasystoles and Allied Arrhythmias.* Grune & Stratton, 1953.

Scherf D & others: On the response of ectopic auricular tachycardias to vagus stimulation. Am Heart J 45:95, 1953.

Scherf D & others: Paroxysmal tachycardia precipitated by atrial and ventricular extrasystoles. Am J Cardiol 11:757, 1963.

Schoonmaker FW, Osteen RT, Greenfield JC Jr: Thioridazine (Mellaril)-induced ventricular tachycardia controlled with an artificial pacemaker. Ann Intern Med 65:1076, 1966.

Schroeder JS: Ambulatory electrocardiographic monitoring: Technique and clinical indications. JAMA 236:494, 1976.

Schulze RA Jr & others: Ventricular arrhythmias in the late hospital phase of acute myocardial infarction: Relation to left ventricular function detected by gated cardiac bloodpool scanning. Circulation 52:1006, 1975.

Seides SF: The electrophysiology of propranolol in man. Am Heart J 88:733, 1974.

Selzer A, Wray HW: Quinidine syncope: Paroxysmal ventricular fibrillation occurring during treatment of chronic atrial arrhythmias. Circulation 30:17, 1964.

Shine KI, Kastor JA, Yurchak PM: Multifocal atrial tachycardia: Clinical and electrocardiographic features in 32 patients. N Engl J Med 279:344, 1968.

Simcha A, Carter RAB: Paroxysmal atrial tachycardia in infants and children. Lancet 1:832, 1971.

Singh BN, Vaughan Williams EM: A fourth class of antidysrhythmic action? Effect of verapamil on ouabain toxicity, on atrial and ventricular potentials, and on other features of cardiac function. Cardiovasc Res 6:109, 1972.

Sinno MZ, Gunnar RM: Hemodynamic consequences of cardiac dysrhythmias. Med Clin North Am 60:69, 1976.

Skinner NS & others: Hemodynamic consequences of atrial fibrillation at constant ventricular rates. Am J Med 36:342, 1964.

Skinner NS Jr & others: Hemodynamic effects of altering the timing of atrial systole. Am J Physiol 205:499, 1963.

Södermark T & others: Effect of quinidine on maintaining sinus rhythm after conversion of atrial fibrillation or flutter: A multicentre study from Stockholm. Br Heart J 37:486, 1975.

Sokolow M: Some quantitative aspects of treatment with quinidine. Ann Intern Med 45:582, 1956.

Sokolow M, Ball RE: Factors influencing conversion of chronic atrial fibrillation with special reference to serum quinidine concentration. Circulation 14:568, 1956.

Sokolow M, Edgar AL: Blood quinidine concentration as a guide in the treatment of cardiac arrhythmias. Circulation 1:576, 1950.

Sokolow M, Perloff D: The clinical pharmacology and use of quinidine in heart disease. Prog Cardiovasc Dis 3:316, 1961.

Sowton E & others: Long-term control of intractable supraventricular tachycardia by ventricular pacing. Br Heart J 31:700, 1969.

Sowton E & others: The suppression of arrhythmias by artificial pacing. Lancet 2:1098, 1964.

Spurrell RAJ: Reciprocation: A mechanism for tachycardias. Am Heart J 91:409, 1976.

Stern S: Treatment and prevention of cardiac arrhythmias with propranolol and quinidine. Br Heart J 33:522, 1971.

Stock JPP: *Diagnosis and Treatment of Cardiac Arrhythmias,* 2nd ed. Butterworth, 1970.

Talbot RG, Julian DG, Prescott LF: Long term treatment of ventricular arrhythmias with oral mexiletine. Am Heart J 91:58, 1976.

Talbot S: Fixed and variable coupling of ventricular extrasystoles. Cardiology 58:117, 1973.

Talbot S, Dreifus LS: Characteristics of ventricular extrasystoles and their prognostic importance. Chest 67:665, 1975.

Talbot S, Greaves M: Association of ventricular extrasystoles and ventricular tachycardia with idioventricular rhythm. Br Heart J 38:457, 1976.

Taylor J, Kosowsky B, Lown B: Complications of procainamide in a prospective antiarrhythmic study. Circulation 44 (Suppl 2):43, 1971.

Ticzon AR, Whalen RW: Refractory supraventricular tachycardias. Circulation 47:642, 1973.

Van Durme JP: Tachyarrhythmias and transient cerebral ischemic attacks. Am Heart J 89:538, 1975.

Vassaux C, Lown B: Cardioversion of supraventricular tachycardias. Circulation 39:791, 1969.

Vaughan Williams EM: Classification of antiarrhythmic drugs. Pages 449–472 in: *Symposium on Cardiac Arrhythmias.* Sandøe E, Flensted-Jensen E, Olesen KH (editors). Astra (Sweden), 1970.

Vedin JA & others: Relations of resting and exercise-induced ectopic beats to other ischemic manifestations and to coronary risk factors: Men born in 1913. Am J Cardiol 30:25, 1972.

Verrier RL, Thompson PL, Lown B: Ventricular vulnerability during sympathetic stimulation: Role of heart rate and blood pressure. Cardiovasc Res 8:602, 1974.

Vetter NJ, Julian DG: Comparison of arrhythmia computer and conventional monitoring in coronary-care unit. Lancet 1:1151, 1975.

Waldo AL & others: Continuous rapid atrial pacing to control recurrent or sustained supraventricular tachycardias following open heart surgery. Circulation 54:245, 1976.

Wallace AG & others: Electrophysiologic effects of quinidine. Circ Res 21:960, 1966.

Watanabe Y, Dreifus LS: Arrhythmias: Mechanisms and pathogenesis. Page 35 in: *Cardiac Arrhythmias.* Dreifus LS, Likoff W (editors). Grune & Stratton, 1973.

Weisberger AS, Feil H: Lanatoside C in the treatment of persistent paroxysmal auricular tachycardia. Am Heart J 34:871, 1947.

Wellens HJ: Pathophysiology of ventricular tachycardia in man. Arch Intern Med 135:473, 1975.

Wellens HJ, Durrer D: Effect of procainamide, quinidine, and ajmaline in Wolff-Parkinson-White syndrome. Circulation 50:114, 1974.

Wellens HJJ & others: Effect of digitalis in patients with paroxysmal atrioventricular nodal tachycardia. Circulation 52:779, 1975.

Wetherbee DG, Brown MG, Holzman D: Ventricular rate response following exercise during auricular fibrillation and after conversion to normal sinus rhythm. Am J Med Sci 223:667, 1952.

Wigle ED & others: Mitral valve prolapse. Annu Rev Med 27: 165, 1976.

Winkle RA, Glantz SA, Harrison DC: Pharmacologic therapy of ventricular arrhythmias. Am J Cardiol 36:629, 1975.

Winkle RA & others: Clinical efficacy and pharmacokinetics of a new orally effective antiarrhythmic, tocainide. Circulation 54:884, 1976.

Winkle RA & others: Treatment of recurrent symptomatic ventricular tachycardia. Ann Intern Med 85:1, 1976.

Wit AL, Hoffman BF, Rosen MR: Electrophysiology and pharmacology of cardiac arrhythmias. 9. Cardiac electrophysiologic effects of beta adrenergic receptor stimulation and blockade. (3 parts.) Am Heart J 90:521, 665, 795, 1975.

Wit AL, Rosen MR, Hoffman BF: Electrophysiology and pharmacology of cardiac arrhythmias. 2. Relationship of normal and abnormal electrical activity of cardiac fibers to the genesis of arrhythmias. B. Reentry. Section II. Am Heart J 88:798, 1974.

Wit AL, Rosen MR, Hoffman BF: Electrophysiology and pharmacology of cardiac arrhythmias. 8. Cardiac effects of diphenylhydantoin. Am Heart J 90:265, 1975.

Wolff L: Clinical aspects of paroxysmal rapid heart action. N Engl J Med 226:740, 1942.

Wu D, Denes P: Mechanisms of paroxysmal supraventricular tachycardia. Arch Intern Med 135:437, 1975.

Yoon MS, Han J, Fabregas RA: Effects of ventricular aberrancy on fibrillation threshold. Am Heart J 89:599, 1975.

Yurchak PM: Differential diagnosis of atrial tachyarrhythmias. Postgrad Med 53:31, April 1973.

Zipes DP, Fisch C: ECG analysis No. 1: Premature ventricular beats. Arch Intern Med 128:140, 1971.

Zipes DP, Fisch C: ECG analysis No. 10: Supraventricular arrhythmias with abnormal QRS complex. Arch Intern Med 130:781, 1972.

Zoll PM: Resuscitation of the heart in ventricular standstill by external electrical stimulation. N Engl J Med 247:768, 1952.

16 . . .
Infective Endocarditis

GENERAL CONSIDERATIONS

Changing Characteristics of Endocarditis

Use of the term infective endocarditis reflects the view that it is no longer appropriate to think of acute and subacute endocarditis as separate diseases or to think only of bacteria as possible causes. Endocarditis now appears in so many forms and is caused by so many different organisms, bacterial (including rickettsial) and fungal (rarely viruses or parasites), that the classic distinction between acute and subacute forms has become blurred and artificial. Some cases are hyperacute, some are chronic, and the range of severity frustrates any attempt at neat classification into 2 types. The same organism may cause either acute or subacute endocarditis depending on its virulence and the status of the host defenses.

The clinical features of infective endocarditis have changed to some degree as a result of factors that play a role both in producing the disease and in modifying its course. While classic cases of subacute bacterial endocarditis due to *Streptococcus viridans* in chronic rheumatically diseased valves still occur, new forms of the disease are seen in which infection occurs in a patient who is already taking one or more antibiotics on a long- or short-term basis. Such patients may have subacute infections with virulent organisms or low-grade infections with exotic organisms not ordinarily encountered in "spontaneously" occurring disease.

The Compromised Host

Alterations in the susceptibility of the host due to corticosteroid or immunosuppressive therapy (or, rarely, congenital deficiency of the immune mechanism) may lower the patient's resistance and make it possible for normally nonpathogenic organisms such as serratia and the fungi to flourish in the bloodstream. However, endocarditis rarely results. An important form of endocarditis occurs as a result of intravenous drug abuse, chiefly with heroin, and following cardiac surgery. Extraneous factors have so altered the course of endocarditis that it is necessary to think in terms of a much wider spectrum of disease than heretofore.

Endocarditis in the Preantibiotic Era

Before antibiotic drugs came into widespread use, subacute infective endocarditis was uniformly fatal within months to about 2 years. Acute infective endocarditis was rare because patients with overwhelming septicemic infections did not live long enough to develop clinical manifestations of cardiac involvement, although vegetations were often seen on the heart valves at autopsy. Soon after penicillin was introduced for the treatment of endocarditis, it became clear that although the infection could usually be brought under control, it damaged the heart valve and was likely to aggravate the valvular disease by causing increased incompetence. This complication was more likely to be important in patients who originally showed minimal hemodynamic changes of valvular disease. The situation in patients with acute endocarditis was similar in that the infection, even if controlled by antibiotic therapy, severely damaged the valve and made it acutely incompetent, leading to acute heart failure that was often fatal. Thus, with the advent of antibiotic therapy, infective endocarditis came to be both a complication and a cause of valvular disease, and the prevention of acute valvular damage and its surgical treatment became almost as important as control of the infection.

Current Status of Endocarditis

Infective endocarditis often is still an insidious disease, not diagnosed during life, tending to occur in patients who are already acutely or chronically ill from other causes. Early diagnosis and early and effective specific antibiotic therapy are vital not only because the chances of eradicating the infection are greater with early treatment but also because the likelihood of damage to the heart valve by the infection increases with the length of time the infection is uncontrolled.

Increase in Frequency of Endocarditis

The increase in the number of patients with atherosclerotic changes as a result of advanced age, the introduction of prosthetic heart valves, the use of immunosuppressive drugs, and the prevalence of intravenous drug abuse have tended to increase the number of patients in whom endocarditis develops insidiously. The increase in the complexity of diagnostic and therapeutic procedures, the large number of patients in whom long-term venous catheterization is used, and the increased numbers of patients treated by peritoneal dialysis and hemodialysis as well as by prolonged use of multiple broad-spectrum antibiotics have provided increased opportunities for organisms to enter the bloodstream and have also increased the variety of organisms to which the patient may be exposed.

Changing Etiology & Symptoms

Many of the classic features of subacute bacterial endocarditis that occurred commonly before the antibiotic era are less frequent now because of antibiotic therapy, which is commonly used for any symptoms resembling "flu." Such treatment suppresses but usually does not eradicate the bloodstream infection. As a result, a new "iatrogenetically subacute" form of endocarditis is seen, with an altered pattern of causative organisms. In the past, *S viridans* was responsible for 90–95% of cases of subacute bacterial endocarditis, but this organism is now responsible for only about half of cases and about one-third of all cases of infective endocarditis. The relative frequency of infections with *Staphylococcus aureus, S albus, Streptococcus faecalis* (enterococcus), gram-negative organisms both aerobic and anaerobic, yeasts, and fungi is increasing at the expense of *S viridans.* Each of these organisms may cause either acute or subacute endocarditis. Infections with certain organisms (eg, bacteroides) are still infrequent, but all rare organisms must now be considered possible etiologic agents.

Complexity of Management

These above-mentioned factors have combined to make infective endocarditis one of the most difficult of all cardiac diseases to manage. Not only is the diagnosis often difficult, but the choice of antibiotic, its route of administration, and the assessment of its effects cause problems. In addition, close observation of the patient during therapy is essential because of the likelihood of development of acute heart failure due to acute valvular damage. Acute cardiac catastrophes, such as dehiscence of valve leaflets or prosthetic valves, perforation of valve cusps, rupture of aneurysms, or abscesses of the myocardium into other cardiac chambers with fistula formation—as well as the ever-present threat of serious systemic embolism—make the management of infective endocarditis a difficult and worrying task. Since emergency cardiac surgery may become necessary at a few hours' notice, it is an advantage to treat the patient at a center where facilities and personnel for open heart surgery are available. The period during which the patient is at risk is long because in some cases it is the fibrosis and shrinkage that occur with healing of the endocardial infection that cause or aggravate the valvular incompetence and are responsible for subacute heart failure.

The Need to Differentiate Acute From Subacute Infective Endocarditis

Although acute infective endocarditis is more fulminant and may be caused by organisms which in the past have produced subacute clinical pictures, the treatment of the 2 conditions is similar although the urgency is greater in the acute forms. Acute infective endocarditis is more fulminant—the course is measured in days or weeks rather than months, as is the case in subacute infective endocarditis. *Staphylococcus aureus* rather than *Streptococcus viridans* is most apt to be the responsible organism, and valve destruction and perforation are more likely to occur quickly, leading to rapidly developing cardiac failure. Prompt, specific treatment is essential. Surgical treatment is more often required because rapid destruction of valves may occur. The prognosis is better in subacute than in acute infective endocarditis because valve destruction occurs more slowly. Acute infective endocarditis may be overlooked because it frequently occurs on a normal valve, whereas subacute infective endocarditis often occurs on previously damaged valves. Murmurs may be absent at the onset of acute infective endocarditis, but valve lesions may result in gross insufficiency of the involved valve even though the infection is controlled by antibiotic therapy.

PATHOGENESIS & PATHOLOGY

The presence of pathogens in the bloodstream creates an opportunity for organisms to be deposited on damaged, roughened valves, such as in congenital or rheumatic lesions; the organisms are enmeshed in deposits of fibrin and platelets on the endothelium of the valve to form irregular vegetations. A typical pathologic illustration of subacute bacterial endocarditis on a rheumatic aortic valve is seen in Fig 16–1. The vegetations vary in size and may become quite large and friable in candidal infections. They may occur on the downstream side of the damaged valve, and small fragments may break off, causing embolization to the systemic circulation in left-sided lesions such as mitral and aortic valve disease and to the lungs in right-sided

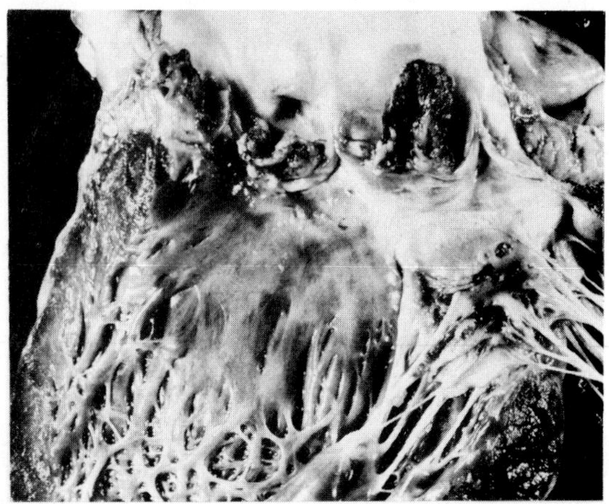

Figure 16–1. Rheumatic aortic valve in a 31-year-old male with *Streptococcus viridans* infection and subacute bacterial endocarditis. (Courtesy of O Rambo.)

lesions, usually on the tricuspid valve. The bacteria may invade the endothelium of the valve but are usually relatively superficial. Effective drug treatment requires penetration of the vegetation in order to reach the bacteria in sufficient concentration to kill them.

Involvement of normal valves. Bacteria and fungi from intravenous injection of infective material (as in "mainline" heroin addicts), from indwelling venous catheters, from infection of arteriovenous shunts, or from bacteria that gain entry during renal dialysis may settle on normal valves, so that Levine's dictum, "No cardiac murmur, no bacterial endocarditis," is no longer tenable. As the bacteria or other organisms become embedded in the fibrin-platelet matrix, further growth of organisms enlarges the vegetation and makes the organisms inaccessible to normal cellular host defenses. Massive bacteremia and infection on the valve may destroy the valve, perforate the leaflets, cause progressive gross incompetence of the involved valves, and allow rapid development or worsening of cardiac failure.

Special valve and congenital factors. Tricuspid lesions are involved in infective endocarditis almost exclusively in intravenous drug users, and the relative frequency of left- and right-sided lesions in such patients varies in different cities and institutions. Pulmonary stenosis, patent ductus arteriosus, ventricular septal defect, and bicuspid aortic valve are the most common congenital cardiac lesions in which endocarditis develops. Infective endocarditis is rare in atrial septal defect (especially in secundum defects).

Precipitating factors. A precipitating factor should always be sought. Dental procedures (extraction or deep scaling), recent instrumentation of the genitourinary tract, gynecologic procedures, or inflammatory gastrointestinal disease sometimes precede the illness. In about half of subacute cases, no cause can be established; fewer cases of acute endocarditis are of unknown cause. In acute infective endocarditis, septicemia due to any cause plus the special situations previously mentioned is often present.

Other factors and influences. Embolism from discharge of fragments of the vegetation into the systemic or pulmonary circulation is responsible for many of the clinical features, as will be noted later. Surgical drainage in addition to antibiotics may be required for metastatic abscesses.

Endocarditis is more apt to occur in patients with mild to moderate valvular disease. For example, it is rare in severe mitral stenosis and infrequent in patients with established atrial fibrillation.

Host defenses with antibody formation, local attempts at repair, and local macrophage infiltration can be seen at autopsy but rarely are adequate in themselves to clear the infection. Age is a factor; most cases occur in young adults, but older and younger persons are not immune to the disease. At present the age distribution is bimodal, with younger individuals most apt to have acute infective endocarditis and older ones subacute endocarditis, probably because of the presence of unoperated rheumatic valvular disease in the older patients. Current data indicate that the median age at onset is 45 years, 25% of patients are over 60 years of age, and only 7% are under 20 years of age (Mills, 1974). For earlier data, see Fig 16–2.

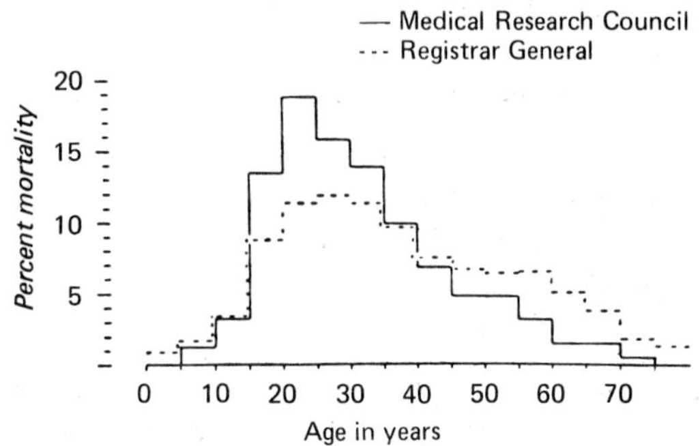

Figure 16–2. The age incidence in 408 cases in the Medical Research Council series, compared with the age incidence in 4531 deaths due to acute or subacute bacterial endocarditis derived from the Registrar General's Reviews 1940-1944. Ages are shown in groups of 5 years. *Note:* The age distribution has undergone a marked shift to the right in the last quarter century. (Reproduced, with permission, from Cates JE, Christie RV: Subacute bacterial endocarditis. Q J Med (New Series) 20:93, 1951.)

CLINICAL FEATURES

1. SUBACUTE INFECTIVE ENDOCARDITIS

Diagnosis

The onset of endocarditis may be chronic and insidious and, unless one searches for infections due to bacteria or fungi in every patient in whom the combination of fever and valvular lesions coexists, the diagnosis can be missed for weeks or months. The presenting symptoms are usually nonspecific and are often attributed to a febrile illness (eg, "flu") because the symptoms include fever, malaise, arthralgia, muscle pains with fatigue, and chills with high fever in the acute varieties. If short-term antibiotic treatment is given, the clinical picture is that of recurrent "flu."

The diagnostic features of endocarditis can be categorized under the headings fever and infection, valvular lesions, and evidence of systemic or pulmonary emboli. If the diagnosis is suspected from the presence of a murmur or valve lesion, fever, and emboli, blood cultures must be obtained.

A. Fever: Fever is the most frequent presenting sign and may appear without apparent predisposing cause or may follow a major or minor surgical procedure. Prostatic and other urogenital operations in men and dilatation and curettage of the uterus, septic abortion, and other gynecologic procedures in women are sometimes precursors of endocarditis, both acute and

Table 16–1. Major arterial emboli diagnosed during life.*

Site of Embolism	Time of Embolism: Before Treatment	During Treatment	After Treatment	Not Specified	Total
Brain	33	22	12	6	73
Eye	7	2			9
Coronary		3	5		8
Spleen	16	10	2	9	37
Kidney	7	1		6	14
Mesentery	1	2	2	1	6
Aortic			1		1
Iliac			1		1
Femoral		1			1
Popliteal	3	1			4
Leg	1	1	1		3
Axillary				1	1
Arm and forearm		1		2	3
Not specified		1		2	3
Total	63	45	24	27	164

*Reproduced, with permission, from Cates JE & Christie RV: Subacute bacterial endocarditis. Q J Med (New Series) 20:93, 1951.

subacute. Weakness, malaise, and loss of weight without fever may occur in debilitated or elderly patients, especially if antibiotics have been given even in small doses, and may occasionally be due to acute renal failure secondary to endocarditis. The symptoms may be overlooked in elderly patients, in whom the diagnosis is often missed or is made only at autopsy. The higher mortality rate in these patients is probably due to delayed diagnosis and thus delayed onset of effective antibiotic therapy. In uremic, elderly, and debilitated patients, fever is often absent.

B. Emboli: Acute systemic embolism may be the presenting symptom and may occur at any time during the course of the disease (Table 16–1). Emboli are usually small except in candida or serratia infections (acute or chronic) and are usually characterized by microscopic hematuria (which may also be due to immune complex disease) or petechiae. Osler's nodes, one of the best-known manifestations of infective endocarditis, were described by Osler in 1893 as ephemeral painful, nodular erythematous spots on the skin, chiefly of the hands and feet. The site where the lesions eventually appear is usually painful first. Although Osler thought that these cutaneous manifestations were probably caused by minute emboli, other investigators have thought that they might be due to an immune mechanism. However, aspirates from the nodes at autopsy reveal pathogenic organisms, and histologic examination reveals a microabscess in the papillary dermis, together with microemboli in the nearby dermal arterioles, making suspect the theory of vasculitis resulting from an immunologic reaction (Alpert, 1976). Nontender nodules on the soles of the feet and the palms of the hands (Janeway's lesion) are thought now to be a hypersensitivity reaction or deposit of immune complex but were formerly thought to be emboli. Emboli to the systemic circulation are uncommon in right-sided valvular lesions of acute endocarditis; the right-sided manifestations are recurrent pneumonia or pulmonary embolism.

1. Small emboli—In left-sided lesions, emboli to the skin may be manifested by splinter hemorrhages in the nails of the fingers or toes (but these may occur in individuals engaged in manual labor). Petechiae (usually on the conjunctiva or hard palate or around the neck and upper trunk) are more definite evidence of embolism. At first they are red and small, but when observed over a period of days they become brown and gradually fade. Hemorrhagic areas with white centers may be seen in the fundi owing to emboli in the nerve fiber retinal layer (Roth spots). These are less common than petechiae. Emboli to the kidney may cause flank pain or microscopic hematuria. Petechiae and microscopic hematuria must be specifically sought every day.

2. Large emboli—Large emboli may involve (1) the cerebral arteries, causing hemiplegia, other central nervous system deficit, neurologic syndromes including headache, psychiatric symptoms, confusion, or sterile meningitis; (2) the coronary arteries, resulting in acute myocardial infarction; or (3) the vasa vasorum, leading to mycotic aneurysms. These last may rupture, often after prodromal symptoms of headache and somnolence if they involve the cerebral arteries. When such prodromal symptoms are present, cerebral angiography should be performed to establish the presence of mycotic aneurysms so that appropriate surgical therapy can be planned. Mycotic aneurysms may appear anywhere, often in branches of the renal artery. Rupture is infrequent, and these lesions are often missed.

3. Septic abscesses—If staphylococci are the infecting organisms in either acute or subacute cases, septic abscesses may develop, especially in the liver, kidney, brain, and spleen, and treatment will be unavailing until the lesion is drained surgically. Septic abscesses may contribute to continued fever and require surgical incision even though the organisms on the endocardium of the valves have been eradicated.

4. Splenomegaly and clubbed fingers—These are less common in acute endocarditis and in subacute cases of short duration. They are usually late signs in untreated patients and, although they were common in the preantibiotic era, are much less common today (approximately 10% of cases). As in any systemic infection, splenomegaly may occur, although it is less frequent when antibiotic therapy is given early in the course of the disease.

C. Immune Complex Nephritis and Renal Emboli: Glomerulonephritis and renal failure are frequently seen in infective endocarditis and were formerly thought to be embolic in origin. More recently it has become evident that the renal lesions are immunologic in origin and are due to the deposit of antigen-antibody complexes and complement on the glomerular basement membrane. Immunofluorescence of renal biopsy specimens demonstrates granular deposits of IgM and C3 in all glomeruli studied (Perez, 1976). The antigen in glomerular deposits corresponds to the organism found in blood cultures.

D. Anemia: Normocytic anemia is common, especially in long-standing infection, and probably accounts in part for the weakness and lassitude seen in patients with chronic infective endocarditis.

E. Cardiac Findings: Symptoms of heart disease such as dyspnea or palpitations develop late in subacute (in contrast to acute) infective endocarditis, and the cardiac origin of the illness may only be suspected if murmurs or a known valvular lesion is present or if embolic manifestations appear.

In subacute infective endocarditis a murmur is almost always present, indicating previous valve involvement of rheumatic or congenital origin. The valve involvement is usually mild to moderate, and patients may not know they have a cardiac lesion. Careful auscultation for the presence of such a lesion is mandatory in suspicious cases, and subacute endocarditis is an important cause of fever of unknown origin in patients in whom cardiac disease is overlooked.

Recently, it has been appreciated that lesions heretofore not considered to be possible predisposing causes of subacute infective endocarditis may in fact be important etiologic factors. These include prolapsed mitral valve (systolic click-murmur syndrome), fibrosis and calcification of the annulus of the mitral valve, and atherosclerosis of the aortic ring and valve. Prolapse of the mitral valve can often be demonstrated by echocardiography (see Chapter 12) or angiography. Echocardiography may also be helpful and occasionally is diagnostic in doubtful cases of vegetations on the aortic valve, especially if they are large (> 5 mm), as in fungal infections (Fig 16–3). Echocardiography is less helpful when endocarditis involves the mitral valve.

Changing murmurs help in diagnosis of acute infective endocarditis when the fulminant valve lesions progress rapidly. They are much less helpful in subacute infective endocarditis when the changing murmurs are probably due in large part to anemia, tachycardia, or other hemodynamic variables that change from one time of examination to another. The abrupt appearance of a diastolic murmur, such as that of aortic insufficiency, is more helpful, as are the developing signs of tricuspid insufficiency in acute infective endocarditis (see below).

Cardiac failure formerly was a late occurrence, as was the development of atrial fibrillation. Untreated patients often died of infection before cardiac failure could develop. Early cardiac failure is frequent today in acute cases, but in subacute cases it may not occur until months after bacteriologic cure, as infection heals and valve lesions worsen (especially aortic valve lesions). Pericarditis is infrequent.

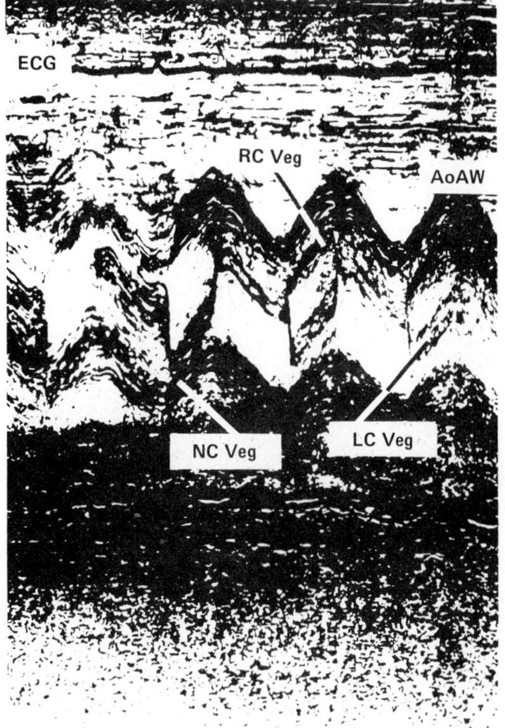

Figure 16–3. Echocardiogram shows dense posteriorly moving echoes indicating aortic valve vegetations in a patient with aortic valve endocarditis. NC, noncoronary cusp; LC, left coronary cusp; RC, right coronary cusp; AoAW, anterior aortic wall. (Reproduced, with permission of the American Heart Association, Inc., from Hirschfeld DS, Schiller N: Localization of aortic valve vegetations by echocardiography. Circulation 53:280, 1976.)

Laboratory Findings: Blood Cultures

The definitive diagnosis is made in suspected cases by finding a positive blood culture, which is discovered in 80–90% of cases where competent laboratory assistance is available. Organisms are discharged into the circulation independently of the time of the fever.

The important principles regarding blood cultures for infective endocarditis are the following:

(1) For subacute cases 2 separate cultures should be obtained daily for 2–3 days. For acute cases, 2–3 cultures are obtained during the several hours of initial clinical work-up.

(2) Both aerobic and anaerobic bacteria, yeasts, and fungi should be sought with appropriate technics.

(3) The cultures must be incubated long enough (1–3 weeks) to allow slow-growing organisms to emerge, and appropriate subcultures must be performed.

(4) At least 2 cultures should yield the same organism to rule out contamination.

(5) Blood cultures must be obtained before antibiotics are started. Alternatively, antimicrobials should be stopped for 3–7 days before drawing blood for cultures.

(6) If cultures are positive, the sensitivity of the organism to various antibiotics, alone and in combination, should be determined as a guide to treatment (see below).

(7) Venous blood is usually adequate. It is rarely necessary to culture arterial blood or bone marrow.

(8) The more meticulous the technic of blood culture, the less frequent the false-negative blood culture report.

2. ACUTE INFECTIVE ENDOCARDITIS

The circumstances in which acute infective endocarditis occurs are discussed above. This section will emphasize the differences between acute and subacute endocarditis but will discuss also the organisms, the involved valve, and the hemodynamic effects.

Diagnosis

The infection is apt to be more abrupt, with higher fever, chills, and the presence of septic abscesses because the predominant organism is usually *S aureus*, even in heroin addicts who infect the mixture injected with organisms already present in the nose, throat, and skin (Table 16–2). In California, *Candida parapsilosis* and *Serratia marcescens* were unusually frequent organisms in 1971–1974 (Mills, 1976). The symptoms of infection usually predominate, and organisms are more easily cultured and identified than in subacute cases. When the lesion is on the tricuspid valve, however, pulmonary complications of "pneumonia," pulmonary embolism, and pulmonary abscess are dominant. X-rays of the chest reveal pleural effusions and changing pulmonary infiltrates of variable size and shape that may recur. The same is true of subacute right-sided lesions, which are rare. Splenomegaly and clubbed fingers are less frequent. The major postmortem lesions in patients with *S aureus* endocarditis are listed in Table 16–3.

A. Emboli: In fungal endocarditis, emboli are more frequent and can be large and disabling. Cerebral embolism may produce hemiplegia, and the possibility of endocarditis must always be considered in patients who develop acute stroke. Smaller emboli, such as petechiae, are less frequent than in subacute bacterial endocarditis, and the same is true of splinter hemorrhages and Osler's nodes. The decreased frequency of systemic emboli in acute infective endocarditis is due to the frequency of right-sided lesions as well as to the rapid downhill course resulting from the severe infection.

Table 16–2. Organisms cultured in heroin-infected endocarditis with positive blood cultures.*

Organism Cultured	Number
Staphylococcus aureus	25
Staphylococcus aureus and *Streptococcus viridans*	1
Staphylococcus aureus and *Enterobacter aerogenes*	1
Staphylococcus aureus and *Candida albicans*	1
Streptococcus faecalis	3
Streptococcus viridans†	3
Pseudomonas aeruginosa†	2
Staphylococcus epidermidis	2
Diplococcus pneumoniae	1
Enterobacter aerogenes	1

*Slightly modified and reproduced, with permission, from Banks T, Fletcher R, Ali N: Infective endocarditis in heroin addicts. Am J Med 55:444, 1973.

†In one patient *Streptococcus viridans* was cultured on one admission but *Pseudomonas aeruginosa* a year later.

Table 16–3. Major postmortem lesions in 39 patients with *Staphylococcus aureus* endocarditis.*

Lesions	Patients	
	Number	Percent
Myocardial abscesses	14	36
Purulent pericarditis	4	10
Pneumonia, lung abscesses, septic infarcts	19	49
Renal abscesses, septic infarcts, nephritis	22	56
Brain abscesses, septic emboli, or infarcts	11	28
With meningitis	6	
Without meningitis	5	
Meningitis	11	28
Without brain involvement	5	
With brain lesions	6	

*Reproduced, with permission, from Watanakunakorn C, Tan JS, Phair JP: Some salient features of *Staphylococcus aureus* endocarditis. Am J Med 54:473, 1973.

B. Cardiac Findings:

1. Changing murmurs and valve findings—The frequency with which acute infective endocarditis occurs on normal cardiac valves makes serial examination more important than is the case in subacute endocarditis. The development of murmurs and evidence of valvular involvement may be noted if the patient is under close observation as the infection on the valve increases and the vegetations become larger. This is especially true of tricuspid insufficiency in heroin addicts, and careful examination may disclose the progressive appearance and lengthening of a tricuspid systolic murmur, made worse by inspiration as right atrial inflow increases with inspiration. A right-sided gallop rhythm may appear, as may the progressive development of a prominent *v* wave in the jugular venous pulse and enlargement of a tender, pulsating liver with right-sided failure. Valvular vegetations can be demonstrated by echocardiography, as shown in Fig 16–4. When acute infective endocarditis involves the aortic valve, the diastolic murmur may be long and soft and the first sound may be soft because of early closure of the mitral valve (see below). The diastolic pressure may be maintained by reflex peripheral arteriolar vasoconstriction, and early mitral valve closure may be a sign of increasing aortic insufficiency. As the magnitude of the aortic regurgitant flow increases, there is a rapid early diastolic rise in left ventricular pressure and left atrial pressure before the onset of systole, causing a prominent Austin Flint diastolic murmur (see Acute Aortic Incompetence, Chapter 13). These findings are not specific for endocarditis. If hemodynamic measurements are made, the crossover of left ventricular end-diastolic pressure and left atrial pressure precedes the Q wave of the ECG instead of slightly following it at

A

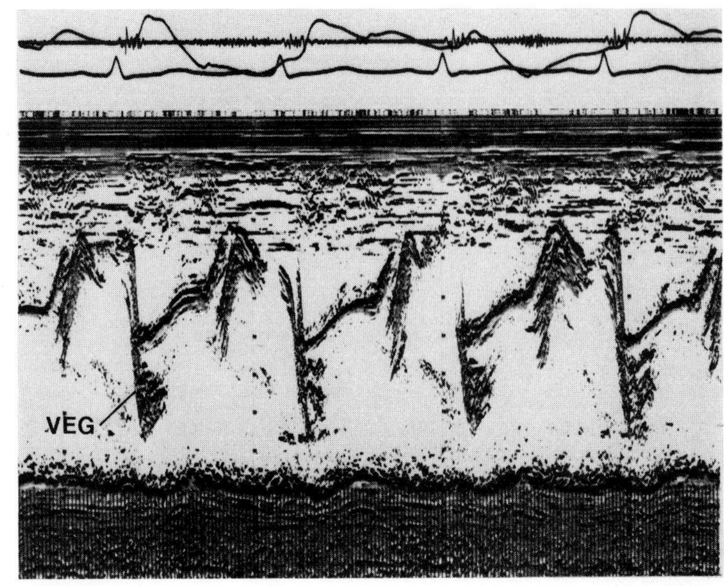

Figure 16–4. *A:* Dense echoes below the tricuspid valve in a patient with acute endocarditis of the tricuspid valve. M mode echocardiogram. (Courtesy of NB Schiller.) *B:* Vegetation on the mitral valve. Real time 2-dimensional echocardiograms. (Courtesy of NB Schiller and NH Silverman.) *C:* Vegetation on the aortic valve. NCC, noncoronary cusp. Real time 2-dimensional echocardiogram. (Courtesy of NB Schiller and NH Silverman.)

B

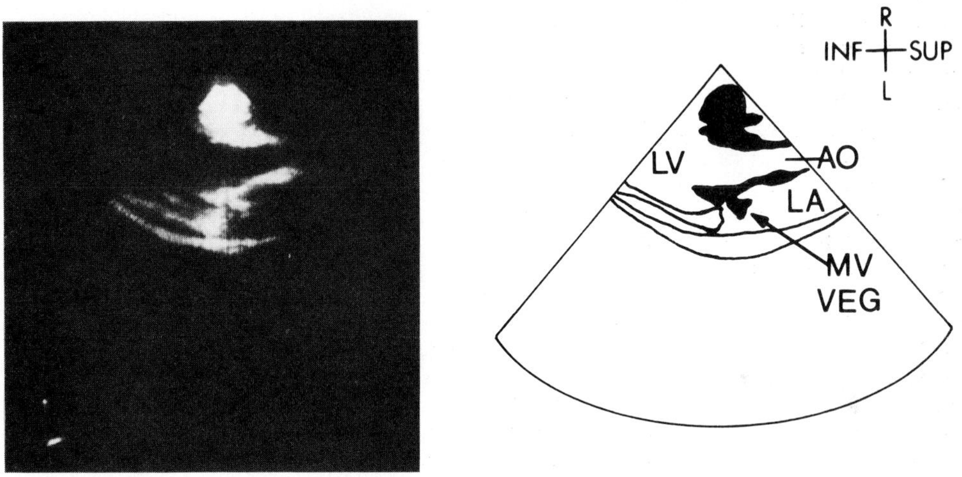

R
INF SUP
L
LV
AO
LA
MV
VEG

C

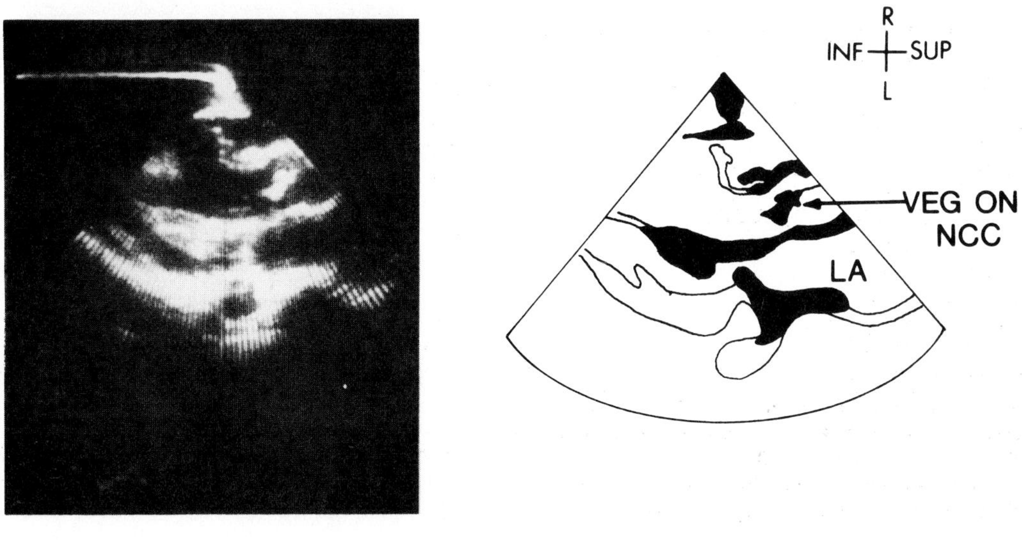

R
INF SUP
L
VEG ON
NCC
LA

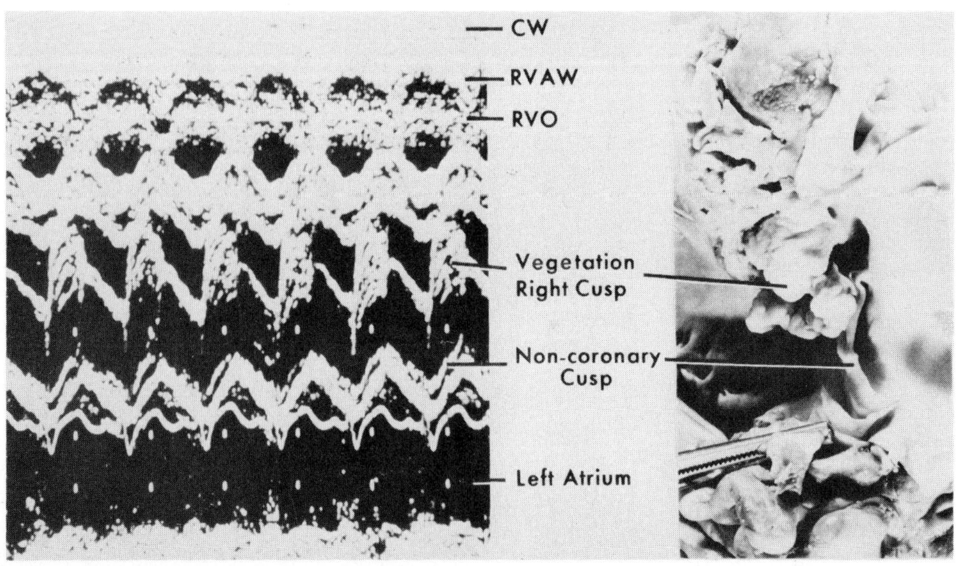

Figure 16–4. (Cont'd.) *D:* Vegetation on the aortic valve shown with anatomic lesion at autopsy. M mode echocardiogram. CW, chest wall; RVAW, right ventricular anterior wall; RVO, right ventricular outflow tract. (Courtesy of NB Schiller.)

the peak or downstroke of the R wave. Early closure of the mitral valve can be clearly demonstrated on echocardiography, when the anterior and posterior leaflets approximate each other well before the onset of the Q wave of the ECG with a normal P–R interval (Fig 16–5). This ominous sign is a harbinger of severe left ventricular failure. The magnitude of the acute aortic insufficiency can also be shown by supra-aortic cineangiography, which shows the left ventricle fully opacified in a single beat of the regurgitant flow.

2. **Cardiac failure**–Cardiac failure is the most feared complication of acute infective endocarditis and may occur with startling rapidity in left-sided lesions, whether mitral or aortic. One cannot use the width of the pulse pressure, the loudness of the murmur, or the size of the left ventricle as a guide to the severity or imminence of left ventricular failure. The left ventricle is often only slightly enlarged, and the ECG may not reveal left ventricular hypertrophy in acute as compared to chronic aortic insufficiency because of the rapid development of aortic or mitral insufficiency (see Chapter 13). Symptoms of pulmonary edema and echocardiographic evidence of marked early closure of a mitral valve lead the physician to suspect perforation or destruction of the aortic valve and indicate the need for valve replacement. Vigorous medical treatment may be needed while the infection subsides so that the sutures will hold. Careful judgment is required to determine the timing of operation if cardiac failure worsens despite control of the infection.

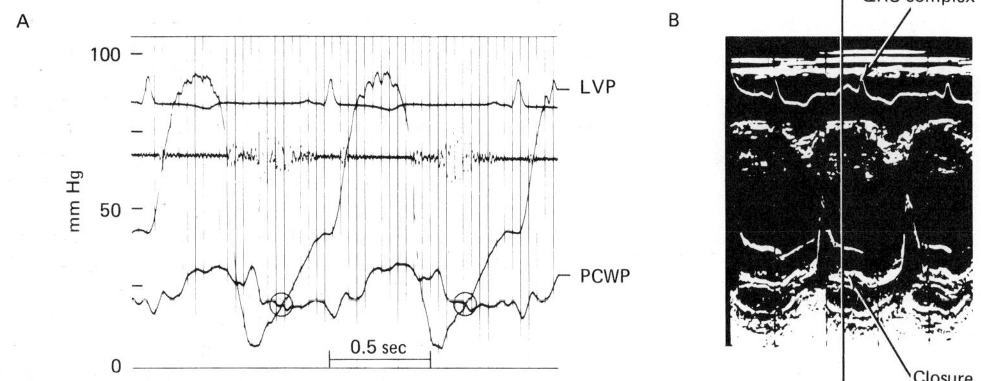

Figure 16–5. *A:* Early closure of the mitral valve. Simultaneous ECG, left ventricular pressure (LVP) and pulmonary capillary wedge pressure (PCWP), and phonocardiogram. Mitral valve closure (circled) occurs when LVP exceeds PCWP, clearly preceding electrocardiographic QRS complex. Phonocardiogram obtained at the cardiac apex demonstrates a middiastolic Austin Flint murmur. (Adapted and reproduced, with permission of the American Heart Association, Inc., from Botvinick EH & others: Echocardiographic demonstration of early mitral valve closure in severe aortic insufficiency: Its clinical implications. Circulation 51:836, 1975.) *B:* Echocardiogram showing mitral valve closure (line) preceding the QRS complex. (Courtesy of NB Schiller.)

3. **Ventricular septum and muscle involvement**— The infection on the aortic valve may spread to the ventricular septum, and abscesses may develop and rupture into the right heart or may interfere with conduction of the cardiac impulse and cause atrioventricular block with or without syncope. Septic abscesses can be suspected if there is sudden development of atrioventricular block or hemiblock. Mitral valve infections may cause septic abscesses of the papillary muscles or destruction of the mitral ring, resulting in flail mitral valves that require prompt surgical correction.

DIFFERENTIAL DIAGNOSIS

Infective endocarditis must be differentiated from all other causes of prolonged and obscure fever (Table 16–4). The diagnosis is based on a positive blood culture in conjunction with the presence of a valve lesion and the absence of diagnostic signs or tests supporting an alternative diagnosis. Infection, neoplasm, and connective tissue disorders are the most common causes of fever of unknown origin (40%, 20%, and 20%, respectively), and these must be excluded.

Table 16–4. Diagnostic categories of fever of undetermined origin.*

Common causes
- Infections
  - Systemic
    - Tuberculosis (miliary)
    - Infective endocarditis (subacute)
    - Miscellaneous rare infections: Cytomegalovirus infection, toxoplasmosis, brucellosis, psittacosis, gonococcemia, chronic meningococcemia, disseminated mycoses
  - Localized
    - Hepatic infections: Liver abscess, cholangitis
    - Other visceral infections: Pancreatic, tubo-ovarian abscesses; empyema of gallbladder; pericholecystic abscess
    - Intraperitoneal infections: Subhepatic, subphrenic, paracolic, appendiceal, pelvic, and other abscesses
    - Urinary tract
      - Pyelonephritis, renal carbuncle, perinephric abscess
      - Prostatic abscess
- Neoplasms
- Collagen-vascular disease

Less common causes
- Granulomatous disease (other than that due to known infectious agents)
- Inflammatory bowel disease
- Pulmonary embolization
- Drug fever
- Factitious fever
- Hepatic cirrhosis with active hepatocellular necrosis
- Miscellaneous uncommon diseases (familial Mediterranean fever, Whipple's disease, etc)

*Reproduced, with permission, from Jacoby GA, Swartz MN: Current concepts: Fever of undetermined origin. N Engl J Med 289:1407, 1973.

The major difficulty in diagnosis occurs when blood cultures are negative, which means that reliance must be placed on associated diagnostic features. This emphasizes the importance of optimally obtained and examined blood cultures.

(1) Bacteremia may be due to pneumonia, septic thrombophlebitis, meningitis, cellulitis, or infected fistulas. There must be evidence of valve lesions as well as emboli before septicemia can be considered to have originated in the heart. Miliary tuberculosis must be kept in mind and serial chest x-rays obtained.

(2) Acute rheumatic fever occasionally is confusing, but only if blood cultures are negative. In acute rheumatic fever the arthralgia or arthritis responds rapidly to salicylates, and there may be erythema marginatum, chorea, or previous beta-streptococcal infection which can be documented by increasing antistreptolysin O titers in the serum.

(3) Neoplasm can be diagnosed by appropriate measures or by biopsy of lymph nodes or bone marrow. If atrial myxoma is suspected, echocardiography and angiography can be diagnostic. (See Chapter 21 for discussion of atrial myxoma.)

(4) Connective tissue disorders must be suspected and diagnosed on the basis of skin or renal lesions, a positive LE cell preparation or antinuclear antibody test, renal biopsy, and negative blood cultures.

PREVENTION OF BACTERIAL ENDOCARDITIS

The American Heart Association has recommended chemoprophylaxis when bacteremia is likely, as with dental extraction or deep scaling, genitourinary instrumentation, and similar procedures (Table 16–5). Some dentists believe that prophylaxis is futile because vigorous chewing may also produce transient bacteremia and continuous prophylaxis to prevent acute rheumatic fever is ineffective or unreasonable.

Beeson (1974) recommends (1) penicillin, 1 million units intramuscularly, plus streptomycin, 0.5 g intramuscularly; or (2) vancomycin, 1 g intravenously immediately before and after urologic or gynecologic procedures, and streptomycin, 0.5 g intramuscularly just before and 6 hours after the procedure.

Chemoprophylaxis at the time of cardiac surgery is universally recommended. It usually consists of penicillin and an aminoglycoside or cefazolin, 1 g of each just 8 and 2 hours before surgery and again 12 hours after surgery. For patients undergoing dental procedures or urologic or pharyngeal surgery, give either (1) procaine penicillin G, 600 thousand units daily intramuscularly for 2 days; or (2) penicillin V, 600 thousand units orally 4 times daily on the day of surgery and for 2 days after surgery. If the patient is sensitive to penicillin, erythromycin, 250 mg orally 4 times daily on the day of surgery and for 2 days after-

Table 16–5. Suggested prophylaxis for gastrointestinal and genitourinary tract surgery and instrumentation and dental procedures. (Adapted from recommendations of the American Heart Association.)

Gastrointestinal and genitourinary tract surgery and instrumentation:

Penicillin plus streptomycin

Give procaine penicillin G, 600 thousand units, mixed with crystalline penicillin G, 200 thousand units, intramuscularly. Administer 1 hour before the procedure and once daily for the 2 days following the procedure.

plus

Streptomycin, 1–2 g intramuscularly 1 hour before the procedure and once daily for the 2 days following the procedure. *Dosage for children:* 40 mg/kg intramuscularly 1 hour before the procedure and once daily for the 2 days following the procedure. (***Caution:*** Dosage must not exceed 1 g/24 hours.)

Ampicillin plus streptomycin

Give ampicillin, 25–50 mg/kg orally or intravenously 1 hour before the procedure and then 25 mg/kg every 6 hours for the remainder of that day and for the 2 days following the procedure.

plus

Streptomycin as above.

Erythromycin plus streptomycin

For patients suspected of being allergic to the penicillins, erythromycin can be given in the dosages set forth under Dental Procedures (below) plus streptomycin as above. Vancomycin can be used as an alternative to erythromycin:

Vancomycin plus streptomycin

Give vancomycin, 0.5 g intravenously 1 hour before the procedure and then 0.5 g intravenously every 6 hours for the remainder of that day and for the 2 days following the procedure. *Dosage for children:* 20 mg/kg 1 hour before the procedure and then 10 mg/kg every 6 hours for the remainder of that day and for the 2 days following the procedure.

plus

Streptomycin as above.

Dental procedures:

Penicillin

1. Intramuscularly: Give procaine penicillin G, 600 thousand units, mixed with crystalline penicillin G, 200 thousand units, 1 hour before the procedure and once daily for the 2 days* following the procedure.
2. Orally: (a) Give penicillin V or phenethicillin, 0.5 g 1 hour before the procedure and then 600 thousand units every 6 hours for the remainder of that day and for the 2 days* following the procedure, or (b) procaine penicillin G, 1.2 million units 1 hour before the procedure and then 600 thousand units every 6 hours for the remainder of that day and for the 2 days* following the procedure.

For patients suspected of being allergic to the penicillins or those receiving continuous *oral* penicillin for rheumatic fever prophylaxis who may harbor penicillin-resistant viridans streptococci, erythromycin may be used as an alternative to penicillin:

Erythromycin†

1. Adults: Give 0.5 g orally 1½–2 hours before the procedure and then 250 mg every 6 hours for the remainder of that day and for the 2 days following the procedure.
2. Children: Give 20 mg/kg orally 1½–2 hours before the procedure and then 10 mg/kg every 6 hours for the remainder of that day and for the 2 days* following the procedure.

*Or longer in the case of delayed healing.

†Erythromycin preparations for parenteral administration are also available.

ward, or vancomycin, 0.5 g every 8 hours intravenously for 1 day, can be given. If the patient is undergoing genitourinary or gastrointestinal surgery and gram-negative bacteremia is likely, kanamycin, 1 g intramuscularly daily, or gentamicin, 120 mg intramuscularly daily, can be used in addition to penicillin.

The available data do not point to a clear choice among the prophylactic regimens described above. There are well-documented cases in which bacterial endocarditis followed a surgical procedure despite an apparently adequate prophylactic regimen.

Prevention of acute endocarditis involves prevention or early treatment of all causes of septicemia that may subsequently affect the cardiac valves; the control of "mainline" drug abuse, which is primarily a social and educational problem; and early recognition of systemic infection in the compromised host. Early recognition and effective treatment of acute endocarditis are mandatory to prevent serious complications and fatalities.

TREATMENT OF INFECTIVE ENDOCARDITIS (Acute, Subacute, Chronic)

General Principles

The cardinal principles of treatment of infective endocarditis are (1) to isolate the infecting organism by obtaining at least 2 positive blood cultures; (2) to determine its susceptibility to various antibiotics, alone and in combination; (3) to choose antimicrobial therapy which is bactericidal and not merely bacteriostatic; and (4) to continue therapy long enough to destroy all the organisms within the vegetation and so to totally eradicate the infection. If septic abscesses are present and do not respond to appropriate antibiotic therapy given long enough, surgical drainage is required if technically feasible. If severe valvular insufficiency develops, along with symptoms of progressive cardiac failure, surgical excision of the involved valve and insertion of a prosthesis must be undertaken with proper timing. The results are less good with tricuspid prostheses than with mitral or aortic ones.

A. Choice of Antibiotic: The choice of antibiotics is based on experience, the results of laboratory sensitivity tests, the status of renal function, and the presence or absence of allergic hypersensitivity to any particular antibiotic, eg, penicillin.

The least toxic but most effective antibiotics, such as the penicillins, are preferable; tetracyclines, erythromycins, lincomycins, and chloramphenicol generally cannot eradicate the infection even if the organism appears to be susceptible in vitro. Aminoglycosides are rarely single drugs of choice but occasionally participate in synergistic drug combinations that provide optimal bacterial action. The objective should be total eradication of the infection. One should choose a regimen shown by experience to result in the highest percentage of cures rather than one which may cure half of cases with oral therapy when parenteral therapy, larger doses, or a longer course of therapy would produce a much higher rate of cure. For example, an infection with *S viridans,* which usually is very sensitive to penicillin, might be cured with 2 weeks of oral therapy, but the likelihood of cure is much greater if one gives the drug parenterally for 3–4 weeks.

The potency of available antibiotics is such that eradication of infection is almost always possible with one drug or a combination of drugs. Deaths are usually due to delayed or inadequate treatment, exotic organisms, septic abscesses, perforation of mycotic aneurysms, or destruction of valves, requiring surgery.

B. Steps in Management:

1. Obtain positive blood culture–It is best to try to withhold therapy until a positive blood culture is obtained so that therapy can be specific. Any complications that occur within a few days before the report of the blood culture are apt to be embolic and probably will not be influenced by immediate therapy. One can therefore withhold drugs unless the patient has a high fever with acute endocarditis, in which case therapy directed to the most common pathogens, *S aureus* and gram-negative organisms, is appropriate until the reports of the blood culture are available and therapy changed accordingly. Unless the clinical situation is urgent, beginning treatment too soon may interfere with the possibility of obtaining a positive blood culture and therefore make specific antibiotic therapy more difficult to select.

2. Parenteral therapy–The antimicrobial agent is best injected as a bolus over a 20-minute period by Volutrol into the intravenous tubing of a continuous intravenous infusion of dextrose and water. Injections should be given every 4–6 hours to avoid deterioration of the antibiotic as well as irritation of the endothelium of the vein receiving the infusion. Some drugs (eg, vancomycin) cause severe pain if given intramuscularly or if extravasation outside the vein occurs; when antimicrobial therapy is required for 4–6 weeks, this is a major factor to be considered, and if there are alternative effective drugs that do not have this disadvantage they should be used. Patients receiving therapy over a period of 4–6 weeks are usually quite comfortable with a slow intravenous drip of glucose and water and intermittent injection of a bolus of antibiotic. The patient can be ambulatory.

3. Duration of therapy–The duration of therapy has always been in some dispute. In general, infection with organisms such as sensitive *S viridans* can be cured in 3–4 weeks, whereas infections with *S aureus* require 5–6 weeks of therapy. The aim of treatment is to cure as many infections as possible, and it is advisable to err on the side of overtreating rather than risk the dangers of stopping too soon and allowing the infection to regain a foothold. Organisms that are more difficult to eradicate, such as candida, may require early surgical

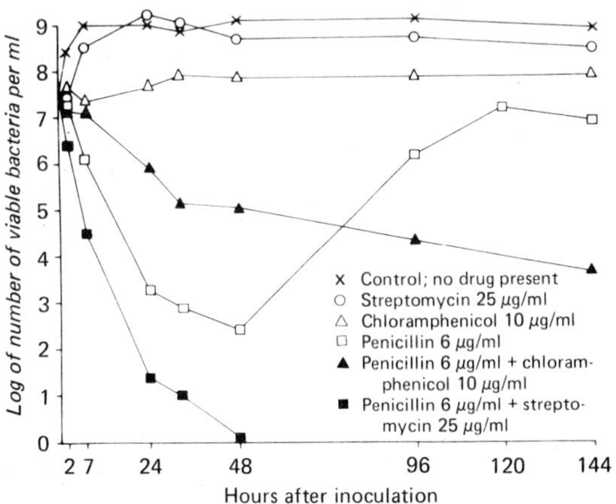

Figure 16–6. The effects of penicillin (6 μg/ml), and chloramphenicol (10 μg/ml), singly and in combination, on a strain of *Streptococcus faecalis* in vitro. The synergistic effect of combined therapy is obvious from the increased bactericidal effect of the combined penicillin and streptomycin (indicated by the dark squares). (Reproduced, with permission, from Jawetz E: Synergism and antagonism among antimicrobial drugs: A personal perspective. West J Med 123:87, 1975.)

excision of the involved valve because drug therapy alone is relatively ineffective.

4. Testing for bactericidal activity–When antimicrobial agents are used singly or in combination, additive or synergistic (Fig 16–6), it is wise to determine if bactericidal concentrations have been achieved by determining the level of serum dilution that is bactericidal for the infecting organism 2 hours after the last dose of the antibiotic. Jawetz (1978) has shown that a dilution of at least 1:8 is desirable in order to assure a satisfactory result. Patients may continue to have occasional fever or embolic phenomena, yet the antibiotic program may be completely effective. Knowing that the serum dilution of ⩾ 1:8 is bactericidal for the organism gives the physician the necessary confidence to continue the antibiotic regimen without changing from one drug to another. It is important to achieve a bactericidal concentration of antibiotics so as not to have the unfortunate experience of giving inadequate therapy for 4–6 weeks only to have to begin all over again when the disease relapses in 1–4 weeks after antibiotics are stopped. Once a course of treatment has been chosen on the basis of all the evidence, it should not be changed without a good reason.

Table 16–6 shows drug selections for various organisms and Table 16–7 their dosage when renal failure is present.

5. Observations during the course of treatment–If a satisfactory antimicrobial regimen has been selected, patients usually begin to feel well within a few days even though occasional fever or embolic phenomena may occur. The subjective feeling of well-being is a very promising therapeutic manifestation, and the converse is also true. A negative blood culture and serum bactericidal activity in adequate dilution (⩾ 1:8) are excellent prognostic features. If the patient continues to have fever, especially with chills, after the start of a regimen which should be effective, the possibility of septic abscesses should be considered; radioactive isotope scans of the liver, kidney, and spleen may be

Table 16–6. Anti-infective chemotherapeutic agents against suspected or proved causes of infective endocarditis.*

Suspected or Proved Etiologic Agent	Drug(s) of First Choice	Alternative Drug(s)
Gram-negative cocci		
Gonococcus	Penicillin[1], ampicillin	Tetracycline[2], spectinomycin
Gram-positive cocci		
Pneumococcus	Penicillin[1]	Erythromycin[3], cephalosporin[4]
Streptococcus, hemolytic groups A, B, C, G	Penicillin[1]	Erythromycin[3]
Streptococcus viridans	Penicillin[1] plus aminoglycoside	Cephalosporin, vancomycin
Staphylococcus, nonpenicillinase-producing	Penicillin[1]	Cephalosporin, vancomycin
Staphylococcus, penicillinase-producing	Penicillinase-resistant penicillin[5]	Cephalosporin, vancomycin, lincomycin
Streptococcus faecalis (enterococcus)	Ampicillin plus aminoglycoside	Vancomycin
Gram-negative rods		
Enterobacter (Aerobacter)	Kanamycin or gentamicin	Chloramphenicol
Bacteroides (except *B fragilis*)	Penicillin[1] or chloramphenicol	Clindamycin
Escherichia		
E coli sepsis	Kanamycin or gentamicin	Cephalosporin, ampicillin
Haemophilus (meningitis, respiratory infections)	Chloramphenicol	Ampicillin, co-trimoxazole[6]
Klebsiella	Cephalosporin or kanamycin	Gentamicin, chloramphenicol
Proteus		
P mirabilis	Penicillin or ampicillin	Kanamycin, gentamicin
P vulgaris and other species	Gentamicin or kanamycin	Chloramphenicol, tobramycin
Pseudomonas		
Ps aeruginosa	Gentamicin or polymyxin	Carbenicillin, amikacin
Serratia, Providencia	Gentamicin, amikacin	Co-trimoxazole[6] plus polymyxin
Gram-positive rods		
Listeria	Ampicillin plus aminoglycoside	Tetracycline
Acid-fast rods		
Nocardia	Sulfonamide[7]	Minocycline
Rickettsiae	Tetracycline	Chloramphenicol

*Modified and reproduced, with permission, from Jawetz E: Chapter 28 in: *Current Medical Diagnosis & Treatment 1978.* Krupp MA, Chatton MJ (editors). Lange, 1978.

[1] Penicillin G is preferred for parenteral injection; penicillin G (buffered) or penicillin V for oral administration. Only highly sensitive microorganisms should be treated with oral penicillin.

[2] All tetracyclines have the same activity against microorganisms and all have comparable therapeutic activity and toxicity. Dosage is determined by the rates of absorption and excretion of different preparations.

[3] Erythromycin estolate and troleandomycin are the best absorbed oral forms.

[4] Cephalothin and cefazolin are the best accepted parenteral cephalosporins; cephalexin or cephradine the best oral forms.

[5] Parenteral methicillin, nafcillin, or oxacillin. Oral dicloxacillin or other isoxazolylpenicillin.

[6] Co-trimoxazole is a mixture of 1 part trimethoprim plus 5 parts sulfamethoxazole.

[7] Trisulfapyrimidines have the advantage of greater solubility in urine over sulfadiazine for oral administration; sodium sulfadiazine is suitable for intravenous injection in severely ill persons.

Table 16–7. Half-life in serum and proposed dosage regimen for various antibiotics used in renal failure.*

	Principal Mode of Excretion or Detoxification	Approximate Half-Life in Serum: Normal	Approximate Half-Life in Serum: Renal Failure†	Proposed Dosage Regimen in Renal Failure: Initial Dose‡	Proposed Dosage Regimen in Renal Failure: Give Half of Initial Dose at Interval of	Significant Removal of Drug by Dialysis (H = Hemodialysis; P = Peritoneal Dialysis)
Penicillin G	Tubular secretion	0.5 hour	6 hours	6 g IV	8–12 hours	H, P no
Ampicillin	Tubular secretion	1 hour	8 hours	6 g IV	8–12 hours	H yes, P no
Carbenicillin	Tubular secretion	1.5 hours	16 hours	4 g IV	12–18 hours	H yes, P no
Methicillin	Tubular secretion	0.5 hour	6 hours	6 g IV	8–12 hours	H, P no
Cephalothin	Tubular secretion	0.8 hour	8 hours	4 g IV	18 hours	H, P yes
Cephalexin Cephradine	Tubular secretion and glomerular filtration	2 hours	15 hours	2 g orally	8–12 hours	H, P yes
Cefazolin	Tubular secretion and glomerular filtration	2 hours	30 hours	2 g IM	24 hours	H, P yes
Kanamycin	Glomerular filtration	3 hours	3–4 days	15 mg/kg IM	3–4 days	H, P yes§
Amikacin	Glomerular filtration	2.5 hours	3 days	15 mg/kg IM	3 days	H, P yes
Gentamicin	Glomerular filtration	2.5 hours	2–4 days	3 mg/kg IM	2–3 days	H, P yes§
Tobramycin	Glomerular filtration	2.5 hours	3 days	3 mg/kg IM	2 days	H, P yes
Vancomycin	Glomerular filtration	6 hours	6–9 days	1 g IV	5–8 days	H, P no
Polymyxin B	Glomerular filtration	6 hours	2–3 days	2.5 mg/kg IV	3–4 days	P yes, H no
Colistimethate	Glomerular filtration	4 hours	2–3 days	5 mg/kg IM	3–4 days	P yes, H no
Tetracycline	Glomerular filtration	8 hours	3 days	1 g orally or 0.5 g IV	3 days	H, P no
Chloramphenicol	Mainly liver	3 hours	4 hours	1 g orally or IV	8 hours	H, P poorly
Erythromycin	Mainly liver	1.5 hours	5 hours	1 g orally or IV	8 hours	H, P poorly
Clindamycin	Glomerular filtration and liver	2.5 hours	4 hours	600 mg IV or IM	8 hours	H, P no

*Reproduced, with permission, from Jawetz E: Anti-infective chemotherapeutic and antibiotic agents. Chapter 28 in: *Current Medical Diagnosis & Treatment 1978.* Krupp MA, Chatton MJ (editors). Lange, 1978.

†Considered here to be marked by creatinine clearance of 10 ml/min or less.

‡For a 60 kg adult with a serious systemic infection. The "initial dose" listed is administered as an intravenous infusion over a period of 1–8 hours, or as 2 intramuscular injections during an 8-hour period, or as 2–3 oral doses during the same period.

§Aminoglycosides are removed irregularly in peritoneal dialysis. Gentamicin is removed 60% in hemodialysis.

helpful as well as repeat blood cultures looking for a second organism possibly missed on the initial cultures. Drug fever is another possibility.

a. **Daily examination**—The patient should be examined daily for the appearance of new murmurs, evidence of cardiac enlargement or cardiac failure, and evidence of embolic manifestations such as petechiae, Osler's nodes, and splinter hemorrhages of the fingernails or toenails. The urine should be examined frequently for microscopic hematuria and casts. The development of pain and friction rub in the left upper quadrant suggests an embolus to the spleen. Pain in the flank associated with hematuria suggests an embolus to the kidney. If the patient develops central nervous system symptoms with headache and somnolence, the possibility of brain abscess or mycotic aneurysm of one of the cerebral arteries should be considered; if the symptoms are severe and progressive, cerebral ultrasonography, angiography, or CT scan should be performed with a view toward localizing an aneurysm whose rupture is imminent.

b. **Check laboratory work**—Renal function should be monitored frequently because it may deteriorate either as a result of renal emboli or because of a hypersensitivity reaction with glomerulitis. The drug regimen should be altered if renal failure is present or develops (Table 16–7). Frequent blood counts should be performed to note the development of progressive normocytic anemia or a marked elevation of the white count that might suggest a septic abscess. Frequent ECGs are desirable to detect the development of intraventricular conduction defects or atrioventricular block suggesting an abscess of the ventricular septum.

Course of the Disease

A. **Valvular Changes:**

1. **Aortic insufficiency**—If the endocarditis involves the aortic valve, careful attention must be paid to signs suggesting worsening of aortic insufficiency. Frequent examination is required to measure pulse pressure and diastolic blood pressure, to note the duration of the diastolic murmur, and to assess the possibility of early mitral valve closure and progressive enlargement of the heart or signs of left ventricular failure, which may be manifested by frank pulmonary edema or by episodic dyspnea. Many of these patients are young adults or adolescents with no previous valvular disease.

2. **Mitral insufficiency**—Progressive enlargement of the left atrium as shown by echocardiographic or radiologic examination, as well as progressive enlargement of the left ventricle may signify serious dysfunc-

tion of this valve (see Chapter 13).

3. **Tricuspid insufficiency**–In acute endocarditis involving the tricuspid valve, the patient should be examined daily for the appearance of signs of tricuspid insufficiency (see Diagnosis, above). (See also Fig 16–4A.)

B. Heart Failure: Progressive destruction of any of the valves associated with either left or right ventricular failure, depending upon the valve involved, should be an indication for serious consideration of cardiac surgery because many of these patients have perforation of the valve leaflets, septal abscess, or rupture of a mycotic aneurysm from the aortic sinus (sinus of Valsalva) into the right heart and can be helped by surgical repair. When heart failure occurs in a patient in whom the infection has not been controlled, a serious dilemma arises; surgery should be considered after maximal efforts have failed to control the infection and to treat the cardiac failure. The presence of pulmonary rales and radiologic evidence of pulmonary venous congestion support the diagnosis of left ventricular failure. Early mitral valve closure is a reliable sign of increasing aortic insufficiency.

Specific Antimicrobial Regimens

A. Subacute Endocarditis Due to *Streptococcus viridans*: Viridans streptococci (usually originating in the oropharynx) are the infecting organism in more than 70% of spontaneously arising cases of typical slow-onset endocarditis. A majority of such organisms are susceptible to 0.1–1 unit/ml penicillin G in vitro. Penicillin G, 5–10 million units daily (in divided doses given as a bolus every 4 hours into an intravenous infusion of 5% dextrose in water), continued for 3–4 weeks, is generally curative. Enhanced bactericidal action is obtained if an aminoglycoside (eg, gentamicin, 3–5 mg/kg/day intramuscularly) is added during the first 10–14 days of treatment. More resistant organisms are occasionally encountered, requiring daily doses of penicillin G of 20–50 million units. Probenecid, 0.5 g 3 times daily orally, further enhances blood levels of penicillin by interfering with its tubular excretion.

B. Endocarditis Due to *Streptococcus faecalis*: This organism causes about 5–10% of cases of spontaneously occurring endocarditis and occasionally also follows abuse of intravenous drugs. Treatment requires the simultaneous use of penicillin and an aminoglycoside. Penicillin G, 20–40 million units daily, or ampicillin, 6–12 g daily, is given in divided doses as bolus injections every 2–3 hours into an intravenous infusion of 5% dextrose in water. An aminoglycoside (streptomycin, 0.5 g every 12 hours, kanamycin, 15 mg/kg/day, or gentamicin, 5 mg/kg/day) selected by appropriate laboratory test for ribosomal susceptibility is injected intramuscularly 2–3 times daily in divided doses. The cell wall inhibitory drug (penicillin) enhances the entry of the aminoglycoside and permits killing of the enterococci. This treatment must be continued for 4–5 weeks. Cephalosporins cannot be substituted for penicillins in this regimen.

C. Endocarditis Due to Staphylococci *(Staphylococcus aureus, S epidermidis)*: If the infecting staphylococci are *not* penicillinase producers, penicillin G, 10–20 million units in divided doses as an intravenous bolus, is the treatment of choice. If the staphylococci produce penicillinase, methicillin, 8–12 g daily, and nafcillin, 8–12 g daily, given as a bolus every 2 hours into an intravenous infusion, are the first choice alternative drugs. In probable or established hypersensitivity to penicillin, the alternative drug is vancomycin, 2–3 g daily in divided doses every 4 hours intravenously. This treatment must usually be continued for 5–6 weeks, and a frequent careful check for metastatic lesions or abscesses must be conducted to avoid reseeding of cardiac lesions from such reservoirs of infectious organisms.

D. Endocarditis Due to Gram-Negative Bacteria: The susceptibility of these organisms to antimicrobial drugs varies so greatly that effective treatment must be based on laboratory tests. Aminoglycosides (gentamicin, 5–7 mg/kg/day, kanamycin, 15 mg/kg/day, amikacin, 15 mg/kg/day, or tobramycin, 5–7 mg/kg/day) are often combined with a cell wall inhibitory drug (cephalothin, 6–12 g/day, cefazolin, 4 g/day, ampicillin, 6–12 g/day, or carbenicillin, 12–30 g/day) to enhance penetration of the aminoglycoside. (See Table 16–7 for methods of administration.) Laboratory guidance is essential not only for drug susceptibility tests but also to establish the presence of sufficient bactericidal activity in serum obtained during treatment. The dosage of aminoglycosides must be adjusted if renal function is impaired as determined by serum creatinine levels and creatinine clearance. Suggested modifications in time-dose regimens for aminoglycosides and other nephrotoxic drugs are given in Table 16–7. Each of these drugs also is capable of causing eighth nerve damage, and the patient should be monitored daily for hearing loss and vestibular function.

E. Endocarditis Due to Yeasts and Fungi: These organisms rarely arise spontaneously but are seen with increasing frequency in abusers of intravenous drugs, after cardiac surgery, or in immunosuppressed individuals. *Candida albicans, C parapsilosis,* and *Torulopsis glabrata* are among those encountered most commonly, but virtually any fungus, including aspergillus and even histoplasma, can be seen. Candida endocarditis is often associated with bulky, friable vegetations which tend to produce massive emboli in large arteries. Candida endocarditis has occurred early after the insertion of prosthetic valves, and the diagnosis may be based on the finding of pseudohyphae in emboli surgically removed from large vessels. It may take 1–3 weeks to grow these organisms in blood cultures.

The drugs most active against yeasts and fungi are amphotericin B (0.5–1.2 mg/kg/day intravenously) and flucytosine (150 mg/kg/day orally). However, these drugs rarely eradicate fungal endocarditis. Early surgical excision of the involved valve tissue during antifungal therapy and the continuation of the latter for several weeks offer the best opportunity for cure.

Prosthetic Valve Endocarditis

Endocarditis on a prosthetic valve occurs in 1–4% of patients and is one of the most disturbing postoperative complications of prosthetic valve surgery. Most cases have involved the aortic valve, but the mitral valve may be infected as well. Infection may occur early, within a month or 2 of surgery; or late, as with any diseased valve. The early onset of infection is thought to be caused by organisms introduced at the time of surgery such as from an infected pump oxygenator, from contamination of the various intravenous lines used during the procedure, or from infected personnel. A postoperative wound infection, especially of the sternum, may be a source of infection of the prosthetic valve. Although only one-third of infections of prosthetic valves occur early (within the first 2 months), the mortality rate is high (70–80%) in the early-onset cases as compared to the more frequent late-onset endocarditis (often many months to a year or so after the valve was introduced); the late-onset cases have a lower mortality rate; the overall mortality rate of all cases of prosthetic valve endocarditis approximates 50–60%. The causes of early death in Wilson's 1975 series were prosthetic valve dysfunction, infection, cardiac failure, and emboli.

Early-onset endocarditis of a prosthetic valve is usually due to *S aureus* or a gram-negative organism, whereas late-onset endocarditis is usually due to *S viridans* or to gram-negative bacilli. Candida infections are most apt to occur early rather than late (Wilson, 1975).

Late-onset endocarditis usually follows one of the common predisposing causes of endocarditis on a damaged valve and pathologically involves the neoendothelium which grows over cloth-covered valves.

It is of interest that on pathologic examination, all patients with prosthetic valve endocarditis have infection located behind the site of attachment of the prosthesis to the valve ring with spread to the neighboring structures. Severe regurgitation of the involved valve follows the prosthetic detachment and may require urgent surgery (Arnett, 1976).

A. Medical and Surgical Treatment: Medical treatment of prosthetic valve endocarditis is most disappointing, and it may be necessary to resect the valve and introduce a new one and combine the procedure with effective antimicrobial therapy. The mortality rate is 50–60% even in properly treated patients, and this emphasizes the difficulty of managing these patients because of the rapidity with which the valve can be dehisced by abscess formation and subsequent progressive cardiac failure. In candida infections, large artery embolism may be the indication for replacing the prosthetic valve.

The high mortality rate may be a function of delayed surgery, allowing destruction of the valve, progressive development of renal and cardiac failure, and development of emboli (especially cerebral) before the patient is operated on again. It is now acknowledged that if medical treatment is not successful, operations should be performed earlier regardless of whether the patient has a prosthetic or homograft valve. Prolonged aggressive antibiotic therapy and early surgical replacement of the infected valve are required if the infection is not rapidly controlled or if there is evidence of rapid destruction of the involved valve with progressive cardiac failure.

B. Prevention: Preventing infection is obviously better than treating prosthetic valve endocarditis; efforts have been made to ensure adequate antibacterial prophylaxis when prosthetic valves are inserted. Since the most common bacteria that cause early-onset prosthetic valve endocarditis are *S aureus* and gram-negative organisms, vigorous therapy with combined drugs is recommended, eg, methicillin, 8–12 g/day intravenously, and gentamicin, 3–5 mg/kg/day intramuscularly, in 3 equal doses for 3 or 4 postoperative days. The results with cephalothin have been poor, and the toxicity of amphotericin B makes its use to prevent the uncommon candida infections unwise. Good studies to establish the most effective prophylactic regimen are not available, but vigorous prophylaxis against the most likely organisms would seem a reasonable course of action.

Prophylaxis of late-onset endocarditis is the same as prophylaxis in the patient with a known rheumatic or congenital heart lesion (see p 507). The predisposing factors are similar, and *S viridans* is the most common organism. Special efforts (eg, prophylactic antibiotics) are necessary to prevent late-onset endocarditis in any patient with a prosthetic valve.

Treatment of Subacute Endocarditis in Patients With Negative Blood Cultures

This is a difficult problem because the physician does not know which organism is causing the endocarditis. In this situation the "best guess" technic is employed, using a combination of penicillin, 20–40 million units, and streptomycin, 0.5 g twice daily intramuscularly, because the most common organisms are *S viridans* and *S faecalis.* This combination may be effective in *S epidermidis* endocarditis. If the patient fails to improve in 1–2 weeks, a trial of other bactericidal drugs is indicated, eg, vancomycin, 0.5 g every 4 hours intravenously. Various aminoglycosides may also be tried as a last resort in the hope that blood cultures obtained initially may reveal an etiologic organism after several weeks. Because of its great frequency in autopsied cases, endocarditis must be assumed to be present in staphylococcal septicemia even if the clinical diagnosis of endocarditis is not certain.

Penicillin Hypersensitivity

For many forms of endocarditis, penicillins have the best record of cure. A history of allergic reaction to penicillin is notoriously unreliable. Only 10–15% of patients with such a history cannot be given penicillin in a situation where it is clearly the drug of choice. All penicillins are cross-reactive, and cephalosporins have a much less successful record than penicillins in the treatment of endocarditis. Therefore, it may be desirable to attempt penicillin treatment in cases of endocarditis where a penicillin-susceptible organism has been recovered, in spite of a past history of penicillin reaction, except one of anaphylaxis.

The following steps are advisable:

(1) Skin tests with penicilloyl-polylysine, native penicillin (1–10 units), and penicillin degraded after prolonged storage in a refrigerator. Unless strong positive reactions are observed within 1 hour, proceed with treatment.

(2) An available airway and a person skilled in its insertion and the use of resuscitation must be at the bedside (preferably in the intensive care unit) for 40–45 minutes. An intravenous infusion of 5% dextrose in water must be in place and running. A syringe with 5 ml of epinephrine 1:1000 must be available at the bedside. A test dose of 100 units of penicillin G is injected into the intravenous tubing with close observation for a possible immediate reaction. If none has occurred in 45 minutes, inject 50,000 units of penicillin G into the tubing and again observe for 40 minutes. Absence of a reaction permits beginning of regular penicillin dosage with the assurance that an immediate life-threatening anaphylactic reaction will not occur.

Delayed, serum sickness type reactions, with skin rashes, angioneurotic edema, fever, or arthritis, may develop in such individuals. Administration of corticosteroids or antihistamines can often suppress these reactions and permit completion of the planned treatment. In extremely penicillin-hypersensitive patients, vancomycin is the best drug.

Procedure After Completion of 4- to 6-Weeks' Course of Treatment

The physician's responsibility does not end with completion of the course of therapy. The only proof of cure is persistence of good health, absence of relapse, and repeatedly negative blood cultures. The patient should be observed at weekly intervals and should keep a daily record of his temperature. Blood for culture should be taken once a week for 2 months. The patient should be examined carefully for evidence of embolic phenomena, splenomegaly, clubbed fingers, and microscopic hematuria. If after 2 months there are no clinical symptoms or signs and the blood cultures have been consistently negative, it is safe to consider that a cure has been achieved. The patient is then seen every month or every other month for another 3 or 4 months to be on the safe side. It is always advisable to keep the cultures of the organism, because, in case of relapse or recurrence, a question will arise with regard to whether the same organism is responsible.

Persistent & Resistant Infection or Development of Cardiac Failure

If effective antibiotic therapy fails to eradicate the infection and positive blood cultures persist or recur, or if adequate combinations of drugs are not bactericidal, one should change the antibiotics, as mentioned previously, and hope to find the combination that will eradicate the organism. This may be difficult in the case of gram-negative or unusual organisms, especially yeasts and fungi, or if the patient has a prosthetic valve. Cardiac failure may develop late as a result of progressive damage with fibrosis of the valve, especially the aortic valve. The development of severe aortic insufficiency may be quite rapid, and surgical replacement with a prosthetic valve is essential. At times, the urgency of surgical replacement is such that patients have had to be operated on within hours of arrival at the hospital. A few such patients have been cured by antibiotic therapy combined with surgical removal of the infected valve. Cardiac failure may progressively worsen even though the infection is eradicated; the physician is then faced with a different situation—a destroyed valve producing cardiac failure—in which case the valve should be replaced because it is destroyed and not because it is infected.

PROGNOSIS

Antibiotic therapy has reduced the mortality rate of infective endocarditis from almost 100% in untreated subacute and acute varieties to about 30% in the former and 20–50% in the latter. This remarkable achievement is best appreciated by physicians who had to deal with endocarditis prior to the antibiotic era. The residual high mortality rate in acute staphylococcal infections is due to the occurrence of septic abscess which may be inaccessible to drainage and to the occasional destruction of valves, thus requiring surgery.

The prognosis in subacute infective endocarditis depends upon the organism involved, its sensitivity to antibiotic agents, the presence of an artificial valve, and the resistance of the host. In sensitive *S viridans* infections, for example, the mortality rate is about 10%. However, with more resistant *S viridans, S aureus,* or gram-negative organisms, the mortality rate increases to 30–40%.

The prognosis depends also upon the class of patient being reported. Deaths are more frequent in elderly debilitated patients, in whom fever may be absent or minimal in the subacute variety and in whom the diagnosis may be delayed or missed because of atypical features of the disease. In *S aureus* endocarditis, for example, there may be a 2- to 3-fold higher mortality rate in older patients as compared to younger ones; most of the unsuspected fatal cases have been in the age group over 70.

The significant residual mortality rate in acute and subacute endocarditis means that the physician should actively seek the diagnosis; obtain blood cultures whenever fever occurs in a patient with valvular disease or in any patient with prolonged fever of obscure origin; and look for septic abscesses that can be surgically drained. Early diagnosis and prompt effective treatment will reduce the mortality rate, and surgical removal of the infected valve may be curative if infection is not controlled by full doses of appropriate antibiotic agents. The emergence of unusual organisms (discussed above) requires knowledge of the therapeutic possibilities of other available antibiotic agents. Cooperation between the infectious disease specialist and the cardiologist is necessary both to eradicate the infection and to recognize when the complications of valve destruction require surgical therapy whether or not infection has been controlled.

The incidence of endocarditis following an aortic homograft valve was 2.6% in 539 patients in the experience of Barratt-Boyes of New Zealand (1969). Early endocarditis occurred in less than 1% and was almost universally fatal. The mortality rate was almost 50% in patients with late endocarditis associated with development of an aortic leak. This incidence of endocarditis is about the same as that following the insertion of Starr-Edwards prostheses (Wilson, 1975).

Continuous prophylactic antibiotics are not required in patients with homograft valves, but "antibiotic cover" is recommended when dental or surgical procedures are required in patients with plastic valves.

• • •

References

Alpert JS & others: Pathogenesis of Osler's nodes. Ann Intern Med 85:471, 1976.

Appel GB, Neu HC: The nephrotoxicity of antimicrobial agents. (3 parts.) N Engl J Med 296:633, 722, 784, 1977.

Arnett EN, Roberts WC: Prosthetic valve endocarditis: Clinicopathologic analysis of 22 necropsy patients with comparison of observations in 74 necropsy patients with active infective endocarditis involving natural left-sided cardiac valves. Am J Cardiol 38:281, 1976.

Banks T, Fletcher R, Ali N: Infective endocarditis in heroin addicts. Am J Med 55:444, 1973.

Barratt-Boyes BG & others: Aortic homograft valve replacement: A long-term follow-up of an initial series of one hundred and one patients. Circulation 40:763, 1969.

Barratt-Boyes BG & others: Homograft valves. Med J Aust 2 (Suppl 1):38, 1972.

Bayer AS & others: Circulating immune complexes in infective endocarditis. N Engl J Med 295:1500, 1976.

Beeson PB, McDermott W (editors): *Textbook of Medicine,* 14th ed. Saunders, 1974.

Botvinick EH & others: Echocardiographic demonstration of early mitral valve closure in severe aortic insufficiency: Its clinical implications. Circulation 51:836, 1975.

Cates JE, Christie RV: Subacute bacterial endocarditis: A review of 442 patients treated in 14 centres appointed by the Penicillin Trials Committee of the Medical Research Council. Q J Med 20:93, 1951.

Chase RM: Infective endocarditis today. Med Clin North Am 57:1383, 1973.

Cliff MM, Soulen RL, Finestone AJ: Mycotic aneurysms: A challenge and a clue. Arch Intern Med 126:977, 1970.

DeMaria AN & others: Echography and phonography of acute aortic regurgitation in bacterial endocarditis. Ann Intern Med 82:329, 1975.

Dismukas WE & others: Prosthetic valve endocarditis: Analysis of 38 cases. Circulation 48:365, 1973.

Dreyer NP, Fields BN: Heroin-associated infective endocarditis: Report of 28 cases. Ann Intern Med 78:699, 1973.

Foster MT Jr, Harrison HE: Bacterial endocarditis. Chapter 8 in: *Infectious Diseases.* Marr JJ (editor). Little, Brown, 1973.

Geraci JE & others: Haemophilus endocarditis: Report of 14 patients. Mayo Clin Proc 52:209, 1977.

Green GR, Peters GA, Geraci JE: Treatment of bacterial endocarditis in patients with penicillin hypersensitivity. Ann Intern Med 67:235, 1967.

Hall B, Dowling HF: Negative blood cultures in bacterial endocarditis: A decade's experience. Med Clin North Am 50:159, 1966.

Hirschfeld DS, Schiller N: Localization of aortic valve vegetations by echocardiography. Circulation 53:280, 1976.

Hutter AM, Moellering RC: Assessment of the patient with suspected endocarditis. JAMA 235:1603, 1976.

Iannini PB & others: Candida precipitins as a diagnostic aid in Candida endocarditis. JAMA 236:2518, 1976.

Jacoby GA, Swartz MN: Current concepts: Fever of undetermined origin. N Engl J Med 289:1407, 1973.

Jawetz E: Anti-infective chemotherapeutic and antibiotic agents. Chapter 28 in: *Current Medical Diagnosis & Treatment 1978.* Krupp MA, Chatton MJ (editors). Lange, 1978.

Jawetz E: Synergism and antagonism among antimicrobial drugs: A personal perspective. West J Med 123:87, 1975.

Jawetz E, Sonne M: Penicillin-streptomycin treatment of enterococcal endocarditis. N Engl J Med 274:710, 1966.

Johnson DH, Rosenthal A, Nadas AS: A forty-year review of bacterial endocarditis in infancy and childhood. Circulation 51:581, 1975.

Kaplan EL & others: Prevention of bacterial endocarditis. Circulation 56:139A, 1977.

Kaye D (editor): *Infective Endocarditis.* University Park Press, 1976.

Lachman AS & others: Infective endocarditis in the billowing mitral leaflet syndrome. Br Heart J 37:326, 1975.

Lerner PI, Weinstein L: Infective endocarditis in the antibiotic era. (4 parts.) N Engl J Med 274:159, 199, 323, 388, 1966.

Mann T & others: Assessing the hemodynamic severity of acute aortic regurgitation due to infective endocarditis. N Engl J Med 293:108, 1975.

Menda KB, Gorbach SL: Favorable experience with bacterial endocarditis in heroin addicts. Ann Intern Med 78:25, 1973.

Mills J, Drew D: *Serratia marcescens* endocarditis: A regional illness associated with intravenous drug abuse. Ann Intern Med 84:29, 1976.

Mills J, Utley J, Abbott J: Heart failure in infective endocarditis: Predisposing factors, course, and treatment. Chest 66:151, 1974.

Moellering RC, Swartz MN: Drug therapy: The newer cephalosporins. N Engl J Med 294:24, 1976.

Nastro IJ, Finegold SM: Endocarditis due to anaerobic gram-negative bacilli. Am J Med 54:481, 1973.

Osler W: Chronic infectious endocarditis. Q J Med 2:219, 1909.

Ostermiller WE Jr, Dye WS, Weinberg M: Fungal endocarditis following cardiovascular surgery. J Thorac Cardiovasc Surg 61:670, 1971.

Parrott JCW & others: The surgical management of bacterial endocarditis: A review. Ann Surg 183:289, 1976.

Perez GO, Rothfield N, Williams RC: Immune-complex nephritis in bacterial endocarditis. Arch Intern Med 136:334, 1976.

Pollack AA & others: Amikacin therapy for serious gram-negative infection. JAMA 237:562, 1977.

Reiner N, Gopalakrishna KV, Lerner PI: Enterococcal endocarditis in heroin addicts. JAMA 235:1861, 1976.

Roy P & others: Spectrum of echocardiographic findings in bacterial endocarditis. Circulation 53:474, 1976.

Seelig MS & others: Candida endocarditis after cardiac surgery: Clues to earlier detection. J Thorac Cardiovasc Surg 65:583, 1973.

Slaughter L, Morris JE, Starr A: Prosthetic valvular endocarditis: A 12-year review. Circulation 47:1319, 1973.

Smith CR & others: Controlled comparison of amikacin and gentamicin. N Engl J Med 296:349, 1977.

Stein PD, Harken DE, Dexter L: The nature and prevention of prosthetic valve endocarditis. Am Heart J 71:393, 1966.

Tumulty PA: Management of bacterial endocarditis. Geriatrics 22:122, 1967.

Vogler WR, Dorney ER, Bridges HA: Bacterial endocarditis: A review of 148 cases, 1948–1960. Am J Med 32:910, 1962.

Watanakunakorn C, Tan JS, Phair JP: Some salient features of *Staphylococcus aureus* endocarditis. Am J Med 54:473, 1973.

Weinstein L, Schlesinger JJ: Pathoanatomic, pathophysiologic, and clinical correlations in endocarditis. (2 parts.) N Engl J Med 291:832, 1122, 1974.

Westenfelder GO, Paterson PY: Life-threatening infection: Choice of alternate drugs when penicillin cannot be given. JAMA 210:845, 1969.

Wilson WR, Washington JA II: Infective endocarditis: A changing spectrum? Mayo Clin Proc 52:254, 1977.

Wilson WR & others: Prosthetic valve endocarditis. Ann Intern Med 82:751, 1975.

Wise JR Jr, Oakley CM, Goodwin JF: Acute aortic regurgitation in patients with infective endocarditis: The distinctive clinical features and the role of premature mitral valve closure. J Maine Med Assoc 63:273, 1972.

17 . . .
Myocardial Disease

MYOCARDITIS & CARDIOMYOPATHY

This chapter discusses myocarditis, cardiomyopathy, and various diseases and clinical states of which disease of the myocardium may be a manifestation. It deals with hypertrophic cardiomyopathy (often called idiopathic hypertrophic subaortic stenosis, or IHSS) under a separate heading because the overall clinical picture and mode of presentation of the patient with hypertrophic cardiomyopathy, with murmurs suggestive of valvular disease, leads the physician to an entirely different set of investigative procedures from those indicated in the management of patients with idiopathic cardiomyopathy, in whom systemic and pulmonary congestion are the principal features.

The common known causes of chronic myocardial disease (ischemic, hypertensive, valvular, congenital, as well as infective endocarditis and syphilis) are discussed in other chapters.

GENERAL CONSIDERATIONS

Diseases of the myocardium form a complex and heterogeneous group of diseases that are somewhat confusing chiefly because they are due to varied causes, not all of them known, but also because the clinical manifestations vary from a trivial illness recognized only by nonspecific ECG abnormalities, mild chest pain, or slight enlargement of the heart to fulminant cardiac failure with severe dyspnea, gallop rhythm, hypotension, tachycardia, recurrent ventricular arrhythmias, and death, which may occur suddenly and unexpectedly. Myocarditis may be acute or chronic, and the acute form may be benign or fulminant. The terms chronic myocarditis and chronic cardiomyopathy are often used interchangeably, since the cause is often unknown and because the inflammatory infiltrate suggests infection ("-itis"). "Chronic idiopathic cardiomyopathy" goes by a variety of names, none of them entirely satisfactory, including Fiedler's myocarditis, idiopathic myocarditis, primary myocardial disease, "vexation of the heart," endocardial myofibrosis, Löffler's syndrome, and alcoholic cardiomyopathy. Myocarditis may be primary in the heart, or the myocardial disease may be secondary to systemic diseases such as the connective tissue disorders.

Some forms of myocardial disease are much more common in tropical and subtropical areas than in temperate climates. The reasons for this geographic distribution are not definitely known, but nutritional factors are thought to be responsible. The diagnosis is often made by exclusion, especially in the case of idiopathic cardiomyopathy, and the physician must consider common diseases in the differential diagnosis that may have unusual clinical features such as ischemic cardiomyopathy, "burned-out" hypertension, rheumatic heart disease (especially aortic stenosis with low cardiac output), and congenital heart disease. Cardiomyopathy is apparently increasing in frequency for reasons that are totally obscure; as congenital and rheumatic heart disease in adults become less common, cardiomyopathy and the acute myocarditides have come to form a larger percentage of cases of cardiac disease.

Myocarditis is often associated with pericarditis (myopericarditis), especially in viral infections. The endocardium and the valves are less often involved except in the case of acute rheumatic fever or endocardial fibrosis. Myocardial disease due to drug toxicity is becoming increasingly common with use of cardiotoxic drugs such as the phenothiazines, doxorubicin, the corticosteroids, emetine, and antimony as well as those that may cause lupus erythematosus, eg, procainamide, hydralazine, and phenytoin.

This chapter is less clearly structured than some of the other chapters in this book because of the variety of cardiac conditions, some of unknown cause, that may occur independently of systemic disease (eg, sarcoidosis and lupus erythematosus), of which cardiac involvement may be only a small part. Some of the entities included in this chapter could as well be discussed in other chapters (eg, sarcoidosis or beriberi heart) but are dealt with here in order to concentrate multisystem entities in one place.

ETIOLOGY & CLASSIFICATION

There is no completely satisfactory classification of the myocardial disorders. Table 17–1 is an attempt at etiologic classification, but many of the diseases are of unknown cause. In such cases the diagnosis must be inferred from the associated systemic features, as in secondary cardiomyopathy and primary viral myocarditis. The most common cause of viral myocarditis is coxsackie B virus, usually type B3 or B5; it is diagnosed by isolating the virus from throat washings, feces, or blood, by a 4-fold increase in serum antibody titers from paired sera, or, in fatal cases, by isolating the virus from the myocardium. Infiltrative diseases such as primary amyloidosis may be difficult to diagnose, but newer immunoelectrophoretic technics and procedures such as rectal or gum biopsy may be helpful. In sarcoidosis, chest x-ray may reveal characteristic hilar adenopathy or pulmonary infiltration or, in advanced disease, right ventricular hypertrophy and cor pulmonale.

Table 17–1. Classification of diseases of the myocardium.

- I. Chronic congestive cardiomyopathy, idiopathic or primary.
- II. Hypertrophic cardiomyopathy.
- III. Acute cardiomyopathy associated with specific diseases:
  - A. Infectious: Usually acute but may be chronic.
    - Viral (especially coxsackie, echo, or poliomyelitis)
    - Mycotic (eg, histoplasmosis, toxoplasmosis, candida)
    - Parasitic (eg, schistosomiasis, trichinosis, trypanosomiasis [acute Chagas' disease])
    - Rickettsial (eg, epidemic typhus, scrub typhus, Q fever)
    - Bacterial (eg, pneumococcus, diphtheria)
  - B. Acute rheumatic fever.
  - C. Acute or subacute myocardial damage due to drugs:
    - Antiarrhythmia agents (eg, digitalis)
    - Antimony
    - Corticosteroids
    - Doxorubicin
    - Emetine
    - Hydralazine
    - Methysergide
    - Phenothiazines
    - Phenytoin
    - Procainamide
    - Tricyclic antidepressants (eg, amitriptyline, imipramine)
- IV. Cardiomyopathy associated with specific metabolic diseases:
  - Thyrotoxicosis
  - Myxedema
  - Alcoholic cardiomyopathy
  - Beriberi heart
  - Nutritional cardiomyopathy
  - Acromegaly
  - Inherited metabolic disorders
- V. Cardiomyopathy associated with recognized chronic diseases, usually of unknown cause:
  - A. Connective tissue disorders:
    - Systemic lupus erythematosus
    - Scleroderma
    - Rheumatoid arthritis
    - Polyarteritis nodosa
  - B. Sarcoidosis.
  - C. Hemochromatosis.
  - D. Amyloid disease.
  - E. Endomyocardial fibrosis.
  - F. Peripartum disease.
  - G. Neurologic disorders (eg, Friedreich's ataxia).
  - H. Chagas' disease.

PATHOLOGY

General Considerations of Pathology

The pathologic features of cardiomyopathy associated with systemic disease are rarely specific. They may be relatively minor and discovered at autopsy in a patient who during life had no clinical manifestations of heart disease. One should clearly distinguish myocarditis recognized only at postmortem from clinically significant disease that produces cardiac symptoms and dysfunction.

Goodwin (1970) has described the heart in congestive cardiomyopathy as large and flabby and the heart in hypertrophic cardiomyopathy as stiff and relatively small. If the patient has widely distributed noncaseating granulomatous disease with hilar adenopathy, the myocardial fibrosis is probably due to sarcoidosis.

Focal or diffuse inflammatory changes resulting from infection may be seen in any of a number of viral infections and may be unassociated with cardiac symptoms or clinical manifestations of acute illness. Varying degrees of myofibrillary hypertrophy, fibrosis, or inflammation involving the myocardial cells or conduction system may be found in any of the conditions causing cardiomyopathy. If cardiac enlargement and cardiac failure are present, the general pathologic findings of cardiac failure may be seen, including chronic passive congestion. Evidence of the primary systemic disease may be seen in other organs.

The pathologic processes in cardiomyopathy and myocarditis may be focal or diffuse; may be a pathologic curiosity at autopsy; or may cause fatal cardiac failure, arrhythmias, or conduction defects.

Common Specific Pathologic Pictures

The following are the most common types of pathologic change seen at autopsy with some examples of the underlying causes that may be responsible. It is of interest that most cases of cardiomyopathy are of unknown cause. When the cause is known, the condition is not usually called simply cardiomyopathy but identified as, for example, hypertensive heart disease.

(1) Infiltration of the myocardium with inflammatory cells of a variety of types, disorganizing their structure and showing "abnormal architecture" (Roberts, 1975), best seen by electron microscopy. (Acute myocarditis, connective tissue disorders.)

(2) Infiltration with infecting organisms. (Acute

viral myocarditis, candida infections, Chagas' disease.)

(3) Focal or diffuse fibrosis of any part of the myocardium or conduction system. (Scleroderma, sarcoidosis, endocardial fibrosis.) When the fibrosis affects the vascular bed of the lungs, pulmonary hypertension, cor pulmonale, and right heart failure may occur.

(4) Arteritis with inflammatory changes in the walls of small arteries as well as perivascular and interstitial infiltration of cells with or without granuloma formation. (Systemic lupus erythematosus.)

(5) Injury to myocardial cells as a result of excessive deposition of various substances. (Immune complexes in lupus erythematosus, fibrils of light chain immunoglobulins in amyloid disease, glycogen in Gierke's disease, calcium in renal failure, iron in hemochromatosis, invasion of myocardial cells from tumors.)

(6) Metabolic changes caused by biochemical substances produced by tumor. (Serotonin or bradykinins in carcinoid syndrome.)

(7) Direct injury of myocardial cells from drugs. (Doxorubicin, digitalis, sympathetic amines, alcohol, methysergide, food or drink additives such as cobalt in cobalt-beer cardiomyopathy.)

(8) Deposition or accumulation of metabolic substances that injure the myocardial cell as a result of enzyme defects. (Serotonin in carcinoid syndrome, inherited metabolic disorders.)

Pathology of Conduction System

In all cases of myocardial disease, the damage to cardiac muscle may interfere with the ventricular conduction system, causing destruction of the sinoatrial or atrioventricular node or large portions of the Purkinje system. Stokes-Adams attacks, arrhythmias, and sudden death are common in such disorders as scleroderma, sarcoidosis, and Chagas' disease, in which fibrosis dominantly involving the conduction system may occur. The inflammatory or fibrotic lesions may interrupt the ventricular conduction system, so that there may be disorders of cardiac impulse formation or distribution in the absence of dysfunction of the cardiac muscle as a whole; the patient may then have symptoms of conduction defect in the absence of cardiac enlargement or cardiac failure, though both may of course be present.

GENERAL PATHOPHYSIOLOGY

The pathophysiologic changes of myocarditis and cardiomyopathy cause clinical cardiac disease in a variety of ways: (1) by impairing myocardial cell contractility as a result of destruction of myocardial cells and decreasing the number of contractile units; (2) by interfering with and restricting filling of the ventricles; (3) by decreasing or increasing cardiac output and cardiac work; (4) by inducing progressive myocardial dilatation and hypertrophy that may lead to cardiac failure; (5) by inducing pericarditis or pericardial effusion, which may lead to cardiac tamponade; (6) by inducing ischemia of the myocardium, which may lead to myocardial necrosis; and (7) by endocardial thrombus formation, leading to embolization.

The resulting impairment of cardiac function usually consists of low output failure with decreased myocardial contractility and increased cardiac volume. Occasionally there may be increased cardiac output, as in thyrotoxicosis, anemia, or Paget's disease of bone. (See discussion of high output failure, Chapter 10.) When impairment of left ventricular function is sufficiently great, the ejection fraction falls below 30% and cardiac failure usually ensues. This is usually progressive and ultimately fatal unless the underlying cause is removed or reversed.

COMMON CLINICAL FINDINGS IN PRIMARY MYOCARDIAL DISEASE

(See below for specific entities.)

The hemodynamic criteria for diagnosis of primary myocardial diseases are outlined in Table 17–2, although cardiac catheterization and coronary angiography are usually not required for diagnosis. The final diagnoses in 99 patients (Harvey, 1964) thought at first to have primary myocardial disease were as follows: primary myocardial disease, 78; arteriosclerotic heart disease, 11; constrictive pericarditis, 3; and others (fibrosarcoma, sarcoidosis, atrial septal defect, collagen diseases, amyloidosis, mitral stenosis, aortic dissection), 7.

In practically no instance of cardiomyopathy—acute or chronic, primary or secondary—is there anything specific about the clinical features so far as they

Table 17–2. Criteria for diagnosis of primary myocardial disease.*

I. Abnormal ventricular function
  A. Hemodynamics
    1. LVEDP† at rest > 13 mm Hg or
    2. LVEDP at rest < 13 mm Hg but exercise LVEDP abnormal
  B. Ventriculogram
    1. Increased end-diastolic volume
    2. Increased left ventricular mass
    3. Abnormal motion pattern
II. Normal selective coronary cinearteriogram
III. No primary valvular disease
IV. No congenital heart disease
V. No hypertension

*Reproduced, with permission of the American Heart Association, Inc., from Kreulen TH, Gorlin R, Herman MV: Ventriculographic patterns and hemodynamics in primary myocardial disease. Circulation 47:299, 1973.

†LVEDP = left ventricular end-diastolic pressure.

relate to the heart itself. The heart can respond to injury in only a few ways: cardiac failure, arrhythmia, conduction defects, embolization, and chest pain.

Symptoms

In acute myocarditis the patient usually presents with an acute febrile illness associated with fever, malaise, arthralgias, chest pain, dyspnea, and palpitations. The patient may have associated pericarditis, with chest pain characteristic of pericardial involvement which is improved by sitting up and worse during swallowing. The chest pain is frequently vague and nondiagnostic. An acute febrile illness with symptoms suggesting cardiac involvement should provoke a meticulous search for signs of heart disease by physical examination, electrocardiography, radiology, and echocardiography. The patient may experience syncope (Stokes-Adams attacks) if conduction defects are present. Cardiac catheterization is rarely performed in acute myocarditis unless the diagnosis is in doubt, in which case the hemodynamic features listed in Table 17–2 may be helpful.

Signs

A. Cardiac Signs: Tachycardia out of proportion to the fever should suggest the diagnosis. There are usually no abnormalities on inspection except for displacement of the cardiac impulse to the left. Palpation may disclose a left ventricular heave. The blood pressure is usually normal. Auscultation may reveal equalization of the first and second sounds, which results in a soft first sound, so-called tictac rhythm. A "functional" systolic murmur due to cardiac dilatation may be present. There may be a gallop rhythm with S_3; and, if definite cardiac failure is present, the patient may have a raised pulmonary venous or jugular venous pressure. The venous pressures are normal in the absence of cardiac failure. Various types of ventricular arrhythmias or atrioventricular conduction defects may be found.

Acute circulatory collapse, with hypotension, cold and clammy extremities, oliguria, and obtundation, may occur when myocardial damage is severe (eg, in severe infections). Emboli and sudden death may occur.

B. Signs of Associated Disease: Signs of the associated disease may be present in the lungs, skin, liver, kidneys, or elsewhere in patients with secondary myocardial disorders.

Electrocardiography

The ECG findings are usually nonspecific. ST–T changes, often in the inferior leads, are the most common abnormalities. If the conduction system is involved by the inflammatory or infiltrative process, the patient may have conduction defects, including partial atrioventricular block. In a young person with acute viral infection, the development of ST–T abnormalities, partial atrioventricular block, and conduction defects should suggest myocarditis; in an older person, ischemic cardiomyopathy will have to be excluded.

X-Ray Findings

The radiologic findings are also nonspecific. The heart may be enlarged and globular, and there may be signs of pericardial effusion in the chest film. Pericardial effusion can be confirmed by the echocardiogram, which shows an echo-free zone between the epicardium of the left ventricle and the chest wall. (See Chapter 18.) With gross cardiac failure there may be pulmonary venous congestion, and with cor pulmonale there may be radiologic signs of pulmonary hypertension and right ventricular enlargement. If the patient has sarcoidosis, there may be hilar adenopathy and pulmonary infiltration. In lymphomatous and malignant disease, the radiologic examination may show evidences of tumor in various parts of the body.

Noninvasive Tests

Echocardiography may reveal enlargement of the left ventricle and may rule out other diseases (eg, hypertrophic cardiomyopathy and mitral stenosis) or E point separation in severe cardiac failure (see Chapter 10).

Cardiac Catheterization

Cardiac catheterization is usually done to rule out surgically treatable lesions in so-called congestive cardiomyopathy (see below) or to differentiate congestive cardiomyopathy from hypertrophic cardiomyopathy or constrictive pericarditis (see Chapter 18). Catheterization and angiography in congestive cardiomyopathy will show a left ventricle of increased volume in diastole, averaging about 200 ml/m^2—in contrast to the average normal of about 80 ml/m^2 (Goodwin, 1970)—with poor pulsations, a decreased ejection fraction (averaging 40%), normal coronary arteries as shown on coronary arteriography, and a symmetric, decreased wall motion without ventricular aneurysm or segmental contraction abnormalities. The left ventricular filling pressure may be raised out of proportion to right ventricular filling pressure, which helps to differentiate congestive or hypertrophic cardiomyopathy from constrictive pericarditis; however, this sign is not completely reliable, because right ventricular failure may occur secondary to left ventricular failure, and the filling pressure may be approximately equal in the 2 ventricles. Right atrial pressures in cardiomyopathy due to amyloidosis and constrictive pericarditis are shown in Fig 17–1. The hemodynamic findings are of prognostic importance, and the prognosis for survival is much less favorable when the ejection fraction is low—especially when it is less than 20% (Feild, 1973).

Prognosis

The cardiac failure of myocardial disease may differ from that due to ischemic cardiomyopathy or severe valvular disease depending upon the cause. In acute viral myocarditis or peripartum cardiomyopathy, for example, cardiac failure may be completely reversible over a period of 1–2 months. In the case of viral myocarditis, it may be recurrent.

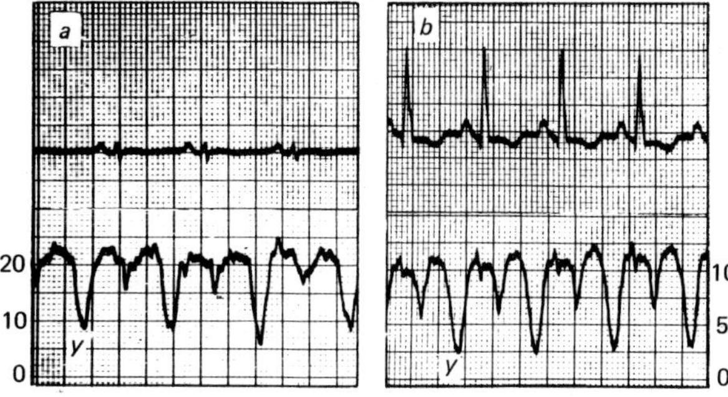

Figure 17–1. Right atrial pressure (lower register) and synchronous ECG (upper register) in *(a)* cardiomyopathy, and *(b)* constrictive pericarditis. Note high venous pressure and steep *y* descent in both conditions, indicating the similarity in the right atrial pressures, in contrast to what some authors have written. (Reproduced, with permission, from Brigden W: Uncommon myocardial diseases: The noncoronary cardiomyopathies. Lancet 2:1179, 1957.)

DISEASES OF THE MYOCARDIUM

IDIOPATHIC CARDIOMYOPATHY

This is a miscellaneous group of diseases of unknown cause, divided on the basis of the clinical and hemodynamic features into 3 types (Goodwin, 1970): (1) congestive cardiomyopathy, with clinical features of cardiac enlargement, increased cardiac volume, and symptoms and signs of congestive failure with poor pump function; (2) hypertrophic cardiomyopathy (see below); and (3) restrictive cardiomyopathy, with infiltrative myocardial disease associated with endomyocardial fibrosis, amyloid disease, scleroderma, hemochromatosis, and other disorders that interfere with left ventricular filling and emptying (decreased distensibility).

Idiopathic congestive cardiomyopathy is a nonspecific diagnosis, and there are no characteristics that differentiate congestive cardiomyopathy from other myocardial diseases with a similar end-point: congestive failure. Excessive alcohol intake over a period of many years is a possible cause in many cases, and acute and subacute myocardial abnormalities have been recognized in patients with a long history of alcoholism. Ischemic cardiomyopathy is responsible for some cases (see Chapter 8). Diabetes affects the small vessels of the heart and may be responsible for vasculitis and heart failure and anginal pains similar to those of large vessel coronary disease. In these instances, the main coronary arteries are often normal, as shown both by coronary arteriography and pathologic examination, although, as discussed in Chapter 8, atheromas may be found at an earlier age in diabetes. The histologically nonspecific nature of fibrosis and hypertrophy of the myocardial fibers has already been noted, and specific causes are unidentified in the great majority of cases. Even endocardial biopsy during left and right heart catheterization has rarely established a cause of cardiomyopathy. Nutritional deficiencies and thiamin deficiency may be aggravating causes.

As newer immunochemical technics are applied to the investigation of congestive cardiomyopathy, some cases may prove to be of specific immunologic origin. Ten of 40 cases reported from the Cameroons were found to have unsuspected serologic evidence of trypanosomiasis as compared to 2% in a random sample of healthy persons in the general population (Blackett, 1976).

Clinical Findings

A. Symptoms: The disease is suspected early in patients who have dyspnea, chest pain, or palpitations. Dyspnea is typical of that seen in cardiac failure (see Chapter 10) and may progress from dyspnea on exertion to orthopnea, paroxysmal nocturnal dyspnea, and pulmonary edema. When right heart failure supervenes, peripheral edema may be a prominent symptom.

The chest pain is nondescript and not typical of angina pectoris. It may be related to pulmonary congestion or, if pleuritic, to pulmonary embolism. Pericardial pain is rare.

Patients who complain of palpitations may have chronic atrial fibrillation or paroxysmal atrial or ventricular arrhythmia. The arrhythmias may be incidental or may dominate the clinical picture. Ventricular premature beats occur in about half of cases; ventricular tachycardia or fibrillation usually occurs late.

Dizziness or syncope may occur from bradyarrhythmia or ventricular conduction defects secondary to fibrosis.

Symptoms of pulmonary or systemic emboli may occur, sometimes dominating the clinical features.

B. Signs: The signs are those of cardiac hypertrophy or cardiac failure (see Chapter 10). The cardiac failure is usually left ventricular with pulmonary rales, left ventricular gallop rhythm, and left ventricular heave which is displaced downward and to the left. If the disease is more advanced, right ventricular and congestive heart failure are found with a raised venous pressure and pulsating neck veins and liver, an enlarged tender liver, and dependent edema of the legs or sacrum. The signs do not differ from those seen in congestive heart failure (see Chapter 10). The blood pressure is usually normal, although the role of burned-out hypertension remains an enigma. Thirty to 40% of patients with cardiomyopathy have a history of hypertension or intermittently raised pressure, but hypertension is not usually present in patients presenting with cardiac failure. It is not known whether this is due to the decreased arterial pressure resulting from associated low cardiac output or the development of coronary disease.

Signs of pulmonary emboli (see Chapter 19) or systemic emboli (see Chapter 20) may be found when these complications occur.

C. Laboratory Findings: There are no specific laboratory findings unless the congestive cardiomyopathy is due to a specific disease such as myocardial ischemia.

D. Electrocardiographic Findings: ECG changes include left ventricular hypertrophy (see Chapter 9), ventricular and atrial arrhythmias (see Chapter 15), conduction defects (see Chapter 14), and nonspecific ST–T abnormalities (see Chapter 8).

E. X-Ray Findings: The x-ray changes are those of cardiac enlargement, chiefly left ventricular, with a large cardiac volume and with pulmonary congestion but without disproportionate left atrial enlargement, calcified valves, or abnormalities of the aorta (see Chapter 10).

F. Echocardiography: Because it is noninvasive, echocardiography is particularly helpful in excluding pericardial effusion (see Chapter 18), aortic stenosis (when murmur is not heard because of severely decreased cardiac output) (see Chapter 13), and mitral valve disease (see Chapter 12) and in estimating left ventricular volume and ejection fraction (see Chapter 10). Massive increases in diastolic volume or decreases in ejection fraction ($< 20\%$) are of bad prognostic import.

G. Hemodynamic Findings and Angiography: The findings are those of a large volume heart with poor contractions and generalized hypokinesia, decreased ejection fraction (usually $\leqslant 30$–40%), increased left ventricular filling pressure, and possibly increased right atrial and right ventricular pressure. These features are described in Chapter 10.

Differential Diagnosis

A. Ischemic Cardiomyopathy: Increased left ventricular volume with decreased ejection fraction and generalized hypokinesia are seen on left ventricular angiography in both idiopathic cardiomyopathy and ischemic cardiomyopathy. The latter may also be associated with greatly increased cardiac volume, but there are usually segmental defects in contraction rather than symmetric hypokinesis.

B. Other Disorders: Other forms of cardiac disease (eg, valvular heart disease), hypertension, and secondary cardiomyopathies are discussed elsewhere in this book.

Treatment

There are no specific measures for idiopathic cardiomyopathy or endomyocardial fibrosis. Treat cardiac failure as outlined in Chapter 10. Anticoagulant and anti-arrhythmia treatment may be valuable in some cases.

Cardiac failure may be severe and unrelenting in idiopathic congestive cardiomyopathy, and the use of intravenous and oral vasodilator therapy should be considered if the usual therapeutic agents fail (see Chapter 10).

Prognosis

Without treatment, the prognosis of idiopathic cardiomyopathy is poor. Even with the best care, survival for only 2–3 years is the rule, although some patients have survived 5–6 years. Prolonged bed rest and intensive treatment of cardiac failure may improve the prognosis. There are no data on whether vasodilator therapy to decrease the impedance against which the left ventricle contracts may prolong life, but this should be attempted if conventional therapy fails and the patient continues to have symptoms and signs of cardiac failure (see Chapter 10).

HYPERTROPHIC OBSTRUCTIVE CARDIOMYOPATHY

Classification & Diagnosis

The use of the term hypertrophic obstructive cardiomyopathy to denote the condition described in this section is not entirely satisfactory. It does not suggest any specific cause, although it does identify the 2 main features of the condition—hypertrophy and obstruction—and indicates that the basic cause lies in the heart muscle. The condition may exist with or without obstruction; the former may be provoked by various maneuvers (see pp 525 and 527).

Many prefer the terms idiopathic hypertrophic subaortic stenosis or asymmetric hypertrophy to describe this disease or group of diseases with various causes. The term idiopathic hypertrophic subaortic stenosis has the disadvantage of suggesting that the disease involves the aorta rather than the ventricle, and it does not cover right-sided lesions. The term asymmetric left ventricular hypertrophy is unsatisfactory both because asymmetry is not an inherent feature of the lesion and because asymmetric hypertrophy may affect either the septum or the ventricle.

Goodwin's classification (1973), as described on p 521, may be confusing with respect to hypertrophic cardiomyopathy. Some patients exhibit features of both congestive and hypertrophic forms. The relationship between hypertrophy and obstruction is also not always clear. Obstruction may be present at all times, may occur intermittently in response to naturally occurring stresses, or may occur only in response to pharmacologic or other stimuli (see p 527).

The cardinal features of hypertrophic obstructive cardiomyopathy are illustrated in Fig 17–2. The hypertrophy, which involves mainly the septum, interferes with systolic emptying of the left ventricle. The anterior leaflet of the mitral valve comes into apposition with the septal muscle, and narrowing of the outflow tract gives rise to the characteristic systolic murmur. The severity of the obstruction varies with the

Cardinal features: *Left ventricular (especially septal) hypertrophy; systolic outflow obstruction; systolic anterior motion of mitral valve; excessive left ventricular emptying.*

Variable factors: *Severity; level of peripheral resistance; low resistance and low blood volume lead to obstruction.*

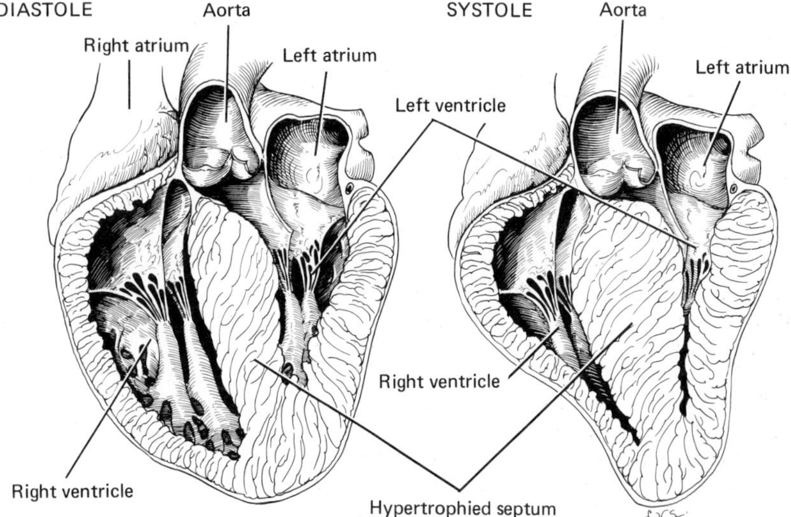

Figure 17–2. Hypertrophic obstructive cardiomyopathy (left lateral view). The cardiac features are displayed.

level of the peripheral resistance, the adequacy of the central blood volume, and the degree of ventricular emptying. In some cases septal hypertrophy involves the right side of the heart in addition to or instead of the left, and a picture resembling that of infundibular pulmonary stenosis is then seen.

Cause

The cause of the condition is unknown. In some cases the disorder is clearly congenital, and familial distribution is also reported. In other cases the condition appears to develop later in life in a patient with a clear history of essential hypertension.

Age & Sex Incidence

The disease occurs with equal frequency in both sexes and is seen in all age groups. The possibility of associated skeletal muscle disease has been raised.

Pathology

Hypertrophic obstructive cardiomyopathy can logically be viewed as a disorder of growth, occurring either in the natural development of the adult left ventricle during childhood or in the process of hypertrophy in response to some stimulus that increases the work of the left ventricle. The 2 processes of hypertrophy and obstruction are interrelated, and it is not always clear which came first in an individual case. For example, in patients with subvalvular aortic fibrous ring stenosis, the secondary ventricular hypertrophy may produce a picture which mimics that seen in a patient with hypertrophic obstructive cardiomyopathy. Pathologic examination of the heart shows abnormally situated and abnormally large muscle bundles, especially in the interventricular septum.

Criteria for Diagnosis

There is no agreement on what criteria are required for diagnosis. The best evidence of obstruction is a significant pressure difference between the body of the ventricle and the subvalvular area or aorta, using a side-hole closed-tip catheter at left heart catheterization (Fig 17–3). Systolic anterior motion of the mitral valve on echocardiography is a valuable sign of obstruction, but its specificity is not clear.

Evidence of hypertrophy can also be obtained in different ways. Pathologic examination of the heart is seldom available, and, since the obstruction may be "variable," the state of the heart at autopsy is not necessarily relevant. Electrocardiography, angiocardiography, and echocardiographic measurement of wall thicknesses in the septal region and at the free posterior wall do not always provide internally consistent information. Emptying of the ventricle that is more complete than normal on angiocardiography is an important feature of the disease, but little is known

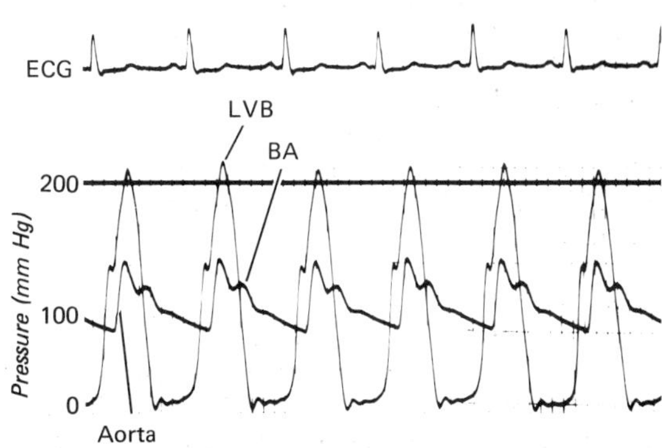

Figure 17–3. Simultaneous brachial arterial (BA) and left ventricular body (LVB) pressure tracings and ECG in a patient with hypertrophic obstructive cardiomyopathy.

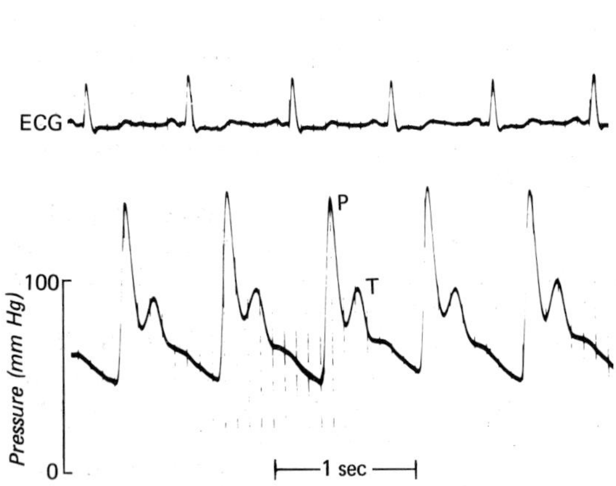

Figure 17–4. Bifid brachial arterial pulse in a patient with hypertrophic obstructive cardiomyopathy. The early percussion wave (P) is followed by a smaller tidal wave (T).

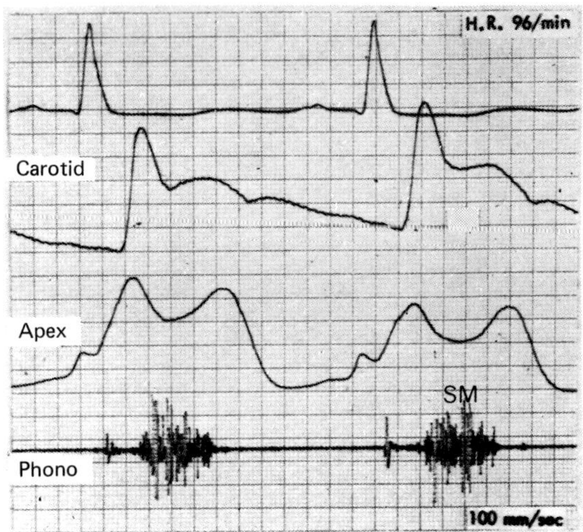

Figure 17–5. ECG, carotid pulse, apexcardiogram (apex), and phonocardiogram of a 36-year-old man with clinical and hemodynamic features of hypertrophic obstructive cardiomyopathy. Blood pressure was 120/50. Note the *a* wave and double humped apical impulse in the apexcardiogram, as well as the position of the systolic murmur (SM) late in systole. (Reproduced, with permission, from Burchell HB: Hypertrophic obstructive type of cardiomyopathy: Clinical syndrome. Pages 29–42 in: *Ciba Foundation Symposium: Cardiomyopathies.* Wolstenholme GEW, O'Connor M [editors]. Little, Brown, 1964.)

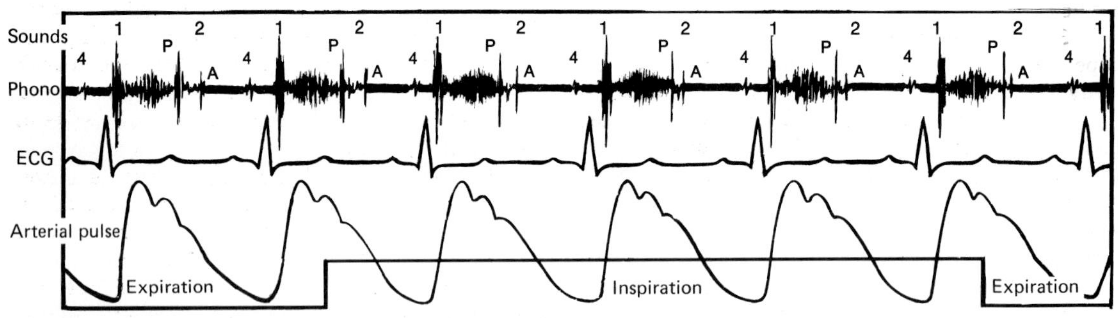

Figure 17–6. Phonocardiogram, ECG, and arterial pulse in hypertrophic obstructive cardiomyopathy. Phonocardiogram shows presystolic gallop, loud first sound, ejection murmur, and soft late A_2 with paradoxic splitting. (Courtesy of Roche Laboratories Division of Hoffman-La Roche, Inc.)

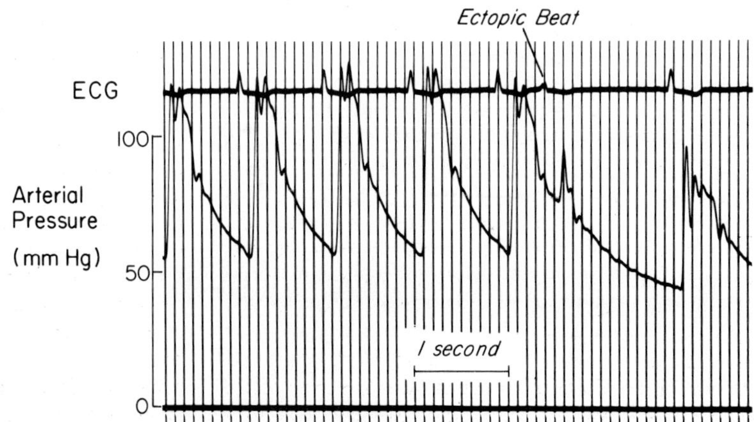

Figure 17–7. Bifid arterial pulse in a patient with hypertrophic obstructive cardiomyopathy showing Brockenbrough's sign, ie, decrease in systolic arterial pressure in a beat following an ectopic beat.

about this aspect of cardiac physiology.

The main problems presented by this clinical entity are in the criteria for diagnosis and in prognosis. Because of the wide variability of the clinical manifestations in different patients, there are wide differences of opinion about the minimum abnormality required to establish the diagnosis. The dangers of creating cardiac neurosis by warning patients with minor or subclinical findings of the possibility of sudden death are obvious.

Clinical Findings

A. Symptoms:

1. History of heart murmur–The presence of a heart murmur is not an uncommon reason for referral to a cardiologist. A spurious history of rheumatic fever is sometimes given because the murmur was heard in childhood, perhaps in association with an episode of sore throat.

2. Dyspnea and chest pain–Dyspnea on exertion and chest pain are the commonest presenting symptoms. The pain is a dull, aching, substernal discomfort and radiates to the arm like angina pectoris. It resembles the pain in other lesions associated with left ventricular hypertrophy in being closely associated with dyspnea. Classic angina in which there is pain without dyspnea, rapidly relieved by rest and nitroglycerin, is less common. Failure of nitroglycerin to relieve chest pain should suggest the diagnosis of hypertrophic cardiomyopathy.

3. Other symptoms–Fatigue, dizziness, and syncope are often reported. The syncope is not necessarily related to the severity of exertion; in fact, it is usually unrelated to exertion and does not carry the dire prognosis that might be expected. Sudden death occurs, especially in familial cases with marked septal hypertrophy, but the frequency of this outcome is not well documented, and it is not directly related to severity.

4. Factors influencing symptoms–The severity of symptoms varies with the state of the circulation. Anything that reduces peripheral resistance, such as a hot environment, pregnancy, standing up suddenly, exercise, or amyl nitrite inhalation, may induce or exaggerate outflow obstruction and bring on symptoms. Left ventricular failure occurs late and may follow the onset of atrial fibrillation. Congestive heart failure occurs but is quite uncommon.

B. Signs:

1. Pulse–The pulse is jerky, with a bifid quality. The rapid initial upstroke is followed by a small tidal wave (Fig 17–4). The outflow obstruction develops after the start of systole, and the initial ejection of blood through an unobstructed outflow tract is responsible for the sharp rise in the pulse wave. As the obstruction develops during systole, it cuts down the rate of ejection and the pulse wave falls off, only to rise again later in systole.

2. Cardiac impulse–The same mechanism accounts for the findings on palpation at the apex of the heart in some cases, where a bifid impulse is felt during systole. In other cases, the apical impulse is bifid for another reason. The hypertrophied ventricle is less compliant than normal, and there is an abnormally forceful left atrial contraction. This produces a palpable presystolic impulse that gives a double apical impulse. When both of these factors are present, there is a triple cardiac impulse that is virtually pathognomonic of the conditions (Fig 17–5).

3. Systolic murmur–There is almost invariably a harsh, long systolic murmur that peaks like other ejection murmurs in mid systole but starts early and may last for almost the whole of systole (Fig 17–4).

4. Other signs–Third and fourth heart sounds are commonly heard, but ejection clicks and aortic diastolic murmurs are quite rare. Mitral incompetence is also present in many cases, making it difficult to decide whether the murmur is pansystolic or ejection in character. In fact, the murmur may be best termed a "pansystolic ejection murmur." Mitral diastolic murmurs may occur, especially when reduced left ventricular compliance interferes with diastolic filling of the left ventricle, and may cause confusion with mixed mitral valve lesions of rheumatic heart disease. Left ventricular contraction may be prolonged, and paradoxic splitting of the second sound is sometimes present (Fig 17–6). Posture has a marked effect on the murmur, and sudden squatting often abolishes or lessens the intensity of the murmur, as it does the obstruction.

5. Effect of an ectopic beat–The peripheral arterial blood pressure is often smaller after a long diastolic pause following an ectopic beat (Brockenbrough's sign; Fig 17–7). The more forceful ventricular contraction (postectopic potentiation) increases the degree of outflow obstruction.

6. Effect of amyl nitrite–Amyl nitrite inhalation and isoproterenol induce or exaggerate the outflow obstruction murmur while phenylephrine relieves obstruction (Fig 17–8). Such studies may help in determining the degree of associated mitral incompetence. Amyl nitrite also brings out the murmur of aortic stenosis, but this murmur is shorter and associated with a slowly rising pulse and should not lead to confusion.

C. Electrocardiographic Findings: ECG evidence of left ventricular hypertrophy or left or (less often) right bundle branch block is almost always present, and the diagnosis is suspect if the ECG is normal. Arrhythmias are common, and Wolff-Parkinson-White forms of ECG abnormality are sometimes seen.

D. X-Ray Findings: Left ventricular hypertrophy can usually be seen on chest x-ray (Fig 17–9), but the cardiac silhouette is often not much enlarged because the hypertrophy takes place at the expense of the left ventricular cavity. The poststenotic dilatation seen in valvular aortic stenosis is absent, and calcification of the aortic valve is not seen on cinefluoroscopy. Left atrial enlargement is seldom marked, and pulmonary congestion may be present if left ventricular failure has occurred. Calcification in the mitral ring is found in about one-fourth of cases.

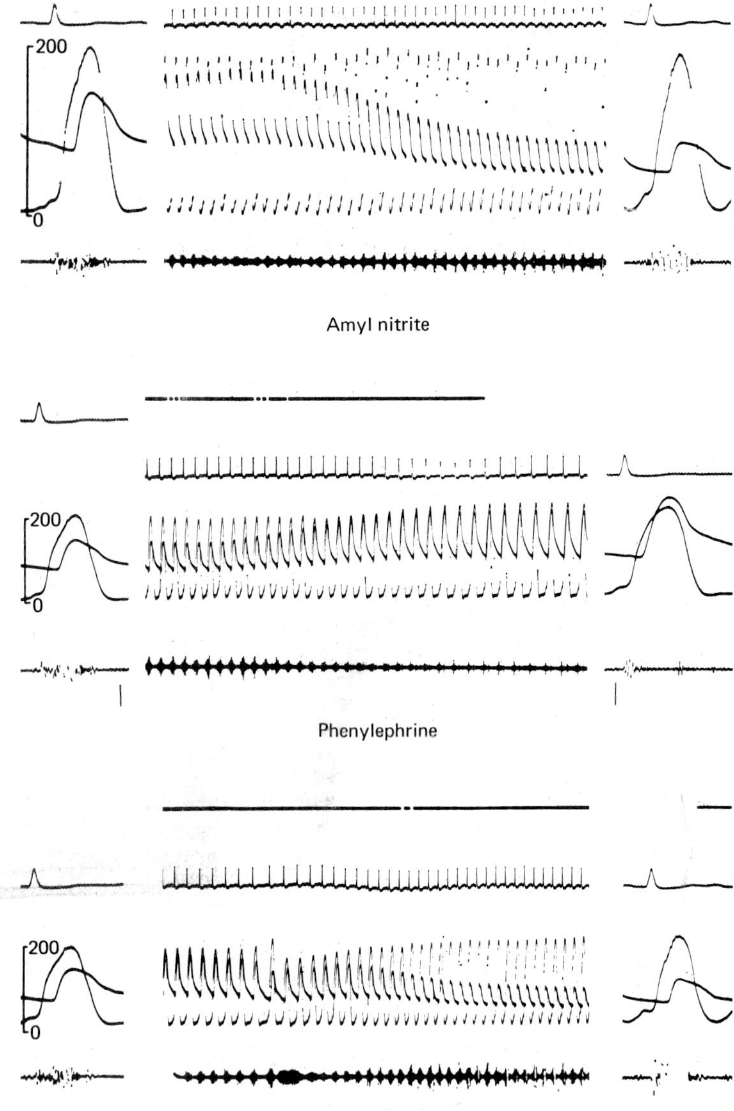

Figure 17–8. Simultaneous left ventricular and femoral artery pressure and phonocardiogram. *Top:* Increase of pressure gradient and systolic murmur with inhalation of amyl nitrite. *Middle:* Abolition of murmur and gradient with phenylephrine. *Bottom:* Increase of gradient and murmur with isoprenaline (isoproterenol). (Reproduced, with permission, from Nellen M in: *Hypertrophic Obstructive Cardiomyopathy.* Wolstenholme G, O'Connor M [editors]. Churchill, 1971.)

E. Special Investigations:

1. Noninvasive investigations—Echocardiography is becoming the principal tool for clinical diagnosis of the disease. The presence of a normal aortic valve, a hypertrophied interventricular septum, and the characteristic systolic anterior motion of the anterior cusp of the mitral valve (Fig 17–10) should leave no doubt about the diagnosis. If anything, the echocardiographic manifestations of hypertrophic obstructive cardiomyopathy may be too sensitive, and the disorder tends to be suspected in otherwise normal persons in whom systolic anterior motion of the mitral valve may be seen after amyl nitrite inhalation. Echocardiography can also provide noninvasive measurements of ventricular thickness and is useful in detecting asymmetric hypertrophy of the heart involving the interventricular septum. It is customary to compare septal measurements with those of the free posterior wall of the left ventricle. A ratio of more than 1.3:1 between the 2 measurements has been said to be diagnostic of the condition, but the specificity of the finding is not yet established.

Echocardiography is rapidly becoming the most practical and satisfactory means of making the differential diagnosis and can obviate the need for cardiac catheterization (see below) in asymptomatic or mild cases. It can also be used to follow the patient and assess the response to treatment.

Indirect arterial pulse tracings and apexcardiograms give evidence of the nature of the bifid impulse.

2. Invasive investigations—Left heart catheterization and left ventricular angiography are indicated in symptomatic cases in order to establish the diagnosis and level of severity as clearly as possible, especially if

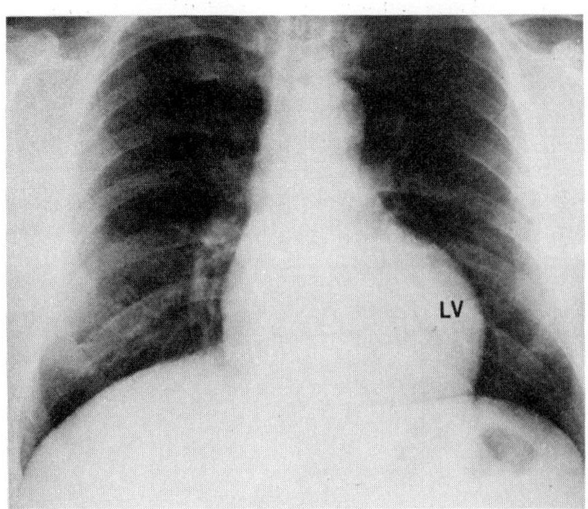

Figure 17–9. Chest x-ray of a patient with hypertrophic obstructive cardiomyopathy showing left ventricular predominance.

surgery is contemplated. Both investigations have greatly increased our knowledge of the mechanics of the lesion.

3. **Pressure tracings**—In patients with clear evidence of obstruction, there is a pressure difference between the body of the left ventricle and the subvalvular chamber. The presence of a murmur does not ensure the presence of a pressure difference. Since the ventricle empties more completely than normal, it is not uncommon for the tip of a left ventricular catheter to become embedded in the interstices of the trabeculae in the body of the ventricle. If an end-hole catheter is used, spurious pressure tracings can be obtained. For this reason, a closed-tip, side-hole (Lehmann) catheter should be used for studies in which the diagnosis is suspected. The outflow chamber distal to the obstruction can often be recognized by the marked disturbance of flow within it. Violent systolic oscillations of pressure are seen that are thought to be due to the rapid acceleration of blood at the site of obstruction. Withdrawal of the catheter from the body of the left ventricle to the outflow area ordinarily shows a pressure difference of 30–100 mm Hg in symptomatic cases, and no further pressure difference is seen on withdrawal across the aortic valve (Fig 17–11).

4. **Provocative tests**—The hemodynamic findings can vary from moment to moment, even when provocative measures are not employed. The effects of ectopic beats on the pressure difference across the obstruction are shown in Fig 17–12. In cases in which there is little or no pressure difference within the ventricle, amyl nitrite inhalation can be used to reduce the peripheral resistance, encourage ventricular emptying, and induce obstruction. Similarly, an infusion of isoproterenol can be used to increase the force of cardiac contraction and bring about the physical signs, as shown in Fig 17–13. The Valsalva maneuver decreases venous return and increases or induces obstruction. In our opinion, such provocative measures should only be used in patients with little or no obstruction, and simultaneous arterial and left ventricular pressure tracings should always be available. In patients in whom obstruction is present, propranolol can be given intravenously to demonstrate the reversibility of the obstruction. However, failure to respond to this measure should not be taken to mean that the drug will not be useful in treatment. Provocative and alleviative studies, while they have been helpful in elucidating the mechanisms involved in the disease, are seldom necessary for diagnosis. The possibility of obtaining false-positive

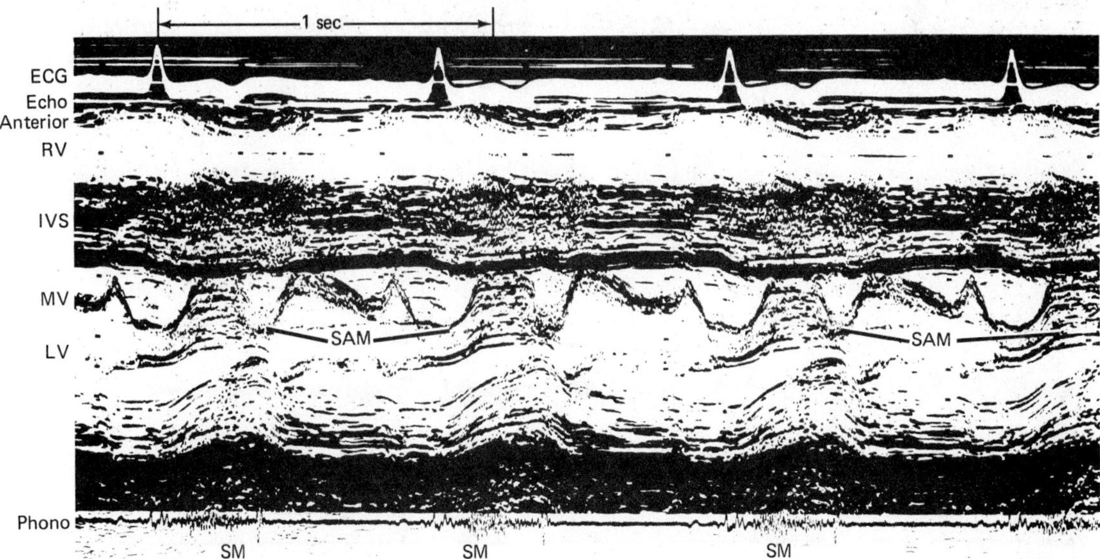

Figure 17–10. Echocardiogram showing systolic anterior motion (SAM) of mitral valve in a patient with hypertrophic obstructive cardiomyopathy. Septal (IVS) thickening and a long systolic murmur (SM) can also be seen. MV, mitral valve; RV, right ventricle; LV, left ventricle. (Courtesy of NB Schiller.)

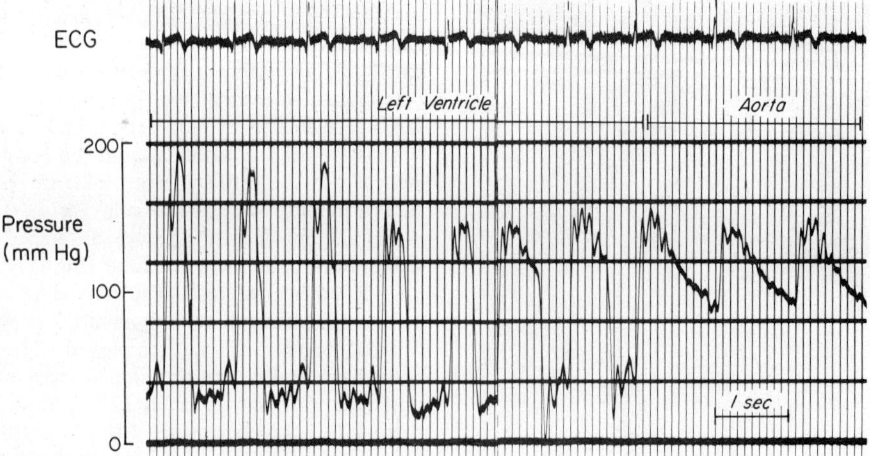

Figure 17–11. Withdrawal pressure tracing from left ventricle to aorta in a patient with hypertrophic obstructive cardiomyopathy. The pressure difference of 50 mm Hg is in the ventricle and not between the ventricle and the aorta.

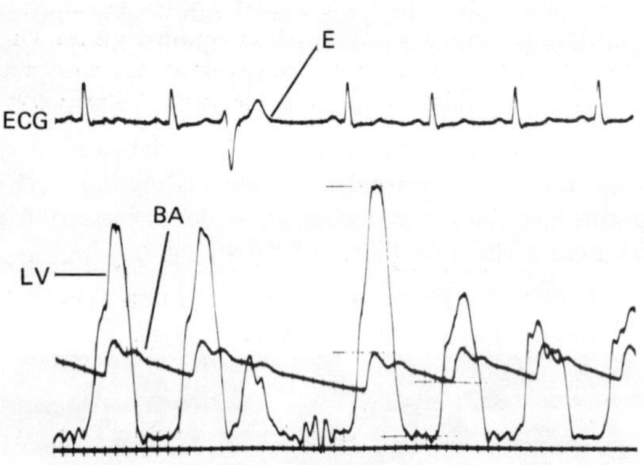

Figure 17–12. Pressure tracings in the left ventricle (LV) and brachial artery (BA) in a patient with hypertrophic obstructive cardiomyopathy. The pressure difference is greater after an ectopic beat.

results with catheter entrapment in the ventricular trabeculae should always be borne in mind.

5. Angiography–Left ventricular cineangiography is a useful confirmation test. The hypertrophied left ventricular muscle mass can be seen to narrow the waist of the ventricle in early systole (Fig 17–14A). The subvalvular region during late systole takes on the appearance of an inverted cone filled with contrast material (Fig 17–14B). The body of the left ventricle is almost completely empty because of the exaggerated "muscle-bound" contraction that has expelled almost all of its contents. The base of the cone is the aortic valve; the posterior surface is the anterior cusp of the mitral valve; and the anterior surface is the hypertrophied interventricular septum. The tip of the cone is the site of the obstruction. Left ventricular angiography also shows mitral incompetence, but care must be taken to exclude spurious incompetence associated with ectopic beats. Angiography can also delineate rings and shelves of tissue below the aortic valve which may be present in some cases. Selective coronary angiography is seldom indicated because the large coronary vessels seen in the disease fill well from aortic injections and are almost always normal.

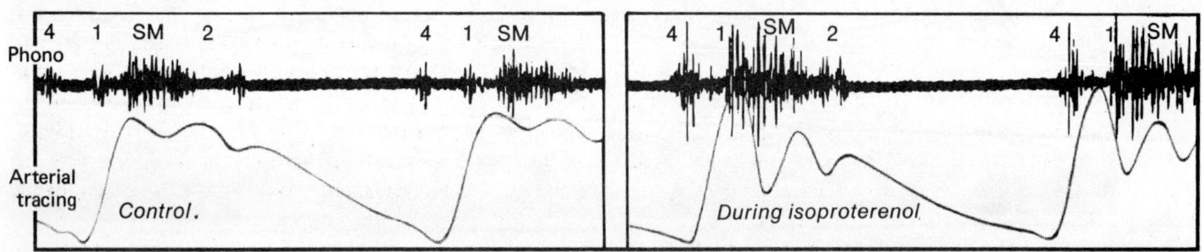

Figure 17–13. Phonocardiogram and external carotid pulse tracing in a patient with hypertrophic obstructive cardiomyopathy. During isoproterenol infusion, the atrial sound (4), the systolic murmur (SM), and the bifid nature of the arterial pulse are more obvious. (Courtesy of Roche Laboratories Division of Hoffman-La Roche, Inc.)

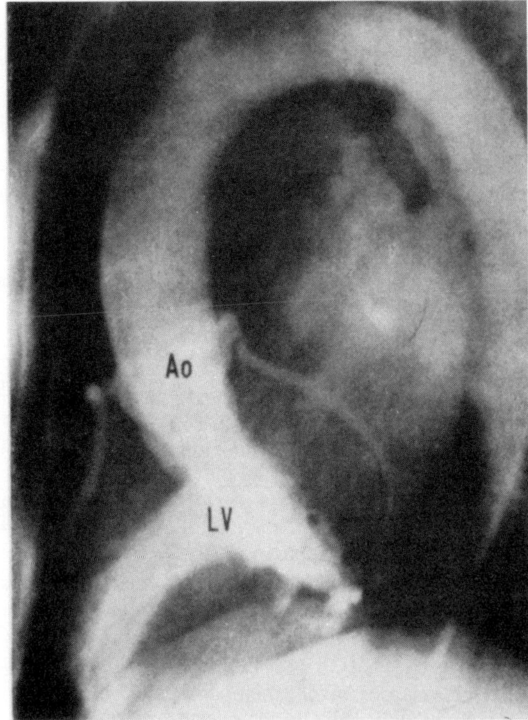

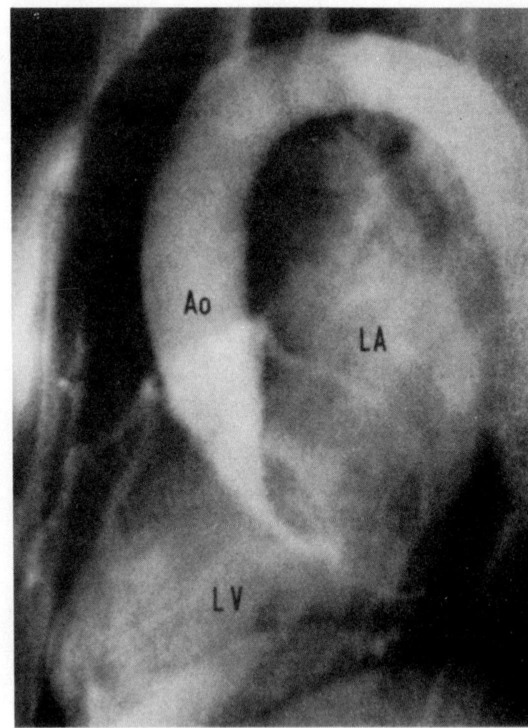

Figure 17–14. Angiographic features of hypertrophic obstructive cardiomyopathy. Single frame of angiogram following injection of contrast medium into the left ventricle in a patient with hypertrophic obstructive cardiomyopathy. In *A*, during early systole, the ventricular body is narrowed by hypertrophied muscle. In *B*, during late systole, the left ventricular body is empty and the cone-shaped shadow of the distal subvalvular chambers is seen. (Reproduced, with permission, from Cohen J & others: Hypertrophic obstructive cardiomyopathy. Br Heart J 26:16, 1964.)

Differential Diagnosis

The physical signs of hypertrophic obstructive cardiomyopathy resemble those of mitral incompetence or ventricular septal defect more closely than those of aortic stenosis. There is, however, left ventricular outflow obstruction in both valvular and subvalvular lesions, and, although the jerky, bifid pulse of obstructive cardiomyopathy is readily distinguished from the anacrotic, slow-rising pulse of aortic stenosis, this lesion does enter into the differential diagnosis in practice. Marked left ventricular hypertrophy is not seen in mitral incompetence or ventricular septal defect, and its presence in a patient with a long, harsh systolic murmur should suggest obstructive cardiomyopathy.

Complications

Atrial fibrillation, ventricular arrhythmias, and sudden death are important complications, and a relationship is presumed to exist between the latter two. Young patients with the familial disease seem most prone to these complications. Left ventricular failure with pulmonary edema may follow the onset of atrial fibrillation. In other cases, left ventricular failure may actually relieve obstruction and help to improve the condition because it leads to cardiac dilatation. Mitral incompetence may be caused by long-term damage to the valve by turbulent flow in the outflow tract. Endocardial fibrosis and thickening are seen in this area and are thought to be due to mechanical trauma.

Treatment

In general, it is sound practice to reserve treatment for patients with symptoms and to follow all patients closely to determine whether their clinical status is stable or worsening.

A. Medical Treatment: Propranolol is the major therapeutic weapon. The initial dosage of 10 mg 3 times daily should be increased to tolerance, and up to 200 mg/day may be needed in some cases. The objective of propranolol therapy is to decrease the force of left ventricular contraction to a level at which the ventricle no longer obstructs its own outflow. Propranolol tends to prevent arrhythmias as a subsidiary benefit, and it is only in patients who have not improved with an adequate trial of propranolol that differences of opinion about treatment exist. Other antiarrhythmia drugs are of nonspecific value.

B. Surgical Treatment: Surgical incision and resection of hypertrophied muscle bundles in the ventricular outflow tract is advocated in some centers; mitral valve replacement has been recommended in others; and even the production of bundle branch block has been suggested as a mode of therapy. It seems likely that the wide spectrum of cases accounts for the differences of opinion about treatment. We are reluctant to advocate surgery until a protracted trial of propranolol, with increasing doses up to more than 200 mg/day if necessary, has been given every opportunity to work. In our experience, muscular incision and resection is the only form of surgical treatment that should be undertaken.

Problems arise when the patient cannot tolerate propranolol (eg, because of asthma). In such cases, overhydration with increased salt and water intake and even salt-retaining steroids (eg, fludrocortisone, 0.1–0.3 mg/day) may be useful.

The question whether to give digitalis often arises in patients with evidence of left ventricular failure. Digitalis has been thought to aggravate obstruction because it increases the force of cardiac contraction. The drug should obviously not be used unless left ventricular failure is present. In our experience, it is not harmful in patients with failure, and its use is not contraindicated. In patients in whom arrhythmia is particularly difficult to control, surgery may be helpful.

Prognosis

The long-term prognosis of hypertrophic obstructive cardiomyopathy is not yet fully established because the condition has only been widely recognized for about 20 years. The sudden deaths of some patients with hypertrophic obstructive cardiomyopathy weigh on the minds of physicians. On the other hand, there seems no doubt that some patients with the disease can live long and relatively asymptomatic lives. We have seen patients in their 50s and 60s with obvious disease in whom a history of a murmur dates back to childhood. It seems possible that the course is more benign when abnormal muscular hypertrophy develops later in life. The specter of sudden death tends to hover over these patients; and, since the disease can run a course of 50 years or more, it seems likely that many years will have to elapse before a clear picture of the prognosis will emerge. In some patients, the characteristic murmur disappears with the onset of left ventricular failure, and the evidence of obstruction disappears as the failing ventricle dilates.

Pregnancy is well tolerated in young women with the disease unless cardiac failure is present.

ACUTE MYOCARDITIS ASSOCIATED WITH SPECIFIC DISEASES

Acute myocarditis is most commonly due to acute rheumatic fever or to one of the type B coxsackieviruses but may also be caused by any other virus, eg, type A coxsackie, echo, poliomyelitis, varicella, mumps, or hepatitis viruses. Myocarditis is present in about 1% of all patients in special infectious disease services in general hospitals in the USA. Most patients with myocarditis and acute exanthems seen on an infectious disease service are free of cardiac symptoms, and signs are discovered only by careful examination (including ECG). The acute exanthems rarely cause cardiac failure or cardiac dysfunction.

Pathology

Cardiac involvement occurs in 5–10% of coxsackievirus infections (Grist, 1974), and the histologic effects are shown in Figs 17–15 and 17–16. The disease may be mild or severe.

Clinical Findings

A. Myocarditis Due to Type B Coxsackieviruses:

1. Symptoms and signs–Fig 17–17 shows the relative frequency of important clinical symptoms and signs in proved coxsackievirus heart disease. Of all the types of coxsackieviruses, types B3 and B5 are most commonly associated with myocarditis in adults. Coxsackievirus myocarditis is usually suspected in adults on the basis of an acute febrile illness with lethargy, chest pain, dyspnea, enlargement of the heart, and nonspecific ST–T changes. There may be obvious signs of cardiac failure in severe cases. Patients often have associated pericarditis; the presence of a pericardial rub in association with ECG abnormalities demonstrates pericardial involvement and distinguishes coxsackievirus infection with myocarditis from other influenzalike syndromes.

The illness usually lasts 1–4 weeks but may persist for months. Multiple recurrences may occur over a period of 1–2 years, but rarely is the condition severe, fulminant, or fatal. Patients who survive are usually completely well months later, but the prognosis must be guarded because chronic cardiac failure has continued over a period of 2–3 years in 5–10% of patients. Some observers believe that coxsackievirus myocarditis may be a cause of idiopathic cardiomyopathy that occurs later in life. The same is true of chronic constrictive pericarditis, but the data are scant and only a few well-documented examples of such patients have been reported. It is rare to observe a transition from acute coxsackievirus myocarditis to either chronic idiopathic cardiomyopathy or constrictive pericarditis.

2. Laboratory findings–The diagnosis is confirmed by virus isolation from throat washings or feces or by the appearance of a 4-fold increase in neutralizing antibody from paired sera during the course of the disease.

3. X-ray findings–The chest film may demonstrate significant cardiac enlargement, often with pleural or pericardial effusion. If the latter is suspected, echocardiography can then establish its presence and magnitude (see Chapter 18).

B. Myocarditis Due to Other Viruses: Myocarditis has been noted frequently, usually by ECG changes or some alteration of heart sounds, as an incidental feature of other viral diseases such as echovirus infection, mumps, poliomyelitis, infectious mononucleosis, measles, and hepatitis. In other rare cases in which myocardial involvement is of clinical significance, the

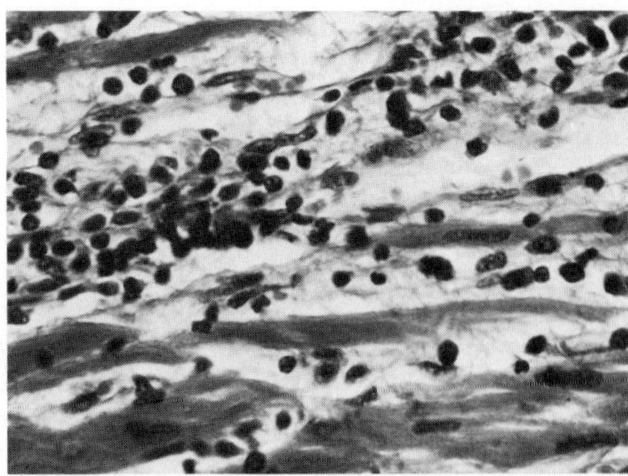

Figure 17–15. Focus of inflammatory cell infiltration in the myocardium in viral myocarditis. H&E stain. (Courtesy of O Rambo.)

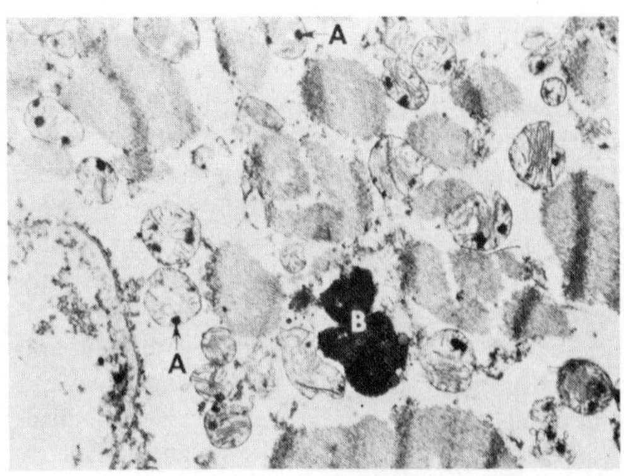

Figure 17–16. Electron micrograph of the myocardium in coxsackie B4 myocarditis showing fragmented myofibrils (B) and swollen mitochondria (A), demonstrating the severity of the acute process. Original magnification of X 25,000 reduced by 36%. (Reproduced, with permission, from Rose HD: Recurrent illness following acute coxsackie B4 myocarditis. Am J Med 54:544, 1973.)

manifestations are gallop rhythm, enlargement of the heart, or other signs of cardiac failure (see Chapter 10). Focal myocardial infiltration may be found on pathologic examination of the heart from patients with many types of viral infections who had no clinical evidence of heart disease during life. There is no doubt that the myocardium is affected in some of these infections without causing any clinical findings that may lead to a diagnosis. One must therefore distinguish between the focal inflammatory infiltrates seen pathologically (Saphir, 1960) and the clinical manifestations of acute myocarditis, which are rare in these viral diseases.

C. Acute Myocarditis Due to Rickettsiae: Rickettsial diseases (Q fever, scrub typhus [Tsutsugamushi disease], Rocky Mountain spotted fever, and epidemic typhus fever) are exceptions to the statement that myocarditis secondary to systemic disease produces few clinical manifestations. Depending on its severity, the infection may result in cardiac or circulatory failure in the second week of disease, but this is rarely a prominent feature. In the Serbian epidemics of 1915, cardiac failure was thought to be the cause of death in a third of fatal cases autopsied. In the Polish epidemic, microscopic lesions (the so-called typhus nodules of myocarditis) were present in all 39 cases autopsied

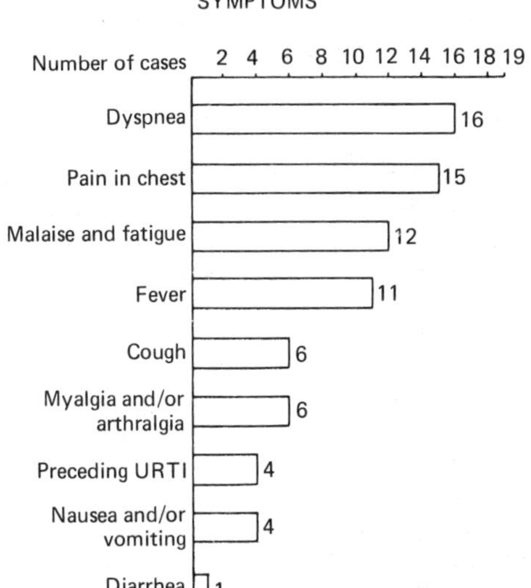

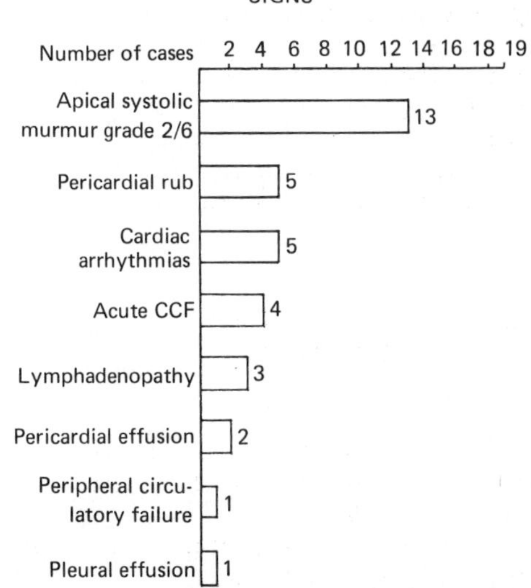

Figure 17–17. Clinical symptoms and signs in 19 proved cases of coxsackievirus heart disease. (Modified and reproduced, with permission, from Sainani GS, Dekate MP, Rao CP: Heart disease caused by coxsackievirus B infection. Br Heart J 37:819, 1975.)

(Strong, 1920). In Q fever there may be tachycardia out of proportion to the fever as well as dyspnea, fatigue, or chest pain suggesting myocardial involvement as with other rickettsial diseases.

Rocky Mountain spotted fever (which also occurs in the New England states) may rarely cause myocarditis, and rickettsiae may be identified by the monocyte culture technic as well as by specific antibody titers, especially complement fixation. Serologic confirmation occurs late in the course of the disease, and one must suspect the diagnosis on epidemiologic and clinical grounds. Q fever can be recognized serologically by the presence of complement-fixing antibodies.

Scrub typhus myocarditis in American troops during World War II was characterized by persistent, apparently unaccountable fatigue, tachycardia, and ECG and radiologic evidence of cardiac involvement requiring prolonged convalescence lasting for months even though the disease occurred in healthy young men. Eventually, all patients recovered completely (Sokolow, 1945).

D. Acute Myocarditis Due to Chagas' Disease: Acute Chagas' disease is usually associated with systemic symptoms. The initial local skin and eye lesions may be associated with acute myocarditis, but the dominant feature of the disease is late chronic cardiac failure or conduction defects. Human African trypanosomiasis has been found pathologically to cause chronic pancarditis as well as valvulitis and lesions of the conducting system (Poltera, 1976). The usual presenting symptoms are neurologic rather than cardiac because meningoencephalitis is frequently associated with the disease. The histologic pattern is similar to that seen in Chagas' disease, but myocarditis is less frequent in infections due to *Trypanosoma gambiense* than in those due to *T cruzi.* The possibility that idiopathic hypertrophy in African countries might be due to undiagnosed trypanosomiasis must await further study in the light of this report, although other authors believe trypanosomiasis is an unlikely cause.

E. Trichinosis: This is a diffuse disease caused by ingestion of the helminth *Trichinella spiralis,* usually from inadequately cooked pork. The worm may be eaten with beef contaminated with infected pork or in infected pork sausages. The organism is destroyed by heating at 60 °C for 30 minutes; using preheated garbage as fodder prevents hogs from becoming infected.

The disease is suspected in a patient with fever, periorbital edema, muscle pains, and eosinophilia who has eaten inadequately heated pork. The larvae spread through the body, but focal inflammatory myocarditis is responsible for some of the deaths.

Myocarditis occurs 3–8 weeks after infection and is suspected on the basis of dyspnea, tachycardia, and ECG changes in conjunction with the general features noted above. The ECG changes are nonspecific, with ST–T changes, sinus tachycardia, and ventricular premature beats. Congestive failure occurs rarely.

The diagnosis is strongly suspected on the basis of severe eosinophilia (often $\geqslant 50\%$) and splinter hemorrhages of the nails and confirmed by complement fixation tests and skeletal muscle biopsy.

Treatment is supportive, plus corticosteroid therapy. The long-term prognosis is good, and chronic cardiac disease is rare.

Differential Diagnosis of Acute Myocarditis

Acute myocarditis due to infection with viruses (eg, coxsackieviruses), protozoa (eg, trypanosomes), or bacteria (eg, pneumococci) must be distinguished from acute toxic myocarditis due to drugs or diphtheria and from myocarditis associated with acute rheumatic fever, connective tissue disorders, and acute glomerulonephritis. ECG changes in viral diseases may be due to acute circulatory failure from infection, metabolic abnormalities such as disturbances in acid-base balance, and hypoxia and not to myocarditis as such.

Nonviral myocarditis is recognized on the basis of the obvious manifestations of the underlying disease, as in diphtheria, rheumatic fever, or pneumococcal pneumonia. Chagas' disease is endemic in South and Central America but rare in the USA, and the diagnosis of acute myocarditis is usually based on epidemiologic evidence as well as the presence of a chagoma at the site of entry of the parasites and recovery of trypanosomes in blood drawn early in the course of the disease. If the patient lives in a thatched hut in which the Triatoma vector lives, the diagnosis should be considered.

Acute rheumatic fever is associated with other major findings such as arthritis and a history of recent streptococcal infection; arthritis is relieved by salicylates, and recent streptococcal infection can be inferred from finding increasing titers of antistreptolysin antibodies in the serum. Diphtheria causes a typical lesion in the throat but may infect the skin also (common in the Orient and Asia), and the organism can be identified from throat and skin cultures. In acute myocardial toxicity from drugs, awareness of the use of drugs, their dosage, and the presence of the disease being treated with drugs helps differentiate myocardial toxicity from acute myocarditis. This may be quite difficult in patients with acute lupus erythematosus with fever, pericarditis, and vasculitis, and specific diagnostic procedures such as lupus erythematosus preparations and serial neutralizing antibody determinations for viral infections may be required to make the differentiation.

Acute glomerulonephritis may present as acute cardiac failure, but the poststreptococcal state, hypertension, and urinary findings should make the diagnosis clear. Hemodynamic findings indicate that "cardiac failure" in acute nephritis is usually due to salt and water retention and not to cardiac failure per se. The cardiac index is often increased, averaging 5.4 liters/min/m^2 at rest and 7.5 liters/min/m^2 with exercise–in contrast to the low cardiac output in acute cardiac failure. The pulmonary capillary wedge pressure is slightly increased at rest but within the normal range after exercise (averaging 15 mm Hg at rest and 18 mm Hg after exercise) (Binak, 1975).

Treatment of Acute Myocarditis*

In the absence of effective specific antiviral therapy, treatment consists of general supportive care and management of cardiac failure, arrhythmias, or conduction defects if they occur. Coxsackieviruses have been recovered directly from the myocardium, and it has been shown in mice that virus multiplication increases when the mice exercise vigorously, with a corresponding increase in mortality rate. Clinical experience suggests that early exercise should be avoided to prevent multiplication of viruses and further impairment of cardiac function.

In nonviral acute myocarditis, treatment is directed toward the underlying cause if possible, as it is with diphtheria or pneumococcal infections. Some patients with candida infections respond to amphotericin B or flucytosine, and a recent report by Ruskin and Remington (1976) indicates that 80% of patients receiving antitoxoplasma chemotherapy (pyrimethamine and sulfonamide) showed marked clinical improvement or complete remission. Most cases of disseminated toxoplasmosis and myocarditis result from infection in immunosuppressed individuals or those that have defects in cellular immunity.

Prognosis

Follow-up of 14 of 19 patients with coxsackie B acute myocarditis by Sainani and associates (1975) revealed no deaths, but 3 patients had chronic heart failure, with enlarged hearts in 2. The remainder had no definite symptoms or signs of myocarditis, but 3 had vague precordial pain with normal chest films and ECGs.

RHEUMATIC FEVER

Rheumatic fever is a subacute or chronic systemic disease which for unknown reasons may either be self-limiting or lead to slowly progressive valvular deformity. Rarely, it is acute and fulminant. It is a much less common disease in the USA now, probably because of effective treatment of beta-hemolytic streptococcal infections, but it is still common in developing countries.

Rheumatic fever and its sequelae used to be the commonest cause of heart disease in people under 50 years of age in the USA, and as a cause of heart disease in people of all ages it ranked third behind hypertension and atherosclerotic coronary disease. The prevalence is probably much less now in developed countries, but the disease is still common elsewhere. Chorea is seen more frequently in females. The peak incidence occurs between the ages of 5 and 15; rheumatic fever is rare before age 4 and after age 50.

*Treatment of myocarditis associated with rheumatic fever is discussed on p 536; treatment of Chagas' disease on p 556.

Etiology

Rheumatic fever is initiated by an infection with group A beta-hemolytic streptococci, appearing usually 1–4 weeks after an episode of tonsillitis, nasopharyngitis, or otitis media. The streptococcal infection is the antigen for the antigen-antibody response resulting in rheumatic fever.

Pathology

The acute phase of rheumatic fever may involve the endocardium, myocardium, pericardium, synovial joint linings, lungs, peritoneum, or pleura. The characteristic lesion is a perivascular granulomatous reaction and vasculitis (Aschoff nodule; Fig 17–18). The mitral valve is attacked in 75–80% of cases, the aortic valve in 30%, and the tricuspid and pulmonary valves in less than 5%. Small pink granules appear on the surface of the edematous valve. Healing may be complete, or progressive scarring due to subacute or chronic inflammation may develop over months or years.

Diagnosis

The diagnosis is more readily made in epidemics of streptococcal infections such as occur in wartime, when the relationship of β-hemolytic streptococcal infections and the subsequent nonsuppurative complications of rheumatic fever are more readily seen. Even mild cases can be recognized under these circumstances. When isolated cases of rheumatic fever occur, the diagnosis is often unsuspected and not made. This may explain the high percentage of patients with rheumatic heart disease who deny a previous history of rheumatic fever.

Children usually have a more fulminant disease than adults and therefore the diagnosis is more easily made. In adults the diagnosis is infrequently made except in "epidemics." The disease "licks the joints and bites the heart" of children, but the reverse is usually true of adults.

The diagnosis may be difficult, with scarcely diagnosable illness. ("Let me see the patient in 5–10 years, and I'll tell you whether or not the current illness was

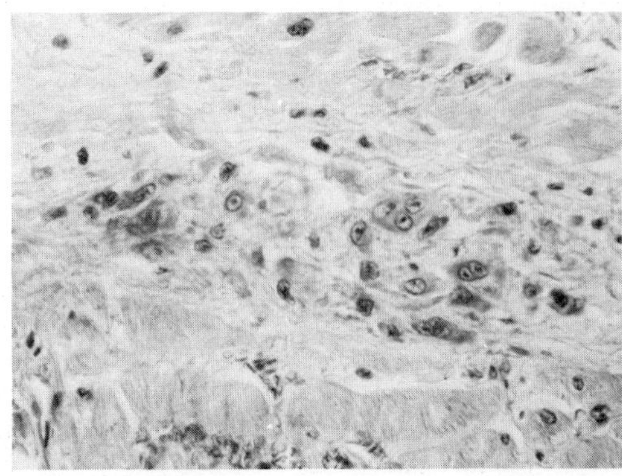

Figure 17–18. Typical multinucleated Aschoff nodule from the atrial appendage in a patient with rheumatic heart disease. Magnification X 100, H&E stain. (Courtesy of O Rambo.)

rheumatic fever.") Or it may be obvious, with all the criteria necessary for diagnosis. Because of the difficulties in interpreting the symptoms, the diagnostic findings have been separated into major and minor criteria, with at least 2 major criteria being necessary for diagnosis. The *major criteria* are peri-, myo-, or endocarditis, chorea, subcutaneous nodules, erythma marginatum, and polyarthritis. The *minor criteria* are fever, malaise, abdominal pain (especially in children), "growing pains," and laboratory findings of leukocytosis, raised sedimentation rate, and evidence of a preceding streptococcal infection (increased titer of antistreptolysin O).

Clinical Findings

A. Symptoms: The disease usually begins with either fever or arthritis in a patient who has recovered from a β-hemolytic streptococcal infection 2–3 weeks previously.

1. Fever—The fever may be low-grade and intermittent, but in severe cases with pericarditis or myocarditis it may be substantial (about 39 °C). It is a "minor" criterion of rheumatic fever because it may be due to many causes. The fever often lasts for weeks or months, in conjunction with general symptoms of malaise, asthenia, weight loss, and anorexia, which may indicate a smoldering rheumatic state but are also characteristic of any chronic active disease.

2. Joint pains—"Growing pains" in joints, periarticular tissues, or muscle systems may be a symptom of rheumatic fever ("polyarthralgia") but are not specific.

3. Arthritis—Arthritis with effusion is characteristically a migratory polyarthritis of gradual or sudden onset which involves the large joints sequentially, one becoming hot, red, swollen, and tender as the inflammation in the previously involved joint subsides. Body temperature rises as each successive joint becomes inflamed. In adults, only a single or a small joint may be affected. The acute arthritis lasts 1–5 weeks and subsides without residual deformity. *Note:* Joint involvement is considered a major criterion only when definite effusion and signs of inflammation are present. This is in contrast to arthralgia, in which pain or stiffness is present without these objective signs. Prompt response of arthritis to therapeutic doses of salicylates is characteristic (but not diagnostic) of rheumatic fever.

Table 17–3. Incidence of symptoms and signs of rheumatic fever in 1000 patients.

Carditis	653
Chorea	518
Arthritis	410
Arthralgia	401
Epistaxis	274
Precordial pain	240
Pericardial rub	130
Abdominal pain	117
Subcutaneous nodules	88
Rash	71

*Reproduced, with permission of the American Heart Association, Inc., from Bland EF, Jones TD: Rheumatic fever and rheumatic heart disease: A 20-year report on 1000 patients followed since childhood. Circulation 4:836, 1951.

4. Peri-, myo-, endocarditis ("carditis")—The symptoms of carditis in rheumatic fever are often slight and must be looked for specifically. The patient does not complain of dyspnea unless cardiac failure is present. Chest pain is usually prominent, either made worse with breathing (pleuritis), related to posture if pericardial (see Chapter 18), or epigastric if there is peritoneal involvement. The interpretation of the symptoms is clarified by signs, ECG, and x-ray findings (see below). The patient may complain of palpitations due to a rapid heart rate, but symptoms of arrhythmia are uncommon.

5. Skin lesions and subcutaneous nodules—The patient may complain of skin lesions or subcutaneous nodules, but these are more frequently found on physical examination (see Signs, below).

6. Chorea—Chorea consists of purposeless jerky movements, continual and nonrepetitive, of the limbs, trunk, and facial muscles. Milder forms masquerade as undue restlessness as the patient attempts to convert uncontrolled movements into seemingly purposeful ones. Facial grimaces of infinite variety are common. These movements are made worse by emotional tension and disappear entirely during sleep. The episode lasts several weeks or occasionally months.

Sydenham's chorea may appear suddenly as an isolated entity with no "minor criteria" or may develop in the course of overt rheumatic fever. Eventually, 50% of patients have other signs of rheumatic fever. Girls are more frequently affected, and occurrence in adults is rare.

B. Signs:

1. General appearance—The patient may seem well or may appear both acutely and chronically ill, with pallor, subdued affect, and general debility.

2. Arthritis—The joints may be normal on examination in patients with arthralgia and growing pains, or reddened and swollen in acute arthritis. Movement of the involved joint or even the weight or movement of bedsheets over the joint is poorly tolerated. There is marked disparity between the often slight effusion and faint blush over the affected joint and the magnitude of the pain. The arthritis may involve only one joint or may "migrate" to involve multiple joints as the patient is examined daily. Often the initial joint improves as a new joint is affected, but occasionally polyarthritis is present.

3. Carditis—The myocardial signs may be minimal or characterized by tachycardia out of proportion to the fever, which persists during sleep and is greatly increased by slight activity; by cardiac enlargement with the cardiac impulse displaced to the left; by pericardial friction rub with or without a raised jugular venous pressure, depending on the presence and amount of pericardial effusion; by painful engorgement of the liver (especially in cardiac failure in children); and by signs of left ventricular failure such as gallop rhythm or pulmonary rales. Cardiac murmurs are infrequent at onset, but with the passage of days careful auscultation may reveal a short, soft middiastolic murmur of mitral valve involvement (Carey-Coombs murmur), a short early diastolic murmur of aortic valve involvement, or a soft pansystolic murmur of mitral incompetence which becomes louder during the course of the disease and is transmitted to the axilla. Short systolic murmurs are common but are due to fever or tachycardia and not to mitral incompetence. The heart sounds may be "tictac," as described in the section on acute myocarditis, and may change in quality on daily examination.

4. **Arrhythmias**–Premature beats may occur but are uncommon; atrial fibrillation and ventricular tachycardia are rare.

5. **Erythema marginatum (annulare)**–This is frequently associated with skin nodules. The lesions begin as rapidly enlarging macules which assume the shape of rings or crescents with clear centers. They may be slightly raised and confluent. The rash may be transient or may persist for long periods.

6. **Subcutaneous nodules**–These are uncommon except in children. The nodules may be few or many; are usually small (2 cm or less in diameter), firm, and nontender; and are attached to fascia or tendon sheaths over bony prominences such as the elbows, the dorsal surfaces of the hands, the malleoli, the vertebral spines, and the occiput. They persist for days or weeks, are usually recurrent, and are clinically indistinguishable from the nodules of rheumatoid arthritis.

7. **Recurrent nosebleeds**–These may be seen on examination. Recurrent epistaxis is believed by some clinicians to be an indication of "subclinical" rheumatic fever.

C. **Laboratory Findings**: These are helpful in 3 ways:

1. **As nonspecific evidence of inflammatory disease**–The sedimentation rate and white count are almost always increased during active rheumatic fever except when chorea is the only clinical sign. Variable leukocytosis and normochromic anemia may appear. Slight proteinuria and microhematuria do not necessarily indicate concomitant glomerulonephritis.

2. **As evidence of antecedent beta-hemolytic streptococcal infection**–A high titer or increasing antistreptolysin O titer indicates recent infection but does not mean that rheumatic fever is present. Throat culture is positive for beta-hemolytic streptococci in 50% of cases of active rheumatic fever.

3. **As strong evidence against the diagnosis**–A low antistreptolysin O titer (50 Todd units) which does not rise on repeated tests tends to rule out rheumatic fever. A normal sedimentation rate is rare in the presence of active rheumatic fever.

D. **Electrocardiographic Findings**: P–R prolongation greater than 0.04 sec above the patient's normal P–R interval is the most significant abnormality; changing contour of P waves or inversion of T waves is less specific. The characteristics are tabulated in Table 17–4.

Table 17–4. ECG abnormalities in 700 cases of rheumatic fever.*

		No.	Percent
Total cases with abnormalities in the ECG		147	21
Of the 147 cases:			
1. Conduction defects		88	60
Partial atrioventricular block	83		
Complete atrioventricular block	3		
Intraventricular block	2		
2. T wave changes		52	35
Inversion $T_{1,2}$ or T_4	17		
Diphasic T_1 and T_4	11		
Flat T_1 and T_4	24		
3. Abnormal rhythms		14	10
Shifting atrial pacemaker	7		
Junctional rhythm	4		
Junctional escape	2		
Atrial fibrillation	1		
4. Miscellaneous		12	8
Marked left axis deviation or right axis deviation	7		
Inversion P_2 and P_3	5		
Duration of atrioventricular block			
Of 76 cases:			
0–4 days		11	15
5–8 days		3	4
9–14 days		39	51
15–21 days		14	18
22–28 days		6	8
Over 3 months		3	4

*Reproduced, with permission, from Sokolow M: Significance of electrocardiographic changes in rheumatic fever. Am J Med 5:365, 1948.

E. **X-Ray Findings**: X-ray of the chest is usually normal but may reveal cardiac enlargement, especially on serial examinations. A grossly enlarged cardiac shadow may rapidly appear if pericardial effusion develops (see Chapter 18).

F. **Special Investigations**: Echocardiograms are diagnostic if pericardial effusion develops but are probably not sensitive enough to demonstrate early valvular involvement. Experience is too limited to make a definite statement regarding the value of echocardiography in early valvular inflammation.

Differential Diagnosis

Rheumatic fever may be confused with the following: rheumatoid arthritis, osteomyelitis, chronic infections, traumatic joint disease, neurocirculatory asthenia or cardiac neurosis, bacterial endocarditis, pulmonary tuberculosis, chronic meningococcemia, meningitis, acute poliomyelitis, connective tissue diseases (eg, disseminated lupus erythematosus), serum sickness, drug sensitivity, leukemia, sickle cell anemia, inactive rheumatic heart disease, congenital heart disease, and "surgical abdomen."

Complications

Congestive heart failure occurs in severe cases. Other complications include cardiac arrhythmias, pericarditis with large effusion, rheumatic pneumonitis, pulmonary embolism and infarction, cardiac invalidism, and early or late development of permanent heart valve deformity.

Prevention of Recurrent Rheumatic Fever

The principles of prevention are to avoid beta-hemolytic streptococcal infections if possible and to treat streptococcal infections promptly and intensively with appropriate antibiotics.

A. General Measures: Avoid contact with persons who have "colds" or other upper respiratory infections. Patients with rheumatic fever do better in a moderate climate where streptococcal infections are less common.

B. Prevention of Infection: Two methods of prevention are now advocated.

1. Penicillin–The preferred method of prophylaxis is with benzathine penicillin G, 1.2 million units intramuscularly every 4 weeks. Oral penicillin (200–250 thousand units daily before breakfast) may be used instead but is less reliable. Prophylaxis is advocated especially for children who have had one or more acute attacks and should be given with particular care during the school year and usually until age 30. Some advise continuing prophylaxis until age 40–45. Adults should receive preventive therapy for about 5 years after an attack. Recurrences are rare in patients receiving prophylactic antibiotic therapy.

2. Sulfonamides–If the patient is sensitive to penicillin, give sulfadiazine, 1 g orally daily throughout the year. *Caution:* Patients receiving sulfonamides should have periodic blood counts and urinalyses. If there is any tendency toward leukopenia, the drug should be stopped immediately and a different drug substituted.

C. Treatment of Streptococcal Sore Throat: Prompt therapy (within 24 hours) of streptococcal infections will prevent most attacks of acute rheumatic fever.

Treatment

A. Medical Treatment:

1. Salicylates–The salicylates markedly reduce fever, relieve joint pain, and may reduce joint swelling. There is no evidence that they have any effect on the natural course of the disease. *Note:* The salicylates should be continued as long as necessary to relieve pain, swelling, or fever. If withdrawal results in recurrence of symptoms, treatment should be reinstituted immediately.

a. Sodium salicylate is the most widely used of this group of drugs. The maximum dose is 1–2 g orally every 2–4 hours to allay symptoms and fever; 4–6 g/day suffice in most adults. In an occasional patient, maximum doses may not be completely effective. There is no evidence that intravenous administration has any advantage over the oral route. Early untoward reactions to the salicylates include tinnitus, nausea and vomiting, and gastrointestinal bleeding. Antacids are usually given with salicylates to reduce gastric irritation. *Caution:* Do not use sodium salicylate or sodium bicarbonate in patients with acute rheumatic fever who have associated cardiac failure.

b. Aspirin may be substituted for sodium salicylate, with the same dosages and precautions. No sodium should be used in the presence of heart failure.

2. Penicillin–Penicillin should be employed at any time during the course of the disease to eradicate streptococcal infections.

3. Corticosteroids–There is no proof that cardiac damage is prevented or minimized by corticosteroids even when given early in large doses. Corticosteroids are effective anti-inflammatory agents for reversing the acute exudative phase of rheumatic fever and are probably more potent for this purpose than salicylates. A short course of corticosteroids usually causes rapid improvement in the acute manifestations of rheumatic fever and is indicated in severe cases with high fever, pericarditis, active myocarditis, rapid heart rate, and painful swollen joints. There may be prompt disappearance of fever, malaise, tachycardia, and polyarthritis. Abnormal ECG changes (prolonged P–R interval) and sedimentation rates may return to normal limits within a week.

A suggested schedule, to be started as soon as severe rheumatic fever is diagnosed, is as follows: Give prednisone, 5–10 mg orally every 6 hours for 3 weeks, and then gradually withdraw over a period of 3 weeks by reducing and then discontinuing first the nighttime, then the evening, and finally the daytime doses. In severe cases the dosage should be increased, if necessary, to levels adequate to control symptoms.

B. General Measures: Bed rest should be enforced until all signs of active rheumatic fever have disappeared. The criteria are as follows: return of the temperature to normal with the patient at bed rest and without medications, normal sedimentation rate, normal resting pulse rate (under 100/min in adults), and return of ECG to normal or fixation of abnormalities. The patient may then be allowed up slowly, but several months should elapse before return to full activity unless the disease was exceedingly mild. Maintain good nutrition.

C. Treatment of Complications:

1. Congestive failure–Treat as for congestive failure, with the following variations:

a. A low-sodium diet and diuretics are of particular value in promoting diuresis and treating failure in acute rheumatic fever.

b. Digitalis is usually not as effective in congestive heart failure due to acute rheumatic fever as in other forms of congestive failure and may accentuate myocardial irritability, producing arrhythmias which further embarrass the heart. Digitalis should be given but with extreme care.

c. When congestive failure and pericarditis with or without effusion are dominant, they often respond dramatically to corticotropin or the corticosteroids, but the anti-inflammatory action may fail to modify subsequent valvular effects. When sodium-retaining hormonal agents are employed, excess sodium intake is prohibited and thiazide diuresis is imperative.

2. **Pericarditis**—Treat as any acute nonpurulent pericarditis. The rheumatic effusion is sterile, and antibiotics are of no value. The general principles include relief of pain, by opiates if necessary, and removal of fluid by pericardiocentesis if tamponade develops. This, however, is rarely necessary. If pericardiocentesis is performed, it should be preceded and followed by a short course of penicillin therapy to prevent infection of the pericardium. Corticotropin and the corticosteroids as well as salicylates should be continued or started, as they seem to have a specific favorable effect in aiding resorption of the fluid.

Prognosis

Initial episodes of rheumatic fever last months in children and weeks in adults. Twenty percent of children have recurrences within 5 years. Recurrences are uncommon after 5 years of well-being and rare after age 21. The immediate mortality rate is 1–2%. Persistent rheumatic activity with a greatly enlarged heart, heart failure, and pericarditis indicate a poor prognosis as shown in Table 17–5; 30% of children thus affected die within 10 years of the initial attack. Otherwise the prognosis for life is good. Eighty percent of all patients attain adult life, and half of these have little if any limitation of activity. Approximately one-third of young patients have detectable valvular damage after the initial episode, most commonly involving the mitral valve. After 10 years, two-thirds of surviving patients will have detectable valvular disease. In adults, residual heart damage occurs in less than 20% and is generally less severe (Engleman, 1954). Mitral insufficiency is the commonest ultimate lesion, and aortic insufficiency is much more common than in children. The influence of corticosteroids on long-term prognosis is still being debated, although the short-term benefit is clear. Twenty percent of patients who have chorea develop valvular deformity even after a long latent period of apparent well-being.

Table 17–5. Fatalities in rheumatic fever in patients with special features.*

Onset (Number of Cases)	10 Years (Fatalities)	20 Years (Fatalities)
Greatly enlarged heart		
70	56 (80%)	57 (81%)
Congestive failure		
207	148 (71%)	152 (80%)
Pericarditis		
130	73 (56 %)	77 (63%)
Nodules		
88	34 (38%)	37 (43%)
Arthritis		
410	91 (22%)	109 (27%)
Chorea		
518	49 (9.4%)	63 (12%)

*Reproduced, with permission of the American Heart Association, Inc., from Bland EF, Jones TD: Rheumatic fever and rheumatic heart disease: A 20-year report on 1000 patients followed since childhood. Circulation 4:836, 1951.

Table 17–6. Causes of death in 301 cases of rheumatic fever and heart disease among 1000 patients after 20 years.*

Rheumatic Heart Disease			
Rheumatic fever		231	(80%)
Congestive failure			
Subacute bacterial endocarditis	26	30	(10%)
Acute bacterial endocarditis	4		
Other causes:			
Cerebral embolism	3		
Sudden and unexpected	10	30	
Uncertain	8		
Unrelated disease or accident	9		
Possible Rheumatic Heart Disease			
Unrelated disease or accident		10	

*Reproduced, with permission of the American Heart Association, Inc., from Bland EF, Jones TD: Rheumatic fever and rheumatic heart disease: A 20-year report on 1000 patients followed since childhood. Circulation 4:836, 1951.

ACUTE MYOCARDIAL DAMAGE DUE TO DRUG TOXICITY

Acute myocardial damage has been seen in the past after the use of a variety of drugs, notably emetine, digitalis, sympathomimetic drugs, arsenic, antimony, amphetamines, and tricyclic antidepressants (amitriptyline, imipramine). Myocardial toxicity is occurring with greater frequency as a result of the use of high doses of multiple drugs in the treatment of serious diseases. Multiple cytotoxic chemotherapy is now being used prior to bone marrow transplants and in the treatment of acute leukemia, lymphoma, carcinoma of the lung and gastrointestinal tract, and connective tissue disorders involving the kidney. Recent observations indicate that about one-fourth of patients (4 out of 15) receiving high-dose multiple chemotherapy may die of acute myopericardial failure during treatment as a result of endothelial injury, pericardial effusion, cardiac failure, and cardiac arrhythmias (Appelbaum, 1976).

Cytotoxic agents, eg, cyclophosphamide (Cytoxan) and doxorubicin (Adriamycin), may produce clinical as well as pathologic myocardial disease; the toxic effects are dose-related and more apt to occur when cytotoxic drugs are used in combination. The total dose of doxorubicin in adults should not exceed 500 mg/m^2 body surface—less in children or if the patient has received radiation therapy to the mediastinum or is receiving concomitant therapy with other potentially cardiotoxic agents.

As with any variety of acute myocardial disease or toxicity, the clinical presentation may be with arrhythmias or conduction defects rather than cardiac failure. Patients receiving emetine (for amebiasis) or antimony (for schistosomiasis) may demonstrate ECG abnormalities without clinical symptoms or signs; it is then desirable to use alternative drugs or proceed with smaller dosages and close observation.

Serial ECGs, chest films, and echocardiograms, cautious restriction of total dosage (see above), and close clinical observation for early evidences of cardiac involvement are advised. Decrease in the height of the R wave is an early sign of cardiac toxicity, and the risk/benefit ratio of continued therapy must be assessed. Cardiac enlargement and cardiac failure may develop slowly or rapidly.

Treatment

Withdraw cardiotoxic drugs and treat cardiac failure and arrhythmias as outlined in Chapter 10.

Prognosis

The prognosis is good if appropriate measures are taken before severe cardiac failure occurs, poor if the offending drug is continued after early cardiac toxicity is manifest. Mild to moderate cardiac failure subsides gradually after the cardiotoxic drug is stopped.

CHRONIC DISEASE OF THE MYOCARDIUM SECONDARY TO KNOWN METABOLIC DISEASE

THYROTOXIC HEART DISEASE

The increase in metabolic rate resulting from excess production of thyroid hormone requires that cardiac output and peripheral blood flow be increased, producing symptoms and signs that may be confused with heart disease. If there is underlying heart disease, the manifestations of cardiac failure in thyrotoxicosis are even more obvious. It may be difficult to distinguish the cardiac disease from the effects of circulatory hyperactivity produced by the increased metabolic rate. There is controversy in the literature about whether thyrotoxicosis per se can cause cardiac failure.

Sandler and Wilson (1959) reported a study of 462 patients with thyrotoxicosis of whom 150 had cardiac involvement. Although many patients with cardiac involvement had no obvious heart disease on first presentation, most of them had ischemic or hypertensive heart disease, and only a few had no evidence of associated heart disease. Half of those with cardiac failure had evidence of previous heart disease. The increased cardiac output and metabolic rate with increased oxygen consumption associated with thyrotoxicosis may precipitate cardiac failure in these patients.

Clinical Findings

A. Symptoms: The predominant symptoms are those of the underlying thyrotoxicosis. Nervousness, agitation, sweating, palpitations, tremor, diarrhea, and weight loss are the usual symptoms. Dyspnea is usually not prominent unless the patient has cardiac failure or underlying cardiac or pulmonary disease. Palpitations due to atrial fibrillation are uncommon before age 40.

There is a clear relationship between the patient's age and the prevalence of atrial fibrillation and cardiac failure. The fact that both fibrillation and cardiac failure are uncommon below age 40 has been cited in support of the argument that thyrotoxicosis does not cause heart failure. The increase in frequency of both with age suggests that thyrotoxicosis unmasks subclinical coronary or hypertensive heart disease but does not *cause* heart disease. Atrial fibrillation and cardiac failure are both related to age; by producing dilatation and hypertrophy, the former may produce cardiac failure even in the absence of heart disease. The presence of atrial fibrillation is particularly serious in older patients with thyrotoxicosis.

B. Signs: Patients may have tachycardia, peripheral vasodilatation, sweating, systolic hypertension with increased pulse pressure, rapid upstroke of the carotid pulse, and flow murmurs in the heart.

1. Predominant cardiac findings–The cardiac manifestations may overshadow the clinical picture of thyrotoxicosis. Manifestations of hyperthyroidism are usually present in these patients but are often overlooked because cardiac symptoms are dominant. One can suspect the diagnosis by noting the warm, moist hands and relatively quick movements which are surprising for a patient in heart failure. There is often a disparity between the vigor of the patient and the symptoms and signs of heart failure.

2. Overlooked thyrotoxicosis–Thyrotoxicosis should always be suspected in patients with unexplained atrial fibrillation or congestive heart failure poorly responsive to digitalis therapy or in patients with systolic hypertension with a wide pulse pressure and a normal or short circulation time. This latter finding is in contrast to the delayed circulation time usually seen in patients with cardiac failure.

3. Absence of thyrotoxic symptoms–In so-called apathetic thyrotoxicosis, the patient is subdued and lacking in energy instead of excited and nervous. There is, however, a disparity between the apathetic facies and hyperactive movements noted on alert examination. It is often helpful to compare the apparent well-being of the patient with the severity of symptoms. Patients with apathetic facies may have tremor, but hyperactive movements are more common. Increased peripheral blood flow with hyperemia often results in what has been called "salmon skin," which is a helpful clinical feature.

4. Cardiac symptoms and signs–Cardiac manifestations may precede obvious evidence of thyrotoxicosis; such manifestations, mainly atrial fibrillation, may precede the other clinical manifestations of thyrotoxicosis by months or years. Careful observation and repeated studies for thyroid disease may permit recognition of the development of thyrotoxic heart disease when it was not obvious at the onset of the atrial fibrillation.

C. Laboratory Findings: Laboratory tests that help in the diagnosis of thyrotoxicosis are summarized in Table 17–7.

Table 17–7. Role of laboratory tests in diagnosis of thyrotoxicosis.*

Test	Normal Range†	Comment
Protein-bound iodine (PBI)	4–8 μg/dl	Classic test now largely supplanted by more specific T_4 test.
Serum thyroxine (T_4) concentration		
Total	4–11.5 μg/dl	Elevated values usually confirm hyperthyroidism unless T_4 binding globulin is also high.
Free	0.8–2.4 ng/dl	Independent of binding globulin.
Serum triiodothyronine (T_3) resin uptake	Female: 24–34% Male: 25–35%	A reflection of available binding sites in T_4 binding globulin. Should be used only in conjunction with measurement of serum T_4 to exclude possibility that increase in total serum T_4 results from increase in T_4 binding globulin.
Serum T_3 concentration	80–100 ng/dl	Considerable variability from laboratory to laboratory. Normal values decrease with advancing age. Absolute concentration of T_3 in serum is invariably elevated in hyperthyroidism and is elevated in association with normal serum T_4 in T_3 toxicosis.
Thyroid suppression	In 24-hour radioactive iodine uptake, decrease to less than 50% of initial value	Useful in some patients if serum measurements are borderline. Will not confirm hyperthyroidism, but a normal test excludes the diagnosis.
Serum thyroid-stimulating hormone concentration (TSH)	5–10 μU/ml	Basal values of no use in diagnosis of thyrotoxicosis. Lack of increase in response to thyrotropin-releasing hormone suggests hyperthyroidism.

*Reproduced, with permission, from Ingbar SH: When to hospitalize the patient with thyrotoxicosis. Hosp Pract 10:45, Jan 1975.
†Values considered normal may differ from laboratory to laboratory.

D. Electrocardiographic Findings: Except for sinus tachycardia, there are no abnormal ECG signs unless atrial fibrillation supervenes or independent cardiac disease is present.

E. X-Ray Findings: The chest x-ray is normal unless cardiac failure has developed, in which case cardiac enlargement with or without pulmonary congestion is present.

F. Special Investigations: Hemodynamic data in 7 hyperthyroid patients revealed tachycardia, a slight increase in mean arterial pressure and cardiac index, a slightly raised left ventricular end-diastolic pressure (averaging 18.7 mm Hg), and a decreased systemic vascular resistance, all of which returned to normal following administration of propranolol (Pietras, 1972).

Differential Diagnosis

Overt thyrotoxicosis is usually so obvious that few diseases should be confused with it. When the clinical picture is incomplete, especially in early cases, the diagnosis can be confusing. Anxiety is one of the most important conditions to be distinguished because of the nervousness, tremor, tachycardia, sweating, and similar symptoms that occur in that state. Evidence of a raised cardiac output, including vasodilatation and warm, moist skin, is important in differentiating thyrotoxic patients from those with anxiety states, in whom there may be increased sweating but a cold and moist skin. Other manifestations of hyperthyroidism, such as unexplained weight loss and diarrhea, may be helpful diagnostic clues. Sleeping tachycardia is an important sign. Other causes of unexplained atrial fibrillation must be excluded if this is the presenting symptom or sign (eg, "silent" mitral stenosis, atrial septal defect, coronary heart disease, left atrial myxoma, infective endocarditis). If weakness and weight loss are the dominant findings, one must exclude neoplasms, various types of myopathies, liver disease, myasthenia, and depression. If cardiac failure due to no apparent cause is the presenting manifestation, one must exclude ischemic coronary cardiomyopathy, idiopathic cardiomyopathy, or cardiomyopathy associated with various systemic disorders (see below) as well as common varieties of cardiac failure that may have obscure features (valvular heart disease, atrial septal defect, "burned-out" hypertension, coronary disease, and cardiac failure resulting from untreated atrial fibrillation with a rapid ventricular rate).

Definitive diagnosis in these "atypical" cases is possible with the use of relatively specific biochemical studies, notably serum T_3, T_4, and, if necessary, radioiodine uptake. These tests may be interfered with by previous iodine intake, either as medication or during radiologic studies using iodine-containing contrast media.

Treatment

The treatment of thyrotoxic heart disease is similar to the treatment of thyrotoxicosis in the absence of cardiac disease, consisting usually of antithyroid drugs such as propylthiouracil or methimazole followed in several weeks by radioiodine. If the thyroid gland is very large, substernal, or multinodular, subtotal thyroidectomy may be the treatment of choice. Antithyroid drugs prevent organic binding of iodide in the thyroid and peripheral binding of triiodothyronine. Radioiodine administration is postponed for several weeks following administration of antithyroid drugs to accomplish this.

If the cardiovascular manifestations, especially tachycardia, are dominant and severe, beta-adrenergic blocking agents such as propranolol may be used to control the rapid heart rate and decrease the cardiac output with exercise. They do not affect the underlying excess thyroid secretion. Oral propranolol is usually adequate in modest doses, usually less than 160 mg/day; it can be given intravenously at a rate no faster than 1 mg/min if the clinical situation dictates rapid reversal of the cardiac symptoms—especially if thyroid storm is thought to be imminent. Younger individuals, however, require larger doses—up to 320 mg/day—and usually require more definitive treatment. Overall thyroid function is not affected by administration of propranolol.

Prognosis

The early diagnosis of thyrotoxicosis may influence the subsequent therapeutic results, which are not as dramatic in thyrotoxicosis as in myxedema and may be less than satisfactory. Twenty percent of the patients studied by Sandler and Wilson (1959) died of congestive heart failure within 1–7 years after starting therapy; complete relief of symptoms occurred in only 40% and was directly related to the disappearance of atrial fibrillation after treatment. In patients in whom sinus rhythm followed treatment with radioiodine, no deaths occurred and all patients with cardiac failure were improved. In patients in whom atrial fibrillation persisted, 20% died, and striking clinical responses were correspondingly less. The current availability of electrical cardioversion for the treatment of atrial fibrillation should improve these results if atrial fibrillation persists after treatment of thyrotoxicosis with radioiodine; cardioversion should be employed in an attempt to establish normal sinus rhythm.

MYXEDEMA & MYXEDEMA HEART

Myxedema heart is a well-known entity described by Zondek in 1918 and stated by Fahr (1925) to be associated with cardiac failure because two-thirds of his patients with myxedema had radiologic enlargement of the cardiac silhouette and he did not distinguish cardiac failure from pericardial effusion. More recent physiologic studies have shown that in most myxedema patients pericardial effusion and not cardiac failure is responsible for the enlarged cardiac shadow seen radiologically. Investigations using echocardiography have shown that some patients have dilatation of the left ventricle without significant pericardial effusion whereas others have dominant pericardial effusion with an essentially normal cardiac shadow, while a third group have a combination of cardiac dilatation and pericardial effusion. The cardiac shadow may be enlarged even after all pericardial fluid has been removed. The cause of the effusion is not clearly understood.

In one large series of cases of myxedema, the disease occurred spontaneously in 40% of patients, but in the remaining 60% it followed either ^{131}I therapy or thyroidectomy. At present, many more cases of myxedema are seen following successful ^{131}I therapy, and it is feared that with the passage of time the numbers will increase. When a patient with thyrotoxicosis improves following administration of ^{131}I, the physician must continue to be alert for the late appearance of myxedema.

Clinical Findings

A. Symptoms: The symptoms of myxedema include weakness, fatigue, dry and puffy skin, hoarseness, thick tongue, and slow pulse. Patients with myxedema heart characteristically complain of exertional fatigue more than dyspnea, angina due to associated coronary disease, and periorbital and peripheral edema. The pulse volume has a small amplitude, with a weak carotid upstroke—in contrast to what would be expected in bradycardia.

Two uncommon symptoms are perhaps not fully appreciated. One is the frequency of paresthesia, which in Wayne's series (1960) was 56% (in others as high as 75%), and perceptive deafness, which occurred in about half of cases in Wayne's series. Another symptom frequently helpful in diagnosis is husky hoarseness. On more than one occasion myxedema has been strongly suspected in a patient with heart disease entirely on the basis of voice. Coarse, dry skin changes may also be obvious and helpful in diagnosis.

B. Signs: The cardiac findings in myxedema are summarized in Table 17–8. That the cardiac manifestations of myxedema are usually due to pericardial ef-

Table 17–8. Cardiac findings in myxedema.*

1. Exertional fatigue, dyspnea, or angina pectoris.
2. Periorbital and peripheral edema.
3. Relative bradycardia.
4. Low voltage of QRS complex, T and P waves on ECG.
5. Enlargement of cardiac shadow with:
   a. Weak and distant heart sounds
   b. Difficulty in finding apex beat
   c. Poor cardiac contraction to palpation and fluoroscopy
   d. Small pulse with slow carotid upstroke in face of bradycardia.
6. Effusions in pericardium, pleura, and peritoneum; tamponade rare.
7. Echocardiography may reveal cardiac enlargement, pericardial effusion, or both.
8. Hemodynamic findings:
   a. Decreased O_2 consumption
   b. Decreased cardiac output
   c. Decreased pulse rate
   d. Normal arteriovenous O_2 difference
   e. Normal response of cardiac output, systemic resistance, and right atrial pressure to exercise.

*Modified and reproduced, with permission, from Sokolow M: Heart disease in patients with thyroid dysfunction: Medical Staff Conference, University of California, San Francisco. Calif Med 109:309, 1968.

fusion rather than cardiac failure is supported by the rarity of clinical congestive failure and the frequency of effusion as shown on echocardiography (see below). Physical signs such as orthopnea, raised venous pressure, enlargement of the liver, and gallop rhythm are usually absent, and, despite an abrupt increase in the size of the heart shadow, pulmonary venous congestion is often absent. Following the removal of pericardial fluid, the cardiac size is usually (not always) found to be normal.

The cardiac border may appear to be enlarged, but the weak and distant heart sounds and the difficulty in palpating the apical impulse make an accurate clinical determination of heart size difficult and should make one suspect hypothyroidism.

The slow pulse may be *only relative* in patients with myxedema. For example, the heart rate may be only 60–70 beats/min, which would be an unusual finding in a patient with cardiomegaly and presumed congestive heart failure.

Patients may have effusions in the pericardial, pleural, and peritoneal cavities; because of the slow development of effusion, large amounts of pericardial fluid may be found (2000–4000 ml).

C. Electrocardiographic Findings: Low voltage of the QRS complex as well as of the T and P waves suggests cardiac failure in patients with myxedema. A typical ECG showing the development and regression of T wave abnormalities in myxedema is presented in Fig 17–19.

D. X-Ray Findings: The cardiac shadow may be enlarged and may be due to cardiac failure, pericardial effusion, or a combination of the two (Fig 17–21).

E. Echocardiography: Echocardiograms are valuable in hypothyroidism in differentiating between enlarged cardiac shadows due to pericardial effusion and those due to left ventricular dilatation (Figs 17–20 and 17–21). Fig 17–20 shows a classic large pericardial effusion and decrease in the size of the heart following thyroxine therapy. Fig 17–21 presents an echocardiogram and serial chest films showing only minimal pericardial effusion but a dilated left ventricle with a wide space between the anterior border of the mitral valve and the ventricular septum. Following thyroxine therapy, left ventricular size becomes normal on chest films as well as echocardiograms.

F. Hemodynamic Data: Patients with myxedema heart do not require catheterization. When catheterization was done in the past for research purposes, patients had a decreased pulse rate, normal arteriovenous

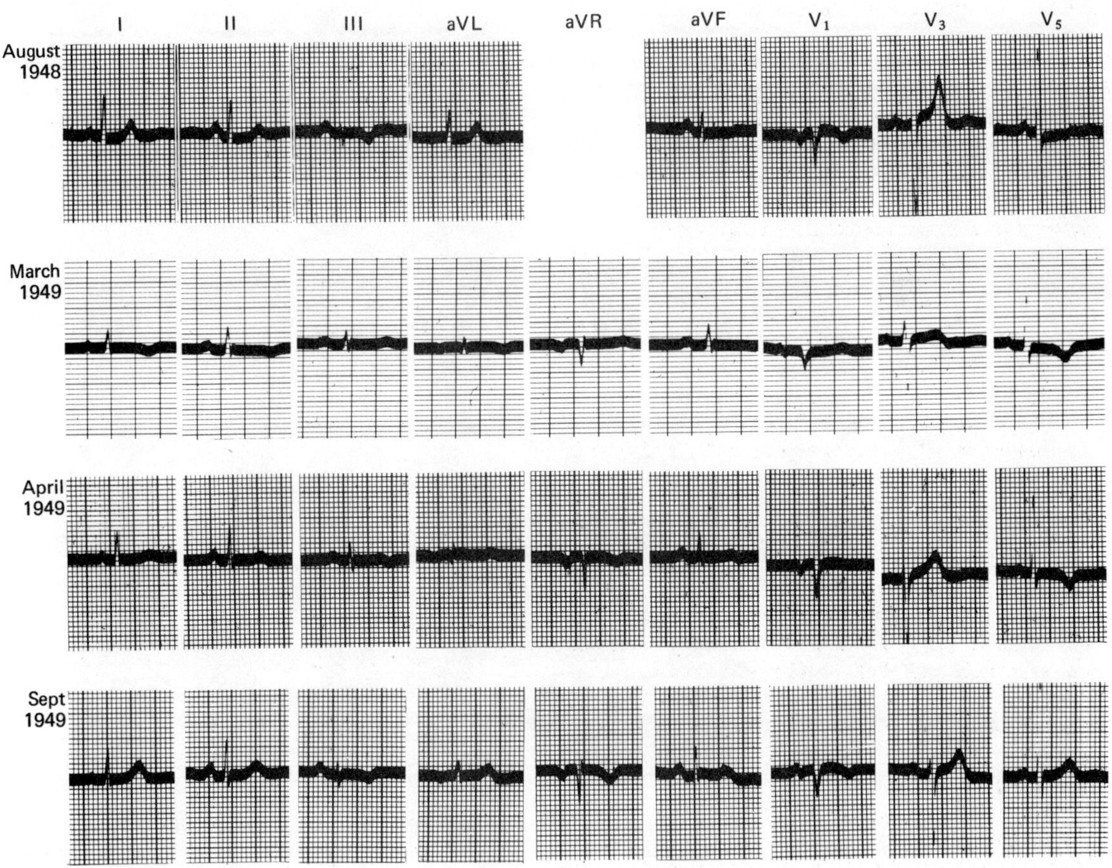

Figure 17–19. Hypothyroidism in a 47-year-old woman following thyroidectomy for hyperthyroidism in September 1948. BMR −51 in March 1949. Note progressive improvement in T waves after thyroid replacement was started in March 1949.

oxygen difference, and a normal response of cardiac output, peripheral resistance, and right atrial pressure to exercise. The cardiac index is low but increases normally with exercise. Systemic vascular resistance is not significantly affected. In one series of cases (Graettinger, 1958), systemic vascular resistance fell rapidly with exercise in patients with myxedema, whereas it did not in patients with congestive failure. Right atrial pressure increased with exercise in patients with cardiac failure but not in patients with myxedema. The cardiac index in myxedema was found to be one-third that seen in patients with thyrotoxicosis.

Differential Diagnosis

The diagnosis of myxedema is frequently missed because the clinical manifestations occur slowly and subtly and may be attributed to aging, ie, as the patient tires more easily and becomes slower in thought and movement. Many patients with a diagnosis of myxedema are treated initially for anemia. Periorbital nonpitting edema, generalized collections of serous fluid, and proteinuria may suggest nephritis. Finally, the diagnosis of cardiomyopathy is often made in myxedematous patients because of the presence of presumed cardiomegaly on radiologic examination.

There may be a delay of 5–10 years between the onset of symptoms and the diagnosis of myxedema.

Treatment

The response to treatment with thyroid hormone is dramatic, but severe angina, acute myocardial infarction, cardiac failure, psychotic reactions, and ventricular tachycardia may develop within 24–72 hours of onset of treatment if one starts with too large a dose of thyroid substance or thyroxine or increases the dose too rapidly. Treatment should be started with no more than 7.5 mg of desiccated thyroid or 2.5–5 μg of triiodothyronine (Cytomel) or synthetic thyroxine. Improvement will occur within days with synthetic compounds, and, unless there is impending coma, there is no urgency about restoring the patient to a euthyroid state.

Prognosis

The enlarged heart shadow usually returns completely to normal after thyroid therapy with complete clinical resolution, often within a month, but relapses may occur rapidly if thyroid therapy is stopped.

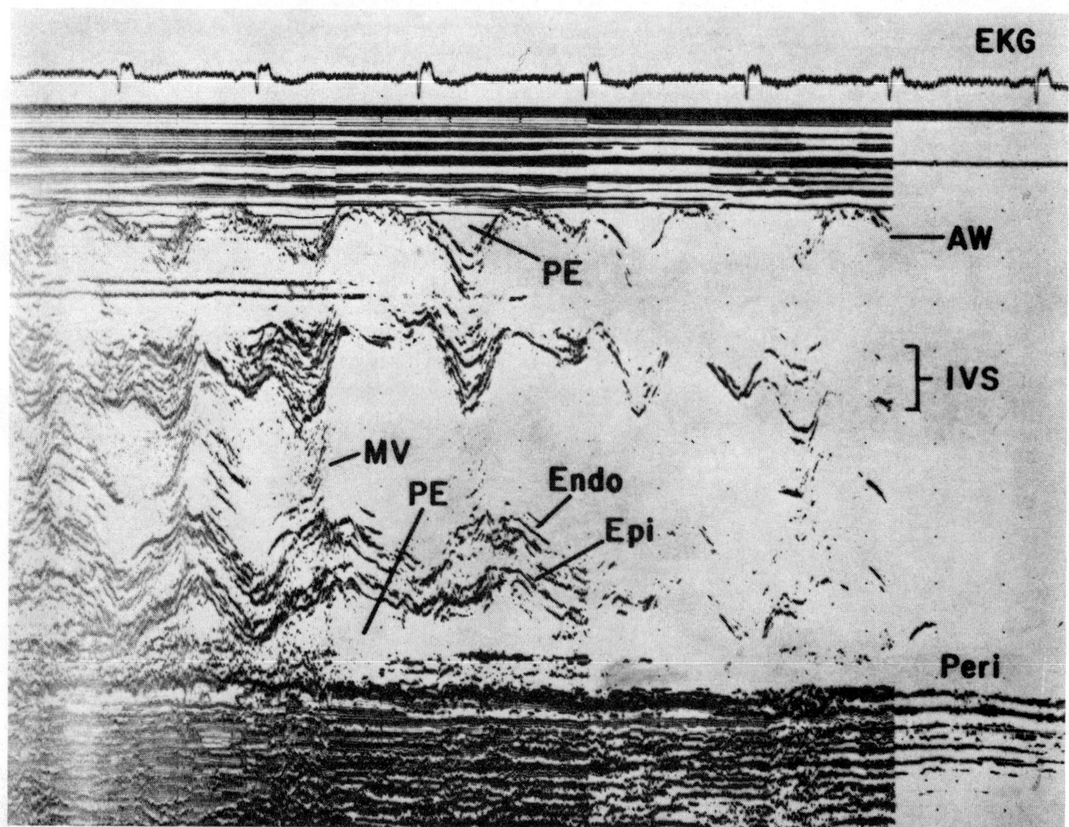

Figure 17–20. Echocardiogram showing the classic features of a large pericardial effusion in a patient with myxedema: a flat pericardium, a large posterior echo-free space, and a smaller anterior echo-free space. PE, pericardial effusion; Endo, endocardium; Epi, epicardium; AW, anterior wall; IVS, interventricular septum; Peri, pericardium. (Reproduced, with permission of the American Heart Association, Inc., from Kerber RE, Sherman B: Echocardiographic evaluation of pericardial effusion in myxedema: Incidence and biochemical and clinical correlations. Circulation 52:823, 1975.)

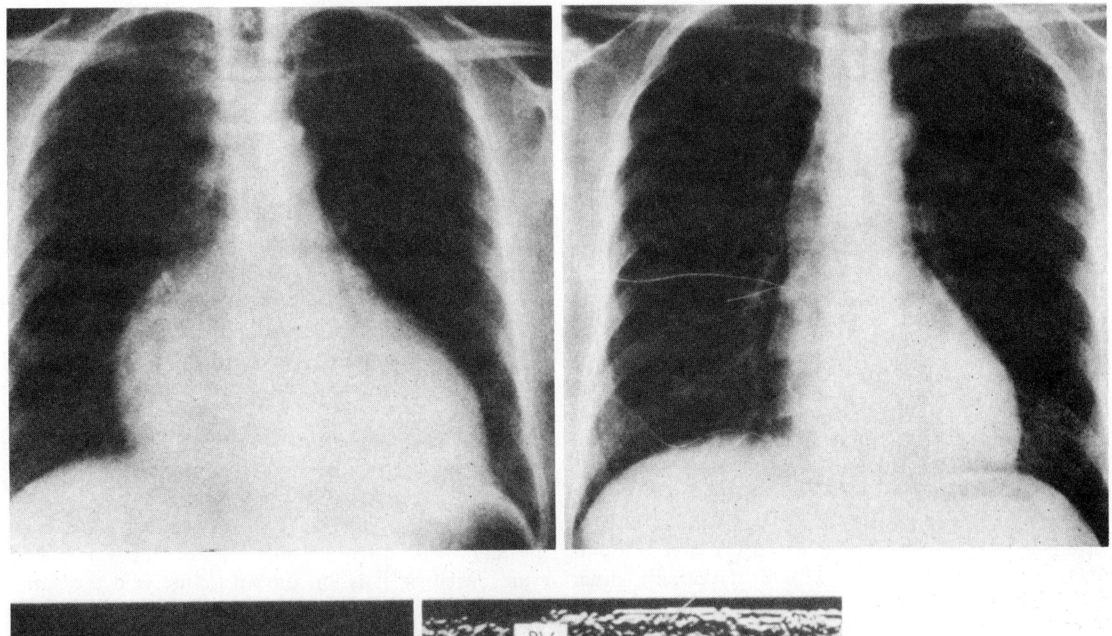

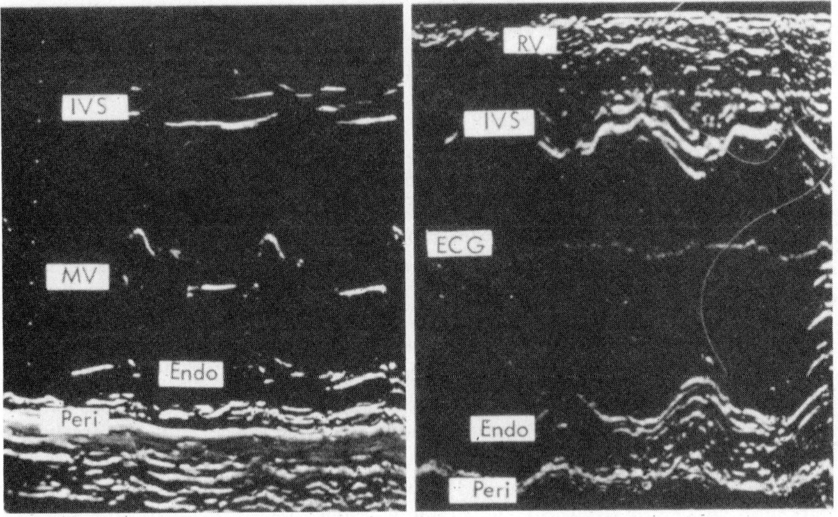

Figure 17–21. *Top:* Chest x-ray studies of patient with hypothyroid cardiomyopathy. ***Left:*** Before therapy, showing pronounced cardiomegaly. ***Right:*** Six months after institution of thyroxine therapy, the heart size has returned to normal. ***Bottom:*** Echocardiograms of patient with hypothyroid cardiomyopathy. ***Left:*** Before treatment, showing the dilated left ventricle (between IVS and Endo) with a short-axis diameter of 6.5 cm (normal: less than 5.4 cm). Motion of interventricular septum and endocardial wall is notably reduced. A small posterior pericardial effusion is present. ***Right:*** After thyroxine replacement therapy. Left ventricular size is now normal (4.2 cm) and motion of the posterior left ventricular wall and interventricular septum are markedly improved. IVS, interventricular septum; MV, mitral valve; Endo, endocardium of posterior left ventricular wall; Peri, pericardium of posterior left ventricular wall; ECG, electrocardiogram; RV, anterior right ventricular wall. (Reproduced, with permission, from Reza MJ, Abbasi AS: Congestive cardiomyopathy in hypothyroidism. West J Med 123:228, 1975.)

ALCOHOLIC CARDIOMYOPATHY*

This is a subject of some controversy because alcohol may produce cardiomyopathy by a primary toxic effect on the heart, by nutritional deficiency (especially of thiamin, as in beriberi heart disease) if the individual does not eat an adequate diet, or as a result of additives (cobalt in cobalt-beer cardiomyopathy). Chronic alcoholics may have intermittent thiamin deficiency or excessive requirements for thiamin, as when they develop fever from infections, or after a high-carbohydrate diet; therefore, a mixed picture of toxic alcoholic cardiomyopathy and nutritional beriberi heart disease may be found. Alcoholic cardiomyopathy may also complicate other types of cardiomyopathy. As Brigden (1972) stated, "There is no

*See also beriberi heart disease, p 545, and nutritional heart disease, p 546.

clear-cut boundary between cardiovascular beriberi and non-thiamin-responsive myocardial disease." Dietary deficiency of protein or calories infrequently causes chronic congestive cardiomyopathy, which is more frequently due to alcohol and should be differentiated from it. In populations afflicted by famine and in prisoners of war examined after a weight loss of about 20 kg, cardiac enlargement, hypoproteinemia, and cardiac failure are rarely seen; cardiac atrophy is much more common (Ramalingaswami, 1968). Endomyocardial fibrosis has been thought by some to be related to inadequate nutrition.

Involvement of the Liver

Alcohol not only affects the cells of the myocardium by direct toxic action; it also affects the cells of the liver, even in patients receiving good diets with adequate vitamins. As a result, patients may present with hepatic involvement as well as cardiac disease, although some patients are able to drink large amounts of alcohol for many years without developing either cardiac or hepatic disease, or one but not the other.

Relationship of Beriberi Heart Disease to Alcoholic Cardiomyopathy

Beriberi heart disease, when clearly related to thiamin deficiency, was described by Wenckebach in 1929 (Wenckebach, 1934) and by Soma Weiss in 1937. High output failure is the dominant clinical feature in most cases, but some had low cardiac output because of delay in treatment. In contrast to the hyperkinetic circulation with tachycardia, raised cardiac output, and warm extremities of patients with beriberi heart disease, the patient with alcoholic cardiomyopathy has signs of low cardiac output, relatively weak pulses of small volume, and cold extremities. The heart is large and bulky, with a markedly decreased ejection fraction. Large doses of thiamin are ineffective in treatment of alcoholic cardiomyopathy, in contrast to beriberi heart disease, but a hyperkinetic circulation (overactive, high cardiac output) can be produced in a week in a chronic alcoholic who develops a fever or abruptly reduces thiamin intake.

Beriberi heart was formerly common in developing countries and found occasionally in the USA before recognition of the need for thiamin replacement and the ready availability of vitamin supplements in patients receiving deficient diets. Alcoholic cardiomyopathy, however, is common where large amounts of alcohol are consumed daily even with adequate nutrition and vitamins. In alcoholic cardiomyopathy with good nutrition (including vitamin supplements), left ventricular dysfunction can often be demonstrated by sophisticated technics before the patient develops clinical symptoms or obvious signs of cardiac enlargement or failure. Most cases of alcoholic cardiomyopathy in the USA are probably due to a direct toxic action of alcohol on the myocardium.

Clinical Findings

The criteria for the cardiac diagnosis of alcoholic cardiomyopathy are similar to those of idiopathic cardiomyopathy or chronic congestive cardiomyopathy, with the exception of the history of alcoholic intake. The typical clinical picture is idiopathic cardiac failure in a man in the early middle years without coronary heart disease, hypertension, valvular heart disease, or congenital heart disease. There is no history of valvular or congenital heart disease but a definite history of large alcohol intake over a period of many years; most patients have drunk more than 250 ml of whiskey or its equivalent every day for at least 10 years. Brigden (1964) has emphasized the importance of alcohol in chronic idiopathic heart disease and believes that it is responsible for at least half of all cases of chronic congestive cardiomyopathy.

A. Symptoms: The onset is usually insidious, with nonspecific fatigue, dyspnea, palpitations, and possibly edema.

B. Signs: There may be cardiac enlargement and evidences of left ventricular failure. When cardiac failure develops, it is low output failure, and the patient usually has all the clinical features of that condition. The cardiac failure is chiefly left ventricular, but there may be right ventricular failure as well, with raised venous pressure, tricuspid insufficiency, and a rapid small pulse. There is usually a left or right ventricular heave, gallop rhythm, murmurs of functional mitral or tricuspid insufficiency and pulmonary rales, enlarged tender liver, and dependent edema. Although the arterial blood pressure may be elevated during the phase of severe failure with compensatory systemic vasoconstriction, the pressure falls to normal when failure is improved with routine cardiac therapy.

C. Electrocardiographic Findings: Abnormalities, especially low voltage of QRS complexes, ST–T abnormalities, and left ventricular hypertrophy, may be present before the development of cardiac failure. Arrhythmias and conduction defects are common.

D. X-Ray Findings: Cardiac enlargement, cardiac failure, and pulmonary congestion may be present.

E. Special Investigations: In addition to left ventricular hypertrophy found clinically and electrocardiographically, as in all cases of cardiomyopathy, patients have enlarged hearts with pulmonary venous engorgement; when studied by coronary angiography and left ventricular cineangiography, the coronary arteries are normal and the ejection fraction is decreased, so that the heart is a large, boggy organ. Echocardiography can demonstrate the large left ventricle with decreased ejection fraction and the mitral valve floating within the left ventricular cavity (Fig 17–22).

Differential Diagnosis

Alcoholic cardiomyopathy must be distinguished from other disorders that produce congestive cardiomyopathy in patients with long histories of excessive alcohol intake. Hypertension is excluded by normal blood pressure after restoration to the compensated state; coronary artery disease by the absence of angina pectoris or myocardial infarction clinically or electrocardiographically and, if necessary, by negative coro-

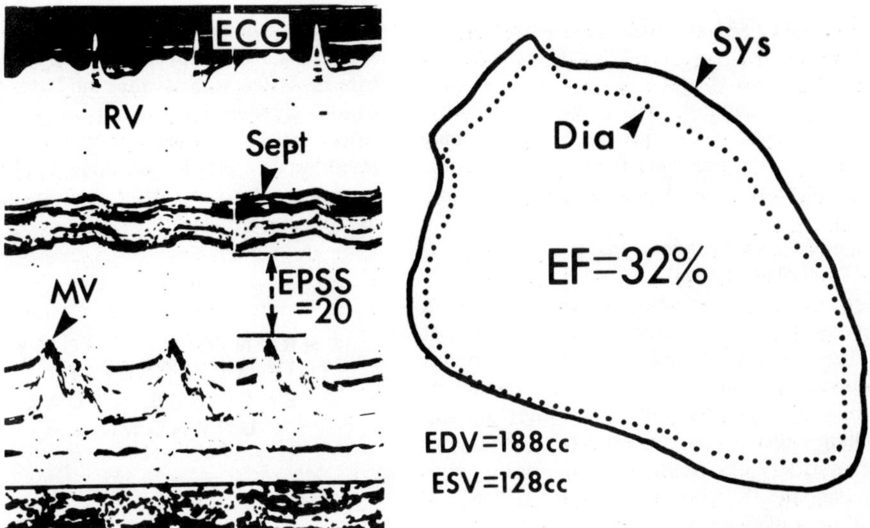

Figure 17–22. Echocardiogram of patient with alcoholic cardiomyopathy demonstrating a decreased ejection fraction of 32%, a large end-diastolic volume, and a wide separation between the anterior portion of the mitral valve leaflet and the ventricular septum. EF, ejection fraction; EDV, end-diastolic volume; ESV, end-systolic volume; MV, mitral valve; RV, right ventricle; Sept, septum; EPSS, end point of mitral valve separated from septum. (Reproduced, with permission, from Massie BM & others: Mitral-septal separation: A new echocardiographic index of left ventricular function. Am J Cardiol 39:1008, 1977.)

nary angiogram; valvular heart disease by the absence of a history of murmurs and by decrease of murmurs when compensation is restored. Congenital heart disease is excluded by a negative history and no abnormalities of congenital heart disease on cineangiograms.

Treatment

Early awareness of the appearance of cardiomyopathy compels complete abstinence from alcohol as the initial and most important step in treatment. Later, abstinence may have only marginal benefit. Bed rest, intravenous thiamin (50 mg)—of minimal or no benefit in the low output stage—and conventional treatment for heart failure are the mainstays of management. If this is not successful, vasodilator therapy (see Chapter 10) is advised. If the disease is not too far advanced, improvement but not complete reversal may be achieved. Burch and his associates (1965) have strongly emphasized the value of many months of bed rest in patients who fail to respond. Prolonged bed rest may be more effective in decreasing cardiac size in alcoholic cardiomyopathy than in other diseases such as ischemic cardiomyopathy. Unfortunately, thromboembolic phenomena and relapse are common.

Prognosis

The heart may become much smaller and all cardiac symptoms may disappear following months of bed rest. However, rapid recurrence of heart failure often occurs when patients become ambulatory. Furthermore, prolonged bed rest increases the hazard of multiple episodes of thromboembolism. The psychologic and economic consequences of prolonged inactivity must also be considered.

BERIBERI HEART DISEASE

In the USA beriberi heart disease is uncommon because thiamin deficiency severe enough to result in beriberi is rare. It is usually seen in malnourished chronic alcoholics. The clinical features and differentiation from non-thiamin-deficient chronic alcoholic cardiomyopathy are included in the preceding section in order to contrast the 2 major ways in which alcohol may cause heart disease. Beriberi is most common in populations and individuals (as in the Orient) who eat thiamin-deficient diets.

Clinical Findings

Patients with beriberi have dyspnea, edema, and right heart failure in combination with warm extremities and bounding pulses characteristic of the high cardiac output state. See Alcoholic Cardiomyopathy (above) for the clinical findings when the low output phase of chronic alcoholic cardiomyopathy supervenes.

Treatment & Prognosis

Beriberi heart disease improves rapidly when large doses (50 mg) of thiamin are given orally or parenterally. The skin temperature falls in hours after parenteral thiamin therapy. Enlargement of the heart and evidences of right heart failure subside within a matter of days to 1–2 weeks, and the syndrome does not occur when adequate thiamin supplements are given.

Beriberi heart disease is reversed by thiamin only when the process is relatively acute and precipitated by an increased demand for thiamin. Chronic alcoholic cardiomyopathy does not respond to thiamin.

NUTRITIONAL HEART DISEASE

As discussed under alcoholic cardiomyopathy, malnutrition with selective deficiency of thiamin may cause beriberi heart disease and is in part responsible for the clinical features of alcoholic cardiomyopathy.

Deficiency of Calories, Proteins, Fats, & Vitamins (Total Malnutrition)

Under conditions of famine or semistarvation in which there are combined dietary deficiencies and not selective ones (as with thiamin), the heart responds with atrophy, interstitial edema, and disappearance of all pericardial fat, but the patient does not develop cardiac failure either of the beriberi type or the chronic congestive variety of chronic alcoholic cardiomyopathy (although the ECG may show nonspecific ST–T changes). Protein deficiency may cause kwashiorkor, a disease usually of children considered to be due to protein deficiency and characterized by hypoproteinemia and generalized edema. Cardiac failure due to protein starvation is uncommon both in children and (especially) in adults, although cardiac output may be decreased. When the diet is abruptly improved, as in liberated prisoners of war, generalized edema simulating cardiac failure may develop because of the abrupt increase in sodium intake associated with the normal diet or perhaps because of transient adrenal insufficiency; diuresis occurs spontaneously in weeks, aided by small amounts of diuretics. There have been no short-term cardiac sequelae.

The coincidence of nutritional deficiency and endomyocardial fibrosis in developing tropical countries in Africa suggests that the latter is due to malnutrition, though this has not been proved and a viral cause has also been postulated. Ramalingaswami (1968) states that in the Bihar famine of 1967 fatal cases showed no mural thrombi or other abnormalities of the endocardial wall.

CHRONIC CARDIOMYOPATHY DUE TO SPECIFIC DISEASE ENTITIES, USUALLY OF UNKNOWN ORIGIN

SARCOIDOSIS

Sarcoidosis is a chronic granulomatous disease of unknown cause affecting chiefly young blacks (average age about 25). Many organ systems are affected, but especially the lungs and the heart. The disease may involve the heart directly and cause ventricular arrhythmias, heart block, and sudden death; autopsy studies show involvement of the heart in about 25% of fatal cases (Fig 17–23). Granulomas in patients with cardiac involvement are most commonly seen in the left ventricle, ventricular septum, and papillary muscles.

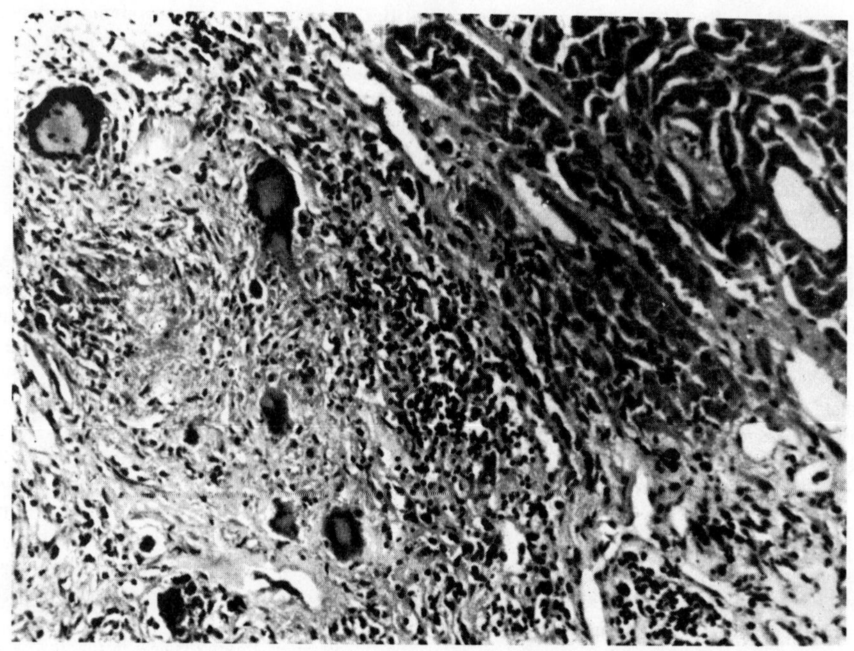

Figure 17–23. Sarcoid granuloma in myocardium with epithelioid cells, multinucleated giant cells, and lymphocytes. (X 350.) (Reproduced, with permission, from Fawcett FJ, Goldberg MJ: Heart block resulting from myocardial sarcoidosis. Br Heart J 36:220, 1974.)

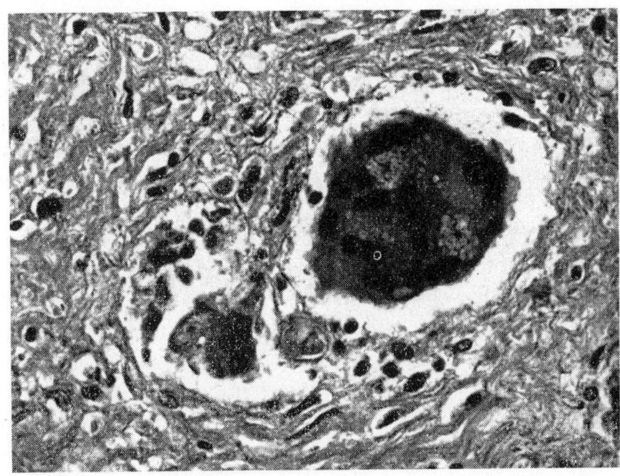

Figure 17–24. Atrioventricular bundle destroyed and replaced by dense fibrous tissue containing numerous giant cells in sarcoidosis. (Magnification X 365, H&E stain.) (Reproduced, with permission, from Porter GH: Sarcoid heart disease. N Engl J Med 263:1350, 1960.)

Clinical Findings

The most common clinical feature—although infrequent in sarcoidosis in general—is cor pulmonale secondary to fibrosis of the interstitial tissues of the lung and small pulmonary arteries resulting in pulmonary hypertension, right ventricular hypertrophy, and ultimately right ventricular failure (see Chapter 19).

A. Symptoms and Signs: The onset is with general symptoms of fatigue and malaise, acute uveitis, hilar adenopathy and nodular and fibrous pulmonary infiltrates on the chest film, and skin lesions, most characteristically erythema nodosum. Other systemic manifestations include hypercalcemia, hyperglobulinemia, and generalized adenopathy. Biopsy of the skin or lymph nodes shows extensive fibrosis and noncaseating granulomatous infiltration without organisms; the same process may affect the heart. Kveim-Siltzbach skin tests are positive in 80% of cases but are of limited value in diagnosis. The endocardium and valves are rarely involved. Cardiac failure is uncommon in sarcoidosis in general but occurs in a third of patients with cardiac sarcoidosis. Pericardial effusion is not uncommon. Roberts (1977), in a large series of patients studied at necropsy, noted ventricular arrhythmias in 45%, cardiac failure in 30%, and sudden death in 65%. Sudden death was the first manifestation of the disease in a third of those who died suddenly. In each, death occurred during exertion. Complete atrioventricular block occurred in 12%. Recurrent tachycardia occurred in about 40% of those who died suddenly.

B. Serial Observations Leading to Treatment:

1. Pulmonary function studies and serial chest films are advised, especially in patients complaining of dyspnea, to demonstrate abnormalities due to pulmonary fibrosis. If pulmonary function studies show progressive abnormalities, steroid therapy may be tried, particularly if the patient has evidences of pulmonary hypertension with right ventricular heave, atrial gallop, a palpable pulmonary artery, or ECG evidence of right ventricular hypertrophy. Serial pulmonary function studies have shown improvement in some cases treated with corticosteroids.

2. Serial ECGs are advised so as not to miss early progressive right ventricular hypertrophy resulting from pulmonary hypertension, as well as to detect involvement of the conduction system, in which case insertion of a pacemaker should be considered in order to prevent Stokes-Adams attacks and sudden death. Corticosteroids are usually ineffective when conduction defects and ventricular arrhythmias dominate the clinical picture.

Most patients, even with obvious sarcoid disease elsewhere, do not have clinical evidences of cardiac dysfunction, although ECG abnormalities—usually atrioventricular conduction delay, right ventricular hypertrophy, or ST–T changes—may be found in the absence of clinical symptoms. In proved sarcoidosis of the heart, complete atrioventricular block has been found in 25% of patients and atrioventricular and intraventricular conduction defects in another 25% (Fig 17–24).

Prognosis

Sudden and unexpected death is the usual outcome in cardiac sarcoidosis. Four of 6 patients died in this way in a series reported by Ghosh and others (1972).

SYSTEMIC LUPUS ERYTHEMATOSUS

Lupus erythematosus is a systemic disease of unknown cause thought to be due to vasculitis secondary to autoimmunity and characterized by deposition of immune complex in the capillaries of visceral organs. The disease was formerly thought to be uncommon, but new diagnostic serologic tests now make it possible to recognize milder diseases sooner. Furthermore, the ominous course described formerly is not the rule, as milder cases are now diagnosed more frequently.

The disorder affects the heart in 10–20% of cases, causing an inflammatory reaction which may be widespread or focal and involving the pericardium as well as the myocardium and, much less commonly, the valves. Chronic renal failure is most common, but patients may have pericardial effusion or cardiac failure.

Table 17–9. American Rheumatism Association diagnostic criteria for systemic lupus erythematosus.*†

Facial erythema
Discoid lupus
Raynaud's phenomenon
Alopecia
Photosensitivity
Oral or nasal ulcers
Arthritis without deformity
Lupus erythematosus cells
Chronic false-positive serologic test for syphilis
Profuse proteinuria
Cellular casts
Pleuritis or pericarditis
Psychosis or convulsions
Cytopenia

*The presence of any 4 during any period of observation has an estimated specificity of 99%.

†Reproduced, with permission, from Decker JL (moderator) & others: Systemic lupus erythematosus: Contrasts and comparisons. Ann Intern Med 82:391, 1975.

Systemic lupus erythematosus is one of the most common causes of pericardial effusion in a university hospital.

Systemic lupus erythematosus has been diagnosed more frequently in the last 25 years for reasons that are not completely clear; the availability of better diagnostic serologic tests may be responsible.

Clinical Findings

The American Rheumatism Association criteria for systemic lupus erythematosus are shown in Table 17–9.

A. Symptoms and Signs: In large-scale serologic surveys designed to identify early manifestations of lupus erythematosus, the disease is often found to be a chronic mild one characterized by a rash, slightly raised arterial pressure, arthritis, Raynaud's phenomenon, myopericarditis, and prompt response to corticosteroid therapy.

Cardiac involvement in active cases is suspected on the basis of evidence of enlargement of the heart, pericardial effusion, and ECG changes. A typical example of T wave inversions characteristic of myopericarditis in systemic lupus erythematosus is shown in Fig 17–25. Hypertension is common and may lead to left ventricular hypertrophy and left ventricular failure.

Other nonsystemic manifestations include a characteristic butterfly malar rash, photosensitivity reaction, Raynaud's phenomenon, arthritis resembling rheumatoid arthritis, and lupus nephritis (focal or diffuse proliferative glomerulitis, membranous glomerular nephropathy). The patient may have pleural effusion as well as central nervous system involvement with seizures, chronic organic brain syndrome (dementia, confusion), aseptic meningitis, reversible psychosis, and peripheral neuritis. Libman-Sacks endocarditis may be found pathologically but is rarely a clinical problem.

B. Laboratory Findings: The diagnosis is confirmed by finding lupus erythematosus cells in the blood and pericardial fluid, a chronic false-positive serologic test for syphilis, antinuclear antibodies in the

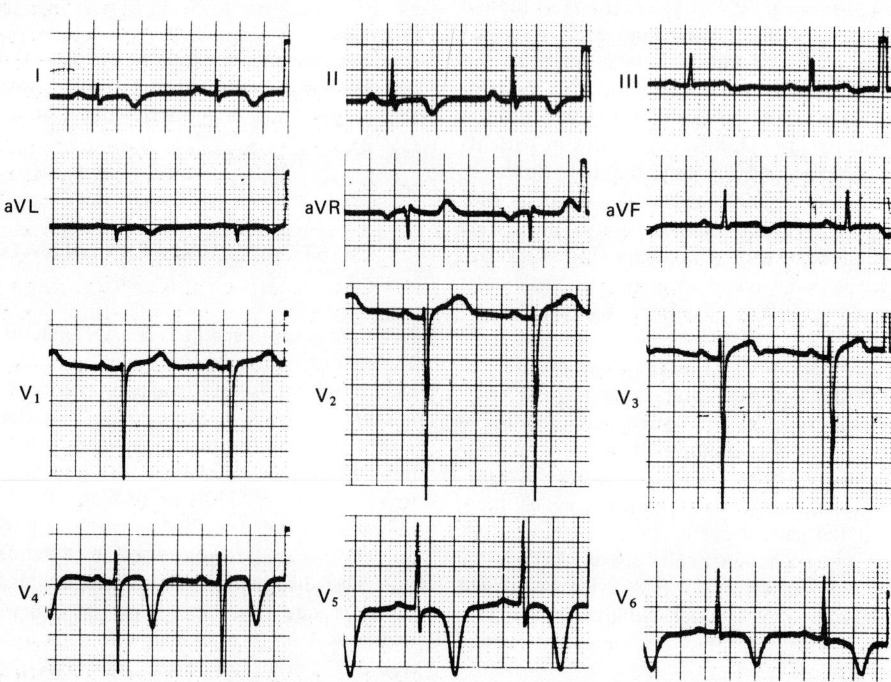

Figure 17–25. T wave inversions characteristic of myopericarditis in a 27-year-old woman with classic clinical lupus erythematosus.

Table 17–10. Causes of death in 36 patients with lupus erythematosus.*

Condition	Patients	
	Number	Percent
Sepsis	14	40
Cardiac disorders	8	20
Cerebrovascular accidents	4	11
Renal failure	4	11
Miscellaneous	6	18
Totals	36	100

*Reproduced, with permission of the American Heart Association, Inc., from Bulkley BH, Roberts WC: The heart in systemic lupus erythematosus and the changes induced in it by corticosteroid therapy: A study of 36 necropsy patients. Am J Med 58:243, 1975.

Table 17–11. Drugs implicated (in descending order of importance) in the induction of a lupuslike syndrome.*

Procainamide	Penicillamine
Hydralazine	Oral contraceptive agents
Isoniazid	Phenothiazines
Sulfonamides	Quinidine
Penicillin	Ethosuximide
Tetracycline	Phenylbutazone
Streptomycin	Phenytoin
Aminosalicylic acid	Mephenytoin
Griseofulvin	Trimethadione

*Reproduced, with permission, from Bardana EJ, Pirofsky B: Recent advances in the immunopathogenesis of systemic lupus erythematosus. West J Med 122:130, 1975.

serum, hypergammaglobulinemia, an increased erythrocyte sedimentation rate, and reduced serum complement. The false-positive serologic test may be one of the first clues to the presence of the disease. Urinalysis reveals proteinuria and the characteristic "telescopic" findings (Krupp, 1943) in which all varieties of cells and casts are found simultaneously in the urinary sediment. Anemia, leukopenia, lymphopenia, and thrombocytopenia are common.

Treatment

Although mild forms of systemic lupus erythematosus may be treated symptomatically, myocarditis and other serious complications of the disease require judicious use of corticosteroids. Prolonged careful clinical and laboratory follow-up may be necessary. Immunosuppressive drugs such as cyclophosphamide or azathioprine are used in resistant cases, but the results are at best marginal; most patients respond to corticosteroid therapy alone.

Prognosis

Sepsis is the most common cause of death in systemic lupus erythematosus, often occurring as a side-effect of corticosteroid therapy. Other causes of death are heart disorders (myocardial infarction, arrhythmias, cardiac failure), progressive renal disease, and central nervous system involvement (see above and Table 17–10).

Early steroid therapy makes it less likely that the kidneys will become involved, so that much longer survival is now possible. The disease may be intermittently active, but at times it is fulminant and responds to administration of large doses of steroids, which often results in severe complications of corticosteroid therapy.

DRUG-INDUCED SYSTEMIC LUPUS ERYTHEMATOSUS

Recently it has been recognized that a variety of drugs such as procainamide, hydralazine, phenytoin, and some of the phenothiazines may cause a syndrome indistinguishable from lupus erythematosus with pericarditis, arteritis, and characteristic serologic changes (Table 17–11). In practically all instances, the syndrome subsides after withdrawal of the drug.

The worst offender is procainamide; at least half of all patients receiving it for about 6 months develop positive serologic changes and ultimately clinical signs of lupus, which disappear slowly when the drug is stopped. The skin and kidneys are usually spared, and the first manifestations may be serologic and hematologic ones. The high frequency with which procainamide produces lupus prevents its use in chronic therapy of arrhythmias; however, since it may take months for the lupus syndrome to appear, the drug may be used during the acute phase for short periods.

Lupus occurs less commonly with hydralazine, particularly in the doses ordinarily prescribed. In patients receiving 200 mg/day or less, lupus is quite uncommon, whereas in the period prior to the availability of other antihypertensive drugs, when doses of 600–800 mg/day were used, lupus was much more frequent.

Phenytoin and isoniazid are uncommon causes of lupus.

SCLERODERMA

The diffuse fibrosis and vasculitis so obvious in the skin, gastrointestinal tract, and lungs in generalized scleroderma may also involve the heart. The clinical cardiac abnormalities in patients with scleroderma are tabulated in Table 17–12. Fig 17–26 shows the typical pathologic features of scleroderma, in this instance

Table 17–12. Clinical cardiac abnormalities in 47 patients with scleroderma.*†

Myocardial Lesion	Severe (13 patients)		Mild (10 patients)		Absent (24 patients)	
Congestive heart failure	11 (85%)		3 (30%)		8 (33%)	
Congestive heart failure without renal or lung involvement	4 (31%)		0		0	
Angina pectoris	3 (23%)		0		0	
Ventricular irritability	8 (62%)		1 (10%)		1 (4%)	
Conduction abnormality	8 (62%)		3 (30%)		6 (25%)	
Right bundle branch block		5		1		3
Left anterior hemiblock		2		2		5
First degree heart block		1		1		1
Complete heart block		3		0		0
Cardiac death	8 (62%)		2 (20%)		1 (4%)	
Sudden death	5 (38%)		1 (10%)		0	
Congestive heart failure	3 (23%)		1 (10%)		1 (4%)	
Constrictive pericarditis	0		0		1 (4%)	
Total with clinical cardiac abnormalities	11 (79%)		4 (40%)		10 (42%)	

*Five patients excluded because of coexisting severe epicardial coronary artery disease.
†Reproduced, with permission of the American Heart Association, Inc., from Bulkley BH & others: Myocardial lesions of progressive systemic sclerosis: A cause of cardiac dysfunction. Circulation 53: 483, 1976.

involving the kidney but similar to that seen in the heart. Perivascular fibrosis is clearly shown. With the exception of right heart failure when the lungs are involved, cardiac failure is uncommon. Left ventricular function is usually normal. The major cardiac lesion is fibrotic destruction of the conduction system and the small coronary arteries. Six of 8 patients studied at postmortem by James (1974) died suddenly as a result of fibrous destruction of the sinoatrial and atrioventricular nodes. Cardiac arrhythmias were frequent in these patients, as would be expected when the conduction system is involved. ECG and clinical features of atrioventricular block, Stokes-Adams attacks, and sudden death are similar to those seen in cardiac sarcoidosis. Serial ECGs are advised in scleroderma heart disease so as to determine when conduction defects have progressed, making it advisable to insert an artificial pacemaker to prevent sudden death.

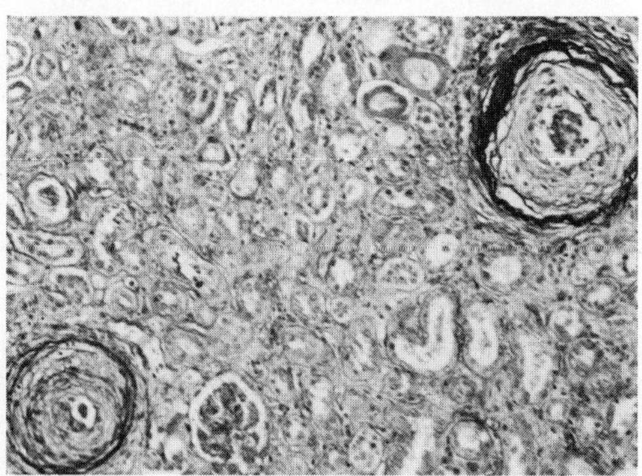

Figure 17–26. Pathologic features of scleroderma of the kidney (similar to myocardium). (Courtesy of O Rambo.)

There is no specific treatment. Supportive treatment includes pacing for conduction defects.

RHEUMATOID ARTHRITIS

Rheumatoid arthritis is a form of connective tissue disorder. Rheumatoid factor is present in the serum, and this finding is associated with other positive serologic tests typical of other varieties of connective tissue disorders such as lupus erythematosus. The frequency of cardiac symptoms and signs in a large group of patients with rheumatoid arthritis is shown in Table 17–13. Rheumatoid arthritis may cause inflammatory changes in the pericardium, myocardium, and aortic valve, producing pericardial effusion and aortic insuf-

Table 17–13. Frequency of cardiac symptoms and signs in 254 patients with rheumatoid arthritis and 254 controls.*

Cardiac Abnormality	Patients With Arthritis	Controls
Congestive heart failure	25	3
Angina pectoris	16	4
Enlargement of left ventricle	48	28
Enlargement of right ventricle	5	0
Atrial enlargement	6	1
Aortic systolic murmur	7	1
Aortic diastolic murmur	4	0
Mitral diastolic murmur	7	1
Totals	118	38

*Reproduced, with permission, from Cathcart ES, Spodick DH: Rheumatoid heart disease: A study of the incidence and nature of cardiac lesions in rheumatoid arthritis. N Engl J Med 266:959, 1962.

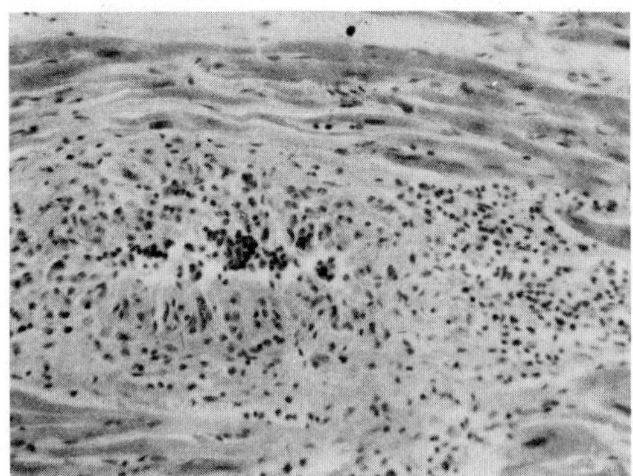

Figure 17–27. Inflammatory infiltrate of the myocardium in rheumatoid arthritis. (Courtesy of O Rambo.)

ficiency as the most common cardiac manifestations. The frequency with which pericarditis is detected is increased if echocardiograms are done on all patients with rheumatoid arthritis. A typical histologic example of rheumatoid vasculitis of the myocardium is shown in Fig 17–27. The process may involve the mitral valve and the myocardium. At autopsy, about a third of all patients with rheumatoid arthritis have evidences of pericarditis, conduction system abnormalities, or aortic valve disease. Clinically, however, only a small percentage of patients–probably less than 5%–have active cardiac disease. Rheumatoid arthritis may be a precursor of amyloid disease of the heart, in which case the amyloid disease dominates the clinical cardiac picture.

ANKYLOSING SPONDYLITIS

Ankylosing spondylitis, once thought to be a variant of rheumatoid arthritis, is now considered a separate disease. It occurs chiefly in men and may cause inflammatory aortic insufficiency, resulting from aortitis (similar to that due to syphilis) and atrioventricular conduction problems. (See Chapter 13.)

HEMOCHROMATOSIS

Hemochromatosis, an excess iron storage disease, can be classified as primary (idiopathic) or secondary (transfusion) hemosiderosis. The former is less common but has triggered considerable research regarding iron absorption, excretion, storage, and control. It has been established that idiopathic hemochromatosis is genetic, transmitted as an autosomal dominant trait. It is rare and occurs spontaneously in the absence of repeated transfusions or hematologic disorders. Iron storage is increased because of enhanced intestinal absorption of iron from the normal 1 mg to 3 mg/day. The mechanisms by which the rate of absorption of iron is controlled are not known, but the increased absorption ultimately leads to overloading of the body cells with iron.

Idiopathic genetic hemochromatosis is much commoner in men, perhaps because of the intermittent blood loss during menstruation and pregnancy in women. Excessive amounts (20–40 g instead of the normal 1–2 g) of iron are retained and stored in the cells in the tissues, especially the liver cells, and provoke a variable fibrotic reaction which may involve the myocardium, interfering with left ventricular function. Iron deposition in the heart does not occur until the liver is first saturated with iron (Buja, 1971). A typical example is shown in Fig 17–28. Ordinary myocardial cells are affected more than the cells of the conductive system.

Secondary hemochromatosis is more common and usually due to multiple blood transfusions (100 or more) in chronic aplastic or hemolytic anemias. The 250 mg of iron in each unit of blood (500 ml) are stored in the body because excretion of iron cannot be increased. Iron is deposited as hemosiderin, leading to the alternative name transfusion siderosis. Rarely, iron loading results from excessive oral intake for many years or from congenital abnormalities of iron metabolism (eg, thalassemia major, transferrinemia, pyridoxine-responsive anemia) (Crosby, 1974).

Iron is deposited in the liver, pancreas, heart, spleen, thyroid, lymph nodes, adrenals, anterior pituitary, joints, gonads, lungs (to a lesser extent), and central nervous system (rarely). It has been described clinically as bronze diabetes in association with cirrhosis, pituitary insufficiency, testicular atrophy, involvement of the heart, and arthropathy with chrondrocalcinosis.

The presenting symptoms and signs of cardiac deposition of iron may be similar to those of any infiltrative cardiac disease, with fatigue, dyspnea, gallop rhythm, ventricular arrhythmias, conduction defects, and signs of heart failure. "The iron heart is not a strong heart but a weak one" (Buja, 1971). The diagnosis can be established by biopsy of the liver, kidney, heart, or skin and the use of stains for stainable iron (hemosiderin) appropriate to the tissues obtained. In skin biopsies, one must use care to exclude melanin.

Cardiac involvement consists of atrial and ventricular arrhythmias, conduction defects, cardiac enlargement, and cardiac failure.

The course of the disease is usually unfavorable unless excess iron stores are removed early by frequent phlebotomies (see below). Early diagnosis can be made if the disease is suspected in every case of unexplained cardiomyopathy, cirrhosis, or diabetes, especially if the skin is an unusual bronze or a grayish tan color. Serum iron is usually normal, but iron-binding capacity is 60–70% (often more) saturated instead of the normal 20–40%.

Treatment & Prognosis

Treatment consists of phlebotomy; it has been

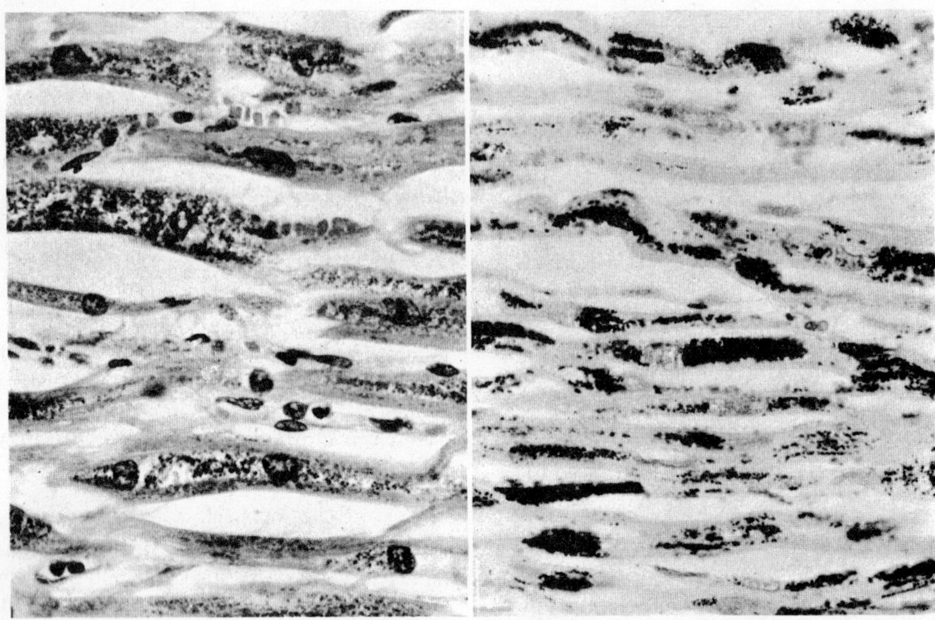

Figure 17–28. Histologic sections of left ventricular myocardium showing extensive iron depositions (dark areas.) *Left:* H&E stain. *Right:* Iron stain. (Magnification, each X 560.) (Reproduced, with permission, from Arnett EN & others: Massive myocardial hemosiderosis: A structure-function conference at the National Heart and Lung Institute. Am Heart J 90:777, 1975.)

estimated that 100 phlebotomies of 500 ml of blood once a week will eliminate the excess iron within 2 years. More rapid removal of blood may produce hypotension or cardiac arrhythmias. The condition can subsequently be controlled by intermittent phlebotomies, maintaining the hemoglobin at about 11 g/dl.

In secondary hemochromatosis resulting from multiple transfusion for the treatment of anemia, phlebotomy cannot be relied on for treatment. One must then attempt to maintain the patient at a somewhat lower hemoglobin level in order to reduce the number of transfusions. Technics to deplete the body stores of iron are only modestly satisfactory but can be attempted, especially a low-iron diet and deferoxamine.

AMYLOID DISEASE

Amyloid disease of the heart has always interested clinicians because of its long history and because it is estimated to be responsible for about 5–10% of cases of cardiomyopathy due to causes other than coronary artery disease. It is usually primary in the heart but may be secondary to other conditions, eg, multiple myeloma, chronic infections, regional ileitis, chronic disorders of connective tissues such as rheumatoid arthritis, or periodic fever (familial Mediterranean fever). The cause is obscure, although recent investigations indicate that a faulty immunologic response may be responsible for increased production by plasma cells and deposition of amyloid protein in the heart, kidney, and other organs of the body. The heart has a "glassy" appearance, and there may be generalized vasculitis involving the liver, spleen, and kidneys as well as the heart. The small vessels of the heart may have amyloid deposits in the walls of the vessels, producing occlusive disease from the vasculitis as well as restrictive disease from the deposition of amyloid. A typical example is shown in Fig 17–29. Fig 17–30 is a typical Congo red stain preparation of amyloidosis from a rectal biopsy. Table 17–14 lists the presenting symptoms and signs of amyloidosis.

Clinical Findings

A. Symptoms and Signs: Amyloid disease of the heart is a restrictive cardiomyopathy and may be confused with constrictive pericarditis. Amyloid disease should be considered in all patients with plasma cell leukemia, multiple myeloma, chronic infections, and long-standing periodic fever. Definitive diagnosis is based on finding amyloid deposits in biopsies of the rectum, liver, or gums (Fig 17–30); of the 3 sites, rectal biopsy is the most reliable of the simple and least painful procedures and most likely to be positive. Subcutaneous fat biopsy may be diagnostic. The oral lesions, in additions to papules, may include macroglossia with a large, firm tongue resulting from amyloid deposition. About half of patients with primary amyloidosis have demonstrable Bence Jones protein in the urine; conversely, only about half of patients with multiple myeloma who have Bence Jones proteinuria have amyloid disease.

Amyloid deposits consisting of fibrils of light

Table 17–14. Presenting symptoms and signs in amyloidosis.*

	Primary (%)	Secondary (%)
Symptoms		
Fatigue	67	65
Weight loss	55	62
Edema	46	41
Dyspnea	30	33
Paresthesias	26	26
Light-headedness or syncope	30	7
Hoarseness	12	16
Gross bleeding	7	11
Pain in involved organ	5	34
Signs		
Liver palpable	45	49
Edema	35	33
Spleen palpable	7	11
Macroglossia	12	26
Lymphadenopathy		
Generalized	8	8
Submandibular	9	11
Purpura	17	15
Hypotension, orthostatic	16	8
Skin lesions (amyloid)	4	8

*Adapted from Kyle RA, Bayrd ED: Amyloidosis: Review of 236 cases. Medicine 54:271, 1975. © 1975 by Williams & Wilkins Co., Baltimore, Md.

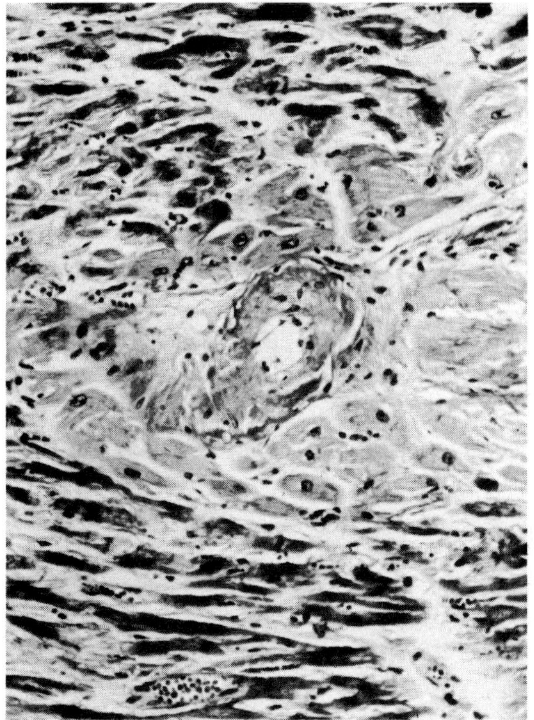

Figure 17–29. Amyloidosis involving the wall of a small artery and surrounding myocardium. Magnification X 150. The dark-staining areas are ischemic myocardial fibers. (Reproduced, with permission, from Castleman B [editor]: Case Records of the Massachusetts General Hospital. N Engl J Med 286:364, 1972.)

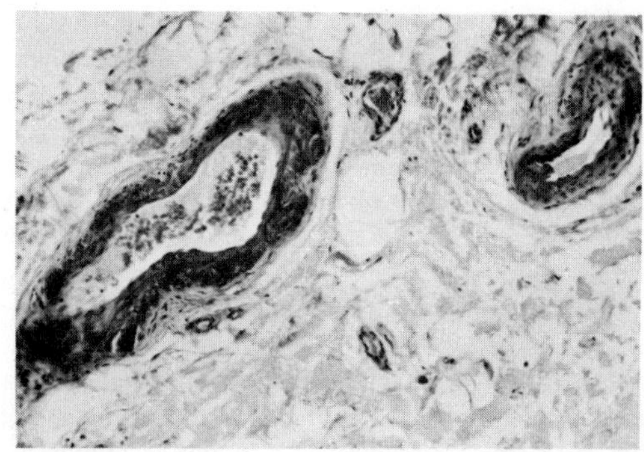

Figure 17–30. Rectal amyloidosis from rectal biopsy. Magnification X 40, Congo red stain. The dark areas are deposits of amyloid in the walls of blood vessels. (Courtesy of O Rambo.)

chain immunoglobulins may be found anywhere in the myocardium; if large and extensive, they may produce restrictive cardiomyopathy. The deposits may be small and scattered, especially in older individuals, and may not give rise to any cardiovascular symptoms or signs. If the amyloid deposits involve the conduction system, eg, the sinus node or the atrioventricular node, the patients may have ventricular arrhythmias or ECG evidence of conduction defects, heart block, and syncope. The severity of amyloid involvement varies considerably; some patients are found to have amyloid deposits at postmortem who have had no cardiac symptoms during life; in other cases, the deposits are sufficiently large to cause heart failure, arrhythmias, and conduction defects.

Progressive renal failure may occur as excess protein is deposited in the basement membrane of the glomeruli.

B. Laboratory Findings: Bence Jones proteinuria is usually associated with multiple myeloma or secondary amyloidosis, although it occurs to a lesser degree in primary amyloid disease, neoplastic diseases, and immunologic disorders such as Waldenström's macroglobulinemia. Bence Jones protein was discovered because it precipitates when heated to moderate temperatures (50–60 °C) but redissolves on further heating to 100 °C and then reprecipitates upon cooling. Other proteins (eg, albumin) precipitate upon heating but do not redissolve.

Recent investigations have shown that Bence Jones proteins are homogeneous light chain polypeptides of immunoglobulins which can be found in both urine and blood; the light chains can be found by electron microscopy or quantitative immunochemistry of the urinary sediment. The autoimmune nature of amyloid disease is supported by the finding that the characteristic protein represents the light chains of immunoglobulins (Glenner, 1973).

The distinction between primary and secondary amyloidosis has become blurred because of the lower incidence of chronic infections and the availability of more precise immunochemical methods (immunoelectrophoresis, immunoassay) of quantifying the light chain polypeptides in the urine and serum that characterize amyloid disease. Furthermore, because renal function—especially the reabsorptive function of the proximal tubule—determines how much of the serum immunoglobulin formed by the plasma cells is excreted in the urine, there may be none in the urine despite excessive amounts of IgM (for example) in the serum.

The amount of light chain polypeptide immunoglobulins excreted in the urine and found in the serum varies in different patients and at different times in the course of the disease, complicating its diagnostic value. The greatest amount is formed and excreted in multiple myeloma, with or without plasmacytoma, but even this is not absolute. Bence Jones proteinuria may be missed on the usual heat test but can be verified if special technics such as immunoelectrophoresis of the concentrated urine specimen to estimate smaller amounts of the protein are used. Sulfoxyl precipitates both albumin and Bence Jones protein but may be useful as a screening test. Some cases of primary amyloidosis are not associated with Bence Jones proteinuria.

C. Electrocardiography: The ECG sometimes arouses suspicion of an infiltrative process in the heart because of low voltage of the QRS complexes.

Treatment

The only treatment is that of the underlying condition causing the amyloidosis, eg, chronic infection. Attempts to treat amyloidosis with cytotoxic agents and corticosteroids have not been successful.

ENDOMYOCARDIAL FIBROSIS & LÖFFLER'S ENDOCARDITIS

These uncommon conditions of unknown cause are considered by most authorities to be a single entity, whereas others believe they are different entities that cannot yet be distinguished by available technics. Whether or not endomyocardial fibrosis and Löffler's endocarditis are identical or distinct pathologic processes, the cardiac lesion consists of endomyocardial fibrosis, myocarditis, endocardial thrombosis, and eosinophilic infiltration. Endomyocardial fibrosis was first described by Davies in Uganda in 1948 and since then has been described elsewhere in tropical Africa and Brazil. Löffler described eosinophilic endocarditis in 1936. Both are infrequent (though they do occur) in the Western world but are among the most common diseases of the myocardium in developing countries. The myocardial lesions of Davies and of Löffler's endomyocardial fibrosis cannot be differentiated by histologic study whether or not eosinophilia is present (Brockington, 1973; Roberts, 1969). The cases with eosinophilia are often associated with leukemia and lymphoma, and these disorders should be looked for. Endomyocardial fibrosis produces a plaquelike thickening of the endocardium which appears grossly as a white lining of the entire endocardium, frequently associated with mural thrombi and systemic or pulmonary emboli. The disease usually affects the endocardium and myocardium of the left ventricle, but the right ventricle may also be involved. Cardiac filling is interfered with, and the patient may present with clinical features of restrictive cardiomyopathy (see above under idiopathic cardiomyopathy) and may be confused with chronic constrictive pericarditis.

The onset of the disease is usually vague and insidious. It occurs in teenagers and young adults in developing countries and in older adults in developed ones. Some patients present with fever, which has led to the view that a viral infection may be the basic cause of the process.

Clinical Findings

When restriction of filling and emptying of the ventricles occurs because of the thick lining of endomyocardial fibrosis, the patient presents with cardiac failure of unknown cause although valvular insufficiencies in tricuspid and mitral areas may produce murmurs suggesting valvular heart disease. When the process affects predominantly the right ventricular endocardium, the patient may have a right ventricular heave and pulmonary hypertension from right ventricular disease, associated pulmonary lesions, or left ventricular failure, followed by tricuspid insufficiency and right ventricular failure; the disease must therefore be differentiated from mitral valve disease and chronic pulmonary disease—as well as congenital heart disease when it occurs in children and teenagers. Pericardial effusion followed by heart failure suggests tuberculous pericarditis, which must be excluded. When the process involves the left ventricle, as is usually the case, the patient may present with clinical and radiologic evidence of left ventricular failure (see Chapter 10). In advanced cases, both right and left ventricular endocardiums are involved and the patient may then have both right and left ventricular failure and pulmonary hypertension. Definitive diagnosis may be made by right and left ventricular cineangiography if the process is advanced. Otherwise, the diagnosis is suspected on the basis of the clinical features but often cannot be distinguished from idiopathic congestive cardiomyopathy with right ventricular failure. Intracardiac calcification is a helpful sign.

Treatment & Prognosis

Treatment is unsatisfactory and is generally only supportive, with conventional therapy for cardiac failure. The prognosis is poor, with the usual survival being a matter of only a few years.

SICKLE CELL DISEASE & CHRONIC ANEMIA

Sickle cell disease can cause cardiovascular manifestations. The anemia may increase the cardiac output, and the tendency of sickle cells to occlude small vessels may narrow the pulmonary or coronary arteries and produce cor pulmonale or angina. When the hemoglobin is less than 6 or 7 g/dl in any type of anemia, cardiac output is increased at rest and systemic vascular resistance is decreased, but the maximal cardiac output with exercise is still less than normal. Because of thrombotic obliteration of the pulmonary arteries that occurs in sickle cell disease, patients may develop right ventricular hypertrophy and pulmonary hypertension and ultimately right heart failure. The left ventricle is usually enlarged (as shown by chest films or echocardiography), which may be due to a combination of chronic anemia and the vascular occlusions that occurs in sickle cell crises. Systolic murmurs are frequent but nondescript; if the anemia is severe, there may be diastolic as well as systolic murmurs. Because of frequent thrombotic involvement of the smaller coronary arteries, patients may have dyspnea and angina; because of the anemia, they may present with a hyperdynamic high output cardiac state (see High Output Failure in Chapter 10).

Treatment consists mainly of hydration with intravenous fluids and symptomatic relief of pain by narcotics. There is no specific therapy of proved value.

CHAGAS' DISEASE
(American Trypanosomiasis)

Chagas' disease of the heart is an acute and chronic myocardial disease due to infection with the protozoon *Trypanosoma cruzi,* transmitted to man in the feces of a Triatoma insect during blood feeding. The insect lives in the thatched roofs of adobe houses in South America, especially Brazil and Argentina, and bites its victims while they sleep. Chagas' disease is a major health problem in central South America, infecting one-third of the people and causing chronic cardiac disease in one-third of those infected. It is rare in the USA although the insect vector has been found in Texas and some of the southern states.

The disease was first described by Chagas in 1909 (Chagas, 1910), and subsequent epidemiologic and clinical studies have documented its endemic nature and clinical importance. The organism does not multiply in the blood but can be obtained by culture in the acute phases. It penetrates cells of various organs and multiplies and spreads, ultimately involving the heart.

Clinical Findings

The disease has acute and chronic phases separated by a latent period of 10–20 years.

A. Acute Phase: The acute phase begins within days after inoculation by the insect and consists of a general febrile systemic reaction plus signs depending on the site of entry of the organism, usually either the eye or the skin. The eye is swollen and discolored, with regional adenopathy (Romaña's sign). Skin inoculation results in a localized lesion called a chagoma (Fig 17–31), similar to a furuncle. During the acute phase, which lasts several months, ECG and radiologic signs of acute myocarditis or pericardial effusion can be demonstrated in approximately one-third of patients. Complement-fixing antibodies appear in the blood in about 2 months (Prata, 1968).

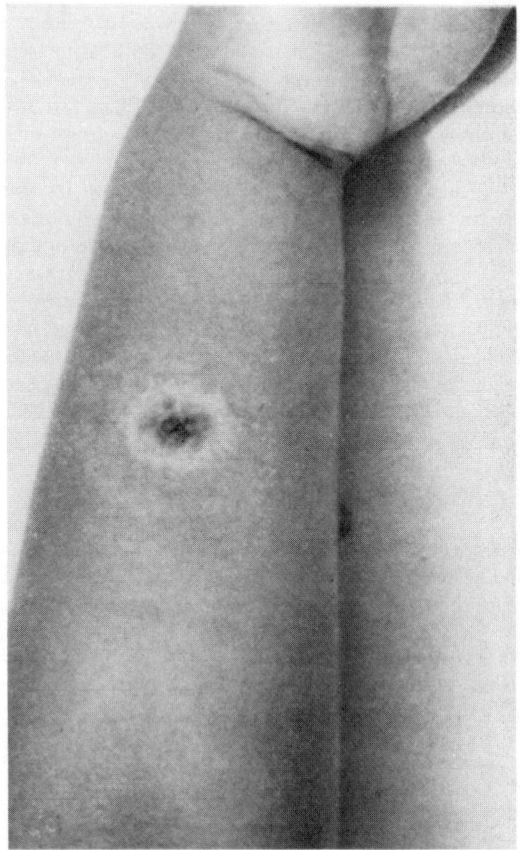

Figure 17–31. Inflammatory chagoma on the skin of the forearm in acute Chagas' disease. (Reproduced, with permission, from Prata A: Chagas' heart disease. Cardiologia 52:79, 1968.)

B. Late Chronic Phase: Many patients have no clinical or systemic manifestations of the acute phase, and the diagnosis is only made many years later when they present with symptomatic atrioventricular or intraventricular conduction defects, chronic congestive cardiomyopathy with or without achalasia and dilatation of the esophagus, and serologic evidence of previous infection by *T cruzi* plus a history of residence in an endemic area.

The chronic cardiomyopathy is nonspecific but resembles idiopathic or chronic congestive cardiomyopathy, with the exception that palpitations and conduction defects are more common and sudden death is a more important cause of death (20%, according to Prata, 1968). In addition to dyspnea, palpitations, and syncope, patients have cardiac enlargement, aneurysms and thromboses of the apexes of both ventricles, and marked enlargement of both atria, seen radiologically or by echocardiography. Systemic or pulmonary emboli are due to intracardiac thrombi. Coronary disease is uncommon, in part because most patients are under 50 years of age.

When the pathologic lesion dominantly involves the conduction system, as it may also in sarcoidosis or scleroderma, the heart may be normal in size but the ECG may show arrhythmia and atrioventricular or intraventricular conduction defects. Complete atrioventricular block may ensue, cause Stokes-Adams attacks, and require artificial pacemakers to prevent sudden death. Cardiac enlargement and cardiac failure occur later, usually within a few years of the onset of heart block.

Treatment

Treatment is symptomatic, with pacemakers for syncope and conventional treatment of cardiac failure and systemic emboli when they occur. The only means of prevention is by improving housing and destroying the insect vector.

PERIPARTUM CARDIOMYOPATHY

Cardiac failure occurring just before, during, or within the first 2 months after delivery, in the absence of any known preexisting cardiac disease or symptoms in the first 2 trimesters of pregnancy, is an uncommon disorder of unknown cause. The relationship to pregnancy is an essential part of the diagnosis, but the disease may be delayed for 1–3 months and the relationship to pregnancy may be overlooked. A high percentage (about 80%) of patients with idiopathic cardiomyopathy in the tropics give a history of onset in relationship to pregnancy (Burch, 1972).

The clinical manifestations may be alarming, with the rapid development of severe cardiac failure with or without pericardial effusion usually shortly after delivery. Severe dyspnea, orthopnea, tachycardia, chest pain, cardiac enlargement, gallop rhythm but no murmurs, pulmonary rales, and pulmonary congestion on the chest film attest to the presence of severe left ventricular failure, although raised venous pressure indicates right ventricular failure as well. Systemic embolism may occur. Transient hypertension may be found at the outset but subsides with treatment of cardiac failure. Preeclampsia-eclampsia and acute glomerulonephritis must be excluded. The ECG shows primary T wave inversions (not secondary to conduction defects) in the left ventricular leads, suggesting acute myopericarditis, with which this disorder is frequently confused. Coronary angiography has been done in a few cases and shows nothing abnormal.

The clinical course usually lasts 3–6 months, and most patients recover following conventional treatment for cardiac failure. Gilchrist (1963) found no evidence of residual cardiac symptoms or signs in 7 patients studied 1–10 years after congestive heart failure. Figs 17–32 and 17–33 illustrate the course in a 32-year-old woman who developed cardiac failure 4 months following delivery of a normal child. X-rays of

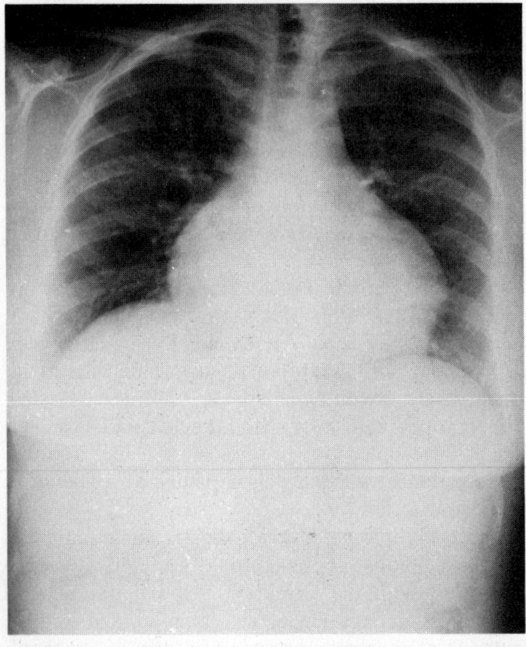

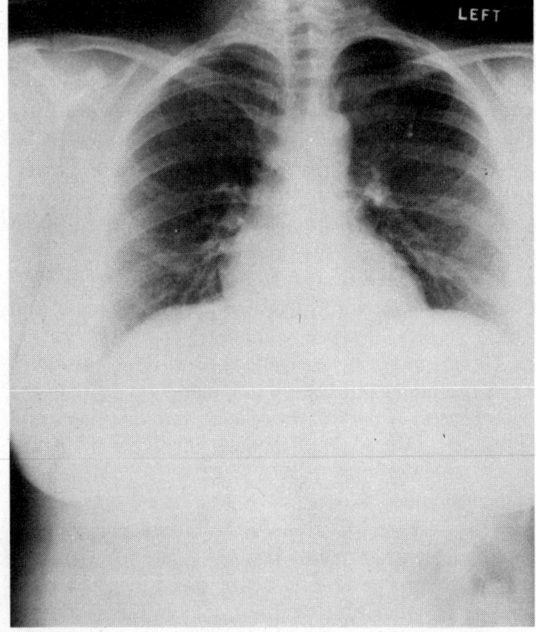

Figure 17–32. *A:* March 15, 1972. Chest films of a 32-year-old woman who developed cardiac failure 4 months following delivery of a normal child. Films show progressive decrease in size of cardiac shadow. Patient was perfectly well by October 1973. *B:* November 7, 1974.

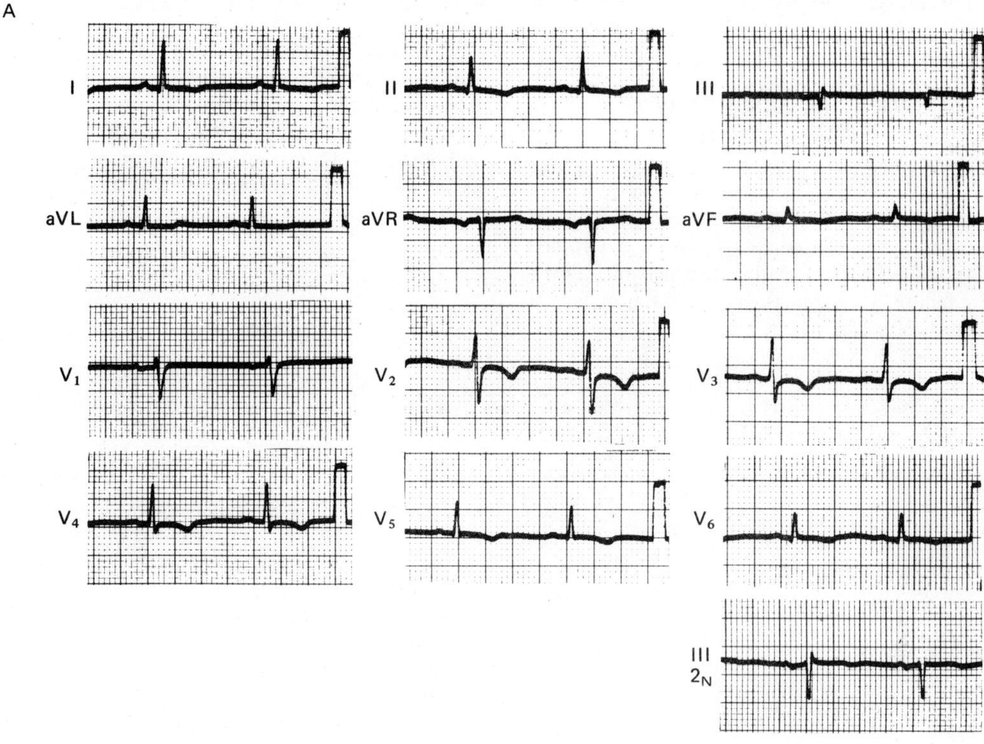

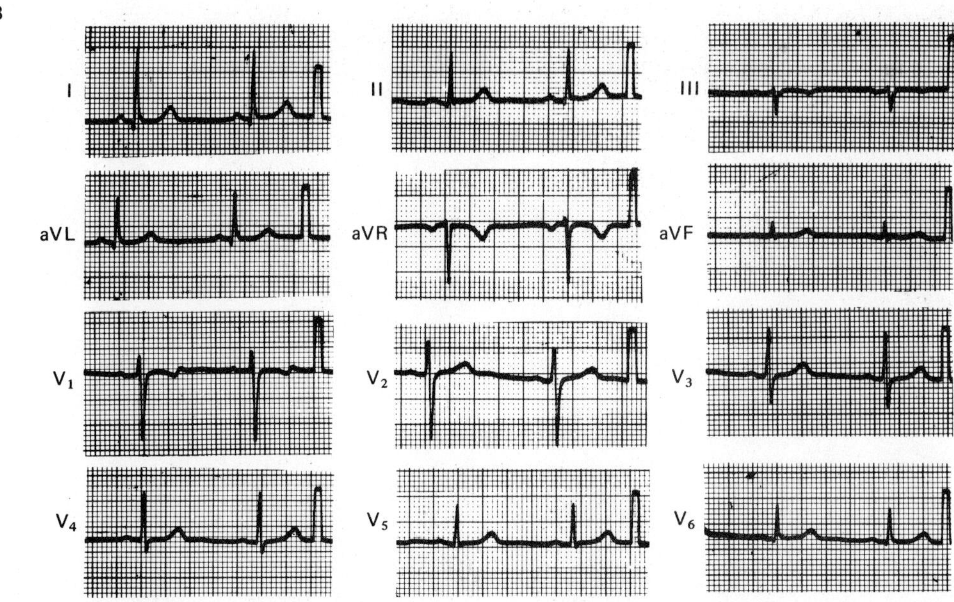

Figure 17–33. *A:* March 15, 1972. ECGs of same 32-year-old woman who developed cardiac failure 4 months following delivery of a normal child reveal regression of ECG abnormalities with diffuse T wave inversions on March 15, 1972. *B:* Completely gone by October 1, 1973.

the chest show progressive decrease in size of the heart shadow (Fig 17–32), and ECGs show regression of electrocardiographic abnormalities (Fig 17–33).

NEUROPATHIC DISORDERS & HEART DISEASE

Neuropathic disorders are a rare cause of heart disease. Patients with Friedreich's ataxia, dystrophia myotonica, and other neuropathic disorders may develop cardiac failure, arrhythmias, and conduction defects with Stokes-Adams attacks.

CARDIAC INVOLVEMENT IN INHERITED DISORDERS OF METABOLISM

These constitute a group of genetically determined enzymatic abnormalities and are only mentioned here for completeness. A comprehensive paper by Blieden and Moller (1974) classifies the disorders and discusses them from the point of view of their basic biochemistry and clinical features.

• • •

References

Idiopathic Cardiomyopathy

Abbasi AS: Echocardiography in the differential diagnosis of the large heart. Am J Med 60:677, 1976.

Adelman AG & others: Current concepts of primary cardiomyopathies. Cardiovasc Med 2:495, 1977.

Blackett K, Ngu JL: Immunological studies in congestive cardiomyopathy in Cameroon. Br Heart J 38:605, 1976.

Borer JS, Henry WL, Epstein SE: Echocardiographic observations in patients with systemic infiltrative disease involving the heart. Am J Cardiol 39:184, 1977.

Brigden W: Cardiomyopathy. Practitioner 190:222, 1963.

Brigden W: Uncommon myocardial diseases: The noncoronary cardiomyopathies. (2 parts.) Lancet 2: 1179, 1243, 1957.

Brooksby IAB, Coltart DJ, Webb-Peploe MM: Progress in endomyocardial biopsy. Mod Concepts Cardiovasc Dis 44:65, 1975.

Bulkley BH & others: Thallium 201 imaging and gated cardiac blood pool scans in patients with ischemic and idiopathic congestive cardiomyopathy: A clinical and pathologic study. Circulation 55:753, 1977.

Burch GE (editor): Cardiovascular Clinics Series. Vol 4: *Cardiomyopathy.* Davis, 1972.

Burch GE, Giles TD: Prolonged bed rest in the management of patients with cardiomyopathy. Page 375 in: *Cardiomyopathy.* Burch GE (editor). Davis, 1972.

Burchell HB: Unusual causes of heart failure. Circulation 21:436, 1960.

Cochrane CG, Koffler D: Immune complex disease. Adv Immunol 16:185, 1973.

Emanuel R, Withers R, O'Brien K: Dominant and recessive modes of inheritance in idiopathic cardiomyopathy. Lancet 2:1065, 1971.

Feild BJ & others: Left ventricular function and hypertrophy in cardiomyopathy with depressed ejection fraction. Circulation 47:1022, 1973.

Fejfar Z: Cardiomyopathies: An international problem. Cardiologia 52:9, 1968.

Fowler NO: The secondary cardiomyopathies. In: *Myocardial Diseases.* Fowler NO (editor). Grune & Stratton, 1973.

Goodwin JF: Congestive and hypertrophic cardiomyopathies: A decade of study. Lancet 1:731, 1970.

Goodwin JF: Hypertrophic diseases of the myocardium. Prog Cardiovasc Dis 16:199, 1973.

Goodwin JF: Prospects and predictions for the cardiomyopathies. Circulation 50:210, 1974.

Goodwin JF, Oakley CM: The cardiomyopathies. Br Heart J 34:545, 1972.

Gould L & others: Nonobstructive primary myocardial disease: Hemodynamic studies in fourteen cases. Am J Cardiol 22:523, 1968.

Greenwood RD, Nadas AS, Fyler DC: The clinical course of primary myocardial disease in infants and children. Am Heart J 92:549, 1976.

Hamby RI: Primary myocardial disease. Medicine 49:55, 1970.

Harvey WP, Segal JP, Gurel T: The clinical spectrum of primary myocardial disease. Prog Cardiovasc Dis 7:17, 1964.

Hatle L, Orjavik O, Storstein O: Chronic myocardial disease. 1. Clinical picture related to long-term prognosis. Acta Med Scand 199:399, 1976.

Hatle L, Stake G, Storstein O: Chronic myocardial disease. 2. Haemodynamic findings related to long-term prognosis. Acta Med Scand 199:407, 1976.

Hickie JB, Hall GV: Cardiomyopathies: Report of fifty cases. Australas Ann Med 9:258, 1960.

Hudson REB: *Cardiovascular Pathology.* Vol 2. Arnold, 1965.

Hudson REB: Pathology of cardiomyopathy. Page 3 in: *Cardiomyopathy.* Burch GE (editor). Davis, 1972.

Kawai C, Takatsu T: Clinical and experimental studies on cardiomyopathy. N Engl J Med 293:592, 1975.

Kreulen TH, Gorlin R, Herman MV: Ventriculographic patterns and hemodynamics in primary myocardial disease. Circulation 47:299, 1973.

Kuller L, Lilienfeld A, Fisher K: Sudden and unexpected deaths in young adults: An epidemiological study. JAMA 198:188, 1966.

Massie BM & others: Mitral-septal separation: A new echocardiographic index of left ventricular function. Am J Cardiol 39:1008, 1977.

Massumi RA & others: Primary myocardial disease: A report of 50 cases and review of the literature. Circulation 31:19, 1965.

Mattingly JW: The clinical concept of primary myocardial disease. Circulation 32:845, 1965.

Mattingly TW, Sjoerdsma A: Cardiovascular manifestations of functioning carcinoid tumors. Mod Concepts Cardiovasc Dis 25:337, 1956.

McDonald CD, Burch GE, Walsh JJ: Prolonged bed rest in the treatment of idiopathic cardiomyopathy. Am J Med 52:41, 1972.

Millward DK, McLaurin LP, Craige E: Echocardiographic studies of the mitral valve in patients with congestive cardiomyopathy and mitral regurgitation. Am Heart J 85:413, 1973.

Oakley CM: The relation between function and causation in cardiomyopathy. Postgrad Med J 51:271, 1975.

Olsen EGJ: Diagnostic value of the endomyocardial bioptome. Lancet 1:658, 1974.

Olsen EGJ: Pathological recognition of cardiomyopathy. Postgrad Med J 51:277, 1975.

Perloff JK: The cardiomyopathies: Current concepts. Circulation 44:942, 1971.

Perlroth MG: Connective tissue diseases and the heart. JAMA 231:410, 1975.

Roberts WC, Ferrans VJ: Pathologic anatomy of the cardiomyopathies: Idiopathic dilated and hypertrophic types, infiltrative types and endomyocardial disease with and without eosinophilia. Hum Pathol 6:287, 1975.

Rossen RM, Alderman EL, Harrison DC: Circulatory response to vasodilator therapy in congestive cardiomyopathy. Br Heart J 38:695, 1976.

Schlant RC: Physiology of idiopathic cardiomyopathies. Page 61 in: *Cardiomyopathy.* Burch GE (editor). Davis, 1972.

Segal JP, Harvey WP, Stapleton J: Clinical features and natural history of cardiomyopathy. Pages 37–57 in: *Myocardial Diseases.* Fowler NO (editor). Grune & Stratton, 1973.

Sekiguchi M, Konno S: Diagnosis and classification of primary myocardial disease with the aid of endomyocardial biopsy. Jpn Circ J 35:737, 1971.

Waagstein F & others: Effect of chronic beta adrenergic blockade in congestive cardiomyopathy. Br Heart J 37:1022, 1975.

Wheeler RC, Abelmann WH: Cardiomyopathy associated with systemic diseases. Page 283 in: *Cardiomyopathy*. Burch GE (editor). Davis, 1972.

Hypertrophic Obstructive Cardiomyopathy

Adelman AG & others: The clinical course in muscular subaortic stenosis. Ann Intern Med 77:515, 1972.

Adelman AG & others: Long-term propranolol therapy in muscular subaortic stenosis. Br Heart J 32:804, 1970.

Beck W: Syphilitic obstruction of coronary ostia successfully treated by endarterectomy. Br Heart J 27:911, 1965.

Bentall HH & others: Surgical treatment and postoperative haemodynamic studies in hypertrophic obstructive cardiomyopathy. Br Heart J 27:585, 1965.

Braunwald E, Aygen MM: Idiopathic myocardial hypertrophy without congestive heart failure or obstruction to blood flow. Am J Med 35:7, 1963.

Brock RC: Functional obstruction of the left ventricle. Guys Hosp Rep 106:221, 1957.

Brockenbrough EC & others: A hemodynamic technic for the detection of hypertrophic subaortic stenosis. Circulation 23:189, 1961.

Bulkley BH, Weisfeldt ML, Hutchins GM: Isometric cardiac contraction: A possible cause of the disorganized myocardial pattern of idiopathic hypertrophic subaortic stenosis. N Engl J Med 295:135, 1977.

De la Calzada CS & others: Effect of acute administration of propranolol on ventricular function in hypertrophic obstructive cardiomyopathy measured by non-invasive techniques. Br Heart J 38:798, 1976.

Epstein SE (moderator, NIH Conference): Asymmetric septal hypertrophy. Ann Intern Med 81:650, 1974.

Epstein SE & others: The role of operative treatment in patients with idiopathic hypertrophic subaortic stenosis. Circulation 48:677, 1973.

Feizi O, Emanuel R: Echocardiographic spectrum of hypertrophic cardiomyopathy. Br Heart J 37:1286, 1975.

Flamm MD, Harrison DC, Hancock EW: Muscular subaortic stenosis: Prevention of outflow obstruction with propranolol. Circulation 38:846, 1968.

Frank S, Braunwald E: Idiopathic hypertrophic subaortic stenosis: Clinical analysis of 126 patients with emphasis on the natural history. Circulation 37:759, 1968.

Goodwin FJ: ?IHSS, ?HOCM, ?ASH: A plea for unity. (Editorial.) Am Heart J 89:269, 1975.

Goodwin JF & others: The clinical pharmacology of hypertrophic obstructive cardiomyopathy. Page 189 in: *Cardiomyopathies.* Wolstenholme GE, O'Connor M (editors). Churchill, 1964.

Goodwin JF: Hypertrophic diseases of the myocardium. Prog Cardiovasc Dis 16:199, 1973.

Henry WL, Clark CE, Epstein SE: Asymmetric septal hypertrophy (ASH): The unifying link in the IHSS disease spectrum. Circulation 47:827, 1973.

Henry WL & others: Mechanism of left ventricular outflow obstruction in patients with obstructive asymmetric septal hypertrophy (idiopathic hypertrophic subaortic stenosis). Am J Cardiol 35:337, 1975.

Larter W & others: The asymmetrically hypertrophied septum: Further differentiation of its causes. Circulation 53:20, 1976.

Morrow AG & others: Operative treatment in idiopathic hypertrophic subaortic stenosis: Techniques and the results of preoperative and postoperative clinical and hemodynamic assessments. Circulation 37.589, 1968.

Nellen M & others: Effects of prompt squatting on the systolic murmur in idiopathic hypertrophic obstructive cardiomyopathy. Br Med J 3:140, 1967.

Perloff JK: Clinical recognition of aortic stenosis: The physical signs and differential diagnosis of the various forms of obstruction to left ventricular outflow. Prog Cardiovasc Dis 10:323, 1968.

Popp RL, Harrison DC: Ultrasound in the diagnosis and evaluation of therapy of idiopathic hypertrophic subaortic stenosis. Circulation 40:905, 1969.

Powell WJ Jr & others: Symptomatic prognosis in patients with idiopathic hypertrophic subaortic stenosis (IHSS). Am J Med 55:15, 1973.

Salzman SH & others: Epinephrine infusion in man: Standardization, normal response, and abnormal response in idiopathic hypertrophic subaortic stenosis. Circulation 43:137, 1971.

Shah PM & others: Echocardiographic assessment of the effects of surgery and propranolol on the dynamics of outflow obstruction in hypertrophic subaortic stenosis. Circulation 45:515, 1972.

Steiner RE: Radiology of hypertrophic obstructive cardiomyopathy. Proc R Soc Med 57:444, 1964.

Stenson RE & others: Hypertrophic subaortic stenosis: Clinical and hemodynamic effects of long-term propranolol therapy. Am J Cardiol 31:763, 1973.

Swan DA & others: Analysis of the symptomatic course and treatment of hypertrophic obstructive cardiomyopathy. Br Heart J 33:671, 1971.

Tajik AJ & others: Idiopathic hypertrophic subaortic stenosis: Long-term surgical follow-up. Am J Cardiol 34:815, 1974.

Walston A: Electrocardiographic and hemodynamic correlations in patients with idiopathic hypertrophic subaortic stenosis. Am Heart J 91:11, 1976.

Whiting RB & others: Idiopathic hypertrophic subaortic stenosis in the elderly. N Engl J Med 285:196, 1971.

Wigle ED & others: Results in ventriculomyotomy in muscular subaortic stenosis. Am J Cardiol 11:572, 1963.

Wolstenholme GEW, O'Connor M (editors): *Hypertrophic Obstructive Cardiomyopathy*. Churchill, 1971.

Acute Myocarditis From Specific Diseases

Abelmann WH: Viral myocarditis and its sequelae. Annu Rev Med 24:143, 1973.

Abelmann WH, Kowalski HJ, McNeely WF: Cardiovascular studies during acute infectious hepatitis. Gastroenterology 27:61, 1954.

Bell RW, Murphy WM: Myocarditis in young military personnel: Herpes simplex, trichinosis, meningococcemia, carbon tetrachloride, and idiopathic fibrous and giant cell types. Am Heart J 74:309, 1967.

Bengtsson E: Acute myocarditis and its consequences in Sweden. Postgrad Med J 48:751, 1972.

Binak K & others: Circulatory changes in acute glomerulonephritis at rest and during exercise. Br Heart J

37:833, 1975.

Castleman B, Scully RE, McNeely BU (editors): Case records of the Massachusetts General Hospital (viral myocarditis). N Engl J Med 286:1100, 1972.

De la Chapelle CE, Kossmann CE: Myocarditis. Circulation 10:747, 1954.

Ebert RV, Stead EA: Circulatory failure in acute infections. J Clin Invest 20:671, 1941.

Fine I, Brainerd H, Sokolow M: Myocarditis in acute infectious diseases. Circulation 20:859, 1959.

Finland M & others: Acute myocarditis in influenza A infections: Two cases of nonbacterial myocarditis, with isolation of virus from the lungs. Am J Med Sci 209:455, 1945.

Gore I, Saphir O: Myocarditis: A classification of 1402 cases. Am Heart J 34:827, 1947.

Grist NR, Bell EJ: A 6-year study of coxsackievirus B infections in heart disease. J Hyg (Camb) 73:165, 1974.

Hakkila J, Frick HM, Halonen PI: Pericarditis and myocarditis caused by toxoplasma: Report of a case and review of the literature. Am Heart J 65:758, 1958.

Hirschman SZ, Hammer GS: Coxsackie virus myopericarditis: A microbiological and clinical review. Am J Cardiol 34:224, 1974.

Lerner AM, Wilson FM, Reyes MP: Enteroviruses and the heart (with special emphasis on the probable role of coxsackieviruses, group B, types 1–5). 1. Epidemiological and experimental studies. Mod Concepts Cardiovasc Dis 44:7, 1975.

Lewes D: Viral myocarditis. Practitioner 216:281, 1976.

Lewes D, Rainford DJ: Symptomless myocarditis and myalgia in viral and *Mycoplasma pneumoniae* infections. Br Heart J 33:613, 1971.

Miller RA, Hastreiter AR: Myocarditis: The acute and chronic acquired primary myocardial disease of infants and children. Am J Dis Child 100:736, 1960.

Monif GRG, Lee CW, Hsiung GD: Isolated myocarditis with recovery of ECHO type 9 virus from the myocardium. N Engl J Med 277:1353, 1967.

Moore CM & others: Varicella myocarditis. Am J Dis Child 118:899, 1969.

Pruitt RD: Acute myocarditis in adult. Prog Cardiovasc Dis 7:73, 1964.

Roberts WC, Fox SM III: Mumps of the heart: Clinical and pathologic features. Circulation 32:342, 1965.

Rose HD: Recurrent illness following acute coxsackie B4 myocarditis. Am J Med 54:544, 1973.

Rosenberg HS, McNamara DG: Acute myocarditis in infancy and childhood. Prog Cardiovasc Dis 7:179, 1964.

Ruskin J, Remington JS: Toxoplasmosis in the compromised host. Ann Intern Med 84:193, 1976.

Sainani GS, Dekate MP, Rao CP: Heart disease caused by coxsackie virus B infection. Br Heart J 37:819, 1975.

Sands MJ Jr & others: Pericarditis and perimyocarditis associated with active *Mycoplasma pneumoniae* infection. Ann Intern Med 86:544, 1977.

Saphir O: Myocarditis: A general review, with analysis of two hundred and forty cases. (2 parts.) Arch Pathol 32:1000, 1941; 33:88, 1942.

Saphir O: Nonrheumatic inflammatory diseases of the heart. C. Myocarditis. Page 779 in: *Pathology of the Heart,* 2nd ed. Gould SE (editor). Thomas, 1960.

Smith WG: Coxsackie B myopericarditis in adults. Am Heart J 80:34, 1970.

Sokolow M, Garland LH: Cardiovascular disturbances in tsutsugamushi disease. US Naval Medical Bulletin, page 1054, 1945.

Strong RP: Anti-typhus campaign in 1915 in Serbia considered in connection with present typhus epidemic in Poland. Int J Public Health 1:188, 1920.

Viruses and heart disease. (Editorial.) Lancet 2:991, 1974.

Weinstein L, Shelokov A: Cardiovascular manifestations in acute poliomyelitis. N Engl J Med 244:281, 1951.

Wenger NK: Infectious myocarditis. Page 167 in: *Cardiomyopathy.* Burch GE (editor). Davis, 1972.

Wenger NK: Myocarditis. Chapter 72 in: *The Heart,* 2nd ed. Hurst JW, Logue RB (editors). McGraw-Hill, 1966.

Wolbach SB, Palfrey FW: Typhus fever. Med Clin North Am 4:1877, 1921.

Woodward TE & others: Specific microbial infections of the myocardium and pericardium: A study of 82 patients. Arch Intern Med 120:270, 1967.

Rheumatic Fever

Bland EF, Jones TD: Rheumatic fever and rheumatic heart disease: A twenty year report on 1000 patients followed since childhood. Circulation 4:836, 1951.

Clarke M, Keith JD: Atrioventricular conduction in acute rheumatic fever. Br Heart J 34:472, 1972.

Combined Rheumatic Fever Study Group: A comparison of short-term, intensive prednisone and acetylsalicylic acid therapy in the treatment of acute rheumatic fever. N Engl J Med 272:63, 1965.

Engleman EP, Hollister LE, Kolb FO: Sequelae of rheumatic fever in men: Four to eight year follow-up study. JAMA 155:1134, 1954.

Feinstein AR, Spagnuolo M: The clinical patterns of acute rheumatic fever: A reappraisal. Medicine 41:279, 1962.

Feinstein AR, Stern EK: Clinical effects of recurrent attacks of acute rheumatic fever: A prospective epidemiologic study of 105 episodes. J Chronic Dis 20:13, 1967.

Feinstein AR & others: Rheumatic fever in children and adolescents: A long-term epidemiologic study of subsequent prophylaxis, streptococcal infections, and clinical sequelae. 6. Cardiac changes and sequelae. Ann Intern Med 60 (Suppl 5):87, 1964.

Markowitz M, Gordis L: *Rheumatic Fever,* 2nd ed. Saunders, 1972.

Schieken RM, Kerber RE: Echocardiographic abnormalities in acute rheumatic fever. Am J Cardiol 38:458, 1976.

Sellers TF Jr: An epidemiologic view of rheumatic fever. Prog Cardiovasc Dis 16:303, 1973.

Sokolow M: Significance of electrocardiographic changes in rheumatic fever. Am J Med 5:365, 1948.

Sokolow M, Snell A: Atypical features of rheumatic fever in young adults. JAMA 133:981, 1947.

Stollerman GH, Rusoff JH, Hirschfeld I: Prophylaxis against group A streptococci in rheumatic fever: The use of single monthly injection of benzathine penicillin G. N Engl J Med 252:787, 1955.

Stollerman GH & others: Jones criteria (revised) for guidance in the diagnosis of rheumatic fever. Circulation 32:664, 1965.

Strasser T, Rotta J: The control of rheumatic fever and rheumatic heart disease: An outline of WHO activities. WHO Chron 27:49, 1973.

Svartman M & others: Immunoglobulins and complement components in synovial fluid of patients with acute rheumatic fever. J Clin Invest 56:111, 1975.

Tompkins DG, Boxerbaum B, Liebman J: Long-term prognosis of rheumatic fever patients receiving regular intramuscular benzathine penicillin. Circulation 45:543, 1972.

UK and US Joint Report: The natural history of rheumatic fever and rheumatic heart disease: Ten-year report of a cooperative clinical trial of ACTH, cortisone and aspirin. Circulation 32:457, 1965.

Wee AST, Goodwin JF: Acute rheumatic fever and carditis in older adults. Lancet 2:239, 1966.

Myocardial Toxicity Due to Drugs

Alarcon-Segovia D: Drug-induced lupus syndromes. Mayo Clin Proc 44:664, 1969.

Appelbaum FR & others: Acute lethal carditis caused by high-dose combination chemotherapy: A unique clinical and pathological entity. Lancet 1:58, 1976.

Bana DS & others: Cardiac murmurs and endocardial fibrosis associated with methysergide therapy. Am Heart J 88:640, 1974.

Blomgren SE, Condemi JJ, Vaughan JH: Procainamide-induced lupus erythematosus: Clinical and laboratory observations. Am J Med 52:338, 1972.

Buja LM & others: Cardiac ultrastructural changes induced by daunorubicin therapy. Cancer 32:771, 1973.

Freeman JW & others: Cardiac abnormalities in poisoning with tricyclic antidepressants. Br Med J 2:610, 1969.

Harrison DT, Sanders LA: Pericarditis in a case of early daunorubicin cardiomyopathy. Ann Intern Med 85:340, 1976.

Jefferson JW: A review of cardiovascular effects and toxicity of tricyclic antidepressants. Psychosom Med 37:160, 1975.

Lefrak E & others: A clinicopathologic analysis of Adriamycin cardiotoxicity. Cancer 32:302, 1973.

Minow R, Benjamin R, Gottlieb J: Adriamycin cardiomyopathy: An overview with determination of risk factors. Cancer Chemother Rep 6:195, 1975.

Morin Y, Coté G: Toxic agents and cardiomyopathies. Page 245 in: *Cardiomyopathy.* Burch GE (editor). Davis, 1972.

Rinehart J, Lewis R, Balcerzak S: Adriamycin cardiotoxicity in man. Ann Intern Med 81:475, 1974.

Smith B: Damage to the intrinsic cardiac neurones by Rubidomycin (daunorubicin). Br Heart J 31:607, 1969.

Tobis J, Das BN: Cardiac complications in amitriptyline poisoning: Successful treatment with physostigmine. JAMA 235:1474, 1976.

Ugoretz RJ: Cardiac effects of doxorubicin therapy of neoplasms. JAMA 236:295, 1976.

Von Hoff DD & others: Daunomycin-induced cardiotoxicity in children and adults: A review of 110 cases. Am J Med 62:200, 1977.

Weinberger A & others: Endocardial fibrosis following busulfan treatment. JAMA 231:495, 1975.

Wilcox RG, James PD, Toghill PJ: Endomyocardial fibrosis associated with daunorubicin therapy. Br Heart J 38:860, 1976.

Thyrotoxic Heart Disease & Myxedema

Davies CE, Mackinnon J, Platts MM: Renal circulation and cardiac output in low-output heart failure and in myxedema. Br Med J 2:595, 1952.

DeGroot WJ: Cardiomyopathy associated with endocrine disorders. Page 305 in: *Cardiomyopathy.* Burch GE (editor). Davis, 1972.

Ellis LB & others: Effect of myxedema on cardiovascular system. Am Heart J 43:341, 1952.

Fahr G: Myxedema heart. JAMA 84:345, 1925.

Graettinger JS & others: Correlation of clinical and hemodynamic studies in patients with hyperthyroidism with and without congestive heart failure. J Clin Invest 38:1316, 1959.

Graettinger JS & others: A correlation of clinical and hemodynamic studies in patients with hypothyroidism. J Clin Invest 37:502, 1958.

Ingbar SH: When to hospitalize the patient with thyrotoxicosis. Hosp Pract 10:45, Jan 1975.

Kerber RE, Sherman B: Echocardiographic evaluation of pericardial effusion in myxedema: Incidence and biochemical and clinical correlations. Circulation 52:823, 1975.

Pietras RJ & others: Cardiovascular response in hyperthyroidism: The influence of adrenergic-receptor blockade. Arch Intern Med 129:426, 1972.

Reza MJ, Abbasi AS: Congestive cardiomyopathy in hypothyroidism. West J Med 123:228, 1975.

Sandler IG, Wilson GM: The nature and prognosis of heart disease in thyrotoxicosis: A review of 150 patients treated with ^{131}I. Q J Med 28:347, 1959.

Sokolow M: Heart disease in patients with thyroid dysfunction: Medical Staff Conference, University of California, San Francisco. Calif Med 109:309, 1968.

Wayne EJ: Clinical and metabolic studies in thyroid disease. Br Med J 1:78, 1960.

Zondek H: As Myxodemherz. Munchen Med Wochenschr 65:1180, 1918.

Alcoholic Cardiomyopathy

Alexander CS: Cobalt-beer cardiomyopathy: A clinical and pathologic study of twenty-eight cases. Am J Med 53:395, 1972.

Brigden W: Alcoholic cardiomyopathy. Page 203 in: *Cardiomyopathy.* Burch GE (editor). Davis, 1972.

Brigden W, Robinson J: Alcoholic heart disease. Br Med J 2:1283, 1964.

Burch GE, De Pasquale NP: Alcoholic cardiomyopathy. Cardiologia 52:48, 1968.

Burch GE & others: Prolonged bed rest in the treatment of the dilated heart. Circulation 32:852, 1965.

Demakis JG & others: The natural course of alcoholic cardiomyopathy. Ann Intern Med 80:293, 1974.

Eliaser M, Giansiracusa F: The heart and alcohol. Calif Med 84:234, 1956.

Kestleloot H & others: Alcoholic perimyocardiopathy. Acta Cardiol (Brux) 21:341, 1966.

Massie BM & others: Mitral-septal separation: A new echocardiographic index of left ventricular function. Am J Cardiol 39:1008, 1977.

McDonald CD, Burch GE, Walsh JJ: Alcoholic cardiomyopathy managed with prolonged bed rest. Ann Intern Med 74:681, 1971.

Mitchell JH, Cohen LS: Alcohol and the heart. Mod Concepts Cardiovasc Dis 39:109, 1970.

Regan TJ & others: Whiskey and the heart. Cardiovasc Med 2:165, 1977.

Rubin E, Lieber CS: Alcohol-induced hepatic injury in non-alcoholic volunteers. N Engl J Med 278:869, 1968.

Spodick DH, Pigott VM, Chirife R: Preclinical cardiac malfunction in chronic alcoholism: Comparison with matched normal control and with alcoholic cardiomyopathy. N Engl J Med 287:677, 1972.

Tobin JR Jr & others: Primary myocardial disease and alcoholism: Clinical manifestations and course of the disease in a selected population of patients observed for three or more years. Circulation 35: 754, 1967.

Beriberi & Nutritional Heart Disease

Alexander CS: Nutritional heart disease. Page 221 in: *Cardiomyopathy.* Burch GE (editor). Davis, 1972.

Aykroyd WR: Beriberi. Ann Nutr Aliment 11:171, 1957.

Hackel DB, Goodale WT, Kleinerman J: Effects of thiamine deficiency on myocardial metabolism in intact dogs. Am Heart J 46:883, 1953.

Ramalingaswami V: Nutrition and the heart. Cardiologia 52:57, 1968.

Swanepoel A, Smythe PM, Campbell JAH: The heart in kwashiorkor. Am Heart J 67:1, 1964.

Weiss S, Wilkins RW: The nature of the cardiovascular disturbances in nutritional deficiency states (beriberi). Ann Intern Med 11:104, 1937.

Wenckebach KF: *Das Beriberi-Herz.* Springer, 1934.

Wharton B, Howells GR, McCance RA: Cardiac failure in kwashiorkor. Lancet 2:384, 1967.

Sarcoidosis

Bashour FA & others: Myocardial sarcoidosis. Dis Chest 53:413, 1968.

DeRemee RA, Andersen HA: Sarcoidosis: A correlation of dyspnea with roentgenographic state and pulmonary function changes. Mayo Clin Proc 49:743, 1974.

Duvernoy WFC, Garcia R: Sarcoidosis of the heart presenting with ventricular tachycardia and atrioventricular block. Am J Cardiol 28:348, 1971.

Fawcett FJ, Goldberg MJ: Heart block resulting from myocardial sarcoidosis. Br Heart J 36:220, 1974.

Fleming HA: Sarcoid heart disease. Br Heart J 36:54, 1974.

Ghosh P & others: Myocardial sarcoidosis. Br Heart J 34: 769, 1972.

Gozo EG & others: The heart in sarcoidosis. Chest 60: 379, 1971.

James DG & others: A tale of two cities: A comparison of sarcoidosis in London and New York. Arch Intern Med 123:187, 1969.

James DG, Neville E, Walker A: Immunology of sarcoidosis. Am J Med 59:388, 1975.

Littner MR & others: The clinical assessment of roentgenographically atypical pulmonary sarcoidosis. Am J Med 62:361, 1977.

Longcope W, Freiman D: A study of sarcoidosis based on combined investigations of 160 cases, including 30 autopsies from the Johns Hopkins Hospital and Massachusetts General Hospital. Medicine 31:1, 1952.

Maycock RL & others: Review: Manifestations of sarcoidosis: Analysis of 145 patients, with a review of nine series selected from the literature. Am J Med 35:67, 1963.

Mitchell DN, Scadding JG: Sarcoidosis. Am Rev Respir Dis 110:774, 1974.

Porter GH: Sarcoid heart disease. N Engl J Med 263:1350, 1960.

Roberts WC, McAllister HA Jr, Ferrans VJ: Sarcoidosis of the heart: A clinicopathologic study of 35 necropsy patients (group I) and review of 78 previously described necropsy patients (group II). Am J Med 63:86, 1977.

Sarcoidosis: Medical Staff Conference, University of California, San Francisco. West J Med 126:288, 1977.

Scadding JG: *Sarcoidosis.* Eyre & Spottiswoode (London), 1967.

Sharma OP: *Sarcoidosis: A Clinical Approach.* Thomas, 1975.

Siltzbach LE & others: The course and prognosis of sarcoidosis around the world. Am J Med 57:847, 1974.

Stein E & others: Asymptomatic electrocardiographic alterations in sarcoidosis. Am Heart J 86:474, 1973.

Systemic Lupus Erythematosus

Bardana EJ, Pirofsky B: Recent advances in the immunopathogenesis of systemic lupus erythematosus. West J Med 122:130, 1975.

Block SR, Christian CL: The pathogenesis of systemic lupus erythematosus. Am J Med 59:453, 1975.

Brigden W & others: The heart in systemic lupus erythematosus. Br Heart J 22:1, 1960.

Bulkey BH, Roberts WC: The heart in systemic lupus erythematosus and the changes induced in it by corticosteroid therapy. Am J Med 58:243, 1975.

Cathcart ES: Current concepts in management of lupus nephritis. Hosp Pract 12:59, May 1977.

Cohen AS & others: Preliminary criteria for the classification of systemic lupus erythematosus. Bull Rheum Dis 21:643, 1971.

Cruickshank B: *Lupus Erythematosus,* 2nd ed. Univ of Southern California Press, 1974.

Decker JL & others: Cyclophosphamide or azathioprine in lupus glomerulonephritis: A controlled trial: Results at 28 months. Ann Intern Med 83:606, 1975.

Decker JL & others: Systemic lupus erythematosus: Contrasts and comparisons. Ann Intern Med 82: 391, 1975.

Dubois EL (editor): *Lupus Erythematosus.* Univ of Southern California Press, 1974.

Estes DE, Christian CL: The natural history of systemic lupus erythematosus by prospective analysis. Medicine 50:85, 1971.

Fessel WJ: Systemic lupus erythematosus in the community. Arch Intern Med 134:1027, 1974.

Grigor RR & others: Outcome of pregnancy in systemic lupus erythematosus. Proc R Soc Med 70:99, 1977.

Hahn BH, Kantor OS, Osterland CK: Azathioprine plus prednisone compared with prednisone alone in the treatment of systemic lupus erythematosus: Report of a prospective controlled trial in 24 patients. Ann Intern Med 83:597, 1975.

Harvey AM & others: Systemic lupus erythematosus: Review of the literature and clinical analysis of 138 cases. Medicine 33:291, 1954.

Hejtmancif MR & others: The cardiovascular manifestations of systemic lupus erythematosus. Am Heart J 68:119, 1964.

Klemperer P, Pollack AD, Baehr G: Pathology of disseminated lupus erythematosus. Arch Pathol 32: 569, 1941.

Krupp MA: Urinary sediment in visceral angiitis (periarteritis nodosa, lupus erythematosus, Libman-Sachs disease): Quantitative study. Arch Intern Med 71: 54, 1943.

Shearn MA: The heart in systemic lupus erythematosus. Am Heart J 56:452, 1959.

Strauer BE & others: Lupus cardiomyopathy: Cardiac mechanics, hemodynamics, and coronary blood flow in uncomplicated systemic lupus erythematosus. Am Heart J 92:715, 1976.

Trimble RB & others: Preliminary criteria for the classification of systemic lupus erythematosus (SLE). Arthritis Rheum 17:184, 1974.

Wolf L & others: Classification criteria for systemic lupus erythematosus: Frequency in normal patients. JAMA 236:1497, 1976.

Scleroderma

Bluestone R & others: Treatment of systemic sclerosis with D-penicillamine: A new method of observing the effects of treatment. Ann Rheum Dis 29:153, 1970.

Bulkley BH & others: Myocardial lesions of progressive systemic sclerosis: A cause of cardiac dysfunction. Circulation 53:483, 1976.

D'Angelo WA & others: Pathologic observations in systemic sclerosis (scleroderma). Am J Med 46:428, 1969.

James TN: De subitaneis mortibus. 8. Coronary arteries and conduction system in scleroderma heart disease. Circulation 50:844, 1974.

Muers M, Stokes W: Treatment of scleroderma heart by D-penicillamine. Br Heart J 38:864, 1976.

Norton WL, Nardo JM: Vascular disease in progressive systemic sclerosis (scleroderma). Ann Intern Med 73:317, 1970.

Oram S, Stokes W: The heart in scleroderma. Br Heart J 23:243, 1961.

Ridolfi RL, Bulkley BH, Hutchins GM: The cardiac conduction system in progressive systemic sclerosis: Clinical and pathologic features of 35 patients. Am J Med 61:361, 1976.

Sackner MA & others: The pathophysiology of scleroderma involving the heart and respiratory system. Ann Intern Med 60:611, 1964.

Scarpelli DG: Clinicopathological exercise. N Engl J Med 293:922, 1975.

Rheumatoid Arthritis & Ankylosing Spondylitis

Berger HW, Seckler SG: Pleural and pericardial effusions in rheumatoid disease. Ann Intern Med 64:1291, 1966.

Bulkley B, Roberts WC: Ankylosing spondylitis and aortic regurgitation: Description of the characteristic cardiovascular lesion from study of eight necropsy patients. Circulation 48:1014, 1973.

Cathcart ES, Spodick DH: Rheumatoid heart disease: A study of the incidence and nature of cardiac lesions in rheumatic arthritis. N Engl J Med 266:959, 1962.

Cryer PE, Kissane J (editors): Rheumatoid arthritis, vasculitis and paroxysmal hypertension. (Clinicopathologic conference.) Am J Med 59:395, 1975.

Kirk J, Cosh J: The pericarditis of rheumatoid arthritis. Q J Med 38:397, 1969.

Kra SJ, Fazzone P: Rheumatoid carditis. Conn Med 34: 247, 1970.

Lebowitz WB: The heart in rheumatoid arthritis (rheumatoid disease). Ann Intern Med 58:102, 1963.

Sokoloff L: The heart in rheumatoid arthritis. Am Heart J 45:635, 1953.

Hemochromatosis

Arnett EN & others: Massive myocardial hemosiderosis: Structure-function conference at National Heart and Lung Institute. Am Heart J 90:777, 1975.

Bomford A, Williams R: Long-term results of venesection therapy in idiopathic haemochromatosis. Q J Med 45:611, 1976.

Buja LM, Roberts WC: Iron in the heart. Am J Med 51: 209, 1971.

Crosby WH & others: Hemochromatosis (iron-storage disease). JAMA 228:743, 1974.

Easley RM & others: Reversible cardiomyopathy associated with hemochromatosis. N Engl J Med 287: 866, 1972.

Edwards CQ & others: Hereditary hemochromatosis: Diagnosis in siblings and children. N Engl J Med 297:7, 1977.

Engle MA, Erlandson M, Smith CH: Late cardiac complications of chronic, severe, refractory anemia with hemochromatosis. Circulation 30:698, 1964.

Feller ER & others: Physiologic studies in the precirrhotic stage of familial hemochromatosis. N Engl J Med 296:1422, 1977.

Finch SC, Finch CA: Idiopathic hemochromatosis, an iron storage disease. Medicine 34:381, 1955.

Forth W, Rummel W: Iron absorption. Physiol Rev 53: 724, 1973.

MacDonald RA: *Hemochromatosis and Hemosiderosis.* Thomas, 1964.

Pollycove M: Hemochromatosis. In: *The Metabolic Basis of Inherited Disease,* 4th ed. Stanbury JB & others (editors). McGraw-Hill, 1978. [In press.]

Powell LW: Changing concepts in hemochromatosis. Postgrad Med J 46:200, 1970.

Rowe JW & others: Familial hemochromatosis: Characteristics of the precirrhotic stage of a large kindred. Medicine 56:197, 1977.

Sherlock S: Hemochromatosis: Course and treatment. Annu Rev Med 27:143, 1976.

Skinner C, Kensmure ACF: Haemochromatosis presenting as congestive cardiomyopathy and responding to venesection. Br Heart J 35:466, 1973.

Treatment of idiopathic haemochromatosis. (Editorial.) Lancet 1:290, 1977.

Amyloid Disease

Aach R, Kissane J (editors): Amyloidosis: Clinical conference. Am J Med 53:495, 1972.

Alinaghi F, Walsh TS, Massie E: Amyloid heart disease. Am J Cardiol 13:750, 1964.

Brigden W: Cardiac amyloidosis. Prog Cardiovasc Dis 7:142, 1964.

Buja LM, Khoi NB, Roberts WC: Clinically significant cardiac amyloidosis: Clinicopathologic findings in 15 patients. Am J Cardiol 26:394, 1970.

Cathcart ES & others: Immunoglobulins and amyloidosis:

An immunologic study of 62 patients with biopsy-proved disease. Am J Med 52:93, 1972.

Chew C & others: The functional defect in amyloid heart disease. Am J Cardiol 36:438, 1975.

Child JS & others: Echocardiogram for amyloid cardiopathy. N Engl J Med 295:960, 1976.

Cohen AS: Amyloidosis. N Engl J Med 277:574, 1967.

Cohen AS: Hereditary amyloidosis. In: *The Metabolic Basis of Inherited Diseases,* 3rd ed. Stanbury J, Wyngaarden J, Fredrikson D (editors). McGraw-Hill, 1972.

Farrokh A, Walsh TJ, Massie E: Amyloid heart disease. Am J Cardiol 13:750, 1964.

Frederiksen T & others: Familial primary amyloidosis with severe amyloid heart disease. Am J Med 33:328, 1962.

Glenner GG, Terry WD, Isersky C: Amyloidosis: Its nature and pathogenesis. Semin Hematol 10:65, 1973.

Isobe T, Osserman EF: Patterns of amyloidosis and their association with plasma-cell dyscrasia, monoclonal immunoglobulins and Bence-Jones proteins. N Engl J Med 290:473, 1974.

Josselson AJ, Pruit RD, Edwards JE: Amyloid localized to the heart: Analysis of 29 cases. Arch Pathol 54:359, 1952.

Kyle RA: Multiple myeloma: Review of 869 cases. Mayo Clin Proc 50:29, 1975.

Kyle RA, Bayrd ED: Amyloidosis: Review of 236 cases. Medicine 54:271, 1975.

Levisman JA & others: Echocardiographic findings in amyloid heart disease. Circulation 51–52 (Suppl 2): 208, 1975.

Meaney E & others: Cardiac amyloidosis, constrictive pericarditis and restrictive cardiomyopathy. Am J Cardiol 38:547, 1976.

Ridolfi RL, Bulkley BH, Hutchins GM: The conduction system in cardiac amyloidosis: Clinical and pathologic features of 23 patients. Am J Med 62:677, 1977.

Rukavina JG & others: Primary systemic amyloidosis: A review and an experimental, genetic, and clinical study of 29 cases with particular emphasis on the familial form. Medicine 35:239, 1956.

Skinner M, Benson MD, Cohen AS: Amyloid fibril protein related to immunoglobulin λ chains. J Immunol 114:1433, 1975.

Solomon A: Bence-Jones proteins and light chains of immunoglobulins. (Second of 2 parts.) N Engl J Med 294:91, 1976.

Westermark P, Stenkvist B: A new method for the diagnosis of systemic amyloidosis. Arch Intern Med 132:522, 1973.

Wright JR & others: Relationship of amyloid to aging: Review of the literature and systematic study of 83 patients derived from a general hospital population. Medicine 48:39, 1969.

Zucker-Franklin D, Franklin EC: Intracellular localization of human amyloid by fluorescence and electron microscopy. Am J Pathol 59:23, 1970.

Endomyocardial Fibrosis & Löffler's Endocarditis

Bell JA, Jenkins BS, Webb-Peploe MM: Clinical, haemodynamic, and angiographic findings in Löffler's eosinophilic endocarditis. Br Heart J 38:541, 1976.

Brockington IF, Olsen EGJ: Löffler's endocarditis and Davies' endomyocardial fibrosis. Am Heart J 85:308, 1973.

Brockington IF, Olsen EGJ, Goodwin JF: Endomyocardial fibrosis in Europeans resident in tropical Africa. Lancet 1:583, 1967.

Chew CYC & others: Primary restrictive cardiomyopathy: Nontropical endomyocardial fibrosis and hypereosinophilic heart disease. Br Heart J 39:399, 1977.

Cockshott WP, Sarić S, Ikeme AC: Radiological findings in endomyocardial fibrosis. Circulation 35:913, 1967.

Davies H, Deuchar DC, Missen GAK: Endomyocardial fibrosis: Two cases with severe pulmonary hypertension presenting in England. Guys Hosp Rep 114:337, 1965.

Davies JNP: African endomyocardial fibrosis. Page 345 in: *Cardiomyopathy.* Burch GE (editor). Davis, 1972.

Davies JNP: Endomyocardial fibrosis in Africans. East Afr Med J 25:10, 1948.

Falase AO, Kolawole TM, Lagundoye SB: Endomyocardial fibrosis: Problems in differential diagnosis. Br Heart J 38:369, 1976.

Löffler W: Endocarditis parietalis fibro-plastica mit Bluteosinophilie, ein eigenartiges Krankheitsbild. Schweiz Med Wochenschr 17:817, 1936.

Parry EHO, Abrahams DG: The natural history of endomyocardial fibrosis. Q J Med 34:383, 1965.

Roberts WC, Buja LM, Ferrans VJ: Löffler's fibroplastic parietal endocarditis, eosinophilic leukaemia and Davies' endomyocardial fibrosis: The same disease at different stages? Pathol Microbiol (Basel) 35:90, 1970.

Roberts WC, Liegler DG, Carbone PP: Endomyocardial disease and eosinophilia: A clinical and pathologic spectrum. Am J Med 46:28, 1969.

Schryer MJP, Karnauchow PM: Endocardial fibroelastosis: Etiology and pathogenetic considerations in children. Am Heart J 88:557, 1974.

Scott ME, Bruce JH: Löffler's endocarditis. Br Heart J 37:534, 1975.

Shaper AG: On the nature of some tropical cardiomyopathies. Trans R Soc Trop Med Hyg 61:458, 1967.

Shillingford JP, Somers K: Clinical and haemodynamic patterns in endomyocardial fibrosis. Br Heart J 23:433, 1961.

Solley GO & others: Endomyocardiopathy with eosinophilia. Mayo Clin Proc 51:697, 1976.

Somers K, Fowler JM: Endomyocardial fibrosis: Clinical diagnosis. Cardiologia 52:25, 1968.

Somers K & others: Hemodynamic features of severe endomyocardial fibrosis of the right ventricle, including comparison with constrictive pericarditis. Br Heart J 30:322, 1968.

Sickle Cell Disease & Chronic Anemia

Neff MS & others: Hemodynamics of uremic anemia. Circulation 43:876, 1971.

Wintrobe MM: The cardiovascular system in anemia: With a note on the particular abnormalities in sickle cell anemia. Blood 1:121, 1946.

Chagas' Disease

Chagas C: Aspecto clinico da nova entidade morbida produzida pelo schizotrypanum cruzi. Brasil-med 24:263, 1910.

De Raadt P, Koten JW: Myocarditis in rhodesiense trypanosomiasis. East Afr Med J 45:128, 1968.

Hutt MRS, Wilks NE: African trypanosomiasis (sleeping sickness). Pages 57–68 in: *Helminthic and Protozoal Diseases with Clinical Correlation.* Rojas HM (editor). Williams & Wilkins, 1971.

Köberle F: Chagas' heart disease: Pathology. Cardiologia 52:82, 1968.

Koten JW, de Raadt P: Myocarditis in *Trypanosoma rhodesiense* infections. Trans R Soc Trop Med Hyg 63:485, 1969.

Laranja FS & others: Chagas' disease: A clinical, epidemiologic and pathologic study. Circulation 14:1035, 1956.

Massumi RA, Gooch A: Chagas' myocarditis. Arch Intern Med 116:531, 1965.

Poltera AA, Cox JN: Owor R: Pancarditis affecting the conducting system and all valves in human African trypanosomiasis. Br Heart J 38:827, 1976.

Prata A: Chagas' heart disease. Cardiologia 52:79, 1968.

Rosenbaum MB: Chagasic myocardiopathy. Prog Cardiovasc Dis 7:199, 1964.

Peripartum Cardiomyopathy

Brown AK & others: Cardiomyopathy and pregnancy. Br Heart J 29:387, 1967.

Burch GE, Giles TD, Tsui CY: Postpartal cardiomyopathy. Page 269 in: *Cardiomyopathy.* Burch GE (editor). Davis, 1972.

Demakis JG & others: Natural course of peripartum cardiomyopathy. Circulation 44:1053, 1971.

Gilchrist AR: Cardiological problems in younger women: Including those of pregnancy and the puerperium. Br Med J 1:209, 1963.

Nagaratnam N, Fernandopulle M: Heart disease of pregnancy and puerperium. Cardiologia 52:121, 1968.

Stuart KL: Peripartal cardiomyopathy. Cardiologia 52:44, 1968.

Walsh JJ & others: Idiopathic myocardiopathy of the puerperium (postpartal heart disease). Circulation 32:19, 1965.

Inherited Disorders

Blieden LC, Moller JH: Cardiac involvement in inherited disorders of metabolism. Prog Cardiovasc Dis 16:615, 1974.

Khosla SN: Heart in Friedreich's ataxia. Am J Med Sci 270:475, 1975.

Perloff JK: Cardiac involvement in heredofamilial neuromyopathic diseases. Page 333 in: *Cardiomyopathy.* Burch GE (editor). Davis, 1972.

Perloff JK, DeLeon AC Jr, O'Doherty D: The cardiomyopathy of progressive muscular dystrophy. Circulation 33:625, 1966.

18 . . .
Pericarditis

Pericardial disease usually also involves the epicardium, often spreading to or from the myocardium. It almost always produces inflammatory changes, which include irritative and mechanical effects in addition to those caused by bacterial, viral, and fungal infections. The clinical manifestations of pericardial disease depend on such factors as the cause of disease, the presence or absence of fluid or fibrosis in the pericardial cavity, and the extent of mechanical interference with cardiac filling caused by fluid or fibrosis. Pericardial disease exhibits a wide spectrum of clinical manifestations and varies in importance from an inconsequential associated finding to a major cardiovascular problem, as in acute myopericarditis. The association between pericarditis and myocarditis is also dealt with in Chapter 17.

Causes of Pericardial Disease

The various causative factors in pericarditis are listed in Table 18–1. The pericardium may be involved in acute bacterial or viral infections such as pneumonia, when infection spreads from the lungs or mediastinum, and in chronic infections such as tuberculosis. Other generalized conditions such as uremia, diffuse lupus erythematosus, scleroderma, serum sickness, radiation therapy, rheumatoid arthritis, or different varieties of lymphoma or other malignancies may involve the pericardium. Although the involvement of the pericardium in these disorders is usually incidental, all these conditions may occasionally cause significant hemodynamic changes (about 10% of cases). Uremia is coming to be an important factor in pericardial disease now that renal dialysis is widely used in the palliative treatment of chronic renal disease. The commonest primary pericardial infections are those due to viruses (eg, coxsackie B virus), but these infections usually also affect the myocardium because epicarditis is also present. When myocarditis predominates, the clinical picture is as described in Chapter 17. Aseptic inflammatory changes are seen following acute myocardial infarction. They are especially noticeable in anteroseptal infarcts in which the necrosis of cardiac tissue involves the surface of the heart and causes changes that are indistinguishable from those due to inflammation. Another form of aseptic inflammation occurs both after myocardial infarction (3–6 weeks) and following cardiac surgery. This is postpericardiotomy syndrome, in which low-grade, probably autoimmune, self-limiting inflammation involves the pericardium and pleura. It was first seen after mitral commissurotomy and was originally thought to represent a recurrence of rheumatic fever. However, it is also seen after operations for congenital lesions.

Blunt or penetrating trauma such as that associated with stab wounds or rib fracture may damage the pericardium and lead to hemopericardium. Hemopericardium also occurs when vascular structures such as the heart or the aorta rupture into the pericardium.

Malignant disease also affects the pericardium, usually causing effusion. Neoplastic involvement of the pericardium may occur either by direct spread or, more rarely by blood-borne means, and the effusion is often large and recurrent. Tumor usually spreads directly by way of the mediastinum, but secondary deposits and even primary tumors of the pericardium (mesoendothelioma and sarcoma) can occur. The accu-

Table 18–1. Causes of pericardial disease.*

1. Infections
   a. Viral (idiopathic): Coxsackie, influenza
   b. Bacterial: Tuberculosis, staphylococcus, streptococcus, pneumococcus, meningococcus
   c. Fungal
   d. Parasitic
2. Hypersensitivity
   a. Collagen diseases: Rheumatic fever, rheumatoid arthritis, systemic lupus erythematosus, scleroderma
   b. Following myocardial infarction: Dressler's syndrome
   c. Postpericardiotomy
   d. Serum sickness
   e. Drug reaction
   f. Idiopathic (viral) relapsing
3. Trauma: Blunt or penetrating
4. Metabolic disorders
   a. Uremia
   b. Myxedema
5. Neoplasm: Lymphoma
6. Aortic dissection
7. Myocardial infarction
8. Cobalt-beer myocardiopathy
9. Radiation therapy
10. Heart failure

*Modified and reproduced, with permission, from Goldman MJ: Pericarditis. West J Med 123:467, 1975.

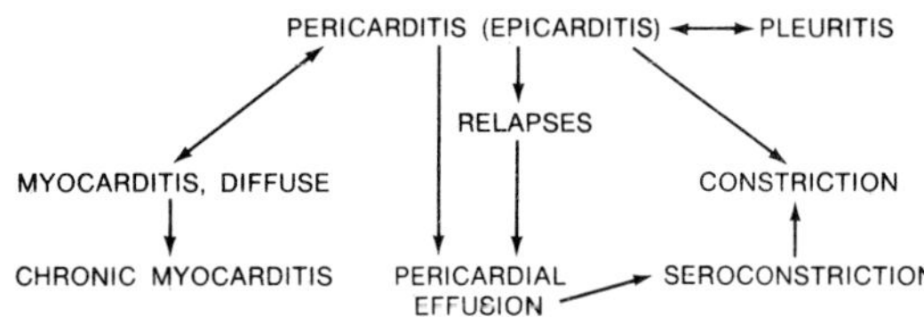

Figure 18–1. Spectrum of pericardial disease. (Reproduced, with permission, from Goldman MJ: Pericarditis. West J Med 123:467, 1975.)

mulation of fluid in the pericardial cavity, seen in heart failure, is due to transudation. In myxedema, enlargement of the cardiac silhouette is usually due to pericardial fluid but may be myocardial enlargement. In tuberculous cases, the infection is more chronic and effusion is relatively common. In some cases, other serous cavities (pleura or peritoneum) are also affected. The disease runs a chronic course, and pain, fever, and myocardial involvement are less prominent than in viral cases.

Clinical Findings

The clinical findings in pericardial disease depend on the severity and cause of the inflammatory process, the amount of accumulated pericardial fluid, and the rate of rise of intrapericardial pressure. The pressure rise in turn influences hemodynamic changes.

The clinical picture of pericardial disease has 3 manifestations: fibrinous (dry) pericarditis, pericardial effusion, and chronic constrictive pericarditis. These different manifestations are interrelated, as shown in Fig 18–1. Spread of the disease to involve the myocardium is not infrequent.

FIBRINOUS (DRY) PERICARDITIS

Clinical Findings

A. Symptoms: Fibrinous pericarditis most commonly occurs in the course of some other disease; thus, the symptoms depend on the cause, and pain is not necessarily a feature. In primary pericarditis caused by viral infection, pain, malaise, fever, and myalgia are the usual presenting symptoms. The pain is often worse with breathing, swallowing, or belching, and it may radiate to the shoulder. It is often substernal and associated with cough. The patient may obtain relief by sitting up and leaning forward or by kneeling on all fours. Pain characteristically decreases or disappears when effusion develops.

The pericarditis that occurs in about 15% of cases of acute myocardial infarction is not generally painful. It is noted about the third day after infarction, is usually transient, and is of little hemodynamic significance except when anticoagulants cause hemorrhage into the pericardial cavity. Postpericardiotomy syndrome, which occurs about 3–6 weeks after cardiac surgery or myocardial infarction, causes pericardial or pleural pain and may be associated with fever. It may be confused with hemorrhagic pericardial effusion due to anticoagulant therapy or postoperative infection.

B. Signs: The most important and often the only sign of fibrinous pericarditis is the development of a pericardial friction rub. In most cases in which pericarditis is secondary to a generalized disease, the only sign of pericardial involvement is a friction rub, which is often variable and transient. Pericardial friction produces a rough, scratchy 2- or 3-component superficial sound which is unrelated to other heart sounds. The components are associated with atrial systole, ventricular systole, and ventricular diastole. Friction can be confused with extraneous stethoscope sounds, with noise caused by hair on the chest, and with murmurs, especially to-and-fro murmurs. Both the bell and the diaphragm of the stethoscope are used to listen for friction rubs, and the patient should not breathe dur-

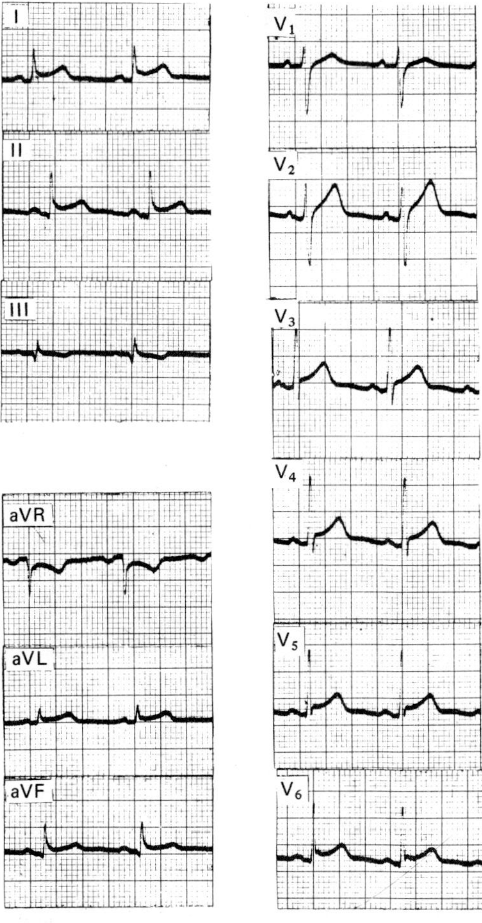

Figure 18–2. Acute pericarditis. ST segment elevation with concave upward curvature is seen in leads I, II, aVL, aVF, and V_{2-6}. Reciprocal ST segment depression is seen in cavity lead aVR. Clinical diagnosis: Acute "benign" pericarditis. (Reproduced, with permission, from Goldman MJ: *Principles of Clinical Electrocardiography,* 9th ed. Lange, 1976.)

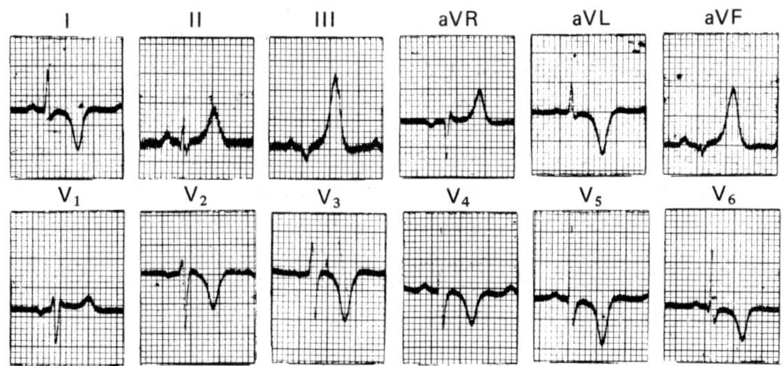

Figure 18–3. Pericarditis (late pattern). Deep, symmetrically inverted T waves in I, aVL, and V_{2-6}. Clinical diagnosis: Acute rheumatic fever in a 25-year-old white man; persistent pericardial friction rub. (Reproduced, with permission, from Goldman MJ: *Principles of Clinical Electrocardiography,* 9th ed. Lange, 1976.)

ing auscultation. Other physical signs in a patient with fibrinous pericarditis are attributed to the basic underlying disease.

C. **Electrocardiographic Findings**: Like the friction rub, ECG signs of pericarditis may be the only evidence indicative of pericardial involvement. Initially, ECG changes consist of ST–T segment elevation in all left ventricular leads (Fig 18–2), with preservation of the upward concavity, in contrast to the acute injury of acute myocardial infarction, in which the ST segment has upward convexity. Return of the ST segment (Fig 18–3) to the baseline in a few days is followed by symmetric T wave inversion. Reciprocal changes are absent except in aVR, and Q waves do not occur. It may be difficult to differentiate pericarditis from nontransmural myocardial infarction at the stage of T wave inversion because epicarditis is present and the presence of other diagnostic features, especially elevated serum enzymes (myocardial band creatine phosphokinase) is required.

D. **X-Ray Findings**: The heart is not necessarily enlarged. Any radiologic changes should be attributed to the underlying disease. If there is associated effusion, the shadow may be enlarged (see Pericardial Effusion, below).

E. **Laboratory Findings**: Leukocytosis of 10–20 thousand is usually seen in viral pericarditis. A raised sedimentation rate is also found regardless of cause. Serologic abnormality due to generalized disease may be present (eg, positive LE cell preparation, presence of antinuclear antibody, or elevated serum creatinine).

Differential Diagnosis

Acute viral pericarditis must be distinguished from acute myocardial infarction. In pericarditis, pain, fever, and ECG changes are present from the onset of illness. In myocardial infarction, pain comes first and is followed a few days later by fever and friction rub. The ECG patterns in pericardial and myocardial disease are contrasted in Fig 18–4. Q waves are not seen in pericarditis. It is almost always possible to make the diagnosis by following the serial changes on the ECG, unless the patient is first seen after the third or fourth day and has nontransmural infarction. Serial ECG examination as well as specific myocardial enzyme studies (myocardial band creatine phosphokinase) should be used to decide whether a patient who is suffering from some generalized disease has ECG changes due to pericarditis or to myocardial infarction. The diagnosis of associated myocarditis may prove difficult, and the distinction between pleural and pericardial inflammation is likewise difficult: The friction rub is related to inspiration in pleural inflammation and is heard during held respiration in pericardial inflammation, but in many cases the friction rub is pleuropericardial and shares the features of both entities.

Viral pericarditis is sometimes difficult to distinguish from tuberculous pericarditis. Viral cases tend to be more acute and are less likely to lead to effusion. Because tubercle bacilli are difficult to find, the fluid should be cultured. Diagnostic pericardiocentesis is indicated. The distinction between the 2 causes has important implications in treatment.

Treatment

The underlying disease should be treated and symptomatic therapy given for the pericarditis. In acute viral pericarditis, salicylates and expectant treatment are usually all that is needed, but corticosteroids may be helpful in severe cases. Corticosteroids are not indicated in tuberculous cases unless given with antituberculosis drugs. In postpericardiotomy syndrome, symptomatic treatment is also all that is necessary in most cases. If the pericarditis fails to clear in a week to

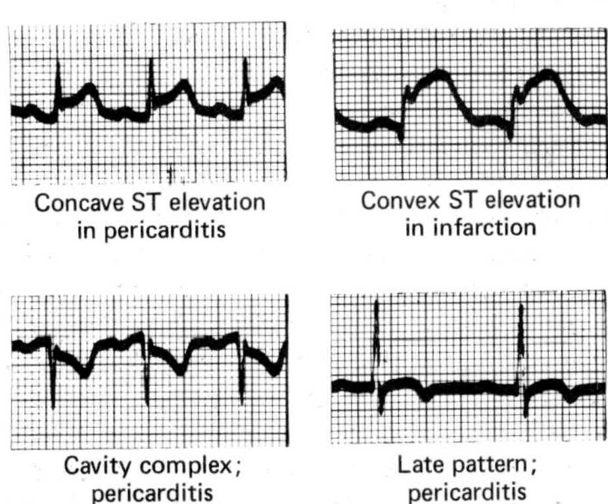

Figure 18–4. Electrocardiographic patterns in pericarditis and infarction. (Reproduced, with permission, from Goldman MJ: *Principles of Clinical Electrocardiography,* 9th ed. Lange, 1976.)

10 days, or if the infection is severe, corticosteroids are often utilized. Although there is no conclusive evidence that they are effective, a trial of treatment may be worthwhile. The disease often becomes worse when corticosteroid treatment is stopped, which suggests that corticosteroids are effective.

Prognosis

The ultimate prognosis in most cases of acute viral pericarditis is excellent, provided that myocardial involvement is minimal. Tuberculous cases respond to specific treatment, which must sometimes be administered without proof of the cause. The relative incidence of viral and tuberculous lesions varies in different areas, and viral lesions are now more common than tuberculous ones in the USA. In a few cases, the disease persists or recurs, and signs of pericardial constriction can develop in a period of weeks to months. This is rare, however. In most cases of fibrinous pericarditis, the prognosis depends more on the underlying disease, and pericardial involvement is only a minor part of the clinical picture. Relapses are common and may constitute a major problem.

PERICARDIAL EFFUSION

The time necessary for fluid to accumulate in the pericardium can vary from seconds (in rupture of a major structure) to weeks or months in chronic infections. It is the *rate* of rise in the intrapericardial pressure that is the most important factor in determining the development of hemodynamic and clinical features of cardiac tamponade. If pericardial fluid accumulates slowly, the pericardium stretches, and there is little rise in pressure and little or no interference with cardiac filling. If the fluid accumulates rapidly or if effusion occurs into a pericardium thickened and noncompliant because of fibrosis, serious interference with cardiac filling can occur with remarkable speed. The compliance of the pericardial cavity is markedly nonlinear, so that although significant amounts of fluid can sometimes accumulate without much rise in pressure, a further slight increase in fluid may produce a considerable rise in pressure as well as symptoms and signs of tamponade.

Clinical Findings

A. Symptoms: Pericardial effusion per se causes no specific symptoms. The pain of pericarditis may disappear when effusion develops. On the other hand, pain may develop with hemopericardium as blood irritates the pericardium.

Acute pericardial tamponade may cause symptoms ranging from anxiety, sweating, dyspnea, dizziness, and syncope to frank shock. The clinical picture ranges in severity from slight circulatory and hemodynamic abnormalities to circulatory collapse. There is no precise point at which tamponade can be said to have occurred.

B. Signs: The physical signs of pericardial effusion depend on the amount of effusion. In the absence of evidence of tamponade, the pulse, pulse pressure, and blood pressure are normal, but the patient may appear anxious, and there is usually some tachycardia. Venous pressure is often raised because pericardial pressure is raised even in the absence of tamponade. Monitoring the venous pressure level is vitally important in management. In difficult cases it is advisable to insert a central venous catheter and obtain serial readings directly.

The heart appears enlarged in pericardial effusion. The cardiac impulse is usually difficult to detect but may be palpable, and an increase in size of the area of cardiac dullness is more readily detected in this than in any other condition. Heart sounds are often distant, and a friction rub may still be audible even though the pain has disappeared and significant effusion has occurred. Murmurs are usually absent, but a pericardial filling sound (pericardial knock) can often be heard about 0.12 sec after A_2 even when tamponade is absent (Fig 18–5). This sound occurs when distention of the heart during ventricular filling halts abruptly. This sign is often masked when there is effusion and is more prominent when constriction is present.

The pulse rate is rapid, and the blood pressure and pulse pressure are low. Pulsus paradoxus, defined as a more than 10 mm or 10% fall in systolic arterial pressure on normal inspiration, can be detected when the blood pressure is measured either by the indirect method or directly (Fig 18–6). Pulsus paradoxus is incorrectly named because it is merely an exaggeration of the normal finding of decreased arterial pressure with inspiration. In tamponade due to effusion or constriction, cardiac volume and the reservoir of blood in the left heart are soon exhausted as blood pools in the lungs during inspiration and starves the left side, reducing cardiac output and arterial pressure. Venous pressure and the nature of the venous pulse are also important. The neck veins usually show a major negative wave at the time of the *y* descent. This constitutes diastolic collapse of the veins and is due to rapid filling of the right heart in early diastole at a time when intracardiac pressure is at its lowest after the end of systole. The sign is not specific for pericardial disease and can be seen in any form of severe right heart failure (Fig 18–7). Another nonspecific physical sign associated with pericardial disease is the Kussmaul sign, an

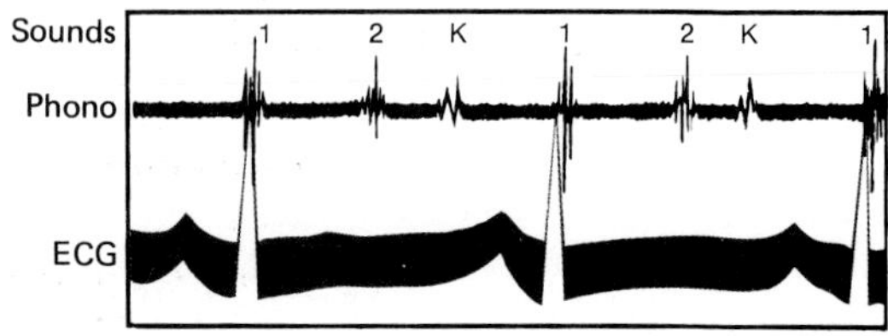

Figure 18–5. Phonocardiogram of typical sharp, early diastolic pericardial knock (K). (Courtesy of Roche Laboratories Division of Hoffman-La Roche, Inc.)

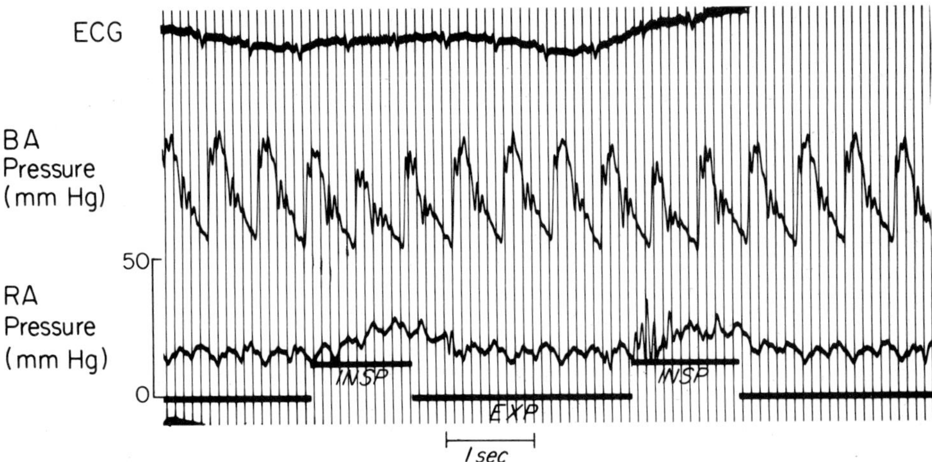

Figure 18–6. Brachial arterial (BA) and right atrial (RA) pressures showing pulsus paradoxus in a patient with constrictive pericarditis and an increase in right atrial pressure on inspiration (Kussmaul's sign). Both the systolic and diastolic atrial pressures rise with inspiration. (See Fig 18–7.)

inspiratory increase in venous pressure (Fig 18–6). When right heart filling is excessive, the increase in venous pressure occurring on inspiration cannot be accommodated in the restricted right atrium, and atrial pressure consequently rises. In classic cases of acute tamponade, the heart is small; consequently, cardiac filling stops abruptly when the heart meets the limits of the tense pericardial cavity. If effusion is moderate, this shock is felt as a palpable diastolic impulse. It is associated with the pericardial knock or filling sound, which generally occurs after the time of an opening snap and before the time of the usual third sound; it can be the loudest sound in the cardiac cycle even when heart sounds are distant because of effusion. When effusion is extensive, murmurs are usually absent and heart sounds may be distant.

C. Electrocardiographic Findings: The T waves are usually low, biphasic, inverted or flat, and the overall voltage low in the limb leads in pericardial effusion. There are no specific ECG changes of tamponade, but electrical alternans is sometimes seen in pericardial effusion.

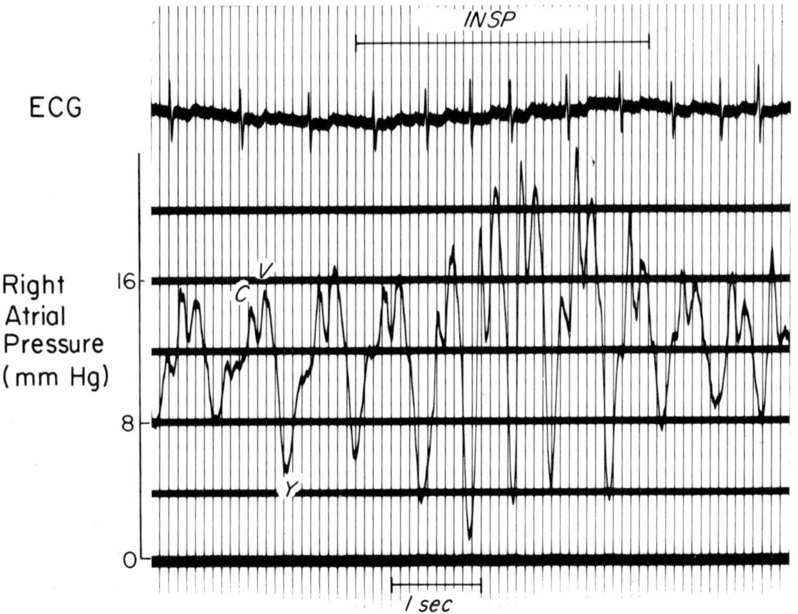

Figure 18–7. Right atrial pressure tracing and ECG in a patient in severe heart failure with atrial fibrillation. Inspiration causes an increase in both the *y* descent and the *cv* peak. The mean pressure is relatively unchanged.

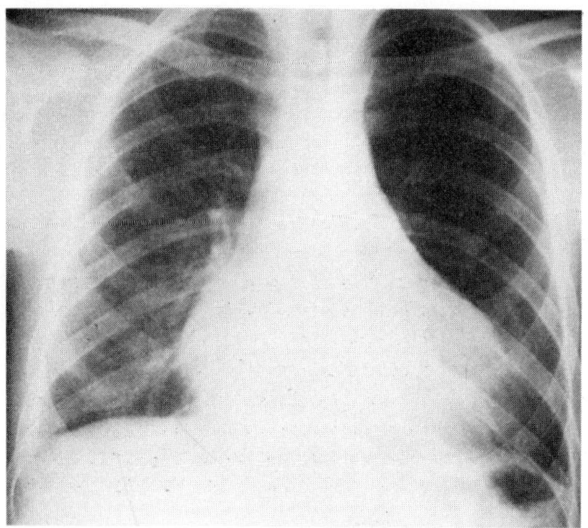

Figure 18–8. Chest x-ray of a patient with pericardial effusion.

D. X-Ray Findings: The cardiac silhouette is enlarged in pericardial effusion and may reach enormous proportions in chronic lesions without affecting cardiac function. The principal problem is to decide whether the heart itself is enlarged. The shape of the cardiac silhouette in pericardial effusion is trangular on posteroanterior view (Fig 18–8). An acute right cardiophrenic angle, clear lung fields, and associated pleural effusion are common. Serial examinations may be useful to determine changes in heart size. The lack of signs of specific chamber enlargement may be helpful. It is important not to confuse the massive cardiac enlargement seen in giant left atrium with pericardial effusion. Since the left atrium forms the right border of the heart in giant left atrium, right heart catheterization and right atrial angiography can produce misleading results and lead to an unnecessary and dangerous attempt at pericardiocentesis, with inadvertent puncture of the heart.

E. Special Investigations:

1. Noninvasive technics–Specific diagnostic tests such as LE cell preparations, thyroid function tests, and renal function tests are indicated in some cases. Tuberculin testing and bacteriologic examination are required if an infective origin is suspected. Pericardial effusion is one of the conditions in which echocardiography is of particular help in diagnosis. The increase in the echofree space between the posterior wall of the left ventricle and the pericardium is more reliable than the equivalent space at the front of the heart. The development of tamponade can be detected from narrowing of the right ventricular outflow tract, especially during expiration, as shown in Fig 18–10. Serial echocardiograms are thus particularly helpful in following the course of the disease. The development of adhesion and fibrosis with thickening of the pericardium as the effusion is absorbed is shown in Fig 18–10.

2. Invasive technics–

a. Catheterization and angiography–Right heart catheterization and right atrial angiography were used in the past to help in the diagnosis of pericardial effusion, but they are less frequently employed now that echocardiography has become available. The finding of a significant–1 cm or more–gap between the catheter tip or the border of the contrast material in the atrium and the edge of the cardiac silhouette suggests the presence of fluid. Some physicians advocate coronary angiography, with injection of contrast medium into the left coronary artery to outline the anterior de-

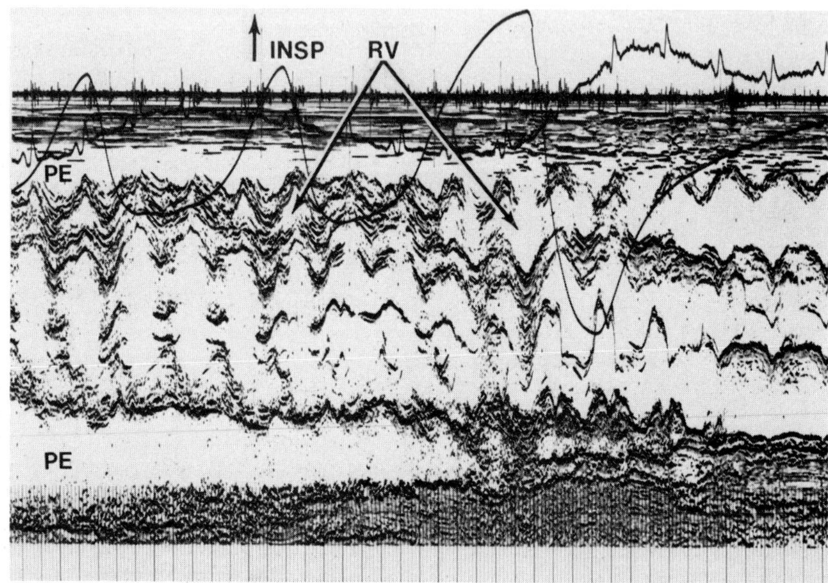

Figure 18–9. Echocardiogram showing cardiac tamponade in a patient with substantial pericardial effusion (PE). The right ventricular cavity (RV) is compressed and almost obliterated; it is seen to enlarge during inspiration. Inspiration (INSP) is upward. (Courtesy of NB Schiller.)

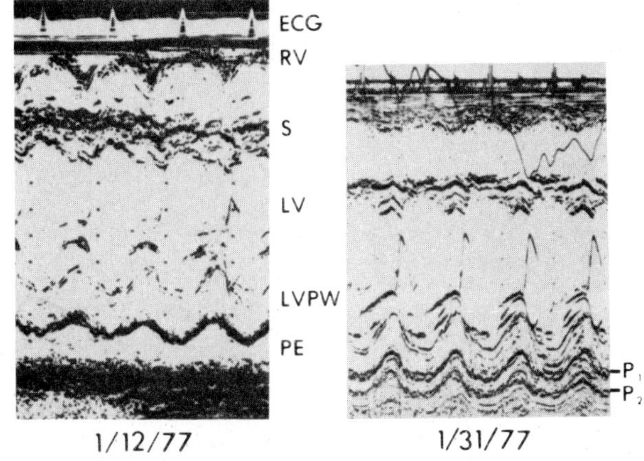

Figure 18–10. Serial echocardiograms in a patient with pericardial effusion showing development of pericardial thickening and fibrosis when the effusion is absorbed. RV, right ventricle; S, septum; LV, left ventricle; LVPW, left ventricular posterior wall; PE, pericardial effusion; P_1 and P_2, visceral and parietal pericardial layer. (Courtesy of NB Schiller.)

scending coronary artery on right anterior oblique view. If there is a significant shadow beyond the filled vessel, pericardial effusion is probably present. Intravenous injection of soluble gases (mainly CO_2) with the patient lying on the left side has also been used for diagnosis. The gas accumulates as a bubble in the right atrium and outlines the right atrial wall to show the distortion due to the presence of fluid or pericardial thickening.

b. **Pericardiocentesis**–Although echocardiography is extremely valuable in indicating the presence and site of pericardial effusion, the ultimate diagnostic procedure is pericardiocentesis, which is needed for diagnostic and often for therapeutic reasons in every case of hemodynamically significant pericardial effusion. The procedure is described on p 116. The data provided by echocardiography help the physician decide whether to tap the pericardium, and pericardiocentesis is seldom indicated if echocardiography is negative.

Differential Diagnosis

Enlargement of the heart due to dilatation or hypertrophy is virtually the only condition which must be distinguished from pericardial effusion, although primary tumor (angiosarcoma) may rarely enter into the differential diagnosis. In some cases there may be effusion in addition to cardiac enlargement. In these cases, the introduction of air into the pericardium at the time of pericardiocentesis serves to indicate heart size and the thickness of the pericardium. Echocardiographic examination has provided significant help in differentiating between pericardial effusion and cardiac enlargement.

Treatment

The treatment of pericardial effusion depends on the cause and on the severity of the hemodynamic effects. If effusion is not great and there are no symptoms, supportive treatment is all that is needed, but if effusion is considerable or recurrent or if signs and symptoms of tamponade are developing, a pericardial tap should be performed. Purulent pericardial effusion should be drained and smear and culture of the fluid obtained for examination; thoracotomy is often necessary to achieve adequate drainage. Serous effusion that occurs in such diseases as tuberculosis, uremia, or malignancy may need to be tapped repeatedly. This is especially true if malignant disease is the cause of the effusion. Chemotherapeutic agents may be instilled into the pericardial cavity after tapping to prevent recurrence of effusion. Many kinds of effusion require no treatment other than measures treating the underlying cause. Acute cardiac tamponade is an acute medical emergency, and the physician must always remain on the alert to prevent its recurrence. Resection of a portion of pericardium for biopsy and extensive pericardiotomy to allow free communication with the pleura may be needed for recurrent effusion in which several taps have failed to relieve symptoms.

Prognosis

The prognosis in pericardial effusion depends on the cause of the disease. Pericardial effusion is seldom a dangerous condition in the absence of tamponade, and repeated pericardiocentesis is seldom necessary for more than a few weeks except in malignant or other major systemic disease.

CHRONIC CONSTRICTIVE PERICARDITIS

This rare insidious disease mimics chronic right heart failure; until recently, it was usually due to chronic tuberculous pericarditis. It is an uncommon sequel to inflammatory disease of the pericardium. (The pericardium may become adherent to the myocardium without causing constriction, and it is the shrinkage associated with fibrosis that is responsible for the constriction.) Tuberculosis is no longer the commonest cause of constrictive pericarditis in the Western world, although it still accounts for most cases in developing countries. In nontuberculous cases the cause sometimes cannot be found, although in some cases, previous viral pericarditis, chest trauma, mediastinal irradiation, connective tissue disease, or uremia may have been present. The chronic inflammatory changes in the pericardial cavity surround the heart with a sheath of tough, unyielding fibrous tissue that interferes with cardiac filling. The actual or effective intrapericardial pressure rises, and the pressure in all heart chambers at the end of diastole rises. The heart is immobilized because it is encased in an unyielding fibrous cage that interferes with its excursion during contraction and relaxation. The more compliant chambers, the atria and the right ventricle, bear the brunt of the burden, but end-diastolic pressures in all cardiac chambers tend to be the same: about 15–25 mm Hg in severe cases. The encasement does not necessarily involve all chambers, but the effective intrapericardial pressure rises on both sides of the heart. Although the effects of the disease are more severe in the more distensible right heart, the left side is almost invariably involved also.

Clinical Findings

A. Symptoms: Swelling of the abdomen and legs is the symptom suggesting a diagnosis of constrictive pericarditis. Dyspnea is not generally prominent but is usually present in all cases to some degree. Anorexia, weakness, wasting, and dyspepsia are seen in advanced cases that have not been properly diagnosed. These symptoms are due to a combination of low cardiac output and marked hepatic congestion. A history of a previous attack of acute or subacute pericarditis is an important feature. The absence of a history of other forms of heart disease is also valuable. Pain is not a prominent feature of the disease. The patient is usually able to lie flat without any problem and does not suffer from paroxysmal nocturnal dyspnea.

B. Signs: The pulse is usually rapid and the blood pressure low. Pulsus paradoxus is present in classic cases of the disease. Its absence points strongly against a diagnosis of pericardial constriction. The heartbeat is irregular in about 30% of cases because of atrial fibrillation. The onset of arrhythmia is related to the age of the patient and the severity of the disease.

The patient appears chronically ill in advanced cases. The neck veins are distended, the venous pressure is markedly raised, and there is a rapid *y* descent. Tamponade and constriction cannot be differentiated on the basis of a consistent difference in venous pulse. A prominent positive systolic wave in the jugular venous pulse argues against a diagnosis of constriction, but diastolic collapse of the venous pulse is not necessarily diagnostic of constriction. In classic cases, cardiac enlargement is not marked, but in practice the heart is usually enlarged. A palpable and audible filling sound (pericardial knock) just before the normal third heart sound is almost invariably present. There is usually no cardiac murmur, and the heart sounds are soft.

Rales may be present at the base of the lung, and the liver is usually markedly enlarged and tender but not pulsating. Ascites tends to be more prominent than ankle edema, and the combination of wasting and edema resembles that seen in advanced right heart failure or cirrhosis of the liver.

C. Electrocardiographic Findings: There are no specific ECG changes. The voltage in the limb and precordial leads tends to be low, and T wave inversion is common. The presence of significant right or left ventricular hypertrophy on ECG contradicts a diagnosis of constrictive pericarditis.

D. X-Ray Findings: The heart is classically not significantly enlarged and shows no specific chamber enlargement. The pulmonary artery is not enlarged, and pulmonary congestion is seldom marked. Redistribution of pulmonary blood flow to the apexes speaks against the diagnosis. X-rays provide the most useful sign distinguishing myocardial disease from pericardial constriction, namely intrapericardial calcification, shown in Fig 18–11. This sign is most commonly seen in tuberculous cases, but it can occur in cases with viral origins. Signs of calcification on x-ray do not necessarily mean that constriction is always present, but if calcification is found, a primary myocardial cause for the patient's disease is unlikely except in tropical (African) endomyocardial fibrosis.

E. Special Investigations:

1. Noninvasive technics—Venous pulse tracings, phonocardiography, and echocardiography are helpful in making the distinction between constrictive pericarditis and primary myocardial disease, but they are not absolutely diagnostic. The abrupt cessation of ventricular filling can be seen on echocardiography and contrasts with the ventricular dilatation and slowed ejection rate seen in cardiomyopathy.

2. Invasive technics—Cardiac catheterization is often performed in an attempt to confirm the diagnosis. Unfortunately, there are no absolute diagnostic hemodynamic features that can help distinguish between constrictive pericarditis and restrictive cardiomyopathy, the principal condition with which con-

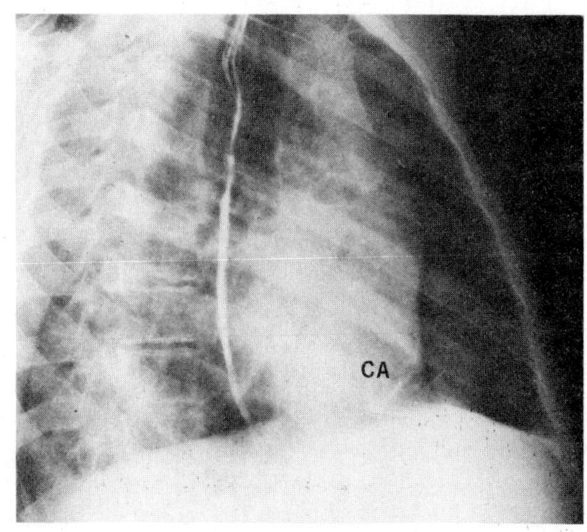

Figure 18–11. Chest x-ray of a patient with constrictive pericarditis showing calcification (CA) in the pericardium. Right anterior oblique view.

strictive pericarditis is confused. The problem of diagnosis is greatest when the level of diastolic pressure in all cardiac chambers is equal. There is little hemodynamic difference between interference with filling resulting from causes outside the heart, those in the heart wall, and those within the cardiac chambers. The hemodynamic features of impaired cardiac filling are shown in Fig 18–12 and include a marked diastolic dip and plateau in the right ventricular pressure tracing (square root sign), a marked diastolic drop in venous pressure, and equalization of end-diastolic pressure in all cardiac chambers. The square root sign is caused by limitation of cardiac filling, and the start of the plateau coincides with the audible filling sound. Pulsus paradoxus is not a specific sign of pericardial disease, and all the hemodynamic manifestations can be seen in patients with restrictive cardiomyopathy as well. These signs also occur in patients with endomyocardial fibrosis of the type seen in tropical Africa. In this condition, there is endocardial rather than pericardial calcification.

Although it is true that the distinction between pericardial and myocardial disease cannot be made with certainty, there are some features that strongly suggest primary myocardial disease. They are disproportionate increase in wedge pressure, low cardiac output, raised pulmonary vascular resistance, marked cardiac enlargement, raised pulmonary arterial pressure (systolic over 50 mm Hg), atrial gallop, marked pulmonary congestion, and a diastolic right ventricular pressure plateau less than 30% of systolic pressure. This last sign actually reflects the low right ventricular pulse pressure in constrictive pericarditis.

Differential Diagnosis

Superior vena caval obstruction should not be confused with constrictive pericarditis because evidence of inferior vena caval obstruction, with hepatic enlargement and ascites, is absent. Similarly, cirrhosis of the liver, in which the jugular venous pressure is not raised, should be readily distinguished. The principal entities with which constrictive pericarditis can be confused are restrictive cardiomyopathy or endomyocardial fibrosis. The distinction is extremely difficult to make; furthermore, pericardial, myocardial, and endocardial fibrosis tend to influence one another because

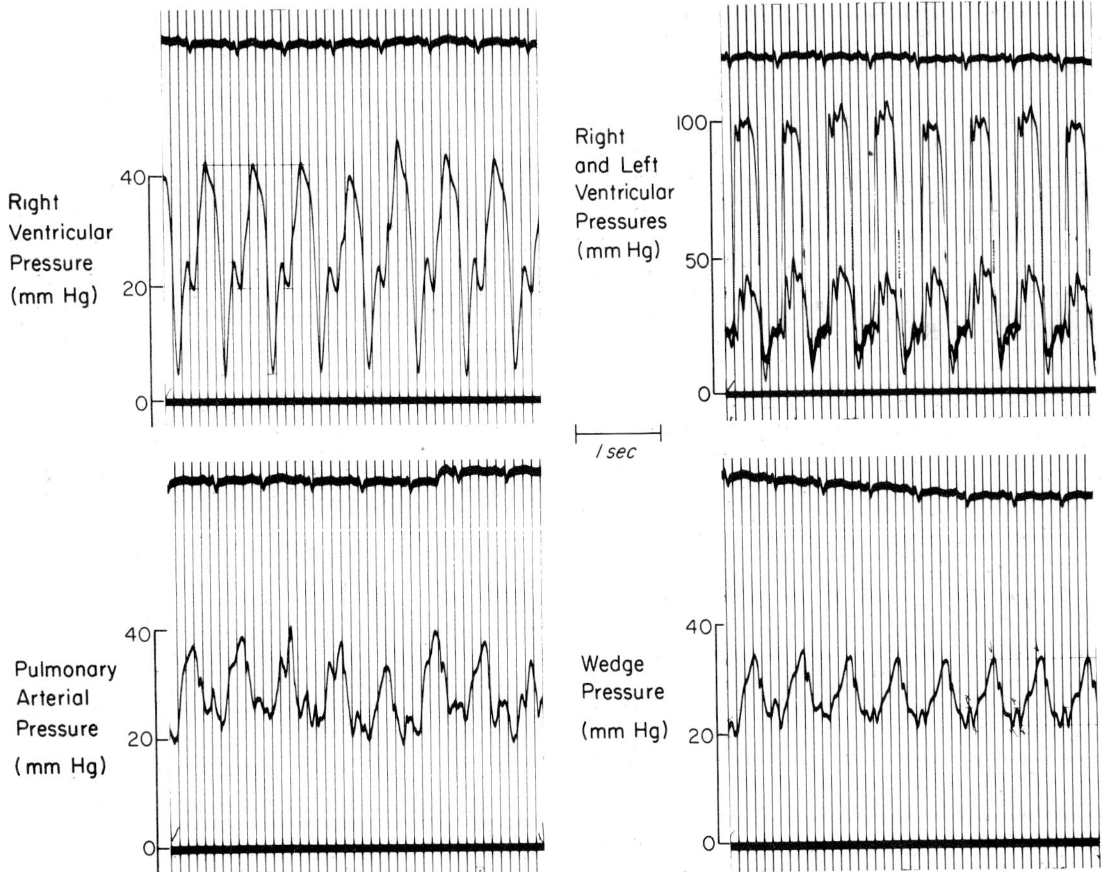

Figure 18–12. Intracardiac pressure tracings from a patient with constrictive pericarditis. The diastolic pressure is elevated to about 20 mm Hg in every chamber. The right ventricular pressure tracing shows a marked diastolic dip followed by a plateau (square root sign).

the fibrotic process tends to spread from one structure to the other. Pericardial fibrosis tends to involve the muscle of the thin-walled right ventricle; similarly, endocardial fibrosis tends to spread to the underlying cardiac muscle. Although exploratory thoracotomy may be indicated in difficult cases, it is harmful in patients with cardiomyopathy and should be avoided if possible.

The response to treatment with digitalis and its derivatives can be helpful. The venous pressure may fall to normal in patients with right heart failure. In contrast, in constrictive pericarditis, the venous pressure remains high in spite of medical therapy.

The lack of any clear differentiating hemodynamic features of constrictive pericarditis has already been mentioned. Of the indicators available, equal diastolic pressures throughout the heart, a high diastolic plateau of pressure in the right ventricle, and low pulmonary arterial pressure are probably the most reliable indicators of pericardial constriction.

Treatment

Surgical resection of the shell of fibrous tissue around the heart is always indicated in symptomatic cases, preferably before marked hepatic enlargement has occurred. The operation is almost always palliative rather than curative since some evidence of restricted motion of the heart is evident after operation, even though symptoms and signs may no longer be present. The operation can be either one of the easiest or one of the most difficult facing the cardiac surgeon. If there is a well-defined plane of cleavage between the fibrotic pericardium and the heart, or even a thin layer of fluid between the thickened pericardium and the heart, pericardial resection can be relatively simple. In most cases, however, especially when the disease is of long standing, the pericardium and the wall of the right ventricle form a single mass of dense fibrous tissue, and dissection is hazardous because of the danger of perforating the right ventricle. The left side of the heart may also be involved; if so, this side should be freed first to avoid pulmonary edema. Considerable judgment is necessary to decide when sufficient tissue has been resected to relieve the obstruction to filling. If too much is removed, the right ventricle tends to dilate, and right heart failure results. Resection of fibrous tissue around the back of the heart is also often needed, and this may be technically difficult. The surgical mortality rate is about 5–10% and varies with the stage of the disease. It is higher in advanced cases. Any resected tissue should be examined histologically, and tubercle bacilli should be sought. If tuberculosis is not diagnosed by pathologic examination, specific diagnosis by other means is indicated, eg, tuberculin testing, sputum examination, or culture of gastric washings.

Restoration of sinus rhythm after operation is indicated in patients with atrial fibrillation or flutter.

Prognosis

The prognosis in constrictive pericarditis is reasonably good. The disease runs a chronic course. In patients in whom the disease is not diagnosed, the chronically raised venous pressure may be tolerated surprisingly well. Cardiac cirrhosis of the liver eventually develops. The principal determinant in prognosis is the success of the surgical treatment.

• • •

References

Beaudry C: Uremic pericarditis and cardiac tamponade. Ann Intern Med 64:990, 1966.

Churchill ED: Decortication of the heart (Delorme) for adhesive pericarditis. Arch Surg 19:1457, 1929.

Comty CM, Cohen SL, Shapiro FL: Pericarditis in chronic uremia and its sequels. Ann Intern Med 75:173, 1971.

Dressler W: The post-myocardial infarction syndrome: A report on 44 cases. Arch Intern Med 103:28, 1959.

Fowler NO, Manitsas GT: Infectious pericarditis. Prog Cardiovasc Dis 16:323, 1973.

Goldman MJ: Pericarditis. West J Med 123:467, 1975.

Lokich JJ: The management of malignant pericardial effusions. JAMA 224:1401, 1973.

Marini PV, Hull AR: Uremic pericarditis: A review of incidence and management. Kidney Int 7(Suppl 2):163, 1975.

Martin RG & others: Radiation related pericarditis. Am J Cardiol 35:216, 1975.

Montgomery JZ & others: Hemodynamic and diagnostic features of pericardial disease. West J Med 122:295, 1975.

Ribot S & others: Treatment of uremic pericarditis. Clin Nephrol 2:127, 1974.

Schiller NB, Botvinick EH: Right ventricular compression as a sign of cardiac tamponade: An analysis of echocardiographic ventricular dimensions and their clinical implications. Circulation 56, 1977. [In press.]

Schrire V: Pericarditis (with particular reference to tuberculous pericarditis). Australas Ann Med 16:41, 1967.

Singh & others: Pericardiectomy in uremia: The treatment of choice for cardiac tamponade in chronic renal failure. JAMA 228:1132, 1974.

Somers K & others: Hemodynamic features of severe endomyocardial fibrosis of the right ventricle, including comparison with constrictive pericarditis. Br Heart J 30:322, 1968.

Spodick DH: Differential diagnosis of acute pericarditis. Prog Cardiovasc Dis 14:192, 1971.

Spodick DH: *Chronic & Constrictive Pericarditis.* Grune & Stratton, 1964.

Veerasamy KG & others: Subacute constrictive uremic pericarditis: Survival after pericardiectomy. JAMA 235:1351, 1976.

White PD: Chronic constrictive pericarditis (Pick's disease) treated by pericardial resection. Lancet 2:597, 1935.

Wood P: Chronic constrictive pericarditis. Am J Cardiol 7:48, 1961.

19 . . .
Pulmonary Heart Disease

The principal site of involvement in pulmonary heart disease is the pulmonary vascular bed. The pulmonary blood vessels, arterioles, capillaries, and veins may be affected by heart disease, leading to pulmonary parenchymal involvement, or by pulmonary disease, leading to cardiac involvement, mainly affecting the right heart. The pulmonary blood vessels themselves may be the primary site of disease, as in schistosomiasis (bilharziasis), primary pulmonary hypertension, pulmonary arteriovenous fistula, or lodging of the emboli in the pulmonary vessels, which interrupts blood supply to the lungs and affects the function of either the right or the left heart. The presence of heart disease has an important effect on the response of the lungs to embolization. The lungs have a double arterial blood supply from bronchial and pulmonary arteries. In normal persons, the lungs do not become infarcted when their pulmonary arterial blood supply is occluded. When the lungs are congested, as is commonly the case in patients with heart disease, pulmonary embolism is followed by pulmonary infarction, leading to hemorrhagic consolidation with obvious pulmonary parenchymal involvement.

The close relationship between heart disease and lung disease is further emphasized by the effects of cigarette smoking. Carcinoma of the bronchus and pulmonary emphysema are closely associated with excessive cigarette smoking. Premature coronary artery disease is also more common in habitual cigarette smokers. Thus, both heart and lung disease are often present in the same patient, and, since dyspnea and chest pain are important symptoms in both heart and lung disease, diagnostic problems, especially those of apportioning the total disability between disease of the heart and disease of the lungs, are particularly frequent.

PULMONARY HYPERTENSION

The development of increased pulmonary arterial pressure (pulmonary hypertension) represents the most important response of pulmonary blood vessels to disease. Pulmonary hypertension may result from primary parenchymal disease of the lungs, from changes in the walls of the blood vessels, or from obstruction to the lumen caused by thrombosis or embolization. The clinical picture varies widely depending on the cause of the pulmonary vascular involvement, but the final common pathway tends to result in right ventricular overload, right ventricular hypertrophy, and right heart failure. The term "cor pulmonale" is used to describe right heart involvement, and cor pulmonale is said to be present when any right-sided abnormality can be demonstrated; frank right heart failure does not have to be present.

Pulmonary circulation in the adult seems to be almost completely passive when compared to the systemic circulation. It behaves as an unreactive, low-pressure, low-resistance, short, high-flow pathway from the heart via the pulmonary arteries to the pulmonary capillary bed, which constitutes the large (100 m^2) site of gas exchange. The fetal, neonatal, and infant pulmonary circulations are less passive and have higher pressures and resistances in relation to their corresponding systemic circulations.

Mechanism of Production of Pulmonary Hypertension

The principal stimuli evoking a response in the pulmonary arterioles are (1) alveolar hypoxia, as occurs with exposure to high altitude, and (2) pulmonary venous hypertension. The site of reaction in both cases is the smooth muscle of the pulmonary arterioles. Both stimuli cause arteriolar vasoconstriction that is at first functional, spasmodic, and reversible; with time, however, the vasoconstriction develops into organic muscular hypertrophy, which is ultimately irreversible. The age at which the patient is first exposed to these stimuli and their magnitude and duration play an important role in determining the response of the pulmonary circulation. Since responsiveness decreases with age, stimuli that have been present since birth or infancy cause more severe and less readily reversible changes. Hypoxia and raised pulmonary venous pressure interact; consequently, pulmonary hypertension is more severe in patients living at higher altitudes who have disorders causing raised pulmonary venous pressure. Similarly, patients with diseased pulmonary vessels are prone to pulmonary embolism, thrombosis, and infarction, all of which aggravate the development of pulmonary hypertension. Thus, pulmonary hypertension tends to be progressive because thrombosis and embolism contribute to further pulmonary vascular obstruction.

Effects of Loss of Lung Tissue

The normal pulmonary circulation is especially capable of handling increased blood flow without much concomitant rise in pressure. The pressure/flow characteristics of pulmonary circulation are thus highly nonlinear, and the use of a single value (pressure/flow in mm Hg/l/min) to describe its resistance is overly simplistic. Increasing flow without increasing pressure implies the opening up of parallel circulatory pathways. It follows that loss of lung tissue, eg, following pneumonectomy, decreases the reserve capacity of the pulmonary vascular bed and increases the tendency for pulmonary hypertension to develop. As progressively larger amounts of lung tissue are removed, the capacity of the pulmonary vascular bed is ultimately reduced to a level at which the normal cardiac output cannot be accommodated without an increase in pulmonary arterial pressure. The principal mechanism causing chronic pulmonary hypertension in chronic lung disease is the loss of lung tissue—loss of arterioles, capillaries, and veins—caused by inflammation, fibrosis, or atrophy. The effects are small initially because the reserve of lung tissue is so large. However, once clinical manifestations of pulmonary hypertension have occurred, the disease tends to be rapidly progressive, since approximately seven-eighths of the pulmonary circulation must be destroyed before any clinical signs of right heart overload develop. In chronic lung disease, alveolar hypoxia, the effects of which are potentiated by hypercapnia and acidosis, causes an additional potentially reversible element of pulmonary hypertension. This element tends to aggravate the strain on the right ventricle, especially in acute exacerbations of bronchitis or pneumonia.

Effects of Increased Left Atrial Pressure

Pulmonary arterial vasoconstriction in response to a rise in left atrial pressure is the most important cause of pulmonary hypertension and right heart failure in patients with heart disease. The mechanism of this reaction is unknown. The magnitude of the response varies considerably in different patients, but younger persons usually show greater changes. Although mitral stenosis is the classic example of a lesion causing raised pulmonary vascular resistance in adults, any longstanding moderate or severe increase in left atrial pressure—eg, left atrial myxoma, aortic valve disease, systemic hypertension, cardiomyopathy, or any combination of causes—can result in raised pulmonary vascular resistance. The response is nonspecific, and the cause of raised left atrial pressure seems to have little effect on the basic disease process. It is not clear whether the increases in pulmonary arterial pressure seen in infants and children with congenital heart lesions involve a similar mechanism in a more reactive pulmonary vascular bed or whether an entirely different mechanism is involved. It is clear that lesions in adults are more readily reversible, either immediately, following infusion of tolazoline or acetylcholine, or more slowly, after surgical relief of the cause of left atrial hypertension. Pulmonary hypertension does not inevitably follow raised left atrial pressure. In some cases, chronic left atrial hypertension causes marked dyspnea and recurrent pulmonary edema without provoking any vasoconstrictive reaction in the pulmonary arterioles.

Pulmonary Hypertension in Patients With Lung Disease

Patients with parenchymal lung disease tend to develop pulmonary hypertension during acute exacerbations of their disease. Thus, during acute episodes of asthma, bronchitis, or pneumonia, the combination of lung disease and alveolar hypoxia leads to an acute rise in pulmonary arterial pressure. The pulmonary arterial pressure may fall to normal when the acute illness subsides, but with time some permanent changes occur, and ultimately the pulmonary hypertension becomes permanent. The rate of progression of right heart involvement varies widely from case to case depending on the nature of the pulmonary parenchymal disease, the frequency of superadded infection, the intensity of the response to hypoxia, and the response to treatment.

Pulmonary Hypertension in Schistosomiasis (Bilharziasis)

Bilharzial heart disease is due to the deposition of ova of Schistosoma (*S japonicum, S mansoni, or S haematobium*) in the lung (Fig 19–1). The condition arises from urinary or intestinal tract infection, and the disease is common in Egypt in agricultural workers in the Nile delta. The ova lodge in the pulmonary arterioles during their migration through the body and produce an inflammatory change which on healing leaves a nodule. The change leads to pulmonary hypertension, right ventricular hypertrophy, and right heart failure. The classic radiologic signs include a large pulmonary artery and diffuse mottling of the lung parenchyma. Beaded nodules in the arterioles have been called bilharzial tubercles (Bedford, 1946).

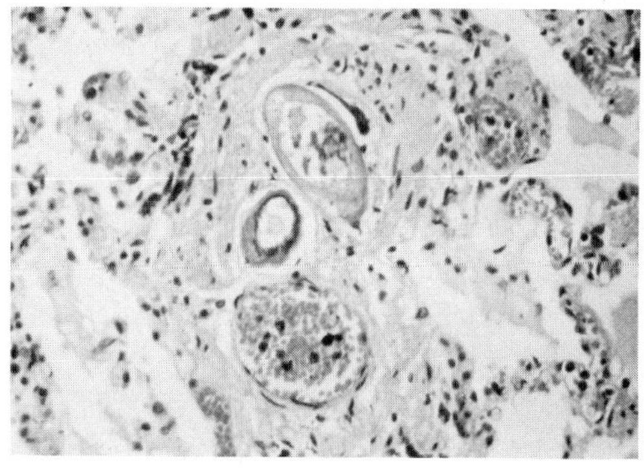

Figure 19–1. Bilharzia in the lung. Note the ova in the arterioles and the inflammatory reaction. Magnification X 40. (Courtesy of O Rambo.)

The clinical picture is one of right heart failure without lung disease and is similar to that in primary pulmonary hypertension. It is not uncommon to see aneurysmal dilatation of the pulmonary artery and marked enlargement of the right ventricle. The disease must be distinguished from other causes of pulmonary hypertension, especially pulmonary heart disease resulting from chronic bronchitis and emphysema, mitral stenosis, and atrial septal defect.

There is no satisfactory treatment when cor pulmonale develops. Antimony is used in the treatment of schistosomiasis, but, because it may itself produce toxic myocardial effects, it is usually contraindicated once heart failure has appeared in these patients. Other compounds which are used but have moderate to severe side-effects are niridazole, stibophen, and hycanthone. Prevention of bilharziasis consists of avoiding wading or swimming in stagnant fresh water in which the snail vector (Planorbis) lives.

Primary Pulmonary Hypertension

In rare cases, pulmonary arterial vasoconstriction occurs without a rise in left atrial pressure, giving rise to a disease known as primary or idiopathic pulmonary hypertension. The condition is commonest in premenopausal women but can occur at any age. The onset is insidious and the course usually relentlessly progressive, leading to death in 2–8 years from intractable right heart failure. The most striking clinical feature is low cardiac output, with weakness, fatigue, dyspnea, palpitations, and edema and ascites developing as right heart failure progresses. Cyanosis is often present and may be peripheral, due to low output, or, rarely, central, in cases in which diffuse fine pulmonary fibrosis (which does not show up on the chest x-ray) interferes with gas exchange. Syncope on effort can occasionally occur. At autopsy, the abnormal pulmonary vascular bed is so frequently seen to be the site of thrombosis and embolism that some have doubted the primary vasospastic nature of this condition.

Thromboembolic pulmonary hypertension can occur as a separate identifiable disease in patients who have repeated episodes of pulmonary embolism that are so frequent that complete resolution does not have time to occur between attacks. It is difficult to differentiate between vasospasm and thromboembolism in the genesis of primary pulmonary hypertension because multiple small pulmonary emboli can trigger reflex changes and may also produce pulmonary vasoconstriction. Pulmonary embolism is seldom the sole cause of chronic pulmonary hypertension but undoubtedly often contributes significantly to the clinical picture in patients with mixed lesions.

PULMONARY ARTERIOVENOUS FISTULA

Pulmonary arteriovenous fistula is a rare but specific form of pulmonary vascular disease. This condition, which is often associated with hereditary hemorrhagic telangiectasia (Osler's disease), consists of congenital arteriovenous malformations in the lungs which give rise to cyanosis, clubbing of the fingers, and a high output state. Venous blood passing through the abnormal channels often causes a bruit; in addition, the blood is not exposed to oxygen in the lungs, so that arterial desaturation occurs which is exaggerated on exercise. Cardiac output is increased, and polycythemia and increased blood volume follow. The condition is most frequently seen in young adults and tends to mimic congenital heart disease. Hemoptysis is a common complication. Resection of the lobe of the lung which is the site of the malformation is the principal treatment. Unfortunately, the lesions are often multiple, and, if this is not detected preoperatively, they sometimes enlarge and cause a recurrence of the condition after operation. The lesions usually show up on plain chest x-rays, as shown in Fig 19–2, and their vascular nature can be readily determined by pulmonary angiography (Fig 19–3).

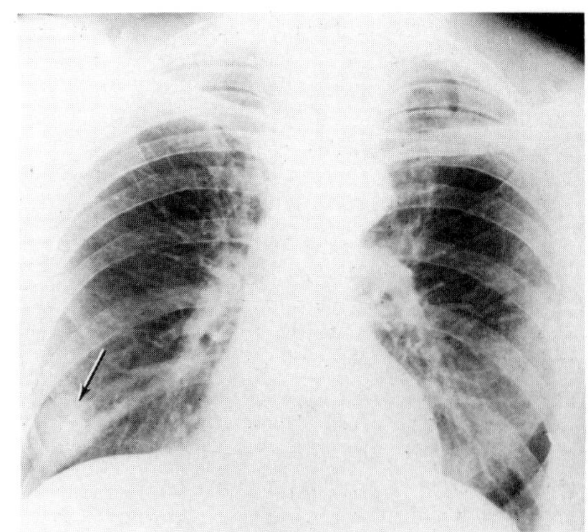

Figure 19–2. Chest x-ray showing a pulmonary arteriovenous fistula in the lower lobe of the right lung.

PULMONARY EMBOLISM

Pulmonary embolism is an important complication of heart disease. Its incidence and significance are extremely difficult to determine. Data based on autopsy findings indicate that pulmonary embolism is extremely common, some studies having found thrombus in pulmonary vessels in over half of patients. The distinction between antemortem and postmortem thrombus may be difficult to make. Agonal embolism and thrombosis in situ in the slow-moving blood of the lungs in moribund patients almost certainly account for many of the thrombi seen at autopsy.

The significance of the thrombotic material found

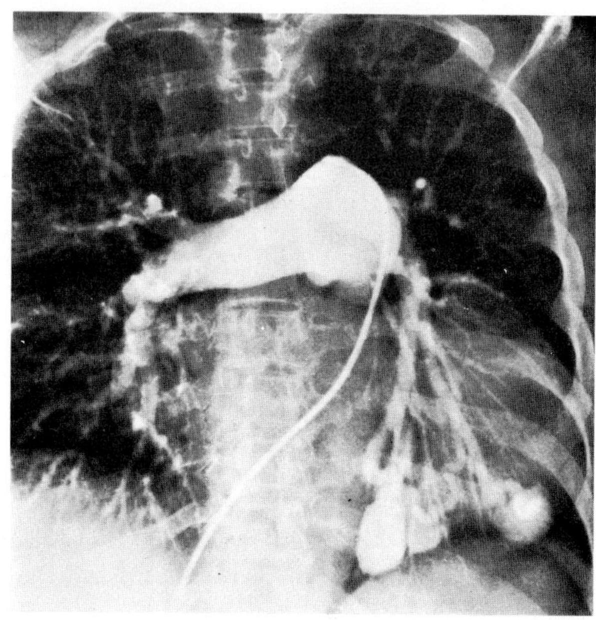

Figure 19–3. Angiogram showing 3 large arteriovenous fistulas in left lower lobe of the lung. (Reproduced, with permission, from Dines DE & others: Pulmonary arteriovenous fistulas. Mayo Clin Proc 49: 460, 1974.)

at autopsy is difficult to determine. In massive pulmonary embolism in which a large mass of red cells, fibrin, and platelets impacts in a main pulmonary artery and causes a sudden fatal obstruction to the circulation, the importance of the event is plainly evident. However, in chronically ill patients with wasting diseases who are comatose for several days, the episode is likely to be masked. Because the illness is terminal, an episode in which thrombus reaches a small- or moderate-sized artery is of lesser importance.

These considerations are not intended to underestimate the importance of pulmonary embolism as a complication but only to show that autopsy studies may not provide a realistic view of the incidence and clinical picture. Pulmonary embolism is insidious, often missed on physical examination, and often misdiagnosed as pneumonia, atelectasis, pleurisy, pulmonary congestion, or edema. The physician should maintain a high index of suspicion because the correct diagnosis may be difficult to make on account of the nonspecific nature of the clinical, radiologic, and electrocardiographic features of the condition.

Obstruction of the pulmonary vascular bed involving the lumen of blood vessels–pulmonary embolism or thrombosis–is more common in patients with heart disease than in those with lung disease. The nature and amount of embolic material, the site of obstruction, and the rate of removal of embolic material all play a part in determining the clinical picture, and the previous state of the pulmonary circulation determines whether the lung undergoes infarction or not. Normal lungs obtain their blood supply from both pulmonary and bronchial arteries. When the lungs are congested, as occurs in heart failure or in prolonged immobilization of comatose patients, bronchial blood flow is not ordinarily sufficient to maintain the viability of lung tissue that has been deprived of its pulmonary arterial blood supply. In such cases of congestion, the affected area of lung is infarcted and consolidated, which deprives it of air and causes a temporary loss of function.

The manifestations of pulmonary embolism vary greatly. Acute massive impaction of several hundred grams of thrombus in the main pulmonary artery can cause acute circulatory collapse or shock, with almost instantaneous death. There can also be repeated showers of multiple microscopic thrombi, eg, schistosome ova in bilharziasis. Small thrombi lodge in the pulmonary arterioles far out in the lungs and cause much more insidious pulmonary changes; in rare cases, right heart failure is the first clinical manifestation. The site of origin of the embolic material is commonly the veins of the legs and pelvis, but fat emboli from the bone marrow following fracture of the long bones also occur. Soft, recently formed thrombus is much more readily lysed than well-organized old thrombus or fat. Thus, the ability of the thrombolytic processes of the body to dispose of embolic material by breaking it up into smaller pieces which lodge in more peripheral parts of the lung constitutes an important and highly variable factor in the clinical course of pulmonary embolism.

The cross-sectional area of the pulmonary arterial bed increases with each division of the pulmonary artery. Consequently, as embolic material moves farther out in the lungs, a progressive increase in pulmonary blood flow, a progressive fall in pulmonary arterial pressure, and relief of right ventricular overload occur. Acute overload of the right heart, like acute overload of the left heart, tends to produce a different clinical picture from that observed in chronic obstruction of pulmonary blood flow. The magnitude of the overload can also vary because the pulmonary embolism may be massive or only moderate. The lodgment of small amounts of embolic material in the pulmonary circulation may well pass unnoticed. There is thus a wide variation in severity of the clinical effects of pulmonary embolism, further complicated by variations in the state of the preexisting pulmonary circulation. It may be several weeks before hypertrophy occurs in the right heart in response to sudden severe pulmonary vascular obstruction. A sudden acute rise in systemic venous pressure, without marked increase in pulmonary arterial or right ventricular pressure, is thus the principal effect of an acute lesion on the right side of the heart. Inadequate left-sided venous return, with an acute fall in left ventricular output, tachycardia, hypotension, shock, and circulatory collapse, dominates the clinical picture, and it may be difficult to determine whether the basic lesion is right-sided or left-sided. In more chronic, less rapidly developing, less severe lesions, right ventricular output can be maintained and the compensatory changes—right ventricular hypertrophy and dilatation—are more obvious.

Right Heart Failure Secondary to Lung Disease

The ultimate result of pulmonary vascular disease is right heart failure. This may be acute, as in massive pulmonary embolism; subacute, as when an acute pulmonary infection occurs in a patient with preexisting moderate pulmonary hypertension; or chronic, as in the end stages of chronic lung disease or primary pulmonary hypertension. The clinical picture varies with the cause of the lung disease, and pulmonary thromboembolism constitutes an important variable factor. The name cor pulmonale has been used to describe the condition, but this term should be used to cover any form of right-sided ventricular abnormality due to lung disease.

Massive Pulmonary Embolism; Acute Right Heart Failure (Acute Cor Pulmonale)

Acute cor pulmonale is seen almost exclusively in association with massive pulmonary embolism. Massive pulmonary embolism usually occurs in apparently healthy persons who may be of any age. The disease affects females more often than males. Patients have usually been recently subject to some minor trauma. Recent normal delivery, hernia operation, minor gynecologic or urologic surgery, varicose vein operation, or some other procedure involving the legs or pelvis is ordinarily the precipitating factor. Loosely adherent, soft, friable thrombus forms undetected in the veins of the legs or pelvis (phlebothrombosis). The thrombus suddenly breaks loose (in classic cases during straining at stool) and lodges at or near the bifurcation of the main pulmonary artery. The patient complains of sudden, severe central chest pain and collapses, often with loss of consciousness. Death can occur within a few minutes if the thrombus is large and does not dislodge. If the thrombus is smaller or moves more peripherally, either spontaneously or in response to pounding on the chest or closed chest massage, acute cor pulmonale rather than sudden death is seen.

Dyspnea, cyanosis, anxiety, impaired consciousness, and all the manifestations of an acute circulatory catastrophe are present. The diagnosis is difficult to confirm in the face of simultaneous emergency and supportive treatment and the general hectic activity involved in managing an acute life-threatening situation. Physical examination may not reveal any specific diagnostic signs. The electrocardiogram and chest x-ray may not be diagnostic in the earliest stages. The ECG will not necessarily show the changes of acute myocardial infarction, which is the most frequent and difficult disorder that must be considered in the differential diagnosis. The ECG changes of acute right ventricular overload can mimic myocardial infarction. Evidence of oligemic lungs, perhaps with an asymmetric increase in translucency, may be seen on radiograms in patients who survive the initial episode by half an hour or more. There may be evidence of arterial hypoxia ($P_{O_2} < 70$ mm Hg), but this finding is nonspecific.

The place of surgical removal of embolic material in the treatment of massive pulmonary embolism has been the subject of controversy in recent years. A confirmed diagnosis of massive pulmonary embolism with accessible thrombus in the main pulmonary artery or its branches is required before surgery is performed. This necessitates emergency pulmonary angiocardiography, preferably done in an operating room in a center equipped to perform cardiopulmonary bypass. Since such facilities are not widely available, less drastic measures must also be instituted. Anticoagulation with heparin (5000–10,000 units intravenously, repeated every 3 hours) can help to break up the thrombus, move it to a more peripheral part of the lung, and prevent extension. Any factor that moves the obstructing thrombus farther down the pulmonary artery may promote the patient's recovery. Even a small increase in the flow of blood to the lungs will sometimes help to provide a venous return to the left heart and will also avoid the development of secondary thrombosis around the embolus. Manipulation of a cardiac catheter in the pulmonary artery may serve to move the thrombus farther down the vessel; turning the patient into various positions and striking forceful blows to the precordium may also help.

Prevention of massive pulmonary embolism is clearly preferable to treatment. Patients with a history of pulmonary embolism, deep venous thrombosis, cerebral thrombosis, or thrombophlebitis should not use oral contraceptives. The morbidity and mortality rate from pulmonary embolism is 4–8 times higher in women who take oral contraceptive drugs. Encouraging patients to move about in bed and allowing them to walk about in their rooms as soon as possible after minor surgery or childbirth have helped to reduce the incidence of massive pulmonary embolism. Subcutaneous heparin injections in low doses (2500–3000 units every 6–8 hours) in the postoperative period or intravenous dextran 70 administered with intravenous fluids after surgery has reportedly been effective in reducing the incidence of fatal massive pulmonary embolism in double-blind studies. Since massive pulmonary embolism occurs in only about one in 100 cases in which it might be expected to develop, specific tests for the presence of deep vein thrombi in the legs, eg, localization of thrombus in the legs by scanning after radioactive fibrinogen injection and Doppler blood velocity studies, are not likely to be helpful. In thrombophlebitis (which is a much more common condition) smaller, more adherent thrombi that provoke local pain, swelling, and signs of inflammation occur. These seldom if ever break loose, and prophylactic measures other than avoiding oral contraceptives are of doubtful value.

Moderate Pulmonary Embolism

The description of massive pulmonary embolism given above concerns cases in which no prior heart or lung disease is present, cardiopulmonary reserve is large, and bronchial arterial blood supply is good. In most cardiac patients, however, these conditions do not exist. The clinical picture in such patients is different. Relatively small emboli that would pass unnoticed in a healthy person cause serious problems, with exacerbation of congestive heart failure or pulmonary infarction, with pain, pleural irritation, hemoptysis, and effusion. The venous stasis and congestion seen in heart failure predispose to thrombus formation not only in the legs but also in the right heart and even in the lungs themselves, so that pulmonary thromboembolic complications are especially common in cardiologic practice. Pulmonary embolism in which a moderate-sized embolus lodges in the lungs and is sufficiently large to occlude the artery leading to a lobe or a lobule is an insidious condition that is often overlooked. Data obtained at autopsy indicate a surprisingly high incidence of thrombi in the lungs (more than 50% of cases), and this suggests that agonal lesions may be common.

Clinical Findings

A. Symptoms: The classic symptoms of a chest pain that is often worse on inspiration, dyspnea, cough, and hemoptysis in susceptible patients such as those with congestive heart failure, mitral valve disease, or myocardial infarction should strongly suggest a diagnosis of pulmonary embolism. Not infrequently, unexplained dyspnea, fever, tachycardia, increase in venous pressure, or worsening of venous congestion provides a clue to the diagnosis, but in many cases the acute episode passes unnoticed.

B. Signs: Physical signs in the lungs depend on the development of consolidation or pleural involvement. Pleural friction rub, impaired movement, dullness to percussion, diminished air entry, and bronchial breathing can be heard, and signs of pleural effusion may develop. Signs of increased pulmonary arterial pressure such as increased right ventricular impulse, increased intensity of the pulmonary valve closure sound, or palpable pulmonary artery pulsation should be sought.

C. Electrocardiographic Findings: The ECG signs of pulmonary embolism are variable. A peaked right atrial P wave may be seen, and atrial arrhythmias, especially fibrillation or flutter, can occur. A change in electrical axis toward the right; right bundle branch block, either complete or incomplete (Fig 19–4); and T wave inversions in the anterior chest leads (V_{1-3}) are seen in about 10–15% of patients. In some cases, Q waves in leads II, III, and aVF mimic posterior myocar-

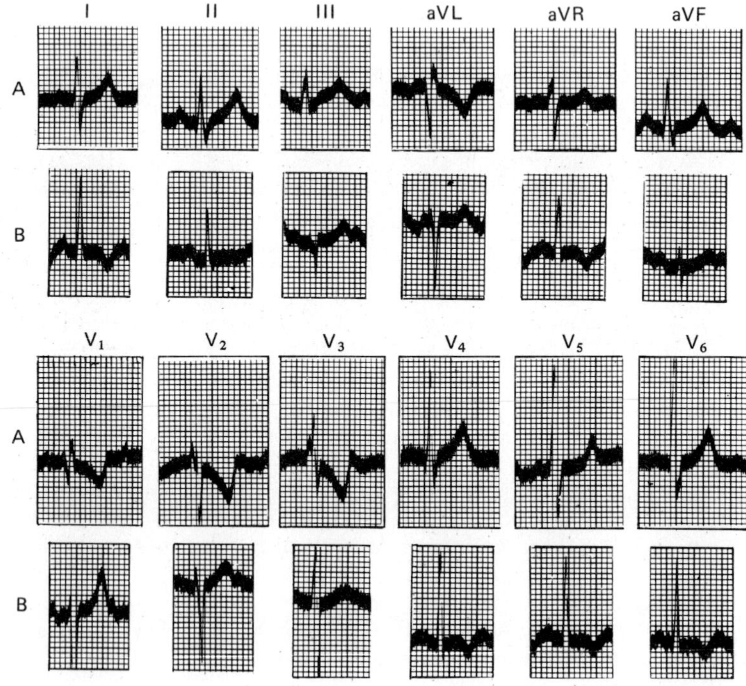

Figure 19–4. Incomplete right bundle branch block as a manifestation of acute right ventricular strain. *A:* The pattern is that of an incomplete bundle branch block (rsr′ complexes with depressed ST segments and inverted T waves in V_{1-3}). *B:* Five days after *(A):* There has been a marked change. The incomplete right bundle branch block is no longer present. In the interval the T waves have become inverted in leads I, aVR, and V_{4-6}. *Clinical status:* At *(A)* the patient had an episode of acute pulmonary infarction. Five days later he had markedly improved. The ECG in *(A)* was a reflection of acute right ventricular strain. The pulmonary hypertension had clinically subsided by *(B)*, and the second ECG demonstrated the abnormalities associated with the basic heart disease, beriberi. (Reproduced, with permission, from Goldman MJ: *Principles of Clinical Electrocardiography*, 9th ed. Lange, 1976.)

dial infarction. In most cases, nonspecific ST changes and slight right axis deviation are seen. Patients with associated coronary disease may show changes indicative of myocardial ischemia.

D. X-Ray Findings: The patient may be too ill for anything except a bedside x-ray, which is often unsatisfactory. Significant pulmonary embolism can occur even with completely clear lung fields, and radiologic evidence of consolidation following pulmonary infarction takes up to 12 hours to develop. The diaphragm tends to be high on the side of the lesion, which is commonly at the base of the lung. A wedge-shaped shadow extending out to the pleural surface is a classic manifestation, as shown in Fig 19–5. The lesion may cavitate later, and pleural effusion at the costophrenic angles or in the interlobular fissures is not uncommon.

E. Special Investigations: Leukocytosis, increased sedimentation rate, increased serum enzymes (lactic dehydrogenase and serum glutamic-oxaloacetic transaminase), and slight increase in indirect bilirubin concentration are seen in many cases. Arterial P_{O_2} is often reduced (less than 70 mm Hg), but the finding is nonspecific. External radioactive scanning following injection of radionuclides such as radioiodinated human serum albumin has proved valuable in patients without a history of prior lung disease. The results of lung scans must be interpreted together with simultaneous or near simultaneous chest x-rays. Pulmonary lesions other than emboli can give rise to clear, unperfused areas on the lung scan, and it is only the finding of an unperfused area in a segment of lung that is clear on the chest x-ray that is significant. Pulmonary emboli can clear so rapidly and can move to the periphery of the lungs so readily that confusion may occur when the radioactive scan and chest x-ray are obtained even a few hours apart.

Pulmonary angiography is a more invasive technic that can be used to demonstrate blockage of the pulmonary vasculature, which may be present although it does not appear on a chest radiogram, as shown in Fig 19–6. The indications for this method of demonstrating occlusive lesions in pulmonary arteries are not clear, but the study should only be performed if the lung scan shows a high probability of pulmonary embolism.

Although angiography is mandatory if thoracotomy is under consideration, performing such a time-consuming, expensive, and potentially dangerous procedure seems unnecessary when treatment with anticoagulants is clearly indicated.

Complications

Secondary thrombus with further blockage of pulmonary vessels, inadequate recanalization, and secondary infection of infected lung tissue are the principal complications of pulmonary embolism. Recurrence of pulmonary embolism is always possible, since pulmonary emoblisms are often multiple. However, complete recovery with full recanalization is the usual outcome, and the complication of chronic thromboembolic pulmonary hypertension is rare. Such chronic hypertension develops only after a long period of several months or years of repeated embolization, possibly with some associated impairment of the thrombolytic mechanisms as well.

Differential Diagnosis

The diagnosis of pulmonary embolism can be extremely difficult, especially in patients who are ill from other causes and in postoperative patients. The condition is so insidious that it should be suspected in any sick patient in whom unexplained deterioration or fail-

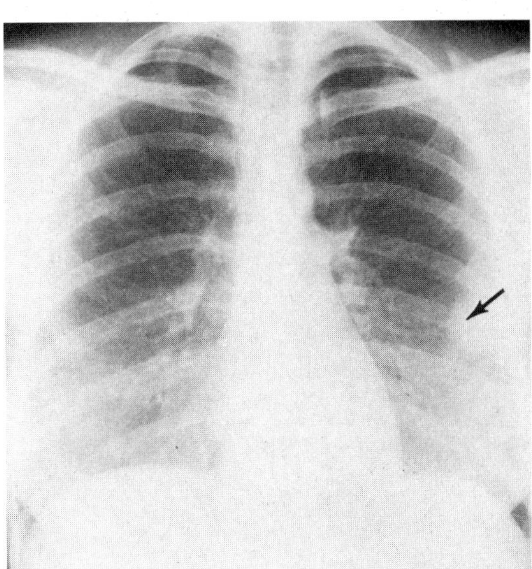
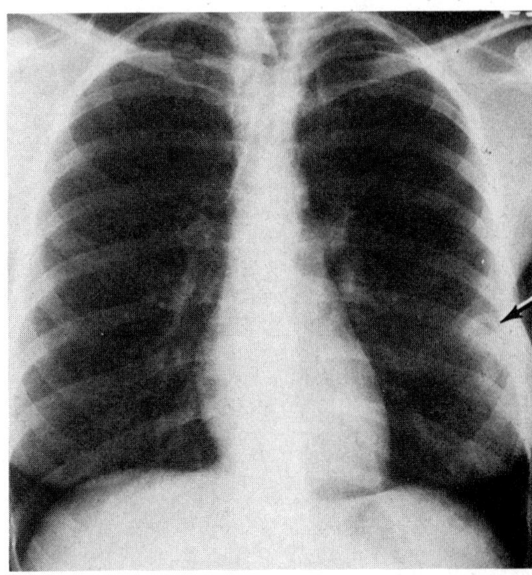

Figure 19–5. Serial chest x-rays of a woman patient with pulmonary infarction. The infarct has formed a cavity in the second (right-hand) x-ray. (Courtesy of G Gamsu.)

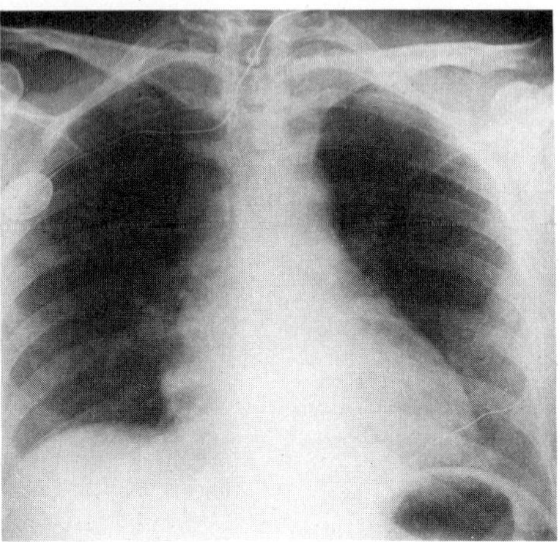

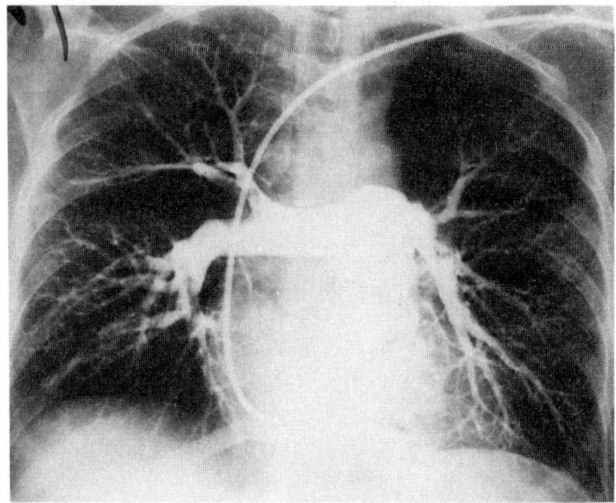

Figure 19–6. Normal chest x-ray *(left)* obtained on the same day as a pulmonary angiogram *(right)*. The angiogram shows significant obstruction to the right and left upper lobes, even though the chest x-ray was normal. (Courtesy of G. Gamsu.)

ure to thrive is detected. The physician must maintain a high index of suspicion in order to make the correct diagnosis. In many cases the diagnosis can be made in retropsect from careful examination of the chart of the vital signs. A sudden increase in heart rate or respiratory rate, followed by an unexplained rise in temperature on the following day, may have occurred in a patient with an obvious pulmonary infarct that was not previously apparent. Intercurrent lower respiratory tract infections can be readily mistaken for pulmonary emboli and vice versa. Likewise, minor, short-lived episodes of acute pulmonary congestion may cause a similar clinical picture. Repeated episodes of embolism tend to differ slightly in their manifestations, whereas recurrent pulmonary congestion tends to produce a series of similar episodes.

Pulmonary embolism enters into the differential diagnosis of almost all forms of lung disease and many varieties of heart disease. It occurs during the course of these diseases and may also be confused with the diseases themselves. Thus, pneumonia and atelectasis (especially if they occur postoperatively) and pleurisy with or without effusion may all be confused with pulmonary infarction. Hemorrhage into the lung is an important feature of pulmonary infarction that is also seen in other conditions such as bronchial carcinoma, tuberculosis, or any disease causing hemoptysis. Acute chest pain in pulmonary embolism can be confused with that occurring in myocardial infarction, spontaneous pneumothorax, pericarditis, aortic dissection, and even upper abdominal disease such as cholecystitis or perforated peptic ulcer.

Treatment

The principal decision in treatment is whether to use anticoagulant therapy. Anticoagulant therapy is more generally accepted in pulmonary embolism than in any other cardiologic disorder. Intravenous heparin (5000–10,000 units intravenously, followed by 5000 units intravenously every 4–6 hours) has become almost standard treatment, followed by warfarin (Coumadin), 30–50 mg on the first day, 10–15 mg on the second day, and a maintenance dose of 5–15 mg, depending on the prothrombin time, on subsequent days. Anticoagulant therapy is generally maintained for 6 weeks to 3 months after an episode of pulmonary embolism.

There are no measures that absolutely prevent the development of pulmonary embolism in cardiac patients, but initiating active leg exercises and breathing exercises, avoiding long periods of bed rest (especially with pressure on the popliteal fossa), and discontinuing the use of oral contraceptives are useful. The physician must exercise care in treating cardiac patients who are in a sitting position. Excessive flexing of the knee and sitting in cramped positions in automobiles and on airplanes predispose to venous stasis. Searching for tender veins in the calves, maintaining a high index of suspicion, and instituting anticoagulant therapy at the first sign of symptoms are important aspects of therapy. In patients with embolism that recurs in spite of anticoagulant treatment, inferior vena caval ligation, either partial or complete, has been advocated. However, this procedure does not necessarily prevent embolism, and it may even provide another site for thrombus formation; it also often leads to edema of the legs. The thrombolytic process is generally so effective that the long-term (6–12 week) prognosis depends on the underlying cardiac condition rather than on the embolism. No specific treatment is needed for pulmonary infarction. Control of pain and antibiotics for the treatment of secondary lung infection may be required. If infarction results in severe hemoptysis, anticoagulant therapy may have to be withdrawn. One of the principal advantages of heparin is that its effects can be neutralized by protamine. There is no entirely satisfactory antidote to warfarin, although treatment with vitamin K is usually attempted.

Prognosis

Pulmonary embolism seldom leads to chronic lung disease. If the patient survives the acute episode, whether it is a massive embolism or a moderate-size one involving pulmonary infarction, the lesion almost invariably heals completely without leaving a scar on the lung. The prognosis in acute massive embolism improves with the passage of time; however, most patients die within the first hour. This important cause of death in previously healthy people accounts for over 40,000 fatalities per year in the USA. In those who survive the first hour, the prognosis improves, partly because of the opportunity for treatment and partly because the embolic material may have broken up and moved to a more peripheral area of the lungs. The body's ability to lyse the thrombus is remarkable, and the speed with which the embolic material can disappear may complicate the diagnosis. In patients with terminal diseases and in those with heart disease, an embolus is often the crucial negative factor leading to death. The development of permanent pulmonary hypertension following pulmonary embolism is extremely rare. Chronic pulmonary hypertension occurs when there are frequent recurrent episodes of embolism with inadequate time between episodes for resolution of the disease process or when there are inadequate thrombolytic mechanisms. It is difficult to ascertain the effect of treatment on the prognosis because of the variable course in untreated cases and the initial difficulty in establishing a firm diagnosis.

RIGHT HEART FAILURE SECONDARY TO CHRONIC LUNG DISEASE

Pulmonary hypertension ultimately leads to right heart failure. The clinical picture depends primarily on the cause of the lung disease.

Chronic cor pulmonale is defined as heart *disease* (rather than heart *failure*) that is secondary to disease of the respiratory system. Right ventricular enlargement secondary to chronic disease of the respiratory system is most commonly due to parenchymal lung diseases such as fibrosis, emphysema, or pneumonia. The clinical picture is little influenced by the underlying cause, which may be pulmonary granuloma, sarcoidosis, scleroderma, pneumoconiosis, or any form of fibrosis, including idiopathic lesions (Hamman-Rich disease). The clinical picture is usually one of recurrent episodes of pulmonary infection or bronchial obstruction leading to temporary increases in the load on the right heart and right heart failure. Any lesion producing alveolar hypoxia causes a vicious cycle because of increased pulmonary arterial pressure due to pulmonary vasoconstriction. This mechanism is involved in alveolar hypoventilation due to weakness or paralysis of the respiratory muscles and also in central nervous disease leading to inadequate pulmonary ventilation. Both these conditions can cause chronic cor pulmonale even when the lungs themselves are normal. Massive obesity, as in the Pickwickian syndrome, can also cause right heart failure; it is another cause of alveolar hypoventilation in which the lungs are normal. Chest wall disorders such as kyphosis and scoliosis may occasionally lead to heart failure but usually only when chest infection is present. Before antibiotic therapy and assisted ventilation were available, the first episode of right heart failure was often fatal in patients who had chronic lung disease secondary to respiratory infection or obstruction. Modern treatment of acute pulmonary failure often leads to recovery but leaves the lungs damaged to a variable degree and often more vulnerable to a recurrent episode of infection. After several episodes of acute right heart failure, the patient reaches a precarious condition in which even minor illnesses such as influenza or an upper respiratory infection can be life-threatening. In such patients, the degree of right heart failure is an indication of the stage of the disease. Arterial hypoxia increases cardiac output by causing systemic vasodilatation and especially by increasing the heart rate. These factors tend to aggravate right heart failure. Since patients with chronic lung disease are often middle-aged and have smoked cigarettes for many years, associated atherosclerotic heart disease is common, and an element of left heart failure is frequently present in addition to right heart failure. Some feel that right heart failure can lead to left heart failure as the enlarging right ventricle displaces the left ventricle backwards, but this is difficult to prove.

Clinical Findings

A. Symptoms: Dyspnea is the primary symptom in patients with chronic cor pulmonale. Coexisting pulmonary and cardiac disease may make it difficult to determine the cause of dyspnea. In the usual case of chronic cor pulmonale, dyspnea is most commonly due to the increased work of breathing resulting from the mechanical effects of the lung disease causing the right heart overload.

However, dyspnea is also seen in the rarest form of chronic cor pulmonale—primary pulmonary hypertension. In this condition, the mechanical properties of the lungs are normal, and some other explanation must be sought to explain the dyspnea. An inadequate systemic cardiac output is thought to cause alveolar hyperventilation, and excessive ventilation, especially during exercise, is thought to be responsible for the dyspnea. Edema of the ankles, abdominal swelling, and right upper quadrant pain due to hepatic congestion are often seen. Palpitations, weakness, syncope, and coldness of the hands and feet also occur in primary pulmonary hypertension.

B. Signs:

1. Noncardiac signs—Patients with arterial hypoxia due to bronchitis tend to exhibit hypervolemia and vasodilatation rather than the vasoconstriction and low output state seen in patients with emphysema and primary pulmonary hypertension. Patients with chronic lung disease have been divided into "blue bloaters," in whom hypoxia, hypervolemia, recurrent bronchitis, and cor pulmonale are prominent, and "pink puffers," in whom hypoxia is absent, hypovolemia and emphysema are common, and cor pulmonale is rare. Similarly, cor pulmonale has been classified as either hypoxic or pulmonary hypertensive, depending on whether a high output or a low output state predominates. Such generalizations are useful in delineating the different mechanisms involved but must not be taken as definitive, mutually exclusive categories.

Cyanosis and clubbing of the fingers are often seen. The cyanosis may be peripheral, due to the low cardiac output in patients with pulmonary hypertension, or central and associated with significant arterial hypoxemia ($P_{O_2} < 60$ mm Hg) and hypercapnia ($P_{CO_2} > 50$ mm Hg) in patients with chronic lung disease or alveolar hypoventilation. Clubbing of the fingers is most frequently seen in patients with chronic pulmonary infections or bronchial carcinoma. Tachycardia and a raised jugular venous pressure with *a* and *v* waves occur. Hepatomegaly, ascites, and edema of the ankles are seen if the patient is in right heart failure.

2. Cardiac signs–Cardiac manifestations depend on the nature of the lung disease. In patients with emphysema, bronchitis, or bronchial obstruction, the cardiac impulse may be difficult to palpate because of overlying lung tissue. The sounds may be distant and murmurs absent. Conversely, in primary pulmonary hypertension, a prominent right ventricular heave below the sternum, a loud pulmonary valve closure component of a closely split second heart sound and ejection click, and a short pulmonary systolic murmur are noted, often with a pulmonary diastolic (Graham Steell) murmur due to pulmonary incompetence. In later stages, a pansystolic high-pitched murmur of tricuspid incompetence is often easily detected.

C. Electrocardiographic Findings: Sinus rhythm is the rule, and the ECG shows evidence of right atrial or ventricular predominance. In patients with severe obstructive lung disease, right atrial hypertrophy may be all that is apparent. ECG changes of right ventricular hypertrophy (Fig 19–7), like the physical signs, are sometimes masked. In patients with marked pulmonary hypertension, the reverse is true, and clear evidence of right ventricular hypertrophy, with P pulmonale, tall R waves, and ST depression with T wave inversion in the right-sided chest leads is prominent, as shown in Fig 19–8.

D. X-Ray Findings: Enlargement of the main pulmonary artery is the most reliable radiologic indication of chronic cor pulmonale. The degree of cardiac enlargement, although obvious in serial radiograms, may be unimpressive, especially in emphysema. Right ventricular and right atrial enlargement are seen in primary pulmonary hypertension, as shown in Fig 19–9. They are notoriously difficult to confirm on chest x-rays, but in advanced cases of cor pulmonale with pulmonary hypertension, both chambers are obviously enlarged. Pulmonary congestion is not seen unless associated left-sided disease is present. In practice, many patients with chronic lung disease have associated left ventricular disease, and it may be difficult to ascertain how much damage has been done by cardiac disease and how much by pulmonary disease. Superimposed pulmonary congestion and intercurrent pulmonary infections further complicate the differentiation of the effects of heart disease from those of lung disease.

E. Special Investigations: Polycythemia with hematocrit levels above 50% is usually present in hypoxic patients. Measurement of arterial blood gas tensions and pH is necessary in acutely ill patients in order to assess the severity of pulmonary failure. Right heart catheterization is indicated in patients with pulmonary

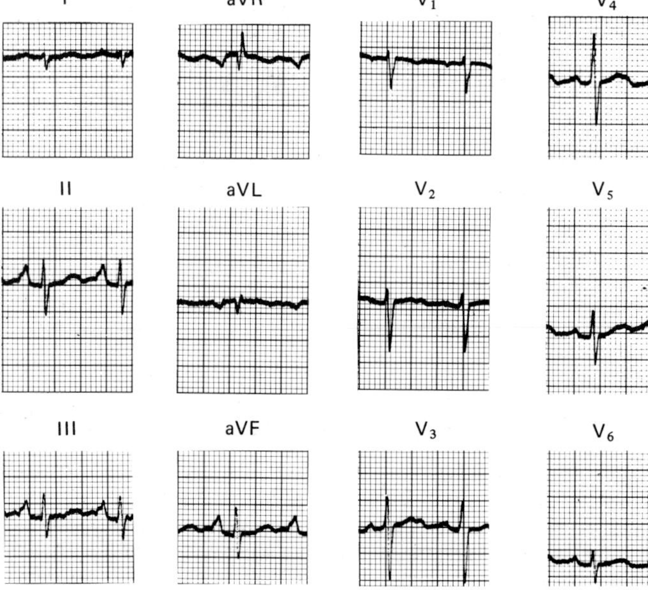

Figure 19–7. Pulmonary emphysema and cor pulmonale. The tall peaked P waves in leads II, III, and aVF are consistent with right atrial hypertrophy. There are small initial QRS forces to the left (r in lead I) with greater terminal forces to the right (S in I). These terminal forces are directed superiorly (S in II, III, and aVF). This is an example of the S_1, S_2, S_3 syndrome. The tracing is consistent with pulmonary emphysema. The prominent P waves are the only positive evidence of right heart overload. (Reproduced, with permission, from Goldman MJ: *Clinical Electrocardiography,* 9th ed. Lange, 1976.)

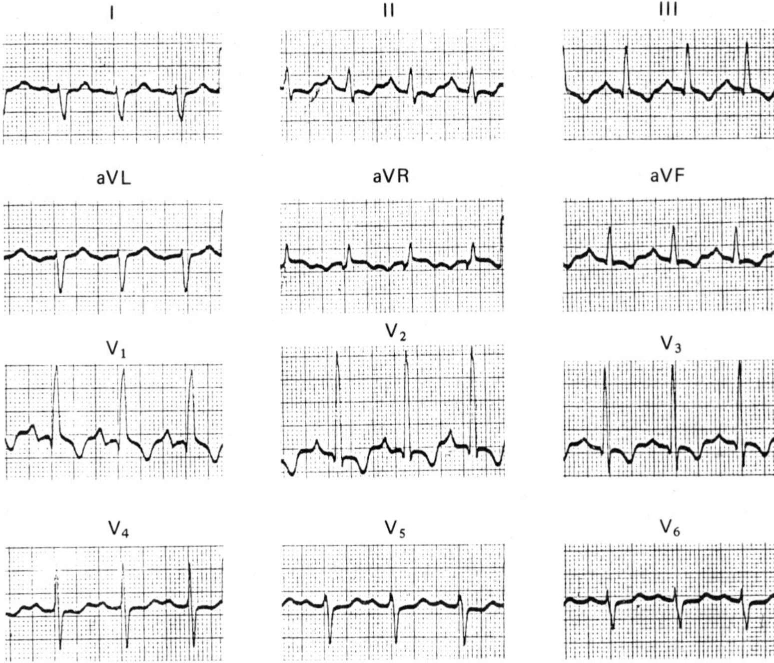

Figure 19–8. ECG from a patient with primary pulmonary hypertension showing severe right ventricular hypertrophy.

hypertension in order to confirm the diagnosis by determining wedge pressure. Such investigations are extremely helpful because lesions repairable by surgery such as mitral stenosis and left atrial myxoma can easily be overlooked during examination. Pulmonary hypertension in association with congenital heart lesions (Eisenmenger's syndrome) may enter into the differential diagnosis, but the presence of right-to-left shunting causing arterial desaturation does not necessarily indicate congenital heart disease, since a foramen ovale can open up in chronic cor pulmonale when right atrial pressure rises above left atrial pressure. The response of arterial blood gas tension and pulmonary vascular resistance to oxygen inhalation or vasodilator agents such as tolazoline (Priscoline) and acetylcholine may be important in directing therapy and determining the reversibility of the condition.

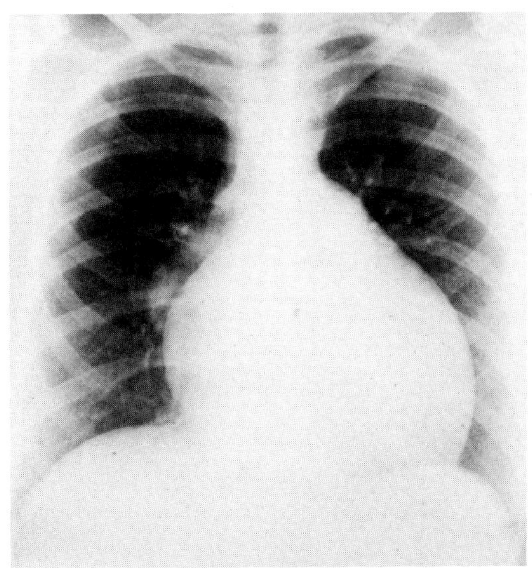

Figure 19–9. Chest x-ray showing cardiac enlargement with prominence of the pulmonary artery, right atrium, and right ventricle in a patient with primary pulmonary hypertension. The lung fields are abnormally translucent in association with reduced pulmonary blood flow.

Differential Diagnosis

Disorders to be differentiated from right heart failure due to lung disease include mitral stenosis, thromboembolic pulmonary hypertension, and Eisenmenger's syndrome. When coincidental pulmonary disease is present, the differential diagnosis can be extremely difficult. Cardiac catheterization is indicated when clear evidence of pulmonary hypertension is found. This diagnosis is suspected more commonly than it is proved, and clinical signs of right heart failure (palpable pulmonary arterial pulsation and loud pulmonary valve closure) tend to be unreliable signs of pulmonary hypertension.

Complications

Right heart failure is such an integral part of chronic cor pulmonale that it is hardly a complication. Similarily, chest infection, pulmonary thrombosis, embolism, and alveolar hypoxia occur so frequently in the course of the disease that they are not really considered complications. Atrial arrhythmias are relatively common in acute exacerbations of pulmonary infection, but chronic atrial fibrillation is rare. Pulmonary valvular incompetence causing an immediate diastolic (Graham Steell) murmur over the pulmonary artery is more a part of the disease than a complication.

Treatment

The prevention of heart failure is of the utmost importance in patients with lung disease. Prevention involves early and vigorous treatment of chest infections, vaccination against influenza, and avoidance of contact with persons who have upper respiratory tract infections. Cigarette smoking is extremely likely to have a serious effect on cardiopulmonary function in patients with cor pulmonale. Every effort should be made to persuade the patient to stop smoking.

The most important principles of therapy are to improve respiratory function, relieve arterial hypoxemia, reduce pulmonary hypertension, and improve right ventricular function.

The patient must first be treated vigorously and effectively for any intercurrent chest infection that is clearly present, or such infection must be carefully ruled out if there are no apparent symptoms. Relief of arterial hypoxia by oxygen therapy with a mask or nasal catheter as described in Chapter 7 is of great help. The dangers of oxygen therapy–abolition of the patient's hypoxic ventilatory drive and hypoventilation with serious CO_2 retention–have been exaggerated. Any tendency toward hypoventilation with oxygen should be remedied by the use of assisted or artificial ventilation via an endotracheal tube, with clearing of the air passages. Opinions differ about the indications for intensive artificial ventilation in patients in pulmonary failure (which is defined as a P_{CO_2} level greater than the P_{O_2} level). Tracheostomy and artificial ventilation with frequent endotracheal suction and fiberoptic bronchoscopy are readily performed in some centers. However, such intensive measures are seldom needed if adequate preventive measures have been instituted and the patient is under optimal long-term supervision. The treatment of right heart failure with digitalis and diuretics is of secondary importance and is seldom effective as a sole treatment regimen. Digitalis has a reputation for ineffectiveness in patients with cor pulmonale, but there is no evidence that it is harmful except when excessive doses are administered in the hope of slowing the heart rate. In older patients in whom there is associated left ventricular disease, digitalis is often of value and should always be tried. Chronic anticoagulant therapy may be of value for patients with obvious thromboembolic complications. Such therapy is also used in patients with primary pulmonary hypertension but without evidence of benefit. The treatment of primary pulmonary hypertension is particularly unsatisfactory, and the patient develops increasingly severe right heart failure in spite of all measures, including corticosteroid therapy, which is often given as a last resort in the hope that some form of collagen disease is responsible for the pulmonary hypertension. Corticosteroids may be of value in the treatment of chronic cor pulmonale associated with connective tissue disorders (eg, scleroderma), but they do not generally help patients who are in right heart failure.

Prognosis

Cor pulmonale is such a late manifestation of pulmonary disease that the prognosis is poor. Pulmonary reserve has been severely compromised by the time a patient develops either hypercapnia secondary to inadequate ventilation or right ventricular enlargement secondary to inflammatory, fibrotic, or degenerative lung disease. The prognosis is best in patients who have a severe pulmonary infection but little or no chronic underlying lung disease. Because such patients cannot be positively identified until after the acute infection has been treated, intensive measures are indicated in emergency situations for patients who have not previously been under the care of a physician. The prognosis in primary pulmonary hypertension is poor. Death in 2–8 years is the rule. Patients with thromboembolic disease live longer because favorable factors such as lysis and organization of thrombi may influence the clinical picture.

DIFFERENTIATION OF HEART DISEASE & LUNG DISEASE

Lung disease and heart disease often coexist. The harmful effects of cigarette smoking predispose to chronic bronchitis and emphysema and also to carcinoma of the bronchus. They also increase the risk of premature coronary artery disease. In consequence, many patients suffer from both cardiac and pulmonary disease, and the 2 compound one another. The hypoxia associated with acute exacerbations of chronic obstructive lung disease increases the cardiac output and increases the load on the heart, which may be already compromised by coronary disease. Conversely, myocardial infarction or left heart failure in a patient with impaired pulmonary function due to emphysema predisposes to acute pulmonary infection leading to pulmonary failure (hypoxia and hypercapnia). Whereas the distinction between pure lung disease and pure heart disease is relatively easy, separating the pulmonary and cardiac elements in mixed lesions is extremely difficult.

Clinical Findings

A. Symptoms: Dyspnea is an important symptom in both heart and lung disease. The dyspnea of lung disease tends to be episodic, being worse at some times than others. It is not infrequently present at rest, when attacks of asthma, bronchospasm, or acute bronchitis occur. It may also be worse on exercise, especially when asthma or bronchospasm is induced by effort. The dyspnea of emphysema produces a basic, permanent, irreversible level of dyspnea. Although the patient's dyspnea may be worse at times, it never remits completely. It is thus important in obtaining a history of dyspnea to find out how much the patient's breathlessness varies from day to day and to concentrate on the level of dyspnea on the patient's "best day." If significant emphysema is present, dyspnea will be present even on the "best day." Conversely, if the patient has a normal exercise tolerance on the best day, then emphysema is not present. The dyspnea of lung disease is associated with the application of increased force to move the lungs and thorax, and the patient is aware of the mechanical problem in breathing. Cardiac dyspnea is less labored unless pulmonary edema is present and is more like the dyspnea of normal effort.

Chest pain occurs in both heart and lung disease. The patient with lung disease complains of a tight constricting feeling across the chest on exertion or at rest when bronchitis or bronchospasm is present. This can usually be distinguished from anginal pain, because it is discomfort rather than pain and usually neither radiates like angina nor is so quantitatively related to exertion. Pleural pain suggests lung disease but can occur in heart disease when pulmonary embolism leads to pulmonary infarction.

Cough occurs both in heart disease and lung disease. Its presence is much more common in lung disease, but pulmonary congestion secondary to raised left atrial pressure can also cause cough. The cough in heart disease is dry and unproductive unless pulmonary edema develops, when profuse watery sputum occurs. The cough of pulmonary congestion often comes on with exercise. Cough with purulent, mucopurulent, rusty, or tenacious sputum is indicative of lung disease. Hemoptysis occurs in both heart and lung disease, and its presence is not often of value in distinguishing heart and lung disease.

B. Signs: In comparison with symptoms, there is much less overlap in physical signs between heart and lung disease. Pleural friction rubs and rales and rhonchi can occur in both. The pulmonary signs associated with pulmonary congestion and edema can be mistaken for those of asthma or bronchospasm, but "cardiac asthma" is not often confused with asthma or bronchitis because of the history of previous attacks in asthma and the presence of obvious signs of mitral or left ventricular disease in patients with pulmonary congestion.

C. Electrocardiographic Findings: The ECG is particularly helpful in distinguishing between heart and lung disease in cigarette smokers. The presence of evidence of left ventricular predominance with ST–T wave changes in the left-sided leads indicates that there is at least some heart disease. Atrial arrhythmias occur in both varieties of disease, but chronic atrial fibrillation is more common in heart disease.

D. X-Ray Findings: Cardiac enlargement is difficult to interpret. The heart is often smaller than normal in patients with emphysema, and hearts of apparently normal size may in fact be enlarged for those particular patients. It is easy to confuse right- and left-sided cardiac enlargement on chest x-rays, and pulmonary infarction can readily be confused with the radiologic findings of pulmonary infection.

E. Special Investigations: One of the principal uses of pulmonary function tests is to distinguish between heart and lung disease. Whereas the vital capacity is reduced in patients with pulmonary congestion, the maximum expiratory flow rates are relatively normal and the flow-volume curves do not indicate significant obstruction. The percentage of the vital capacity expelled in the first second is greater than 70 in heart disease but is less than 70 in patients with significant obstruction due to lung disease. In difficult cases, the measurements of lung compliance, lung and airway resistance, and lung volume may be required to detect the large lung volumes, high resistance, and normal or increased compliance in emphysema. The frequency dependence of compliance and resistance characteristic of chronic lung disease are also helpful diagnostic points. Air trapping on expiration and large closing volumes are also characteristic of obstructive lung disease.

Arterial blood gas measurements should be made if there is any doubt. The hypoxia and hypercapnia ($P_{O_2} < 70$ mm Hg, $P_{CO_2} > 45$ mm Hg) often seen in lung disease are rare in heart disease except when pulmonary edema is present. In difficult cases, cardiac catheterization with measurement of pulmonary vascular resistance and full pulmonary function studies are likely to be needed to separate the effects of lung disease from those of heart disease.

• • •

References

Adams WR, Veith I (editors): *Pulmonary Circulation.* Grune & Stratton, 1958.

Allison PR & others: Pulmonary embolism. Thorax 15:273, 1960.

Bedford DE & others: Bilharzial heart disease in Egypt: Cor pulmonale due to bilharzial pulmonary endarteritis. Br Heart J 8:87, 1946.

Bell WR, Simon TL: A comparative analysis of pulmonary perfusion scans with pulmonary angiograms. Am Heart J 92:700, 1976.

Bell WR, Simon TL, DeMets DL: The clinical features of submassive and massive pulmonary emboli. Am J Med 62:355, 1977.

Bergofsky EH & others: Cardiorespiratory failure in kyphoscoliosis. Medicine 38:263, 1959.

Burwell CS & others: Extreme obesity associated with alveolar hypoventilation: A Pickwickian syndrome. Am J Med 21:811, 1956.

Christie RV: Emphysema of the lungs. Br Med J 1:143, 1944.

Clagett GP, Salzman EW: Prevention of venous thromboembolism in surgical patients. N Engl J Med 290:93, 1974.

Comroe JH Jr: *Physiology of Respiration,* 2nd ed. Year Book, 1974.

Crane C & others: The management of major pulmonary embolism. Surg Gynecol Obstet 128:27, 1969.

Dalen JE, Dexter L: Pulmonary embolism. JAMA 207:1505, 1969.

Dexter L: Thromboemboli as a cause of cor pulmonale. Bull NY Acad Med 41:981, 1965.

Dines DE & others: Pulmonary arteriovenous fistulas. Mayo Clin Proc 49:460, 1974.

Eberlein TJ, Carey LC: Comparison of surgical managements for pulmonary emboli. Ann Surg 179:836, 1973.

Fleming HA, Bailey SM: Massive pulmonary embolism in healthy people. Br Med J 1:1322, 1966.

Fletcher CM & others: The diagnosis of pulmonary emphysema in the presence of chronic bronchitis. Q J Med 32:33, 1963.

Goldsmith RS: Infectious diseases: Metazoal. Chapter 26 in: *Current Medical Diagnosis & Treatment 1977.* Krupp MA, Chatton MJ (editors). Lange, 1977.

Gray FD: *Pulmonary Embolism: Natural History and Treatment.* Lea & Febiger, 1966.

Humphries JO, Bell WR, White RI: Criteria for the recognition of pulmonary emboli. JAMA 235:2011, 1976.

McDonald IG & others: Major pulmonary embolism: A correlation of clinical findings, haemodynamics, pulmonary angiography, and pathological physiology. Br Heart J 34:356, 1972.

McIlroy MB, Apthorp GH: Pulmonary function in pulmonary hypertension. Br Heart J 20:397, 1958.

Miller GAH, Hall RJC, Paneth M: Pulmonary embolectomy, heparin and streptokinase: Their place in the treatment of acute massive pulmonary embolism. Am Heart J 93:568, 1977.

Oakley C, Somerville J: Oral contraceptives and progressive pulmonary vascular disease. Lancet 1:890, 1968.

Rudolph A & others: Effects of tolazoline hydrochloride (Priscoline) on circulatory dynamics of patients with pulmonary hypertension. Am Heart J 55:424, 1958.

Shepherd JT & others: Clinical physiological and pathological considerations in patients with idiopathic pulmonary hypertension. Br Heart J 19:70, 1957.

Short DS, Bedford DE: Solitary pulmonary hypertension. Br Heart J 19:93, 1957.

Wagenvoort CA, Wagenvoort N: *Pathology of Pulmonary Hypertension.* Wiley, 1977.

Westlake EK & others: Carbon dioxide narcosis in emphysema. Q J Med 24:155, 1955.

Wilhelmsen L, Hagman M, Werko L: Recurrent pulmonary embolism: Incidence, predisposing factors and prognosis. Acta Med Scand 192:565, 1972.

Wood P: Pulmonary hypertension. Br Med Bull 8:348, 1952.

20 . . .
Diseases of the Aorta & Systemic Arteries

The diseases described under this heading include syphilitic aortitis and aneurysm, arteritis involving arteries of different sizes, systemic embolism, and systemic arteriovenous fistula. Arteritis and systemic embolism occur in a wide variety of diseases, and the accounts in this chapter deal mainly with the cardiologic aspects. Systemic embolism is also discussed in the chapters dealing with the forms of heart disease in which embolism occurs.

SYPHILITIC CARDIOVASCULAR DISEASE

Pathology

The basic lesion in the tertiary form of syphilis which affects the cardiovascular system is endarteritis obliterans. The primary site of disease is the thoracic aorta, and endarteritis of the vasa vasorum weakens the media and causes swelling and scarring of the intima, giving rise to the characteristic "crow's foot" or "tree bark" markings seen at autopsy. The changes in the intima can narrow the ostia of the coronary vessels and also affect the aortic valve cusps. The weakening of the media leads to dilatation of the aorta, which, in addition to causing fusiform or saccular aneurysms in the thoracic aorta, leads to aortic valve ring dilatation and progressive aortic incompetence. Syphilitic disease produces changes similar to those seen in patients with aortic incompetence due to other causes. However, calcification and stenosis of the valve do not occur, and infective endocarditis is rare.

Clinical Findings

Syphilitic heart disease has become much rarer in the past 50 years since effective treatment of primary syphilis has been widely available. When it does occur, the disease is less florid, and instead of causing symptoms in persons 40–60 years of age, cardiovascular syphilis now affects older persons. Consequently, atherosclerotic lesions almost always coexist with syphilitic lesions. Atherosclerotic aneurysms are described in Chapter 9. In contrast to syphilitic aneurysms, they are usually fusiform rather than saccular and are much more likely to involve the descending aorta. Syphilitic aneurysms of the thoracic aorta act as space-occupying, expanding, cardiovascular "tumors" that compress and erode surrounding structures. They occur more commonly in men by a factor of 3:1. Their clinical manifestations vary with the site of the aneurysm. Aneurysms of the ascending aorta classically produce physical signs; aneurysms of the arch of the aorta cause symptoms; and aneurysms of the descending aorta cause pain or are asymptomatic.

A. Symptoms: Symptoms appear late in cardiovascular syphilis, and significant abnormalities may be found in asymptomatic patients. Pain in the chest is the most important symptom of aortic aneurysm. In descending thoracic aortic lesions, pain is caused by erosion of the vertebral column, and it is constant, boring, severe, and worse at night. Ascending aortic lesions involving coronary ostia may cause angina pectoris with pain at rest or during exercise. The angina occurs as the result of interference with coronary blood flow. Ascending aortic lesions may occur with or without aortic incompetence. Pain may also arise from aortic lesions that do not involve the coronary vessels; this pain is attributed to stretching of aortic tissue. The symptoms associated with aneurysms of the arch of the aorta stem from pressure on surrounding structures and include cough due to pressure on the trachea or left bronchus, hoarseness due to pressure on the left recurrent laryngeal nerve, dysphagia due to pressure on the esophagus, swelling of the neck and face due to superior vena caval compression, and hemoptysis. This last manifestation may be the final symptom when the aneurysm ruptures into the bronchial tree.

B. Signs: The signs of aortic aneurysm may be attributable to the lesion, as in visible or palpable pulsation localized to the right of the sternum, which is more specific than pulsation in the suprasternal notch and may be seen with minor aortic dilatation. Signs caused indirectly by involvement of neighboring structures include the wide pulse pressure and water-hammer pulse of aortic incompetence, jugular venous distention and facial edema due to superior vena caval obstruction, Horner's syndrome (enophthalmos, meiosis, and ptosis) due to sympathetic nerve compression, and tracheal tug. This latter sign is elicited by standing behind the patient and pulling the larynx upwards; the "tug" of the aneurysm pulls the cervical structures down with each heartbeat. Cardiac enlargement, which is often massive, results from aortic incompetence. The immediate diastolic murmur of aortic incompetence is heard to the right of the sternum. The aortic valve closure sound is often high-pitched and has a tambour drumbeat quality even in the absence of an aneurysm or aortic incompetence. Aortic systolic murmurs are commonly heard, both with and without aortic incompetence, and they should not be taken as evidence of aortic stenosis. Signs of left ventricular failure may be present in patients with aortic incompetence. Associated neurologic signs of central nervous system syphilis are common and help point out the syphilitic cause of the aortic aneurysm.

C. Electrocardiographic Findings: There are no specific syphilitic changes on the ECG. Left ventricular hypertrophy occurs in response to aortic incompetence. Left bundle branch block and ischemic ST and T wave changes can occur in older persons.

D. X-Ray Findings: Aortic dilatation is often visible in patients with aortitis without aneurysm formation. Aortic aneurysms give rise to abnormal shadows on the chest x-ray which vary enormously from case to case. An example of an aneurysm of the arch of the aorta is shown in Fig 20–1. To distinguish between aneurysms and other tumors is difficult. Transmitted pulsations are not readily distinguished from the direct expansile pulsation of an aneurysm. Lack of pulsation does not exclude the possibility of an aneurysm because thrombus formation may obliterate the cavity and leave a solid tumor. Oblique views should always be obtained. Cinefluoroscopy provides a permanent record of the lesion for comparison with later studies. Calcification should be sought in the wall at the origin of the ascending aorta, where it is virtually pathognomonic of a syphilitic lesion. Calcification in the aortic arch and knuckle is much more common and is indicative of atherosclerosis. Syphilitic calcification is thin, beaded, and eggshell-like. It is usually seen best on the left anterior oblique or lateral view, as shown in Fig 20–2. When the descending aorta is involved, erosion of the thoracic vertebral column should be sought on the lateral view. Syphilis virtually never involves the abdominal aorta because syphilitic and abdominal aneurysms are mutually exclusive.

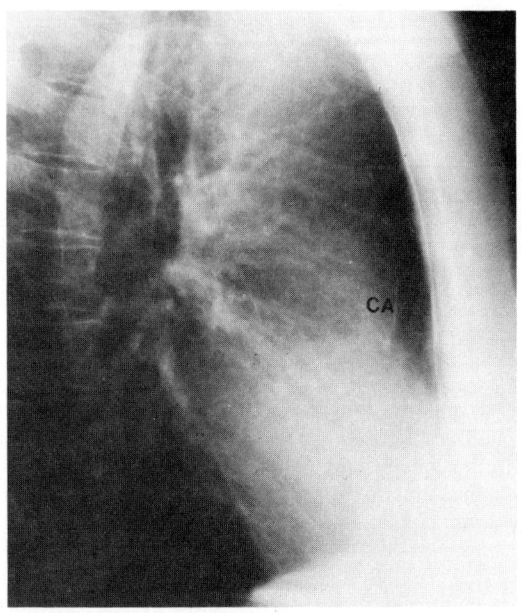

Figure 20–2. Lateral chest x-ray showing linear calcification (CA) of the ascending aorta in a patient with syphilitic aortitis.

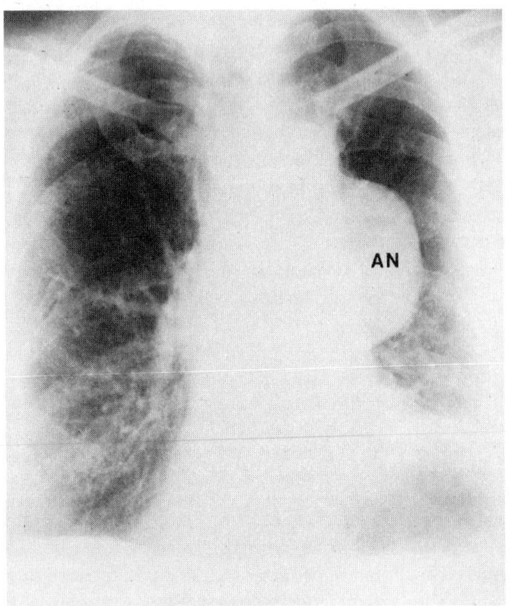

Figure 20–1. Chest x-ray showing a syphilitic aneurysm of the arch of the aorta (AN).

E. Special Investigations: Positive serologic tests for syphilis, either past or present, are most helpful in the diagnosis, but negative tests do not exclude the possibility of syphilitic disease any more than a positive test indicates that a given lesion is syphilitic. An elevated blood sedimentation rate is almost always seen when syphilitic cardiovascular disease is active and untreated. Cardiac catheterization and angiography are indicated if surgical treatment is contemplated. Angiography may be needed to distinguish aneurysms from other intrathoracic tumors; the procedure is generally well tolerated. The possibility of associated neurosyphilis should not be overlooked. Lumbar puncture should be performed in order to detect cerebrospinal fluid abnormalities associated with tertiary syphilis, tabes, or general paresis.

Differential Diagnosis

The differential diagnosis of syphilitic lesions is often difficult. Syphilitic aneurysms can be confused with intrathoracic tumors and cysts, and their luetic origin cannot always be proved. Atherosclerotic aneurysms can also occur; these are more likely to dissect than syphilitic aneurysms. Although positive serologic tests are of great value, they do not always indicate the true cause of the lesion. Furthermore, mixed lesions also occur. If there is any doubt about the diagnosis, eg, when a dilated aorta is found in a patient with weakly positive serology, a course of penicillin should be given.

Treatment

If syphilitic disease is active or progressive and especially if serologic tests are positive, antisyphilitic treatment with penicillin is indicated before any surgical measures are undertaken. Older remedies such as potassium iodide by mouth may be helpful in the control of pain and pressure symptoms. Penicillin treatment for syphilitic cardiovascular disease should be undertaken in the hospital, if possible, because of the possibility of a Jarisch-Herxheimer reaction. This involves a sudden acute allergic response attributed to massive death of spirochetes. It causes swelling of the aortic endothelium and may occlude the coronary ostia. Initial treatment should use a small (10,000 unit) test dose of penicillin combined with corticosteroids (eg, prednisone, 10–20 mg every 6 hours) for the first few doses. The treatment of choice for cardiovascular syphilis is benzathine penicillin G, 7.2 million units total, divided into weekly doses of 2.4 million units by intramuscular injection for 3 successive weeks. Alternative treatment consists of aqueous procaine penicillin G, 9 million units total, administered as 600,000 units a day by intramuscular injection for 15 days. In patients who are allergic to penicillin, tetracycline, 500 mg orally 4 times a day for 30 days, is recommended, or erythromycin, 500 mg orally 4 times a day for 30 days.

Surgical resection of syphilitic aneurysms and aortic valve replacement for aortic incompetence should always be considered. Direct surgery for ostial coronary lesions may be necessary. If the patient is asymptomatic and the disease shows no evidence of progression, the patient's progress should be monitored. The results of valve replacement in syphilitic lesions are similar to those obtained in operation on lesions due to other causes. The aorta in patients with syphilis holds sutures securely, and the tissues tend to be less friable than in Marfan's syndrome. The older operations that wrapped aneurysms and introduced materials to promote thrombus formation are no longer indicated, and resection with the insertion of Teflon grafts is now the treatment of choice.

Complications

Almost all the manifestations of syphilitic cardiovascular disease can be regarded as complications since endarteritis obliterans of the vasa vasorum, which is the basic lesion, has no direct effects, and expansion of the aorta is a secondary effect. Rupture of the aorta into any hollow thoracic structure is a late complication that is inevitably fatal. Thrombosis in association with stasis is common, but secondary embolism is rarer than in atherosclerotic lesions. Cardiac arrhythmias, complete heart block, infective endocarditis, and acute aortic dissection seldom occur. It should be remembered that the primary lesion is aortic and that cardiac involvement is almost always secondary, although gummatous myocarditis may be seen at autopsy.

Prognosis

The prognosis in syphilitic cardiovascular disease has greatly improved with better treatment of primary and secondary syphilis. Inadequately treated patients rather than untreated ones form the majority of cases. In partially arrested syphilitic disease, the patient develops a lesion in later life that progresses more slowly and carries a better prognosis. When the aortic valve is diseased, with significant aortic incompetence, the prognosis is worse. It is also worse when the aortic arch is involved in aneurysm formation because of the large number of vital structures that can be readily affected. The cause of death in patients with cardiovascular syphilis is now usually atherosclerotic in origin, and death in middle age (age 40–60) is rare.

ARTERITIS

Arteries of various sizes may be involved in an inflammatory process that can be either idiopathic or part of some generalized systemic disease. A clinical classification of the various vasculitis syndromes is presented in Table 20–1. The 3 types of lesions that produce arteritis as their main manifestation are temporal arteritis, aortic arch arteritis (Takayasu's disease),

Table 20–1. Clinical classification of vasculitis syndromes, indicating the wide variety of conditions in which the conditions may occur.*

Usually characterized by necrotizing vasculitis	
Temporal arteritis	Henoch-Schönlein purpura
Wegener's granulomatosis	"Classic" polyarteritis nodosa
Aortic arch arteritis	
Occasionally complicated by necrotizing vasculitis	
Rheumatic diseases	**Hypersensitivity**
Rheumatoid arthritis	Serum sickness
Systemic lupus erythematosus	Drug allergy
Dermatomyositis	Amphetamine abuse
Rheumatic fever	**Paraproteinemias**
Infections	Essential cryoglobulinemia
Hepatitis B	Multiple myeloma
Acute respiratory infections	Macroglobulinemia
Streptococcal infections	**Others**
Poststreptococcal glomerulonephritis	Dermal vasculitis
	Ulcerative colitis
Bacterial endocarditis	Cogan's syndrome
Respiratory diseases	Colon carcinoma
Löffler's syndrome	
Asthma	
Serous otitis media	

*Reproduced, with permission, from Christian CL, Sergent JS: Vasculitis syndromes: Clinical and experimental models. Am J Med 61:385, 1976.

and polyarteritis nodosa. In the other diseases, either the other manifestations predominate or the arteritis is a pathologic feature found on histologic examination.

The term temporal arteritis is not specific but refers to a form of arteritis that is usually associated with giant cell formation and involves the cranial arteries of older persons. Although the temporal arteries are a readily accessible site of lesions, their involvement is not inevitable, and the clinical picture overlaps that of Takayasu's disease.

Takayasu's disease (pulseless disease) is a form of arteritis that classically affects the aorta and its major branches, especially those leading to the head and upper limbs. Giant cell formation may be seen histologically, and smaller arteries can also be involved. Thrombosis of major vessels and embolization are the major manifestations. After several major aortic branches have been occluded, the pressure in the remaining vessels rises, because the heart pumps into a restricted vascular bed. This leads to cardiac hypertrophy and ultimately to left ventricular failure.

Polyarteritis nodosa is a multisystem disease of unknown cause that is usually considered one of the connective tissue disorders but is primarily a diffuse vasculitis with aneurysm formation involving the small arteries throughout the body. Diffuse vasculitis may occur as a variant of polyarteritis nodosa. James (1966, 1977) has noted that small coronary arteries varying from 0.1–1 mm in diameter may be involved, producing angina pectoris, myocardial infarction, and left ventricular failure with ventricular arrhythmias. The lesions in polyarteritis nodosa can occur anywhere in the body. The kidney, heart, gastrointestinal tract, lungs, and central nervous system are commonly affected. Because of the variability of the site and severity of the individual lesions, the clinical features can mimic almost any disease.

Clinical Findings

A. Symptoms: The symptoms of arteritis vary widely with the site of the lesion. In temporal arteritis, the principal presenting symptom is headache with a throbbing swelling over the affected artery. Fever, malaise, visual disturbance–blurring of vision or even sudden blindness–or neurologic disturbances are commonly seen. In other cases, the disease is more general, and arthralgia, abdominal pain, or chest pain may be the presenting symptom. In Takayasu's disease, the effects of sudden occlusion of a major vessel may be the first manifestation, eg, limb pain, hemiplegia, or sudden blindness. The presenting symptoms of polyarteritis nodosa are extremely variable.

B. Signs: The signs of arteritis, like the symptoms, vary widely. As an example, the major clinical features in 107 cases of Takayasu's disease are shown in Table 20–2. Loss of the pulse of a major vessel and a bruit over a vessel are the commonest signs, and systemic hypertension is also a prominent feature. Systemic hypertension is also common in polyarteritis nodosa; in consequence, cardiac enlargement, fundal changes, and proteinuria are often seen. The age of the patient varies in the different forms of arteritis. Temporal arteritis commonly occurs in women over age 50, whereas Takayasu's disease is most frequently seen in young women 20–30 years of age. Polyarteritis nodosa is more common in men than in women and occurs at any age.

C. Electrocardiographic Findings: ECG changes resulting from hypertension, with left ventricular hypertrophy and ST–T wave changes, may be seen. In some cases, actual myocardial infarction occurs, with consequent ECG changes.

D. X-Ray Findings: The heart is not infrequently enlarged, and signs of pulmonary congestion or infarction may develop.

E. Laboratory Findings and Special Investigations: Leukocytosis, perhaps with eosinophilia, is not uncommon. The sedimentation rate is raised, and tests of renal function often show impairment. Biopsy of an easily accessible lesion constitutes the most important means of establishing the diagnosis. The classic picture of arteritis may be found in any organ, and examples are shown in Figs 20–3 and 20–4. Skin, muscle, and

Table 20–2. Major clinical features of patients with Takayasu's arteritis.*

	No. of Cases	Percent
General symptoms	84	78
Asthenia	60	56
Weight loss	24	22
Fever	20	18
Cardiovascular		
Dyspnea on exertion	78	72
Paroxysmal dyspnea	20	18
Palpitations	47	43
Angina pectoris	12	11
Intermittent claudication	32	29
Pulse deficit	103	96
Vascular bruits	101	94
Valvular bruits		
Mitral regurgitation	6	5
Aortic regurgitation	8	7
Heart failure	38	35
High blood pressure	78	72
Neurologic		
Headaches	61	57
Syncope	14	13
Hemiplegia	8	7
Visual disturbances	9	8
Abnormal fundi†	44	41
Abdominal		
Vomiting	21	19
Diarrhea	10	10
Pain	8	7
Miscellaneous		
Arthralgias	57	53
Palpable cervical nodes	28	26

*Modified and reproduced, with permission, from Lupi-Herrera E & others: Takayasu's arteritis: Clinical study of 107 cases. Am Heart J 93:94, 1977.

†Keith-Wagener classification of fundi.

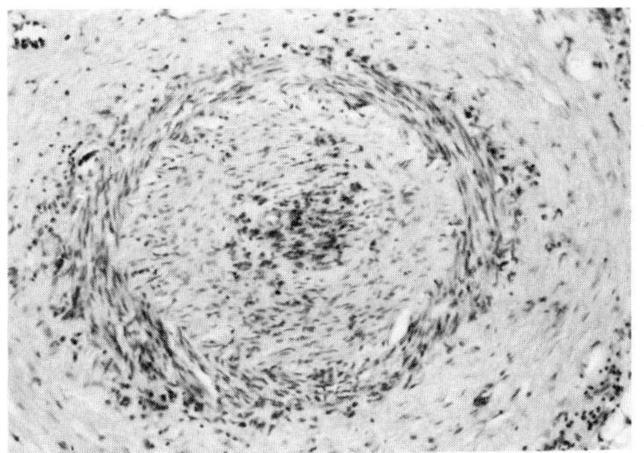

Figure 20–3. Mesenteric occlusive vasculitis in a patient using amphetamines to excess. (Magnification X 40, H&E stain.) (Courtesy of O Rambo.)

renal biopsy are often used. In difficult cases, help can sometimes be obtained from selective angiography. For example, mesenteric angiography may demonstrate multiple small aneurysms on the arteries to the gut.

Differential Diagnosis

The differential diagnosis of arteritis covers almost the entire range of medicine. The possibility of arteritis must be borne in mind with any patient in whom more than one organ system is involved.

Complications

Blindness, hemiplegia, myocardial infarction (left heart failure), renal failure, and systemic embolization are some of the more severe complications of arteritis. Almost any complication can occur, and the diseases generally run a steadily progressive course.

Treatment

The treatment of arteritis is unsatisfactory. Corticosteroids are commonly used and there is evidence that they can prevent and even reverse blindness in some cases. If hypertension is a feature, the blood pressure should be reduced with antihypertensive drugs (see Chapter 9). Immunosuppressive drugs (eg, azathioprine) have been used, particularly in polyarteritis nodosa, but their effectiveness is not established.

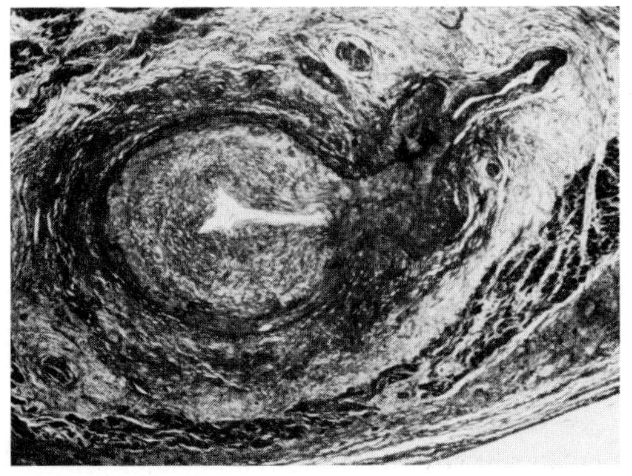

Figure 20–4. Inflammation in a coronary artery of a patient with polyarteritis nodosa. (Courtesy of O Rambo.)

Prognosis

The prognosis is poor, especially when renal or left heart failure occurs. Most patients die within 5 years.

SYSTEMIC EMBOLISM

Systemic embolism is an important complication of a number of heart diseases, including valvular and congenital heart disease, infective endocarditis, and myocardial infarction, which have been discussed elsewhere in this book. This section deals with embolism that is apparently unrelated to heart disease as well as embolism that has an established cardiac cause. It also deals more extensively with the manifestations and treatment of systemic embolism affecting particular parts of the systemic arterial bed.

Factors Promoting Thrombosis

The 3 factors promoting thrombosis in the left side of the heart and great vessels are stasis, changes in composition of the blood, and endothelial damage. Stasis is associated both with dilatation of such chambers as the left atrium, left ventricle, and aorta and with ineffective contraction, as occurs in atrial fibrillation and myocardial infarction. Changes in composition of the blood may be due to hemoconcentration, polycythemia, or an increase in the number or stickiness of platelets, as occurs in certain blood diseases. Endothelial damage is usually the result of inflammation (using the term in its widest sense to include trauma, ischemic necrosis, mechanical damage, and infections). The role of drugs, especially oral contraceptive agents, is also important in the development of thrombosis. Such drugs increase blood lipids and platelet stickiness and have been demonstrated to increase the chances of thromboembolism.

The Nature of Embolic Material

Not all embolism is due to the accumulation of thrombotic material. Emboli composed of microorganisms, especially fungi from exuberant vegetations, can cause important damage. Valve tissue, artificial valve material, pieces of tumor (as in left atrial myxoma), foreign bodies (eg, in drug addicts), calcium, and aggregates of platelets and fibrin from heart valves or atheromatous lesions may cause embolism.

The clinical consequences of embolism vary widely. This fact is explained by the great variety of materials forming the embolus and by the differences in the age and size of the thrombus that breaks off to form the embolus. Fresh red thrombus is the commonest form of embolic material. Because it is often readily lysed by the defense mechanisms of the body, in many cases the clinical effects of embolism, although severe and dramatic at onset, are relatively short-lived and are followed by complete or almost complete recovery. In contrast, if organized thrombus, calcium, tumor material, or a large mass of candida organisms constitutes the embolus, the obstruction to the blood vessel is permanent.

The State of the Arterial Bed

The state of the arterial bed where the embolus lodges is an important variable in the clinical picture. Healthy young persons with normal blood vessels and a well-marked capacity to develop good collateral circulation withstand embolism better than do older, more atherosclerotic persons in whom degenerative changes have already occurred. Thus, age and age-related disease influence the clinical effects of embolism. Local spasm of the embolized vessel can also suddenly occur in response to the impact of the embolus, and such spasms aggravate the acute manifestations of an embolus. The role played by secondary thrombosis in exacerbating the damage also varies, and in some cases thrombosis of the vein accompanying the embolized artery leads to secondary pulmonary embolism. If the embolus contains viable virulent organisms, abscesses may occur. If the organisms are less virulent, they may simply weaken the wall of the artery, and a mycotic aneurysm may form, as in some forms of infective endocarditis.

Specific Sites of Embolism

Many emboli lodge in sites where they provoke no clinical manifestations. Skeletal muscles harbor emboli without any signs of disease. The kidneys are also capable of accommodating emboli, and scars from infarcts that have occurred at various times are occasionally seen at autopsy in patients who have died of congestive heart failure. The liver with its double arterial blood supply is seldom if ever the site of infarction except in polyarteritis nodosa. The visceral manifestations of embolism generally occur as infarction, with death and necrosis of tissue, which is clinically recognizable only when the infarction is large or strategically placed or when it interferes with organ function. The central nervous system is the prime site for embolism that is likely to cause symptoms and signs. Even here, however, areas of infarction are found at autopsy in patients who had no clinical manifestations of any lesion.

A. Cerebral Embolism:

1. **In patients with heart disease**—Embolic material lodged in the brain produces the most serious and dramatic clinical manifestations of embolism. The onset is instantaneous, often with loss of consciousness or convulsions. Neurologic damage is most severe at onset. Hemiplegia, aphasia, and loss of vision are the commonest acute severe manifestations. Almost any clinical neurologic picture can occur, but an instantaneous, dramatic onset is the most characteristic feature. Spasm of the cerebral vessels and cerebral edema tend to make initial damage seem greater than it is, and recovery of function, although variable, is frequently remarkably rapid and surprisingly complete.

The physician's course of action in treating a patient who has just suffered a cerebral embolism depends on the certainty of the diagnosis of cerebral embolism. If the physician has not seen the patient before, the heart should be examined carefully for evidence of valvular disease, and a history of possible heart disease should be elicited from relatives. The possibility of expectant treatment is greater when the diagnosis is confirmed. Head injury, subarachnoid hemorrhage, cerebral thrombosis, and intracerebral hemorrhage must be ruled out, and the patient must be closely watched for evidence of clinical deterioration or recovery. The foot of the bed should be raised and oxygen administered by face mask. The addition of CO_2 to act as a cerebral vasodilator has been advocated, but there is little or no evidence that this procedure is beneficial. Systemic vasodilators should be avoided because they tend to reduce cerebral perfusion pressure. Lumbar puncture is indicated if there is any doubt about the diagnosis. The cerebrospinal fluid is seldom if ever hemorrhagic in cases of embolism. Cerebral angiography is not indicated since embolectomy is never performed in cases of spontaneous cerebral embolism involving intracranial vessels. The place of anticoagulant therapy in the treatment of cerebral embolism is not clear. Hemorrhage into the area of infarction and secondary thrombosis around the site of embolism can occur and exacerbate neurologic damage. The most logical course is to continue anticoagulant therapy if the patient has already been given anticoagulants and to withhold it in all other cases. In comparison with the prognosis in cerebral hemorrhage or cerebral thrombosis, the prognosis in cerebral embolism without anticoagulant therapy is sufficiently good that striking evidence of therapeutic benefit would be necessary to justify the use of anticoagulants in all patients.

Rehabilitation of the patient should be started as soon as possible. Improvement in nervous system function tends to occur at an exponentially decreasing rate over a 2-year period after the episode of embolism. Complete or almost complete recovery occurs in over 80% of patients with mitral valve disease who suffer cerebral embolism from left atrial thrombus. However, recovery seldom occurs if endocarditis is the cause of the embolus. The management of patients with mitral disease in whom cerebral embolus has occurred is not altered by the embolus. Mitral valve surgery is performed if indicated but not solely because of the embolus. The indications for restoration of sinus rhythm by cardioversion are similar to those in patients without embolism.

Embolism is, if anything, more common after valve replacement than before the operation, and restoration of sinus rhythm is likely to be only temporary unless the atrial fibrillation is of recent onset. Another embolus may well occur when atrial fibrillation recurs. Anticoagulant therapy is recommended by many, but it does not always prevent embolism. Because of the danger of hemorrhage into the area of infarction, an embolus involving the cerebral circulation in a patient who has been given full doses of anticoagulants is likely to be more serious than in a patient who has not received anticoagulants.

2. In patients without heart disease—A different form of cerebral embolism frequently occurs in patients with atherosclerotic lesions involving the vessels of the head. In this case, the clinical picture is different from that seen in patients with heart lesions. The emboli are smaller and much more likely to be multiple, and the entire clinical picture is much more insidious, causing symptoms that have been labeled as transient ischemic attacks. Small aggregations of platelets and thrombi form on ulcerative atherosclerotic lesions in moderate-sized arteries such as the internal carotid or vertebral artery. Pieces of these thrombi dislodge and move to other areas, giving rise to repeated episodes, which resemble each other and always involve vessels distal to the lesion. Dizziness, sudden vertigo, weakness or paralysis, faintness, loss of speech, and sudden blindness are the common presenting features. A systolic bruit should be listened for in the neck and a full neurologic examination performed. Every attempt should be made to see the patient during an attack, when central nervous system abnormalities are more likely to be detected. The clinical picture is likely to be confused with that of arrhythmia, aortic stenosis, senile dementia, or central nervous system disease rather than that associated with embolism from thrombotic material accumulated in the heart.

Cerebral angiography is required for diagnostic purposes, and surgical treatment of extracranial lesions is indicated in addition to anticoagulant therapy. This treatment differs from that of cerebral embolism in patients with heart disease. In those patients, because the thrombus is larger and can lodge anywhere in the body, cerebral angiography is not indicated, and anticoagulant therapy may be dangerous.

B. Coronary Embolism: Coronary embolism presents a clinical picture that is indistinguishable from that of myocardial infarction due to atherosclerosis. Embolism presumably can occur without infarction and pass unnoticed in young patients and persons with excellent collateral blood supply. The onset of coronary embolism is instantaneous, and syndromes in which there is a gradual onset of chest pain are not seen. ECG changes develop in the usual manner, and the clinical course is usually benign if the source of the embolus is left atrial thrombus. The reason is that, in such cases, the embolic material (fresh red thrombus) is readily lysed. Embolism with calcific material in patients with aortic valve disease carries a much poorer prognosis. The treatment is similar to that in patients with lesions due to an atherosclerotic cause; in most cases, a period of rest under observation is all that is required. Management of the underlying heart disease is not altered by the occurrence of an embolus. The patient's status is reviewed and appropriate action initiated without using the embolus as an indication for any specific procedure.

C. Peripheral Embolism Involving the Extremities: It is rare for embolism involving the arms to cause symptoms sufficient to warrant treatment. Exceptions occur when the embolic material is not thrombus. In such cases embolectomy may be indicated. The commonest sites of embolization requiring urgent treatment are the external iliac and femoral arteries. If the embolus lodges farther down the leg, collateral circulation through the profunda femoris artery is usually sufficient to maintain adequate circulation unless significant atherosclerosis is also present. Femoral arterial occlusion usually causes an acute, severe pain in the leg, with loss of sensation, pallor, and a cold, pulseless limb.

The severe ischemic pain provides the most important indication for surgical treatment. The femoral artery is readily accessible in the groin, and the dangers of damaging distal tissues are negligible. It is not necessary to localize the site of the embolus accurately by means of angiography because balloon-tipped (Fogarty) catheters can be passed up and down the vessel and used to extract thrombus from areas not directly accessible through the incision. Any embolic material should always be saved for bacteriologic and histologic examination. The diagnosis of atrial myxoma has occasionally been accomplished by this means, and the nature of the infecting organism in endocarditis has been established by analysis of embolic material.

Surgical exploration should be undertaken as soon as possible after diagnosis. It can be conveniently carried out under local anesthesia. In the period before operation the limb should be kept cool in order to slow the metabolic processes. Meperidine (50–150 mg intramuscularly) should be given for relief of pain. Problems may arise if the patient is not seen until some time after an acute episode. Embolectomy can be beneficial even as long as a week after an acute episode, and the length of time that has elapsed since the embolism should not necessarily be taken as a contraindication to surgical exploration. In cases seen shortly after the acute episode, anticoagulation can be delayed until after operation. If surgery is not to be undertaken, anticoagulation with heparin should be given (5000–10,000 units intravenously every 4–6 hours), followed by warfarin (Coumadin), 30–50 mg on the first day, 10–15 mg on the second day, and a maintenance dose of 5–15 mg, depending on the prothrombin time, on later days. The heparin should be stopped on the third day when the prothrombin time is prolonged.

The prognosis following embolism in the leg depends mainly on the degree of atherosclerosis and consequently on the age of the patient. The prognosis is worse in patients with mural thrombi following myocardial infarction and in those with endocarditis. Intermittent claudication following the acute episode occurs occasionally, but in younger patients in whom the source of embolus is left atrial thrombus, recovery is usually complete.

D. Other Sites of Embolism: Mesenteric embolism causes severe epigastric pain of acute onset, with or without acute circulatory collapse. Mesenteric embolism must be differentiated from other acute abdominal emergencies. Melena occurs within a few hours, followed by paralytic ileus with vomiting and abdominal distention. Surgical exploration with bowel resection is often performed, but the results are not uniformly good. As with all other forms of systemic embolism, expectant treatment can sometimes give good results, especially if the embolus moves to a more distal site and blood flow is thereby restored. Anticoagulant therapy is contraindicated because hemorrhage into the gut is almost always present.

Renal embolism seldom causes significant difficulties. Hematuria and renal colic associated with the passage of blood clots or dull flank pain due to the embolus itself are the commonest manifestations. Acute renal failure is rarely seen. Renal embolism may be followed by hypertension (see Chapter 9). Studies of renal function and renal angiography in patients with mitral stenosis and systemic hypertension have shown evidence of segmental renal ischemia, and embolism should be considered when systemic hypertension is seen in association with mitral valve disease—especially when atrial fibrillation is present.

Splenic embolism may cause left upper quadrant pain and tenderness and may be associated with perisplenitis, a friction rub, and pain that is worse on inspiration. Mild analgesics are usually all that are required.

Investigation of Causes of Embolism

It is not uncommon for the patient to present with one or more acute episodes and symptoms highly suggestive of embolism. There may be no obvious signs of heart disease to account for the episodes. Careful examination of the heart reveals no evidence of valvular disease. The heart is not enlarged and the ECG is within normal limits. In such cases cardiac catheterization, pulmonary angiography, and complete examination of the left heart chambers are often performed, especially in order to rule out a lesion that is amenable to surgery, such as left atrial myxoma. In our experience, such studies have not as yet shown that a previously unsuspected intracardiac cause was responsible for embolism, but such cases have been reported.

Ulcerative atheromatous lesions in the aorta or in the carotid artery should also be considered as possible causes. If the lesions are confined to some specific part of the circulation, a lesion in the artery supplying that area (eg, a vessel in the head) may be suspected as the cause. In most cases in which the cause is not immediately obvious and emboli involve more than one area, an explanation is not found. Paradoxic embolism via a patent foramen ovale is sometimes suggested as a cause, but this is difficult to prove or disprove until autopsy. Embolism has always been a common postmortem finding in both the systemic and the pulmonary circulations. In dying patients circulation is often extremely sluggish in the period just before death. Small nodular thrombotic (marantic) lesions are not uncommonly found on the heart valves at autopsy, particularly in patients dying of malignant disease. However, these lesions are clinically unimportant because they are virtually impossible to diagnose during life and because they do not give rise to embolism.

SYSTEMIC ARTERIOVENOUS FISTULA

A systemic arteriovenous fistula provides a low-resistance pathway through which blood can flow from the high-pressure arterial bed into the low-pressure venous system. The volume flow rate through the fistula depends on the size of the communication and on the height of the arterial pressure above the venous pressure. If a normal blood flow is to be maintained to perfuse the body in the presence of a fistula, the cardiac output must be increased by an amount equal to the fistula flow. The fistula flow thus constitutes a constant unremitting load on the heart, and, if the fistula is large or if cardiac function is impaired, heart failure is likely to develop.

Systemic arteriovenous fistulas may be congenital, as in hemangiomatous lesions, or traumatic. The trauma may be due to stab or gunshot wounds that establish a communication between an artery and its adjacent vein, often in a limb. In some cases the trauma is surgical and inadvertent, and a fistula forms after an operation. Nephrectomy, cholecystectomy, and laminectomy are among the more common operations in which this complication occurs. In other cases, the systemic arteriovenous fistula is purposely created to provide ready access to a blood vessel with high flow for the treatment of renal failure by hemodialysis.

Pathophysiology

A systemic arteriovenous fistula is a prime cause of a high output state (see Chapter 10). A high output state also occurs in pregnancy, thyrotoxicosis, anemia, beriberi heart disease, and generalized Paget's disease of bone. The extra load on the heart resulting from a high output state gives rise to a number of secondary effects which become more important as the patient becomes older or cardiac function deteriorates.

When there is a systemic arteriovenous fistula, the baroreceptor mechanisms act to maintain a normal arterial blood pressure. The tendency for the arterial pressure to fall as blood leaks out of the arterial bed leads to tachycardia, increased cardiac output, and vasoconstriction in other beds which, unlike the fistula, are capable of responding to sympathetically mediated peripheral vasoconstriction. The increased cardiac work constitutes a constant extra load on the heart that varies with the size of the fistula. Although the load is well tolerated if the fistula is small and the patient is young, problems arise when the fistula is large (30% increase in resting output) or when age-related changes such as atherosclerosis or hypertension are present. When the load on the heart is so great that adequate perfusion of the body—especially the kidneys—cannot be maintained, a form of heart failure called high output failure develops.

High output failure. Some increase in blood volume occurs in any arteriovenous fistula that is large enough to increase the resting cardiac output significantly. When renal perfusion is inadequate, further increase in blood volume with salt retention and edema occur. This increases the load on the heart. The left ventricular and later the right ventricular end-diastolic pressures rise, and the patient develops heart failure. The picture that results is remarkable in that the peripheral vasoconstriction, weak pulse, and hypodynamic cardiac impulse with cool extremities and peripheral cyanosis seen in low output failure are replaced by a bounding pulse, warm moist palms, a hyperdynamic cardiac impulse, warm limbs, and pink skin. The acuteness of the onset of the load, its magnitude, and its duration are important variables determining the clinical picture.

Clinical Findings

A. Symptoms: The patient is sometimes aware of the flow through the fistula, which gives rise to a buzzing sensation localized to the affected area. Palpitations, fatigue, and dyspnea are seen, but, in general, exercise tolerance is well maintained, because the fall in systemic resistance with exercise tends to decrease the fistula flow. The patient may notice that the skin near the fistula is warmer than normal and notice overgrowth of blood vessels around the site of the lesion.

B. Signs: The pulse is bounding and the heart rate increased. The pulse pressure is increased and the skin warm and moist. If the fistula is in a limb, that limb often grows to be longer than the opposite one, and tortuous varicose veins develop near the site of the fistula. Increased venous pressure occurs late in the disease. The heart is often enlarged, with a hyperdynamic cardiac impulse and a loud first sound. Third and fourth heart sounds may be heard, and a systolic murmur not infrequently develops in association with the increased stroke volume. A palpable and audible bruit is also detectable over the site of the fistula. This sign is of most help when the fistula is in the abdomen or back. If the fistula is accessible and can be occluded by manual compression, its clinical significance can be assessed. If the fistula is significant, its occlusion raises the systemic vascular resistance and provokes a baroreceptor response. This consists of bradycardia and peripheral vasodilatation. The fall in heart rate on occlusion and the increase on release (Branham's sign) constitute the best means of assessing a fistula at the bedside. In older patients and those with renal failure, this simple test is less reliable, and a significant fistula can be present in a patient in whom Branham's sign is negative.

C. Electrocardiographic Findings: Tachycardia and minor changes indicative of left ventricular overload (high-voltage QRS complexes and ST–T wave changes in the left ventricular leads) are seen. Significant hypertensive changes may be present in patients undergoing dialysis.

D. X-Ray Findings: The heart is usually enlarged, with a left ventricular configuration, and serial chest x-rays are valuable in demonstrating progressive enlargement. Pulmonary congestion is only seen in the late stages, when heart failure is present.

E. Special Investigations: Blood volume is increased in most cases of fistula of significant degree, and mild anemia is seen because it is the plasma volume that is raised. Echocardiography shows the left ventricle to be dilated and overactive, with evidence of excessive wall motion. Cardiac catheterization is not indicated for diagnosis, but if it is performed, the intracardiac pressures are found to be relatively normal and the cardiac output raised.

Differential Diagnosis

Systemic arteriovenous fistula must be distinguished from other forms of high output state, eg, pregnancy, thyrotoxicosis, beriberi, anemia, and Paget's disease. Heart failure due to hypertensive or atherosclerotic disease or cardiomyopathy may be confused with or associated with the effects of a fistula, especially in patients undergoing hemodialysis. The possibility that the fistula is playing a part in cardiac problems must always be kept in mind in such patients, especially when the stress of anemia is added. In addition, the development of heart failure after a surgical operation should raise the possibility that an arteriovenous fistula has been accidentally created.

Complications

A fistula may become infected, leading to endarteritis with subsequent hemorrhage or embolism. The fistula may progressively increase in size as the abnormal blood vessels grow in response to increased flow through them, or spontaneous thrombosis of the fistula may occur. Heart failure is the most important complication, and the purpose of treatment is to prevent its development.

Treatment

Any arteriovenous fistula that is of clinical significance—one causing bradycardia on occlusion or one large enough to increase heart size—should be closed if possible. Traumatic fistulas and those accidentally created at surgery are usually readily dealt with surgically, but hemorrhage may be difficult to control at operation. Congenital malformations with arteriovenous fistulas often recur after surgical attempts to eradicate them. Fistulas that are created to facilitate hemodialysis may have to be reduced in size if they cause too large a cardiac load; if they become thrombosed, another fistula may have to be created.

Treatment of high output failure with digitalis and diuretics is generally less effective than in the treatment of low output failure, and elimination of the fistula or at least reduction of its size is the treatment of choice.

Prognosis

The prognosis of systemic arteriovenous fistula

depends on the ease with which its cardiovascular effects can be eliminated. The results are worst in patients with large congenital malformations. The prognosis of patients with renal failure undergoing hemodialysis should not be influenced by the fistula. A fistula large enough to provide an adequate route for dialysis can be achieved without compromising cardiac function in almost every case.

• • •

References

Christian CL, Sergent JS: Vasculitis syndromes: Clinical and experimental models. Am J Med 61:385, 1976.

Cohen SM & others: Cardiac output and peripheral bloodflow in arteriovenous aneurysm. Clin Sci 7:35, 1948.

Conn DL & others: Immunologic mechanisms in systemic vasculitis. Mayo Clin Proc 51:511, 1976.

Crane C: Atheromatous embolism to lower extremities in arteriosclerosis. Arch Surg 94:96, 1967.

Cryer PE, Kissane J (editors): Multiple arterial occlusions in a young woman. Am J Med 59:837, 1975.

Dale WA (editor): *Management of Arterial Occlusive Disease.* Year Book, 1971.

Edwards EA: Acute peripheral arterial occlusion. JAMA 223:909, 1973.

Ehrenfeld WK, Hoyt WF, Wylie EJ: Embolization and transient blindness from carotid atheroma. Arch Surg 93:787, 1966.

Fogarty TJ, Cranley JJ: Catheter technic for arterial embolectomy. Ann Surg 161:325, 1965.

Fogarty TJ & others: A method for extraction of arterial emboli and thrombi. Surg Gynecol Obstet 116:241, 1963.

Ghose MK, Shensa S, Lerner PI: Arteritis of the aged (giant cell arteritis) and fever of unexplained origin. Am J Med 60:429, 1976.

Gomes MMR, Bernatz PE: Arteriovenous fistulas: A review and 10-year experience at the Mayo Clinic. Mayo Clin Proc 45:81, 1970.

Hamilton CR Jr, Shelly WM, Tumulty PA: Giant cell arteritis: Including temporal arteritis and polymyalgia rheumatica. Medicine 50:1, 1971.

Hemodynamic consequences of an arteriovenous fistula: Medical Staff Conference, University of California, San Francisco. Calif Med 117:38, Oct 1972.

Holman E: *Arteriovenous Aneurysms.* Macmillan, 1937.

Holsinger DR, Osmundson PJ, Edwards JE: The heart in periarteritis nodosa. Circulation 25:610, 1962.

Hoye SJ & others: Atheromatous embolization: A factor in peripheral gangrene. N Engl J Med 261:128, 1959.

Hunder GG & others: Daily and alternate-day corticosteroid regimens in treatment of giant cell arteritis: Comparison in a prospective study. Ann Intern Med 82:613, 1975.

James TN: Small arteries of the heart. Circulation 56:2, 1977.

James TN, Birk RE: Pathology of the cardiac conduction system in polyarteritis nodosa. Arch Intern Med 117:561, 1966.

Jones E, Bedford DE: Syphilitic angina pectoris. Br Heart J 5:107, 1943.

Klein RG & others: Large artery involvement in giant cell (temporal) arteritis. Ann Intern Med 83:806, 1975.

Love WS, Werner CG: Observations upon syphilis of the heart, coronary ostia and coronary arteries: With special reference to the myocardial lesions noted in stenosis of the coronary ostia. Am J Syphilis 18:154, 1934.

Lupi-Herrera E & others: Takayasu's arteritis: Clinical study of 107 cases. Am Heart J 93:94, 1977.

Roberts WC, Wibin EA: Idiopathic panaortitis, supra-aortic arteritis, granulomatous myocarditis and pericarditis. Am J Med 41:453, 1966.

Rose GA, Spencer H: Polyarteritis nodosa. Q J Med 26:43, 1957.

Schrire V: Arteritis of the aorta and its major branches. Australas Ann Med 16:33, 1967.

Strachan RW: The natural history of Takayasu's arteriopathy. Q J Med 33:57, 1964.

Szilagyi DE & others: Peripheral congenital arteriovenous fistulas. Surgery 57:61, 1965.

Thompson JE & others: Arterial embolectomy: A 20-year experience with 163 cases. Surgery 67:212, 1970.

Wylie EJ, Ehrenfeld WK: *Extracranial Occlusive Cerebrovascular Disease: Diagnosis and Management.* Saunders, 1970.

21 . . .
Cardiac Tumors & Miscellaneous Forms of Heart Disease

CARDIAC TUMORS

Cardiac tumors are more frequently metastatic than primary. While pathologic evidence of cardiac or pericardial involvement can be found in about 10% of autopsies in patients with malignant disease, the incidence of clinical manifestations is less. As shown in Table 21–1, the site of the primary is most often in the lung or the breast, indicating that the tumor is likely to spread locally to involve the heart or pericardium. Various types of lymphoma also tend to involve the heart, again mainly by spread from the mediastinum. Metastases seldom affect left ventricular function, although when pericardial effusion occurs, the patient may show manifestations of pericardial tamponade. The most common primary malignant tumors involving the heart are sarcomas of various types. The most common benign tumor of the heart is a myxoma–usually left atrial myxoma–although the right atrium may be involved and, more rarely, the ventricle.

A cardiac tumor may obstruct blood vessels in the region of the heart; may interfere with atrial or ventricular filling, either within or outside the cardiac chambers; or may involve the pericardium.

Clinical Findings

A. Symptoms: The presenting symptoms in patients with cardiac tumors are often bizarre and confusing. Posturally variable dyspnea, cough, and syncope can occur. Chest pain is not infrequent, and evidence of systemic or pulmonary congestion with dyspnea or edema is sometimes seen. In patients with metastases, there is often no clinical clue to involvement of the heart in the patient's history.

B. Signs: Evidence of pericardial involvement may be found with pericardial friction or increased venous pressure. In myxoma there are often changing murmurs, perhaps influenced by posture. The tumor is often pedunculated and is mobile, and the degree of obstruction to blood flow varies with posture and varying hemodynamic events. The patient may thus have a diastolic murmur in one body position but not in another. Careful search for evidence of embolism is always important, and the recovery of embolic material for histologic examination is sometimes of diagnostic value. In some cases of myxoma, systemic signs such as fever, tachycardia, and clubbing of the fingers are seen.

C. Electrocardiographic Findings: There are no specific ECG changes in cardiac tumors. High-voltage P waves have been reported in rare cases of myxoma, and P mitrale is sometimes seen. If pulmonary hypertension develops, there may be right ventricular hypertrophy on the ECG.

D. X-Ray Findings: Bizarre outlines of the cardiac

Table 21–1. Prevalence of cardiac and pericardial metastases and relative frequency of site of primary tumor.*

Source	Autopsies	Metastasis	Primary Tumor (Percent)					Total
			Lung	Breast	Lymphoma	Melanoma	Other	(Percent)
Scott & Garvin (1939)	1082	118 (10.9%) cardiac and pericardial	35	14	14	4.2	. . .	67.2
Prichard (1951)	4375	146 (3.3%) cardiac and pericardial	11	15	12	12	. . .	50
Lamberta & others (1951)	1032	31 (3.0%) pericardial	73	6	. . .	. . .	20	99
DeLoach & Hagues (1953)	980	137 (13.9%) cardiac and pericardial	16	8	46	9	. . .	79
Cohen & others (1955)	315	65 (20.6%) cardiac and pericardial	19	35	15	8	. . .	77
Nakayama & others (1965)	765	74 (9.7%) cardiac and pericardial	27	19	19	8	. . .	73

*Modified and reproduced, with permission, from Lokich JJ: The management of malignant pericardial effusions. JAMA 224:140, 1973. © 1973, American Medical Association.

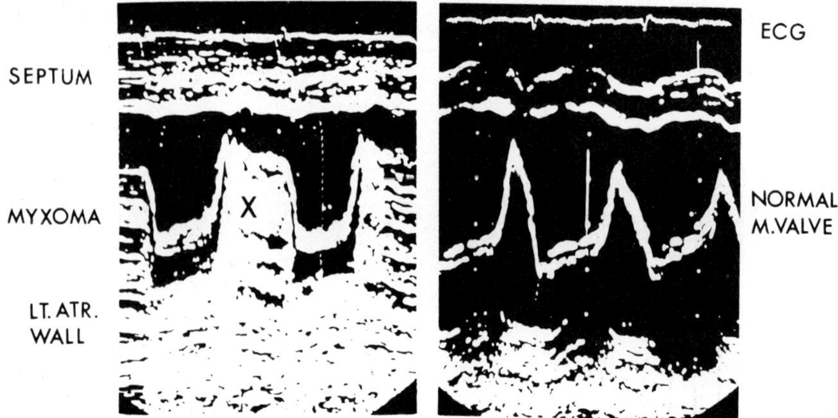

Figure 21–1. *Left:* Preoperative echocardiogram showing mass of echoes (X) posterior to the anterior mitral valve cusp in diastole continuous with the left atrial wall. In systole, no such echoes are present. Posterior descent of anterior mitral cusp is restricted. *Right:* In postoperative echocardiogram, mass of echoes posterior to the anterior mitral valve cusp is no longer present, and descent of the cusp in diastole is normal. Atrial fibrillation is present. (Reproduced, with permission, from Srivastava TN, Fletcher E: The echocardiogram in left atrial myxoma. Am J Med 54:136, 1973.)

shadow and enlargement of the heart shadow due to pericardial effusion should be sought. Left atrial enlargement is seen in left atrial myxoma in many cases.

E. Laboratory Findings and Special Investigations: A raised sedimentation rate, anemia, and raised serum globulin are sometimes seen in myxomas. Echocardiography can be helpful in showing dense multiple echoes posterior to the anterior mitral valve leaflet in diastole. Pre- and postoperative echocardiograms in a patient with left atrial myxoma are shown in Fig 21–1. The results of echocardiography are not always so dramatic, and the tumor can be missed. Full studies with right and left heart catheterization and angiography are always needed before exploration is undertaken. Raised atrial or venous pressures on the right or left side are usually found, and in left atrial myxoma pulmonary congestion with perhaps a raised pulmonary vascular resistance is common. The tumors are usually slow-growing, and the disease is therefore insidious. Angiography is most useful in diagnosis. Left atrial myxoma can often be seen on left ventricular angiography. The small amount of mitral incompe-

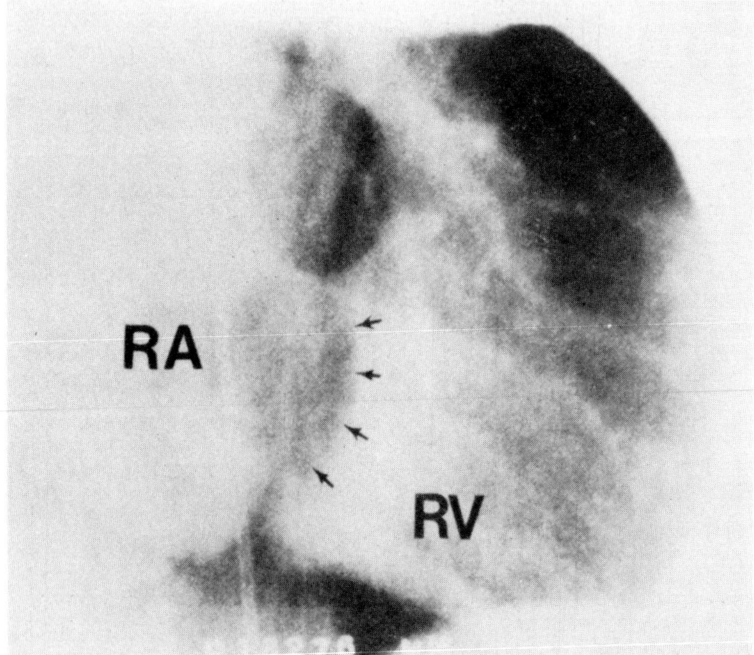

Figure 21–2. Right atrial angiocardiogram in 30-degree right anterior oblique view. Arrows indicate edge of filling defect. RA, right atrium; RV, right ventricle. (Reproduced, with permission, from Berman ND & others: Angiographic demonstration of blood supply of right atrial myxoma. Br Heart J 38:764, 1976.)

tence that often accompanies left ventricular injections of contrast material may outline the tumor, and the motion of the myxoma as it moves up and down with the heartbeat can sometimes be seen. Examples of angiograms in patients with right atrial (Fig 21–2) and left atrial (Fig 21–3) myxomas show how filling defects can be demonstrated. In patients with other forms of primary or secondary tumors, pericardiocentesis is often responsible for the establishment of the diagnosis when malignant cells are demonstrated in the fluid.

Differential Diagnosis

Left atrial myxoma is most likely to be confused with rheumatic disease of the mitral valve. The episodic nature of the symptoms and signs and the presence of systemic manifestations are the most useful features in diagnosis. Other primary or secondary tumors involving the heart can be confused with pericardial disease, with myocarditis or cardiomyopathy, or with valvular heart disease in some instances. The systemic manifestations of myxoma bring to mind many differential diagnoses, eg, infective endocarditis, connective tissue disorders, occult malignancy, and chronic infections.

Treatment

Surgical removal of a right or left atrial myxoma is usually curative, although the tumor may rarely recur. Malignant cardiac tumors are usually fatal

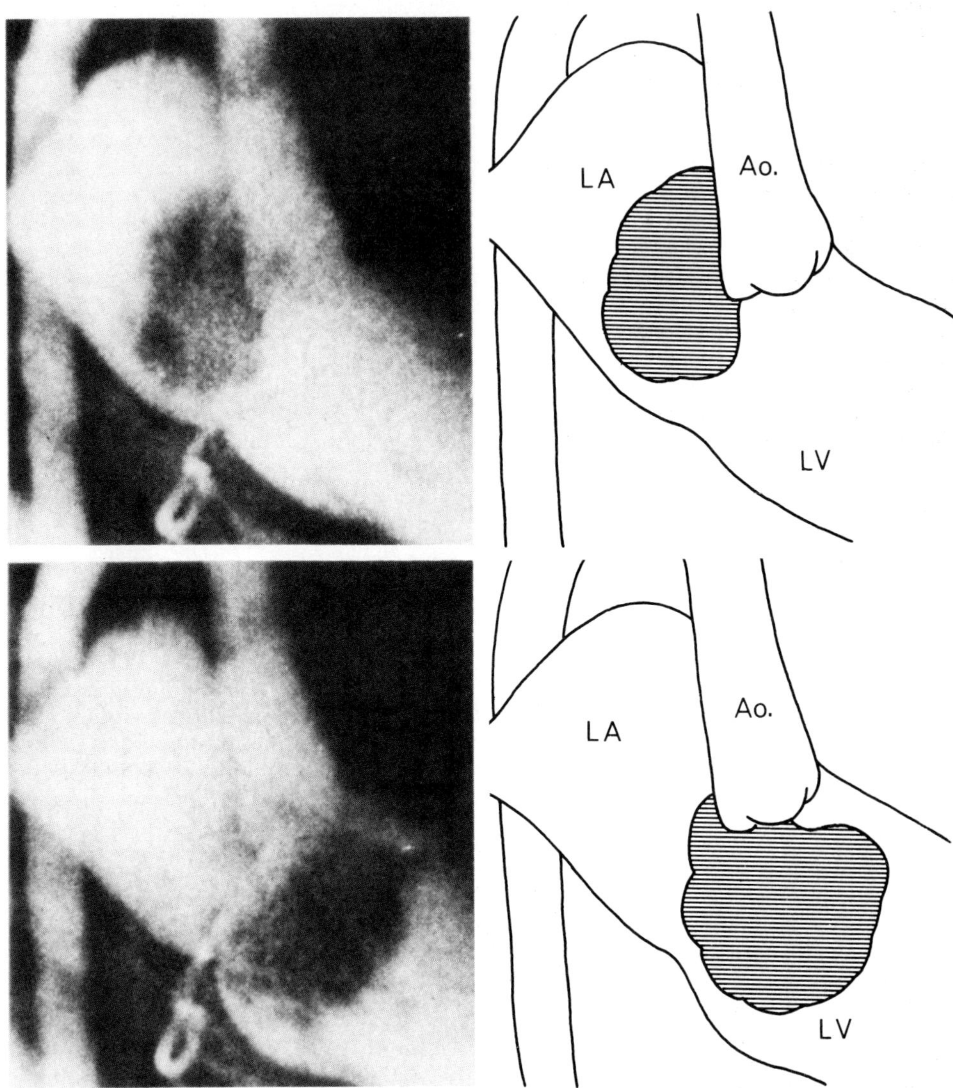

Figure 21–3. Two frames from a cineangiogram accompanied by explanatory drawings. In systole, the myxoma is in the left atrium; in diastole, it floats into the left ventricle. (Reproduced, with permission, from Selzer A, Sakai FJ, Popper RW: Protean clinical manifestations of primary tumors of the heart. Am J Med 52:9, 1972.)

whether they are metastatic or primary angiosarcomas. Malignant pericardial effusion from metastatic disease usually requires systemic chemotherapy combined with local instillation of chemicals or radiotherapy (or both) to the pericardium.

Prognosis

Without treatment, patients with atrial myxoma may gradually develop worsening symptoms of pulmonary or systemic venous congestion as the tumor grows. Sudden death may occur if the mitral valve becomes totally obstructed. Pulmonary emboli in right atrial myxoma may lead to severe pulmonary symptoms and, if repeated, to pulmonary hypertension and right heart failure. Systemic emboli from left atrial myxoma may lead to hemiplegia, loss of a limb, or other severe vascular occlusions. Systemic symptoms of fever, arthralgia, and fatigue may cause chronic invalidism until one of the major cardiac or embolic catastrophes occurs.

HYPOTENSION

Hypotension should be regarded as a symptom rather than a disease. Since gravity is the most significant force affecting the cardiovascular system, it is not surprising that hypotension is ordinarily more apparent when the patient stands upright and that the compensatory mechanisms maintaining arterial pressure are more severely stressed in the standing than in the recumbent position.

Causes of Hypotension

Hypotension results from inadequate cardiac output, as in myocardial infarction; from inadequate circulating blood volume; or from failure of the normal reflex mechanisms that maintain a constant arterial pressure. All these factors operate in a number of disorders, and several may combine in a given patient to cause the primary symptom of hypotension–dizziness or faintness–which is made worse when the patient suddenly stands up.

Disturbances of blood volume are clinically more common than disturbances of reflex control of the circulation, and they stem from 2 factors. One is a decrease in plasma or red cell volume due to hemorrhage, fluid loss, diarrhea, vomiting, unrecognized internal hemorrhage, dehydration, excessive diuresis, or excessive sweating; the other is a change in capacity of a blood-filled compartment (heart, arteries, capillaries, or veins).

Decreased blood volume as a cause of hypotension is particularly striking in adrenal insufficiency disorders, eg, Addison's disease and hypopituitarism. Wasting disorders of the bowel associated with diarrhea and anemia are also commonly associated with hypotension, and a sudden episode of faintness with hypotension is often the first manifestation of gastrointestinal hemorrhage.

Abnormalities of reflex control of arterial pressure usually result from disease of the central nervous system and its autonomic pathways. Disease may also affect the peripheral parts of the autonomic nervous system via innervation of blood vessels that are particularly susceptible to the effect of drugs.

Clinical Features

The clinical picture of hypotension associated with an inadequate blood volume is dominated by the effects of the compensatory mechanisms that are mediated by the autonomic nervous system. These effects cause anxiety, weakness, palpitations, tachycardia, restlessness, vasoconstriction, sweating, pallor, and cold extremities. In contrast, in hypotension associated with autonomic nervous system disease, the patient faints, with few or no accompanying symptoms. Dizziness and dimness of vision usually give little warning of impending loss of consciousness. Recovery is rapid when cerebral blood flow is restored with the patient in the recumbent position.

Hypotension Associated With Inadequate Blood Volume

A. Vasovagal Attacks and Fainting: The commonest form of hypotension is that seen in simple fainting. A sudden muscular vasodilatation mediated by cholinergic sympathetic nerves results in an acute fall in effective blood volume owing to sudden pooling of blood in peripheral areas of the body (normally the legs). Simple fainting occurs in normal subjects and may also be provoked by disease, especially myocardial infarction with or without pain. Fainting may also occur during cardiologic investigations. The vagus nerve plays an important part in the mechanism of fainting, and simple faints are sometimes called vasovagal attacks. The primary stimulus to simple fainting may be physical or psychic. Trauma, pain, or stimulation of vagal afferents–especially in the ascending aorta near the right coronary ostium–may cause hypotension, even in recumbent subjects. Fear, the sight of blood, observing trauma to others, or seeing other people faint may all cause hypotension. Premonitory symptoms include feeling alternately hot and cold, yawning, sweating, and an uneasy or sinking feeling in the epigastrium. The patient looks pale and develops bradycardia before the ultimate sudden acute muscular vasodilatation occurs.

B. Prevention and Treatment of Fainting Attacks: Fainting attacks can be aborted by lying down or raising the legs or by administering intravenous atropine (0.4–0.8 mg). A tendency to faint is aggravated by all the factors causing low blood volume and also by a hot environment, prolonged standing, an empty stomach, pregnancy, suddenly standing up, nervousness, and novel surroundings. Fainting seldom occurs spontaneously in supine subjects, but it can readily be provoked during arterial puncture or coronary artery catheterization. If the patient has lost consciousness, recovery may take 15–45 minutes. The earlier restorative measures are instituted, the sooner recovery occurs. Raising the legs and administering atropine are specific remedies. Vasoconstrictive drugs such as norepinephrine and angiotensin have no place in treatment.

Bradycardia is the most important indication that reflex factors are involved in syncope in patients with hypotension. Dramatic improvement occurs after the administration of atropine in patients with myocardial infarction in whom reflex hypotension has occurred. A short period of cerebral and cardiac hypoperfusion is relatively harmless in healthy young subjects, but disastrous consequences may result in older atherosclerotic patients with cerebral or coronary arterial disease and in those with aortic or pulmonary stenosis. Cerebral and myocardial infarction may result, and ventricular arrhythmia may occur during periods of marked vagal bradycardia. The role of simple vasovagal attacks causing sudden death in patients with heart disease is not known.

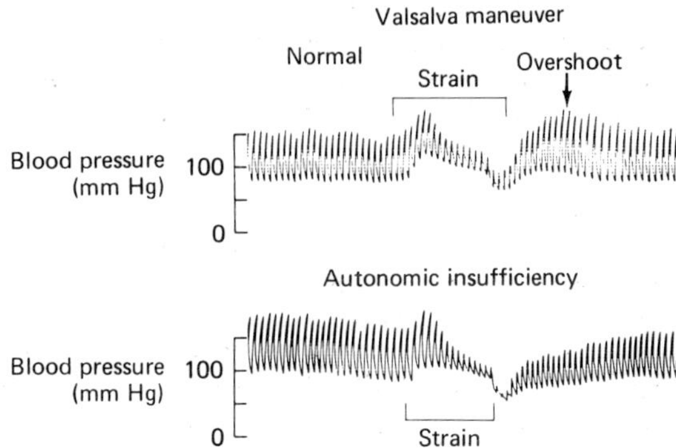

Figure 21–5. Arterial pressure tracings from a normal subject and a patient with tabes dorsalis and autonomic nervous system insufficiency. There is a greater fall in pressure during the period of strain and no overshoot on release of pressure in the patient with autonomic nervous system insufficiency.

Hypotension Associated With Abnormal Reflex Control Mechanisms

A. Autonomic Insufficiency: Postural (orthostatic) hypotension due to disturbances of autonomic nervous system control is seldom seen in patients under age 50. It occurs in patients with diabetes mellitus or uremia associated with peripheral neuropathy, in tabes dorsalis, and in various types of degenerative central nervous system disease involving the basal ganglia. It also causes Shy-Drager syndrome, which resembles parkinsonism. At least 2 of the classic triad of symptoms–postural hypotension, impaired sweating, and loss of sexual function with impotence in men–are usually present. No associated disease is found in about one-third of cases. The diagnostic physical finding is a progressive fall in arterial pressure when the patient is standing or when the lower body is subjected to suction, as shown in Fig 21–4. There is little or no accompanying increase in heart rate. In the lower body suction procedure, the subject lies flat, with the legs and pelvis enclosed in an airtight box. Pressure in the box is reduced by sucking air out of the system at a rate sufficient to maintain a desired level of pressure around the legs.

A lack of overshoot in arterial pressure also occurs after Valsalva's maneuver, as shown in Fig 21–5. This finding should be sought in direct arterial pressure tracings because it cannot always be accurately assessed in noninvasive bedside studies using indirect methods. Sympatholytic (antihypertensive) drugs, diuretics, tranquilizers, potassium depletion, and primary aldosteronism also impair circulatory reflex reactivity. In some cases, myocardial infarction causes unexplained loss of autonomic nervous system function; in rare cases, autonomic insufficiency is seen in acute viral infections.

B. Treatment of Autonomic Insufficiency: The treatment of postural hypotension due to autonomic insufficiency consists of eliminating any factors that tend to reduce blood volume or impair circulatory reactivity. In addition, active measures to expand blood volume should be instituted. Such simple reme-

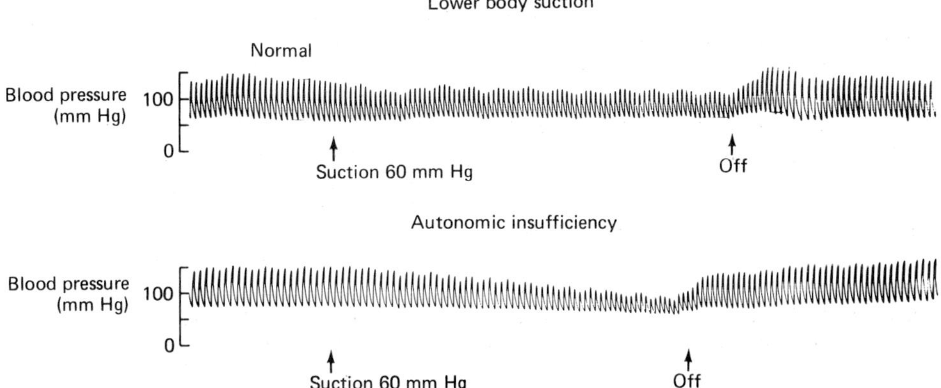

Figure 21–4. Arterial pressure tracings from a normal subject and a patient with autonomic insufficiency showing the effects of negative pressure applied to the lower body. There is a progressive fall in blood pressure and no overshoot when the pressure is released in the patient with autonomic insufficiency.

dies as increasing salt intake and raising the head of the bed to provide a constant stimulus to the autonomic nervous system control mechanisms during sleep often help. Avoiding sudden changes in posture and stopping or decreasing medication such as antihypertensive drugs, sedatives, and alcohol, which impair circulatory reactivity, may also improve symptoms. Blood volume expansion by means of fludrocortisone acetate and prevention of the shifting of large volumes of blood to the legs by means of elastic lower-body stockings should be reserved for patients in whom simple measures have failed. It should be remembered that the primary function of autonomic nervous system reflex control is to limit rises in arterial pressure and that patients with autonomic insufficiency are frequently hypertensive in the supine or head-down position. The measures taken to prevent hypotension in the standing position often result in hypertension in the supine position. When autonomic insufficiency is due to central nervous system disease, paralysis of the nervous control system is almost inevitably irreversible. Treatment is basically palliative, and the prognosis depends on the underlying pathologic process. Patients whose heart rates change in response to posture, exercise, and other stimuli live longer than those with fixed heart rates.

NEUROCIRCULATORY ASTHENIA
(Cardiac Neurosis)

The functional cardiac disorder known as neurocirculatory asthenia is also called effort syndrome, disordered action of the heart, soldier's heart, and Da Costa's syndrome. This condition causes the most difficulty during wartime, when conscription mobilizes apparently healthy men who develop symptoms either during military training or during actual combat that make them entirely unfit for military service. Da Costa first described the condition in the American Civil War; Thomas Lewis in World War I and Paul Wood in World War II were both involved in defining and diagnosing the condition. A similar clinical picture is seen in civilian life, but in that context the symptoms vary from patient to patient.

Clinical Findings

The spectrum of cases is wide, with incapacity varying from mild to severe. The condition has usually been present before military service and is found in men, women, and children. Wood stressed the psychologic aspects of the disorder and considered the condition to be a form of anxiety neurosis. Physicians sometimes unwittingly contribute to the patient's neurotic tendency by stressing the need for rest in patients with heart disease. The patient becomes fearful of exercise, and the combination of anxiety and inactivity is particularly likely to produce the clinical picture of cardiac neurosis. Occasionally, prolonged enforced bed rest in suspected cases of rheumatic fever may lead to cardiac neurosis. The physician must guard against the possibility of causing or aggravating neurotic tendencies, especially in young persons.

A. Symptoms: Dyspnea on exertion or on exposure to threatening situations is the predominant symptom, and all symptoms are aggravated by mental or physical stress. The breathlessness often involves an inability to get a deep enough or satisfying breath. Other symptoms, in the order of frequency, are weakness, palpitations, fatigue, cold sweating (especially of the palms), nervousness, dizziness, noncardiac pain in the left chest, headache, tremulousness, sighing, flushing, cramps, paresthesias, dryness of the mouth, vasovagal fainting, insomnia, increased frequency of micturition, diarrhea, and anorexia. Although some of these symptoms may be indicative of organic cardiac disease in certain circumstances, they are also readily recognized as symptoms of an anxiety state.

B. Signs: The patient is often thin and of asthenic build. A distaste for physical activity and a rapid resting heart rate are usually present. Blood pressure may be increased if the patient is excited when examined, but persistent hypertension is not found. The heart rate increases readily with exercise or when the patient stands up after lying down or squatting. Return of the heart rate to normal after exercise is delayed. Hyperventilation and tachypnea are common, particularly with stress, but no abnormal physical signs other than occasional ejection systolic murmurs are found on examination. The presence of hemodynamically insignificant organic heart disease, a trivial "functional" murmur, or insignificant ECG changes may complicate the picture, and it may be extremely difficult to decide which problems are functional in nature.

C. Electrocardiographic Findings: The ECG is usually normal apart from sinus tachycardia, although ST segment changes simulating ischemia may be seen.

D. X-Ray Findings: Chest x-ray shows a normal or reduced heart size.

E. Special Investigations: An exercise test may be useful in demonstrating disproportionate tachycardia, hyperventilation, and tachypnea. Cardiac catheterization reveals normal pressures and a cardiac output that is often raised.

Differential Diagnosis

Active rheumatic fever, rheumatic carditis, anemia, thyrotoxicosis, systemic arteriovenous fistula, tuberculosis, pleurisy, influenza, or any high output state must be differentiated from neurocirculatory asthenia. The diagnosis of effort syndrome probably includes more than one condition; with time, various different syndromes will probably be identified. There is almost certainly a relationship between effort syndrome and poor physical conditioning. Modern life in the Western world has meant a low average level of physical activity for the general population. Physical inactivity tends to produce a physiologic state resembling that seen in effort syndrome. Prolonged bed rest, debilitating illness, or simple inactivity all reduce exercise tolerance, cause disproportionate tachycardia, and result in marked tiredness after effort. Physical training programs are capable of altering the response to exercise. In Sweden, a group of patients identified as having "vasoregulatory asthenia" underwent a training program which resulted in significant improvement in symptoms and exercise tolerance.

The physiologic "defect" in untrained persons is a failure in the mechanisms distributing cardiac output to different parts of the systemic circulation. Muscular exercise involves a marked increase in muscle blood flow. As a compensatory mechanism, perfusion of nonessential parts of the systemic circulation (skin, kidneys, other viscera, and nonexercising muscles) is ordinarily reduced. If nonessential perfusion is maintained, the total cardiac output for a given work load is greater than normal; a higher pulse rate and limited exercise tolerance result. Training programs can reduce both cardiac output and heart rate at submaximal loads and increase the subject's maximal exercise performance. The arteriovenous oxygen difference at a given work load consequently increases. The statement that training increases the amount of oxygen extracted by the muscles is not correct. The arteriovenous oxygen difference is increased because a larger proportion of cardiac output perfuses the exercising muscles, and blood draining exercising muscles is low in oxygen content.

Treatment

Like patients with any form of neurosis, those with cardiac neurosis respond poorly to treatment such as exercise training programs, and they are not generally treated sympathetically by physicians. It is possible that some patients will be shown to have enzymatic defects in their muscles and that the present consensus that the condition is entirely psychologic will be proved false. The clinical manifestations so closely resemble those of sympathetic nervous system overactivity that propranolol should be given a trial in gradually increasing doses up to 200 mg/day.

Prognosis

Patients with cardiac neurosis can usually lead relatively normal lives if they are not subject to stress. There is no evidence that cardiac neurosis shortens life. Patients who develop symptoms while in the armed forces usually recover when they return to civilian life. However, some patients persist in self-imposed chronic invalidism.

ABNORMAL POSITION OF THE HEART

Cause of Abnormal Position of the Heart; Associated Conditions

Displacement of the heart interferes with physical examination more than it impairs function of the heart. Abnormalities on the ECG and chest x-ray due to displacement of the heart are also confusing and often suggest more serious abnormalities than are actually present. Abnormal position of the heart may be due to congenital abnormalities, as in dextrocardia, dextroversion, or absence of the left pericardium. It may be due to lung disease, which either pushes or pulls the heart and mediastinal contents to one side, or to abnormalities of the thoracic cage, which may be congenital or acquired. There may be associated congenital abnormalities in the heart itself, especially when chest deformity is congenital. Chest deformity also occurs as a result of congenital heart disease. Cardiac hypertrophy in children with a soft cartilaginous thorax tends to produce a bulge in the left upper chest, which is seen well in ventricular septal defect. The developing thorax becomes fixed in its abnormal shape, and the deformity persists into adult life. The heart itself may be normally situated, but the great vessels may be abnormal, as in right-sided aortic arch or absence of the left pulmonary artery, which may occur as isolated lesions or with Fallot's tetralogy. A left-sided superior vena cava may persist, either alone or with a right superior vena cava, and the inferior vena cava may enter the right atrium in an abnormal position. These lesions are seen with atrial septal defects but can also occur alone.

Dextrocardia & Dextroversion

The heart may be situated in the right side of the chest either because of mirror image dextrocardia or because of dextroversion. Dextrocardia is usually associated with complete situs inversus involving the abdominal viscera; it is also found with other congenital heart anomalies. In dextroversion, the cardiac chambers are on the correct side, but the heart is twisted and lies more to the right and more in the right side of the chest than normal. Dextroversion is also associated with congenital heart lesions. The position of the heart per se has no effect on its function.

Displacement Due to Lung Disease

The heart can be either pulled to one side by fibrosis or collapse of the ipsilateral lung or pushed by pleural effusion or pneumothorax to the contralateral side. The mediastinal contents are shifted as one unit, and the function of the heart is seldom if ever affected. The largest displacement is seen in patients who have undergone pneumonectomy, and bizarre radiologic findings appear when overdistention of the remaining lung leads to herniation of the lung to the opposite side of the thorax.

Displacement Due to Abnormalities of the Thoracic Cage

Displacement of the heart due to pectus excavatum and kyphoscoliosis may cause physical findings suggestive of heart disease. Since associated congenital heart lesions are common, the diagnosis is often difficult. Depression of the sternum may be associated with abnormalities of the position of the thoracic spine. These abnormalities narrow the anteroposterior diameter of the thorax. In this case, the heart may appear enlarged on the posteroanterior view and narrowed on the lateral view. Systolic ejection murmurs, wide splitting of the second sound, and even diastolic murmurs can occur. The ECG may show an incomplete right bundle branch block, and the large cardiac shadow on the posteroanterior view with a prominent right ventricular outflow tract may suggest atrial septal defect. In some cases, atrial septal defect is actually present, as in Figs 21–6 and 21–7. In kyphoscoliosis (Fig 21–8), the heart is often rotated, usually toward a right anterior oblique position. The outflow tract is thus abnormally prominent. The ECG shows clockwise rotation of the heart as a result of cardiac displacement, and it is often difficult to be sure that the heart is normal. Patients with chest deformity not infrequently complain of symptoms similar to those of effort syndrome, eg, dyspnea, palpitations, sweating, fatigue, noncardiac pain, and nervousness. In the large majority of cases, there is no underlying heart disease and no specific cardiac treatment is indicated. If the chest deformity is severe, operation may be indicated for cosmetic repair of pectus excavatum. Orthopedic treatment of kyphoscoliosis should not be influenced by cardiac considerations.

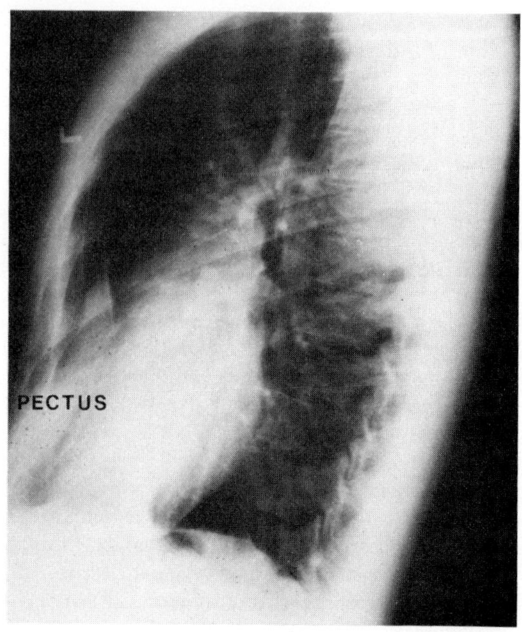

Figure 21–7. Lateral chest x-ray of a patient with pectus excavatum and atrial septal defect. The depression of the sternum (pectus) can be seen. The heart does not appear to be enlarged on this view (cf Fig 21–6).

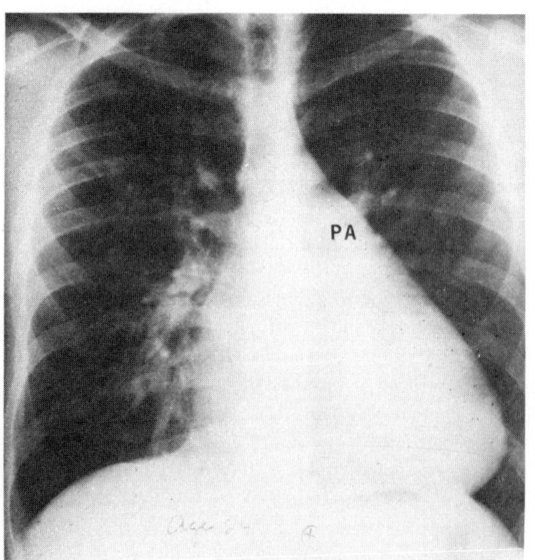

Figure 21–6. Posteroanterior chest x-ray of a patient with pectus excavatum and atrial septal defect. The pulmonary artery (PA) is prominent, and the heart appears to be greatly enlarged.

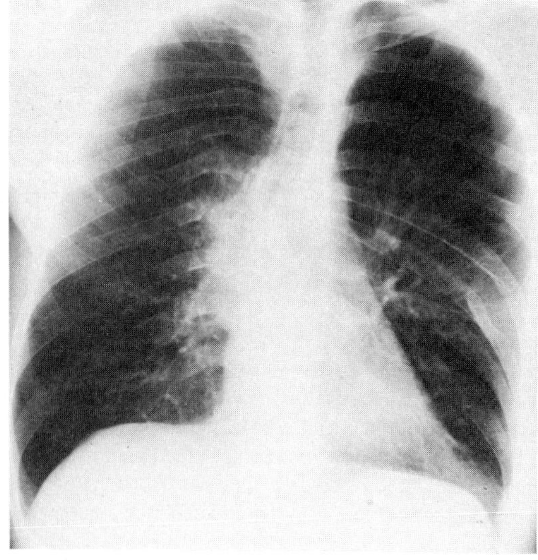

Figure 21–8. Chest x-ray of a patient with kyphoscoliosis showing rotation of the heart toward the right anterior oblique position. (Courtesy of G Gamsu.)

• • •

References

Bannister R, Ardill L, Fentem P: An assessment of various methods of treatment of idiopathic orthostatic hypotension. Q J Med 38:377, 1969.

Bergofsky EH & others: Cardiorespiratory failure in kyphoscoliosis. Medicine 38:263, 1959.

Berman ND & others: Angiographic demonstration of blood supply of right atrial myxoma. Br Heart J 38:764, 1976.

Biglieri EG, McIlroy MB: Abnormalities of renal function and circulatory reflexes in primary aldosteronism. Circulation 33:78, 1966.

Brigden W, Sharpey-Schafer EP: Postural changes in peripheral blood flow in cases with left heart failure. Clin Sci 9:93, 1950.

Cohen ME, White PD: Neurocirculatory asthenia: 1972 concept. Milit Med 137:142, 1972.

DaCosta JM: On irritable heart: A clinical study of a form of functional cardiac disorder and its consequences. Am J Med Sci 61:17, 1871.

Fenoglio JJ Jr, McAllister HA Jr, Ferrans VJ: Cardiac rhabdomyoma: A clinicopathologic and electron microscopic study. Am J Cardiol 38:241, 1976.

Glancy DL, Morales JB, Roberts WC: Angiosarcoma of the heart. Am J Cardiol 21:413, 1968.

Goodwin JF: The spectrum of cardiac tumors. Am J Cardiol 21:307, 1968.

Grant RT: Observations on the after-histories of men suffering from the effort syndrome. Heart 12:121, 1925.

Greenwood WF: Profile of atrial myxoma. Am J Cardiol 21:367, 1968.

Harbold NB, Gau GT: Echocardiographic diagnosis of right atrial myxoma. Mayo Clin Proc 48:284, 1973.

Harvey WP: Clinical aspects of cardiac tumors. Am J Cardiol 21:328, 1968.

Heath D: Pathology of cardiac tumors. Am J Cardiol 21:315, 1968.

Hedors E, Mogensen L: Atrial myxoma: 12 cases operated in Stockholm 1954–1973. Eur J Cardiol 2:101, 1974.

Kerber RE, Kelly DH, Gutenkauf C: Left atrial myxoma: Demonstration by stop-action cardiac ultrasonography. Am J Cardiol 34:838, 1974.

Lewis T: *The Soldier's Heart and the Effort Syndrome.* Hoeber, 1919.

Lokich JJ: The management of malignant pericardial effusions. JAMA 224:1401, 1973.

McIlroy MB, Bates DV: Respiratory function after pneumonectomy. Thorax 11:303, 1956.

Miller JJ & others: Primary cardiac tumors: Surgical considerations and results of operation. Circulation 45 (Suppl 1):134, 1972.

Otsuki Y & others: Angiosarcoma of the heart: Report of a case and review of the literature. Acta Pathol Jpn 23:407, 1973.

Peters MN & others: The clinical syndrome of atrial myxoma. JAMA 230:695, 1974.

Petsas AA & others: Echocardiographic diagnosis of left atrial myxoma: Usefulness of suprasternal approach. Br Heart J 38:627, 1976.

Pitt A & others: Myxoma of the left atrium. Circulation 36:408, 1967.

Selzer A, Sakai FJ, Popper RW: Protean clinical manifestations of primary tumors of the heart. Am J Med 52:9, 1972.

Sharpey-Schafer EP: Circulatory reflexes in chronic disease of the afferent nervous system. J Physiol (Lond) 134:1, 1956.

Srivastava TN, Fletcher E: The echocardiogram in left atrial myxoma. Am J Med 54:136, 1973.

Steiner RE: Radiologic aspects of cardiac tumors. Am J Cardiol 21:344, 1968.

Strohl KP: Angiosarcoma of the heart: A case study. Arch Intern Med 136:928, 1976.

Valsalva AM: *De Aure Humana: Traj ad Rhenum.* Utrecht. G. Vand Water 84, 1707.

Wagner HN Jr: Orthostatic hypotension. Bull Johns Hopkins Hosp 105:322, 1959.

Waxler EB, Kawai N, Kasparian H: Right atrial myxoma: Echocardiographic, phonocardiographic, and hemodynamic signs. Am Heart J 83:251, 1972.

Wood PH: DaCosta's syndrome. (3 parts.) Br Med J 1:767, 805, 845, 1941.

Worton CM: Primary malignant tumors of the heart. Cancer 2:245, 1949.

22...

Heart Disease in Pregnancy

INTRODUCTION

Heart disease in pregnancy has become a less important clinical problem in the developed countries in recent years because valvular and congenital heart diseases are now recognized and treated prior to childbearing age. Rheumatic heart disease, especially mitral stenosis, accounts for about 90% of cases of heart disease in pregnant women, but most of these women have mild valvular disease because those with more severe types have had surgical treatment. Acute rheumatic fever, the precursor of rheumatic valvular heart disease, is much less common today than was the case 20–30 years ago, in part because of antibiotic (chronic penicillin or sulfonamide) prophylaxis against streptococcal infections and in part because of prompt treatment of streptococcal infections when they do occur. The prevalence in developing countries is difficult to determine, but, because cardiac surgery is less frequently performed in those countries, the clinical problem of management of pregnancy in women with severe mitral stenosis still arises.

Congenital heart disease is now recognized at a much earlier age as a result of greater availability of neonatal and pediatric cardiac care units. With the exception of the infrequent Eisenmenger syndrome, in which shunt defects are associated with severe pulmonary hypertension, severe congenital heart disease is treated surgically before childbearing age. Awareness of the importance of rubella in the first trimester of pregnancy and its prevention by immunization before pregnancy occurs has resulted in a marked decrease in the incidence of rubella in early pregnancy, one of the common causes of congenital heart disease. The authors are not aware that the incidence of congenital heart disease has indeed decreased in recent years, but the frequency of the problem of untreated congenital heart disease in pregnancy is less now; even before the advent of open heart surgery, it was responsible for only 3–5% of all cases of heart disease in pregnancy.

CLASSIFICATION

Pregnant patients with heart disease can be divided into 2 general categories. The first category consists of women with preexisting heart disease in whom the physiologic load imposed by pregnancy increases the work of the heart. In such cases, if the reserve capacity of the heart is compromised, the heart may fail.

The second category is made up of women with disease induced by pregnancy, eg, preeclampsia-eclampsia, peripartum cardiomyopathy, thromboembolic disease causing multiple pulmonary emboli and pulmonary hypertension, and dissection of the aorta or of a coronary artery.

Preexisting heart disease is usually valvular or congenital, but other types must be recognized also. Hypertension, mitral valve prolapse, and hypertrophic cardiomyopathy all may occur in women of childbearing age. Coronary heart disease is sufficiently rare at this age that it does not cause a clinical problem except in women with severe juvenile onset diabetes mellitus or homozygous genetic hypercholesterolemia. Coronary heart disease may appear in the 20s in these conditions.

PHYSIOLOGIC CHANGES IN THE MOTHER AS A RESULT OF PREGNANCY

The most striking cardiovascular change in pregnancy is an increase in the cardiac output of about 30% by the third or fourth month, usually due to increased stroke volume because the heart rate increases only slightly—about 10 beats/min. Oxygen consumption increases to a lesser extent—about 20% (Metcalfe, 1974). Systemic vascular resistance decreases despite the raised cardiac output because of the arteriovenous fistula-like pregnant placenta and possibly as a result of increased prostaglandin production. There is a marked increase in total body water of about 7 liters, of which 75% is extracellular, reaching a maximum in the second trimester. Plasma volume and red cell volume also increase in normal pregnancy. The increased

Table 22–1. Effect of pregnancy on maternal circulatory and respiratory functions.*

Function	Change
Heart rate	Slow increase of 10 beats/min from 14–30 weeks. Rate maintained at this level to 40 weeks.
Arterial blood pressure	Systolic unchanged until the 30th week. Diastolic slightly reduced (period of maximal pulse pressure).
Venous blood pressure	Arms: No change. Legs: Gradual marked increase between 8–40 weeks.
Cardiac output	Increase of 30–50% by the 32nd week; decline to 20% increase at 40 weeks.
Total body water	Increased between 10–40 weeks.
Plasma and blood volume	Rise of 15% between 12–32 weeks; slight decline to 40 weeks.
Red cell mass	Augmented 10–15% between 8–40 weeks.
Vital capacity	Rises 15% by the 20th week; decline of 5% by 40 weeks.
Oxygen consumption	Increased 15% between 16–40 weeks.
Circulation time	Decreases from 13 to 11 sec by 32nd week, then returns to 13 sec by 40th week.
Glomerular filtration rate	Increases 30–50% by second trimester.

*Modified and reproduced, with permission, from Benson RC: *Handbook of Obstetrics & Gynecology*, 6th ed. Lange, 1977.

extracellular fluid is to only a slight extent the result of increased aldosterone secretion, which is but modestly raised in most pregnancies. Plasma renin and angiotensin are increased, yet the blood pressure in most normal pregnancies not only does not rise but actually falls, especially in the first and second trimesters. Body weight increases an average of about 10 kg (Table 22–1).

The glomerular filtration rate increases up to 30–50% above normal during normal pregnancy, although it decreases in preeclampsia. This results in a greatly increased filtered load of sodium, all of which is reabsorbed or excreted except for a small amount which is progressively retained, so that by the end of pregnancy approximately 500 mEq of sodium are retained in the extracellular fluid volume and in the developing fetus. Tubular sodium reabsorption greatly exceeds the amount that can be attributed to aldosterone, and the mechanism for the very large increase is not known. The role of progesterone has been studied because it increases at least 300-fold during pregnancy, antagonizes aldosterone, and causes excretion of sodium in normal women, perhaps by decreasing renovascular resistance and thus renin secretion. It undoubtedly influences blood volume changes of pregnancy.

The relative increase in plasma and blood volume in comparison to red cell mass accounts for the hemodilution and fall in hemoglobin during pregnancy, which often is confused with true anemia.

Because the physiologic changes occur early in pregnancy, by the beginning of the second trimester, patients with cardiac disease may develop symptoms of cardiac failure early in pregnancy if their cardiac reserve is severely limited, and in such cases intervention such as therapeutic abortion can be performed per vaginam. The load of pregnancy continues throughout the entire period of gestation, and some patients may tolerate pregnancy well until the last 1–2 months despite the fact that the load has been present all through pregnancy.

In the latter part of pregnancy, the position of the mother is quite important in influencing cardiac output, which is reduced in the supine position (by mechanically obstructing the inferior vena cava and decreasing venous return) and increased in the lateral position.

Oxygen consumption at rest increases progressively during pregnancy, whereas cardiac output increases in the first and second trimesters and for unknown reasons falls in the last several weeks of pregnancy. Burwell (Circulatory..., 1954) has proposed that this discrepancy is due to the arteriovenous fistula-like function of the placenta. The high output state resembles that seen in arteriovenous fistulas, and the patient has a hyperdynamic cardiac impulse, a raised venous pressure, dilated and pulsating digital arteries, a warm skin, and decreased systemic vascular resistance. The importance of the uterine and placental blood flow has been emphasized by Page (1939, 1953), who believes that impairment of perfusion of these organs may be important in the development of preeclampsia.

PHYSIOLOGIC CHANGES WITH LABOR & THE PUERPERIUM

In addition to marked changes in arterial and pulse pressure and in pulse rate with uterine contractions during labor, cardiac output increases with each contraction, especially in the supine position.

Most of the hemodynamic changes return to normal by 10 days after delivery. With the exception of peripartum cardiomyopathy, cardiac complications of pregnancy are rare after the tenth day.

CARDIAC COMPLICATIONS OF PREGNANCY

As indicated previously, the cardiovascular load of normal pregnancy is large, but most normal women and women with mild valvular or congenital heart disease or hypertension tolerate pregnancy without difficulty. If cardiac function is impaired in the prepregnant state (New York Heart Association class III or IV) or worsens in the first few weeks of pregnancy, cardiac complications progressively increase. Patients who have had cardiac failure in a previous pregnancy are more apt to develop cardiac failure in the current pregnancy.

The most serious varieties of heart disease complicating pregnancy are severe mitral or aortic stenosis, Eisenmenger's syndrome, and severe coarctation of the aorta. In the presence of these more severe varieties of cardiac disease, cardiac failure may be anticipated as pregnancy continues and may cause serious problems at the time of delivery.

DIFFICULTY IN DIAGNOSIS OF HEART DISEASE IN PREGNANCY

The recognition of cardiac disease or of early cardiac failure may be difficult in pregnant women, especially if they have not been seen prior to pregnancy. The increased blood volume, cardiac output, and hyperdynamic cardiac state may cause cardiac ejection murmurs, raised venous pressure, hyperdynamic cardiac impulse, physiologic S_3, symptoms of dyspnea, and, especially later in pregnancy, edema due to sodium retention. These normal physiologic changes of pregnancy must be recognized as such and not attributed to cardiac disease or cardiac failure. Vital capacity does not normally change during pregnancy, and a decrease indicates developing pulmonary venous congestion. A measurement of basal vital capacity should be obtained early in pregnancy so as to interpret changes; a single test is not valid.

Recognition of the underlying cardiac disease is based on the same cardinal clinical features that characterize the diagnosis in the nonpregnant state, and the reader should refer to the respective sections regarding the various cardiac diseases.

MANAGEMENT OF CARDIAC DISEASE IN PREGNANCY

As indicated previously, cardiac failure is uncommon in patients who, before pregnancy, had minimal symptoms and good cardiac reserve, with class I or II impairment (New York Heart Association criteria). If the limitation was more severe prior to pregnancy and patients were in class III or IV, or if they had a history of cardiac failure in a previous pregnancy, or if they had one of the severe varieties of cardiac disease mentioned on p 6—and especially if symptoms increase in the first trimester of pregnancy and are not controlled by medical therapy—therapeutic abortion should be performed unless the patient has strong objections. If the cardiac symptoms are less severe or if they appear later in pregnancy, treatment should consist of bed rest, restriction of sodium intake, digitalis, and antihypertensive agents if the patient is hypertensive (see Hypertension in Pregnancy). Bed rest throughout the remainder of pregnancy may allow a woman to maintain the pregnancy and avoid the development of cardiac failure. The fetal mortality rate is increased in patients who develop cardiac symptoms during pregnancy, possibly because of impaired placental perfusion, and management of the pregnant cardiac patient should also include careful examination of the fetal heart sounds and fetal movements.

SURGICAL PROCEDURES DURING PREGNANCY

Patients with surgically curable cardiac lesions such as severe mitral stenosis, severe coarctation, or infective endocarditis with rapidly developing cardiac failure have been operated on during pregnancy with only a slightly increased mortality rate. The fetal mortality rate has been higher, but not excessively so. It is obviously preferable to delay definitive surgery until after delivery or, even better, to perform it before pregnancy; but in some instances the patient is first seen during pregnancy with severe cardiac failure, and cardiac surgery may be undertaken. With improvement in the treatment of cardiac failure and the availability of better inotropic and vasodilator agents, the need for cardiac surgery in pregnancy has become considerably less.

HYPERTENSION IN PREGNANCY

The management of hypertension, whether from hypertensive disease of pregnancy (preeclampsia), preexisting hypertension, or the hypertension of coarctation, is important because of the hazard of aortic dissection and cardiac failure in the presence of hypertension. It is estimated that at least half of all cases of dissection of the aorta in women occur during pregnancy, not all of them in women with hypertension.

Management of Delivery in Women With Heart Disease

It is controversial whether cardiac patients should be delivered by cesarean section or vaginal delivery. Physiologic studies are quite difficult during labor because of the rapid fluctuations of cardiac output, blood pressure, pulse rate, and adrenergic impulses associated with the anxiety of labor. The consensus is that in most patients with cardiac disease, if the patient tolerates pregnancy to term, the vaginal delivery, with deliberate rupture of the membranes if the cervix is dilated, combined with the use of low forceps, causes less physiologic disturbance and is tolerated better than cesarean section. Furthermore, although the physiologic and circulatory changes of cesarean section are often relatively slight when a skilled anesthesiologist and gynecologic surgeon are available, it is better to avoid an abdominal operation if possible.

Sterilization, especially if cesarean section has been performed, is recommended if the patient has an inoperable underlying disease and cardiac failure has occurred during pregnancy unrelated to acute reversible events such as atrial fibrillation, acute respiratory infection, thyrotoxicosis, severe anemia, or intercurrent disease. If the patient has a cardiac condition that is amenable to cardiac surgery and operation can be performed months after delivery, or if the cardiac symptoms have been precipitated by reversible and perhaps nonrecurrent situations such as those mentioned previously, sterilization should not be performed because many women deliver normal infants after the underlying cardiac condition has been corrected surgically.

PREGNANCY IN PATIENTS WITH CARDIAC PROSTHESES

Although it was just stated that patients with valvular prostheses may tolerate pregnancy well, the hazard of anticoagulant therapy must be considered in the management of such patients. The hazards of stopping anticoagulants must also be kept in mind, because even with cloth-covered valvular prostheses systemic emboli may develop. If anticoagulants are not used, therefore, the patient is at risk of systemic emboli. If anticoagulants *are* used, especially the coumarin anticoagulants, hemorrhage may occur, and there is some evidence that these agents may be teratogenic. Despite these risks, women with prosthetic heart valves have continued to receive oral anticoagulants throughout pregnancy. There has been a high incidence of spontaneous abortions, but with careful hematologic control hemorrhagic complications have been fewer than expected. In general, however, it is recommended that early in pregnancy subcutaneous heparin injection twice daily should be used for anticoagulation because it is considered safer than oral anticoagulant therapy. The proper treatment is not agreed on, and the use of homografts for valve replacement in women likely to become pregnant should be considered to obviate the need for anticoagulation. Homograft tissue valves in the past were not favored because of the high incidence of late deterioration and paravalvular leaks, but recent changes in sterilization of the valve have resulted in a greatly decreased incidence of such leaks, making homograft replacement preferable in young women who desire to become pregnant.

GENERAL MEASURES IN MANAGEMENT OF PREGNANCY IN WOMEN WITH HEART DISEASE

As is true of all pregnant women, those with heart disease should get adequate rest and nutrition, with correction of anemia and thyrotoxicosis if present, and should avoid alcohol and tobacco abuse and excessive sodium intake or weight gain. Rest increases uterine, placental, and renal blood flow. In the presence of cardiac disease, factors other than pregnancy (eg, severe exercise) that increase the work of the heart should be decreased or eliminated. There is controversy about the use of diuretic agents such as the thiazides in patients who gain excessive weight or develop edema; in general, it is best to avoid drugs and rely on diet and a low sodium intake to prevent excessive weight gain and edema. (See Hypertensive Disorders of Pregnancy, below.)

The physician should bear in mind the natural dilutional decrease in hemoglobin that occurs in pregnancy, and iron therapy should not be given for the hemodilution of pregnancy unless the hemoglobin is less than 10–11 g/dl. In patients who have valvular or congenital heart disease, antibiotic prophylaxis to prevent infective endocarditis must be given before delivery, although infective endocarditis following delivery is uncommon.* Respiratory infections must be treated promptly, and extra bed rest and decrease in sodium intake should be part of the treatment. The sodium retention (of unknown mechanism) of acute respiratory infections may precipitate pulmonary edema in patients with mitral stenosis, and such patients should avoid contact with persons with upper respiratory infection even though this is difficult to achieve. In older pregnant patients with mitral stenosis, adequate treatment of atrial fibrillation with digitalis may prevent pulmonary venous congestion.

PROGNOSIS OF PREGNANCY IN WOMEN WITH HEART DISEASE

Most patients with cardiac disease tolerate pregnancy surprisingly well and can be managed without interruption of pregnancy if modern methods of treating cardiac failure and arrhythmias are available. The exceptions are severe mitral or aortic stenosis, severe coarctation of the aorta, and Eisenmenger's syndrome. Good prenatal care, awareness of the cardiac functional capacity of the patient prior to pregnancy, and appropriate surgical treatment when indicated may prevent cardiac problems during pregnancy. Unpredictable factors such as respiratory infections, atrial fibrillation, and other arrhythmias may complicate what otherwise appears to be a relatively straightforward clinical situation, and the physician should be alert for the development of these complications and treat them promptly and appropriately. Severe cardiac complications are uncommon today and probably will become even less so for the reasons given in the introductory paragraphs to this chapter.

*See Chapter 16 for prophylaxis for genitourinary procedures.

HYPERTENSIVE DISORDERS OF PREGNANCY

Hypertension during pregnancy may be independent of pregnancy, as occurs in essential hypertension, pheochromocytoma, or coarctation of the aorta, or it may be a complication of pregnancy such as occurs in preeclampsia or eclampsia. The latter 2 are collectively referred to in the older literature as toxemia of pregnancy. The differentiation between essential hypertension and toxemia of pregnancy with preeclampsia depends upon the period during pregnancy when raised blood pressure occurs. In essential hypertension, raised arterial pressure either precedes pregnancy or occurs early in pregnancy, before the last trimester, whereas preeclampsia is characterized by a normal blood pressure prior to pregnancy or early in pregnancy but a rise in pressure in the last trimester. Preeclampsia may complicate essential hypertension, in which case the blood pressure is raised early in pregnancy, and later in pregnancy the pressure increases substantially and is associated with proteinuria and edema. Pheochromocytoma and coarctation of the aorta are independent processes and are diagnosed and treated as discussed in Chapters 9 and 11.

1. ESSENTIAL HYPERTENSION

Essential hypertension is relatively uncommon (about 5%) in the USA and elsewhere in the Western world in young women, as contrasted with a prevalence of about 20% for individuals in their 40s and 50s. If a measurement above 140 mm Hg systolic or 90 mm Hg diastolic on a single reading is considered to constitute hypertension, as many as 20% of young women may have elevated pressures. As discussed in Chapter 9, there is no sharp division between normal blood pressure and hypertension, and lability of pressure is characteristic of all individuals whether they are normal or hypertensive. The problem is complicated in pregnant women because vasodilatation produces a fall in pressure in the second trimester, perhaps as a result of the increased production of prostaglandins or other peptides. The magnitude of the fall can be significant, so that individuals seen for the first time in the second trimester may be considered to be normotensive even though observations before and after pregnancy indicate that the individual is indeed hypertensive. The diagnosis of essential hypertension must be made almost exclusively on the basis of the arterial pressure itself, because in the age range of the usual pregnant patient vascular complications are uncommon unless the hypertension is severe, and ECG and examination of the ocular fundi and heart usually show no abnormalities. If the hypertension is severe, and if vascular complications such as fundal abnormalities, cardiac enlargement, left ventricular hypertrophy, or impairment of renal function are present during the first few months of pregnancy, the likelihood of a significant rise of pressure in the last trimester with the development of preeclampsia and an increased probability of fetal death may indicate the need for therapeutic abortion.

Essential hypertension in pregnancy does not differ greatly from essential hypertension in nonpregnant women, and the decision regarding treatment depends on the severity of the hypertensive disorder and the associated cardiovascular complications. Slight elevations of pressure in the absence of symptoms or of vascular abnormalities require close observation, but the decision regarding drug treatment can be delayed until after the postpartum period. Fetal death is more frequent in patients with more severe hypertension, but the availability of potent antihypertensive drugs makes it possible to control the elevated blood pressure, with resultant improvement in maternal and fetal prognosis.

Management of Essential Hypertension in Pregnancy

The medical treatment of hypertension in pregnancy is similar to that in the nonpregnant woman (see Chapter 9). Treatment must begin at an early stage, not only to prevent vascular complications but also to prevent preeclampsia. General measures such as rest, sodium restriction, and diuretics may be sufficient to lower the pressures to normal in most cases of mild to moderate hypertension. If the hypertension is more severe, medications such as methyldopa and hydralazine can be used. Methyldopa has been used extensively during pregnancy, with excellent control of blood pressure and with only a 10% fetal mortality rate in severely hypertensive women. Hydralazine can be used orally or parenterally; in the latter instance, the blood pressure falls in 15–30 minutes. Hydralazine can be combined with methyldopa and thiazide diuretics to control the average case of essential hypertension. The major problem with the ordinary moderately hypertensive patient is the increased likelihood of development of preeclampsia, which occurs in 10–20% of cases. Unless the hypertension is severe, it is advisable to discontinue or decrease antihypertensive drugs 2–3 days before delivery. Data on the effects of treatment of hypertension on the newborn infant are limited, but adverse effects are uncommon.

Induction of labor and management of delivery should be similar to those of cardiac disease in pregnancy. Vaginal delivery is usually quite satisfactory, with early rupture of the membranes and the use of low forceps to shorten the duration of labor. A small number of patients first develop a raised arterial pressure in the postpartum period. The course of the condition is usually benign, and one should withhold treatment for 3–6 months unless complications occur or the diastolic pressure rises alarmingly (to about 110–120 mm Hg).

Prognosis

The prognosis of essential hypertension in pregnancy is usually good unless preeclampsia-eclampsia supervenes. Even then it is quite good unless the preeclampsia is severe or eclampsia with convulsions develops. Control of blood pressure with modern antihypertensive drugs has made therapeutic abortion unnecessary in most cases, although cesarean section late in pregnancy is preferable to drugs if severe preeclampsia or convulsions occur. Malignant hypertension or cardiac or renal failure discovered early in pregnancy may warrant therapeutic abortion, especially if the patient has preexisting renal disease. The differentiation of renal disease due to chronic glomerular nephritis or chronic pyelonephritis from essential hypertension is difficult if renal impairment is present when the patient is first seen. In addition to benefit to the mother, antihypertensive therapy with methyldopa results in a significantly improved fetal outcome due largely to a decreased number of spontaneous abortions in the second trimester of pregnancy (Redman, Lancet 2:753, 1976). Both in terms of birth weight and general health, the surviving infants of mothers treated with methyldopa were similar to those whose mothers were not treated.

2. PREECLAMPSIA-ECLAMPSIA

The term toxemia of pregnancy is in a sense obsolete, since no toxins have been discovered to produce the clinical syndrome of hypertension, edema, and proteinuria developing in the last trimester of pregnancy. What has been called toxemia of pregnancy is a continuum extending from the mildest forms of preeclampsia to severe eclampsia with multiple severe convulsions. Preeclampsia occurs in about 5% of all pregnancies if one includes toxemia without preceding hypertension and toxemia associated with hypertension. The figure is higher–up to 10%–if toxemia with pyelonephritis is added, but the disorder has gradually declined in incidence in the past several decades (see Prognosis), possibly as a consequence of better prenatal care. Eclampsia is much less frequent, occurring in about 0.1% of pregnant women.

Etiology

The cause of preeclampsia is unknown, and many theories have been offered without universal acceptance even though the condition has been extensively studied for many years. Certain facts are clear, however. The condition is more frequent in the first pregnancy, in patients with preexisting hypertension, in twin pregnancies, in patients with a history of preeclampsia, in patients with hydatidiform mole, and in some populations of black women. One theory offered by Page (1939) is that preeclampsia results from impaired uteroplacental perfusion; this is supported by the observation that during preeclampsia, plasma volume, glomerular filtration rate, and uterine and placental blood flow decrease about 25% in recumbency. The gravid uterus has a poorer arterial blood supply in preeclampsia as compared to the nongravid or normal pregnant uterus, which has an abundant blood supply from the uterine, ovarian, and other arteries. Preeclampsia has been produced in animals by reducing the uterine blood flow by constricting the uterine arteries, and this is perhaps the strongest argument for uteroplacental impairment of perfusion as an etiologic factor. The role of renin has been emphasized by some because renin is produced by the uterus and chorion as well as by the kidney; but this theory has not been universally accepted because, although the plasma levels of renin, renin substrate, and angiotension II and aldosterone are raised in normal pregnancy, plasma renin and aldosterone are lower in pregnancy associated with hypertension than in normal pregnancy (Finnerty, 1958).

Renal & Hepatic Changes in Preeclampsia

The proteinuria that occurs as part of the characteristic triad of hypertension, edema, and proteinuria in preeclampsia is considered to be of glomerular origin. Renal biopsies have shown endothelial swelling, narrowing of the lumen of the capillaries, deposits of fibrin in the glomeruli, and evidences of intravascular coagulation. Renal biopsies by Petrucco (1974) have shown a significant correlation between the clinical severity of preeclampsia and the density and pattern of IgM and IgG deposition in the glomeruli of the kidney. The typical electron microscopic appearance of renal biopsy specimens in preeclampsia is fibrin and immunoglobulin deposition in the capillary loops, especially deposition of IgM and complement. Complement is found to be strongly deposited within the walls of afferent and efferent arterioles. Similar deposition of fibrin, immunoglobulins, and complement was found by Arias (1976) in the livers of preeclamptic but not normal pregnant women by means of immunofluorescent studies of liver biopsies, as shown in Fig 22–1.

These results support the hypothesis that an immunologic mechanism may be responsible for the renal and hepatic lesions of preeclampsia, with a primary vascular disorder similar to the transplant rejection mechanism involving the antibody system. Antiplacental antibodies may be produced that result in deposition of immunoglobulins and complement in the kidney. This hypothesis has not been fully accepted but opens a new avenue of possible mechanism of action of the preeclamptic process.

The severity of preeclampsia and eclampsia may be related to the magnitude of the deposition of the immunoglobulins, but the mechanism by which this is accomplished is at present obscure.

Clinical Findings

Preeclampsia is defined as a syndrome encountered in the second half of pregnancy characterized by at least 2 of 3 cardinal manifestations. The following is quoted from Page (1953):

1. A rather abrupt increase of blood pressure amounting to 30 mm or more systolic and 15 mm or more diastol-

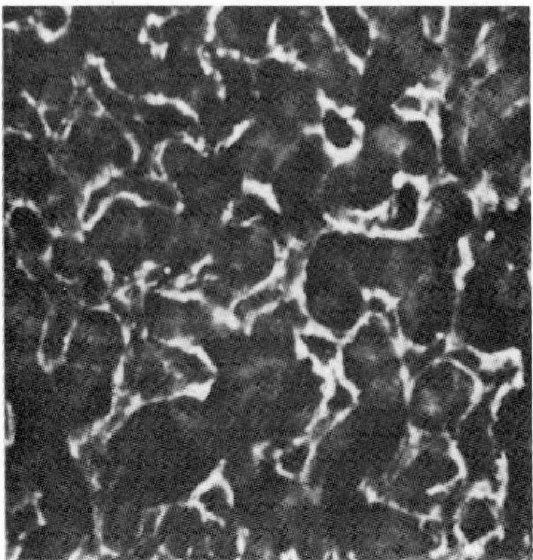

Figure 22–1. Diffuse staining of hepatic sinusoids with fluorescent antiserum to fibrinogen. (Reproduced, with permission, from Arias F, Mancilla-Jimenez R: Hepatic fibrinogen deposits in pre-eclampsia: Immunofluorescent evidence. N Engl J Med 295:578, 1976.)

ic after the 26th week of pregnancy.

2. The appearance (or sudden increase) of proteinuria of at least 0.5 g/day; and
3. Edema in the upper half of the body.

Any 2 of these must be manifest on 2 occasions at least 6 hours apart. If convulsions occur in addition to the above criteria, the case is classified as eclampsia.

Generalized edema is common in pregnancy and when present in the lower half of the body is not considered diagnostic of heart failure. The increased tubular reabsorption of sodium and water causes edema in the upper half of the body which may precede the appearance of proteinuria and hypertension. Benson (1977) estimates that 6–7% of all pregnant women in the USA develop toxemia and that only 5% of this total group develop convulsions with eclampsia. The progression of preeclampsia to eclampsia is an ominous development, and approximately 5–10% of patients with eclampsia die of the disease. Page (1953) estimates that there are approximately 1500 maternal deaths each year and about 15,000 fetal deaths. Deaths from preeclampsia are rare.

Apart from the clinical manifestations of weight gain, edema in the upper half of the body, proteinuria, and hypertension, patients with preeclampsia may develop headache, drowsiness, visual disturbances, dyspnea, and, if the hypertension is severe, pulmonary edema and cardiac failure. Cerebral hemorrhage is the cause of death in about 10% of patients with eclampsia who die. Acute tubular necrosis is an uncommon cause of death but may occur in severe toxemia. Hypotension may develop because of adrenocortical insufficiency, but this is uncommon except in severe eclampsia with hemorrhage and necrosis in the adrenal glands.

Clinical Course

The onset of preeclampsia may be gradual or sudden, and the diagnosis may be difficult to establish in the early stages. Patients may develop edema that is similar to the edema of a normal pregnancy. The proteinuria may be slight, and the elevation of blood pressure may be slight and variable. Any one of these findings should cause the physician to observe the patient more closely. In mild cases, restriction of activity and sodium may be sufficient to reverse the process by increasing uterine, renal, and placental blood flow, but if proteinuria increases or if the blood pressure rises—and especially if the patient develops symptoms such as blurred vision, decreased urine output, or a rapid gain in weight—the patient should be considered to have preeclampsia and should be hospitalized. Examination of the ocular fundi is often helpful; a "shimmering edema" of the retina is said to be characteristic of toxemia, but this finding has not been universally accepted. Papilledema, hemorrhages, and exudates are rare but may occur. Page (1953) states that the development of a generalized boring headache is the most reliable symptom of an impending convulsion and should be the immediate indication for more intensive hospital therapy, including termination of pregnancy.

Prevention of Preeclampsia-Eclampsia

Because the mechanism is not known, preventive methods are empirical and consist of advice regarding prenatal care, good protein nutrition, counseling to recognize the earliest development of preeclampsia, bed rest and sodium restriction when manifestations first appear, recommendations against subsequent pregnancies in patients who have had severe preeclampsia or eclampsia, and the use of antihypertensive drugs to control preexisting hypertension in patients who become pregnant.

Although eclampsia is infrequent, it is one of the common causes of death in pregnant women, and the cardiologist or internist shares with the obstetrician the responsibility for care of the patient once preeclampsia develops. Delivery when signs of impending convulsions (see above) appear is the best preventive treatment for eclampsia. Eclampsia does not occur after the uterus is emptied.

Management of Preeclampsia

As indicated previously, bed rest and sodium restriction are usually adequate to reverse the process in mild preeclampsia, and, if the edema is generalized, thiazides may be added. Many authorities now believe that thiazides should not be used because they may exaggerate the diminished plasma volume in patients with preeclampsia, perhaps as a result of decreased plasma aldosterone or poor perfusion of the kidney. The mechanism is unclear. If preeclampsia does not subside after a few days of hospital therapy, the pregnancy should be interrupted by cesarean section unless the patient is near term, in which case labor should be induced. The infant mortality rate is greater the longer the preeclampsia persists or the worse it gets. The transition from severe preeclampsia to eclampsia with convulsions is one of degree rather than of kind. It is preferable to interrupt the pregnancy by cesarean section if it appears that convulsions, muscular twitching, severe headache, epigastric pain (vascular crisis), or visual disturbances are imminent.

Management of Eclampsia

If convulsions occur, the clinical situation is much worse. As stated previously, the maternal mortality rate is 5–10% and the fetal mortality rate about 20–25%. The tonic and clonic convulsions of eclampsia should be managed by use of intravenous magnesium sulfate (which has proved safe and effective but is of uncertain mechanism), by absolute rest in bed, by constant nursing care, and by avoidance of anything that disturbs the patient and may precipitate a convulsion. Sedatives and the central nervous system depressant magnesium sulfate should be used to control the convulsions, and delivery should be postponed until the convulsions can be stopped. Antihypertensive drugs should be used if the blood pressure is elevated to 115 mm Hg diastolic or more. Some patients with eclampsia have cerebral edema rather than hypertension as the mechanism of their convulsions, and nonspecific therapy with magnesium sulfate is therefore preferred by obstetricians. For reasons that are not clear, eclampsia is less frequent today. Modern antihypertensive therapy may ultimately prove to be desirable, but we know of no random clinical trial comparing magnesium sulfate with antihypertensive drugs. If the patient is oliguric, intravenous fluids should be used with caution. Pregnancy should not be terminated unless the patient is in good condition and has had no convulsions for 24–48 hours.

Prognosis

As indicated previously, maternal deaths are infrequent and decreasing in frequency in preeclampsia. Toxemia is more frequent in patients with preexisting essential hypertension or renal disease than in patients who were normotensive before pregnancy.

Despite the rarity of maternal deaths in preeclampsia, the fetal mortality rate is 2–3 times as high if the mother had preeclampsia than in normal pregnancy. Preeclampsia is more frequent (13–46% in various reports) in patients with preexisting hypertension. About half of cases of eclampsia that occur in multiparous women are preceded by hypertension. Sodium and water retention may cause pulmonary edema and cardiac failure in preeclampsia and eclampsia, especially if a high sodium intake or intravenous fluids are given in the presence of oliguria. Otherwise, pulmonary edema is infrequent. The prognosis of mild preeclampsia is good with bed rest and sodium restriction, but if the condition progresses to one associated with increase of weight, edema, proteinuria, and hypertension, termination of pregnancy should be instituted promptly before convulsions occur. There is a difference of opinion whether permanent hypertension is more frequent in patients who have toxemia of pregnancy. Chesley (1976) has completed a 25- to 35-year follow-up of eclamptic women and concludes that primiparous women with this syndrome (70% of the total) do not have an increased incidence of hypertension or cardiovascular deaths. However, multiparous women who survive eclampsia have a worse prognosis and an incidence of cardiovascular deaths almost 3 times the expected number.

Convulsions greatly increase the hazards of toxemia, with cerebral hemorrhage, pulmonary edema, and adrenal hemorrhage or necrosis being the major causes of death. Interruption of pregnancy in severe preeclampsia usually prevents convulsive eclampsia, and symptomatic treatment of convulsions allows termination of pregnancy by cesarean section if necessary, reducing the maternal and fetal mortality rate. Patients with a history of severe preeclampsia or eclampsia should be discouraged from having further pregnancies and even advised to undergo sterilization. This is because 20–40% of patients with preeclampsia or severe toxemia have a recurrence in subsequent pregnancies, although the mechanism is not known.

• • •

References

Arias F, Mancilla-Jimenez R: Hepatic fibrinogen in pre-eclampsia: Immunofluorescent evidence. N Engl J Med 295:578, 1976.

Barnes AC, Kumar D: Significance of cardiovascular alterations in preeclampsia-eclampsia: A review. Mod Concepts Cardiovasc Dis 33:841, 1964.

Benson RC: *Handbook of Obstetrics & Gynecology,* 6th ed. Lange, 1977.

Bryans CI, Torpin R: A follow-up study of two hundred and forty-three cases of eclampsia for an average of 12 years. Am J Obstet Gynecol 58:1054, 1949.

Bullock JL, Harris RE, Young R: Treatment of thyrotoxicosis during pregnancy with propranolol. Am J Obstet Gynecol 121:242, 1975.

Burch GE: Heart disease and pregnancy. Am Heart J 93:104, 1977.

Burwell CS: Circulatory adjustments to pregnancy. Bull Johns Hopkins Hosp 95:115, 1954.

Burwell CS: The management of heart disease in pregnant women. Bull Johns Hopkins Hosp 95:130, 1954.

Carey HM: Toxaemias of pregnancy. Chapter 9, pages 239–271, in: *Practical Obstetric Problems,* 4th ed. Donald I (editor). Lippincott, 1969.

Chesley LC: Plasma and red cell volumes during pregnancy. Am J Obstet Gynecol 112:440, 1972.

Chesley LC, Annitto JE, Cosgrove RA: The remote prognosis of eclamptic women: Sixth periodic report. Am J Obstet Gynecol 124:446, 1976.

Cutforth R, MacDonald CB: Heart sounds and murmurs during pregnancy. Am Heart J 71:741, 1966.

Daniel DG, Campbell H, Turnbull AC: Puerperal thromboembolism and suppression of lactation. Lancet 2:287, 1967.

Epstein FH: Late vascular effects of toxemia of pregnancy. N Engl J Med 271:8, 1964.

Finnerty FA Jr, Buckholz JH, Tuchman J: Evaluation of chlorothiazide in the toxaemias of pregnancy. JAMA 166:141, 1958.

Gilchrist AR: Cardiological problems in younger women: Including those of pregnancy and the puerperium. Br Med J 1:209, 1963.

Gordon H: Toxaemia of pregnancy. Chapter 8, pages 274–296, in: *Obstetric Therapeutics.* Hawkins DF (editor). Bailliere Tindall, 1974.

Gray MJ: Use and abuse of thiazides in pregnancy. Clin Obstet Gynecol 11:568, 1968.

Greiss FC, Rich JR: The uterine vascular bed: Adrenergic receptors. Obstet Gynecol 23:209, 1964.

Handin RI: Thromboembolic complications of pregnancy and oral contraceptives. Prog Cardiovasc Dis 16:395, 1974.

Hytten FE, Leitch I: *The Physiology of Human Pregnancy,* 2nd ed. Blackwell, 1971.

Ibarra-Perez C & others: The course of pregnancy in patients with artificial heart valves. Am J Med 61:504, 1976.

Kumar D: Chronic placental ischemia in relation to toxemias of pregnancy: Preliminary report. Am J Obstet Gynecol 84:1323, 1962.

Ladner E & others: Dynamics of uterine circulation in pregnant and nonpregnant sheep. Am J Physiol 218:257, 1970.

Landesman R & others: Reserpine in toxemia of pregnancy. Obstet Gynecol 9:377, 1959.

Lindheimer MD, Katz AI: Renal function in pregnancy. Obstet Gynecol Annu 1:139, 1972.

Lindheimer MD, Katz AI: Sodium and diuretics in pregnancy. Med Intelligence 288:891, 1973.

Llewellyn-Jones D: The "toxaemias" of pregnancy. Essential hypertension in pregnancy. Chapters 25 and 26 in: *Fundamentals of Obstetrics and Gynaecology.* Vol 1. Llewellyn-Jones D (editor). Faber & Faber, 1969.

MacGillivray I: Hypertension in pregnancy. Chapter 8, pages 235–256, in: *Modern Trends in Obstetrics–4.* Kellar RJ (editor). Butterworth, 1969.

MacGillivray I: Salt and water balance in normal and toxaemic pregnancy. Pathol Microbiol (Basel) 24:639, 1961.

MacGillivray I, Buchanan TJ: Total exchangeable sodium and potassium in nonpregnant women and in normal and pre-eclamptic pregnancy. Lancet 2:1090, 1958.

Mahon WA, Reid DWJ, Day RA: The in vivo effects of beta-adrenergic stimulation and blockade on the human uterus at term. J Pharmacol Exp Ther 156:178, 1967.

Mendelson CL: The management of delivery in pregnancy complicated by serious rheumatic heart disease. Am J Obstet Gynecol 48:329, 1944.

Metcalfe J, Ueland K: Maternal cardiovascular adjustments to pregnancy. Prog Cardiovasc Dis 16:363, 1974.

Page EW: *The Hypertensive Disorders of Pregnancy.* Thomas, 1953.

Page EW: The relation between the hydatid moles, relative ischemia of the gravid uterus, and the placental origin of eclampsia. Am J Obstet Gynecol 37:291, 1939.

Petrucco OM & others: Immunofluorescent studies in renal biopsies in pre-eclampsia. Br Med J 1:473, 1974.

Pettifor JM, Benson R: Congenital malformations associated with the administration of oral anticoagulants during pregnancy. J Pediatr 86:459, 1975.

Pitts JA, Crosby WM, Basta LL: Eisenmenger's syndrome in pregnancy: Does heparin prophylaxis improve the maternal mortality rate? Am Heart J 93:321, 1977.

Pollak VE, Nettles JB: The kidney in toxemia of pregnancy: A clinical and pathologic study based on renal biopsies. Medicine 39:469, 1960.

Redman CWG & others: Fetal outcome in trial of antihypertensive treatment in pregnancy. Lancet 2:753, 1976.

Redman CWG & others: Plasma-urate measurements in predicting fetal death in hypertensive pregnancy. Lancet 2:1370, 1976.

Scott JR, Beer AE, Stastny P: Immunogenetic factors in pre-eclampsia and eclampsia: Erythrocyte, histocompatibility, and Y-dependent antigens. JAMA 235:402, 1976.

Shnider SM & others: Vasopressors in obstetrics. 2. Fetal hazards of methoxamine administration during obstetric spinal anesthesia. Am J Obstet Gynecol 106:680, 1970.

Sims EA: Pre-eclampsia and related complications of pregnancy. Am J Obstet Gynecol 107:154, 1970.

Szekely P, Snaith L: *Heart Disease and Pregnancy.* Livingstone, 1974.

Ueland K, Novy MJ, Metcalfe J: Cardiorespiratory responses to pregnancy and exercise in normal women and patients with heart disease. Am J Obstet Gynecol 115:4, 1973.

Walters WAW, Lim YL: Changes in the maternal cardiovascular system during human pregnancy. Surg Gynecol Obstet 131:765, 1970.

Willson JR: The recognition of the early toxemias of pregnancy. Med Clin North Am 39:1781, 1955.

Willson JR, Beecham CT, Carrington ER: Diseases of the circulatory system and blood during pregnancy. Toxemias of pregnancy. Chapters 20 and 26 in: *Obstetrics and Gynecology,* 4th ed. Willson JR, Beecham CT, Carrington ER. Mosby, 1971.

23...

Cardiac Disease & the Surgical Patient

INTRODUCTION

Anesthesia and general surgery are a hazard to all patients, especially infants and young children, but the risk in patients in good preoperative physical condition is low in contrast to those with serious cardiac disease. With modern anesthesia, electrocardiographic and blood pressure monitoring, and the ready availability of potent therapeutic agents in the event of untoward developments, cardiac problems are usually minimal unless the preoperative cardiac state was precarious because of known cardiac disease. As a result, middle-aged and elderly individuals with or without known cardiac disease are often referred for preoperative assessment in order to estimate the added risk of anesthesia and surgery and the need for special prophylactic or preoperative treatment.

RISKS OF ANESTHESIA & SURGERY

The risks to any surgical patient include both anesthetic and surgical complications, many of which are preventable. Unexpected hemorrhage, acidosis, impaired ventilation, hypercapnia, decreased systemic vascular resistance, decreased cardiac contractility and conduction, cardiac arrhythmias (with or without increased release of catecholamines), and hypotension with or without a decreased blood volume (such as may occur from hemorrhage)—all interfere with cardiovascular function. Some anesthetic agents such as cyclopropane increase adrenergic activity to the cardiovascular system, whereas others such as halothane reduce cardiovascular sympathetic tone. Anesthetic agents decrease the force of cardiac contraction and may decrease cardiac output. Release of catecholamines may induce arrhythmia or hypertension. Drugs that inhibit the sympathetic nervous system may induce hypotension and reduced systemic flow that impair coronary perfusion, especially in patients with preexisting coronary atherosclerotic lesions. Muscle-relaxing drugs may induce bradycardia and release large amounts of potassium from injured muscles following trauma.

Each hazard producing respiratory or cardiac problems poses a greater risk in patients who have underlying cardiac disease. Cardiac arrest with ventricular fibrillation is the most feared event and is principally due to excessive blood loss, hypotension, accidental administration of potassium or its release by muscle-relaxing drugs, airway obstruction as a result of laryngeal spasm or aspiration of gastric contents, difficulty in intubation at the onset of the surgical procedure, or hypoxemia and acidosis secondary to impaired ventilation. These complications can be minimized by preoperative evaluation and by prophylactic continuous monitoring of cardiovascular variables, eg, arterial pressure, ECG, and intermittent evaluation of blood gases. Preoperative placement of an endocardial right ventricular pacemaker should be done in patients who have Stokes-Adams attacks or bifascicular block with episodes of dizziness or syncope. Meticulous anesthetic and surgical technic combined with prompt recognition and treatment of any complication that may arise decreases the hazard to the patient. Postoperative sodium and water retention may occur causing disturbances in fluid and electrolyte balance.

URGENT VERSUS ELECTIVE SURGERY

Because of the increased hazard of general surgery in the cardiac patient, especially in those with coronary heart disease, the physician must answer certain questions to ascertain when the risks of surgery exceed the risks of the underlying disease and when the reverse is true. Key questions that must be answered are the following: (1) Is the operation urgent or elective? (2) If elective, does the patient have cardiac disease? (3) What is the risk of the underlying surgical disease if surgery is not performed? (4) What additional risk does the heart disease impose on the surgical procedure? (5) Is the surgical diagnosis correct, or could the symptoms, such as abdominal pain, be a manifestation of cardiac disease and not a surgical disease?

URGENT SURGERY

Urgent operations must be done regardless of the underlying cardiac disease and include conditions that threaten life or limb, eg, gross hemorrhage, strangulated hernia, perforation of the bowel or gallbladder, acute bowel obstruction, proximal aortic dissection, ruptured aortic aneurysm, and arterial embolism. The presence of heart disease does not mean that the patient will not tolerate the surgical procedure; one should not withhold a lifesaving procedure merely because of the presence of heart disease.

CARDIAC CONDITIONS MASQUERADING AS SURGICAL ILLNESSES

Gastrointestinal symptoms, including acute abdominal pain, may so dominate the clinical picture that heart disease is not recognized or, if recognized, is not thought to be responsible for the symptoms. Early evidence of cardiac failure is often overlooked because it is overshadowed by the gastrointestinal symptoms. The most common causes of diagnostic confusion are the following:

(1) Angina pectoris or myocardial infarction presenting with dominant epigastric pain.

(2) Fairly abrupt right heart failure presenting with right upper quadrant pain simulating gallbladder disease. This is particularly apt to occur in patients with tight mitral valve disease who develop atrial fibrillation or in patients with mild right heart failure following exercise.

(3) Slowly developing right heart failure, which may present with nonspecific gastrointestinal symptoms of anorexia, nausea, a sensation of heaviness and fullness after meals, and perhaps vomiting. These lead to weight loss and may seem to justify a diagnosis of carcinoma of the upper gastrointestinal tract. If there are no murmurs, the diagnosis of heart disease is often missed.

(4) Pulmonary infarction presenting as jaundice, leading to a diagnosis of biliary tract disease.

(5) Right heart failure or constrictive pericarditis presenting as ascites.

(6) Dysphagia, which may be the presenting symptom in a variety of heart diseases, eg, mitral stenosis with large left atrium, pericarditis, aortic aneurysm, aortic dissection, or anomalies of the aortic arch.

(7) Acute rheumatic fever, which may present with acute abdominal pain, especially in children.

(8) Acute abdominal pain, which may result from acute myocardial infarction or emboli to the splenic, renal, or mesenteric arteries in infective endocarditis or atrial fibrillation. Surgical treatment may be required secondarily if gangrene of the bowel occurs.

(9) Nausea and vomiting, which may occur in cardiac failure, especially as a result of digitalis therapy.

Space does not permit a discussion of the differential diagnosis of these conditions, but one should search for positive diagnostic evidence of heart disease: (1) A history of angina pectoris, dyspnea on effort, orthopnea, or previous ventricular arrhythmias or atrial fibrillation or flutter. (2) Cardiac enlargement with a left or right ventricular heave, with or without characteristic murmurs. (3) Evidence of right heart failure, with increased venous pressure, enlarged and tender liver, and edema or ascites. Orthopnea, decreased vital capacity, and rales and gallop rhythm may be present in left ventricular failure. (4) Signs of myocardial necrosis with fever, tachycardia, or enzyme changes. (5) Typical serial ECG changes of ischemia, infarction, hypertrophy, pericarditis, etc. (6) Radiologic evidence of cardiac enlargement or pulmonary venous congestion.

Considering the possibility of heart disease during the diagnostic process often leads to a better examination and appropriate therapy.

PREOPERATIVE EVALUATION OF THE SURGICAL PATIENT WITH KNOWN OR SUSPECTED CARDIOVASCULAR DISEASE

A thorough history and physical examination combined with a resting ECG, chest x-ray, and noninvasive procedures such as a treadmill exercise test are usually sufficient to diagnose obvious cardiac disease. Twelve- to 24-hour ECG monitoring may be required if the patient has unexplained symptoms of dizziness, syncope, weakness, chest pain, or palpitations in order to determine the presence of cardiac arrhythmias, heart block, or ischemic ST depression.

See p 623 for discussion of drugs that the patient might be taking and that might influence the general state of health or the outcome of operation.

RECOGNITION OF HEART DISEASE

The presence of heart disease is recognized on the basis of symptoms, significant murmurs, an enlarged heart, evidence of cardiac failure, hypertension, conduction defects, atrial fibrillation or flutter, or ventricular arrhythmias. A history of angina pectoris or previous myocardial infarction, Stokes-Adams attacks, cardiac failure, intermittent claudication, or cerebral ischemic attacks may alert the physician to the possibility of cardiac disease. A history of antihypertensive treatment or treatment for cardiac failure may be obtained.

Preoperative ECGs are often valuable but may be difficult to interpret. A patient with known previous myocardial infarction may have a normal ECG; even more importantly, a patient with "unstable angina" may have a normal ECG. Conversely, grossly abnormal changes may be due to an old healed infarct and are therefore of minor importance in deciding whether or not elective surgery should be performed. A baseline ECG is advisable to interpret postoperative changes. An ECG may also show evidence of digitalis therapy, electrolyte disturbances, conduction defects, or arrhythmias. In general, a stable abnormality on the ECG in the absence of cardiac failure or a change in the pattern of angina pectoris indicates that the patient will probably tolerate surgery almost as well as a normal individual. Such a patient with a healed previous myocardial infarction has an added mortality risk of about 3–5%.

The most important contraindications to elective surgery are recent angina pectoris, a crescendo change in the pattern of angina pectoris in recent weeks or months, unstable angina, acute myocardial infarction, severe aortic stenosis, a high degree of atrioventricular block, untreated cardiac failure, and severe hypertension.

SPECIFIC DISEASE PROBLEMS

1. CORONARY HEART DISEASE

The usual patient seen for preoperative evaluation is an older individual with possible coronary heart disease. The physician should search for a history of recent change in the character of the anginal pain, pain at rest, unstable angina, or the possibility of recent myocardial infarction. If known coronary disease is stable, without change in the pattern of pain or in serial ECGs; if there are no symptoms or signs of cardiac failure; and if at least 6 months have elapsed since myocardial infarction, the surgeon can proceed if the indications for surgery are clear and definite.

Emergency surgery must often be done despite a recent myocardial infarction, but the mortality rate is high. Important but not lifesaving surgery is best delayed at least 3 weeks if possible. Purely elective surgery should be postponed for 3–6 months whenever possible.

In patients with known coronary heart disease, the added risk of a new myocardial infarction, as indicated previously, decreases as the time interval following the previous myocardial infarction lengthens. It averages about 5–6% when surgery is performed at least 6 months after the myocardial infarction, but the diagnosis of a new myocardial infarction during or following operations is often difficult because of medication for postsurgical pain and the relative diagnostic unreliability of postoperative serum enzymes except for MB (myocardial band) creatine phosphokinase isoenzymes. The mortality rate is about 30% if a new infarct occurs during or after surgery. A new myocardial infarction is more common with operations on the chest and upper abdomen than in those involving the pelvis or lower abdomen and is more apt to occur on the second or third postoperative day than on the day of operation. For this reason, postoperative patients with known or suspected coronary heart disease should be monitored by daily ECGs and MB creatine phosphokinase isoenzyme determinations in order to determine whether a new infarction has occurred. Older individuals without known coronary heart disease may have flattening of the T waves in the left ventricular leads postoperatively but rarely have deep inversions of the T wave, ischemic ST depression, or new Q waves. Development of the last 3 suggests myocardial ischemia or infarction. Ventricular arrhythmias (see below) are more common during and following surgery when coronary heart disease is present; if the patient is known to have angina pectoris, continuous ECG monitoring is recommended, and the physician should pay careful attention to the possible development of hypoxia, hypotension, and acidosis. If the patient has severe atherosclerosis elsewhere (eg, aortoiliac) and borderline left ventricular function, a flow-directed catheter should be introduced preoperatively to allow intermittent measurements of pulmonary artery diastolic or "wedge" pressure, cardiac output, and blood gases. As noted previously, any indication of an acute change in the preoperative condition, such as unstable angina, means that elective surgery should be postponed, usually for at least 3 months.

2. HYPERTENSION

Patients with uncomplicated chronic hypertension, even with left ventricular hypertrophy and an abnormal ECG, tolerate surgery without a significantly increased mortality rate if there are no evidences of coronary heart disease or cardiac failure and if renal function is normal. Unless the diastolic pressure exceeds 110 mm Hg, it is best to decrease or even stop antihypertensive medication for 2–3 days before surgery and to be certain, if thiazides have been used, that the body potassium has been replenished.

Anesthesiologists have found that the catecholamine depletion that follows adrenergic depleting drugs (eg, reserpine, methyldopa, and guanethidine) or beta-adrenergic blocking drugs (eg, propranolol) can be managed satisfactorily if the drug dosage is tapered for several days prior to surgery and if the anesthesiologist is forewarned and prepared to counteract hypotension or bradycardia, which are the 2 most common complications of these therapeutic agents.

3. ARRHYTHMIAS

Chronic atrial fibrillation with a well-controlled ventricular rate does not increase the risk of surgery, nor does an asymptomatic isolated right or left bundle branch block. Bifascicular block in asymptomatic patients does not require prophylactic pacing but does require close observation. Second or third degree atrioventricular block is a warning sign, especially if associated with left or right ventricular conduction defects; a transvenous electrode catheter should be inserted into the right ventricle before the surgical procedure and the patient monitored, with a pacemaker available in case ventricular standstill occurs. Infrequent atrial or ventricular premature beats usually do not require special treatment, can often be relieved with simple sedatives such as phenobarbital, and may disappear while anesthesia is being given. ECG monitoring during anesthesia and surgery has shown that ventricular arrhythmias are infrequent unless there is underlying left ventricular disease or unless catecholamine release is excessive as a result of ventilatory problems.

If ventricular premature beats preoperatively are frequent and from multiple foci, or if they occur in salvos, surgery can be delayed and the ectopic ventricular beats suppressed with drugs such as quinidine, 200–400 mg orally 2–4 times daily, or procainamide, 250–500 mg orally 3 or 4 times daily. If the clinical situation is more urgent, or if it is considered unsatisfactory to delay surgery for 2–3 days to obtain the effect from oral drugs, lidocaine, 2% solution (20 mg/ml), 50–100 mg intravenously, followed by an intravenous infusion of 1–2 mg/min, will usually quickly abolish the premature beats.

If the premature beats are unifocal and infrequent, they should not be treated with antiarrhythmia drugs but monitored by continuous electrocardiography. If salvos of ventricular beats or complex arrhythmias develop, intravenous lidocaine should be used.

4. VALVULAR HEART DISEASE

Severe aortic stenosis, tight mitral stenosis, and severe coronary ostial involvement due to syphilitic aortitis are the 3 major "valvular" conditions in which general surgery presents a considerably increased hazard. An aortic systolic murmur not associated with evidence of severe aortic valvular disease or significant left ventricular hypertrophy does not increase the mortality rate. Mitral insufficiency is usually tolerated well, but tight mitral stenosis, especially if the patient has sinus rhythm, may result in acute pulmonary edema if the patient abruptly develops atrial fibrillation during surgery.

5. CONGENITAL HEART DISEASE

In the absence of cardiac failure, ventricular septal defect and atrial septal defect usually pose no particular problems or extra hazard. Pulmonary hypertension with Eisenmenger's syndrome carries a significantly increased mortality risk, and surgery should be performed only upon urgent indications. Patients with coarctation of the aorta and patent ductus arteriosus should have their congenital lesions repaired before undergoing elective general surgical procedures. Mild pulmonary stenosis is not a contraindication to elective surgery, but severe pulmonary stenosis is a contraindication because of the hazard of acute right heart failure and a reversed shunt through the foramen ovale or a small atrial septal defect. Patients with tetralogy of Fallot are relatively poor surgical risks because of the polycythemia and because of the possibility of contraction of the infundibulum of the right ventricle with resulting decrease in pulmonary blood flow.

6. CARDIAC FAILURE

Patients with mild cardiac failure whose symptoms and signs are controlled with digitalis and diuretics have only a slightly increased risk from general surgery provided ordinary activity does not cause symptoms. Patients who have dyspnea even when walking on level ground, orthopnea or nocturnal dyspnea, and signs of cardiac failure such as gallop rhythm, increased venous pressure, and rales are at a significantly increased risk, and surgery should be delayed if possible. Cardiac failure should be treated adequately before surgery. It is desirable to have the patient's condition stabilized for at least a month before surgery and to avoid digitalis toxicity and potassium depletion by diuretics. Diuretics and digitalis can then be withheld for a few days before surgery. Digitalization of a patient with cardiac hypertrophy but no heart failure is probably unwise because of the hazard of digitalis toxicity, including arrhythmias. Although digitalis has a positive inotropic action even in normal hearts, clinical evidence of benefit from the drug has not been demonstrated when it has been given to patients with hypertrophy but no failure. If there is a question about whether or not heart failure is present preoperatively, a period of bed rest and restricted dietary sodium may be adequate treatment.

MANAGEMENT OF KNOWN CARDIAC DISEASE PRIOR TO GENERAL SURGERY

If the preoperative assessment reveals known cardiac disease or severe hypertension, especially in the presence of acute symptoms, anemia, an unstable state, serious ventricular arrhythmias, heart block, or cardiac failure, these conditions should be managed before the surgical procedure is undertaken. The treatment of any cardiac condition discovered in the preoperative evaluation should be along the lines of treatment discussed elsewhere in this book and should not differ substantially in the patient with an elective surgical condition as compared with a nonsurgical patient. Careful judgment is required in patients with more urgent surgical conditions, and delay in surgery for as long as possible may be indicated until the cardiac status is somewhat improved. If the surgical condition is urgent, the ability of the physician to treat the cardiac problem may be limited, and surgical treatment must take precedence even though the risk is seriously enhanced.

If the patient has severe valvular or coronary heart disease correctable by cardiac surgery, or if transient cerebral ischemic attacks indicate carotid stenosis with episodic neurologic deficit, surgical treatment of the correctable lesion should precede elective general surgery in order to avoid pulmonary edema, cardiac arrest, or hemiplegia, which may follow the increased demands resulting from general surgery. In such cases, carotid occlusive disease should be treated first. Fortunately, unexpected severe cardiac disease is uncommon in the patient scheduled for elective surgery, so the psychologic and other disturbances incident to cancellation of scheduled operations are reduced. Middle-aged or elderly patients suspected of having heart disease should be admitted to the hospital for a few days before scheduled surgery to allow effective diagnosis and management of any cardiac problem that is unexpectedly elicited. Alternatively, this preoperative evaluation can be done on an outpatient basis if there are no symptoms or important physical findings of cardiovascular disease.

SPECIAL PRECAUTIONS

In addition to conducting a preoperative surgical evaluation for any heart condition that should be managed before elective cardiac or other surgery, the physician should take special precautions if patients are receiving general treatment that may require modification because of the intended surgery. As a rule, anticoagulants should be stopped, although some surgeons have reported good results without stopping anticoagulants. Patients who have had intensive or prolonged corticosteroid treatment, even if it has been stopped for several months, should be identified, and supplementary corticosteroids should be administered (up to the equivalent of 200–300 mg of hydrocortisone per day preoperatively and for several days postoperatively). Patients receiving long-acting insulin for diabetes mellitus should be given regular insulin, and frequent analyses of urine, blood sugar, and ketones should be performed. Any hypersensitivity to drugs, especially antibiotics, should be determined so that patients will not receive them inadvertently. The administration of sodium-containing fluids should be carefully controlled during the preoperative, intraoperative, and postoperative periods because of the known sodium and water retention that follows general surgical operations. Sodium retention is probably due to hemodynamic and perhaps hormonal influences on the nephron. Water retention is due to increased secretion of ADH and not to increased aldosterone levels or decreased glomerular filtration rate. Sodium retention occurring postoperatively or arising from the use of intravenous sodium-containing fluids may precipitate pulmonary edema, and the speed and volume of the infused fluid should be regulated with this hazard in mind. If there is preoperative anemia or extensive blood loss during surgery, red cell mass rather than whole blood should be given slowly, and the patient should be supine and closely watched. If dyspnea, rales, or raised jugular venous pressure appears, the patient should be placed in the semi-Fowler position to decrease the pulmonary blood volume and the infusion slowed or stopped.

MONITORING IN THE PRESENCE OF SEVERE CARDIAC DISEASE

If urgent surgery is required in the patient with severe coronary disease, aortic stenosis, mitral stenosis, or atrioventricular block, the patient should be monitored directly by a flotation catheter. The intra-arterial blood pressure and pulmonary artery pressure (or, preferably, the pulmonary wedge pressure) should be intermittently recorded and blood gas measurements periodically determined. A temporary transvenous right ventricular pacemaker should be inserted when indicated to allow prompt institution of pacing in the event complete heart block develops. Emergency cardiac drugs and facilities for defibrillation should be readily available.

The choice and details of anesthesia are best left to the anesthesiologist, who must be alerted to any possible problems that might occur and informed of any medications the patient has taken even if they have recently been discontinued, such as digitalis, diuretics, antihypertensive agents, corticosteroids, insulin, propranolol, anticoagulants, or tricyclic antidepressants.

• • •

References

Aberman A, Fulop M: The metabolic and respiratory acidosis of acute pulmonary edema. Ann Intern Med 76:173, 1972.

Angelini P & others: Cardiac arrhythmias during and after heart surgery. Prog Cardiovasc Dis 16:469, 1974.

Ayres SN, Grace WJ: Inappropriate ventilation and hypoxemia as causes of cardiac arrhythmias: The control of arrhythmias without antiarrhythmic drugs. Am J Med 46:495, 1969.

Civetta JM, Gabel JC: Flow directed-pulmonary artery catheterization in surgical patients: Indications and modifications of technic. Ann Surg 176:753, 1972.

Dripps RD, Strong MJ, Price HL: The heart and general anesthesia. Mod Concepts Cardiovasc Dis 32:805, 1963.

Driscoll A & others: Post-operative myocardial infarction. N Engl J Med 264:633, 1961.

Giardina EG, Heissenbuttel RH, Bigger JT Jr: Intermittent intravenous procaine amide to treat ventricular arrhythmias: Correlation of plasma concentration with effect on arrhythmia, electrocardiogram, and blood pressure. Ann Intern Med 78:183, 1973.

Hahnemann Symposium on cardiovascular pulmonary problems before and after surgery. 3. Shock and electrolyte disturbances. Am J Cardiol 12:587, 1963.

Hurst JW, Logue RB: *The Heart, Arteries and Veins,* 3rd ed. McGraw-Hill, 1974.

Hurst JW & others: Management of patients with atrial fibrillation. Am J Med 37:728, 1964.

Katz JD & others: Pulmonary artery flow-guided catheters in the perioperative period: Indications and complications. JAMA 237:2832, 1977.

Katz RL, Bigger JT Jr: Cardiac arrhythmias during anesthesia and operation. Anesthesiology 33:193, 1970.

Katz RL, Epstein RG: The interaction of anesthetic agents and adrenergic drugs to produce cardiac arrhythmias. Anesthesiology 29:763, 1968.

Laragh JH: Ethacrynic acid and furosemide. Am Heart J 75:564, 1968.

Logue RB: Medical management in noncardiac surgery. In: *The Heart, Arteries and Veins,* 3rd ed. Hurst JW (editor). McGraw-Hill, 1974.

Lowenstein E, Bland JHL: Anesthesia for cardiac surgery. Chapter 4 in: *Cardiac Surgery,* 2nd ed. Norman JC (editor). Appleton-Century-Crofts, 1972.

Marriott HJL: Differential diagnosis of supraventricular and ventricular tachycardia. Geriatrics 25:91, 1970.

Mauney FM Jr & others: Post-operative myocardial infarction. Ann Surg 172:497, 1970.

Moore ED: Common patterns of water and electrolyte change in injury, surgery and disease. (4 parts.) N Engl J Med 258:277, 325, 377, 427, 1958.

Mundth ED, Austen WG: Postoperative intensive care in the cardiac surgical patient. Prog Cardiovasc Dis 11:229, 1968.

Oaks WW, Moyer JH (editors): *Pre- and Postoperative Management of the Cardio-pulmonary Patient.* Grune & Stratton, 1970.

Perlroth MG, Hultgren HN: The cardiac patient and general surgery. JAMA 232:1279, 1975.

Price HL: *Circulation During Anesthesia and Operation.* Thomas, 1967.

Raftery EB: Diagnosis and management of myocardial infarction during anesthesia. Proc R Soc Med 66:1209, 1973.

Reitemeier RJ: Electrolytic imbalance: Problems associated with gastrointestinal surgery. Med Clin North Am 46:1001, 1962.

Sagar S & others: Efficacy of low-dose heparin in prevention of extensive deep-vein thrombosis in patients undergoing total-hip replacement. Lancet 1:1151, 1976.

Salem MR & others: Cardiac arrest related to anesthesia: Contributing factors in infants and children. JAMA 233:238, 1975.

Samet P: Cardiac arrhythmias: Hemodynamic sequelae of cardiac arrhythmias. Circulation 47:399, 1973.

Schamroth L: How to approach an arrhythmia. Circulation 47:420, 1973.

Shimosato S, Etsten BE: Effect of anesthetic drugs on the heart: A critical review of myocardial contractility and its relationship to hemodynamics. In: *A Decade of Clinical Progress.* Fabian L (editor). Davis, 1971.

Wesler S, Blumgart HL: Management of the cardiac patient requiring major surgery. Circulation 23:121, 1961.

Williams JF Jr, Morrow AG, Braunwald E: The incidence and management of "medical" complications following cardiac operations. Circulation 32:608, 1965.

Index

T